Don't go to the cosmetics counter without me.

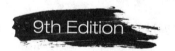

9th Edition

A unique, professionally sourced guide to thousands of skin-care and makeup products from today's hottest brands. Shop smarter, look beautiful, and discover which products really work.

Paula Begoun

with Bryan Barron
and the Paula's Choice Research Team

Contributing Authors: Bryan Barron and Desiree Stordahl
Contributing Editor: Nathan Rivas
Editors: John Hopper, Stephanie Parsons, and Elaine Trumpey
Art Direction, Cover Design, and Typography: Erin Smith Bloom and Moya Laigo
Printing: R.R. Donnelley
Research Director: Bryan Barron
Research Assistants: Heather Hampton and Tracy VanHoof

Copyright © 2012, Paula Begoun
Publisher: Beginning Press
1030 SW 34th Street, Suite A
Renton, Washington 98057

Ninth Edition Printing: October 2012

ISBN: 978-1-877988-35-6
10 9 8 7 6 5 4 3 2 1

This book is distributed to the United States book trade by:
Publishers Group West
1700 Fourth Street
Berkeley, California 94710
(510) 809-3700

And to the Canadian book trade by:
Raincoast Books Dist. Ltd.
2440 Viking Way
Richmond, British Columbia, V6V1N2 CANADA
(604) 633-5714

And in Australia and New Zealand by:
Peribo Pty Limited
58 Beaumont Road
Mount Kuring-gai NSW 2080 AUSTRALIA
(02) 9457 0011

COSMETICSCOP.COM

Expert Advice
Got expert research-supported information on every major skin-care and makeup topic, all written in a succinct, engaging style.

More Product Reviews
Find out whether the latest skin-care and makeup products are worth buying.

Share With Us!
From Facebook to our radio show, we invite you to join the discussion.

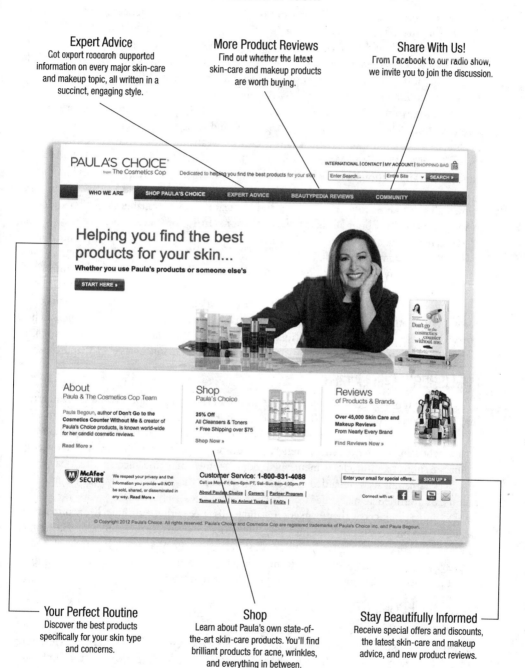

Your Perfect Routine
Discover the best products specifically for your skin type and concerns.

Shop
Learn about Paula's own state-of-the-art skin-care products. You'll find brilliant products for acne, wrinkles, and everything in between.

Stay Beautifully Informed
Receive special offers and discounts, the latest skin-care and makeup advice, and new product reviews.

FROM THE PUBLISHER

Paula Begoun is the best-selling author of Don't Go to the Cosmetics Counter Without Me, The Original Beauty Bible, Don't Go Shopping for Hair Care Products Without Me, and Blue Eyeshadow Should Be Illegal. She has sold millions of books, educating women about the facts and secrets the beauty industry doesn't want them to know. Paula also spearheaded the creation of the world's most extensive database of product reviews at CosmeticsCop.com.

Paula is internationally recognized as a consumer advocate, covering the cosmetics industry and educating women throughout the world. She is called upon regularly by reporters and producers from television, newspapers, magazines, and radio as a cosmetics industry expert. She has appeared on hundreds of talk shows over the years, including The View, The Dr. Oz Show, Dateline NBC, Good Morning America, 20/20, Today, CBS Morning News, Hard Copy, Canada AM, and National Public Radio, and made more than a dozen appearances on Oprah.

Today, with the success of Paula's websites, CosmeticsCop.com and PaulasChoice.com, women all over the world consider Paula and her team the most reliable source for straight-forward information about all their beauty questions. In 1996, Paula launched her own line of skin-care products called Paula's Choice. This distinctive line of products, available online at PaulasChoice.com, is renowned for its effectiveness for a wide range of skin concerns, from acne to wrinkles. While Paula is proud of her line, she realizes that there are vast numbers of product options for women to consider. As a result, she and her team continue to provide their readers with substantiated and documented studies and analysis about skin-care and makeup products from other lines based on the team's extensive research and years of experience. In her reviews and critiques, it is clear that Paula continues to maintain her evenhanded approach to offering readers an unprecedented assortment of smart choices for their cosmetic purchases.

PUBLISHER'S DISCLAIMER

The intent of this book is to present the author's ideas and perceptions about the market-ing, selling, and use of cosmetics. The author's sole purpose is to present consumer information and advice regarding the purchase of makeup and skin-care products. The information and recommendations presented strictly reflect the author's opinions, perceptions, and knowledge about the subject and products mentioned. Some women may find success with a particular product that is not recommended or even mentioned in this book, or they may be partial to a skin-care routine Paula and her team have reviewed negatively. It is everyone's unalienable right to judge products by their own criteria and to disagree with the authors. More important, because everyone's skin can, and probably will, react to an external stimulus at some time, any product can cause a negative reaction on skin at one time or another. If you develop skin sensitivity to a cosmetic, stop using it immediately and consult your physician. If you need medical advice about your skin, it is best to consult a dermatologist.

ACKNOWLEDGMENTS

There are no words that can adequately express the challenge and commitment required for writing a book of this scope and nature. The energy and resourcefulness needed to research, compile, review, write, and edit is an almost endless undertaking. If it were not for my team of Bryan Barron, Desiree Stordahl, Nathan Rivas, Heather Hampton, and Tracy VanHoof this book would not have been possible. Their perseverance and devotion to completing the project go beyond anything I could have hoped for. Not only did they meet deadline after deadline, they did it with an accuracy and exactness that exceeded my every expectation. Without their feedback, patience, and contributions, this book would have been a very good idea but an absolutely unconquerable task.

DEDICATION FROM PAULA

To Bryan Barron, my co-author and co-writer:

Thank you for always making me look good in print! For 12 years you have been my voice when I can't speak, my words when I can't write, my reason when I'm off on a rant, my resolve when I think I can't take another cosmetics company's BS, and my brains when I fumble at making sense of yet one more research paper. As you know all too well, and as your fingers cramp arched over your computer's keyboard, I couldn't and wouldn't have done any of this without you.

With endless appreciation and gratitude, from your co-author and co-writer, Paula Begoun.

CHAPTER ONE

Begin to Be Beautifully Informed

HOW I BECAME A COSMETICS COP

I often marvel at how I happened into this unusual occupation. It's not as if you can answer an ad for this kind of job, and clearly the cosmetics industry and beauty magazines aren't interested in hiring someone to do what I do. Yet, from when I started more than 30 years ago, it was clear I had a passion for the world of cosmetics, and thankfully there was a demand from consumers for this kind of information. After three decades of research and experience, including having sold millions of books, with translations in seven languages, I'm certainly glad I gave up my day job working at cosmetics counters, and eventually became The Cosmetics Cop.

I'm frequently asked what started my career, and I often wonder the same thing myself. I'm fairly certain my inspiration began when I was very young, struggling for years with debilitating, painful eczema over most of my body. If that weren't bad enough, at the age of 11, I began my battle with acne. Even now, both of these issues linger, although each is now under control, thanks to products I've formulated to manage these skin concerns. As you would imagine, I spent a good deal of my childhood and teen years at dermatologists' offices, cosmetics counters, or drugstores, trying every possible treatment or product that promised to give me "normal" skin. It never happened. If anything, my skin just got worse. I felt helpless, trying to find products that would work, but I kept trying and trying hoping the next product would be the answer.

Getting back to what led me to become The Cosmetics Cop. In 1977, I took my first job at a department-store makeup counter to supplement my income as a freelance makeup artist (I always had a knack for doing makeup). As a young makeup artist in Washington, DC, I built up a list of political and celebrity clients and did quite well for myself, both financially and professionally. I found the artistry of creating beautiful makeup styles for women intriguing. However, as with any business, it had its difficulties. During one of the less busy seasons, I applied at a department-store cosmetics department in Silver Spring, Maryland. Amazingly (to me anyway), they weren't interested in my industry experience; they hired me on the spot because I looked the part—nice makeup and well-dressed, but I was told I needed to be "retrained" to sell their products, *especially* so in their approach to skin care.

Even then, I knew something was awry with the business of beauty, particularly in the skin-care arena and the advertising claims being made. I struggled for years with oily skin and blemishes, and my own personal experience long-since had proved that astringents didn't close pores, products claiming not to cause breakouts made me break out, and products that promised to be great for my skin only made it more red and irritated. I didn't yet know all the technical details of why skin-care and makeup products failed abysmally to live up to their claims; I just knew they didn't work as claimed. More often than not, the claims made about what products would do rarely matched their performance, and while it seemed certain to me that much of the cosmetics industry grossly misrepresented its products, at the time I had no way to confirm my suspicions.

On my first day at the department store, I worked behind the Calvin Klein and Elizabeth Arden cosmetics counters. With no previous training or information about either brand, I was told to sell the products. I did the best I could. Unfortunately, my idea about how to help customers was completely different from that of the other salespeople and, more important, different from that of the line's manager.

My first mistake was telling several customers not to bother using an astringent because alcohol-based products wouldn't stop oil production, it would only create more problems like red, flaky, irritated skin. By the end of the second day, the woman working next to me was mortified. She called in the line representative, who made it clear that I should keep my personal opinions to myself and just sell the products—I said I would do my best. This was only my second day! Things had to get better, I thought. They didn't.

The two lines I was assigned to sell didn't always have the best makeup colors or skin-care products for every woman I talked to, so I suggested products from other lines a few inches away that I thought were better. The cosmetics manager told me, "All you need to tell the customer is what is superior about our products, not someone else's. Besides, customers never ask questions because they trust we know what we're talking about." Still, I refused to mislead my customers. Not surprisingly, a few weeks later, I was out of a job.

Shortly after my brief stint in the department store, I read *The Great American Skin Game* by Toni Stabile. It changed my life. This landmark book conveyed in clear, concise terms the processes and techniques the cosmetics industry uses to sell hope to gullible and uninformed consumers. In fact, Stabile was largely responsible for proposing many present-day Food and Drug Administration (FDA) regulations, including mandatory ingredient lists on all retail beauty products. It was a life-changing event for me.

Although it sounds a bit melodramatic, I couldn't continue selling products I knew to be a waste of money or just plain bad for the skin. I'll never forget the moment I looked at the Clinique toner I was using and one of the ingredients high up on the ingredient label was acetone. That's nail polish remover! I didn't need to be a chemist to realize acetone isn't good for any skin-care concern.

Consumers (including myself) deserved better. I wasn't anti-beauty—just the opposite—but I was (and am still) anti-hype and anti-misleading information. Thus, I took my first steps on a long career path, beginning with owning my own cosmetics stores in 1980 and working as a TV news reporter at a local Seattle TV station. Then, in 1985, I started my own publishing company, and wrote 18 books on the beauty industry, which in turn led to creating and owning my own skin-care and makeup company in 1995, Paula's Choice.

Why did I create my own line of products? In part, it was due to pressure from friends and family nagging me to make products that didn't have all the "buts" of the other products I reviewed. They would say, "You always write 'this product is good but …'—but it's too expensive, but it has too much fragrance, but it's in unstable packaging." Initially, I was resistant yet over time, I had to agree: I knew I could make state-of-the-art products that left out all the "buts" and were loaded with skin-beneficial ingredients.

Though I'm a bit reluctant to admit it, I also started my own line of products because I didn't want to write any more books; they were just getting bigger and bigger, each one requiring exhaustive research and energy. It seemed easier to put what I knew about skin care in my own products. Obviously, my passion for writing books hasn't gone away!

My goal from the start has been to do whatever it takes to find and expose the truth behind the ads and the unbelievable claims thrown about by the cosmetics world. After all, one good sales pitch about an "exclusive formula" or a "revolutionary new" skin-care product, and your pocketbook could easily be lighter—by $100 to $500—for a 1-ounce jar of standard cosmetic ingredients, or for new "miracle ingredients" that have no capability of living up to their claims.

I know that I can't stop the cosmetics industry from force-feeding women around the world an endless stream of products along with misleading or outright false claims and information. However, I also know there are enough women (and, increasingly, men) who are interested in seeing the "un-retouched" picture behind the advertising and cosmetics counter to motivate me to continue to do what I do. Sharing this reality with you enables me to help you feel and look more beautiful in the end.

Do I hate the cosmetics industry? Hardly. I am in constant awe of what well-formulated beauty products can do. What I do hate are the ludicrous claims, disproportionate prices, and products that can hurt skin or mislead consumers into taking poor care of their skin.

IT TAKES A VILLAGE!

You may wonder how I'm able to put together a book of this magnitude on my own. Although I used to handle all of the writing and research myself, over the years I've come to my senses and have been fortunate enough to assemble an amazing team to participate in accomplishing what most would say is the impossible. As a result, each edition of my book has moved to a new level of excellence that provides an unparalleled source of information about skin care and makeup that I am proud to share with the world! Without question, this book would not be possible without the hard work and dedication of the entire Paula's Choice Research Team. I have personally trained each of them, and they have taken my instruction and personal philosophy to new heights of dedication and responsibility.

Together, we search out and analyze endless studies on skin care and ingredients, pore over fashion magazines, spend hours upon hours researching products, and make repeated trips to cosmetics counters to ensure our reviews are as accurate and helpful as possible.

I always say it takes a village of enthusiastic and educated people to do the work we do at Paula's Choice, but perhaps even more so to compile a book of this nature—not to mention the thousands of additional reviews available on CosmeticsCop.com. Through it all, my team and I remain steadfast in our mission to provide current and insightful information about skin care and makeup to help you find the best products possible, regardless of your budget, whether they're from Paula's Choice or from another brand.

WHO DO YOU BELIEVE?

I struggle with how best to help you learn the difference between fact and fiction when it comes to taking care of your skin. I'm clearly asking you not to believe what other sources are telling you, but rather to believe me, even though I do have my own skin-care and makeup line. The potential for conflict of interest on my part is obvious. However, I started my mission of researching and evaluating skin-care and makeup products 15 years before I started my own line. I wrote several books revealing the facts and providing insights into every aspect of skin, hair, and makeup before I began formulating my own products in 1995.

My hope is that you will trust the work my team and I do because of the extensive research on which we base our conclusions and because of the unbiased advice we provide. I think you will see just by thumbing through this book that my team and I make balanced recommendations, not only for my own products but also for products from other lines. No other cosmetics company recommends products other than their own, even when the company owns other lines. When I think about it, perhaps the real conflict of interest is that I own my company AND I recommend products from companies other than my own.

It is part of my soul to share with you what I know, and I am passionate about my product line, Paula's Choice. I know it's controversial, but there is nothing else I can do when I know there are countless sources, ranging from doctors to women's magazines, advertisements, cosmetics salespeople, home shopping channels, aestheticians, and companies claiming to be all natural or organic, that either are being completely dishonest, or just don't know the facts.

At the very least, you need to know there is a universal, duplicitous knowledge in the cosmetics industry. They know all too well that you are being obscenely overcharged for what is easily replaced by another far less costly product that is often better formulated.

Regardless of whether or not you agree with everything this book has to say, you will at least have someone else's voice in your ear saying, "Here is research or data proving that this product won't work" or is "bad for your skin" or "Consider this other far less expensive, and better formulated product" or "It isn't worth the money, but at least the product is good for your skin." Then you can make up your own mind about what works best for you. I believe this is far better than basing a decision on the thousands of never-ending false and misleading claims that prevail in the cosmetics industry.

THE SAME WORLDWIDE

My Paula's Choice products sell in 57 countries around the world. As a result, I have done media interviews and speaking engagements in places such as Jakarta, Indonesia; Seoul, Korea; Stockholm, Sweden; Mexico City, Mexico; Singapore; Sydney and Melbourne, Australia; Kuala Lumpur, Malaysia; Amsterdam, The Netherlands; Moscow, Russia; Taipei, Taiwan; Toronto, Canada; and, of course, in almost every major city in the United States.

What I've learned is that the business of beauty is so universally crazy that there is no part of the world where the cosmetics industry works any differently, where the products are any better (not in India, China, Japan, Italy, France, or the United States), or the claims any less far-fetched. Another observation is that no matter where I've been in the world, women are no less obsessed with looking younger and having picture-perfect skin. As a result, women (and female beauty reporters) ask me the same questions everywhere I go.

Women want to know why a product they bought didn't work. Why their deep wrinkles didn't go away? Why their red marks from acne didn't fade? Why their skin wasn't lifted? Why their skin discolorations didn't change? Why they still are breaking out or are just starting to break out? Why they still have dry, flaky skin after buying so many products promising to make things better? Why their skin is so red and irritated? What is the best skin-care ingredient? Do I know about a recent product launched with some miracle ingredient currently advertised or in an infomercial? What about celebrity-endorsed products?

What usually happens during my presentation is I see a look of understanding wash over the audience as they begin to grasp how the cosmetics industry has repeatedly duped them.

What women everywhere want is to take the best care of their skin, to look younger, to have an even skin tone, no breakouts, and on and on. In each country I visit, without fail, beauty ideals revolve entirely around youth and flawless skin. And, because skin color or race isn't a skin type, well-formulated products can make a beautiful difference, just as the bad ones can make matters worse, no matter who you are or where you live. I guarantee this book will help you get closer to your goal of having the skin you want more than anything else you can do. Start here…

CAN YOU HAVE HEALTHY, BEAUTIFUL SKIN?

The answer is YES! Aside from avoiding sun exposure, the primary way to achieve healthy beautiful skin is with well-formulated skin-care products. Cosmetic corrective procedures also can help, but good skin care should be your first line of defense. Of course, you must be realistic—there are no miracles. You can obtain the best skin possible for your skin type and age, but you also have to accept that we are all going to get older, there are genetics and unique health concerns to contend with, menopause will take a toll, and skin disorders like acne or rosacea happen. Skin-care products can't stop any of that, but they can make a huge difference in improving matters. Understanding the limitations and knowing what's possible will not only save you money, but also save you (and your skin) from one disappointment after another.

It is fascinating how much the amount of documented and peer-reviewed research on skin-care and cosmetic ingredients has grown over the past several years. Serious investigation has increased exponentially on all fronts—from why antioxidants, anti-irritants, skin-identical (repairing) ingredients, and cell-communicating ingredients are so important for all skin types, to how skin ages, wrinkles, heals; how hormones impact skin function; and which treatments are effective for blackheads and acne. It also has given us a much better understanding of how sun and oxygen destroy skin, why irritation is harmful for skin, and what is realistic in dealing with these factors.

Perhaps most significant is that skin-care formulations have improved exponentially from when I first started looking carefully at formulas. Yet, for all this progress, I am still disheartened at how much remains the same when it comes to misleading claims, poor formulations, products that contain ingredients that can hurt skin, and products that are priced with nothing more in mind than tempting women into believing expensive means better. Now it's time to cut through the hype, because wasting money isn't pretty!

KNOWING FACT FROM FICTION WILL SAVE YOUR SKIN

You've probably heard the saying that if you repeat a lie often enough it can become fact. That is how much of the beauty industry works—particularly in salons, spas, cosmetics counters, fashion magazines, and even doctors' offices. Throughout this book you will learn the facts about what research says is best for your skin in ways that will surprise you, and often give you dramatic results (almost overnight), especially once you stop using products that are bad (or just useless) for your skin.

You will learn why a skin-care product in jar packaging is a complete waste of money, why many skin-care products cause inflammation (which ages your skin), why many natural ingredients cause irritation and destroy collagen, why irritating ingredients can trigger more oil production in the pore, and so on.

To get started, let me set the record straight on one of my favorite examples of a beauty industry lie that is wasting your money and probably making matters worse for your skin: **You don't need a separate eye cream for the eye area**.

It's true. There is no need to use a separate eye cream around the eye area for wrinkles, sagging, or dark circles. The same ingredients that work on your face for those concerns work just as well for the eye area, and there isn't a shred of research anywhere in the world showing that isn't 100% accurate.

In reality, a well-formulated facial moisturizer that treats skin discolorations, wrinkles, and other aspects of aging also works for the eye area. In fact, it can work even better because most eye creams don't contain sunscreen, whereas many moisturizers do. If you're using an eye cream during the day that doesn't have sunscreen, it leaves your eye area vulnerable to the sun's skin-darkening and aging influences. It's shocking to some, but a facial moisturizer will work just as well—and that's what you are buying with eye creams anyway, just at a higher price for a smaller package.

Despite this well-documented information, most women accept eye creams as a standard necessity because of the incessant brainwashing from all corners of the cosmetics industry. But this is only one instance of the prevalent insanity surrounding beauty products, as we'll explain throughout this book. We'll guide you through how to look at the products you are using, and evaluate the research we present so you can find the best products for your skin and put them together to form an effective skin-care routine!

WHY AN ANTIWRINKLE CREAM CAN'T WORK BETTER THAN BOTOX

Antiwrinkle creams won't replace dermal fillers, laser resurfacing, chemical peels, face-lifts, or plastic surgery. It's not that there aren't brilliant skin-care products you can use to make a huge difference in your skin, but none of them can provide the results you get from a medical cosmetic corrective procedure. No skin-care product out there can completely stop or reverse the complex physiological processes that cause wrinkles—and dry skin does NOT cause wrinkles, and slathering on moisturizers won't change this fact. Here are some of the factors our skin "faces" with time.

Sun damage. DON'T SKIP THIS INFORMATION! I know sun protection doesn't sound miraculous and you probably think you've heard it all, but research shows we aren't using it sufficiently. For all skin types, wherever you are in the world, this is the most important information we can share!

Aside from just growing older, the biggest source of wrinkles, sagging, dark spots, and overall aging skin is UV exposure, and the research about the harm it causes to your skin can fill a skyscraper. Once you understand the implications of sun damage, you will see your skin from a completely new perspective. Everything from collagen loss, elastin destruction, brown discolorations, to skin cancer (after all, the sun is a major carcinogen) is what you can look forward to by not being sun smart.

Sun damage is cumulative—you can wear sunscreen all summer long, but if you skip the winter months, even the best antiwrinkle creams and treatment won't make much, if any, difference in your skin. Research shows that inadequate sun protection will cause a cascade of damage to your skin, including wrinkles and other telltale signs of aging.

Perhaps most startling to me is the recent research showing that sun damage begins within the *first* minute unprotected skin is exposed to the daylight—even on a cloudy day or in a geographic location that doesn't get much daylight!

Research also shows that 90% of us are either not using sunscreen regularly, are applying it incorrectly, or still don't understand why tanning in any measure is a serious problem for skin. (Sources: *Pediatrics*, March 2011, pages 791–817; *Photochemical and Photobiological Sciences*, December 2011, pages 155–162; *Biopolymers*, March 2012, pages 189–198; *Archives of Dermatological Research*, January 2006, pages 294–302; and *British Journal of Dermatology*, December 2005, Supplemental, pages 37–46).

Fat pad depletion and gravity-influenced movement of the face. The fat pads of the cheek, forehead, and jaw move down and inward on the face as the skin becomes less supple and because of simple gravity. There are 21 "fat compartments" in the face alone—and each changes at a different rate, with the eye area and jaw line deteriorating the fastest. (Sources: *Ophthalmic and Plastic Reconstructive Surgery*, September 2011, pages 348–351; *Plastic and Reconstructive Surgery*, December 2011, pages 747–764, and February 2009, pages 695–700; *Journal of Drugs in Dermatology*, November-December 2006, pages 959–964; *Dermatologic Surgery*, August 2006, pages 1058–1069; and *Annals of Plastic Surgery*, March 2004, pages 234–239).

Loss of estrogen due to menopause or illness. Estrogen is a genuinely youth-giving hormone and women start losing it after the age of 40, either naturally or due to surgery or illness. Once estrogen loss kicks in, the "aging" your skin already has undergone from years of cumulative sun damage starts to accelerate. Loss of estrogen causes the skin to thin as skin cell generation slows; the skin starts to produce extra enzymes that break down collagen; and increased water loss occurs as the skin stops making hyaluronic acid, ceramides, and other substances that keep it protected and supple. Loss of estrogen also causes the elastin fibers in your skin to irreversibly harden (Sources: *American Journal of Clinical Dermatology*, October 2011, pages 297–311; *Experimental Gerontology*, October 2010, pages 801–813; *Climacteric Journal of the International Menopause Society*, August 2007, pages 289–297; and *Experimental Dermatology*, February 2005, page 156).

Genetics. The genes you inherit may hinder or help, a great deal or only a little. Greater levels of melanin in darker skin tones lessen the effect of sun damage, thinner faces age faster because there is less bone structure to support the skin, and the amount of skin-protective substances your skin produces are just some of the genetic factors beyond your control (Sources: *Current Problems in Dermatology*, 2007, volume 35, pages 28–38; and *Journal of Investigative Dermatology*, February 2006, pages 277–282).

Bone loss. As the skeletal support structure of the face loses density and bulk, it provides less architectural support for the skin, and that causes skin to sag faster. Bone loss (where the bones lose their density) accelerates each year after menopause (Sources: *Menopause International*, September 2011, pages 76–77; *Facial Plastic Surgery*, October 2010, pages 350–355; and *Plastic and Reconstructive Surgery*, January 2011, pages 374–383).

Cell senescence. This takes place in skin cells as they eventually lose the capacity to divide and re-create themselves. The result is thin, inelastic, dry skin and generally impaired skin function. Known as the "Hayflick phenomenon," this process is named after Dr. Leonard Hayflick, who identified the condition in 1965. You may have heard or read that exfoliation, whether from AHAs (alpha hydroxy acids) or BHA (beta hydroxy acid), speeds the Hayflick phenomenon, which is a preprogrammed genetic human phenomenon of how many preset times a cell reproduces before it no longer can reproduce. It's not true: AHAs and BHA have no influence whatsoever on the Hayflick response. Such a notion flies in the face of physiology because AHA and BHA exfoliants (and manual exfoliants for that matter) deal only with the superficial, top layers of dead skin; they do not affect the live skin cells beneath (Sources: *Dermatology*, August 2007, pages 352–360; *Molecular Biology Reports*, September 2006, pages 181–186; and *Cell Cycle*, September 2004, pages 1127–1129).

Combination of all these factors: No cosmetic or skin-care product can address all these physiological issues and problems. A combination of well-formulated skin-care products and medical treatments can achieve incredible results, but to imagine that a single miracle cream can do this all by itself is just not realistic. Anyone who tells you differently is either lying to you or just ignorant of the facts. You can choose to spend your money on such products, but I guarantee you will be disappointed with the (lack of) results.

THE TRUTH BEHIND 15 OF THE BIGGEST BOGUS BEAUTY CLAIMS

Aside from the fact that no skin-care product can work better than Botox to get rid of wrinkles, there are many other outrageous claims that show up on all types of products, in all price ranges, regardless of where you shop. Chances are you've bought products partly based on these claims. We've all done it. We're tempted into a purchase because we want so desperately to believe that what's on the packaging is true. But when you know the truth you'll be less likely to end up disappointed or disillusioned—or having wasted your money!

1. Safe for Sensitive Skin, Hypoallergenic, or Ophthalmologist-Tested

Why it's meaningless: "Hypoallergenic," "Safe for Sensitive Skin," and "Ophthalmologist-Tested" imply that a product is unlikely or less likely to cause allergic or sensitizing reactions and, therefore, is better for sensitive or allergy-prone skin. However, there are no accepted testing methods, ingredient restrictions, regulations, guidelines, rules, or procedures of any kind, anywhere in the world, for determining whether or not a product qualifies as being hypoallergenic or safe for the sensitive eye area. **A company can label their product "hypoallergenic," "safe for sensitive skin," or "ophthalmologist-tested" because there is no regulation that says they can't.** We have reviewed plenty of products labeled in this manner that contain problematic ingredients that can trigger allergic or sensitizing reactions, even for those with no previous history of sensitivity.

What to look for instead: Follow the recommendations in this book and on CosmeticsCop.com to learn what the products you are using contain and whether or not those ingredients are good for allergy-prone or sensitive skin.

2. Won't Clog Pores or Noncomedogenic

Why it's meaningless: If you struggle with breakouts, most likely you've purchased products claiming to be noncomedogenic (the technical term for "won't clog pores"), and then found out they made your breakouts worse, or made your skin feel oily. The truth is you can't trust any product that makes claims of "noncomedogenic" (or the less common "nonacnegenic") because there is no approved or regulated standard for these statements. The only research that exists in that area is more than 40 years old and it looked at only a handful of skin-care ingredients used in their pure form in animal experiments, and none of that has anything to do with how these ingredients work in a real skin-care product on real human skin.

The same is true for the claim "won't clog pores"; without guidelines in place, even the thickest, greasiest moisturizer around could make the "doesn't clog pores" claim.

What to look for instead: If you're prone to breakouts and clogged pores, **look for products that have a liquid, gel, serum, or lotion consistency** when shopping for skin-care and makeup products. Thinner textures are less likely to clog pores or worsen breakouts than thicker ingredients that can "get stuck" in pores. Many women with oily skin and breakouts have great results using a well-formulated toner as their "moisturizer" during the day, followed by a lightweight moisturizer with sunscreen or a liquid foundation with sunscreen. At night, a light gel-texture moisturizer is a great option for oily skin.

3. Our studies show…

Why it's meaningless: In the world of cosmetics there's an entire business built on claim substantiation. Essentially, a cosmetics company looking to make specific claims for their product hires an outside company to devise a test that is designed specifically to prove the claims. So, whether they're looking to state their product makes skin 40 percent firmer or provides a 25 percent reduction in wrinkles, the study is set up beforehand to make sure it supports the desired claim. Furthermore, when a study is paid for and controlled by the company, a clear bias is present. As a result, these types of studies are rarely done double-blind (meaning neither the study officials nor the participants know who's using what), are not peer-reviewed, and often bypass many of the scientific principles and standards that reliable, published research is held to in order to be taken seriously.

The next time you see stories about test results showing younger-looking skin, on new cell growth, or a claim that sounds too good to be true, regardless of who is making the claim, ask yourself: How many times have I heard this "perfect skin in a bottle" message before? Is this "story" about only a single study, or are there any corroborating studies? Does it sound too good to be true? Where is the entire study? What did it really test? Did they compare the results with the results of other ingredients? Can I see those studies? Sadly, answers to these questions are hard to come by and usually lead to a dead end. Not surprisingly, cosmetics companies rarely provide that information to us when we ask these same questions!

All of this means that the phrase "Our studies show…" is far more about marketing than effectiveness. Almost without exception the details on how the study was conducted are not made public. We only hear about the results, so you must take the company's word for it. It's not unlike a parent telling children to clean their room—as many parents have discovered, unless kids know you're going to inspect their work afterward, a "clean" room is likely still a mess, and you can't simply trust what you are told. It would be nice if we could rely on cosmetics companies to behave better than children, but when it comes to the business of claim substantiation, you always need to look under the proverbial bed to see what's hidden beneath!

What to look for instead: For the most part, ignore all "Our studies show…" claims and focus on what the published research has to say about the key ingredients in the products you're considering. This is especially important for anti-aging products because their claims, despite seemingly impressive statistics, quickly veer into fantasyland.

4. Cosmeceuticals are Better for Skin

Why it's meaningless: The word "cosmeceutical" was invented by cosmetics companies to describe cosmetic products that they claim have some level (proven or not) of pharmaceutical action that goes beyond standard cosmetic ingredients. There is absolutely no truth to this claim; it is false advertising at its best. Yet, when you come across the term, you may think the product is somehow better for your skin than "regular" cosmetics. The fact is, "cosmeceutical" is just a trumped-up word that has no legal or recognized meaning as to what ingredients these products should contain versus the content of "non-cosmeceutical" cosmetics. Any skin-care product can be labeled "cosmeceutical", regardless of its ingredients.

A skin-care product touting the "cosmeceutical-grade" label, or sometimes "pharmaceutical grade," is not subject to formulary standards nor must companies selling such products prove that they are, indeed, superior in any way. Ironically, we have seen dozens of products labeled "cosmeceutical" that are poorly formulated, come in jar packaging that won't keep ingredients stable once the product is opened and exposed to air, and are absurdly overpriced for what you get.

What to look for instead: Look for products that have been highly rated in this book or on CosmeticsCop.com. You can be assured that the hundreds of products we've assigned a "BEST" rating to contain proven ingredients that work to address a wide range of skin-care concerns, depending on their categories (anti-aging, cleanser, exfoliant, sunscreen, etc.), whether or not they are labeled "cosmeceutical".

5. Dermatologist-Tested or Dermatologist-Formulated

Why it's meaningless: When doctors started putting their names on skin-care products that they endorsed and/or formulated, the allure of a physician's recommendation became a popular trend in the cosmetics industry. Yet, "dermatologist-tested" doesn't mean anything if you can't see the details of the studies to support their claims. Dozens of dermatologists are hired every year by cosmetics companies to do "studies," and, of course, the results of the so-called studies are always positive. There has NEVER been a negative study published by any physicians about the products they sell or about a cosmetics company's products they represent, not anywhere in the world of dermatology and plastic surgery. That fact alone should make you highly skeptical of the dermatologist-tested or dermatologist-formulated claims.

What to look for instead: Forget dermatologist endorsements. This isn't to say there aren't knowledgeable or trustworthy dermatologists out there—the danger is when dermatologists fall into the same marketing traps as the rest of the cosmetics industry. If you're in such a situation (and you'll know because the doctor or his/her staff won't be recommending any other products, just pushing the products they sell), turn around and run as fast as you can from the overpriced products they sell and from the often unethical information they provide about their products. Well-formulated skin-care products are about ingredients that research has proven effective, that are non-irritating for your skin, and that are packaged in airtight containers that keep those key ingredients stable. Those are the elements that will truly make a difference in the health and appearance of your skin, regardless of whether or not "dermatologist-approved" appears on the label.

6. Specially Formulated for Mature Skin

Why it's meaningless: Simply put, age is not a skin type. Yet, the cosmetics industry assumes mature skin is dry skin, and that once women get past a certain arbitrary age, all of a sudden they all need the same extra-moisturizing product formulations. If you believe what many cosmetics companies and fashion magazines say, you'd think that everyone over the age of 50 has the same skin type!

The truth is that women over the age of 50 have different skin types, just like women of all ages, and their skin concerns are not all the same. Lots of women over 50 have oily skin, breakouts, rosacea, sensitivity, and so on, just like women of any age. "Mature skin" isn't automatically dry skin, any more than acne-prone skin is only for teens. (Indeed, some women in their 50s find themselves struggling with breakouts for the first time, often due to hormonal changes.)

Plus, there are no special formulary standards that make products labeled "for mature skin" any better than products formulated for other skin types or concerns. More often than not, the only aspect of products labeled for mature skin is that they tend to be thick and heavy, which is not appropriate for everyone over the age of 50.

What to look for instead: It's all about the ingredients and following a consistent skin-care routine that addresses the needs of YOUR skin type and YOUR skin concerns, regardless of your age. The section in this book, "How to Put Together a Skin-Care Routine," is a great place to learn what your routine should include and why each step is beneficial when you're using beautifully formulated products.

7. "Patented Secrets" or "Patented Ingredients"

Why it's meaningless: There is no such thing as a "patented secret"; that's an oxymoron. The only way to *obtain* a patent is to *divulge* the complete contents of the product and its intended use. Another thing. Patents have absolutely nothing to do with a product's effectiveness, or ineffectiveness. All a patent does legally is attribute a formulation or ingredient designation for a specific purpose (such as wrinkles, acne, exfoliation, or skin lightening) specified by the person who owns the patent; it has nothing to do with whether or not those ingredients can do what the person claims, or anything at all for your skin. Patents also do not indicate or validate the quality, reliability, price, or usefulness of a product, nor does a patent mean that certain established ingredients can't be used by other companies for other purposes (Source: United States Patent and Trademark Office, www.uspto.gov).

What to look for instead: Just forget this one. Don't ever let the claim of "patent" convince you of anything ever again.

8. Natural Ingredients and Essential Oils Are Better for Skin

Why it's meaningless: Whatever preconceived notion someone might have, or whatever media-induced fiction someone might believe, about natural ingredients being better for the skin; it's not true. There is no factual basis or scientific legitimacy for that belief. The definition of "natural" is not only hazy, but also loosely regulated, so any cosmetics company can use it to mean whatever they want it to mean. Just because an ingredient grows out of the ground, or from a tree, or is found in nature doesn't make it automatically good for skin. The reverse is also true: Just because an ingredient is synthetic doesn't make it bad.

"Consumers should not necessarily assume that an 'organic' or 'natural' ingredient or product would possess greater inherent safety than another chemically identical version of the same ingredient," said Dr. Linda M. Katz, Director of the FDA's Office of Cosmetics and Colors, to the *New York Times*, November 1, 2007. "In fact, 'natural' ingredients may be harder to preserve against microbial contamination and growth than synthetic raw materials."

"But people should not interpret even the USDA Organic seal or any organic seal of approval on cosmetics as proof of health benefits or of efficacy," said Joan Shaffer, USDA spokesperson. The National Organic Program is a marketing program, not a safety program. Steak may be graded prime, or vegetables labeled organic, but that has no bearing on whether they are guaranteed safe to eat.

Along the same line, there is nothing "essential" about essential oils. Essential is merely a term that companies apply to most fragrant oils to give them an aura of being important for skin, when often just the opposite is true. This is one of the most consistent out-and-out lies that won't go away in the cosmetics industry. Scientific and medical journals, including those that specialize in plants for alternative medicine, have exhaustively established that fragrance, whether natural or synthetic, is problematic for skin. For any company to suggest that products containing such volatile ingredients as rose, orange, pine, or lavender oils are gentle, helpful, or hypoallergenic is not just misleading—it's harmful for skin (Sources: *Dermatitis*, December 2011, pages 327–329; *Acta Dermato-Venereology*, 2007, volume 87, issue 4, pages 312–316; *Dermatology*, 2002, volume 205, number 1, pages 98–102; *Contact Dermatitis*, December 2001, pages 333–340; *Toxicology and Applied Pharmacology*, May 2001, pages 172–178; and www.ams.usda.gov/nop/FactSheets/Backgrounder.html).

9. This is the Best Ingredient for Skin

Why it's meaningless: Skin is the largest organ of the body, and like any other organ, it needs a complex assortment of beneficial nutrients to thrive, far more than any one ingredient can provide. Think about it just like your diet: Spinach has a great deal of nutritional value, but if you eat only spinach, you soon will become unhealthy and malnourished.

Whether you are dealing with acne, sun protection, antiwrinkle products, rosacea, blackheads, or skin discolorations, your skin needs an array of ingredients to be healthy, to heal, and to stay younger. Despite this, endless cosmetics companies constantly launch new products claiming they contain some new miracle ingredient, and telling you that IT is the final answer for your skin. It's a false claim; rationally, how can every ingredient be a miracle? And if the most recent product a cosmetics company launches contains THE miracle ingredient that "really works," why would there ever be a need for another?

What to look for instead: The truth is there is no single best ingredient for skin. In fact, many work better when combined with others; therefore, the more beneficial ingredients there are in a skin-care product the better it is for your skin. Rather than chasing down the next miracle ingredient, shop for products loaded with proven, beneficial ingredients!

10. Skin Adapts, So You Need to Change to New Products Every Now and Then

Why it's meaningless: Your skin doesn't adapt to skin-care products, any more than your body adapts to a healthy diet. If broccoli and grapes are healthy for you, they are always healthy for you, and they will continue to be healthy, even if you eat them every day. The same is true for your skin: As long as you are applying what is healthy for your skin (and avoiding negative external factors such as not protecting it from the sun), it remains healthy.

What to do instead: If you are using great products for your skin type and skin-care concerns, and nothing has changed for your skin, there is no reason to switch products. You may want to consider something new and different, but don't simply change products because you think you have to do so.

11. To Take the Best Care of Your Skin, Just Use What You Like

Why it's meaningless: Many women have problems with their skin because they often like what isn't good for them. For example, you may like getting a tan, but that will most certainly cause wrinkles and skin discolorations, and may cause skin cancer. You may like smoking cigarettes, but that will cause cell death, and the growth of unhealthy, malformed skin cells. You may like the daytime moisturizer you are using, but if it doesn't contain sunscreen, your skin will age much faster due to sun damage. Or, you may like the fact that your moisturizer comes packaged in a jar, but because most state-of-the-art ingredients, especially antioxidants, plant extracts, vitamins, and many cell-communicating ingredients, deteriorate in the presence of air, the jar packaging will not keep them stable, short-changing your skin (not to mention your wallet) soon after the product is opened.

Think about it like your diet, if you just ate what you liked you might eat chocolate cake and ice cream all day long (I know I would)! If you didn't know better from the abundant research about what is good to eat and what is bad to eat and you were asked to choose between spinach and cheesecake, you would assuredly choose the cheesecake every time. The reason we don't (or try not to) is because we know the difference and have learned to make better choices. The same should apply to your skin-care regimen.

What to use instead: You should use products for beneficial reasons; that is, they should have the best formulas possible for your skin type so you can have truly healthy and younger skin. And you should like those products, too, because the choices available satisfy a wide range of personal preferences.

12. Dry Skin is Caused by a Lack of Water

Why it's meaningless: Dry skin is not caused by your skin not having enough moisture; rather, it's because the skin is unable to prevent moisture loss. Adding more moisture to the skin is not necessarily a good thing. If anything, too much moisture, like soaking in a bathtub, is bad for your skin because it disrupts the skin's outer barrier (the intracellular matrix) by breaking down the substances that keep skin cells functioning normally and in good shape. Dry skin is about maintaining a healthy water balance, which requires products that protect your skin from moisture loss.

What to do instead: Concentrate on putting together the best skin-care routine possible with well-formulated products for your skin type that reinforce the skin with barrier repair ingredients such as glycerin, cholesterol, ceramides, hyaluronic acid, lecithin, non-fragrant plant oils, and others. Once you do this, your skin will be able to stay hydrated and smooth. For more details, please see Chapter 5, *Targeted Solutions for Dry Skin.*

13. Your Skin Requires a Special Nighttime Moisturizer

Why it's meaningless: The ONLY difference between a daytime moisturizer and a nighttime moisturizer should be that the daytime version contains a broad-spectrum sunscreen. What you often hear cosmetics salespeople say is that the skin needs different ingredients at night than during the day because the skin is repairing itself while you sleep. In truth, skin is repairing itself and producing new skin cells every nanosecond of every day and every night. There is absolutely no research showing that your skin needs special ingredients at night versus the daytime (except that at night you don't need sunscreen). This is a fabricated notion that has no basis in fact.

Helping skin repair itself in as healthy a manner as possible doesn't change based on the time of day. Skin needs a generous amount of antioxidants, cell-communicating ingredients, and skin-identical ingredients all day and all night.

What to do instead: During the day, use a well-formulated sunscreen; at night, use a well-formulated moisturizer appropriate for your skin type. "Well-formulated" means loaded with the ingredients all skin types need to become and stay healthy: antioxidants, skin-repairing ingredients, cell-communicating ingredients, and anti-irritants.

14. Skin Produces Too Much Oil Because It Is Dry and Needs More Moisture

Why it's meaningless: Oily skin is hard to control because it's the result of genetically determined hormonal changes in your body, and you simply cannot control this genetic predisposition topically. Androgens—the male hormones—are responsible for oily skin and they are present in both men and women. Oily skin can become dry because most products sold to deal with oily skin contain drying, irritating ingredients, which eventually can make oily skin worse! If your skin is best described as dry on top but oily underneath, you're likely using products that are too drying or irritating.

What to do instead: Follow a routine that meets the needs of oily skin, which will absolutely reduce oil production while preventing and eliminating dry, flaky areas. For more details, see Chapter 7, *Targeted Solutions for Oily Skin*.

15. The Ultimate Beauty Lie: Expensive Means Better

Why it's meaningless: The amount of money you spend on skin-care products has nothing to do with how your skin looks. In other words, spending more money does not automatically mean that you are getting more effective products and ingredients. It all comes down to the formula, and you will find good and bad products in all price ranges. An expensive cleanser by La Mer or Perricone MD is not necessarily better for your skin than an inexpensive cleanser from Neutrogena. And the opposite is true as well: Just because a product is inexpensive doesn't make it worse or ineffective. Spending less doesn't hurt your skin, and spending more doesn't necessarily help it. What counts is the formulation. It's a simple truth, but one often ignored!

What to do instead: Don't worry about this; this book will help you find the best products, regardless of price!

IT'S WHAT'S INSIDE THAT COUNTS

My team and I are endlessly asked about ingredients in skin-care products, and especially, which ingredient is the "*very* best." Because there are thousands of ingredients that show up in skin-care products, there is no all-inclusive way to sum up which are the best. The good news is that there are hundreds of great ingredients, but we also know there are dozens of ingredients that are a serious problem for skin.

To make it easier for you to learn about and become familiar with what you'll find on ingredient lists, we maintain an extensive online Cosmetic Ingredient Dictionary, which you can access by visiting CosmeticsCop.com. Please refer to it for details on what an ingredient is or does, or when you hear a claim about a specific ingredient that has miraculous properties for skin. You will be amazed at how legitimate research rarely matches what a cosmetics company wants you to believe.

DON'T GO TO THE COSMETICS COUNTER WITHOUT COSMETICSCOP.COM, EITHER!

All of the reviews in this edition of *Don't Go to the Cosmetics Counter Without Me* are also available online at CosmeticsCop.com. There you'll find reviews for an additional 200 cosmetics lines as well as several features that make it easier than ever to understand exactly the pros and cons of the products you are using or considering. Millions of consumers all over the world use our reviews to find the best products available without spending a fortune. Be sure to check out CosmeticsCop.com for informative articles on skin care and makeup, plus details on all of the latest ingredients and new products.

CHAPTER TWO

What Your Skin Never Needs

WHY YOU MIGHT NOT HAVE THE SKIN YOU WANT

There are many reasons you may not have the skin you want: sun damage, your genetics, skin disorders, aging, hormone loss, health issues, and pollution. All these things, to one degree or another, generate inflammation inside and outside the body via a complex, endless process of molecular deterioration called free-radical damage.

In addition to what inflammation does internally to the body to cause aging and disease, the same progressive deterioration is taking place on your skin. Over time, this perpetual event creates and re-creates inflammation that destroys the aspects of skin that keep it young, healthy, even-toned, firm, and smooth. Inflammation is just bad news no matter how you look at it.

While all the facets of life mentioned above play havoc with your body and your skin due to the inflammation they trigger, what you put on your skin can have the same effect, and often is a significant factor in what can go wrong. Skin-care products can cause irritation, which in turn produces inflammation that results in problems. To take the best care of your skin, it is vital that you understand what you need to address your skin type and your skin concerns, but it is equally important to know what your skin **doesn't** need. That's critical because the very skin-care products you are using may worsen the problems you are trying to correct!

After more than 30 years of reviewing skin-care products, it is still shocking to us how many of the products women buy to treat a specific skin condition actually make matters worse. For example, you may not realize that the products you've purchased claiming to control oily skin often contain ingredients that make skin even more oily. Products claiming to be oil-free often contain ingredients that nonetheless make skin feel greasy. Products claiming they won't cause breakouts may contain pore-clogging, emollient ingredients that make breakouts worse, even though they don't sound like they will, just because we don't recognize the names on the ingredient label. Countless skin-care products contain irritating ingredients that further damage your skin with each use, and that's what this chapter is about.

IRRITATION IS YOUR SKIN'S WORST ENEMY

We cannot stress this enough: Irritation and inflammation are bad for your skin—really, really bad! Daily assaults, such as unprotected sun exposure, splashing the face with hot water, and applying skin-care products that contain irritating ingredients, generate an irritant/inflammatory effect. These types of attacks result in the skin's inability to heal, the breakdown of collagen and elastin, and the weakening of skin's outer protective layer, among many other complications.

For those with oily skin, irritation triggers nerve endings in the pore that activate androgen production, the hormone that increases oil production and makes pores bigger! None of that is good, not for any skin type.

It turns out that much of what we know about skin aging, wrinkles, skin healing, and acne derives from our better understanding of the skin's inflammatory reaction to sun exposure (UV radiation), pollution, cigarette smoke, and even irritation from skin-care products. These all trigger an inflammatory process that leads to the accumulation of damage to the skin, in turn resulting in deterioration of collagen and elastin, depletion of disease-fighting cells, and free-radical damage (Sources: *Biochemical Society Transactions*, April 2011, pages 688–693; *Journal of Dermatological Science*, May 2010, pages 85–90; *Biogerontology*, 2001, volume 2, number 4, pages 219–229; *Clinical Dermatology*, September-October 2004, pages 360–366, *Dermatology*, January 2003, pages 17–23, *Journal of Investigative Dermatology*, July 2003, pages 20–27; *British Journal of Dermatology*, July 1998, pages 102–103; *Ageing Research Reviews*, June 2002, pages 367–380; and *Journal of the International Union of Biochemistry and Molecular Biology*, October-November 2000, pages 279–289).

IRRITATION: THE SILENT KILLER

It would probably be easier for those who smoke cigarettes to stop smoking if the damage it was causing on the inside showed itself instantly on the outside. Regrettably, that isn't the case. Interestingly, the same thing can be said for skin.

Women often think their skin-care products aren't hurting their skin because they don't feel or see any negative reactions. However, although we may not see or feel damage taking place from the things we put on or do to our skin, damage is taking place nonetheless, beneath the surface, and it eventually will show up on the surface, and it won't be pretty.

You can get a clearer idea of how this hidden, underlying damage from irritating skin-care routines or products takes place by imagining what happens to skin in reaction to unprotected sun exposure. The sun is a major cause of free-radical damage and inflammation that causes brown spots, wrinkling, skin cancer, and other degenerative issues. Yet, other than the rare occasion when you are sunburned, you don't feel or even see the damage done to your skin from the sun, not until years later. Even more shocking is that the damaging rays of the sun can penetrate windows—now that really is a silent killer!

FRAGRANCE: SMELLS LIKE TROUBLE FOR YOUR SKIN

We are all attracted to a pleasing fragrance. In fact, the first thing most women do when testing just about any skin-care product is smell it. As nice as it is to have a product with a wonderful aroma, it just doesn't make for good skin care. Whether the fragrance in the product is from a plant or a synthetic source, with very few exceptions, fragrance is a problem for skin.

The way most fragrance ingredients impart scent is through a volatile reaction, which causes irritation and some amount of inflammation. Research has established that fragrances in skin-care products are among the most common cause of sensitizing and allergic reactions. That means daily use of products that contain a high amount of fragrance, whether the fragrance ingredients are synthetic or natural, causes chronic irritation that can damage healthy collagen production, lead to or worsen dryness, and impair your skin's ability to heal. Fragrance-free is the best way to go for all skin types.

Unfortunately, your nose can't tell from how a product smells whether or not it contains irritating fragrance ingredients. Many beneficial skin-care ingredients (antioxidants, for example) have a natural fragrance, and some of them even smell great! It is not easy to distinguish between the potent antioxidants that actually reduce inflammation and the ingredients that are added solely to make you "shop with your nose" and that can cause irritation. Like anything in skin care, the basic information is on the ingredient label, but because those ingredients read like a college chemistry course, they can be a challenge to decipher—another reason why you need our reviews! (Sources: *Inflammation Research*, December 2008, pages 558–563; *Skin Pharmacology and Physiology*, June 2008, pages 124–135, and November-December 2000, pages 358–371; *Journal of Investigative Dermatology*, April 2008, pages 15–19; *Journal of Cosmetic Dermatology*, March 2008, pages 78–82; *Mechanisms of Ageing and Development*, January 2007, pages 92–105; and *British Journal of Dermatology*, December 2005, pages S13–S22.)

EVERYONE HAS SENSITIVE SKIN

Most of us, to one degree or another, have sensitive skin, meaning our skin reacts to the environment and to the things we put on our skin. Regardless of your skin type or concerns, irritation, which inflames the skin, is always damaging, regardless of the source. Lots of things irritate our skin, some we can avoid and some we can't.

No matter how you think your skin reacts to different aspects of the environment or to the products you use, we are all at risk of damage from irritation and the resulting inflammation.

That means, whether you know it or not, you have sensitive skin, and you need to keep this in mind if you are going to take the best possible care of your skin. It is essential that you take the same precautions that those with sensitive skin take. (Identified as having sensitive skin means you see the result of irritation on the surface of your skin—remember irritation and the inflammation it causes can be happening under the skin even if you don't see it on the surface.) What are these precautions? There is really only one, and it goes for all skin types: Treat your skin as gently as you possibly can. Whether you think of your facial skin as normal, oily, dry, or acne-prone, you still must be gentle and avoid things that cause irritation as much as possible.

YOU HAVE TO BE GENTLE

Everyone will react to one degree or another to irritating skin-care ingredients, for the overall health of your skin (and because irritation is so terrible for skin), anything you can do to treat yours gently is a very good thing. We mention this many times throughout this book, not just to be repetitive, but so it really sinks in—being gentle is truly that important.

Always keep in mind that treating skin gently and using well-formulated non-irritating skin-care products encourages normal collagen production, maintains a smooth and radiant surface, helps skin protect itself from environmental damage, reduces oil production, and makes pores smaller.

Never use the following prime offenders: Overly abrasive loofahs or scrubs (aluminum oxide crystals, walnut shells, or pumice), toners containing irritating ingredients (alcohol, menthol, witch hazel; the latter often is mixed with alcohol, but is also irritating on its own), fragrance (both natural and synthetic), bar soaps/cleansers, hot water, or steaming the skin (including saunas/steam rooms).

COMMON IRRITATING INGREDIENTS TO AVOID

The common ingredients that are of greatest concern when they appear at the beginning of an ingredient list include alcohols, often listed as sd alcohol, alcohol denatured, or isopropyl alcohol. (Note: Ingredients such as cetyl alcohol, although "alcohol" is part of the name, are emollients and are not a problem for skin.) Other irritating ingredients include peppermint, menthol, eucalyptus, fragrances (there are too many of these to list), citruses, lavender, and overly-drying cleansing agents such as sodium lauryl sulfate. (Note: sodium laureth sulfate is fine.) (Sources: *Inflammation Research*, December 2008, pages 558–563; *Skin Pharmacology and Physiology*, June 2008, pages 124–135, and November-December 2000, pages 358–371; *Journal of Investigative Dermatology*, April 2008, pages 15–19; *Journal of Cosmetic Dermatology*, March 2008, pages 78–82; *Mechanisms of Ageing and Development*, January 2007, pages 92–105; and *British Journal of Dermatology*, December 2005, pages S13–S22).

Skin Type versus Skin Concern

THE DIFFERENCE BETWEEN SKIN TYPE AND SKIN CONCERN

One of the more confusing aspects of developing a skin-care routine is finding products that work for your skin type while simultaneously addressing your skin-care concerns. It's important to understand exactly what you should be using for each and why, but therein lies the confusion. The issue is that some products are for your skin type and some are for your skin concerns and sometimes products can address both needs. When shopping for a skin-care concern, like brown spots or acne, you should match the treatment to your skin type to find the right products for both.

First, determine your skin type (i.e., normal to dry, oily, combination); this lets you know which formulations work best to address the everyday needs of your skin type so you can put together a basic skin-care routine. That basic routine should include a cleanser, toner, AHA (alpha hydroxy acid) or BHA (beta hydroxy acid) exfoliant, daytime moisturizer with sunscreen, and a moisturizer without sunscreen to use at night. From there, you can identify your skin concerns and then determine what additional targeted solutions are necessary. For example, a concern such as clogged pores can be addressed beautifully by one of the products in your basic skin-care routine, such as a BHA exfoliant. Or, if you have brown spots, you'll want to add a skin-lightening treatment to your regular routine, which will address the discolorations in a more targeted manner than merely using an AHA or BHA exfoliant.

KNOWING YOUR SKIN TYPE IS IMPORTANT

Once you know your skin type, you will have a clearer understanding of which product formulations work best for you. For example, if you have oily skin you want to avoid overly-emollient or greasy formulations at all costs. Conversely, if you have dry skin you will want formulations with a creamier, richer base.

Not sure of your skin type? Keep in mind that almost everyone at some time or another has combination skin. That's because the center area of your face has more oil glands, so you are more likely to be oily or have clogged pores in this "T-zone." Likewise, it is typical for some areas of your face (the eye area, around the nose) to be more reactive to skin-care products and the environment.

Even more important is to realize that you can have more than one skin type: sensitive and dry, oily and blemish-prone, dry and sensitive with acne. The more you know about everything that affects different skin types, the more you'll be able to help your skin finally look and feel as normal as possible!

WHAT INFLUENCES SKIN TYPE

Almost anything can influence skin type—both external and internal elements can and do influence the way your skin looks and feels. To evaluate your skin type, consider some of the factors below. Keep in mind it's possible your skin is simply reacting to influences that are easily isolated and treated—meaning they are within your control to change:

- Hormones
- Skin disorders
- Genetic predisposition
- Smoking and secondhand smoke
- Medications
- Diet
- Your skin-care routine
- Stress
- Unprotected/prolonged sun exposure
- Pollution
- Climate

WHAT CAN CAUSE A SKIN TYPE YOU DON'T WANT

It probably isn't hard to see how smoking, sun damage, diet, and genetics can negatively and dangerously affect your skin. What many people don't realize is that the products they use can be worsening or even creating the very skin issues they are trying to resolve. In other words, what you apply to your skin may be causing a skin type you don't want, or intensifying what you don't like about your skin type!

For example, many products for treating acne contain high amounts of alcohol or other irritating ingredients (peppermint, menthol, citrus) which dry and irritate your skin, triggering more oil production and more blemishes!

You'll never know your actual skin type if you use products containing ingredients that create the very problems you don't want. Another example: If you are using products that contain irritants, you can create dry skin and still make your oily skin worse (think dry skin on top, oily underneath). Alternatively, if you use overly-emollient or thick-textured products along with a drying cleanser, you can clog pores, prevent skin cells from exfoliating (which makes your skin look dull), and make your skin feel oily in areas (i.e., combination skin). If you over-scrub, you can damage the barrier (surface), causing more wrinkles and dry (or worsen already dry) skin.

HOW TO DETERMINE YOUR SKIN TYPE

Once you've ruled out the controllable factors (sun exposure, smoking) that affect your skin type and rid your routine of problematic products (poor formulations, jar packaging, irritating ingredients), you'll be able to determine your skin type more clearly.

Before you get out your mirror and have a close look, it's best to wash your face with a gentle cleanser, apply a state-of-the-art gentle toner (loaded with antioxidants and skin-repairing ingredients), and apply a moisturizer appropriate for your skin type (gel or liquid for oily skin, lightweight lotion or serum for normal skin, a more emollient version for dry skin). Then, wait two hours to see what your skin does without additional products or makeup. The chart below is a general guide to how skin behaves depending on its type—you may see any combination of the descriptions below happening on your face. It bears repeating: Anyone's skin can have multiple "types," and these types can change due to hormonal cycle, season, stress levels, and other factors.

Skin Behavior	Skin Type*				Skin Concern*				
	Oily	Combination	Acne or Blemish-Prone*	Dry to Very Dry	Normal	Eczema	Sun-Damaged	Aging/Wrinkles	Sensitive/Rosacea
Some areas are oily and some areas are dry; may also be sensitive		✓							
Most areas appear dry, flaky, matte, or feel tight; may also be sensitive				✓					
Redness, with or without bumps, (but not pimples)									✓
Mild to moderate breakouts, sometimes around hormone cycles; may also be sensitive			✓						
Lines evident around eyes, mouth, and/or cheeks; may also be sensitive								✓	
Some fine lines and/or skin discolorations; may also be sensitive							✓		
Some areas have red, dry, flaky patches that swell, burn, or itch						✓			
Four hours after cleansing, skin has excess oil; may also be sensitive	✓								
No signs of oiliness or dryness; may also be sensitive					✓				

*May also be a concern

CHOOSING THE RIGHT PRODUCTS FOR YOUR SKIN TYPE

When you discover what your genuine skin type is, you will make better decisions about the type of products to include in your skin-care routine. While all skin types can benefit from the same basic product types (cleanser, toner, exfoliant, sunscreen, and moisturizer), the texture of these products will differ based on your skin type. However, regardless of your skin type, all products must be gentle and include the same beneficial ingredients: antioxidants, skin-repairing, skin-identical, cell-communicating, anti-irritants, salicylic acid (BHA) or alpha hydroxy acid (AHA) exfoliants, and so on. Here is how it works:

- If you have normal to oily skin, the skin-care products you use should contain minimal to no emollients or thickeners, and either be in a liquid or gel base or gel-like serum.
- If you have normal to dry skin, the base of your products should be slightly emollient and the texture a lotion, lightweight cream, or serum.
- If you have combination skin (oily in some areas and dry in others), then you must mix and match products, using the ones appropriate for each area, because a single formula won't work for you. Over time, using the correct skin-care products can eliminate extreme combination skin, and simplify your routine.
- If you have dry skin, use products with a more emollient, creamy, or balm-like base.

The primary thing to remember is that all skin types benefit from the same types of gentle products and essential ingredients; the only difference is the base texture of the product. Following is a chart of how it works.

Product Texture/Base	Skin Type				
	Oily	Combination	Blemish-Prone	Dry	Normal
Lotion		✓	✓	✓	✓
Cream				✓	✓
Gel	✓	✓	✓		✓
Serum	✓	✓	✓	✓	✓
Liquid	✓	✓	✓		✓
Powder	✓		✓		

For detailed information on why you need specific skin-care products, what each does, and what results you can expect, please see Chapter 10, *Putting It All Together: The Best Skin Care Routine for You.*

SOLVING SKIN-CARE CONCERNS

Now that you have the basics, you can take it a step further and focus on treating your skin-care concerns more specifically. This is really about what specialty treatment products you may need over and above the basics we discussed above to take care of your skin. There are specific treatment products, both prescription and non-prescription, targeted toward acne, rosacea, blackheads, very oily skin, advanced sun damage, wrinkles, eczema, and so on. Those needs, along with your basic skin-care requirements, are explained in the following chapters.

CHAPTER FOUR

What Every Skin Type Needs

UNIVERSAL NEEDS FOR ALL SKIN TYPES

Unless you have a serious skin disorder, everyone—and we mean everyone—needs the following products and ingredients, regardless of their skin type or concerns. Ingredients or formulations that affect a product's texture or that target specific skin concerns such as acne or skin lightening may differ, but the universal beneficial ingredients (antioxidants, skin-repairing, and cell-communicating) remain the same. In other words, regardless of your skin type or skin concern, EVERYONE needs well-formulated cleansers, toners, sunscreens, exfoliants, and moisturizers that have the same types of beneficial ingredients. What differs is the feel of the formula (i.e., gels for oilier skin, creams for drier skin). The skin-improving ingredients, such as antioxidants, remain the same across the board.

Think about it like your diet: No matter who you are or where you are in the world, the same foods are either healthy or unhealthy for you. Salmon is good, refined sugar is bad; leafy greens are good, trans fats are bad; excessive alcohol is bad, but moderate alcohol intake can be good; and on and on. You may not like salmon, but there are alternatives you can eat that will be healthy for you. The same is true for your skin: The categories of great ingredients such as skin-repairing substances and antioxidants are the same for everyone.

A GENTLE CLEANSER IS ESSENTIAL

Regardless of your skin type, you must use a gentle cleanser. Research proving that you should cleanse the skin gently, regardless of skin type, is now well established. This is the basic first step for everyone, with normal to oily, dry, or blemish-prone skin. Let us repeat: No matter what your skin type, it is unhealthy and damaging to your skin to use cleansers that are harsh or drying.

Expensive cleansers are a huge waste of money. They will not make your face any cleaner, and they are no more gentle than less expensive water-soluble cleansers. In fact, there is only a handful of standard cleansing agents used in cleansers, and they are the same across the cosmetics spectrum, regardless of price. In reality, there are good and bad cleansers in all price ranges!

One more point: The wrong cleanser can cause problems for your skin. For example, a cleanser that is too moisturizing for your skin type can create blemishes and make your skin feel greasy or oily. A cleanser that is too drying can create combination skin, because drying up skin doesn't stop or change the amount of oil your oil glands produce. This is where the texture of a product and the specific ingredients come into play.

Thankfully, drying cleansing agents are being used less and less in facial cleansers since the first editions of this book were published, but there still are products that include them. For example, they are still present in many bar soaps/cleansers, which typically are far more drying than water-soluble cleansers with gentle cleansing agents, but that can also be true for lotion or liquid cleansers.

Bar soaps/cleansers are problematic for all skin types. The ingredients that keep bar cleansers/soaps in their solid form can clog pores (think of the soap scum that builds up on your tub, this also happens to your skin) and the cleansing agents in bar cleansers/soaps are almost always drying and irritating, and you now know how damaging that is for skin.

Essential Point: **Use a gentle, water-soluble cleanser that removes most types of eye makeup without irritating the eye, and doesn't dry out skin or leave it feeling greasy.** (Sources: *International Journal of Dermatology*, August 2002, pages 494–499; *Cosmetic Dermatology*, August 2000, pages 58–62; *Cutis*, December 2001, volume 68, number 5, Supplemental; *Skin Research and Technology*, February 2001, pages 49–55; *Dermatology*, 1997, volume 195, number 3, pages 258–262; and *Journal of the American Medical Association*, April 1980, pages 1640–1643).

USE A GENTLE EYE-MAKEUP REMOVER

Removing all your eye makeup is more important than you think. Leaving behind traces of eyeshadow or mascara at night while you're sleeping can cause irritation that increases puffiness and, over time, wrinkling. If you wear minimal to light makeup or no makeup at all, a water-soluble cleanser for cleansing your face and eyes can be enough to remove makeup. For those who apply foundation, concealer, eyeshadows, eye pencils, and mascara (especially long-wearing formulas), it takes more diligence to cleanse and get them off your skin completely. In those cases, a gentle makeup remover, containing no fragrance or coloring agents, needs to be part of your nightly routine. Begin by washing your face with a gentle, water-soluble cleanser and remove as much makeup as you can this way, so you minimally pull at the skin. Pulling and tugging skin weakens the elastin fibers, increasing the potential for sagging. Gently massaging a cleanser over the face and eyes and then rinsing prevents tugging and pulling, which is far better for your skin. Then you can remove the last traces of makeup with a gentle makeup remover and soft cotton pad or cotton swab, always pulling and tugging as little as possible. Remember—be gentle!

CONSIDER A GREAT TONER

Toners have become a confusing category of skin-care products. Because of misperceptions, many fashion magazines, dermatologists, and even cosmetics salespeople advise against using a toner, or simply dismiss toners as an optional step. That is disappointing, because a well-formulated toner can provide truly amazing benefits for your skin.

Once you understand how toners work, and know what ingredients are included in the toners we rate as best for skin, you'll see why they are an essential step for achieving the healthy, radiant glow you want.

What we now know is that your skin needs a range of ingredients that restore and repair its surface after it is cleansed. Skin can never get too much of these important ingredients: antioxidants and skin-repairing substances such as glycerin, fatty acids, and ceramides. **The right toner can give your skin a healthy dose of what it needs to look younger, fresher, and smoother, right after cleansing and throughout the day.**

There are so many poorly formulated toners on the market that, without this book, finding the right toner for your skin would be nearly impossible. Many toners are alcohol-based, or are little more than eau de cologne, containing primarily fragrance and hardly any beneficial skin-care ingredients.

However, when a toner is in a gentle solution, loaded with beneficial ingredients, such as antioxidants and skin-repairing and cell-communicating ingredients, you will be giving your skin exactly what it needs to feel nourished, calmed, and soft after cleansing.

If you have oily or blemish-prone skin, you need to be especially careful when shopping for toners. Almost without exception, the toners that claim to be specifically for these skin types and concerns are not going to help, because they usually contain irritants, such as alcohol, witch hazel, and/or menthol, that hurt your skin's healing process. That means red marks won't fade, the likelihood of more breakouts increases, and excess oil production is stimulated at the base of the pore; plus, it will create a dry, flaky surface intermingled with oil. Yuck!

The toners that are best for oily or blemish-prone skin are those whose ingredients help repair the skin's surface, make skin feel smoother, reduce enlarged pores, and contain cell-communicating ingredients that train pores to handle excess oil in a more efficient manner. For combination to oily skin, especially during the summer or in warmer climates, a well-formulated toner may be the only "moisturizer" your oily skin needs, but more about that in a moment!

A Great Exfoliant Can Give You Smoother Skin Overnight

Even if you cleanse, tone, and apply a sunscreen in the morning and a moisturizer at night (that you've chosen from either The Paula's Choice Team's recommendations or from Paula's Choice), there's still one thing missing that could make all the difference in the world to get you the skin you want: a well-formulated exfoliant! Without question, almost everyone can benefit from daily use of a well-formulated AHA (alpha hydroxy acids, such as glycolic and lactic acids) or BHA (beta hydroxy acid is another term for salicylic acid) product.

Why Exfoliation Is So Beneficial For Skin

Skin naturally sheds (exfoliates) millions of skin cells each day. When this natural shedding slows or stops due to sun damage, dry skin, oily skin, genetics, loss of estrogen, or skin disorders, the results are unmistakable: dull, dry, or flaky skin; clogged pores; blemishes; white bumps; and uneven skin tone. An AHA or BHA exfoliant steps in to help put everything in balance again. When you gently get rid of these built-up skin cells you can unclog pores, reduce or stop breakouts, smooth out wrinkles, and even make dry, dull skin disappear!

A gentle exfoliant really can make skin look younger overnight. How is that possible? Think about the skin on your heels before you get a pedicure. The built-up layers of dead, callused skin on your heels looks dry, rough, discolored, and scaly, and deep lines are obvious. Once you remove that layer and apply a moisturizer, your heels immediately look smooth and unwrinkled! Of course what causes calluses on your feet is different from what causes skin cells to build up on your face, and you can't be that rough on your face without damaging the skin—but the same benefit you get from exfoliating your heels also holds true for your face; you just have to be far more gentle. With a well-formulated AHA or BHA exfoliant, that's easy to do!

What's the difference between an AHA and BHA? Both AHAs and BHA are brilliant options for exfoliating the surface of the skin, with extensive research demonstrating their ability to reduce blemishes, build collagen, smooth the skin's surface, reduce wrinkles, and even provide some tightening of the skin. Each has its own special qualities, which you'll want to consider when deciding which one to use.

- **AHAs (primarily glycolic, lactic, or polyhydroxy acids) are preferred for sun damage and dryness** because they exfoliate on the surface of the skin, and have the added benefit of also improving skin's moisture content.
- **BHA (salicylic acid) is preferred for oily, acne-prone skin and for treating black-heads and white bumps** because BHA has the ability to unclog oily pores and normalize the lining of the misshapen pore that contributes to acne.
- **BHA has anti-inflammatory and antibacterial action.** Two interesting properties of BHA explain why it works well for any inflammatory disorder, such as acne, rosacea, or general redness. The reason is that salicylic acid is related to aspirin (aspirin is acetylsalicylic acid) and salicylic acid shares aspirin's anti-inflammatory properties. It is important to mention that an AHA formulated with anti-irritants can provide the same benefit, but by themselves, AHAs do not have anti-inflammatory properties, and AHAs cannot penetrate clogged pores or treat acne as BHA can.
- **If your skin is sun-damaged, and you're also struggling with acne or clogged pores, add a BHA product to your routine.** You'll get the benefit of exfoliating the surface of the skin and the extra benefit of exfoliating inside the pore to improve its shape and prevent clogs.
- **Using AHA and BHA at the same time:** If you'd like to use an AHA and BHA at the same time, doing so is an option, although not necessary. Some people find they work well when they're applied at the same time, or one as part of their morning routine and the other in the evening, but either one should be able to do the job all by itself, either once or twice a day.

HOW DO I USE AN AHA OR BHA?

- Apply the AHA or BHA product after cleansing your face and applying your toner. You can apply it immediately after the toner or you can wait until the toner has dried. You can use an AHA or BHA product once or twice a day.
- You can apply the AHA or BHA product around the eye area, but not on the eyelid or directly under the eye because you don't want to get it in your eye. You can mix a bit of the AHA or BHA into the moisturizer you use around your eye.
- Next, you can apply any other product in your routine, such as moisturizer, serum, eye cream, sunscreen, and/or foundation. If you prefer to wait until the AHA or BHA product has dried, that's fine, but not necessary.
- If you're using a topical prescription product such as Renova, other retinoids, or any of the topical prescription products for rosacea, apply the AHA or BHA first.
- The best AHA and BHA products are listed at the end of this book and on Cosmetics-Cop.com.

SHOULD YOU USE A SCRUB TO EXFOLIATE?

Scrubs are certainly an option for exfoliating your skin, but they have limitations and present concerns that may make it best to avoid them. Scrubs deal only with the top, superficial layer of skin, while most of the layers of built up, dead, sun-damaged skin go far below what you can see on the surface.

What is most problematic is that many scrubs contain scrub particles that have a rough, uneven texture that can damage skin as it abrades the surface, causing tiny tears that disrupt the skin's barrier. Scrubs often cause more problems than they solve.

Another issue is that many scrubs have thick, relatively waxy formulations or contain more cleansing agents than your primary cleanser, adding potential irritation and/or pore-clogging ingredients to skin. Using a scrub also adds another product (expense and complication) to your routine, without providing much benefit in return. There are a handful of scrubs we do recommend for those of you who prefer them, but ultimately you get more benefit from using a daily AHA or BHA exfoliant plus a gentle washcloth with your cleanser for a bit of manual exfoliation.

What about using a battery-powered brush like the clarisonic to exfoliate?

If you want to try manual exfoliation for your skin, consider one of the battery-powered rotating brushes such as the Clarisonic. You also can use a gentle washcloth with your daily cleanser, which works just as well to exfoliate the surface of skin as any cosmetic scrub you can buy. (A gentle washcloth and daily cleanser is Paula's personal choice.) As a bonus, washcloths are softer (thus more gentle) and, unlike some facial scrubs, they don't contain pore-clogging ingredients that aggravate oily, acne-prone skin. The most important consideration is not to over-scrub because it damages skin and creates more problems than it solves. Keep in mind it is easy to overdo it with powered cleansing brushes. The resulting inflammation of over-scrubbing may initially make pores and wrinkles seem less apparent, but over time, the irritation isn't worth those brief benefits.

CAN YOU EXFOLIATE TOO OFTEN?

Exfoliating your skin is great, and once you find a product that works best for your skin type, deciding how often to use it takes experimentation. For many people twice a day works best, for others just once a day, every other day, or for some only once a week.

You may have heard that exfoliating with AHAs or BHA may have a negative effect on skin cell production (i.e., on live skin cell production). Exfoliating does not negatively affect how skin generates healthy cells in the lower layers of the skin because AHAs or BHA are not absorbed past the surface layers of dead skin. If anything, exfoliating dead skin cells on the surface of skin can improve collagen production, increase skin's ability to hold moisture, and allow pores to function normally! (Sources: *Journal of Cosmetic Science*, June 2008, pages 175–182, and March-April 2006, pages 203–204; *Free Radical Biology and Medicine*, May 17, 2008; *Archives of Dermatologic Research*, April 2008, pages S31–S38, and June 1997, pages 404–409; *Journal of Cosmetic Dermatology*, March 2007, pages 59–65, and September 2006, pages 246–253; *International Phytotherapy Research*, November 2006, pages 921–934; *Aesthetic and Plastic Surgery*, May-June 2006, pages 356–362; *Skin Pharmacology and Physiology*, May 2006, pages 283–289; *Journal of Dermatology*, January 2006, pages 16–22; and *International Journal of Cosmetic Science*, February 2005, pages 17–34.)

YOU MUST USE SUNSCREEN 365 DAYS A YEAR

When it comes to protecting your skin from the sun, what you don't know and possibly aren't doing will cause wrinkles, sagging, brown skin discolorations, dull-looking skin, and potentially even skin cancer. While many women clamor for and purchase the latest antiwrinkle cream or serum, all of that is meaningless if you aren't using an effective sunscreen every day of your life (even in the winter, even if it isn't sunny outside). Whether you tan or not (though any amount of tanning is destroying your skin), the damaging rays of the sun are taking a toll that begins the moment your skin sees daylight.

If you are exposed to the sun, even for as little as a few minutes every day—and that includes walking to your car or a bus, or sitting next to a window during the day (the sun's damaging UVA rays can penetrate through clear window glass)—regardless of the season, that exposure adds up over the years, and the accelerated aging it causes can show up as early as your 20s.

Aside from the abundant scientifically valid studies proving how damaging sun exposure is to skin, you can do your own research by comparing the skin on parts of your body that rarely, if ever, see the sun with the skin on parts of your body that are exposed to the sun daily. If you are over the age of 40 or even younger, and you've been regularly tanning, you will notice that the areas that get minimal sun exposure (such as your backside, inside of your arm, breasts, middle back, and thighs) don't appear dry or thin-skinned, don't show brown discolorations, and don't have wrinkles or any of the other common signs of "aging." Meanwhile, the skin that is chronically exposed to the sun without protection looks "older," and has more skin problems than the skin you have protected in some manner. You may not see the damage now, and you might love getting a tan, either from the sun or from a tanning bed, but the damage will show up as prematurely aged skin.

WHAT IS A WELL-FORMULATED SUNSCREEN?

Medical boards around the world recommend using a sunscreen with a sun-protection factor (SPF) of at least 15, but without question, more is better because most of us aren't applying enough. The SPF number is only a measure of protection from the sun's burning rays—known as UVB radiation. Yet it is equally dangerous for your skin to not have UVA protection (UVA rays are responsible for aging and, like UVB, increased cancer risk). Unfortunately, there are many sunscreens that don't contain UVA-protecting ingredients to protect against the entire UVA spectrum.

The rating system and the ingredients needed for UVB protection are well established and relatively universal across countries. For UVA protection, what is accepted around the world are the following ingredients, and they must be listed as **active ingredients: zinc oxide, titanium dioxide, avobenzone (sometimes listed as Parsol 1789 or butyl methoxydibenzoylmethane), Mexoryl SX (ecamsule), or Tinosorb (Tinosorb is available only in products sold outside the United States).** These UVA protection ingredients are generally agreed upon internationally, but if one of them is not listed on the active ingredient list, then it doesn't count—it is not sufficient for it to be listed on the list of regular or "other" ingredients. Let us repeat: If it's not on the active list, then you are not applying adequate UVA protection, and that is dangerous for your skin.

You must apply sunscreen liberally! That means that using an expensive sunscreen can be dangerous if it discourages you from applying it generously. For specifics on sun-protection, including SPF ratings and UVA versus UVB protection, refer to the "Sun Essentials" section at CosmeticsCop.com; there is no single issue in skin care more important than this.

Bottom Line: There is no such thing as a "safe tan" or just "getting a little color," whether from the sun or a tanning bed. In fact, tanning beds are far more dangerous than the sun. Any change in skin color from the sun or from tanning beds means that your skin is being seriously damaged, and all the anti-aging products in the world can't counter that kind of damage.

Essential Point: **Being smart about exposing your skin to the sun and using a well-formulated sunscreen is the most important part of any skin-care routine, especially if your goal is to avoid or minimize wrinkles and other signs of aging** (Sources: *Photodermatology, Photoimmunology, and Photomedicine*, December 2011, pages 318–324; and *Cancer Epidemiology, Biomarkers, and Prevention*, March 2005, pages 562–566).

SUN AND THE VITAMIN D CONTROVERSY

Vitamin D is the one essential nutrient that the body creates from routine, direct sun exposure. But, before you skimp on the *sunscreen* and head outdoors to bask in the sun as you might have read you should do, you need to know the pros and cons of getting this important vitamin from the sun, compared to being sun smart and taking a vitamin D supplement.

Following are vitamin D facts:

- The body itself produces Vitamin D only from exposure to the sun.
- Not having enough vitamin D stored in your body is a serious health issue and an alarming number of people are vitamin D deficient, especially in parts of the world with limited sunshine in the winter.
- Normal levels of vitamin D protect our bodies in numerous ways, including bone health, immune disorders, and reduced occurrence of some cancers, and ongoing research is revealing even more ways vitamin D protects our overall health.
- There are two types of vitamin D: ergocalciferol (commonly known as D2) and cholecalciferol (vitamin D3). Cholecalciferol often is referred to as natural vitamin D because it is the type your body makes upon exposure to sunlight.
- The sun's UVB rays (the rays from the sun that cause sunburn) stimulate vitamin D production, not the UVA rays.

THE VITAMIN D AND SUNSCREEN DILEMMA

What's the dilemma? If exposure to sunlight is the best way to get vitamin D, then what about the damage sun exposure causes? Unprotected sun exposure causes premature aging of the skin, heightens the risk of skin cancer, macular degeneration, and DNA abnormalities, and gets in the way of the body's ability to heal. Swapping one health concern for another is not good medicine for anyone. This dilemma has made the issue of sun exposure controversial and complicated.

The question is: **Can our bodies create vitamin D if we regularly use sunscreen and seek shade?** According to many researchers, the answer is that most likely sunscreen and seeking shade does not block vitamin D production in the body. Despite news stories to the contrary, several large, controlled studies have shown that vitamin D deficiency does not result from ongoing, regular sunscreen use. But there also are studies that counter that point of view.

It is important to understand that wearing sunscreen and seeking shade doesn't explain the entire problem of vitamin D deficiency. Most people don't use sunscreen on a regular basis and they almost never apply enough of it, or reapply it as they should, to get the SPF benefit on the label. That means that during the day, depending on where you live, if you are outside, your skin is getting enough sunlight to enable your body to make sufficient vitamin D.

You may have read that 15 or 30 minutes of unprotected sun exposure a day will create all the vitamin D you need, but there is limited evidence showing that to be the case, especially considering that there are varying amounts of sunlight in different parts of the world and at different times of the year, so you should not rely on that number. For example, 30 minutes of sun exposure at noon during the winter months in London, Paris, Moscow, Seattle, or Toronto won't do you much good.

Despite the conflict, the facts are you need vitamin D and you need to protect your skin from the sun every day. Our strong recommendation is to have the best of both worlds by doing the following: **1. Do NOT give up sunscreen and do not give up being sun smart!** That means you need to seek shade, cover up as much of your body as you reasonably can, wear sunglasses, and wear hats. **2. Have your vitamin D levels tested at your next doctor's appointment and achieve adequate levels of vitamin D from supplements, as recommended by your doctor.** Doing these two things you can be truly healthy without having your skin suffer the aging and potentially cancerous consequences of unprotected sun exposure.

TANNING BEDS

The fear of not getting enough vitamin D and an obsession for having tanned skin is causing an alarming increase in the use of tanning beds. Many tanning salons advertise that they provide the added benefit of increasing vitamin D levels in the body; some even go so far as to say that it eliminates depression. Neither is remotely the case, and this is some of the most damaging information imaginable for your skin.

Aside from the terrible risks associated with using tanning beds, they cannot produce vitamin D in the body. As it turns out, UVB rays are responsible for stimulating vitamin D in the body, and tanning beds emit almost entirely UVA rays!

In terms of depression, there is indeed a small amount of research showing that tanning beds do produce a feeling of euphoria for some people, but that doesn't mean it is a healthy effect. It would be like recommending someone smoke cigarettes because it can have a calming effect, or recommending someone get drunk because it can make them feel happier. Feeling better from something that is hurting you is a mistake, one for which you will pay with your health and appearance in the long run, which is ultimately very depressing (Sources: *The British Journal of Dermatology*, August 2010, Epublication, and October 2005, pages 706–714; *Osteoporosis International*, August 2010, Epublication; *Mayo Clinic Proceedings*, August 2010, pages 752–757; *Current Rheumatology Reports*, October 2005, pages 356–364; *The Journal of Steroid Biochemistry and Molecular Biology*, Epublication, July 19, 2005; *Photochemistry and Photobiology*, Epublication, February 1, 2005; *Experimental Dermatology*, December 2004, page 11; *The Journal of the American Osteopathic Association*, August 2003, pages 3–4; *American Journal of Clinical Dermatology*, March 2002, pages 185–191; *Dermatology*, January 2001, pages 27–30; *British Medical Journal*, October 1999, page 1066; and naturaldatabase.com).

WHY EVERYONE NEEDS A GREAT ANTI-AGING "MOISTURIZER"

With all the anti-aging, antiwrinkling, lifting, firming, nourishing, organic, works-like-Botox eye cream, neck cream, and throat cream products touting their miracle formulations, it's hard to know where moisturizers fit into the picture. In actuality, regardless of the name or claim, "moisturizers," or whatever the industry calls them in terms of their antiwrinkle benefit, whether they are in cream, lotion, serum, or even liquid form, must meet the same requirements of anti-aging and anti-aging treatments. They must supply the skin with ingredients that help maintain its structure, help build collagen and firmer skin, reduce free-radical damage (environmental assaults on the skin from sun, pollution, and air), help cells function more normally, and overall help your skin look and act younger. For all skin types, and we mean all skin types, when you use moisturizers containing the well-researched groups of ingredients that can do these things, they are as close to "anti-aging," or "antiwrinkling," or "repairing" as any skin-care product can be, regardless of the name on the label (or the price).

What are these spectacular anti-aging ingredients? They are antioxidants, skin-repairing ingredients, cell-communicating ingredients, and anti-irritants. You should treat your skin to these ingredients twice daily, at night in your nighttime moisturizer and during the day in your sunscreen, because they are critical for taking optimal care of your skin. Anything less is a waste of your money and a serious detriment to your skin. You also can and should get these essential ingredients and benefits from other products in your routine, such as toners, serums, and exfoliants.

SHOULD YOU USE A LOTION, CREAM, GEL, SERUM, OR LIQUID?

While all skin types benefit from a wide range of antioxidants, cell-communicating ingredients, anti-irritants, and skin-repairing ingredients, they don't all benefit from products with the same thickness or texture. Your skin type dictates whether you should use a gel, cream, lotion, serum, or liquid. Think of it like a healthy meal: The salad and entrée should contain the same kinds of healthy foods, but the preparation is about your personal preference and dietary restrictions.

As a general rule, those with oily or combination skin will prefer lighter-weight lotions, gels, serums, or liquids. Those with dry skin usually prefer creams or more emollient formulations to make up for what their oil glands don't provide or what dry, arid climates exacerbate. Those with blemish-prone skin generally do better with moisturizers that have a thinner consistency, such as a liquid or gel. For blemish-prone or oily skin types, a well-formulated toner may be the only "moisturizer" your skin needs, because a well-formulated toner will contain beneficial ingredients that are similar to those in a "moisturizer."

DO YOU NEED A DIFFERENT MOISTURIZER FOR DAYTIME AND NIGHTTIME?

Putting aside the claims, hype, and misleading information you may have heard, the only real difference between a daytime and nighttime moisturizer is that the daytime version should contain a well-formulated sunscreen. Regardless of the time of day, your skin needs all the current state-of-the-art ingredients we describe in the previous and following paragraphs. Your skin doesn't do special healing at night, nor is it more "receptive" to nutrients, despite what you might have heard from a cosmetics salesperson or read in a fashion magazine. There isn't a shred of evidence showing that the skin needs specific ingredients at night that it doesn't need during the day; the only difference is that during the day you need a reliable sunscreen!

ALL SKIN TYPES NEED SKIN-REPAIRING INGREDIENTS

The term "skin-repairing ingredients" in this book refers to the substances between skin cells that keep them connected and help maintain the skin's fundamental structure. Without an intact protective barrier, skin suffers from myriad problems, including increased sun damage, inflammation, redness, increased breakouts, collagen breakdown, and dryness. There are many ingredients that have the ability to repair the skin's protective outer layers, including ceramides, lecithin, glycerin, polysaccharides, hyaluronic acid, sodium hyaluronate, sodium PCA, amino acids, cholesterol, phospholipids, glycosphingolipids, glycosaminoglycans, vitamin C, and many more. All of these give the skin what it needs to keep its cells intact—and there is no "best," despite what is advertised on TV, magazines, celebrity endorsements, or the Internet. Just like broccoli isn't the only healthy food your body needs, the skin has complex needs as well.

When a moisturizer contains a combination of these ingredients (with no single one being more important than another), it helps reinforce the skin's natural ability to function normally, improves the skin's texture, eliminates dry skin, increases the skin's ability to heal, and builds collagen among other benefits.

ALL SKIN TYPES NEED ANTIOXIDANTS

Antioxidants are perhaps the most essential part of any state-of-the-art anti-aging "moisturizer" (again, regardless of the name on the label). An immense body of research continues to show that antioxidants are a potential panacea for skin's ills, and ignoring their benefit while shopping for moisturizers (or any products with names like "anti-aging" or "anti-wrinkle" or "treatment") means you'll be shortchanging your skin. What makes antioxidants so intriguing is that they seem to have the ability to reduce or prevent some amount of the oxidative damage that works against the skin's normal functions, such as collagen production and preservation, and healthy cell formation—while also preventing some amount of the degenerative effects caused by sun exposure.

The number of antioxidants that can show up in a skin-care product is almost limitless. But, despite endless cosmetics companies launching new miracle ingredients on a constant, unrelenting basis, **there is no single best antioxidant**. In fact, many work well together and thus a "cocktail approach" to antioxidants is preferred. These vital elements for skin can range from coenzyme Q10, grape seed extract, green tea, soybean sterols, superoxide dismutase, vitamin C (ascorbyl palmitate and magnesium ascorbyl palmitate), and vitamin E (alpha tocopherol, tocotrienols) to pomegranate, curcurmin, turmeric, and on and on and on.

Although antioxidants have a great ability to intercept and interrupt free-radical damage, it is ironic that they share a particular weakness: They deteriorate when repeatedly exposed to air (oxygen) and sunlight. Ironic, yes, but it's actually a testament to how antioxidants work in the presence of oxygen and light. In defending skin cells, antioxidants destroy themselves and the free radicals that are generated by oxygen and light. Because of this fact, an antioxidant-laden moisturizer packaged in a jar or clear (instead of opaque) container will start losing its antioxidant benefit soon after opening. This means you should seek out moisturizers with antioxidants and other beneficial ingredients that are packaged in opaque tubes or bottles, and check to be sure the opening through which the product is dispensed is small, thus also minimizing the formula's exposure to air.

The effect of air and light on products that contain antioxidants is well known and accepted in the cosmetics industry. Despite this, however, many companies continue to sell products packaged in jars—even those that are priced in the hundreds of dollars. The truth is that consumers are attracted to "fancy" or expensive-looking jars, and cosmetics companies know this. As long as women continue to buy products in jars and clear packaging, the cosmetics industry will continue to sell them (Sources: *Clinics in Dermatology*, November-December 2008, pages

614–626; *Skin Therapy Letter*, September 2008, pages 5–9; *Journal of Drugs in Dermatology*, July 2008, pages S7–S12; *Dermatologic Therapy*, September-October 2007, pages 322–329; *Dermatologic Surgery*, "The Antioxidant Network of the Stratum Corneum," July 2005, pages 814–817; *Journal of Pharmaceutical and Biomedical Analysis*, February 2005, pages 287–295; and *Cosmetic Dermatology*, December 2001, pages 37–40).

ALL SKIN TYPES NEED CELL-COMMUNICATING INGREDIENTS

"Cell-communicating ingredients" are significant because they have a direct impact on helping skin cells function as younger healthy cells would. Medical journals refer to these as "cell-signaling" substances—but we think "cell-communicating" is more descriptive of what they do in relation to skin care.

Whereas the antioxidants described above work by interfering with a chain-reaction process that results in free-radical damage, cell-communicating ingredients have other valuable effects. These benefits include the ability to tell a skin cell to look, act, and behave better, more like a normal healthy skin cell, and to stop other elements from telling the cell to behave badly or abnormally (caused by such things as unprotected sun exposure or genetics).

Cell-communicating ingredients are vital because antioxidants on their own lack the ability to "tell" a damaged skin cell to behave more normally. Years of unprotected, or insufficiently protected, exposure of skin to the sun causes abnormal skin cell production due to ongoing damage to cellular DNA. Usually the skin regenerates itself with normal, round, even, and intact skin cells, but when damaged cells reproduce, the new cells are uneven and flat, and function inadequately. This is where cell-communicating ingredients (such as niacinamide, retinol, some peptides, and adenosine triphosphate) have the potential to help restore healthy skin-cell production.

Every cell has an almost immeasurable series of receptor sites for different substances. These receptor sites are the cell's communication hookups. When the right ingredient for a specific site shows up, it attaches itself to the cell and transmits information. In the case of skin, this means telling the cell to start doing the things a healthy skin cell should be doing. If the cell accepts the message, it then shares the same healthy message with other nearby cells in a continuing process.

As long as there is an open receptor site and an appropriate, healthy signaling substance is present, a lot of beneficial communication takes place. However, a cell's communication network is more complex than any worldwide telephone system ever made. The array of receptor sites and the substances that can make a connection comprise a huge, complex, and varied group, with limitations and convoluted pathways about which we are still finding out. As far as skin care is concerned, the area of antioxidant research is still in its infancy. No doubt, you will be hearing more and more about cell-communicating or cell-signaling ingredients used in skin-care products, despite the lack of solid research. The good news is that, theoretically, this area of skin care is incredibly exciting (Sources: *Cold Spring Harbor Perspectives in Biology*, April 2011, pages 3–4; *Microscopy Research and Technique*, January 2003, pages 107–114; *Nature Medicine*, February 2003, pages 225–229; *Journal of Investigative Dermatology*, March 2002, pages 402–408; *International Journal of Biochemistry and Cell Biology*, July 2004, pages 1141–1146; *Experimental Cell Research*, March 2002, pages 130–137; *Skin Pharmacology and Applied Skin Physiology*, September-October 2002, pages 316–320; and signaling-gateway.org).

ALL SKIN TYPES NEED ANTI-IRRITANTS

Anti-irritants are other vital elements for effective skin-care formulations. Regardless of the source, irritation is a problem for all skin types, yet even if you are using the best skin-care products for your skin type, environmental factors make irritation and the resulting inflammation it causes almost impossible to avoid.

Anti-irritants are incredibly helpful because they allow skin extra healing time, reducing the problems caused by the environment and other sources of skin damage. Anti-irritants include substances such as allantoin, aloe, bisabolol, burdock root, chamomile extract, glycyrrhetinic acid, grape extract, green tea, licorice root, oat kernel, vitamin C, white willow, willow bark, willowherb, kelp, and many, many more. Their benefit for skin should be strongly considered because they are that rare thing—a case where too much of a good thing really is better!

CHAPTER FIVE

Targeted Solutions for Dry Skin

ADDING MOISTURE?

It might seem logical to assume that the opposite of rough, flaky, tight-feeling dry skin would be "wet" skin that is smooth, soft, and supple-feeling, but that isn't the case. In reality, too much water can be a serious problem because it disrupts the skin's protective barrier, breaking down the substances that keep skin cells bonded together. When these substances are in generous supply, they keep the outer layer of skin intact, smooth, soft, and moist. When these substances are depleted, dryness sets in, and no matter how much moisture you give your skin or how much water you drink, it will never be enough to eliminate dry skin.

On the surface moist, healthy skin is only 10% to 30% water, while the lower layers of skin are about 75% water. Unfortunately, the lower layers of skin cannot efficiently supply the surface layers with water, which is why drinking excess water doesn't have any real impact on dry skin. You can drink all the water you want, but if you have a tendency toward dryness or if you live in an arid environment and aren't using well-formulated products to replace the substances your skin is missing, you will still struggle with dry skin.

It also doesn't help to drench your skin with water from the outside. You could soak in your bathtub for hours, but that absolutely doesn't have any moisturizing benefit. Ironically, submerging skin in water can cause dryness or make dry skin worse because the healthy substances in the skin break down when placed in water, even when soaking for a relatively short period of time.

What is thought to be taking place when you have dry skin is that the substances in skin that keep it intact (technically called the skin's intercellular matrix) have become depleted, and along with a dry environment and/or use of harsh, drying skin-care products, you end up with dry skin. As mentioned, it's not just that the skin doesn't have enough water, but also that it doesn't have the ability to retain the right amount of water in skin because it lacks the skin's natural substances to do this.

Think about it this way: Children rarely have dry skin unless they have a specific skin disorder. Their young skin contains abundant substances that keep it intact, allowing the skin to keep the balance of water it needs so it stays looking moist, plump, and healthy.

There are genetic factors, hormone changes, and health issues that can weaken and disrupt the outer layers of adult skin, but sun damage by far is the biggest external culprit. Coming in a close second to these skin-damaging factors are the products we use and/or how we treat our skin. When we use skin-care products laden with drying, irritating ingredients, it disrupts the outer layers of skin and degrades the skin's protective substances as well. This more often than not leads to dry skin, among other issues.

Adding to this problem is the constant exposure to arid climates—dry air blasting from heaters or air conditioners in our homes and offices—that make it almost impossible to keep water in our already-impaired outer layers of skin.

In short, vital substances are depleted from our skin, making water loss inevitable, which causes dry skin. Preventing those vital substances from breaking down or replacing and restoring them is a primary way to minimize and/or prevent dryness. To do this you must have an effective skin-care routine that includes products specific for dry skin (meaning products with emollient textures) along with ingredients that restore the surface layers of skin, as described in Chapter 4, *What Every Skin Type Needs* (Sources: *Journal of Investigative Dermatology*, 2003, pages 275–284; and *Textbook of Aging Skin*, 2010, Dr. Howard Maibach et al., publisher Springer Verlag).

Help your skin avoid being dry with these vital steps:

- **If you can, add a humidifier** in your home, bedroom, or workplace. Another way to add water to the air is to fill your bathtub with hot or tepid water and let it sit. This will fill the air with much-needed moisture in the winter. It is surprising how beneficial this can be for your skin.

- **Use gentle cleansers from head to toe.** Harsh or drying cleansers and bar soaps of any kind will create dry skin or make matters worse. Our favorite body washes are listed in the Best Products section of CosmeticsCop.com.

- **Avoid immersing your skin in water** for long periods. This includes taking long showers.

- **At night, apply an effective AHA or BHA exfoliant** to your skin. Thickened, built-up layers of dead skin cells, which can result from sun damage, genetics, or other factors, not only make your skin look dry and feel rough, but also, even when you can't see this buildup, block moisturizers from being properly absorbed into the skin. Gently exfoliating these layers of skin and then applying a well-formulated moisturizer can change your skin overnight.

- **Every morning**, whether you think you need it or not, apply an emollient moisturizer with an SPF 15 or greater, and greater is better, that has at least one of the following UVA-protecting ingredients listed as active: avobenzone (also called butyl methoxydibenzoylmethane or Parsol 1789), Tinosorb, Mexoryl SX (ecamsule), titanium dioxide, or zinc oxide. It also should include the same beneficial ingredients as your nighttime moisturizer, as discussed below. (Remember, the only difference between a daytime and nighttime moisturizer is that the daytime version should have sunscreen.)

- **At night, an emollient moisturizer** made with plant oils, skin-repairing ingredients, antioxidants, and cell-communicating ingredients will restore your skin, putting the essential substances back into your skin so that it can stay moist.

- **For very dry skin**, apply a layer of olive oil or other plant oil, such as safflower, almond, or canola, over your nighttime moisturizer as an extra treatment. A quick note: Argan oil, emu oil, or any other plant oil touted as a miracle ingredient for dry skin is nothing more than marketing silliness. You can save your money by not getting caught up in the latest "fad" ingredients! Also, avoid irritating ingredients, including fragrant plant oils such as lavender, citrus, sandalwood, bergamot, and others, because their fragrance components cause irritation that hurts your skin's ability to be healthy.

Targeted Solutions for Wrinkles, Sagging, & Aging Skin

WHAT YOU USE CAN DRAMATICALLY CHANGE YOUR SKIN

You can obtain dramatic results from a state-of-the-art skin-care routine, but you have to be realistic. Skin-care ingredients and products, no matter how beneficial they are, who is selling them, or what claims they assert, cannot replace what plastic surgeons or cosmetic dermatologists can do. The combination of cosmetic procedures and a great anti-aging skin-care routine is what makes a dramatic difference in how your skin looks with each passing year. Simply put, neither one can do it all by themselves.

The plan we present below will improve the overall appearance of your skin almost immediately by supplying it with gentle, effective, restorative, and normalizing ingredients that have a proven record for helping wrinkled, aging, sagging skin look and act younger. Providing such benefits to skin on a daily basis will enhance your skin's health and appearance, encourage collagen production, and help generate normalized skin cells, which altogether means greatly reduced visible signs of aging and sun damage, as well as some amount of skin tightening.

With that in mind, the basic place to start is by following a targeted plan that provides what your skin needs to repair itself and function optimally.

Use a gentle cleanser and well-formulated toner! Don't forget that a gentle cleanser is an important start to any skin-care routine. If you are using drying or irritating cleansers, everything else you do will have to fight against the damage they cause.

A well-formulated toner loaded with antioxidants, skin-repairing ingredients, anti-irritants, and cell-communicating ingredients also plays an important role in your cleansing routine. No cleanser or toner will eliminate wrinkles, but the two combined begin your skin-care routine by reducing irritation and inflammation and restoring skin. This allows the healing process and the normal function of skin to take place—and that's the beginning of younger-looking skin!

Use an effective AHA or BHA product. All of us have some amount of sun damage and most of us have a lot of sun damage, either because we didn't know about sun protection until later in life or because we didn't really know how often or how to apply sunscreen. Even with the best protection and sun avoidance, a percentage of the sun's rays still gets through, not a lot, but enough to take a toll over time.

One significant consequence of sun damage is that the outer layer of skin becomes thickened, discolored, rough, wrinkled, saggy, and uneven. The best way to help shed these built-up layers of abnormal, dead, unhealthy skin is to use a well-formulated alpha hydroxy acid (AHA) or beta hydroxy acid (BHA) exfoliant. Once you add this to your skin-care routine, you can literally see improvement overnight. There is also a good deal of research showing that exfoliating skin with a well-formulated AHA or BHA can help your skin build collagen (Sources: *Journal of Dermatology*, January 2006, pages 16–22; *Journal of Dermatological Treatment*, April 2004, pages 88–93; *Plastic and Reconstructive Surgery*, April 2005, pages 1156–1162; *Dermatologic Surgery*, February 2005, pages 149–154; and *Experimental Dermatology*, December 2003, pages 57–63).

Use a state-of-the-art sunscreen whose formula goes far beyond the basics. There is no debate: Sun exposure ages the skin. Sun protection is the cornerstone of any skin-care routine and sunscreen is the ultimate, quintessential anti-aging skin-care product you can use. Look for a product rated SPF 15 or greater (and greater is better because most of us aren't applying enough) and make sure it has one of the following ingredients listed as active to ensure adequate protection from UVA rays: avobenzone (also known as Parsol 1789 or butyl methoxydibenzoylmethane), titanium dioxide, zinc oxide, Mexoryl SX (ecamsule), or Tinosorb. And apply it like you mean it! Every day, 365 days a year, apply it liberally, and don't forget your hands, arms, and chest because they too will look older sooner if you don't protect them!

Beyond that, it is extremely beneficial if the sunscreen you choose is also loaded with antioxidants, anti-irritants, cell-communicating ingredients, and ingredients that mimic the structure and function of healthy skin. Abundant and ever-expanding scientific research is proving that antioxidants boost sunscreen's effectiveness, and they play a role in mitigating sun damage by reducing the free radicals and skin inflammation that sun exposure generates (Sources: *Experimental Dermatology*, January 2009, pages 522–526; *Journal of the American Academy of Dermatology*, June 2005, pages 937–958; *Photodermatology, Photoimmunology, and Photomedicine*, August 2004, pages 200–204; and *Cutis*, September 2003, pages 11–15).

Consider using a product containing retinol (retinol is the technical name for vitamin A) or a topical prescription version that contains the active derivative of vitamin A, such as **Retin-A**, **Renova**, **Avita** (drug name tretinoin), or **Tazorac** (drug name tazarotene). Tretinoin and tazarotene are prescription-only topical treatments for improving the appearance of sun-damaged (wrinkled and discolored) skin. These vitamin A drugs have the ability to return abnormal skin-cell production back to some level of normalcy—think of them as the gurus of cell-communicating ingredients. The result is an improvement in skin's collagen production, which makes skin smoother and offers a modest but noticeable decrease in the depth and appearance of wrinkles. When used with daily sun protection, they also help prevent future wrinkles.

Retinol, which is a cosmetic skin-care ingredient, can have the same benefit as the prescription versions, because it is converted to tretinoin as it is absorbed into the skin.

Keep in mind that although retinol and prescription derivatives of retinol can be important for skin, one special ingredient is never enough. Skin requires many beneficial ingredients to be younger, healthier, firmer, and less wrinkled, including antioxidants, skin-repairing ingredients, anti-irritants, and other cell-communicating ingredients.

There are other cell-communicating ingredients to consider as well, such as niacinamide and some peptides, but the research on those ingredients in relation to wrinkles and anti-aging is not as extensive as it is for retinol and its derivatives (Sources: *Journal of Drugs in Dermatology*, January 2012, pages 64–69; *Journal of Dermatology*, November 2009, pages 583–586; *Clinical Interventions in Aging*, 2008, pages 71–76; *Cutis*, February 2005, pages 10–13; and *Mechanisms of Ageing and Development*, July 2004, pages 465–473).

Apply well-formulated, emollient, state-of-the-art antiwrinkle/anti-aging moisturizers and serums. These are fundamental. As described in Chapter 4, a brilliant moisturizer/serum/lotion/gel/cream/anti-aging/antiwrinkle product can go a long way toward improving skin's texture, enhancing its radiance, and creating a smoother, younger, more supple appearance. By "well-formulated," we mean a product of any kind that is loaded with antioxidants, skin-repairing ingredients, anti-irritants, and cell-communicating ingredients. All of these combined help your skin generate new collagen, create normalized skin cells, and lessen further damage. Make sure the packaging will keep the beneficial ingredients inside stable once the product is opened. Look for opaque tubes or bottles with pump applicators or small openings, and avoid clear packaging and jars of any kind.

If you have oily skin, a feather-light lotion, gel, or liquid with these ingredients works beautifully; if you have combination or slightly dry skin, a lightweight lotion or serum will be the answer; and if you have dry skin, a cream or rich lotion will be perfect.

CHAPTER SEVEN

Targeted Solutions for Oily Skin

THE RIGHT PRODUCTS REALLY CAN KEEP OIL UNDER CONTROL

If you struggle with the daily annoyance of a shiny face that you feel resembles an oil slick, you know how difficult it is to get oily skin under control. Adding to this dilemma is the fact that many of the products claiming to eliminate shine and reduce oil actually make matters worse because they contain ingredients that irritate your skin and trigger more oil production!

Oily skin is hard to control completely because it's the result of genetically determined hormones in your body, and you simply cannot control those hormones with topically applied skin-care products. Specifically, androgens, male hormones that are present in both men and women, are responsible for stimulating oily production.

Androgens stimulate oil production, and although that truly has benefit for your skin, it is a problem when the androgens stimulate too much oil production, more than the pore can handle. When your pores produce too much oil they enlarge to accommodate the excess production. Overabundant androgens also can cause the pore lining and the surface of the skin to thicken, which blocks oil from getting out of the pore, and that can result in blackheads and other blemishes.

CARING FOR OILY SKIN

The first step in caring for oily skin is to take a critical look at your current skin-care routine. Using products with drying or irritating ingredients may seem like a good idea because they make your skin tingle and feel less oily initially, but in the end these kinds of products with irritating ingredients are always a bad idea for skin.

Irritating or drying ingredients only make matters worse because they actually trigger more oil production directly in the oil gland! You must avoid products that contain irritating ingredients at all costs. The research about this is clear, so please, follow our recommendations closely—you cannot always tell when a product is irritating and inflaming your skin, because irritation is not always obvious on the surface of skin (Sources: *Clinical Dermatology*, September-October 2004, pages 360–366; *Dermatology*, January 2003, pages 17–23; *Journal of Investigative Dermatology*, July 2003, pages 20–27; and *British Journal of Dermatology*, July 1998, pages 102–103).

Products that make your skin tingle (such as those containing menthol, mint, eucalyptus, and lemon) or products that make your skin feel instantly dry and matte (such as those containing alcohol or witch hazel) may feel like they are helping, but tingling and a tight dry feeling are signs of irritation/inflammation, and that is always bad for skin. Tingling and drying out is a clear message from your skin telling you it is being irritated, and if you have oily skin it will simply stimulate more oil production by triggering androgens, the hormones responsible for producing oil directly in the pore! And that doesn't even take into account the damage being done to the surface of the skin and hurting the skin's ability to heal. The cumulative damage will end up causing more problems. Simply put: Tingling and dryness are not desirable effects!

Think of it this way, blemishes are not wet, so drying them out isn't the goal. The goal is to absorb oil in a manner that doesn't damage the skin!

Products that contain pore-clogging or emollient ingredients can make oily skin worse. As a rule, ingredients that keep bar products in solid form (such as bar cleansers and soaps or stick foundations), or ingredients that give moisturizers and lotions a rich emollient, thick texture are likely to clog pores and look greasy on your skin.

Those with oily skin still need all the beneficial ingredients of antioxidants, skin-repairing ingredients, cell-communicating ingredients, and anti-irritants, but those ingredients should be delivered in only a liquid, serum, gel, or very thin, matte-finish lotion formulation.

THE ESSENTIAL SKIN-CARE ROUTINE FOR OILY SKIN

The following essential skin-care guidelines—cleanse, tone, exfoliate, A.M. sun protection, P.M. hydration, and absorb excess oil—will help you take control of your skin so you'll see less oil, smaller pores, and fewer breakouts.

1. Gentle, effective cleanser: Using a gentle, water-soluble cleanser twice daily that cleans your skin without causing dryness is the core of your skin-care routine. Ideally, the cleanser should rinse without leaving a hint of residue and should not contain drying cleansing agents or any other irritating ingredients. Irritation is always a problem for oily skin, as it not only damages the surface of the skin but also stimulates oil production directly in the pore.

2. State-of-the-art toner: Using an alcohol-free and irritant-free toner loaded with antioxidants, skin-repairing ingredients, and cell-communicating ingredients in a soothing, weightless liquid base is an important next step to complete the cleansing process. Toners that contain these kinds of ingredients help skin heal, minimize large pores by reducing inflammation, and remove the last traces of makeup, which if left on can lead to clogged pores. For some skin types, this may be the only "moisturizer" your skin needs.

3. A well-formulated BHA gel or liquid exfoliant: Those with oily skin tend to have an extra-thick layer of built-up dead skin cells on the surface of the skin, and the pores tend to have a thickened lining. Effectively exfoliating the surface of the skin and inside the pore is one of the best ways to remove that buildup, reduce clogged pores and white bumps, and make skin feel smoother.

The best exfoliating ingredient for oily skin is salicylic acid (BHA). Salicylic acid exfoliates not only the surface of your skin but also inside the pore, thus improving pore function and allowing oil to flow easily to the surface, so it doesn't get backed up and plug the pore. In addition, regular use of a BHA exfoliant will help fade the red marks from past blemishes faster, and it also has anti-aging benefits for skin. Another benefit of salicylic acid is that it has anti-inflammatory properties, so it reduces irritation, which helps to calm oil production and increase collagen production and overall skin health.

4. Liberally applied daytime sun protection: Even if you have oily skin, a sunscreen is essential for preventing wrinkles and reducing red marks. If you've avoided sunscreens because the ones you've tried are too greasy or too occlusive, experiment with the ones we recommend in Chapter 15, *The Best Products*. If you wear makeup, consider applying a matte-finish liquid foundation rated SPF 15 or greater and a pressed powder with SPF 15 or greater. That combination will give your skin protection without adding a separate sunscreen underneath. (But don't forget to apply a regular moisturizer with sunscreen to your neck, arms, hands, and chest so they stay young, too.)

5. Lightweight skin-beneficial ingredients at night: At night, a lightweight liquid, gel, or serum will give your skin the essential ingredients all skin types need to function in a normal, healthy manner, such as antioxidant, cell-communicating, and skin-repairing ingredients. Niacinamide is an especially interesting ingredient for oily skin because there is research showing it can normalize pore function. Niacinamide also plays a role in helping encourage an even skin tone.

6. Targeted treatments that absorb excess oil: As you begin to get your oily skin under control, it's likely you still will need to use oil-absorbing products, maybe weekly, biweekly, or even daily. This is an optional step, but many with oily skin find it helpful. Options for controlling oil include blotting papers during the day, and there are primers on our Best Products lists that can absorb excess oil and keep your face relatively shine-free without irritating your skin. Applying an oil-absorbing mask with an irritant-free formula, either once a day or every other day, is also a consideration, as are mattifying products designed to keep oily skin at bay for several hours (Sources: *Mediators of Inflammation*, October 2010 Epublication; *Experimental Dermatology*, October 2009, pages 821–832, and June 2008, pages 542–551; *American Journal of Clinical Dermatology*, volume 10, supplement, 2009, pages 1–6; *Expert Opinion in Pharmacotherapy*, April 2008, pages 955–971; *Journal of Investigative Dermatology*, November 2006, pages 2430–2437; and *International Journal of Cosmetic Science*, February 2005, pages 17–34).

CHAPTER EIGHT

Targeted Solutions for Acne/Blemishes

CLEARING UP THE FRUSTRATION OF ACNE

Acne is essentially an inflammatory disorder caused by interaction among a whole series of physiological triggers that ends in the eruption of a blemish. Understanding how to stop this sequence of events from taking place, along with reducing inflammation, will let you begin to create a successful skin-care routine.

The five major factors (and a theoretical one currently being researched) that contribute to the formation of blemishes are:

1. First and foremost, overproduction of oil by the sebaceous (oil) gland, which is triggered by androgens (the oil gland is an important activation site of androgens).

2. Irregular or excessive shedding of dead skin cells, both on the surface of the skin and inside the pore.

3. Buildup of a specific bacteria in the pore called *Propionibacterium acnes*.

4. Irritation from various factors (including skin-care products) that stimulate oil production directly in the oil gland and increase inflammation.

5. Sensitizing reactions to cosmetics, specific foods (rarely), or medicines that increase inflammation.

6. Some research points to the actual sebum produced by the oil gland as being defective in some way that causes it to become sticky. This stickiness impedes its movement out of the pore lining, causing clogs. Exactly how this condition can be improved is not yet known, although there already are some companies selling products they say will change this condition.

Fundamentally, the above describes how a blemish occurs: Each hair follicle grows from a sebaceous (oil) gland that secretes an oily, firm wax called sebum. The pilosebaceous duct or unit, more commonly referred to as a pore, is the structure that the oil gland and hair follicle share. When things are going well, the sebum smoothly leaves the pore and imperceptibly melts on the skin's surface, helping to keep the skin surface moist and smooth. When things aren't going well, when sebum and dead skin cells plug the pore, bacteria run amok, causing inflammation and swelling, and that's how a blemish starts to form.

Now that you know what causes the problem, the all-important question is: What can you do to control these symptoms? Can you slow down oil production? Can you prevent skin cells from building up and clogging the pore? How do you inhibit or kill the bacteria that cause the inflammation and redness? Can you help skin produce healthy sebum? Well, depending on the severity of your acne, the answer is yes, to all of the above—you can! (Sources: *Expert Opinions in Pharmacotherapy*, April 2008, pages 955–971; and *International Journal of Cosmetic Science*, June 2004, pages 129–138.)

TARGETED SOLUTIONS FOR CLEARING BLEMISHES

Cleansing the face: Use a gentle, water-soluble cleanser. One of the most common myths in the area of skin care is that a cooling or tingling sensation means that a product is "working," which couldn't be further from the truth. That feeling is actually your skin responding to irritation, and products that produce that tingling sensation can damage the skin's healing process, make scarring worse, trigger excess oil production, and encourage the growth of bacteria that cause pimples. Using cleansers that contain pore-clogging ingredients (like bar soaps/cleansers) also can make matters worse. The essential first step is to find a gentle, water-soluble cleanser, such as those on our Best Cleansers list at the end of this book (Source: Dermatologic Therapy, February, 2004, supplement, pages 16–25 and 26–34).

Exfoliating: Use a 1% to 2% beta hydroxy acid (BHA) product or an 8% to 10% alpha hydroxy acid (AHA) product to exfoliate the skin. For all forms of breakouts, including blackheads, BHA is preferred over AHA because BHA is better at cutting through the oil inside the pore, and penetrating the pore is necessary to exfoliate the pore lining. BHA also has anti-inflammatory properties that are vital to healing red swollen blemishes. Another plus is that BHA has antibacterial properties to help kill the acne-causing bacteria.

For some people (including those allergic to aspirin) who can't use BHA, an AHA is the next option. There are limitations to AHA in fighting acne, but in combination with a benzoyl peroxide product you can get very good results as well.

A topical scrub, a battery-powered rotating face brush like the Clarisonic, or a washcloth are options for mechanical exfoliation and extra cleansing, especially if you are wearing heavy makeup. This can definitely be helpful for some people, but it does not in any way take the place of an effective BHA or AHA topical exfoliant. Manual scrubs work only on the very surface of the skin, and when it comes to blemishes it is vital to change what is happening directly in the pore.

If you do use a scrub, cleansing brush, or washcloth, never overdo it because too much abrasion can disrupt the skin's ability to heal, and the irritation from this will worsen your acne. **Remember, you cannot scrub acne away!** (Source: *Cosmetic Dermatology*, October 2001, pages 65–72.)

Kill acne-causing bacteria and reduce inflammation: Benzoyl peroxide is considered the most effective over-the-counter choice for a topical disinfectant/anti-inflammatory ingredient to fight blemishes. Among benzoyl peroxide's attributes is its ability to penetrate into the hair follicle to kill the problem-causing bacteria, while also reducing inflammation, which is key. Furthermore, it doesn't pose the problem of bacterial resistance that occurs with some prescription topical antibacterial/antibiotic treatments.

There aren't many other over-the-counter options for disinfecting the skin. Sulfur is a good disinfectant, but it is also extremely drying and irritating, and can make matters worse by damaging the skin's ability to heal.

Tea tree oil has a small amount of research showing it to be an effective disinfectant, but there is little to no research showing it as a decent alternative. *The Medical Journal of Australia* (October 1990, pages 455–458) compared the efficacy of 5% tea tree oil with that of 5%

benzoyl peroxide for the treatment of acne. The conclusion was that "both treatments were effective in reducing the number of inflamed lesions throughout the trial, with a significantly better result for benzoyl peroxide when compared to the tea tree oil. Skin oiliness was lessened significantly in the benzoyl peroxide group versus the tea tree oil group." Unfortunately, most products on the market contain little more than a 1% concentration of tea tree oil, not the 5% strength used in the study, and this was only one study, sponsored by the company selling tea tree oil (also called melaleuca).

For some people, a topical disinfectant may be enough to get their acne under control, but that is not always the case. Using a topical antibacterial in combination with an exfoliant gives you a powerful weapon in winning the battle against blemishes. It is one of those steps you will have to experiment with to see what works for you (Sources: *Skin Pharmacology and Applied Skin Physiology*, September-October 2000, pages 292–296; *American Journal of Clinical Dermatology*, April 2004, pages 261–265; *Journal of the American Academy of Dermatology*, November 1999, pages 710–716; *Dermatology*, 1998, pages 119–125; *American Journal of Clinical Dermatology*, April 2004, pages 217–223; *Cosmetics & Toiletries Magazine*, March 2004, page 6; and *Infection*, March-April 1995, pages 89–93).

Absorb excess oil: As you begin to get your oily skin under control, it's likely you still will need to use oil-absorbing products, maybe weekly, biweekly, or even daily. This is an optional step, but many with oily skin find it helpful. Options for controlling oil include using blotting papers during the day, as well as other targeted treatment products that absorb excess oil and keep your face relatively shine-free. Applying an oil-absorbing mask that contains no irritants once a day or every other day is also a consideration.

Prescription forms of vitamin A (retinoids): Aside from exfoliating with BHA to improve the shape of the pore as mentioned above, prescription options for doing this include Retin-A (tretinoin), Differin (adapalene), and Tazorac (tazarotene). There is an immense amount of research showing these to be effective in treating acne. Depending on your skin's tolerance, you can use a prescription retinoid product twice per day. You also could try using one only at night, and then use a BHA or AHA during the day. Another option is to apply the BHA or AHA first and then apply the retinoid. Talk to your doctor and experiment to see which frequency, combination, and sequence of application works best for your skin (Source: *Journal of the American Medical Association*, August 11, 2004, pages 726–735).

Note: Benzoyl peroxide negates the effectiveness of most retinoids (such as Retin-A and Tazorac); therefore, you cannot use these two products at the same time. To get the benefits of both, you can use benzoyl peroxide in the morning and the retinoid in the evening. The exception to this rule is Differin (adapalene), which remains stable and effective when used with benzoyl peroxide (Source: *British Journal of Dermatology*, October 1998, page 139).

Have an aesthetician remove stubborn blemishes or do it yourself: Because blemishes can be stubborn, it often is necessary to remove the swollen raised white part of the blemish you can see. It is easy to do this yourself, but you must follow the guidelines discussed below so you don't scrape or damage your skin; after all, scabs are no more attractive than pimples.

Diet: Acne's possible relationship to diet in the past has come and gone with little to no agreement as to whether or not it's true. While advice that consuming greasy foods or chocolate leads to acne has not held up under research, recent studies, including two large controlled trials, reported that cow's milk intake increased acne prevalence and severity. Other studies demonstrated a positive association between a high-glycemic-load diet (sugars and refined carbohydrates) as increasing the risk of acne. Avoiding milk and simple sugars or following a low-glycemic-load diet could make a difference for some people and may be worth experimenting with to see how it works for you.

Oral antibiotics: If topical exfoliants, retinoids, and antibacterial agents don't provide satisfactory results, an oral antibiotic prescribed by a doctor is an option to kill stubborn, blemish-causing bacteria. Several studies have shown that oral antibiotics, used in conjunction with topical tretinoin or topical exfoliants, can control or reduce many acne conditions.

As effective as oral antibiotics are, they should be a near-last resort, not a first line of attack, because oral antibiotics can produce unacceptable long-term health problems. Despite this fact, some dermatologists tend to give the negative side effects of oral antibiotics short shrift and prescribe them as if they were nothing more than candy for their acne patients. Oral antibiotics are anything but candy. They kill the good bacteria in the body along with the bad, and that can lead to health problems. A more worrisome side effect is that the acne-causing bacteria can become immune to the oral antibiotic. However, there are new low-dose oral antibiotics that seem to work well over the long term and that don't have the risk of causing antibiotic resistance (Sources: *Cutis*, August 2008, pages S5–S12; and *International Journal of Dermatology*, January 2000, pages 45–50).

Improving the quality of the oil produced by the oil gland: Some researchers are studying a theory that suggests that the actual makeup of the sebum can cause acne. If the fatty acids and other components of sebum are not normal, it can become thick and sticky, so it has a harder time exiting the pore. As you can imagine, if this theory is true, it would lead to clogged pores. This is why some people think women with dry skin have acne, despite not having oily skin. The problem isn't the increase in oil production that's causing blemishes, but rather the thick, sticky quality of the sebum not allowing it to flow normally to the surface.

This sounds plausible, but it still is just a theory, and no one has identified exactly what part of the sebum may be out of whack. There are a few researchers who think increased levels of cholesterol in the body can increase the viscosity of sebum, leading to clogged pores, but this theory doesn't explain why some people with normal cholesterol have acne and some with high cholesterol don't. Nevertheless, it doesn't hurt to consider balancing your body's level of good and bad lipids by improving your diet. A healthy diet also reduces inflammation throughout your body, and that is helpful for acne as well. Aside from a healthy diet, theoretically, applying niacinamide/nicotinic acid topically may help because it can possibly improve sebum content.

When all else fails: If your breakouts persist after you've tried the options described above, it may be necessary to consider more serious treatments, such as hormone blockers or birth control pills designed to reduce breakouts, or isotretinoin.

Oral isotretinoin is the only option that can potentially cure breakouts; all the other methods merely reduce the problem or keep it at bay. More than 50% of the people who take this vitamin A drug for one round never break out again, and it eliminates oily skin altogether. Those odds are increased significantly for people who take it a second time. However, isotretinoin (formerly sold by the brand name Accutane) is a serious drug with serious side effects, especially in terms of liver function and potential fetal deformity if you take it while pregnant or become pregnant while taking it. This is something to discuss at length with your physician, but for those with chronic or cystic acne, it can be the only relief that works (Sources: *Skin Therapy Letter*, March 2004, pages 1–4; *Expert Opinion on Drug Safety*, February 2004, pages 119–129; and *Journal of the American Medical Association*, August 2004, pages 726–735).

GO AHEAD, POP THAT PIMPLE

The white to red swollen appearance of a blemish is maddening, and research shows it's an emotionally devastating experience, as anyone who has acne will tell you. Using great skin-care products is vital to reducing or stopping breakouts, but what do you do when a blemish shows up?

You've heard people say "never pop a pimple," offering only vague reasons why you shouldn't. They're wrong. In reality, if you know what you're doing, popping a pimple reduces inflammation, scarring, healing time, and gets rid of the ugly white bump. Learning when and how to remove a blemish properly is essential, because leaving a whitehead (or blackhead) sitting there on your face is just not realistic for most of us.

1. Buy a comedone (blemish) extractor (available from Paula's Choice as well as from drugstores and Sephora). Here's what it looks like:

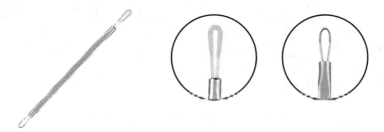

2. Cleanse your face with a gentle water-soluble cleanser first, but do NOT use cold or hot water because that only makes the blemish redder—don't make a pimple angrier than it is already—and hurts the skin's ability to heal.

3. Lightly and extremely gently massage the skin with your cleanser, using a soft, wet washcloth to remove dead skin cells. This makes extracting the pimple easier, but don't overdo.

4. Dry your skin gently. Do not use the comedone extractor or squeeze when your skin is wet because it's more vulnerable to tearing and creating a scab, which can cause scarring.

5. Center the opening of the comedone extractor over the pimple. Then gently (and we mean really gently) and with very little pressure (and we mean very little pressure) push the comedone extractor down on the whitehead and move it across the pimple. That should release the contents.

6. You may have to repeat this once or twice, but that's it.

Remember to be gentle; the goal is to remove the whitehead without creating a scab or damaging the surrounding skin (scabs are no better to look at than a pimple). If you overdo it, you will create a scab and risk scarring.

After your gentle extraction, you must follow up with a 2.5% or 5% benzoyl peroxide product and/or a 1% or 2% salicylic acid (BHA) product. These will help to immediately reduce inflammation, disinfect, and help prevent further breakouts.

Targeted Solutions for Blackheads

STUBBORN AND PERSISTENT BLACKHEADS

Much of what is true for acne is also true for blackheads, with only a few exceptions. The primary difference between a blackhead and a pimple is that the blackhead results from the oil clogging the pore at the surface, whereas a pimple results from a clog at the base of the pore. The oil clogged at the surface of the pore is exposed to air, which causes it to turn black; hence, a blackhead.

In summary, blackheads result primarily from the following:

1. Overproduction of oil by the sebaceous (oil) gland caused by androgens, which are male hormones that both men and women have. The oil gland itself is an activation site of androgens.

2. Irregular or excessive shedding of dead skin cells, both on the surface of the skin and inside the pore, prevents oil from moving normally to the surface of the skin.

3. Irritation from various factors (including skin-care products) that stimulate androgen production directly in the oil gland, causing more oil to be produced.

4. There currently is some research that points to the actual sebum produced by the oil gland being defective in some way, causing it to become sticky, which impedes its movement out of the pore, causing clogs. At this time, there isn't enough research to determine how to correct this problem, if indeed it does exist, but eating an anti-inflammatory diet low in cholesterol is certainly one way to approach it.

To start getting rid of blackheads, you need products that reduce excess oil production by improving the shape of the pore lining; reduce and absorb excess oil; remove dead, built-up surface skin cells that aren't shedding normally; and carefully remove the black plug.

THEY JUST WON'T GO AWAY

Many people say they've tried everything, but their blackheads won't go away. Unfortunately, blackheads tend to be stubborn no matter what you do. Often, however, the problem persists or becomes worse because of the skin-care routine you are using. Here's what you may be doing wrong:

- Many products claiming to address blackheads contain irritants (such as alcohol, peppermint, menthol, lemon, lime, and eucalyptus), which actually increase oil production by stimulating androgen production directly in the pore, making matters worse!

- Trying to remove blackheads with scrubs is a mistake—you cannot scrub blackheads away. Blackheads, although they result from clogs at the surface, still are too deep within the pore to be removed by scrubbing the surface of the skin; they will come back almost immediately. Over-scrubbing and the irritation it causes can lead to more oil production, plus redness and flaky skin.

- Bar soaps and bar cleansers are a problem for fighting blackheads because the very ingredients that keep these bar cleansers in their bar form can clog your pores. Your skin might feel squeaky clean, but that feeling is drying and irritating to skin, which can trigger more oil production. Plus, the film left behind on the skin from the ingredients in the bar (think of the film soap leaves behind on your tub) can further clog pores.

- Using moisturizers that are too emollient for your skin type is a problem for blackhead-prone areas, even if your skin is also dry. Always choose skin-care products appropriate for your skin type. If you have oily skin, as much as possible use only gel, light fluid lotion, or liquid skin-care products, because most of the ingredients that give emollient lotions or creams their thick consistency can clog blackhead-prone pores in oily skin types.

- For stubborn blackheads, you must manually (gently) remove the blackhead. Otherwise, it won't go away, no matter what else you do.

- Using benzoyl peroxide as a way to get rid of blackheads is a typical mistake. Benzoyl peroxide is a treatment for acne because it kills the acne-causing bacteria that live in the pore. Bacteria neither affect nor cause blackheads, so benzoyl peroxide is useless and won't have any benefit. If you have both blackheads and acne, it is fine to use the benzoyl peroxide over the blackhead-prone areas, assuming acne is also present on these parts of your face.

TARGETED SOLUTIONS FOR GETTING RID OF BLACKHEADS

The secret to solving any persistent skin problem is to use the right products and to use them consistently. The following describes what you can do to reduce and maybe even eliminate your blackheads.

Cleansing the Face: Use a gentle, water-soluble cleanser. Using harsh cleansing agents causes irritation, which can trigger excess oil production in the pore. Avoid bar soaps/cleansers!

Exfoliating: Use a 1% to 2% beta hydroxy acid (BHA) product or an 8% to 10% alpha hydroxy acid (AHA) or polyhydroxy acid product to exfoliate the skin. For all forms of breakouts, including blackheads, BHA is preferred over AHA because BHA is better at cutting through the oil and getting inside the pore. Penetrating the pore is necessary to exfoliate the pore lining. However, some people (including those allergic to aspirin) can't use BHA; if that's the case, an AHA is the next best option. BHA also has anti-inflammatory properties that are vital to healing red, swollen blemishes (Source: *Cosmetic Dermatology*, October 2001, pages 65–72).

A topical scrub, a battery-powered rotating face brush, well-formulated scrub, or a washcloth are options for mechanical exfoliation and extra cleansing, especially if you wear heavy makeup. This can definitely be helpful, but it does not take the place of an effective BHA or AHA topical exfoliant. The process that causes blackheads takes place primarily in the pore itself, so dealing only with the surface (as scrubs do) has limited benefits. If you do use these types of manual exfoliants, be careful never to overdo it because too much abrasion can disrupt the skin's ability to heal.

Absorb Excess Oil: Because excess oil is part of the problem, controlling oil plays a significant role in minimizing or eliminating blackheads. Options for controlling oil include using blotting papers during the day and using targeted treatment products that absorb excess oil and keep your face relatively shine-free. Applying an oil-absorbing mask that contains no irritants once a day or every other day is also a consideration, especially for reducing superficial blackheads.

Prescription forms of vitamin A called retinoids: Aside from exfoliating with BHA to improve the shape of the pore, as mentioned above, prescription options for doing this include Retin-A (tretinoin), Differin (adapalene), and Tazorac (tazarotene).

Have an aesthetician remove stubborn blackheads or do it yourself: Because blackheads can be stubborn, it often is necessary to remove the portion of the clog you can see (the blackhead) in order to free the entire plug. It is easy to do this yourself, but you must follow the guidelines presented below so you don't scrape or damage your skin.

HOW TO EXTRACT BLACKHEADS YOURSELF

Can you remove blackheads yourself? Yes! Extremely stubborn blackheads can and should be removed, but only by gently squeezing them out of the pore. Using a comedone extractor and light-handed squeezing can help a great deal.

Follow these steps for gentle, at-home blackhead extraction:

1. Wash your face with a gentle, water-soluble cleanser and follow with a well-formulated toner. It is helpful to use a soft washcloth as long as you do not over-scrub to remove the very top part of the clog (you can't deep clean a pore).

2. Place a slightly warm (not hot), wet washcloth for about one minute over the area you want to squeeze to soften the clog, and then pat the area dry.

3. Use a comedone extractor. First, center it over the blackhead and gently press down and pull forward at the same time.

4. Next, to get more of the blackhead out, use a tissue over each finger (to prevent slipping and accidentally tearing your skin) and then apply even, soft pressure to the sides of the blackhead area, gently pressing down and then up around the affected pore.

5. Repeat this process only once. If nothing happens, it means you cannot remove the blackhead with this first treatment, and continuing will most likely cause a wound and scabbing. You can try again in a couple of days.

6. Follow up with a well-formulated BHA (salicylic acid) exfoliant to reduce inflammation and improve pore function.

Remember: Never pinch, scrape, poke, press, or squeeze too hard. A scab is no prettier than a blackhead! (Sources: *The New Ideal in Skin Health: Separating Fact from Fiction*, Carl Thornfeldt and Krista Bourne, 2010, page 61; *Seminars in Cutaneous Medicine and Surgery*, September 2008, pages 170–176; *Expert Opinion in Pharmacotherapy*, April 2008, pages 955–971; *Dermatologic Surgery*, January 2008, pages 45–50; *Clinical Dermatology*, September-October 2004, pages 367–374; and *Global Cosmetic Industry*, November 2000, pages 56–57.)

Targeted Solutions for Skin Lightening

CAN YOU LIGHTEN SKIN COLOR OR BROWN DISCOLORATIONS?

You can absolutely lighten brown skin discolorations, and to a lesser extent you can lighten your overall skin color if that's your goal. Regardless of your ethnic background or skin color, eventually most of us will struggle with some kind of pigmentation problem, caused by sun damage or hormones. In many parts of the world, due to societal or cultural ideals, women want a lighter complexion. Regardless of your reasons, depending on your expectations, you can gain results from skin care products, both cosmetic and prescription. The question is how much difference will you see?

Your natural skin color is determined by how much melanin you have in your skin and how it's distributed. Melanin is the substance in skin cells responsible for the color of skin; the less melanin, the lighter your skin color; the more melanin, the deeper your skin color. Melanin is formed through a series of reactions in the body involving the amino acid tyrosine and the enzyme tyrosinase. Sun damage, hormones, and some diseases alter the biological process that stimulates natural melanin, causing it to overproduce in some areas.

Any amount of sun damage over time causes skin to have an overall yellowish or ashen brown or a dark-toned pallor, or it can cause "freckle-like" brown patches (once called liver spots, although they have nothing to do with the liver) that will proliferate and grow larger if the problem isn't addressed.

Although the sun is a major factor in causing brown discolorations, both in patches and/or in overall skin color, such discolorations also can result from birth-control pills, pregnancy, estrogen replacement therapy, certain diseases, and genetics. Even if skin discolorations are caused by something other than the sun, unprotected sun exposure will make matters worse.

Regardless of the reason or cause, there are many products and ingredients you can choose to lighten brown skin discolorations or lighten your skin tone. When it comes to selecting treatments for these areas, the most important thing to realize is that it takes experimenting to find what works for you. But, it's important also that you experiment only with products containing the ingredients that research proves work as intended.

SO MANY PRODUCTS, SO MUCH DISAPPOINTMENT

Skin-lightening products abound in the cosmetics industry, and their promise of making skin color lighter or whiter or lightening brown skin discolorations is worldwide. The names of this vast array of products are compelling, often with the conspicuous word "whitening" on the front of the label, typically accompanied by claims that they have "natural" formulas containing a random assortment of plant extracts with supposed skin-lightening properties.

In reality, most of these formulas are a waste of money, and cannot possibly live up to the claims on the label because they don't contain ingredients that can inhibit melanin production or improve skin cell production, or they don't contain enough of the proven ingredients that do work to have an impact. If you have purchased these kinds of products, you already know that's true—unless you happened to buy one that had a well-formulated sunscreen, which will gain and maintain some amount of lightening results simply by preventing excess melanin production.

The information that follows is an overview of what research shows works for the purpose of improving brown skin discolorations or lightening overall skin color. Of course, you must consider the skin-lightening products mentioned in the Best Products chapter to ensure you are getting effective formulations. Wasting money is not pretty, and neither is using products that have little to no hope of providing visible improvement.

WHAT WORKS?

There are five things that you can do to reduce the melanin that causes brown discolorations and darker overall skin color: (1) sunscreen and sun avoidance to block the primary cause of increased melanin production; (2) AHA or BHA exfoliant to shed the buildup of dead, overly pigmented skin cells; (3) melanin-inhibiting ingredients to interrupt the enzyme that triggers melanin formation; (4) retinoids (derivatives of vitamin A or vitamin A itself) to stimulate healthy skin cell composition; and (5) laser or intense pulsed-light medical procedures that target melanin concentrations in the skin and destroy them.

Doing all of these things, in combination, will deliver the best results if your goal is to reduce brown discolorations and improve overall skin tone.

TARGETED SOLUTIONS FOR LIGHTENING BROWN DISCOLORATIONS OR SKIN COLOR

1. Use sunscreen. Perhaps no other aspect of skin care can prevent, reduce, and potentially eliminate sun-induced or hormone-related skin discolorations better than diligent use of a sunscreen rated SPF 15 or greater (and greater is often better), especially because many of us don't use enough to get adequate protection. Along with the SPF number, which tells you about the level of UVB protection a sunscreen provides, a sunscreen also must contain one or more of the following UVA-protecting ingredients listed as active: avobenzone (butyl methoxydibenzoylmethane, or Parsol 1789), Mexoryl SX (ecamsule), Tinosorb, titanium dioxide, or zinc oxide. Using any other skin-lightening product or receiving a medical treatment without also using a sunscreen is a waste of time and money.

Over and above anything else you do, nothing is as important for preventing and reducing skin discolorations or lightening skin tone as avoiding direct sun exposure and using sunscreen 365 days a year.

2. Exfoliate with a well-formulated AHA or BHA exfoliant: This is an extremely important way to improve the general appearance of your skin and skin tone. Shedding built-up layers of dead, overly-pigmented skin cells almost instantly makes skin look more even and restores some amount of natural skin color.

3. Use a product that contains melanin-inhibiting ingredients. To treat the brown spots you already have or to lighten your overall skin color, a product with melanin-inhibiting ingredients such as hydroquinone or other alternatives is indispensable. This is one more way, besides sunscreen, to block or interrupt the physiological process that produces excess melanin and, therefore, lighten the color of your skin.

Any discussion of lightening skin or dark spots with an ingredient that blocks melanin must include a discussion of hydroquinone and the controversies over its use. Hydroquinone has been the decades-long gold standard for inhibiting melanin production. Over-the-counter hydroquinone products contain 0.5% to 2% concentrations; 4% concentrations are available, but only from physicians or by prescription. Over the past several years, research has questioned hydroquinone's safety, particularly in association with oral consumption. Animal studies and other in vitro evaluations have demonstrated problems, including mutagenic reactions. However, that's got to do with ingestion; there is a large amount of research showing that there is no associated reaction when applied topically. What is certain is that when it comes to skin lightening, hydroquinone is incredibly effective, and everything else being studied as an alternative always uses hydroquinone as the comparison because hydroquinone is what researchers know works.

Ironically, hydroquinone is found naturally in some plants, such as bearberry and mulberry, which is why they are being used as skin lighteners; they break down into hydroquinone when applied on the skin. From any perspective, skin lightening is a complicated issue, and when it comes to hydroquinone there are opinions on both sides of the aisle.

Clearly, there are those who want to find alternatives to hydroquinone, and there are options. The most popular and relatively well-researched are azelaic acid, arbutin, bearberry, kojic acid, N-acetyl glucosamine, licorice extract (glycyrrhetinic acid), resveratrol, mulberry, niacinamide, soy, vitamin C, *Arctostaphylos patula*, and *Arctostaphylos viscida*. There is limited research on these options and there is even less research showing how much (what concentration) of these ingredients is needed to produce results. So, at this point, alternatives to hydroquinone are still a bit of a guessing game for the consumer.

A relatively new option for inhibiting melanin production is lignin peroxidase, which is derived from a fungus. Trademarked Melanozyme, and contained in a product called Luminaze (*$120 for 1 fl. oz.*), to be effective, must be activated by hydrogen peroxide, which is achieved by the product's dual-chamber packaging dispenser. The product directions indicate to apply step 1 followed by step 2, rather than dispensing both sides at once. The research about this product and the doctors touting it are for the most part on the payroll of a company that either sells the product or sells the ingredient; therefore, these professional endorsements are not independent or objective by any standard. However, this product deserves mention, even though it doesn't even remotely take the lead over any of the other choices mentioned above.

4. Another consideration is a retinoid. Retinoid is the technical name for vitamin A derivatives or vitamin A itself (also called retinol). The most effective are those in prescription-only medications, such as Renova or Retin-A, along with generic options (the active ingredient is tretinoin) or retinol, which is the entire vitamin A molecule. Retinoids are effective because they boost the production of healthy skin cells.

5. Laser and Intense Pulsed-Light Treatments. Even if you are diligent about using all these methods, dark spots and brown discolorations don't always respond as well as we'd like; they can be stubbornly persistent. As a result, intense pulsed-light (IPL) devices and laser medical treatments have become popular. Offered by dermatologists, plastic surgeons, and medical spas, IPL devices have incredible potential for making a significant difference that topical treatments just cannot provide. However, you still will need topical treatments to maintain the results.

Inevitably, the question becomes which laser or IPL is the best one for brown discolorations? The answer? There isn't a best. It is impossible to select which of the dozens of lasers or IPLs is the best one for your skin tone. These types of devices are more about the skill and experience of the physician rather than which machine is the best. Most of the marketing material you read about any new or existing laser or IPL machine available is really just that: marketing. Every laser or light machine has numerous settings that should be tested and adjusted for each patient. That is, the same machine wouldn't necessarily use the same setting for multiple people, even if what's being treated is the same. When looking for a procedure to deal with your brown discolorations, realize it is the knowledge of your physician that matters most, not the specific machine (Sources: *Dermatologic Surgery*, May 2011, pages 572–595; *Aesthetic Plastic Surgery*, August 2010, pages 486–493; and *Journal of the American Academy of Dermatology*, May 2008, pages 719–737).

COMBINATION THERAPY

One skin-lightening product/treatment is not enough to achieve all that you want in lightening skin color or fading dark spots. Diligent and consistent use of sunscreen, an AHA or BHA exfoliant, a melanin-inhibiting product, a retinoid, and potentially a laser or IPL medical treatment are all needed to make dramatic improvements. This guideline will give you the best of all possible worlds for reducing and even eliminating skin discolorations and appreciably lightening skin color. There aren't any miracles. The research about this issue is well documented as to what really works and what doesn't. If you fall for marketing gimmicks and claims, you will end up wasting money and wasting your time, and not getting the results you want (Sources: *The British Journal of Dermatology*, December 2010, pages 1157–1165; *Critical Reviews in Toxicology*, November 2007, pages 887–914, and March 1999, pages 283–330; *Food and Chemical Toxicology*, November 2006, pages 1940–1947; *Journal of the European Academy of Dermatology and Venereology*, August 2006, pages 781–787; *International Journal of Dermatology*, February 2005, pages 112–115; Cutis, April 2008, pages 356–371; *Journal of Cosmetic Laser Therapy*, September 2006, pages 121–127; *American Journal of Clinical Dermatology*, July 2006, pages 223–230; *Journal of the American Academy of Dermatology*, May 2006, pages S272–S281; and *Journal of Natural Products*, November 2002, pages 1605–1611).

Putting It All Together: The Best Skin-Care Routine for You

Aside from knowing your skin type and concerns, you also must know which products work together best for you, and in what order to use them. The information below is a guideline you can follow to assemble an Essential Skin-Care Routine (whether using products from Paula's Choice or from other brands), along with Advanced Skin-Care Routines that include options to treat your specific concerns step-by-step.

Before you get started, keep in mind these three basic skin-care facts:

1. For best results, unless you are having a reaction to the products you are using, **you must follow your skin-care routine consistently.** Most products don't provide instant results; it takes consistent application to obtain benefits. Just as a healthy diet doesn't improve your body overnight, starting a great, new skin-care routine won't, for the most part, improve your complexion overnight.

2. **It takes experimenting to find the skin-care routine that works for you.** It isn't enough to just find a great product; you also must discover the right combination of products, choosing from the best product formulations available!

3. **Any skin-care routine for any skin type must include sunscreen.**

YOUR ESSENTIAL SKIN-CARE ROUTINE

This simple, step-by-step routine covers the basic types of products everyone should use and the order in which to use them every day. These steps apply regardless of your skin type (oily, dry, normal, or combination).

Essential Routine: MORNING

1. Cleanser
2. Toner
3. Exfoliant
4. Moisturizer with sunscreen rated SPF 15 or greater

Essential Routine: EVENING

1. Cleanser
2. Toner

3. Exfoliant

4. Moisturizer

YOUR ADVANCED SKIN-CARE ROUTINE

The Advanced Routine includes treatment products you can add to your Essential Routine to target your personal skin-care concerns, such as acne, red marks, wrinkles, sun damage, brown spots, or rosacea.

For example, if your sole concern is dry skin, you'll do fine following the Essential Routine. However, if you have dry skin and wrinkles or oily skin and wrinkles and breakouts, you will want to follow the Advanced Routine for best results.

Advanced Routine: MORNING

1. Cleanser

2. Toner

3. Exfoliant

4. Treatment (i.e., serum)

5. Moisturizer with sunscreen rated SPF 15 or greater

6. Targeted solutions

Advanced Routine: EVENING

1. Cleanser

2. Toner

3. Exfoliant

4. Treatment (i.e., serum)

5. Moisturizer

6. Targeted solutions

STEPS FOR YOUR ESSENTIAL OR ADVANCED SKIN-CARE ROUTINE

The following chart provides key details and answers common questions about how each type of product works, their order of application, and what results you can expect. Keep in mind that if you have multiple skin-care concerns, you may need to add more than one treatment or targeted products to your Advanced Routine. For complete details, please see the Expert Advice section of CosmeticsCop.com.

Skin-Care Product	What is this for?	Why do I need this?	What results will I see?
Cleanser **(Essential & Advanced step)**	A gentle, water-soluble cleanser removes debris, oil, and makeup.	Rinsing with water is not enough to clean your face. When your face is clean, it allows the other products you use to work even better, morning and evening.	With a gentle cleanser, your skin will look and act healthier, feel smoother, and be ready to receive maximum benefit from your other products.
Toner **(Essential & Advanced step)**	Well-formulated toners smooth, soften, and calm skin, while removing the last traces of makeup. They also add vital skin-repairing ingredients after cleansing.	Toners with skin-repairing ingredients hydrate and replenish the skin's surface immediately after cleansing. They also help reduce redness and dry patches.	Your skin will feel softer and look smoother, and redness will be reduced. Those with oily skin will see smaller pores over time. Daily use will give your skin what it needs to function in a younger, healthier way.
Exfoliant **(Essential & Advanced step)**	AHA or BHA exfoliants gently remove built-up dead skin cells, revealing new skin. **AHAs exfoliate the surface of skin; BHAs exfoliate the surface of skin and inside the pores.**	Sun damage causes the surface of the skin to become abnormally thick. Acne and oily skin complicate this further. Exfoliating eliminates this buildup, which otherwise will cause clogged pores, uneven skin tone, dullness, and deeper wrinkles.	**Overnight your skin will look radiant, smoother, and younger (really)!** Daily exfoliation with a well-formulated AHA or BHA exfoliant will unclog pores, reduce redness, blackheads,* and breakouts,* diminish wrinkles, build collagen, and improve uneven skin tone. *BHA is best for blackheads and breakouts.*
Targeted solution, if needed: **Acne Treatment**	After exfoliating with an AHA or BHA exfoliant, an acne treatment with benzoyl peroxide kills acne-causing bacteria and helps reduce redness. This is not needed if blackheads are your sole concern.	When acne is your concern, research shows that topical treatment with benzoyl peroxide is an essential step for achieving clear skin. It is a key step in an Advanced Routine for those struggling with breakouts.	With consistent use of an acne treatment, you will see fewer breakouts and a reduction in large, red, swollen blemishes, **reducing, and possibly eliminating, your acne.**
Targeted solution, if needed: **Skin-Lightening Treatment**	Used at least once daily, skin lighteners gradually reduce, and in some cases eliminate, brown (dark) spots and discolorations.	Using a skin-lightening product as part of an Advanced Routine reduces the overproduction of melanin, the skin pigment that causes brown spots and discolorations.	After 8–12 weeks of daily use, you will see discolorations fade. **Your skin tone will be more even and radiant.** To maintain results, ongoing use is necessary.
Anti-Aging/Antiwrinkle Treatment **(typically products labeled "serum")**	Applied morning and evening, serums filled with antioxidants and other anti-aging ingredients protect your skin from environmental damage, including sun damage* and pollution. *When used with a sunscreen rated SPF 15 or greater.*	The best treatment serums with antioxidants improve your skin in numerous ways, from reducing redness to stimulating healthy collagen production and improving the appearance of wrinkles. They are an integral part of an Advanced Routine.	Immediately, your skin will feel smoother and look radiant. **With twice-daily use, signs of damage will fade and your skin will look and behave healthier and younger.**
Anti-Aging/ Antiwrinkle Moisturizer with Sunscreen	This important morning step keeps your skin shielded from sun damage. It must have an SPF 15 or higher rating, and offer broad-spectrum protection.	Broad-spectrum sunscreens with antioxidants are necessary whether you are using an Essential or Advanced Routine. They protect your skin from sun exposure, which is the #1 cause of wrinkles, brown spots, and other signs of aging.	Protecting your skin from further sun damage allows it to generate younger, healthier skin cells. This is the critical step to having radiant skin. **You will see fewer signs of aging!**
Anti-Aging/ Antiwrinkle Moisturizer	All skin types benefit from moisturizers that contain the types of ingredients research has shown help your skin look healthier and younger.	Used daily as part of an Essential or Advanced Routine, moisturizers (cream, lotion, gel, or liquid texture) improve your skin's healthy functioning and keep it feeling smooth and soft. You can (and should) use them around the eye area.	When you use the right moisturizer for your skin type, you will see smoother, glowing skin that's hydrated and healthier. **This will replace dry, dull, or flaky skin with skin that looks and acts younger!**

CHAPTER TWELVE

How We Do Our Reviews

AN OVERVIEW OF HOW WE RATE PRODUCTS

Rating a wide variety of cosmetic products is a rigorous, complex process. Establishing criteria that will let our readers truly distinguish and differentiate a terrible product from a great one, or a good product from one that's mediocre, requires exact and consistently applied guidelines. Moreover, these guidelines must be substantiated with published research that used clear criteria and meticulous scientific methods. These are exactly the criteria I've created with my team for each product type reviewed in this book.

First—and above all—**you need to know that my team and I do not base any rating decision on our personal experience with a product**. In other words, just because we like the way a cleanser or a moisturizer feels on our skin, we know it doesn't mean that thousands of others will feel the same way about it. Our personal feelings or reactions won't help you evaluate whether a product may hurt your skin or live up to any part of the claims highlighted on the label. Not to mention it would be impossible to do a comparative analysis of thousands of products for a range of different skin types and concerns, which is why it has never been done by anyone in the world.

All the ratings for the skin-care products in this book are based primarily on the formulation of the individual product, in combination with what research says works (or doesn't work) for skin. We have consulted countless published, peer-reviewed studies about the ingredients in the product, and have considered the possible resulting interactions with each other and with your skin. We also evaluate these formulas based on published cosmetics chemistry data about ingredient performance and consistency. From that, we can assess a product's potential for irritation, dryness, breakouts, sensitivities, greasiness, and other issues of texture and performance.

We evaluate makeup products more subjectively than skin-care products with regard to their application, color selection, texture, and, most important, how they compare to similar products from other lines. Formulation is also a consideration for makeup products, but predominantly for claims made in regard to skin-care benefits and for any SPF-rated makeup product. Ingredient lists for makeup (such as foundations and powders) applied all over the face are scrutinized for irritants and whether they contain fragrance.

This rating process is more challenging than we can describe, because even if we think a company is absurdly overcharging for its products or is exceedingly dishonest in its claims and advertising, and no matter how unethical it seems, it does not prevent us from saying that a product of theirs is good for a particular skin type or concern. Instead, we often write, "This is a good product, but what a shame the price is so absurd and the claims so ridiculous!"

As with the previous edition of this book, we use a far more stringent standard for excellence for every category of product. Great ratings are no longer awarded to ordinary, perfunctory products with mediocre, standard, or even good formulations. For example, if a product makes claims about containing antioxidants or anti-irritants, then it better contain a convincing amount of these ingredients.

OUR SKIN-CARE REVIEWS

We evaluate skin-care products almost exclusively on the basis of content versus claim. For example, if a product claims to be good for dry, sensitive skin, it cannot contain irritants, skin sensitizers, drying ingredients, and so on.

We also ask the following questions to determine if a product can measure up to its claims, based on established and published research:

1. Given the ingredient list, and based on published research—not just on what the cosmetics company wants you to believe—can the product really do what it promises?

2. How does the product differ from similar types of products?

3. If a special ingredient (or ingredients) is showcased, how much of it is actually in the product, and is there independent (not company-sponsored) research verifying the claims for it?

4. If there is a special ingredient in the product with research supporting its effectiveness, are there other ingredients that work as well or better?

5. Does the product contain problematic fragrances (including volatile fragrance ingredients), sensitizing plant extracts, topical irritants, or other questionable ingredients that could cause problems for skin?

6. How far-fetched are the product's claims?

7. Based on what's known about the ingredients it contains, is the product safe? Are there risks such as allergic reactions, increased sun sensitivity, insufficient sun protection, or potentially harmful ingredients?

We wish we had the space to challenge and explain every single exaggerated claim and lofty explanation that accompanies the products listed in this book, but there is just not enough room (or time) to tackle that prodigious task. We cover most of the distortions and some of the hyperbole about products and ingredients in the reviews and in the Cosmetic Ingredient Dictionary section at CosmeticsCop.com.

OUR MAKEUP REVIEWS

Makeup products are unique because before you can make a judgment about performance, you must personally test them. The ingredients in makeup products are taken into consideration but, barring known irritants, what matters most is texture, application, and performance. For example, whether or not a pressed power has a silky soft finish, a foundation meant to be matte stays matte, the foundation colors relate to real skin color, or the eye and brow pencils go on smoothly without a greasy, smeary finish, and so on. Beyond our criteria, I rely on my more than 20 years as a professional makeup artist and my team's past and ongoing makeup experience to help establish guidelines for the quality of a product and its application.

We also use our extensive database of makeup reviews to perform comparative analyses based on our criteria for each product grouping. For example, if mascara claims to be waterproof, does it really stay on if you've been crying or swimming, and how does it compare to the waterproof mascaras currently rated as best? We also ask many of the same questions we ask about skin-care products, but our focus is mostly on actual performance and not cumulative benefit, which is critical with skin-care.

HOW CAN WE REVIEW SKIN-CARE PRODUCTS WITHOUT USING THEM FIRST?

Many people wonder how we can judge the value of a skin-care product by its label. We've been asked, "Wouldn't that be like judging the taste of a food just by the ingredients in it? What about tasting it yourself?" Taste is necessary information, but it is even more important to know that what you taste is good for you, and you simply can't determine if something you are eating is good for you by taste. It is no longer wise for any of us to consume a food without a clear understanding of how much fat, cholesterol, sodium, coloring agents, or calories it contains, which is exactly why foods sold in the United States and many other countries require standardized nutrition facts labels. Without that information, regardless of the taste, you could, over time, be causing yourself harm.

Even more to the point, no one must try an approved antibiotic to know it will fight infection, take a birth control pill to know it will prevent pregnancy, or have a heart attack to know there are medications and procedures that will save lives. The research is what tells us what we need to know. That is how we approach skin care.

We will help you navigate the ingredients that help skin or hurt skin, and whether or not the formulas are appropriate for your skin type. From there, you can sort through the jungle of choices, basing your decisions on facts and not on advertising mumbo jumbo or impossible promises.

DUE DILIGENCE

I cannot stress enough how much time and effort my staff and I put into gathering our information. We are diligent about making sure we incorporate accurate and precise information and/or research for all the products we review. To accomplish this, the first order of business with every edition is to contact every cosmetics company whose products we're reviewing and ask them (nicely) for whatever data or facts they can send regarding their products and claims. Most cosmetic brands we contacted weren't willing to send us anything about their company or their products, let alone details about the "research" or the "studies" they use to substantiate their claims. Some even asked that they not be included in this book, which begs the question, what are they trying to hide?

I do want to thank the companies that did send us their information. While we may not agree with them on the quality of all their products or their advertising claims, we appreciate their willingness to be forthcoming about their formulations.

The following companies were extremely helpful in providing information for this book: Arbonne, Aveeno, CeraVe, Clean & Clear, Derma E, La Roche-Posay, Make Up For Ever, Murad, N.Y.C. Color, NYX, Obagi, Olay, RoC, Sephora, St. Ives, and Vichy.

UNDERSTANDING THE RATING SYSTEM

We use face symbols (✔☺ = best product, ☺ = good product, ☺ = average product, and ☹ = poor product) alongside text ratings of BEST, GOOD, AVERAGE, and POOR so you can quickly see how products are rated. We also use $$$ symbols when needed for an at-a-glance comparison of expensive and inexpensive choices. What we consider expensive versus inexpensive takes into account the cosmetics industry's average retail price in each category as well as other attributes of the product, including the quality of its packaging, its size, and formula.

With each new edition of this book, our criteria for assigning product ratings have become more and more stringent. We want you to know your skin deserves only the best products based on proven results, not false promises. With the ratings and studies cited in this book, you're finally going to be able to find products that take the absolute best care possible of your skin!

When evaluating a product, we rely on published research on the effectiveness of the ingredients and formulation. For skin care, aesthetic attributes such as texture and finish weigh less heavily on the rating, unless these features make the product significantly less appealing. For example, if a product is clumpy, waxy, or sticky, that factors into our rating.

For the most part, a skin-care product's texture and finish comes down to personal preference, and our indication of which skin types a product is best for takes general preferences into account. For example, someone with oily skin shouldn't use a thick, creamy moisturizer and someone with dry skin shouldn't use a product with a dry, matte finish.

You also will find that the skin types we indicate a product is best for often differ from what the cosmetics company recommends. Using published research, we evaluate product formulas, and the different skin types' response to those ingredients.

Although we often are tempted, we do not base our ratings on what we personally like or don't like because our preferences have nothing to do with whether or not a product will work for your skin type and your preferences. We also never take into consideration reviews that appear on other websites, as this would be a problem for many reasons. First, people often like products that aren't good for them, as we explain throughout this book. Second, in many cases, advertisers, not facts, generate the reviews on other websites. They may be fun to read, but they aren't truly reliable.

Here's how our product ratings break down.

✓☺ **BEST** and ✓☺ **BEST $$$**. These ratings designate products that are the best of the best in their respective categories; the $$$ indicates that a product is on the expensive side of the price scale. The price tag is not related to quality; it is strictly there for your budgetary consideration. Our BEST rating is judiciously assigned whenever a product exceeds the criteria for a product in its category, with minimal to no concerns, and surpasses the formularies of comparable products.

For this edition of *Don't Go to the Cosmetics Counter Without Me*, the "Best Products" list includes only products that receive these superior ratings, categorized by the type of product as well as skin type and related skin concerns. This reduces the number of best products in each category (which makes shopping easier) and assures you that you're getting what our team's experience and substantiated research indicates are truly state-of-the-art products, regardless of how much you choose to spend.

☺ **GOOD** and ☺ **GOOD $$$**. This rating designates a product that meets the criteria for a great formulation established for its category, and we recommend it because of reliable performance or interesting formulary characteristics, or, in the case of makeup, application and wearability. Products with our GOOD rating are a consideration, although they fall short of the formulas in our BEST group. The price tag is not related to quality; it is there strictly for your budgetary consideration.

☺ **AVERAGE**. This rating indicates an OK, but unimpressive, product whose formula is ordinary and/or dated, and not near the level of excellence that your skin deserves. It also may contain a mixed bag of good and some bad ingredients. For makeup, it means the application and wearability is questionable, especially considering there are far superior alternatives. For skin care, an average rating doesn't mean it's a bad product, but that it lacks the state-of-the-art ingredients your skin needs to be younger, clearer, and healthier.

☺ **AVERAGE $$$**. This rating indicates an ordinary, dated product whose excessive price makes it a ludicrous consideration. We also use this rating to identify a product that has a great formula, but whose packaging won't keep the ingredients stable. For makeup, it means there are far better options to consider, so there's no need to settle for less, especially when the product is also overpriced.

☺ **POOR**. This rating is for products we absolutely do not recommend. It reflects a product that's truly a poor choice for skin from almost every standpoint, including, but not limited to, dated formulation, performance, application, and texture, as well as the potential for irritation, collagen breakdown, skin reactions, and breakouts. Because we give this rating only to products we'd never recommend, we do not assign such products a "$$$" designation. After all, regardless of your budget, you should never use a product with this rating, even if you can afford it.

WHEN YOU DISAGREE WITH US

Please be aware that you may not and need not agree with all of our reviews to benefit from the information in this book. For any one of a dozen reasons (personal preference, different expectations, actual usage such as once a week versus twice a day), a product we dislike may work well for you. Alternatively, just the opposite can be true: You may hate a product we rate highly. Regrettably, we cannot account for how millions of women will feel or react to a specific product or account for what happens when you use some good products and some bad or have an allergic reaction (which is completely different from having an irritant reaction) or experience breakouts.

Most Common Questions Answered

NATURAL VERSUS SYNTHETIC INGREDIENTS: WHICH IS BETTER?

To sum it up succinctly, "natural" does not mean good and "synthetic" does not mean bad. Each group has its shortcomings and strengths, but we would no sooner accept any plant as automatically being good for our skin than we would walk naked through a patch of poison ivy assuming that because it's a plant, it must be OK.

"Natural" simply defines the source of the ingredient; it tells you nothing about the ingredient's effectiveness or risks. For example, menthol and peppermint have a natural source, but both are serious skin irritants and a problem for skin. Ingredients like silicone and stearyl alcohol are synthetic, but they are remarkably silky-soft ingredients, vital to an enormous array of cosmetic formulations. Sodium lauryl sulfate is a detergent cleansing agent derived from coconut, but it tends to be more sensitizing than other cleansing agents, so the natural orientation isn't helpful.

"Synthetic" merely tells you that the ingredient was created in a laboratory (although technically that's true for plant extracts as well because it takes quite a bit of manipulation to get a plant into a skin-care product you can use), and although that kind of origin may not sound as nice as "picked from a field," it often means that the resulting ingredient is more "pure" and more stable than a natural ingredient. Natural ingredients contain hundreds of known and unknown components, and not all of those components are good for skin. In addition, the ingredients used to "extract" the plant extract—that is, the chemical processes used to extract the oil or other natural substance from the plant—are usually synthetic and unnatural.

This is not to suggest that plants have no benefits in skin-care products, because they do. However, the notion that any plant is better for skin than a comparable synthetic ingredient is unsubstantiated. Depending on the specific plant, it can have a positive effect, a negative effect, or both positive and negative effects on your skin. Meanwhile, to imply that a tincture of a plant (or an extracted component of it) of the kind used in reported research can have the same effect on skin when mixed into a cosmetic product in teeny, fractional amounts is, more times than not, a stretch of the imagination.

HOW CAN I TELL IF A PRODUCT WILL CAUSE BREAKOUTS?

Why does it seem nearly impossible to find products that won't cause breakouts? It's because many products, even those claiming to be oil-free, suitable, or even beneficial, for acne, oily skin, or blemish-prone skin, actually contain ingredients that trigger breakouts. That's not fair—we agree with you—but it's true, and many of us know this from experience.

So, how can you tell if a product will cause your skin to break out with pimples or black-heads? Unfortunately, most people find it difficult, if not impossible, to differentiate among the products or ingredients that increase blemishes and those that do not.

There is a great deal of evidence that specific ingredients can trigger breakouts and there are lists of pore-clogging ingredients. However, the analysis of any ingredient with regard to breakouts rarely takes into account the ingredient's concentration, or how the ingredient interacts with others in the formula. For example, a tiny amount of an ingredient in a skin-care product isn't the same as a 100% concentration that might have been used in lab tests. Moreover, there are thousands of cosmetic ingredients to consider, and the lists you may have seen on the Internet never examine the whole picture.

Here are a few general precautions and guidelines that will help you in finding products that are far less likely to cause blemishes:

- Avoid products with thick, overly-creamy textures, or any products that come in stick form. The ingredients used to give a skin-care or makeup product a thick or solid texture are more likely to clog pores, creating a perfect environment for blemishes to grow.

- Gels, light serums, liquids, or fluid lotions are types of products that are far less likely to clog pores and cause breakouts.

- Oils of any kind do not actually clog pores, but they do make your skin feel greasy. That adds to the excess oil your skin already produces, thus exacerbating the conditions that lead to more blemishes.

WHICH SKIN-CARE PRODUCTS ARE SAFE TO USE DURING PREGNANCY?

Although it is always important for you to check with your own physician for recommendations about what skin-care products you should or shouldn't use during pregnancy, as a general rule, most skin-care products such as cleansers, toners, moisturizers, eye creams, scrubs, serums, and lip balms that do not contain over-the-counter ingredients regulated by the FDA are fine for use throughout your pregnancy. However, prescription and over-the-counter skin-care ingredients are a different issue.

We're often asked about whether products containing benzoyl peroxide, hydroquinone, sunscreen actives, or salicylic acid are safe to use during pregnancy or while nursing. Unfortunately, many doctors don't have a ready answer, leaving mothers-to-be frustrated and confused. We consulted the American College of Obstetricians and Gynecologists regarding the products about which we are asked most often. Here is what they had to say:

- **Hydroquinone** has not been tested on animals or humans in regard to its use during pregnancy, so there is no information to assess your risk. It is best to avoid using hydro-quinone during pregnancy or while you are breast feeding.

- **Benzoyl peroxide** is an excellent ingredient to combat blemishes and is considered safe in low concentrations (5% or less) when you are pregnant.

- **Salicylic acid (BHA)** is a superior exfoliant for skin, but when used in high concentra-tions for professional peels, it is considered a risk when you are pregnant due to its relation to aspirin. However, the small percentages present in skin-care products (2% or lower) are considered safe. As an alternative, you can use glycolic acid or lactic acid (AHA) exfoliants while pregnant.

- **Sunscreen actives**, as demonstrated in animal studies, are not known to be a risk during pregnancy. Despite fears incorrectly promoted in the media by a few fringe groups intent on scaring women about cosmetics, the American College of Obstetricians and Gynecologists has not found any of the alleged fears about sunscreen ingredients to be substantiated by medical research. As a result, daily sunscreen use is strongly recommended by dermatologists. If you find your skin is more sensitive during pregnancy, consider using sunscreens with the gentle mineral actives titanium dioxide and/or zinc oxide.

- **Prescription retinoids** (e.g., Renova, Retin-A, Differin, Tazorac, and generic tretinoin) and over-the-counter products with retinol should be avoided during pregnancy and while nursing. Although the link is more about oral vitamin A intake, the risks of topical application during pregnancy remain questionable, and most physicians err on the side of caution, so they advise avoidance.

- **"Cosmeceutical" ingredients** such as vitamin C, peptides, and niacinamide are considered safe for use during pregnancy.

- **Prescription topical antibiotics** such as erythromycin and clindamycin are considered safe for use during pregnancy to control acne; however, topical antibiotics are not the most research-supported way to manage acne, whether you're pregnant or not.

- **Prescription and over-the-counter forms of azelaic acid** are considered safe for use during pregnancy. This ingredient helps improve browns spots, acne, and rosacea.

- **Prescription metronidazole (brand names include MetroCream and MetroGel)** is considered safe for managing rosacea during pregnancy.

Although the information above isn't meant to be exhaustive, it should give you a clear idea of what's OK to use during pregnancy and what should be avoided. Most important, you can achieve your skin-care goals during pregnancy, and that's sure to put your mind at ease! If you're ever in doubt about a product, always consult your physician and follow his or her advice.

WHEN SHOULD I THROW OUT A PRODUCT?

We all have beauty products in the back of a drawer or at the bottom of a makeup bag we know should be thrown out. So what stops us? Perhaps we feel like we're wasting money or that we might need that product one day or maybe, just maybe, it will come back in fashion. Unfortunately, keeping old products around is a gamble. Preservatives in products last only so long after opening, and the ingredients have a limited shelf life as well. The trouble is, aside from products that are over-the-counter drugs, such as sunscreens and anti-acne medicines, there are no expiration dates on product packaging, nor are there any requirements for them to be there (except for products sold in the European Union [EU], but we'll get to that in a moment). It's left up to consumers to know when it's time to say goodbye to old products, yet often we just can't let go. However, it's important to toss away products that have long passed their prime.

In an attempt to bring some clarity and consistency, the EU's cosmetics regulatory branch devised a system, represented by an open jar with a number followed by the letter "M." The "M" refers to the Latin word "menses," meaning "month" in English. This symbol establishes how long the product will last after it is opened, commonly known as the Period After Opening (PAO) date. While not required in the United States or Canada, it is mandatory on makeup and skin-care products sold in the 25 EU nations. There are only a few exclusions, such as aerosol containers or single-use products. The purpose of this symbol is to give consumers an idea of how long the product can be safely used (or used "without causing harm") after it is opened.

As good as that sounds, the EU did not establish a system for cosmetics companies to determine a PAO date, so the cosmetics companies make it up themselves. As a result, the PAO date doesn't take into account how the consumer uses the product or how it is stored. For example, if you leave a product in your car on a hot summer day the product degrades more quickly than if stored in normal conditions. Also, products in jar packaging don't last as long as they do in packaging that minimizes exposure to air and keeps your fingers out of it.

In short, establishing a specific date after which a cosmetic product may not be stable, beneficial, or safe is an educated guess. Besides, how many of us document (or even remember) the date when we began using a cosmetic product?

Here's what to keep in mind: As a rule products that contain water as one of the first ingredients have the shortest shelf life after opening because water encourages the growth of bacteria and other microbes. Also susceptible to bacterial contamination are products that are packaged in jars or products with a preponderance of plant extracts, vitamins, or antioxidants. In terms of plant extracts, think about how long produce lasts in your refrigerator—not very long!

Products that contain almost no water (such as powders or lipsticks) last the longest, because it is difficult for bacteria to grow in these kinds of products. Last, if your product is labeled "preservative-free," you should definitely take extra precautions because, without some kind of preservative system, bacteria, fungi, and mold can flourish easily.

Bottom line: Creams, lotions, serums, gels, and liquids should be used up or thrown out after six months to one year. Eyeshadows, blushes, lip pencils, lipsticks, or balms last up to 18 months. For products used around the eye area, like mascaras and liquid or gel eyeliners, four to six months is the general rule. And remember, never share eye-area cosmetics with others, as cross-contamination can and does happen.

SHOULD I AVOID PRODUCTS WITH PARABENS?

You may have run into websites or product lines claiming they don't contain parabens because of how supposedly harmful they are. That's nonsense. Just to be clear, we have no conflict of interest when it comes to parabens because very few Paula's Choice products contain them.

Parabens are a very popular group of preservatives used in many types of beauty products. They may come in the form of butylparaben, ethylparaben, isobutylparaben, methylparaben, or propylparaben. They're controversial because they have been distantly linked (meaning in limited studies and with only a handful of subjects or animal studies) to breast cancer due to their weak estrogenic activity and their presence in breast-cancer tumors, as well as to low sperm-count rates in men. As shocking as that sounds, it is irrelevant when it comes to cosmetics because when parabens are absorbed through the skin, they break down and are no longer estrogenic. It's further meaningless because tumors are composed primarily of water; should we consider water, therefore, carcinogenic, simply because it is present in a tumor? Or should we stop drinking water to avoid tumor formation? Of course not.

It is important to realize that parabens are used in food products as well, and this, not cosmetics, is most likely the source of their impact on the body. What is surprising to some is that parabens actually have a "natural" origin. Parabens form from an acid (p-hydroxy-benzoic acid) found in raspberries and blackberries ... so much for the widely held belief that natural ingredients are the only answer for skin-care products!

No one has any idea (or has evaluated) whether it is the consumption of parabens or their application to the skin that is responsible for their presence in human tissue. In addition, no one knows what the presence of parabens in human tissue means.

In terms of the low male sperm count in relation to parabens, research published in Birth Defects Research, Part B, *Developmental and Reproductive Toxicology*, April 2008, pages 123–133, concluded that parabens had no effect on sperm count in an in vivo experiment (meaning it was done on real men).

As a point of reference, and just to keep the concern over parabens in perspective, it is important to realize that parabens are hardly the only substances that have estrogenic effects on the body. The issue is that any source of estrogen, including the estrogen our bodies produce or the types associated with plant extracts like soy, may bind to receptor sites on cells, either strongly or weakly. This either can stimulate the receptor to imitate the effect of our own estrogen in a positive way, or can generate an abnormal estrogen response. It is possible that a weak plant estrogen can help the body, but it is also possible for a strong plant estrogen to make matters worse. For example, there is research showing that coffee is a problem for fibrocystic breast disease, possibly because coffee exerts estrogenic effects on breast cells

A study conducted at the Department of Obstetrics and Gynecology at Baylor College of Medicine in Houston, Texas, investigated the estrogenic effects of licorice root, black cohosh, dong quai, and ginseng "on cell proliferation of MCF-7 cells, a human breast cancer cell line...." The results showed that "Dong quai and ginseng both significantly induced the growth of MCF-7 cells by 16- and 27-fold, respectively, over that of untreated control cells, while black cohosh and licorice root did not" (*Menopause*, March-April, 2002, pages 145–150). Another study concluded that "Commercially available products containing soy, red clover, and herbal combinations induced an increase in the MCF-7 [breast cancer] proliferation rates, indicating an estrogen-antagonistic activity...." (*Menopause*, May-June 2004, pages 281–289). Despite this evidence, when was the last time you read a media report or received a forwarded e-mail about the breast cancer risk from soy or ginseng? (Sources: *Journal of Applied Toxicology*, July 2008, pages 561–578; *Cosmetics & Toiletries*, January 2005, page 22, January-February 2004, pages 1–4, September-October 2003, pages 285–288, and April 2003, pages 51–56; *Journal of the National Cancer Institute*, August 2003, pages 1106–1118; *Food Chemistry and Toxicology*, October 2002, pages 1335–1373; *Journal of the American Medical Women's Association*, Spring 2002, pages 85–90; *Annals of the New York Academy of Science*, March 2002, pages 11–22; and *American Journal of Epidemiology*, October 1996, pages 642–644).

SILICONES IN SKIN-CARE PRODUCTS

Silicones are a fascinating, popular group of ingredients used in skin-care and hair-care products. Many cosmetic lines, including Paula's Choice, use silicones (such as dimethicone, cyclohexasiloxane, and cyclopentasiloxane among dozens of others) because they are a brilliant group of ingredients that have an amazingly silky, light texture and a natural ability to protect and heal skin. Silicones also provide superior hydration and smoothing. Chances are if you marvel at how silky-smooth your skin feels after applying a skin-care product, it contains silicones. Ditto for how smooth your hair feels after applying hair-care products with silicones.

Claims that silicones in any form cause or worsen acne or suffocate skin are absolutely not true; in fact, just the opposite is true. Silicones are used extensively by physicians to heal wounds and burns because of their unique ability to keep moisture in the skin without occlusion while protecting it from infection and other damage. There is also a good deal of research showing that silicones can heal certain types of scarring. It is regrettable that some companies have chosen to scare people away from silicones in skin-care products, despite what research makes abundantly clear. Of course, these companies want you to believe that their products are perfect and everyone else's are harmful. Once again, Paula's Choice is the only company willing to say there are lots of great products from other lines, depending on the formulations and based on published research on the ingredients (Sources: *Surgical Dressing*, emedicine. com, May 9, 2011, http://emedicine.medscape.com/article/1127868-overview#a1; *Journal of Burn Care and Research*, January 2012, pages 17–20; and *Burns*, February 2009, pages 70–74).

SULFATES AREN'T A PROBLEM, EITHER

Many consumers are scared about sulfates in their skin- and hair-care products. In truth, misinformation is the problem, not the sulfates. Yet, once organizations and companies build up fears about certain cosmetic ingredients and those fears get promoted in the media, there is almost no going back. That has been the case for many brilliantly effective and safe ingredients for skin and hair, including mineral oil, parabens, and now sulfates. We know it is almost impossible to stop rumors and myths, but we still want to present our readers with the facts.

First, to get the conflict of interest part out of the way, Paula's Choice uses sulfates in our cleansers; however, we also have some cleansers that contain alternative cleansing agents. When it comes to whether or not to use a cleanser with sulfates, the focus should be on the overall formula, not just the presence of sulfates alone.

Here are the facts: Sulfates are used mostly as cleansing agents, and the ones that have become the scapegoats of the cosmetics industry include sodium lauryl sulfate, ammonium lauryl sulfate, and sodium laureth sulfate. In reality, there is absolutely no research showing they are a problem in skin-care or hair-care products, other than causing irritation, but that is also true for the sulfate-free cleansing agents some cosmetics companies advertise they are using as alternatives to sulfates. Whether or not any kind of cleansing agent will cause irritation depends on the concentration and on the other ingredients present in the formula. When we evaluate a cleanser, we look for formulas without harsh cleansing agents or irritating ingredients. As long as you follow our recommendations, as presented in this book, you don't need to worry about the presence of sulfates in a product. We've got you covered based on science, not scare tactics.

In reality, not all sulfates are the same, and there are plenty of sulfates that are completely safe and beneficial in skin-care and hair-care formulations. More to the point, sulfate-free alternatives also can be extremely drying and irritating when left on skin for long periods of time under occlusion, but that's not how they are used, either. There is no need to jump on the sulfate-free bandwagon just because it's the new buzzword "safety" claim. More often than not, waves of fear surrounding specific ingredients are more about a company developing a new marketing angle to sell new products. Following what published research has to say is far more beneficial for your skin, not to mention the peace of mind when you have facts, not fabrications (Sources: *International Journal of Toxicology*, July 2010, pages 151S–161S, and December 1999, pages 371–382; *Journal of Cosmetic Science*, March-April 2009, pages 143–151; *Journal of the American Academy of Dermatology*, January 2005, pages 125–132; *Contact Dermatitis*, January 2003, pages 26–32; *International Journal of Cosmetic Science*, December 1999, pages 371–382; Food and Drug Administration, fda.gov; American Cancer Society, cancer.org; Environmental Protection Agency, epa.gov; and Health Canada, http://hc-sc.gc.ca/index-eng.php).

CHAPTER FOURTEEN

Product-by-Product Reviews

ALBA BOTANICA

Strengths: Inexpensive; good cleansers; some good moisturizers; nice lip balms without sunscreen; one excellent lip balm with sunscreen; almost all the facial and body sunscreens provide sufficient UVA protection; mineral sunscreens are available; outstanding self-tanner.

Weaknesses: The natural ingredients in some of the products are natural irritants; jar packaging won't keep air-sensitive ingredients stable; most of the lip balms *with* sunscreen lack sufficient UVA-protecting ingredients; no effective AHA or BHA options; no products to effectively manage acne; no skin-lightening options.

For more information and reviews of the latest Alba Botanica products, visit CosmeticsCop.com.

ALBA BOTANICA CLEANSERS

☺ GOOD **Even Advanced Sea Lettuce Cleansing Milk** *($10.99 for 6 fl. oz.)* is a standard, but good cleansing lotion for normal to very dry skin not prone to blemishes. This doesn't rinse easily without the aid of a washcloth, but it does remove makeup quite well. Although the absence of detergent cleansing agents may appeal to those with sensitive skin, the inclusion of fragrance and a couple of potentially irritating plant extracts should give them pause.

☺ GOOD **Even Advanced Sea Mineral Cleansing Gel** *($10.99 for 6 fl. oz.)* is a very good water-soluble cleanser for normal to slightly dry or oily skin. The plant extracts are indeed from the sea, but your skin isn't going to notice one way or the other because they're rinsed off. What counts are the standard non-natural ingredients that do cleanse skin, remove makeup, and reduce excess oil. Although this contains alcohol and some fragrance ingredients (limonene is an example) the amounts are low enough to not be much cause for concern. Still, as with any cleanser, use caution when applying around the eyes.

☺ GOOD **Hawaiian Facial Wash Deep Cleansing Coconut Milk** *($12.95 for 8 fl. oz.)* is a very standard, but good, detergent-free cleansing lotion for normal to dry skin not prone to blemishes. It removes makeup efficiently but does not rinse well without the aid of a washcloth. The coconut, papaya, and other tropical plants barely amount to enough for your skin to notice a benefit of any kind.

☺ GOOD **Natural Acnedote Deep Pore Wash** *($9.95 for 6 fl. oz.)* contains 2% salicylic acid, which is a great ingredient for exfoliation and absolutely can penetrate into a pore to reduce blemishes and blackheads. However, in a cleanser it has minimal to no effect on breakouts because it is rinsed down the drain before it has a chance to go to work in your pores. For those who like the aura of natural ingredients, there are several in this cleanser; regrettably, some of the plant extracts are problematic for your skin. Although Alba Botanica did include some soothing plant extracts, ideally every plant extract should be soothing and healing, especially for acne-prone skin because redness and inflammation are persistent issues. Although some of the ingredients listed present problems that make the claims a bit bogus, this is still a good water-soluble cleanser for normal to oily skin. This is capable of removing makeup and rinses without a residue. On balance, it deserves its rating, although it doesn't cleanse "deeper" than other water-soluble cleansers.

☺ AVERAGE **Hawaiian Facial Cleanser Pore Purifying Pineapple Enzyme** *($12.95 for 8 fl. oz.)* is an option for normal to dry skin not prone to blemishes. Don't bank on the enzymes in this product being able to cleanse your skin because they are unstable in almost any product. The lotion texture removes most types of makeup, but you may need a washcloth to make sure you've removed everything. Pineapple and papaya can be skin-irritants, but it's unlikely you'll leave this cleanser on your skin long enough for the enzymes to function as exfoliants or irritants.

ALBA BOTANICA EYE-MAKEUP REMOVER

☺ AVERAGE **Even Advanced Eye Makeup Remover** *($7.95 for 4 fl. oz.)* is a dual-phase formula (silicone is one phase, cleansing agents and water the other) that you must shake before each use. This relatively gentle formula contains numerous types of algae that function as water-binding agents (although algae has no effect on makeup removal). Despite the attractive price, the downside is the small amount of alcohol and the fragrance ingredient hexyl cinnamal. These ingredients cause irritation, which is especially bad near the eye.

ALBA BOTANICA TONERS

☺ AVERAGE **Even Advanced Sea Kelp Facial Toner** *($10.99 for 6 fl. oz.)* is composed primarily of water, glycerin, and aloe. This alcohol-free toner is a lackluster option for all skin types. The sea ingredients have water-binding properties but antioxidants are in relatively short supply, and this toner could use more skin-repairing ingredients, too. Still, this came close to earning a better rating—if only it didn't contain potentially irritating witch hazel and grapefruit extracts!

☹ POOR **Hawaiian Facial Toner Complexion Balancing Hibiscus** *($12.95 for 8.5 fl. oz.)* is ironic because the natural ingredients included in this products are its weakness, at least in terms of causing skin irritation without benefit. The main offenders are witch hazel, arnica, and bergamot oil. Without them, this would have been a great option for all skin types.

☹ POOR **Natural Acnedote Deep Clean Astringent** *($9.95 for 6 fl. oz.)* is not a great anti-acne toner because it contains a skin-confusing blend of irritating and helpful ingredients (and your skin deserves only beneficial ingredients). The amount of alcohol is a deal breaker by any standard of good skin care, as we explain in the Appendix, and the fragrant plants only make matters worse.

ALBA BOTANICA EXFOLIANT & SCRUBS

☺ AVERAGE **Hawaiian Facial Scrub Pore Purifying Pineapple Enzyme** *($13.99 for 4 fl. oz.)* is a mild facial scrub that is a suitable option for normal to dry skin. The pineapple poses a slight risk of irritation, and the enzymes don't have the best track record for exfoliation, especially in a rinse-off product. The jojoba beads have a soft abrasive effect, but in the end you'll get better results just using a washcloth (or, even better, a well-formulated AHA or BHA product).

☹ POOR **Even Advanced Sea Algae Enzyme Facial Scrub** *($11.49 for 4 fl. oz.)* is needlessly abrasive due to the main scrubbing agent—crushed walnut shells. Although natural, the shape of walnut shells cannot be easily controlled. That means you're getting fragments with rough or pointed edges that can tear at skin, disrupting its protective barrier. If that weren't bad enough, this scrub also contains pumice and corncob powder for more scrub action. It also isn't easy to rinse!

☹ POOR **Natural Acnedote Face & Body Scrub** *($9.95 for 8 fl. oz.)* contains ground-up walnut shells as the abrasive agent, and that makes it an even bigger problem for those struggling with acne. When acne is present, a scrub is never the best way to go, whether it's natural or not.

Walnut shells, when ground up, have irregular, often sharp edges that can tear the skin, hurting the skin's ability to heal and causing more redness. That's not good for skin that already is suffering from breakouts. If this were a leave-on product, the 2% salicylic acid included could offer benefit, but in a scrub it is just rinsed down the drain. If you have acne, a far better option for skin is a gentle salicylic acid–based, leave-on product. Paula's Choice RESIST Weightless Body Treatment with 2% BHA is a unique product to consider for breakouts from the neck down.

☹ POOR **Natural Acnedote Invisible Treatment Gel** *($9.95 for 0.5 fl. oz.)* has too many irritants and too few benefits. The amount of alcohol is a deal-breaker by any standard of good skin care because alcohol causes free-radical damage, hurts the skin's ability to heal, increases oil production, and causes flaking and dry patches. This also contains arnica and lavender extracts, neither of which is helpful for acne. Natural or not (and this product does contain many natural ingredients), this isn't the antidote for your acne.

ALBA BOTANICA MOISTURIZERS (DAYTIME & NIGHTTIME), EYE CREAMS, & SERUMS

☺ GOOD **Hawaiian Eye Gel Revitalizing Green Tea** *($17.95 for 1 fl. oz.)* is a very good, lightweight gel moisturizer for slightly dry skin anywhere on the face. It contains a good mix of antioxidants, water-binding agents, and some anti-irritants. The cucumber and kelp have no effect on toning or changing wrinkles in any way, shape, or form. Besides, if kelp and cucumber were wrinkle smoothers, why not just apply the pure ingredients (which are available at the grocery or health food stores) to your wrinkles rather than the tiny amounts found in skin-care products? By the way this fragrance-free gel is supposed to be for those with wrinkle-prone skin, but given that no one's skin is wrinkle-proof, this product technically could be recommended for everyone.

☺ GOOD **Un-Petroleum Multi-Purpose Jelly** *($6.99 for 3.5 fl. oz.)*. Despite what this product's name implies, there is nothing wrong with using petroleum jelly (Vaseline) as a moisturizer over very dry areas such as heels, knees, and elbows. Petroleum jelly has been around for more than 100 years and has a proven safety and efficacy record (Sources: *American Family Physician*, October 2008, pages 945–951; and *Acta Dermato-Venereologica*, November-December 2000, pages 412–415). That said, this product is a good alternative balm for dry to very dry skin on the face, lips, or body, but it is exceedingly basic, containing mostly castor seed oil, coconut oil, and wax. It's nice that Alba left out fragrance of any kind, meaning that your skin has little to no risk of irritation.

☺ AVERAGE **Hawaiian Moisture Cream Smoothing Jasmine & Vitamin E** *($19.49 for 3 fl. oz.)* contains a potentially irritating amount of jasmine and has jar packaging, which won't help keep the antioxidants and plant extracts this contains stable during use. Those shortcomings don't make this a must-have moisturizer, but as far as similar products from natural lines go, we've certainly seen formulas that are worse.

☺ AVERAGE **Hawaiian Oil-Free Moisturizer Refining Aloe & Green Tea** *($19.49 for 3 fl. oz.)* contains thickening agents that may be problematic for oily or blemish-prone skin, even though it is oil-free. This has merit as a moisturizer for normal to slightly dry skin and it contains some good water-binding agents. Considering the relatively significant antioxidant content, it's a shame it's in jar packaging; that's what keeps this from earning a higher rating. See the Appendix to learn why jar packaging is a problem for antioxidant-rich products.

☺ AVERAGE **Very Emollient Sunblock Mineral Protection, Facial SPF 20** *($10.99 for 4 fl. oz.)* contains fragrant plant extracts. If these weren't included, this facial moisturizer with pure mineral sunscreens would be a slam-dunk for sensitive skin. As is, it's not an easy recommendation because the lavender presents problems for all skin types. What a shame, because this absolutely provides broad-spectrum protection and its base formula (which is indeed "very emollient") is wonderful for dry skin.

☹ POOR **Even Advanced Sea Lipids Daily Cream** *($16.99 for 2 fl. oz.)* is an emollient moisturizer that falls below standard, not only because its jar packaging compromises the efficacy of the plants and antioxidants it contains, but also because it contains arnica and pellitory (the latter is listed by its Latin name of *Anacyclus pyrethrum*). Arnica can be a significant skin-irritant, and as for pellitory root, according to the website naturaldatabase.com, "Application of pellitory to skin may stimulate nerve endings and result in redness and irritation, which is felt as a hot, burning sensation." That's not something you'd want to do to your skin ever, let alone "daily."

☹ POOR **Even Advanced Sea Moss Moisturizer SPF 15** *($16.99 for 2 fl. oz.)* is a daytime moisturizer with sunscreen that does not include the ingredients needed to shield your skin from the sun's entire range of damaging UVA rays, which is essential for anti-aging benefits (see the Appendix for details). This also contains fragrance ingredients known to cause irritation; this risk is compounded when they're combined in a product that contains synthetic sunscreen actives such as this.

☹ POOR **Even Advanced Sea Plus Renewal Night Cream** *($16.99 for 2 fl. oz.)* won't make anyone's skin ageless, especially not without a sunscreen. Moreover, this emollient moisturizer contains a smattering of problematic ingredients for all skin types, including pellitory, arnica, and the controversial ingredient DMAE. For detailed information on DMAE, please refer to the Cosmetic Ingredient Dictionary at CosmeticsCop.com. The amount of irritating plants in this product puts skin at greater risk for irritation that causes collagen breakdown (meaning it's not going to help you look ageless). More bad news is that the jar packaging won't keep the beneficial antioxidants and the many plant ingredients in this moisturizer stable during use (see the Appendix for details). All told, this is no more of a solution for ageless beauty than vitamin C is a cure-all for the common cold.

☹ POOR **Natural Acnedote Oil Control Lotion** *($15.50 for 2 fl. oz.)* is an oil-control moisturizer with a thin, lotion texture, but it doesn't contain ingredients known to keep oil in check. That means you can expect to see shine shortly after applying this; an "all day matte finish," as claimed, isn't even a distant possibility. What about the 2% salicylic acid (BHA) this contains? Although it contains a high enough amount and the pH of this product is low enough for the salicylic acid to function as an exfoliant, the formula contains some irritating ingredients likely to make oily skin (and breakouts) worse. Of particular concern are the plant extracts melissa and parsley. Melissa, also known as balm mint, creates a tingle, and that tingle means your skin is being irritated. Parsley can cause a phototoxic reaction when skin is exposed to sunlight (Source: naturaldatabase.com). These irritants can stimulate more oil production, which is the opposite of what this product is supposed to do. In short, it's not recommended over a well-formulated BHA product, which you'll find on our Best BHA Exfoliants list at the end of this book.

ALBA BOTANICA SUN CARE

✓☺ BEST **Very Emollient Sunblock Mineral Protection, Fragrance Free SPF 30** *($10.99 for 4 fl. oz.)* is an emollient formula that is great for dry skin, the sunscreens are mineral-based and provide broad-spectrum protection, and the formula is fragrance-free. Consider this a winning combination for anyone with dry, sensitive skin, including those struggling with rosacea. The shea butter, plant oils, and plant extracts provide an antioxidant boost that helps the skin further defend itself from sun damage. Last, the tiny amount of benzyl alcohol is not cause for concern.

✓☺ BEST **Very Emollient Sunblock Mineral Protection, Kids SPF 30** *($10.99 for 4 fl. oz.)* is nearly identical to Very Emollient Sunblock Mineral Protection, Fragrance Free SPF 30 above. As such, the same review applies.

☺ GOOD **Hawaiian Sunscreen Soothing Aloe Vera SPF 30** *($10.99 for 4 fl. oz.)* is not "natural," despite the name. Almost all the actives are synthetic, except for titanium dioxide. Synthetic sunscreens aren't bad ingredients, but they shouldn't be in a sunscreen sold as "natural." That said, this is a very good option for normal to dry skin. It contains 2% titanium dioxide (not the best amount for UVA protection, but better than nothing); its soft, creamy texture makes it easy to apply and it is water-resistant. Alba Botanica includes some antioxidants, always a plus, although they also include a couple of plants and fragrance ingredients that are potentially problematic. The small amount of titanium dioxide keeps this from earning our highest rating. The amount of alcohol is not cause for concern.

☺ GOOD **Very Emollient Sunblock Natural Protection, Facial SPF 30** *($10.99 for 4 fl. oz.)* is nearly identical to the Hawaiian Sunscreen Soothing Aloe Vera SPF 30 above, and the same review applies.

☺ GOOD **Very Emollient Sunblock Natural Protection, Fragrance Free SPF 30** *($10.99 for 4 fl. oz.)* is nearly identical to Very Emollient Sunblock Natural Protection, Facial SPF 30 above. As such, the same review applies.

☺ GOOD **Very Emollient Sunless Golden Tanning Without The Sun** *($10.99 for 4 fl. oz.)* includes dihydroxyacetone to turn your skin color, just as with most self-tanners. It also contains a small amount of erythrulose, a self-tanning ingredient that works more slowly than dihydroxyacetone. What sets this self-tanning lotion for normal to dry skin apart from others are the many emollient plant oils and antioxidants. Those additions are helpful and make this worth considering as something more than just a self-tanner—and the price is great! What's not so great and keeps this self-tanner from earning our highest rating is the inclusion of several fragrance ingredients that pose a risk of irritation. The risk is low, and likely the fragrance helps cover up the after-smell some self-tanners have, but it would be better for your skin without these additions.

☺ AVERAGE **Hawaiian Revitalizing Green Tea SPF 45** *($10.99 for 4 fl. oz.)* is nearly identical to several other SPF 45 sunscreens from Alba Botanica. The only difference between these sunscreens is the marketing angle, with this option being geared toward those who want green tea, even though all SPF 45 sunscreens from Alba Botanica contain this antioxidant—we know, how weird is that? There's not much lavender in here, but that, along with the less-than-generous amount of titanium dioxide (a 2% concentration minimally gets by for UVA protection), keeps this from earning a higher rating. Note: This contains several fragrance ingredients that pose a risk of irritation. Although they're present in low amounts, combined with the synthetic sunscreen actives, their irritation potential is heightened.

☺ AVERAGE **Very Emollient Sunblock Natural Protection, Kids SPF 45** *($10.99 for 4 fl. oz.)* contains a blend of synthetic and mineral actives, just like lots of sunscreens marketed to adults. There is nothing about this sunscreen's formula that makes it better for kids. This sunscreen contains synthetic sunscreen ingredients, which will definitely sting and burn if it gets too close to (or into) your eyes. Marketing angles aside, this provides reliable, water-resistant protection with titanium dioxide on hand to shield your skin from UVA rays (though the amount of it is a bit disappointing). The average rating is due to the inclusion of lavender, an ingredient all skin types should strive to avoid, especially when out in the sun (see the Appendix for details). There isn't a lot of lavender in this sunscreen, but Alba Botanica and many other brands offer sunscreens without lavender, so why take the chance?

☺ AVERAGE **Very Emollient Sunblock Natural Protection Pure Lavender SPF 45** *($10.99 for 4 fl. oz.)* is identical to other Alba Botanica Very Emollient sunblocks above. The only difference is the marketing angle, with this option being geared toward those who want lavender. We're not sure who thinks lavender is a good sunscreen ingredient, but here it is nonetheless. The thing is, lavender isn't a great ingredient for any skin type (we explain why in the Appendix). There's not much lavender in here, but that, along with the less-than-generous amount of titanium dioxide (a 2% concentration, which minimally gets by for UVA protection), keeps this from earning a higher rating. This sunscreen also contains several fragrance ingredients (listed at the end of the ingredient statement) known to cause irritation.

☺ AVERAGE **Very Emollient Sunblock Natural Protection, Sport SPF 45** *($10.99 for 4 fl. oz.)* is marketed to sports enthusiasts. With that aside, it is nearly identical to Alba Botanica's Very Emollient Sunblock Natural Protection, Kids SPF 45. Isn't it interesting how two very different groups (kids and active adults) are supposed to use the same sunscreen, yet the kid-related claims are replaced here with claims about exercise and perspiration—just what the sports-minded are looking for. This sunscreen is just fine for use during sports activities for those with normal to dry skin; it is water-resistant and includes titanium dioxide for decent UVA protection, along with synthetic sunscreen ingredients. As with any sunscreen, you must reapply this after exercise or excessive perspiration, and after toweling off. Be careful because the synthetic sunscreen ingredients can sting if they get in your eyes, which is likely if you apply it to your face and you begin to perspire. It also contains lavender, an ingredient that all skin types should strive to avoid, especially when you are out in the sun. There isn't a lot of lavender in this sunscreen, but Alba Botanica and many other brands offer sunscreens without lavender, so why take the chance? By the way, the lavender also negates the company's fragrance-free claim for this sunscreen.

☺ AVERAGE **Natural Very Emollient Sunscreen Mineral Protection Aloe Vanilla SPF 30** *($10.99 for 4 fl. oz.)*. This sunscreen contains the mineral actives of titanium dioxide and zinc oxide, and so provides reliable broad-spectrum protection. Normally, we'd recommend such sunscreens for sensitive or rosacea-affected skin, but in this case the inclusion of fragrance ingredients (eugenol, geraniol, and others) negates that thumbs-up. If sensitivity is not your concern, this is still a fairly gentle and, as stated, effective sunscreen. It is best for those with normal to very dry skin not prone to breakouts. As with most mineral-based sunscreens, this requires thorough blending to minimize the white cast these actives can leave behind. Despite the gentleness of the active ingredients, think twice before exposing your skin to fragrance ingredients known to be irritating. There are plenty of mineral sunscreens that do not contain these problematic extras.

☹ POOR **Hawaiian Coconut Dry Oil with SPF 15 Natural Sunscreen** *($10.99 for 4.5 fl. oz.)* contains synthetic active ingredients, so you can ignore the "natural" part of this spray-on sunscreen's name. We guess Alba Botanica was hoping you wouldn't notice. It's not that synthetic sunscreen ingredients are bad, but a cosmetics company shouldn't be misrepresenting them in this manner. There really is no reason to consider this sunscreen anyway: It fails to provide sufficient UVA protection because it doesn't contain ingredients that provide that benefit (titanium dioxide, zinc oxide, ecamsule, Mexoryl SX, avobenzone, or Tinosorb). Plus, it is loaded with fragrant oils that are proven skin-irritants. What an all-around disappointment!

ALBA BOTANICA SPECIALTY SKIN-CARE PRODUCTS

☺ AVERAGE **Even Advanced Deep Sea Facial Mask** *($11.49 for 4 fl. oz.)* would be a much better choice for normal to oily skin if it did not contain several emollients and plant oil. None of these ingredients are needed for oily skin, and their presence hinders the absorbent quality of the clay, leaving your skin more confused than revitalized. Those with dry skin will find this too absorbent, which makes it an OK option only if your skin is normal (in which case you wouldn't need a mask like this). Don't worry if you're confused by all this; so are we, which is why this is a superfluous product to consider for any skin type.

☺ AVERAGE **Hawaiian Facial Mask Pore-fecting Papaya Enzyme** *($13.99 for 3 fl. oz.)* is not really Pore-fecting; however, if you leave this seaweed- and papaya-based mask on your skin long enough, the enzymes might have some effect as exfoliants. However, the jar packaging hinders their already limited stability, and pure papaya, along with the enzyme derived from it, papain, can be irritating. AHAs can be irritating, too, but at least they have considerable research proving their benefits when used topically at concentrations that are low enough to make the result worth the minor irritation. If you're curious to try this mask and decide to sidestep the stability issue, it is suitable for all skin types.

ALBA BOTANICA LIP CARE

✓☺ BEST **Very Emollient Sunblock Lip Care SPF 25** *($2.50 for 0.15 fl. oz.)* contains lots of natural ingredients (actually, most lip balms can make this claim), but for a line that espouses natural, it's odd that Alba Botanica opted for three synthetic sunscreen actives. The sunscreen also includes zinc oxide for reliable UVA protection, making this one of the best and most cost-effective lip balms with sunscreen around. The base formula isn't special, but it contains a blend of oils and waxes that work to prevent moisture loss and reduce chapping. The formula has a slight tint to offset the white cast inherent from sunscreens that contain zinc oxide.

☺ GOOD **Clear Lip Gloss** *($4.99)* is a standard, scented non-sticky lip gloss packaged in a squeeze tube with a slanted-tip applicator. The formula delivers plenty of moisture as well as a high-gloss shine. It's available in an array of fruity scents and flavors that will encourage lip-licking, which can lead to chapping. If you can resist that temptation, this is a very good and reasonably priced clear lip gloss option that gives your lips the moisture they need and the shine you want.

☺ GOOD **Coconut Cream Lip Balm** *($2.99 for 0.15 fl. oz.)* is good if you like coconut, because you'll be getting a lot of it in this coconut oil and coconut-flavored lip balm. Thankfully free of irritants such as menthol and peppermint, it is a good, emollient lip moisturizer that contains a small but varied blend of antioxidants.

☺ GOOD **Passion Fruit Nectar Lip Balm** *($2.99 for 0.15 fl. oz.)* is very similar to Coconut Cream Lip Balm, except this option has a passion fruit flavor instead of coconut. It is a good lip balm for mild to major cases of chapped lips, and it contains a small but varied blend of antioxidants.

☺ GOOD **Pineapple Quench Lip Balm** *($2.99 for 0.15 fl. oz.)* is very similar to Coconut Cream Lip Balm, except this option has a pineapple flavor instead of coconut.

☹ POOR **Unpetroleum Cherry SPF 18 Lip Balm** *($2.75 for 0.15 fl. oz.)* lacks the UVA-protecting ingredients of titanium dioxide, zinc oxide, avobenzone, ecamsule, or Tinosorb and is not recommended. It also contains PABA, a UVB sunscreen whose use has fallen out of favor due to its tendency to cause allergic reactions.

☹ POOR **Unpetroleum Tangerine SPF 18 Lip Balm** *($2.75 for 0.15 fl. oz.)* is nearly identical to Unpetroleum Cherry SPF 18 Lip Balm above, and the same review applies.

☹ POOR **Unpetroleum Vanilla SPF 18 Lip Balm** *($2.75 for 0.15 fl. oz.)* is nearly identical to Unpetroleum Cherry SPF 18 Lip Balm above, and the same review applies.

ALMAY

Strengths: An excellent assortment of foundations with sunscreen; very good powders, liquid eyeliner, and mascaras; inviting and well-organized in-store displays.

Weaknesses: Company discontinued all of their skin-care products with the exception of makeup removers; despite their hypoallergenic claims, many products contain potentially ir-ritating and sensitizing ingredients; mediocre blush and eyeshadows; Intense i-color products are mostly gimmicky.

For more information and reviews of the latest Almay products, visit CosmeticsCop.com.

ALMAY MAKEUP REMOVERS

☺ GOOD **Moisturizing Eye Makeup Remover Liquid** *($5.99 for 4 fl. oz.)* is a standard, mineral oil–based liquid that efficiently removes eye makeup, though not without leaving a greasy residue. The gentle, fragrance-free formula is best used prior to cleansing.

☺ GOOD **Moisturizing Eye Makeup Remover Pads** *($5.99 for 80 pads)* consist of a mineral oil–based, fragrance-free solution steeped in pads. They work well to remove makeup but can leave a greasy residue if not rinsed.

☺ GOOD **Oil-Free Eye Makeup Remover Liquid** *($6.29 for 4 fl. oz.)* works well to remove most eye makeup. The lack of silicone or oils makes it a poor choice to remove waterproof mascara.

☺ GOOD **Oil-Free Eye Makeup Remover Pads** *($5.99 for 80 pads)* are nearly identical to the Oil Free Eye Makeup Remover Liquid above, only in pad form, so the same review applies.

☺ GOOD **Oil-Free Makeup Remover Towelettes** *($5.99 for 25 towelettes)* are essentially a gentle, water-soluble cleanser in pre-moistened cloth form. This basic formula will remove a light makeup application but is not capable of removing mascara, long-wearing foundation, or lip color. It is best for normal to slightly dry or slightly oily skin.

☺ GOOD **$$$ Oil Free Makeup Eraser Sticks** *($5.49 for 24 sticks)*. Almay has placed its longstanding, fragrance-free Oil-Free Makeup Remover into sticks whose hollow centers house the liquid. Each end of the stick is outfitted with a cotton swab, and once you snap the stick as directed, the liquid flows onto the tip, ready for use. Although convenient and effective (except for removing waterproof formulas), this ends up being an expensive and time-consuming way to remove eye makeup. You can use any eye makeup remover with regular cotton swabs (or a cotton pad) and get the same results. These sticks are an option for use while traveling, but for daily use at home, the cost quickly adds up.

ALMAY FOUNDATIONS

✓☺ BEST **Clear Complexion Makeup** *($13.99)* is a foundation that promises to "heal blemishes." It contains salicylic acid as the anti-acne active, but in an amount that is too low (0.6%) and at a pH that is too high (pH 6) to be helpful for skin. Even though the salicylic acid in this makeup won't help with blemishes, this still offers an enviably smooth, liquid texture that blends onto skin with ease, providing light to medium coverage and a natural matte finish. It is a great example of how beautiful a foundation can look on the skin. Nine shades are available, and almost all of them are exquisite. Only Warm should be viewed with caution as it may be too peach for some medium to tan skin tones. There are no options for very light or dark skin tones. One caution: Because of the salicylic acid, this product should not be used around the eyes or on the eyelids. This foundation is one to try if you have normal to very oily skin.

✓☺ BEST **Nearly Naked Liquid Makeup SPF 15** *($10.99)* is easily one of Almay's best liquid foundations. Its lightweight cream texture blends superbly, setting to a smooth matte finish that enhances skin without looking flat, fake, or the least bit unnatural. Well suited for someone with normal to oily skin, it offers sheer to light coverage and excellent sun protection from its in-part titanium dioxide and zinc oxide sunscreen. More good news: The nine shades are beautifully neutral, with options for fair to tan skin tones.

✓☺ BEST **TLC Truly Lasting Color 16 Hour Makeup SPF 15** *($12.49)* will not remain looking "just-applied" for the full 16 hours (and definitely not over your oily areas), but don't let the exaggerated claim keep you from trying this fantastic foundation. The silky texture is a pleasure to blend, and provides medium coverage that layers well over trouble spots. Gentle, effective sun protection is assured from the blend of titanium dioxide and zinc oxide, while the smooth matte finish helps keep excess oil in check (just not all day) without looking chalky. The nine mostly neutral shades are indicative of what Almay usually produces, which is good. There are no options for dark skin tones, and the lightest shades may present some trouble for fair skin due to overtones of pink and yellow, but they're still worth considering. Avoid the too-peach Warm.

✓☺ BEST **Smart Shade Smart Balance Skin Balancing Makeup SPF 15** *($13.99)*. This liquid foundation with titanium dioxide and zinc oxide as the only sunscreen ingredients is Almay's second version of their Smart Shade makeup. The original formula, with the same name, is still available, at least for now; the only differences are the price (this one costs more) and the claims Almay makes. That version is reviewed on CosmeticsCop.com. This improved second version not only carries on the skin-matching pigment technology claim of its predecessor, but also adds the claim of being able to sense where skin is oily or dry, and act accordingly. We've seen this claim before, and it never works. Simply put, there's no way a makeup can know where skin is dry or oily and then be able to deposit the right ingredients to improve these disparate conditions. Where would the moisturizing ingredients go when the oil-absorbing ingredients are "activated," and vice versa?

In terms of moisturizing, this silky foundation provides little moisture; the ingredients are primarily about absorbing oil and moisture. It goes on smoothly, blends readily, and sets to a soft matte finish that becomes powdery a short time later. The finish is incredibly skin-like, making this one of the most natural-looking foundations available. Coverage goes from sheer to light. The shades are said to self-adjust to each level (light, medium, and dark), depending on your skin tone. They can't really do that, of course, but the shades are versatile enough to work for most people with light to slightly tan skin. Note: This foundation dispenses white with small colored specks. The specks "burst" as you blend, and the whiteness disappears, so there's no ghostly look to be concerned about. This foundation is best for normal to oily skin.

☺ GOOD **Line Smoothing Makeup SPF 15** *($13.99)* offers excellent UVA protection thanks to its titanium dioxide and zinc oxide sunscreen. It has a slightly thick, initially creamy texture that blends smoothly, provides light to medium coverage, and has a satin matte finish. We disagree with Almay's claim that this formula "hydrates all day" because it contains minimal ingredients with substantial moisturizing properties for skin. The nine shades are mostly neutral and include options for fair to tan skin. Beige and Warm suffer from a noticeable peach cast, and are the only shades to avoid. This foundation is best for normal to slightly dry skin and, contrary to its name, doesn't do much to smooth the appearance of lines.

☺ GOOD **Smart Shade Anti-Aging Makeup SPF 20** *($13.99)*. Almay claims that this liquid foundation can "fight the signs of aging" and in one respect that's true, because Almay included sufficient broad-spectrum sun protection, which will keep your face shielded from the effects of the sun's harmful, aging rays. In this formula, sunscreens zinc oxide and titanium dioxide do double duty because they also impart a good amount of opacity, which makes building this up to medium coverage a breeze. Unlike the original Smart Shade SPF 15, this leaves a satin finish that borders on shiny. While this formula is suitable for normal to oily skin, the finish may not suit very oily skin as well as the original version's matte finish.

Here's how the Smart Shade premise works: As you dispense each shade, it appears grayish white. As you blend, it turns into a flesh tone. Each shade blends well and does not streak or look "dotted" on skin, though its initial appearance is admittedly startling. Almay has divided the shades by depth of skin color. The Light shade fares best because it is the most neutral, and is a versatile option for fair to light skin. Light/Medium is acceptable for medium skin tones, but is too peach for lighter skin, while Medium has a rosiness that makes it unsuitable for most skin colors. However, if one of the better shades works for you, this is certainly worth an audition. One more comment: although this anti-aging makeup contains some intriguing ingredients for improving skin's appearance and healthy functioning, most are present in amounts too small for skin to notice. All of them are listed after the sodium chloride, which is typically 1% or less.

☹ AVERAGE **Wake Up Hydrating Make Up SPF 13** *($12.99)* is a loose-powder foundation with a pure titanium dioxide sunscreen that falls short of the basic worldwide standard of SPF 15, which is a disappointment at the outset. It has a distinct "wet" feel on your skin when applied, which is supposed to indicate that the powder is hydrating, but the wet feeling dissipates quickly. Unless a product has ingredients that can retain the water in your skin, the evaporation taking place actually makes your skin drier. If anything, the ingredients in this powder are absorbent, and will only make your skin drier, not hydrated. Gimmicks aside, this is simply a basic powder foundation with sunscreen that provides light coverage and looks best layered with two blended coats. Once the powder sets, it leaves a sheer gold shimmer behind, which isn't the best for all-over makeup application, especially not for daytime, and it definitely won't make oily or combination skin look matte.

ALMAY CONCEALERS

☺ GOOD **Clear Complexion Concealer** *($7.99)* contains, like all of Almay's Clear Complexion products, salicylic acid. It's present here at 1%, but the pH is over 4, so it won't exfoliate skin and can't help to reduce blemishes and blackheads. This is still a worthwhile liquid concealer that provides medium coverage and a soft, somewhat dry matte finish. It's an option for concealing blemishes or red spots, but be aware of the salicylic acid and keep it away from the eyelid area. All three shades are recommended.

☺ GOOD **Smart Shade Concealer SPF 15** *($8.99)*. This concealer gets its "smart" name from the claim that it "transforms into your ideal shade." But if that were really true, wouldn't just one master shade suffice because it would "transform" for everyone? Almay offers three shades, so they don't seem to believe their own claim! Aside from the hokey name, this concealer has a slightly liquid texture that provides more slip than necessary, so it's somewhat tricky to get it placed just where you want it because it tends to spread too easily. The formula takes longer to set than it should. It ends up having a soft matte finish capable of medium coverage, but you may notice minor creasing under the eyes and fading by the end of the day. Two of the three shades are good and well suited for light skin tones; avoid Medium, which is quite peachy. The smartest part of this concealer is its titanium dioxide and zinc oxide sunscreen, which is why this is worth considering despite the other shortcomings. It is an excellent choice for use around the eye area, especially if your foundation or daytime moisturizer with sunscreen proves irritating when applied around the eyes.

☺ GOOD **Wake Up Under Eye Concealer** (*$8.99*). This liquid concealer has a moisturizing effect that does a good job of diminishing fine lines (temporarily, of course), and its finish imparts a subtle luminosity to brighten up the under-eye area. Among the shades, Light is nearly translucent, while Light/Medium and Medium provide sheer coverage with pink undertones. The squeeze-tube features a built-in brush applicator that helps eliminate wasted product, but you'll need to use your finger or a sponge to facilitate blending. The major drawback for this concealer is that it doesn't do a very good job of concealing. It is too sheer to camouflage dark circles, and that won't make you look more awake.

☺ AVERAGE **Line Smoothing Concealer SPF 10** (*$9.99*) works beautifully as an under-eye concealer thanks to its fluid, smooth application, just the right amount of slip, and soft matte finish. The sole sunscreen active ingredient is titanium dioxide, a gentle choice for a product meant to be used around the eyes, but it's disappointing that the SPF rating is not 15. Three shades are available, all excellent.

☺ AVERAGE **Nearly Naked Cover-Up Stick** (*$7.79*) pales in comparison to Almay's other concealers, but still has merit for someone with dry skin. The coverage this lipstick-style concealer provides is not "Nearly Naked" and it tends to crease into lines under the eye, though that can be reduced by setting it with powder. The wax content of this concealer makes it inappropriate for use over blemishes. Three shades are available, each suitably neutral.

☹ POOR **Clear Complexion Concealer + Treatment Gel BlemishHeal Technology** (*$9.99*) is a dual-sided concealer and acne treatment that comes with a clear salicylic acid spot treatment on one end and a stick concealer on the other. The anti-acne treatment claims it can heal acne blemishes, and although it's medicated with anti-acne salicylic acid, the pH is too high for it to be effective. The formula also contains a high amount of alcohol, which makes it too irritating for all skin types (see the Appendix to find out why irritation is bad for skin). The stick concealer end doesn't fare much better, providing only medium coverage that's fleeting and tends to slip into lines, even after it sets to a satin finish. The three shades are only suitable for light to medium skin.

ALMAY POWDERS

✓☺ BEST **Line Smoothing Pressed Powder** (*$13.49*) feels silky, goes on sheer and exceptionally smooth, and makes normal to dry skin look polished, not powdered. The slight satin finish of this powder won't exaggerate wrinkles, but powders (this one included) don't do much to smooth their appearance, either. That doesn't mean this outstanding option isn't worth considering, and if you have light to medium skin, the three shades are geared for you.

✓☺ BEST **Nearly Naked Loose Powder** (*$11.99*) promises a "flawless, natural-looking finish" and delivers! This talc-based powder has an ultra-silky texture that feels weightless and sets makeup without looking flat or dry. All three shades are suitable for most skin tones since they are translucent. Someone with very oily skin will likely want a more absorbent powder, but all other skin types will appreciate what this has to offer.

☺ GOOD **TLC Truly Lasting Color Pressed Powder SPF 12** *($12.99)* lacks sufficient UVA-protecting ingredients (titanium dioxide, zinc oxide, avobenzone [also called butyl methoxydibenzoylmethane], Tinosorb, Mexoryl SX [also known as ecamsule]). Although it's not a pressed powder to consider if you want broad-spectrum sun protection, it has a beautiful, creamy feel that slips over skin and blends to a natural yet polished finish. You may be tempted by Almay's claim of 16-hour wear for this product, but anyone with oily skin will find they need a touch-up before lunch. In terms of wearability, however, this powder does hold up well throughout the day as far as not pooling into pores or looking streaked but that's true of many top-rated powders (some with great SPF protection). Among the three shades (suitable for light to medium skin), you'll find Medium and Light/Medium appear a bit peach in the compact, but both look softer and more neutral on skin. The rating for this pressed powder does not apply to its deficient sunscreen.

☺ AVERAGE **Clear Complexion Pressed Powder** *($12.49)* claims to clear blemishes with salicylic acid (present at 0.6%), but since a pH value cannot be obtained in a powder, it won't work for that purpose. The formula is talc-based and the texture is unusually dry, though it doesn't look chalky on skin. It contains cornstarch, which aids in absorbing excess oil without feeling heavy. Three sheer shades are available, and all have merit.

☹ POOR **Smart Shade Smart Balance Pressed Powder** *($13.99)*. If this pressed powder could adapt to match your skin tone after application as claimed, it would be a good thing, because it's impossible to determine which shade is right for you just by looking at the packaging—they all look exactly the same! All the shades have a light base with white swirls and dark spots of color that are meant to join together when applied and somehow adjust to your skin tone, and to everyone else's as well. The truth: Makeup cannot magically adjust to the color of your skin because it doesn't know what skin color you have. In reality this is a very dry pressed powder that looks somewhat chalky on skin. Even more disappointing is that it offers little coverage and minimal oil absorption.

ALMAY BLUSHES & BRONZER

☺ GOOD **Smart Shade Blush** *($8.99)* is said to be so smart, it blushes for you—thanks to shade-sensing "smart beads" that transform to your ideal blush color. Available in Pink, Berry, or Natural tone, each offers very soft, sheer color that requires several layers to really register as blush. The liquid texture is surprisingly easy to blend, and sets quickly to a soft matte finish. This blush cannot adjust to your skin tone; however, like any color cosmetic, the way it looks on your skin will be (to varying degrees) different from how the same shade looks on someone else's skin. Almay is taking the ordinary and trying to make it sound customized; all they've created is a good liquid blush for normal to oily skin (Note to those with large pores: This does not magnify them or make them look "dotted with color").

☺ AVERAGE **Powder Blush** *($9.99)* is a below-standard pressed-powder blush that comes in an attractive range of shades and has a reasonably smooth application. The problem is the sparkly particles woven into each shade. They don't do this blush any favors, are distracting in daylight, and tend to flake.

☺ AVERAGE **Smart Shade Bronzer** *($8.99)* is nearly identical to the Smart Shade Blush above, except the color saturation is stronger, so you need less per application to produce noticeable results. Best for normal to oily skin, the main drawback is the color itself, which tends toward orange regardless of your skin tone.

Buying skin-care products packaged in jars? See the Appendix to learn why that's a bad idea.

ALMAY EYESHADOWS

☺ AVERAGE **Intense i-Color Powder Eye Shadow Kits** *($7.49)* presents a collection of four eyeshadow trios, each with shades meant to complement your eye color (a misguided notion, but we'll get to that in a moment). The texture of these shadows is smooth yet powdery, so unless you're careful some flaking is imminent and application can be messy. These go on quite soft, and every shade has an obvious shine that borders on overpowering the underlying color of the eyeshadow itself. The finishes come in smoky, satin and shimmer, but all deposit noticeable shine. The trios for green eyes and blue eyes should mostly be avoided because eyeshadow is not about matching your eye color, it's about shading and shaping the eye area. Even if your goal is to enhance your eye color, to do that effectively you would choose contrasting, not matching, shades. For example, if you want to make white look whiter, you don't put another shade of white next to it, you pair it with a dark shade, like slate or black. Applying blue eyeshadow when you have blue eyes means you're adding color that will visually compete with your eyes, whereas brown shades, or pale peach, caramel, or taupe colors will enhance them. It really is that simple. These trios from Almay are intended to make eyeshadow shopping easier but end up not helping in the least. They just point women back to a makeup theory that hasn't made it into the fashion magazines since the 1970s.

ALMAY EYE & BROW LINERS

✓☺ BEST **Liquid Eyeliner** *($7.29)* remains one of the very best liquid liners at any price. It goes on smoothly and easily, creating a dramatic line—thin or thick—without flaking, chipping, or looking crinkled. Two shades (classic brown and black) are available, both with all-day longevity.

☺ GOOD **Brow Defining Pencil** *($7.49)* is ultra-thin and does not require sharpening. It has a suitably dry texture that demands a soft touch while applying, but that's precisely what it takes to get the best results from this long-lasting brow enhancer. The three shades are terrific, including a great option for blonde (but not white-blonde) eyebrows.

☺ GOOD **Eye Liner** *($7.99)* is a very good, automatic, retractable pencil with a smooth application that is only slightly prone to smudging. As claimed, this pencil is waterproof. In fact, it requires an oil- or silicone-based makeup remover to get it to come off completely.

☺ GOOD **Intense i-Color Liquid Liner for Eyes** *($7.49)* has a brush and application that are nearly identical to Almay's Liquid Eyeliner, except that each of the four shades are loaded with iridescence. The cool factor of this eyeliner is that the shades alter in changing light (for example, Raisin Quartz is a metallic purple that takes on a brownish cast in certain light). The negative is that this much shine so close to the lashes is distracting, and not flattering if wrinkles are noticeable. Still, teens and twenty-somethings will find this a fun departure, and it does last.

☺ AVERAGE **Liquid Eyeliner Pen** *($7.49)* comes in three classic shades—brown, black brown, and black—and delivers a bold line of color that dries quickly. The downside is that the color tends to dissipate throughout the day, resulting in uneven wear. Even though the flexible felt-tip applicator is pointed at the end, the overall shape makes it very difficult to apply a thin line.

ALMAY MASCARAS

✓☺ BEST **One Coat Lengthening Mascara** *($5.99)* has a misleading name because it takes more than one coat to achieve results, but this superior mascara thickens as well as it lengthens! It applies cleanly, and wears and removes well.

✓☺ BEST **One Coat Nourishing Mascara Triple Effect** *($7.99)* is marvelous. It has a dual-sided brush that maximizes length, curl, and thickness, although if you get too enthusiastic while applying, it can go on somewhat heavy and uneven. The brush side with the longer bristles quickly lengthens and separates lashes, while the opposite side has short, closely packed bristles to add thickness and drama. The formula keeps lashes soft, which makes it easy to remove with a water-soluble cleanser, making this a top choice. Of course, there is nothing in it that is nourishing for your lashes.

☺ GOOD **Get Up & Grow Mascara** *($7.99)* has a wide, curvy brush with bristles that deposit color on every single lash. In fact, you get impressive definition, fullness, and length from this mascara, allowing you to create a glamorous look in just a few strokes. What keeps this mascara from earning our best rating is that it tends to flake a bit by the end of the day. Such a shame from a mascara that was almost love at first swipe! As for the "grow" portion of the name—this mascara does not contain anything that will help your lashes grow. The company claims the formula keeps your lashes conditioned so they'll grow longer, but conditioning hair has nothing to do with making hair grow; even if it did, there aren't enough conditioning agents in here to make a difference.

☺ GOOD **One Coat Nourishing Mascara Thickening Waterproof** *($5.99)* applies beautifully and makes lashes noticeably longer and thicker, though we disagree with Almay's claim of "100% thicker lashes." Still, it wears well, is waterproof, and doesn't make lashes feel stiff or brittle.

☺ GOOD **One Coat Thickening Mascara** *($5.99)* has an inaccurate name because this mascara lengthens better than it thickens. Slight clumping is apparent, but it brushes through easily, and this isn't a stubborn formula to remove.

☹ AVERAGE **One Coat Dial Up Mascara** *($8.49)*. If you remember Maybelline's Dial-A-Lash from the 1980s, then you already know the gimmick behind Almay's Dial Up Mascara. By turning the dial at the base, you control the size of the opening where the brush comes out of the container. A smaller opening means that more of the mascara is wiped off when the brush comes out, a larger opening means that less mascara is wiped off; that is, the smaller the opening the less mascara remains on the brush, the bigger the opening the more mascara is on the brush. This is an effective method for controlling the amount of mascara on the brush, giving you the potential to create looks that range from natural to dramatic with one product. But, when it comes to mascara, too much on the brush can spell instant trouble, so keeping it dialed down (i.e., a smaller opening) ultimately produces better results. The rubber-bristled brush is flexible and nicely shaped, but the formula itself is too wet to make this an easy, one-coat wonder. Even though it takes a couple of careful coats to keep lashes from clumping, the result is lashes that have lots of thickness and moderate length. Disappointingly, after the lashes dry they feel stiff and somewhat brittle.

☹ POOR **Intense i-Color Mascara with Light Interplay Technology** *($7.49)*. With a huge plastic-bristled brush and a somewhat goopy texture that tends to clump and smear, this mascara just can't compete with other similarly priced mascaras at the drugstore. Almay's gimmick of "light interplay technology" to bring out your natural eye color means infusing shimmery gold, green, blue, or purple hues into the mascara. How flecks of purple or gold sparkles mixed into black mascara can intensify the color of brown eyes is beyond us. As far as we can tell, the only thing you're intensifying is your chances of getting glitter in your eye!

ALPHA HYDROX

Strengths: A good selection of well-priced, effective AHA products using glycolic acid; excels with skin-lightening and retinol products; a small but workable selection of cleansers.

Weaknesses: Moisturizers with oxygenating ingredients; reliance on jar packaging for some products with antioxidants.

For more information and reviews of the latest Alpha Hydrox products, visit CosmeticsCop.com.

ALPHA HYDROX CLEANSERS

✓☺ BEST **Foaming Face Wash** *($7.49 for 6 fl. oz.)* is a water-soluble cleanser with a slight foaming action. Expect this to do a sufficient job removing makeup and consider it recommended for all skin types except very oily. Foaming Face Wash is also fragrance-free.

☺ GOOD **Nourishing Cleanser** *($8.49 for 4.5 fl. oz.)* contains a couple of vitamins and skin-conditioning agents that aren't all that helpful in a cleanser because they are rinsed from skin so quickly. This is otherwise a standard but good water-soluble cleanser suitable for all skin types, except very oily. The tiny amount of corn and soybean oil should not pose a problem for those with blemish-prone skin.

ALPHA HYDROX TONER

☹ POOR **Toner Astringent for Normal to Oily Skin** *($6.99 for 6 fl. oz.)* lists alcohol as the second ingredient, followed by witch hazel and, shortly thereafter, menthol. This toner is not recommended (and, if you're curious, the pH is too high for the glycolic acid to function as an exfoliant). See the Appendix to learn why irritation is bad for all skin types.

ALPHA HYDROX EXFOLIANTS & SCRUBS

☺ GOOD **AHA Souffle** *($15.49 for 1.6 fl. oz.)* includes 12% glycolic acid formulated at a pH of 4, which makes this effective for exfoliation. The lightweight but substantial-feeling cream base is basic, but although a few antioxidants are included, the jar packaging will quickly render them ineffective. This is still an effective AHA option for normal to dry skin.

☺ GOOD **Enhanced Cream 10% Glycolic AHA Anti-Wrinkle** *($10.99 for 2 fl. oz.)* is nearly identical to the AHA Souffle above, minus the antioxidants (which is fine considering this product is also packaged in a jar) and with a slightly thinner texture. The other difference is the amount of glycolic acid, which is 10% in this product.

☺ GOOD **Enhanced Lotion 10% Glycolic AHA Anti-Wrinkle** *($11.99 for 6 fl. oz.)* remains the best AHA bargain Alpha Hydrox offers. The standard lotion formula contains 10% glycolic acid at a pH of 4, making it an effective option for exfoliating normal to dry skin. There isn't much else of note to discuss, but if you're looking for a good AHA product with a lotion texture, this is one to try.

☺ GOOD **Oil-Free Formula 10% Glycolic AHA Anti-Wrinkle** *($10.99 for 1.7 fl. oz.)* features 10% glycolic acid at a pH of 4 in a lightweight gel base that is indeed oil-free. This is an excellent option for those with oily to very oily skin seeking an AHA product. Keep in mind that if your oily skin is accompanied by blackheads and blemishes, BHA (salicylic acid) offers greater benefits.

☺ GOOD **Sensitive Skin Cream 8% Glycolic AHA** *($9.29 for 2 fl. oz.)* is a very good, fragrance-free AHA exfoliant that contains 8% glycolic acid formulated at a pH to ensure it functions as an exfoliant. Although this offers the multiple benefits of using an AHA exfoliant, it is not rated higher due to the lack of other anti-aging ingredients such as antioxidants and skin-repairing substances. Their absence makes this a less desirable though still effective option that's OK for normal to dry skin. Those with sensitive skin should proceed with caution, as 8% glycolic acid can be too much. If you have sensitive skin and want to try this exfoliant, apply it every other night for the first few weeks and pay attention to how your skin responds.

☺ AVERAGE 14% AHA Swipes ($16.99 for 24 pads) are for those who prefer to use an effective AHA product in pad form, rather than a cream, gel, or lotion. If that's you, then this is a product worth considering, though it's not without drawbacks that you need to know about. The AHA content is higher than usual, but this is still an option if your skin can tolerate this amount; however, 14% AHA is definitely not for everyone and the research on daily use of AHA concentrations above 10% is lacking. If you're one of those people who believes that if a little is good then a lot is better, or if you have very advanced sun damage, then this is an OK option. It is good that Alpha Hydrox included anti-irritants, but not so good that they formulated with methylchloroisothiazolinone and methylisothiazolinone as the preservatives, because they're contraindicated for use in leave-on products. Still, you can swipe a pad over your face, let the solution sit for several minutes, and then rinse with water to remove. Otherwise, because of the preservatives used, we do not recommend leaving the pad solution on your face overnight.

☹ POOR **Intensive Serum, 14% Glycolic AHA** ($18.99 for 2 fl. oz.). This AHA exfoliant in serum form contains 14% glycolic acid, an amount that can definitely produce noticeable results in skin, especially since this product's pH is within range for the glycolic acid to exfoliate. Also on hand are soothing anti-irritants, which is good because for many 14% glycolic acid will be too much (research on routine topical use of AHAs generally recommends concentrations not exceed 10%). Although this AHA serum has a lot going for it, the preservative blend Alpha Hydrox chose is one that's known to be sensitizing. In fact, it is generally not recommended for use in leave-on products (Sources: *Contact Dermatitis*, November 2011, pages 276–285; and October 2006, pages 227–229). Unfortunately, this misstep means Intensive Serum is an exfoliant we cannot recommend.

☹ POOR **Acne Spot Serum** ($10.99 for 0.5 fl. oz.) is loaded with alcohol (listed as ethanol), which is a shame for this anti-acne product. The 2% concentration of salicylic acid and pH of 3.2 guarantee exfoliation and blackhead reduction, but it comes at the cost of irritating already inflamed skin, not to mention that the irritation will trigger more oil production in the pore. The anti-irritants included aren't enough to counteract the damaging effects of the alcohol.

☹ POOR **Eye and Upper Lip Cream** ($9.99 for 0.65 fl. oz.). The eye area and upper lip area are definitely two of the most age-prone places on the face, but this product isn't the antiwrinkle answer. It's a basic emollient moisturizer that contains a decent amount of vitamin E, a basic antioxidant addition to most cosmetics formulations. The amount of lactic acid is too low for it to function as an exfoliant, though it does have some benefit as a water-binding agent. This product contains comfrey extract, which isn't something to use near the eye, or anywhere else for that matter. Topical application of comfrey has anti-inflammatory properties, but it is recommended only for short-term use and only then if you can be sure the amount of pyrrolizidine alkaloids (a toxic component of the plant) is less than 100 micrograms per application—something that would be impossible to determine without sophisticated testing equipment, making comfrey an ingredient to avoid. The alkaloid content makes it a potential skin-irritant (Sources: *Chemical Research in Toxicology*, November 2001, pages 1546–1551; and *Public Health Nutrition*, December 2000, pages 501–508).

ALPHA HYDROX MOISTURIZERS (DAYTIME & NIGHTTIME), EYE CREAMS, & SERUMS

☺ GOOD **Retinol ResQ** *($14.99 for 1.05 fl. oz.)* ranks as one of the top retinol products available in any price range though the formula is getting to be a bit dated, so its rating was downgraded a bit. Still, for the money, this remains worth considering. Alpha Hydrox uses packaging that keeps the retinol stable and they also included antioxidant vitamins E and C along with an anti-irritant. The fragrance-free base formula is quite thick and preferred for normal to very dry skin not prone to blemishes. On balance, a greater array of antioxidants plus some proven skin-repairing ingredients would propel this back to being a top pick.

☺ AVERAGE **Night Replenishing Cream** *($10.49 for 2 fl. oz.)* is a very basic, emollient, fragrance-free moisturizer for dry to very dry skin. Alpha Hydrox recommends this for use around the eyes, and it is suitable for that purpose.

☹ POOR **Oxygenated Moisturizer** *($14.99 for 2 fl. oz.)* claims to oxygenate skin while stimulating collagen production, but providing oxygen to intact, otherwise healthy skin is detrimental because it causes free-radical damage (Sources: *Aging Cell*, June 2007, pages 361–370; *Journal of Pharmaceutical Sciences*, September 2007, pages 2181–2196; and *Human and Experimental Toxicology*, February 2002, pages 61–62). Alpha Hydrox used peroxidized corn oil in the form of TriOxygen-C, a patented ingredient that is also used in the Neoteric line for treating diabetic skin ulcers (Neoteric is the parent company of Alpha Hydrox). Although this ingredient's function is beneficial for supplying oxygen and promoting healing of ulcers, the physiological process that skin enacts to heal wounds is vastly different from treating wrinkles or supplying oxygen to unwounded skin. Both repeated use of any peroxidized substance and delivering extra oxygen to skin are damaging (Sources: *Journal of Reconstructive Microsurgery*, May 2007, pages 225–230; *Plastic and Reconstructive Surgery*, May 2007, pages 1980–1981; and *Cell Tissue Bank*, 2000, volume 1, issue 4, pages 261–269).

☹ POOR **Sheer Silk Moisturizer SPF 15** *($14.99 for 1 fl. oz.)* contains an in-part zinc oxide sunscreen, which is excellent. However, the peroxidized corn oil is cause for concern because oxidizing oil can lead to free-radical damage when applied over intact skin.

ALPHA HYDROX SPECIALTY SKIN-CARE PRODUCTS

✓☺ BEST **Spot Light Skin Lightener Fade Cream** *($9.99 for 0.85 fl. oz.)* is a well-formulated, skin-lightening product that combines 2% hydroquinone with 10% glycolic acid in a base with a pH of 3.3, all in packaging that will keep the hydroquinone stable. The light-weight lotion base is suitable for normal to slightly dry or dry skin, and the only thing missing is a selection of state-of-the-art skin-identical ingredients and more antioxidants (vitamin E is included). Still, this remains one of the better options for those who want to lighten sun- or hormone-induced brown skin discolorations, and the glycolic acid works in tandem with the hydroquinone to improve skin's appearance and texture.

ARBONNE (SKIN CARE ONLY)

Strengths: A small selection of basic but effective cleansers and masks.

Weaknesses: Consistent and pervasive use of volatile fragrant oils that are irritating, allergenic, and/or photosensitizing for skin; disappointing Intelligence line; no effective AHA or BHA products; no skin-lightening or effective anti-acne products; only one sun-care product that does not contain problematic ingredients; Arbonne salespeople tend to use blatant scare tactics to convince consumers theirs is the only brand of "safe" cosmetics when that is far from the truth.

For more information and reviews of the latest Arbonne skin-care products, visit CosmeticsCop.com.

ARBONNE CLEANSERS

☺ AVERAGE $$$ **RE9 Advanced Smoothing Facial Cleanser** *($40 for 3 fl. oz.)* is an extremely standard, and we mean astonishingly standard, cleanser that is overpriced for what you get. It is merely a water-soluble, detergent-based foaming cleanser for normal to oily skin. It works well to remove excess oil and makeup, but it doesn't have a smoothing effect; if anything, applying some of the ingredients, such as orange peel oil and sodium C14-16 olefin sulfonate, on skin is irritating and, therefore, anything but smoothing. As far as the standard cleansing agents, countless other cleansers share the same base, and we're talking about cleansers that cost about $10 for three times as much product, and those products leave out the problematic ingredients. Arbonne did add a few interesting ingredients, such as vitamins and plant extracts that can be anti-irritants, but their benefit is merely rinsed down the drain.

☹ POOR **Clear Advantage Clarifying Wash Acne Medication** *($16.50 for 3.5 fl. oz.)* uses salicylic acid as its active ingredient, but in a cleanser its benefit for blemish-prone skin is wasted. Even though the salicylic acid may have an impact on skin before rinsing, this water-soluble cleanser is not recommended because of the peppermint it contains.

☹ POOR **FC5 Hydrating Cleanser + Freshener** *($25 for 4 fl. oz.)* is a plant-enriched cleansing lotion that is not recommended because it contains far too many irritating ingredients, none of which are beneficial for skin. The biggest culprits are the fragrant citrus oils and sandalwood. None of these ingredients is recommended for use on the face, and they're especially problematic to use around the eyes! In addition, the price is borderline insulting, especially when you consider that what you're getting for the extra money could be a problem for your skin. One other point: The FC5 products from Arbonne are marketed as being natural; well, they contain many synthetic ingredients, and so are about as natural as polyester.

☹ POOR **FC5 Purifying Cleanser + Toner** *($25 for 4 fl. oz.)* is a water-soluble cleansing gel that foams so it's designed to be better for normal to oily skin. The cleanser and toner adds the menthol derivative menthyl lactate to the list of offending ingredients. Overall, this is not recommended. Please see the Appendix to learn why irritation is so bad for all skin types.

ARBONNE EYE-MAKEUP REMOVER

☺ AVERAGE $$$ **Eye Makeup Remover** *($22 for 3.7 fl. oz.)* is marginally effective and overpriced for what you get. Plus, it contains a couple of plant extracts that are a problem for use so close to the eye, which adds up to a below-average way to take off your makeup.

ARBONNE TONERS

☺ AVERAGE $$$ **RE9 Advanced Regenerating Toner** *($35 for 1.7 fl. oz.)* lists witch hazel water as the second ingredient in this poorly formulated toner. Alcohol is also high up on the list and that is never a good ingredient for skin. It is frustrating that the mix of plant extracts and antioxidants present are both beneficial (vitamin C) and problematic (orange peel oil). That means the good antioxidants spend their time fighting the effects of the irritating plants instead of devoting their energy toward improving your skin. Not only is the formula questionable, the price tag is outlandish for such a tiny amount of product with very little going for it. Used daily, you'd be buying more toner each month, which adds up to $420 a year!

☹ POOR **Clear Advantage Clarifying Toner Acne Medication** *($16.50 for 4 fl. oz.)* lists witch hazel as its second ingredient and that, coupled with the peppermint and other plant extracts known for their allergenic potential (dandelion, anyone?), makes this a clear problem, not an advantage, for all skin types. See the Appendix to find out why irritation is bad for all skin types.

ARBONNE SCRUB

☹ POOR **FC5 Exfoliating New Cell Scrub** *($28 for 4 fl. oz.)* is chock-full of problematic plant extracts and also contains a host of irritating fragrant oils. Bamboo extract is the abrasive agent, while benzyl nicotinate is a stimulant-type ingredient that causes increased circulation, which plays a part in the lingering redness after using this scrub. For the health of your skin, please don't subject it to this damaging scrub; the irritation kills cells and breaks down collagen, counter to what anyone concerned with looking younger should be doing to their face.

ARBONNE MOISTURIZERS (DAYTIME & NIGHTTIME), EYE CREAMS, & SERUMS

☺ AVERAGE **$$$ Prolief Natural Balancing Cream** *($34 for 2.5 fl. oz.)* is similar to Arbonne's PhytoProlief reviewed below, and the same review applies.

☺ AVERAGE **$$$ RE9 Advanced Age-Defying Neck Cream** *($82 for 1.7 fl. oz.)* is designed specifically for the neck, which definitely shows signs of aging, right along with the face. The signs of aging on the neck typically are more pronounced because the skin is thinner and it has less supportive elements (e.g., bone, fat, muscles, cartilage). Despite this, the neck doesn't require a special product and we've yet to see a neck cream whose formula is truly different from that of standard facial moisturizers. We've also never seen a single worthwhile study indicating that the neck needs special skin-care ingredients that other parts of the body do not. Adding to the foolish claim that this is somehow special for the neck, it is also an extremely dated (not advanced) formula that has the misfortune of being packaged in a jar. That means you're not only compromising hygiene with each use, but also that the few plant extracts it does contain will not remain stable. The amount of orange peel oil is potential cause for concern because orange peel oil is a major source of the fragrance chemical limonene, which is known to cause contact dermatitis on exposure to air (Sources: *Chemical Research in Toxicology*, March 2010, pages 677–688; *Contact Dermatitis*, December 2009, pages 337–341, and November 2006, pages 274–279). Although that's not good news, more so than any single factor is that this neck cream is a waste of time and money.

☺ AVERAGE **$$$ RE9 Advanced Corrective Eye Creme** *($55 for 0.5 fl. oz.)* is an emollient eye cream suitable for dry skin, but it contains some ingredients that you shouldn't apply near the eyes. Examples are fragrant orange oil along with plant extracts such as clover and rosemary. These ingredients have some benefit for skin, but their irritating chemical constituents make them less desirable when compared with many other plant extracts and oils. Many of this eye cream's truly advanced ingredients are listed after the problematic plant extracts, which isn't what you want to see in a product that costs this much. And why does a product meant for use so close to the eyes contain irritating fragrance ingredients like limonene and linalool? This is a perfect example of how eye creams rarely differ or are better for the eye area than moisturizers identified for the face. See the Appendix to learn why you don't need an eye cream.

☺ AVERAGE **$$$ RE9 Advanced Intensive Renewal Serum** *($58 for 1 fl. oz.)* lists water as the first ingredient, which isn't what you want to see in a serum that costs this much. If proof exists that this can lift and firm skin, Arbonne isn't showing their complete study to anyone and certainly not to the Paula's Choice Research team. This is most likely classic cosmetics industry claim substantiation that Arbonne paid for with the expectation that the test results would be favorable. It occurs all the time in the world of skin care, most likely because we are so prone to fall for the claims and we never ask to see the science behind them. Aside from water, the heart of this serum's formula is silicones and film-forming agents—the same ingredients that show up in countless serums. The amount of film-forming agents may make your skin feel a bit tighter, but no firming or lifting is taking place. Skin-care products, even the beautifully formulated ones, cannot fight the effects of gravity and other factors (such as bone loss and skin's continued growth as we age) that cause skin to sag. Lots of ingredients can create firmer skin by stimulating healthy collagen production, but this one gets tripped up by including several known and potentially irritating ingredients, all listed after the ingredients that published research has proven to have benefit for aging skin. One more point: The ingredients in here that sound like AHAs (i.e., sugar cane and lemon fruit extract) have no research showing they have any exfoliating properties. Also, the teeny amount of salicylic acid present can't exfoliate skin either. This ends up being an average, overpriced serum for normal to oily skin—and at any price your skin deserves brilliant, not average!

☹ POOR **Clear Advantage Clarifying Lotion Acne Medication** *($16.50 for 1.7 fl. oz.)* proved frustrating because it came so close to being a slam-dunk option. This lightweight lotion contains 1% salicylic acid and has a pH low enough to allow it to work as an exfoliant. However, because Arbonne insists on portraying a natural image, several plant extracts were included, too. The problem? Most of them are either irritating or allergenic for skin (Source: naturaldatabase.com). What a shame! Some soothing plant extracts are included, too, but their benefit is canceled out by the problematic extracts.

☹ POOR **FC5 Hydrating Eye Creme** *($30 for 0.5 fl. oz.)* is loaded with fragrant oils, which is a problem, especially in the eye area. Some of the citrus oils are known to cause a phototoxic reaction when skin is exposed to sunlight, and that's not the way to make delicate skin around the eyes stronger or more resistant to signs of aging! Even without the irritants, this is as boring a moisturizer as you can get. By the way, despite Arbonne positioning their FC5 products as natural, all of them contain their share of synthetic ingredients. This eye cream contains two types of acrylate-based film-forming agents that, in the amounts used, can be irritating for use around the eyes. See the Appendix to find out why, in truth, you don't need an eye cream.

☹ POOR **FC5 Moisturizing Night Creme** *($42 for 1.7 fl. oz.)* is a mixed bag of beneficial ingredients for dry akin and a series of fragrant, irritating plant ingredients that make this moisturizer a problem for all skin types. The second ingredient is lemon verbena, a known irritant (Source: naturaldatabase.com). Even without the lemon verbena, the several citrus oils and various fragrance ingredients it contains are potent irritants. Arbonne claims they use fresh mango cell extracts, but there is absolutely no research showing what that means for skin, not to mention that they won't be "fresh" when they are mixed into a skin-care product. There is nothing in here that will keep skin young. One other point: This comes packaged in a jar, so even if you wanted to believe Arbonne's ludicrous claims about the plant extracts, the extracts are all sensitive and won't remain stable in jar packaging. See the Appendix for more details on why jar packaging is a problem.

☹ POOR **FC5 Nurturing Day Lotion with SPF 20** *($39.50 for 1.7 fl. oz.)*. Considering the natural positioning of the FC5 products, it's strange that Arbonne opted to include synthetic sunscreen actives rather than minerals like titanium dioxide. At least they included avobenzone so you get reliable UVA protection. That's great, but the ordinary base formula and the inclusion of several fragrant oils known to cause irritation are disappointing. The citrus oils can cause skin to become discolored when exposed to sunlight, and even though this daytime moisturizer contains an effective sunscreen, why take the risk? There are lots of moisturizers with sunscreen that best this formula, including many that sell for half the price (e.g., Avon, Olay, Neutrogena, Mary Kay, and Paula's Choice).

☹ POOR **FC5 Oil-Absorbing Day Lotion SPF 20** *($39.50 for 1.7 fl. oz.)* claims a "fresh matte appearance," but the tiny amount of cornstarch in this daytime moisturizer with an in-part avobenzone sunscreen isn't enough to absorb much oil. This is even truer when you consider the emollient thickening agents that precede it on the list. You may think this would be better for normal to dry skin, but it isn't recommended for any skin type because it contains several fragrant oils known to cause skin irritation. Some of the citrus oils in this product are capable of causing a phototoxic reaction when skin is exposed to sunlight. The irritants it contains damage healthy collagen production and hurt skin's healing process—two things you don't want if your goal is looking younger and seeing fewer wrinkles!

☹ POOR **FC5 Skin Conditioning Oil** *($12 for 0.5 fl. oz.)* is a moisturizer for very dry skin that is composed primarily of plant oils. Although plant oils have benefit for dry skin, moisturizing with oils doesn't give dry skin the range of ingredients it needs to improve as much as it could. Blending plant oils with ingredients such as glycerin, ceramides, and cell-communicating ingredients, like niacinamide or retinol, is a better way to go. FC5 Skin Conditioning Oil contains many antioxidant-rich plant oils, but there are also fragrant plant oils and extracts included as well, which adds up to a problem for your skin. The fragrant plant oils cause irritation that hurts your skin's healing process and its ability to produce healthy collagen. Please see the Appendix for details on why irritation is so bad for you skin, even if you cannot see or feel it happening.

☹ POOR **Intelligence Rejuvenating Cream** *($35 for 2.2 fl. oz.)* would have been an excellent, ultra-emollient moisturizer for someone with dry to very dry skin if it did not contain irritating citrus oils along with clary and cardamom oils.

☹ POOR **PhytoProlief Natural Balancing Cream** *($34 for 2.5 fl. oz.)* is an emollient moisturizer for dry skin that also contains the hormone progesterone. The progesterone raises medical concerns that should not be promoted under the guise of skin care from a sales team that has no medical experience whatsoever. This isn't the type of product you should be buying at a friend's Arbonne party! Why? Because there is no way to know how much progesterone you'd be applying and whether or not you even need it. Although this product functions well as a moisturizer, the issue of progesterone isn't one to take lightly, even if you find yourself in the throes of menopause (in which case you should be discussing hormone replacement therapy with your doctor, not a cosmetics salesperson, even if it's your friend). This is not rated with a happy face because it contains comfrey (listed as *Symphytum officinale*), a plant extract with toxic components that, while most problematic if ingested, can still present problems for skin if used daily.

☹ POOR **RE9 Advanced Instant Lift Gel** *($46 for 1 fl. oz.)*. The concept of this gel moisturizer is to make skin quickly feel tighter and firmer. It does that, but before we explain how, you need to know that simply making skin feel tighter isn't the same as actually tightening loose skin. In other words, don't expect to see lifted skin—this lightweight moisturizer cannot combat the effects of gravity, bone loss, and other biologic occurrences that lead to skin sagging. What makes skin feel temporarily tighter is the ingredient pullulan. This natural ingredient is a starch derived from a specific strain of yeast. In much the same way you can temporarily smooth a wrinkled shirt with starch, you can, though to a far lesser degree, do the same for skin. The effect is short-lived and no one's going to mistake you for being 10 years younger than your real age, but it can provide a bit of assistance. The problem is that doing so with this product also exposes your skin to irritants, including a high concentration of orange peel oil.

Orange peel oil is a major source of the fragrance chemical limonene, which is known to cause contact dermatitis on exposure to air (Sources: *Chemical Research in Toxicology*, March 2010, pages 677–688; *Contact Dermatitis*, December 2009, pages 337–341, and November 2006, pages 274–279). This isn't an advanced way to care for your skin, and it's really disappointing that the most intriguing ingredients (the ones that do have some good research establishing their antiwrinkle abilities) are barely present.

☹ POOR **RE9 Advanced Night Repair Creme** (*$85 for 1 fl. oz.*) contains lemon verbena as one of the main ingredients in this moisturizer and that isn't good news. The oil from this plant contains volatile ingredients known as terpenes, which are skin-irritants known to cause contact dermatitis (Source: naturaldatabase.com). This also contains an extract from the rose geranium plant, which has no benefit for skin, but is definitely an irritant. Both of these ingredients will quickly be made less potent thanks to the jar packaging, as will all the other plant extracts and antioxidants in this faulty moisturizer. All told, this has far too many problems to be helpful for aging skin, and the inclusion of toxic lavender oil also is a step in the wrong direction.

☹ POOR **RE9 Advanced Restorative Day Creme SPF 20** (*$50 for 1 fl. oz.*) is pricey and we're concerned that the cost of this daytime moisturizer with an in-part zinc oxide sunscreen may keep women from applying it as liberally as they should. Applied to face and neck as directed, you'd be using this up within a month if your goal is to attain the stated SPF rating. A year later, you would have spent $600 for your daily moisturizer. Ouch! Expense aside, an even bigger ouch factor is the formula. The sunscreen portion is fine, but the base contains a mix of helpful and problematic plants. Orange oil and St. John's Wort are the biggest offenders; the latter can cause a phototoxic reaction when skin is exposed to sunlight—and remember, no sunscreen can block 100% of the sun's rays (Source: naturaldatabase.com). Adding to the troubles with this moisturizer is the fact that the most intriguing ingredients are barely present. This isn't much of a collagen-supporting formula, at least not if you look past the sunscreen element.

ARBONNE SUN CARE

☹ POOR **BefoRE Sun Damage Control Water Resistant Sunscreen SPF 30** (*$28 for 6 fl. oz.*) has the ability to protect skin from UVA and UVB rays while remaining water-resistant (though even water-resistant sunscreens require reapplying after swimming or perspiring). It's also loaded with a selection of skin-friendly ingredients, which is why it's so disheartening to find that this otherwise stellar sunscreen also includes so many irritating fragrant oils. In addition to their irritating properties, bergamot and lime oils can cause a phototoxic reaction (Source: naturaldatabase.com) and topical application of lavender oil causes skin-cell death (Source: *Cell Proliferation*, June 2004, pages 221–229).

☹ POOR **BefoRE Sun Made in the Shade Self-Tanner SPF 15** (*$28 for 6 fl. oz.*) lacks sufficient UVA-protecting ingredients and contains several irritating fragrant oils, none of which are helpful for skin. Countless self-tanners exist that turn skin brown without this risk of irritation. See the Appendix to find out why irritation is a problem for all skin types.

ARBONNE LIP & SMILE CARE

☺ GOOD **BefoRE Lip Saver SPF 30** (*$8 for 0.17 fl. oz.*) is the only product in Arbonne's sun line worth trying. This oil–based lip balm protects with an in-part avobenzone sunscreen and also contains two forms of antioxidant vitamin C. The amount of arnica extract is likely too low to be a concern for irritation, but it keeps this product from earning a Best Product rating.

ARBONNE SPECIALTY SKIN-CARE PRODUCTS

☹ POOR **Clear Advantage Acne Spot Treatment** *($22 for 0.4 fl. oz.)* is medicated with 2% salicylic acid. Although salicylic acid is an excellent ingredient for fighting acne, its effectiveness depends on being formulated in a pH range of 3–4. That's not what you're getting here, so the salicylic acid cannot work effectively to clear or prevent breakouts. As for the claim of this being able to help fade red marks from acne, it could do that if the salicylic acid were able to function as an exfoliant. Encouraging skin-cell turnover via exfoliation can help these stubborn marks fade faster than they normally would. Arbonne included a tiny amount of anti-inflammatory plant extracts, but likely not enough to make a noticeable difference in such marks. With some slight formulary tweaks, this would be a very good option for blemish-prone skin.

☹ POOR **FC5 Deep Cleansing Mask** *($32 for 3 fl. oz.)*. The clay in this mask is said to be "glacial clay," which simply means old clay from a lake in the north that has been or routinely is frozen. How is that special for your skin? It isn't. Clay is clay, and all clays have absorbent properties that are useful for oily skin. Although clay has its benefits, those with combination or oily skin are bound to experience problems from this mask because the absorbent clay is joined by emollient thickeners, which those with oily skin (and breakouts) should avoid. The worst aspects of this mask are the numerous fragrant oils and plant extracts. We understand that these ingredients will increase this mask's appeal for those seeking natural skin care, but the fact is most of the natural ingredients Arbonne chose to include can cause irritation. Please see the Appendix to learn why irritation is bad for all skin types, especially oily skin.

☹ POOR **FC5 Intense Hydration Mask** *($32 for 3 fl. oz.)* contains many irritating ingredients that won't help your skin, and that is truly a shame. Intermixed with the irritants are several emollients, antioxidants, and skin-repairing ingredients that dry skin needs to look and feel better. There's no reason to give your skin good ingredients from a product that also causes needless irritation. The fragrant plant oils and some of the plant extracts in this mask hurt your skin's healing process, stunt its ability to produce healthy collagen, and can cause free-radical damage that leads to further signs of aging. That isn't our idea of "intense" skin care!

☹ POOR **RE9 Advanced Cellular Renewal Masque** *($65 for 1.7 fl. oz.)* is a mixed bag that presents your skin with more problems than benefits. It is supposed to exfoliate gently, and it does contain ingredients that can do that (glycolic and salicylic acids) along with natural ingredients (sugar cane and citrus extracts) that are meant to exfoliate, but there is no research to support this. Although the glycolic and salicylic acids are worthwhile exfoliants, their efficacy depends on the pH of the formula—and in this case the pH is too high for either to exfoliate skin. This also contains papaya and pineapple enzymes, also meant to exfoliate, but these ingredients are unstable, especially when packaged in a jar, which is how this product is packaged. See the Appendix to learn why jar packaging is a problem. The biggest problem this mask presents is irritation. It contains several fragrant plant oils plus the potent skin-irritant menthol.

☹ POOR **Revelage Concentrated Age Spot Minimizer** *($45 for 0.5 fl. oz.)* is supposedly a concentrated version of Arbonne's Revelage Intensive Pro-Brightening Night Serum, but other than having a lighter texture, the formula isn't any more concentrated with ingredients capable of diminishing discolorations. This overpriced product has the same pros and cons as the Intensive Pro-Brightening Night Serum reviewed below.

☹ POOR **Revelage Intensive Pro-Brightening Night Serum** *($60 for 1 fl. oz.)* is supposed to improve the appearance of age spots and other discolorations plus brighten your skin with "scientifically studied" ingredients, which is a meaningless comment because most cosmetics ingredients have been "scientifically studied" in some way at some point (even water has been extensively "studied"). Two ingredients in this serum for dry skin may improve skin discolorations: acetyl glucosamine and the vitamin C ingredient ascorbyl glucoside. Neither has a great deal of research confirming efficacy when compared to the gold standard skin-lightening ingredient hydroquinone. Companies like Estee Lauder, Paula's Choice, and Olay also have products that contain these ingredients for less money. Ordinarily, we'd state that a product like this is worth trying, but the formula contains several irritating ingredients your skin doesn't need. In particular, nutmeg oil is problematic due to its many volatile fragrant components, but there's also a form of resorcinol and fragrant jasmine, which add to the irritant potential of the nutmeg oil (Source: naturaldatabase.com).

AVEDA

Strengths: Effective use of beneficial plant oils and extracts in some products; one of the few lines that offers a lip balm and sheer lip tint whose sunscreen includes adequate UVA protection; excellent moisturizing mask options; superior tinted moisturizer with sunscreen; good concealer; terrific brushes; refillable compacts.

Weaknesses: Several products contain irritating essential oils or fragrant components known to cause sun sensitivity or skin-cell death; disappointing Enbrightenment line; substandard cleansers and irritating toners; so-called treatment products that can irritate skin; foundations whose SPF rating falls below the minimum of 15; no blush options; several lip color products that contain irritating fragrant oils.

For more information and reviews of the latest Aveda products, visit CosmeticsCop.com.

AVEDA CLEANSERS

☹ POOR **All-Sensitive Cleanser** *($21 for 5 fl. oz.)* remains a poor choice for sensitive skin due to the irritating witch hazel extract it contains. As a main ingredient that's part of the "plant tea" Aveda uses for this cleanser, it presents too great a risk of irritation for all skin types. What a shame, because Aveda added some soothing plant extracts and this has a smoothing, lotion-like texture that cleanses gently and removes makeup. Interestingly, the preservatives Aveda chose are generally not recommended for sensitive skin due to their higher-than-average risk of causing, you guessed it, a sensitized reaction. These preservatives are of lesser concern in a rinse-off product like this, but there are gentler options that would have made this a better bet for truly sensitive skin.

☺ GOOD $$$ **Enbrightenment Brightening Cleanser** *($35 for 4.2 fl. oz.)* is a very basic water-soluble cleanser whose main cleansing agent is combined with a fatty alcohol to produce copious foam. As for the claims, any well-formulated cleanser will do exactly what this one says it will do. The difference is that many other cleansers do it without causing irritation to skin from fragrance and fragrance ingredients, and without the exorbitant price. The amount of salicylic acid this contains is too low for it to affect a single skin cell, plus it's rinsed away before it can initiate any kind of cell turnover. This cleanser is best for normal to oily skin and is capable of removing makeup.

☺ GOOD $$$ **Green Science Perfecting Cleanser** *($35 for 4.2 fl. oz.)* is aptly described as milky. It's a cleansing lotion sold as being the starting point to get "maximum benefit" from Aveda's Green Science products, but it almost goes without saying that this cleanser doesn't prepare skin in any special way for maximum, or even minimum, benefits. That said, with one exception (that being fragrance ingredients known to cause irritation), this is a very good cleanser for dry to very dry skin not prone to breakouts. It works quickly to remove makeup, but may require using a washcloth to avoid a residue and get all your makeup off. The small amount of fragrance ingredients isn't likely to be too troublesome, though this would be better without them.

☺ GOOD $$$ **Outer Peace Foaming Cleanser** *($27 for 4.2 fl. oz.)* is a liquid-to-foam, water-soluble cleanser that contains gentle detergent cleansing agents along with several anti-irritant plant extracts. Salicylic acid is also present, but only a tiny amount, which is rinsed off before it has a chance to work. The amount of alcohol is insignificant, but the salicylic acid means this should not be used around the eyes. This cleanser contains tamanu oil, which is reputed to contain a fatty acid (calophyllic acid) said to have an antimicrobial action on skin. There is no substantiated information about tamanu oil's effect on acne, although there is some research showing it has wound-healing effects (Source: *International Journal of Cosmetic Science*, December 2002, pages 341–348), but fighting blemishes is completely different from healing wounds. All other claims about tamanu oil's benefit for skin are anecdotal, but its polyphenol content makes it a suitable antioxidant—just not in a cleanser where it is rinsed down the drain, along with the salicylic acid, before it has a chance to work.

☹ AVERAGE $$$ **Botanical Kinetics Purifying Creme Cleanser** *($21 for 5 fl. oz.)* would be a much better lotion-style cleanser without the witch hazel extract, but the emollient ingredients keep it from being a significant problem for the normal to dry skin types that this cleanser is best for.

☹ POOR **Botanical Kinetics Purifying Gel Cleanser** *($21 for 5 fl. oz.)* has a considerable amount of lavender and rosemary, two irritants that tarnish this otherwise standard and effective water-soluble cleanser. Several fragrant components (including eugenol and geraniol) are a problem when used around eyes or mucous membranes.

AVEDA EYE-MAKEUP REMOVER

☺ GOOD **Pure Comfort Eye Makeup Remover** *($16 for 4.2 fl. oz.)* is a water-based, gentle makeup remover that's essentially a modified version of a water-soluble cleanser. This isn't too effective for removing long-wearing makeup, but it's good news that all the plant extracts used have soothing rather than irritating qualities.

AVEDA TONERS

☹ AVERAGE **Botanical Kinetics Skin Firming/Toning Agent** *($20 for 5 fl. oz.)* is a spray-on toner that contains a rather high amount of fragrant rose extract along with a repairing ingredient, alcohol, and a tiny amount of salicylic acid. This is minimally beneficial for skin, and really more akin to misting it with fragrance than the range of ingredients you'll find in well-formulated toners. This toner isn't firming and, while it may feel refreshing, your skin will look better and act younger if you use one of the options on our Best Toners list.

☺ GOOD $$$ **Tourmaline Charged Exfoliating Cleanser** *($29 for 5 fl. oz.)* is a rich, foaming cleanser that uses jojoba beads to gently polish the skin as you wash. This cleanser contains a skin-friendly assortment of nonirritating plant and nut oils, making it a great choice for parched, flaky skin during the winter months. It does contain fragrance and fragrant components along with salicylic acid, but those ingredients would be more of a problem if this product was used around the eyes, and a scrub-type cleanser shouldn't be used in that area anyway.

☹ POOR **Botanical Kinetics Toning Mist** *($20 for 5 fl. oz.)* lists peppermint as the second ingredient and also contains witch hazel and alcohol, along with fragrant plant extracts with

---

👁 Did you know you don't need an eye cream? It's true! See the Appendix to find out why.

no established benefit for skin. This toner is not recommended. See the Appendix to learn why irritation is a problem for all skin types.

☹ POOR **Enbrightenment Brightening Treatment Toner** *($42 for 5 fl. oz.)* is a surprisingly well-formulated toner for all skin types because it contains a potentially efficacious amount of vitamin C along with plant extracts that research (although limited) has shown do have an effect on improving skin tone and discolorations. The amount of salicylic acid is too low for it to be effective, plus this toner's pH is above 4, so exfoliation won't occur, but that could have been overlooked to some extent if everything else were up to par. So, why is it rated Poor? The amount of rosemary extract is too large to ignore; the smell is unmistakable—you could spread this on bread with some olive oil and salt and have a tasty snack—OK, not really, please don't try this at home. In addition, this contains potentially irritating fragrance ingredients that all skin types are better off without.

☹ POOR **Green Science Replenishing Toner** *($39 for 4.2 fl. oz.)* lists rosemary leaf extract as its second ingredient. Although rosemary has potent antioxidant ability, it also contains volatile constituents that will irritate skin. Given the number of antioxidants that don't cause problems for skin, there's no reason to compromise with a product like this. It also contains the sensitizing preservative methylisothiazolinone. Overall, the amount of rosemary extract is unfortunate, because this toner contains a great mix of cell-communicating and moisturizing ingredients.

AVEDA EXFOLIANTS & SCRUBS

☺ AVERAGE $$$ **Tourmaline Charged Radiant Skin Refiner** *($40 for 3.5 fl oz.)* is a scrub that uses bamboo powder and chalk (calcium carbonate) as the abrasive agents. It's a fairly grainy scrub, and one that should be used with caution, if at all. Despite containing some moisturizing ingredients and antioxidants, scrubs simply aren't as effective for exfoliation as well-formulated AHA or BHA exfoliants. Choosing a scrub over an AHA or BHA exfoliant is denying your skin the multiple benefits scrubs simply cannot provide. Note: The tourmaline has no established benefit for skin; even if it did, you'll rinse this scrub off before it can work its alleged magic.

☹ POOR **Botanical Kinetics Exfoliant** *($9.50 for 1.7 fl. oz)* has a workable pH of 3, but the amount of salicylic acid it contains is too small for it to function as an exfoliant. This contains several irritating plant extracts, including lavender, witch hazel, and balm mint. See the Appendix to find out why irritation is so bad for all skin types.

AVEDA MOISTURIZERS (DAYTIME & NIGHTTIME), EYE CREAMS, & SERUMS

☺ AVERAGE $$$ **Tourmaline Charged Hydrating Creme** *($37 for 1.7 fl. oz.)* has a frustrating blend of beneficial and problematic ingredients, and the most helpful ingredients (the many antioxidants in this moisturizer) are hindered by jar packaging. This is an OK moisturizer for normal to dry skin, but the tiny amount of eugenol is potentially problematic. By the way, there's only a dusting of tourmaline in this product, though that's just fine because it has no effect on skin.

☹ POOR **All-Sensitive Moisturizer** *($33 for 5 fl. oz.)* This product claims to be aroma-free, which is meaningless when it comes to taking care of your skin. Irritation doesn't always have an aroma; a product's aroma doesn't necessarily tell you if it's going to be good or bad for your skin. That is exactly the problem with this moisturizer from Aveda. While it doesn't emit a noticeable fragrance, the second ingredient is lavender extract, which presents enough problems for skin to rate it in the top ten of irritants. That's not good for any skin type, especially sensitive skin. See the Appendix to find out why irritation is so bad for skin. As far as moisturizing goes this does have some good emollients, but it lacks potent antioxidants known for combating free-radical damage and encouraging healing.

☹ POOR **Botanical Kinetics Hydrating Lotion** *($33 for 5 fl. oz.)* is a basic, highly-fragranced moisturizer fraught with problematic ingredients, including significant amounts of lavender, rosemary, and comfrey, along with lesser amounts of fragrant components (such as eugenol) that are skin-irritants. Eugenol is particularly egregious. It is a major component of clove oil, and research has shown the eugenol content of clove causes skin-cell death, even when low concentrations of clove (0.33%) were applied to cultured skin cells (Source: *Cell Proliferation*, August 2006, pages 241–248).

☹ POOR **Enbrightenment Brightening Correcting Creme** *($55 for 1.7 fl. oz.)* contains brightening components that have the potential to lighten skin discolorations, but they end up falling under a dark cloud due to the jar packaging. Continual exposure to light and air will cause the active constituents in most of these ingredients to break down, and that leaves you with an expensive, ordinary moisturizer that isn't worth a fraction of the cost. Further trouble comes from the amount of irritating rosemary leaf extract, a plant that has potent antioxidant properties, but its unmistakable fragrance also contains irritating chemicals. This has a lush, emollient texture, but so do many other moisturizers that contain more intriguing ingredients and are packaged to keep those critical ingredients stable.

☹ POOR **Enbrightenment Brightening Correcting Lotion** *($53 for 1.7 fl. oz.)* contains a skin-irritating amount of fragrant rosemary leaf extract—the smell is potent and you'll feel a tingle as soon as you apply it—and that makes this too irritating for all skin types. Add to that several fragrance ingredients and things go from bad to worse. There is no reason to consider this product over several other skin-lightening products, even if you're looking for all-natural, because this product certainly doesn't qualify unless you define the term "skin-lightening" to mean no results at all other than what moisturized skin can produce.

☹ POOR **Enbrightenment Brightening Correcting Serum** *($50 for 1 fl. oz.)* contains a form of vitamin C that limited research has shown to be effective against hyperpigmentation when combined with niacinamide, which is absent from this product. What this does contain that makes it a poor contender if you're looking to help your skin is irritating rosemary leaf extract and several volatile fragrance ingredients. Rosemary has potent antioxidant properties, but the chemicals responsible for its unique scent are not what anyone's skin needs—not when the goal is to reduce inflammation. Normally we'd look past the rosemary extract because most companies don't include much of it, but in this case, the smell is potent and that spells trouble for your skin (though it would be great emanating from your oven on whatever you were roasting). One more comment: the amount of salicylic acid is too low for it to benefit skin, plus the pH is over 4, so exfoliation is unlikely to occur.

☹ POOR **Green Science Firming Eye Creme** *($45 for 0.5 fl. oz.)* makes over-the-top claims about the argan oil it contains. This oil comes from tree nuts native to Morocco, and is said to be rich in vitamin E and linoleic acid. Of course, Aveda also mentions the native Moroccan Berbers, natives who've supposedly used this oil for centuries for medicinal and cosmetic purposes. That must mean it's something special (though keep in mind other natural ingredients, such as lead, were also used for cosmetic purposes until we learned how harmful it can be), but what does published research have to say about argan oil? Not much. The only study concerning topical application of argan oil has shown its oil-controlling, not moisturizing, properties. The remaining body of research has to do with the oil's benefits when consumed orally, and includes studies related to prostate cancer, the circulatory system, and cancer. We do know that argan oil contains beneficial components, including essential fatty acids and the antioxidants vitamin E and ferulic acid. In that sense, argan oil can be considered a reliable antioxidant, though not necessarily any better than other plant oils such as olive or pomegranate (Sources: *Journal of Cosmetic Dermatology*, June 2007, pages 113–118; *Cancer Investigation*, October 2006, pages 588–592; *Clinical Nutrition*, October 2004, pages 1159–1166; and *European Journal of Cancer Prevention*, February 2003, pages 67–75). In the case of this eye cream, jar packaging will not keep the argan oil and other antioxidant ingredients stable once it is opened. In addition, the amount of rosemary extract in this eye cream and the inclusion of Thai ginger oil (also known as plai oil) makes this too irritating for skin. The science may be green, but that doesn't guarantee smart skin care (Source: *Biotechnology and Applied Biochemsitry*, May 2008, pages 61–69)! See the Appendix for more details on jar packaging and to learn why you don't need an eye cream.

☹ POOR **Green Science Firming Face Creme** *($55 for 1.7 fl. oz.)* is nearly identical to Aveda's Green Science Firming Eye Creme above, save for a slightly lighter texture. Otherwise, the same review applies. What a shame because several ingredients in this moisturizer are a boon for dry to very dry skin.

☹ POOR **Green Science Lifting Serum** *($50 for 1 fl. oz.)* makes over-the-top claims about the argan oil it contains as discussed in the review for Aveda's Green Science Firming Eye Creme. In the case of this serum, although it contains several beneficial ingredients, the amount of rosemary extract is cause for concern, while the plai oil (also known as Thai ginger) is a significant irritant. The synthetic fragrances don't help matters either, and aren't in the least "green" ingredients. Lastly, there is no research anywhere showing that the peptides in here will help increase skin cell turnover rate, especially not on the surface of skin—that's what a well-formulated AHA or BHA product does, something Aveda's skin care range is missing. Estee Lauder, Clinique, and Paula's Choice offer much more sophisticated serum formulas without irritants.

☹ POOR **Green Science Line Minimizer** *($85 for 1 fl. oz.)* makes over-the-top claims about the argan oil it contains as discussed in the review for Aveda's Green Science Firming Eye Creme. In the case of this water-based serum, the amount of rosemary extract is cause for concern, as is the plai oil. Also known as Thai ginger, plai oil is similar to common ginger, which means it retains this plant's volatile components that can cause skin irritation. This serum also contains several irritating synthetic fragrance ingredients (not exactly green by anyone's standards) and is really unimpressive compared to the best "wrinkle-filling" products available. For example, Good Skin's Tri-Aktiline Instant Deep Wrinkle Filler is superior to this product, not only because of its formula but also because it apparently actually does fill in superficial lines (though the effect is temporary). And the Good Skin product costs less than half of what Aveda is charging for this product.

☹ POOR **Tourmaline Charged Radiance Fluid** *($40 for 1 fl. oz.)* would have been a worthwhile serum-type moisturizer for all skin types were it not for the inclusion of alcohol (it's the second ingredient) and clary extract, along with a list of unnecessary irritants—oils of peppermint, lavender, geranium, marjoram, orange, and lemon peel. Please see the Appendix to learn why alcohol is a problem for everyone's skin. This does contain tourmaline, which has no proven benefit for skin. If Aveda's statements that tourmaline increases the efficacy of the other ingredients combined with it was true, that would mean the many problematic ingredients in this product would be even more irritating.

AVEDA LIP CARE

☺ GOOD **Lip Saver SPF 15** *($8.50 for 0.15 fl. oz.)* includes an in-part avobenzone sunscreen and is an outstanding emollient lip balm that's packaged ChapStick-style. The ratio of plant oil and jojoba esters to wax produces a softer-texture lip balm that leaves an attractive sheen on lips. The only drawback is the flavor, which is composed of cinnamon and clove. The amounts of these ingredients aren't enough to warrant avoiding the product, but it would have received a Best Product rating without them.

☹ AVERAGE **$$$ Nourish-Mint Renewing Lip Treatment** *($16)* is a glossy lip balm in lipstick form. The colorless formula feels great over chapped lips, and helps prevent moisture loss, just like most well-formulated lip balms. There are no ingredients in this product that plump lips over time; the only reason to consider it over less expensive balms is if you want a noticeably glossy finish and a spearmint flavor (which may prove irritating).

AVEDA SPECIALTY SKIN-CARE PRODUCTS

✓☺ BEST **$$$ Tourmaline Charged Radiance Masque** *($31 for 4.2 fl. oz.)* is a very good moisturizing mask for normal to dry skin. Although this mask's claims of boosting skin's radiance due to the tourmaline it contains are unproven, it isn't a problem for skin. As with all moisturizing masks, the longer it is left on the skin the better your results will be, especially if your skin is dry.

☺ GOOD **$$$ Deep Cleansing Herbal Clay Masque** *($22 for 4.4 fl. oz.)* is as standard a clay mask as it gets. Although it has enough emollients to make it more "comfortable" than many other clay masks, the emollients are more suited to normal to dry skin than oily skin. Clay is not cleansing in the least, though it can absorb oil from skin.

☹ AVERAGE **$$$ Outer Peace Acne Relief Lotion** *($40 for 1.7 fl. oz.)* is a lightweight, matte-finish BHA lotion that contains 0.5% salicylic acid and has a pH of 3.9, meaning that exfoliation will occur, but not very much. With the 0.5% concentration, this product is only marginally effective. It would be better for blemish-prone skin if the salicylic acid were present in at least a 1% concentration, and for more stubborn acne 2% would be preferred.

☹ AVERAGE **$$$ Outer Peace Acne Spot Relief** *($29.50 for 0.5 fl. oz.)* ranks as an effective, but needlessly expensive, BHA lotion that comes with a frustrating balance of positives and negatives. It's great that the 2% salicylic acid is in a base with a pH of 3.7, which will allow exfoliation to occur. It's not so great that Aveda included alcohol, an ingredient that can exacerbate problems for those battling acne. The amount of alcohol isn't much, but this product would have earned a Best Product rating without it.

☹ AVERAGE **$$$ Outer Peace Cooling Masque** *($37 for 4.2 fl. oz.)* is a needlessly expensive clay mask, which doesn't contain anything that brings peace to acne-prone skin. Like all clay masks, this can absorb excess oil and leave skin feeling smooth and looking, at least for the short term, matte. There is more alcohol and preservative in this formula than potentially beneficial plants, and the fragrance can be irritating due to the volatile components it is composed of.

☹ POOR **Enbrightenment Brightening Intensive Massage Masque** *($45 for 4.2 fl. oz.)* is good if you have dry skin and want an overnight treatment. Despite that, there are more reasons to leave this pricey mask on the shelf, chief among them being the amount of fragrant (really fragrant, as in hard to miss) rosemary leaf extract. The irritant potential of this plant far exceeds the positive potential of any of the beneficial ingredients in this mask, all of which are present in lesser amounts.

☹ POOR **Intensive Hydrating Masque** *($22 for 5 fl. oz.)* brings the skin a mixed bag of helpful and potentially harmful ingredients and, despite the name, isn't all that hydrating (you won't think so if your skin is dry to very dry). The amount of lavender extract is likely too problematic to make this worthwhile for even occasional use, especially given the selection of moisturizing masks whose formulas best this one without troublesome ingredients.

☹ POOR **Outer Peace Acne Relief Pads** *($31.50 for 50 pads)* contains 1.5% salicylic acid, but the pH of the base is too high for it to exfoliate skin. Also, the amount of alcohol in this solution is too irritating for all skin types, not to mention that the alcohol cancels out the anti-irritant effect of the much smaller amounts of plant extracts. See the Appendix to find out how alcohol makes oily, blemish-prone skin worse, not better.

AVEDA FOUNDATION

✓☺ BEST **$$$ Inner Light Mineral Tinted Moisture SPF 15** *($28)* is an outstanding tinted moisturizer that uses titanium dioxide as its sole sunscreen active. It has a smooth, creamy texture that hydrates skin while leaving a satin finish, and is suitable for normal to dry skin, offering sheer coverage and a hint of color. Seven shades are available and they are all excellent. Aspen is a real find for someone with fair skin. The "mineral" portion of the name is just Aveda capitalizing on the craze for all things mineral. Note: Aveda calls out bergamot and lavender as being components of this tinted moisturizer's fragrance. The amount of fragrance in this product isn't high, and the amounts of these problematic plant extracts are most likely too low to be cause for concern.

AVEDA CONCEALER

☹ AVERAGE **Inner Light Concealer** *($18)* is a liquid concealer with an initially moist texture that quickly sets to a matte finish, so it must be blended quickly. If you try to apply this in a sweep of color, it goes on somewhat choppy, providing spotty, rather than smooth, even coverage. It works far better if you apply it in dots over the areas where you need it, and then buff it out so you can get natural-looking coverage capable of concealing dark circles (without creasing) and minor redness. Among the six shades, only Bamboo is questionable because it has a slightly orange cast. The others are winning neutrals, with Mahogany a standout for dark skin. Although this concealer has a matte finish, a slight amount of shine is evident. It's a minor issue, but one you should be aware of if you want to avoid shine.

AVEDA POWDER

☺ GOOD **$$$ Inner Light Mineral Pressed Powder** *($20 for 0.24 fl. oz)* is a talc-free pressed powder with a silky texture that feels creamier than most yet remains sheer on skin. Three very good shades are available; however, there are no options for dark skin tones. Keep in mind that because the minerals that comprise this powder have shine, their effect on skin is quite prominent—not really what you want if you're using powder to control or minimize shine.

☹ AVERAGE **$$$ Inner Light Mineral Dual Foundation** *($24)*. There's nothing that makes this pressed powder foundation more "mineral" than any other. The talc-free formula contains mica, which creates a slightly drier but still smooth texture and imparts noticeable shine, something that's not the best for a natural look in daylight. It maintains a soft matte (in feel) finish and is easy to blend, providing sheer to light coverage when used dry. Aveda claims it can be used wet, too, but as with most powder foundations, this method of application can promote streaks and look uneven. Mostly beautiful soft, neutral shades are offered, with options for light (but not very light) to dark skin tones. Watch out for the Carob shade (the darkest color); it has slightly ash overtones that can make dark skin look dull and muddy.

This powder foundation is best for normal to slightly dry or combination skin. Note: This is not recommended for sensitive skin because it contains fragrance and fragrance ingredients known to cause irritation. This is also why it is not rated higher. There are many pressed powder foundations (such as those from M.A.C. or Laura Mercier) that omit fragrance of any kind.

AVEDA BRONZER

☺ AVERAGE **$$$ Uruku Bronzer** *($24)* comes as a duo compact with one shade slightly darker than the other. There are two sets, Amazonia and Brazilian Sun (the darker of the two), and both are flattering hues with good color intensity. Despite the intensity, this bronzer has a surprisingly sheer, even application and it blends smoothly. Unfortunately, it's overly shimmery for the face, taking the appearance of a tan "glow" a few steps too far. For a more natural bronze look, there are better options, and for less money.

AVEDA EYESHADOWS

☺ GOOD **Petal Essence Single Eye Color** *($12)* retains its silky texture and smooth, flake-free application (quite a feat considering every shade has some amount of shine). The range of colors has been reduced, likely so Aveda can launch seasonal eyeshadow colors, but most of the mainstays are workable, depending on how much shine you want. Only Vinca is too purple to work for anything other than pulling focus from what eyeshadow is meant to enhance: the eyes.

☺ GOOD **$$$ Petal Essence Eye Color Trio** *($24)* manages to apply evenly despite a dry texture, although the colors go on sheer and each has a soft to intense shine. If you want a softer look (even from the darkest colors) and don't mind shine, there are some well-coordinated sets to consider. Best among them are Plum Mist, Earth Rose, Black Tulip, Copper Haze, Golden Jasper, and Gobi Sands.

AVEDA EYE & BROW LINER

☺ AVERAGE **Petal Essence Eye Definer** *($14)* is nothing special, just a nice selection of standard, needs-sharpening pencils with an appropriate dry finish that is minimally prone to smudging.

AVEDA LIP COLOR & LIPLINERS

☺ GOOD **$$$ Nourish-Mint Sheer Mineral Lip Color** *($16)* has "mineral" in the name to capitalize on the refuses-to-die trend of mineral makeup. Formula-wise, this sheer lipstick differs little from most others. It has a slightly firmer texture (due to less oil) than Aveda's Nourish-Mint Smoothing Lip Color, and all the shades have a slight shimmer. Like the original Nourish-Mint, this contains some good antioxidants, but the fragrant components, including eugenol, may cause irritation.

☺ GOOD **$$$ Nourish-Mint Smoothing Lip Color** *($14)* is a creamy lipstick that almost crosses the line to greasy, but its lack of slickness helps it stay anchored to lips (for about as long as most creamy lipsticks last). The soft gloss finish and range of shades are attractive, though only the burgundy-to-red shades leave any sign of a stain. Surprisingly, no mint oils or extracts are listed, and this doesn't make your lips tingle upon application. However, this does contain small amounts of fragrant components (including eugenol) and is flavored in part by spearmint. These add-ons may cause irritation, and that keeps this from earning the top rating.

☺ GOOD **$$$ Uruku Color Gloss** *($16)* is a good lip gloss with an attractive selection of soft, translucent colors. The thin, smooth texture doesn't last all that long, but it does impart a sheer gloss finish that avoids being sticky.

☺ GOOD $$$ **Uruku Lip Pigment** *($16)* offers five shades in a creamy/rich finish or a sheer/translucent finish, including some with shimmer. Surprisingly, even the sheer versions of this lipstick impart a significant amount of color, ranging from pink to mauve to red. Uruku Lip Pigment goes on smooth and feels moisturizing from the second you put it on. The only downfall is that it doesn't have great staying power. All things considered, however, this lipstick is a good option for a sheer appearance.

☹ POOR **Lip Shine** *($16)* is a tube-type lip gloss with a light, slick texture. It leaves a smooth, glossy sheen and offers some great colors, but the inclusion of peppermint, anise, cinnamon, and basil oils add up to lip irritation, which dims this gloss's otherwise polished prospects.

☹ POOR **Nourish-Mint Rehydrating Lip Glaze** *($18)* is a thick lip gloss with minimal slip, which impedes smooth, even application. Its strong mint flavor isn't good news because the irritation it causes can make dry, chapped lips worse. Skip this one.

AVEDA MASCARA

☺ AVERAGE **Mosscara** *($18)* claims its conditioning formula is helped by the inclusion of Iceland moss, yet there is not enough moss in it to cover a twig, let alone condition lashes. This is an ordinary mascara formula that produces average length and minimal thickness, but it's hardly exciting or worth considering over the best Maybelline or L'Oreal mascaras.

AVEDA FACE & BODY ILLUMINATOR

☺ GOOD $$$ **Petal Essence Face Accents** *($24 for 0.3 fl. oz.)* combine three stripes of shimmer powder in one pressed-powder pan. The various color combinations are all workable whether applied separately or blended together, and each goes on sheer, imparting more shimmer than pigment.

AVEDA BRUSHES

✓☺ BEST **Flax Sticks** *($55-$65)* are made with unbelievably soft and functional synthetic hair. Ever the environmentally conscious company, Aveda has provided brush handles that are composed of recycled wood and flax. We found the handles to be a bit awkward due to their squared edges, but that's a minor quibble for an overall superior brush collection. Flax Sticks come in two collections, the **Daily Effects Brush Set** *($65)* and the **Special Effects Brush Set** *($55)*, both of which contain solid options, especially for those who prefer synthetic hair. Also worth checking out is the **Inner Light Foundation Brush** *($40)*. Aveda's less impressive brushes include **Envirometal Retractable Lip Brush** *($16)* and **Uruku Bronzing Brush** *($40)*. The lip brush's thin tip is tricky to work with unless you have very small lips, while the Bronzing Brush has a head so large that controlled application is needlessly difficult.

AVEDA SPECIALTY MAKEUP PRODUCTS

☺ AVERAGE $$$ **Color Options Eye Shadow Transformer** *($25)* is meant to intensify powder eyeshadow or to allow the eyeshadow to be used as a liquid eyeliner. Plain tap water on a brush does the same thing, so why spend money on this ancillary product? Good question, and there's no compelling reason to open your pocketbook. Not surprisingly, the main ingredient in this product is ... water. Aloe, glycerin, and a preservative comprise the remainder of this overpriced, unnecessary product.

AVEENO (SKIN CARE ONLY)

Strengths: Very good range of sunscreens that include avobenzone for UVA protection; good baby-care products (reviewed on CosmeticsCop.com).

Weaknesses: Well-intentioned but ineffective anti-acne products; reliance on a single showcased ingredient (typically soy) that makes their anti-aging products less enticing than the competition; no products to address hyperpigmentation; no toners.

For more information and reviews of the latest Aveeno products, visit CosmeticsCop.com.

AVEENO CLEANSERS

☺ GOOD **Positively Ageless Daily Exfoliating Cleanser** ($9.99 for 5 fl. oz.) is a standard, detergent-based cleanser that also contains polyethylene (plastic beads) for a topical scrub action. That's about all there is to this product, and it's an option for all but very dry skin—as long you don't expect to look ageless after using it.

☺ GOOD **Positively Radiant Cleanser** ($7.49 for 6.7 fl. oz.) is a very good, water-soluble cleanser for all skin types except very dry. The soy sterol and soy protein look good on the label, and they do have water-binding properties, but their benefit is negligible in a product that is quickly rinsed from skin.

☺ GOOD **Smart Essentials Pore Purifying Facial Wash** ($6.99 for 6 fl. oz.). This water-soluble cleanser isn't more purifying than any other, but it's a good, inexpensive option for those with normal to oily or combination skin.

☺ AVERAGE **Clear Complexion Cleansing Bar** ($3.29 for 3.5 fl. oz.) contains 0.5% salicylic acid (BHA) in a soap-free bar cleanser, but the pH is too high for the BHA to be effective as an exfoliant and it would be rinsed down the drain before it could have an effect on skin anyway. Bar cleansers can be drying, though this one is gentler than most; it could work for someone with normal to oily skin who doesn't have blemish-prone skin.

☺ AVERAGE **Moisturizing Bar** ($3.29 for 3.5 fl. oz.) is an oat flour–based bar cleanser that is certainly less troublesome for skin than traditional bar soap. However, because the ingredients that keep this in bar form can leave a residue on skin, this isn't preferred to a well-formulated, water-soluble cleanser.

☺ AVERAGE **Positively Radiant Daily Cleansing Pads** ($7.49 for 28 pads). Aveeno boasts about the soy in these dual-textured pads, but there isn't enough of it to amount to a single bean. The water-based formula is composed of mild detergent cleansing agents. However, the cleansing agents' mildness means they won't do a thorough job of dissolving makeup and removing excess surface oil. Unlike several other cleansing cloths/wipes, this product does need to be rinsed. Left on the skin, it leaves a slightly sticky finish, and the strong fragrance from these pads isn't what you'd want to leave on your skin all day or night.

☺ AVERAGE **Ultra-Calming Foaming Cleanser** ($7.49 for 6 fl. oz.) uses feverfew extract, which Aveeno maintains will reduce facial redness and calm skin. According to published research, feverfew is a problem for skin because it causes contact dermatitis (Sources: naturaldatabase.com; *Medicinski Pregled*, January-February 2003, pages 43-49; and *Contact Dermatitis*, October 2001, pages 197–204). However, this cleanser contains only a tiny amount of feverfew extract and so poses less of a problem, especially because it isn't left on the skin. With a gentle base and an array of skin-identical ingredients (though these are not particularly helpful for skin in a cleanser), this is a good option for normal to slightly dry skin. This cleanser is fragrance-free.

☹ POOR **Clear Complexion Daily Cleansing Pads** *($7.69 for 28 pads)* contain a mere 0.5% salicylic acid (BHA), which isn't enough to combat blemishes or stubborn blackheads, plus the pH of the solution is too high for the BHA to exfoliate. These contain the detergent cleansing agent sodium C14-16 olefin sulfonate, which is more drying than most and generally should be avoided. Although it's present here with milder detergent cleansing agents, it is still potentially too drying for most skin types.

☺ AVERAGE **Clear Complexion Foaming Cleanser** *($7.49 for 6 fl. oz.)* is a standard, detergent-based, water-soluble cleanser that contains 0.5% salicylic acid. Such a small amount of salicylic acid (BHA) is only somewhat effective against breakouts, though even if it could have an effect, it would be rinsed down the drain before it had a chance to do anything. This fragranced cleanser contains enough of the drying cleansing agent sodium C14-16 olefin sulfonate to make it a problem for almost all skin types.

AVEENO EXFOLIANTS & SCRUBS

☺ GOOD **Skin Brightening Daily Scrub** *($6.59 for 4.2 fl. oz.)* doesn't entice with lots of needless frills. Instead, this standard, effective scrub goes about its business of allowing you to polish your skin while also providing a cleansing action. It is suitable for all skin types except very dry.

☺ AVERAGE **Smart Essentials Daily Detoxifying Scrub** *($6.99 for 5 fl. oz.)* is an ordinary, highly fragranced scrub that cannot detoxify your skin; there are no toxins lurking in your skin that can be scrubbed away or exorcised. This an OK option for normal to oily skin.

AVEENO MOISTURIZERS (DAYTIME & NIGHTTIME), EYE CREAMS, & SERUMS

☺ AVERAGE **Clear Complexion Daily Moisturizer** *($16.79 for 4 fl. oz.)* has enough enticing claims to fulfill the wish list of anyone suffering from bouts of dryness and breakouts. However, this 0.5% BHA lotion shortchanges blemish-prone skin with too little salicylic acid, despite an effective pH of 3.7. That's discouraging, and things don't perk up since this is also an extremely ordinary lightweight moisturizer with nary an antioxidant or state-of-the-art repairing ingredient to be found. This fragranced product will do little to nothing to clear skin or help with blemishes you may already have.

☺ AVERAGE **Positively Ageless Lifting & Firming Eye Cream** *($27.19 for 0.5 fl. oz.)* is an incredibly average moisturizer for slightly dry skin anywhere on the face. As far as extraordinary goes, it's extraordinary only if you believe Aveeno's claims about an ingredient it uses known as tetrahydroxypropyl ethylenediamine. According to Aveeno's sister company RoC (both owned by Johnson & Johnson), this ingredient has been clinically proven (of course, the results of these clinical studies are not available for public scrutiny and they were done by J&J) to tighten epidermal cells, resulting in a lifted, firmed appearance. Technical information about tetrahydroxypropyl ethylenediamine indicates it functions as a neutralizing agent and helps adjust the pH of water-based products. There is no independent, peer-reviewed research demonstrating it to be effective for sagging skin, unless by tightening they mean constricting due to irritation. Any tightening effect this ingredient has on skin cells would be due to the inflammation that occurs if a product is too alkaline or too acidic. But that would be a temporary effect, not even related to the results possible from surgical procedures or a particularly healthy impact on the skin.

☺ AVERAGE **Positively Ageless Reconditioning Night Cream** *($19.49 for 1.7 fl. oz.)* is a basic but effective moisturizer suitable for normal to slightly dry skin, and Aveeno is banking on the mushroom extracts to produce ageless results. Both species used, reishi (*Ganoderma lucidum*) and *Lentinula edodes*, better known as shiitake, have research concerning their benefits when consumed as food, but there is no research showing them to be effective when used topically on skin (Source: naturaldatabase.com). Both mushrooms have antioxidant properties (Source: *Journal of Agricultural and Food Chemistry*, October 2002, pages 6072–6077), but that benefit will be short-lived because of this product's jar packaging. See the Appendix to learn why jar packaging is a problem.

☺ AVERAGE **Positively Ageless Restructuring Treatment Cream** (*$19.99 for 1.7 fl. oz.*) is sold with several anti-aging claims, but the problematic formula and the jar packaging aren't capable of making them come true. At best, this is an OK lightweight moisturizer for normal to dry skin. It contains a fairly good mix of antioxidants, but the jar packaging won't keep them stable once you begin using this product. Please see the Appendix for details on why jar packaging is a problem. Note: the amount of glycolic acid in this product is too low for it to function as an exfoliant.

☺ AVERAGE **Positively Ageless Youth Perfecting Moisturizer SPF 30** (*$20.49 for 2.5 fl. oz.*) is an OK lightweight daytime moisturizer with sunscreen for normal to oily or combination skin. It contains stabilized avobenzone for reliable UVA (think anti-aging) protection and the formula wears well under makeup. Your skin will benefit from the mushroom-based antioxidants this contains, but the formula would be better if it contained a range of plant- and vitamin-based antioxidants. Also needed to help skin look and act younger is a range of skin-repairing and cell-communicating ingredients, so, despite the good broad-spectrum sun protection, this product doesn't offer much else of significance for younger skin. It does contain fragrance.

☺ AVERAGE **Positively Radiant Daily Moisturizer SPF 15** (*$16.79 for 4 fl. oz.*) is an average daytime moisturizer with sunscreen for normal to combination skin. It provides sufficient UVA (think anti-aging) protection via avobenzone, but the lightweight base formula lacks a good range of antioxidants and repairing ingredients to help skin look and act younger. The "natural light diffusers" referred to in the claims are about the mineral pigment mica. Mica adds shine, it doesn't diffuse anything, and shine isn't skin care. There's nothing wrong with adding mica to a moisturizer, but don't expect it to transform how your skin looks. Note: Despite claims of being gentle enough for sensitive skin, that's not the case. Not only is fragrance a problem for sensitive skin, but the active sunscreen ingredients can cause sensitivity, too. Those with sensitive skin should look for sunscreens with titanium dioxide or zinc oxide as the sole active ingredients. And, of course, fragrance-free formulas are superior for any skin type.

☺ AVERAGE **Positively Radiant Daily Moisturizer SPF 30** (*$16.99 for 2.5 fl. oz.*) has a lighter-weight, drier-finish formula than the other Positively Radiant Daily Moisturizers, as well as offering longer sun protection, still with an in-part avobenzone sunscreen. It's an OK option for normal to slightly oily skin, assuming you don't mind the soft shine it leaves on skin.

☺ AVERAGE **Smart Essentials Anti-Fatigue Eye Treatment** (*$11.99 for 0.27 fl. oz.*). Southernwood (another name for the plant wormwood) extract is listed by its Latin name *Artemisia abrotanum*. It is the active ingredient in the alcoholic drink absinthe. Consuming wormwood via absinthe offers a mix of pros and cons for your health, with the cons dominating (e.g., kidney failure and brain damage are possible outcomes of excess wormwood consumption). With no research proving it does anything helpful for your skin, a "smarter" choice would have been to include plant extracts that have proven benefit, such as antioxidants or anti-irritants; but again, any potential benefits are rinsed down the drain. This is very much a "why bother?" product; check out Clinique's All About Eyes Serum for a better version of a lightweight hydrating gel applied via a metal roller-ball applicator. But note that this recommendation is due to the roller-ball packaging that can help massage away minor puffiness, not because you need a special product for the eye area.

☺ AVERAGE **Smart Essentials Daily Nourishing Moisturizer SPF 30** *($15.59 for 2.5 fl. oz.)*. This daytime moisturizer with sunscreen is an average formula for normal to dry skin. The best part is that it contains stabilized avobenzone for reliable UVA (think anti-aging) protection. Given the name, this product should've been a lot smarter!

☺ AVERAGE **Smart Essentials Nighttime Moisture Infusion** *($15.59 for 1.7 fl. oz.)* is a basic, ordinary formula that's not the smartest choice for dry skin because it will definitely leave someone with dry skin needing more to feel hydrated and smooth. It also lacks any skin-rejuvenating ingredients such as antioxidants or skin-healing ingredients. If signs of aging are a concern, this is hardly an essential choice.

☺ AVERAGE **Ultra-Calming Daily Moisturizer SPF 15** *($16.79 for 4 fl. oz.)* is recommended for its in-part avobenzone sunscreen, though we wouldn't call that or the other active ingredients in this moisturizer "ultra-calming." Many people tolerate the sunscreen agents in this product well, but a product positioned as "calming" would be better with just titanium dioxide and/or zinc oxide for sun protection. These mineral sunscreens have almost zero risk of causing irritation, which is what someone dealing with facial redness or rosacea should be considering. It also contains fragrance—another faux pas for an "ultra-calming" product—and the formula lacks antioxidants. If calming isn't your expectation, this sunscreen is an option, just not an exciting one.

☺ AVERAGE **$$$ Ageless Vitality Elasticity Recharging System, Day SPF 30** *($42.99)*. This two-part system consists of a daytime moisturizer with sunscreen and a serum. The combination of these products is said to stimulate elastin repair or produce new elastin. Lots of companies make this claim because producing healthy elastin is important for skin. Elastin fibers provide support and give skin its ability to bounce back after being manipulated. As elastin becomes damaged from genetic, environmental (sun exposure) aging, gravity, muscle laxity, fat movement, and hormonal loss, it changes skin's structure and the fibers become too weak for skin to snap back as it once did. The result? All of those factors contribute to loss of firmness and sagging skin.

Can this or any of Aveeno's other Age Vitality kits rescue your skin from sagging? Of course not. Assuming these duos could generate more elastin, that is only one aspect of what causes skin to sag and skin-care products can't change that. Just like with Neutrogena Clinical and RoC Brilliance (both of which, like Aveeno, are owned by Johnson & Johnson), all the Ageless Vitality products come with a silicone-based gel (labeled "**Biomineral Concentrate**") that contains minerals and vitamin E. Aveeno plays up the natural angle and the angle that the Biomineral Concentrate (you get 4 small tubes of this for a grand total of 0.32 ounce) "recharges" skin's elasticity. When combined with the moisturizer included in this set, the Biomineral Concentrate is supposed to restore energy to elastin-deficient skin.

Biomineral Concentrate contains copper and zinc. There is research pertaining to copper and its dual role in skin: wound-healing and altering the matrix metalloproteinases (MMP) that contribute to collagen depletion. Applying ingredients that work against this damage is helpful, but this is not the only way to improve aging skin. Zinc is believed to play a co-factor role with copper when it comes to repairing damaged elastin in skin, but again, it's not the only game in town and it does not replace anything a cosmetic dermatologist can do to improve

---

♠ Irritating ingredients are a problem for all skin types. Find out why in the Appendix.

skin or what other skin-care products can provide (Sources: *Connective Tissue Research*, January 2010, Epublication; *Experimental Dermatology*, March 2009, pages 205–211; and *Veterinary Dermatology*, December 2006, pages 417–423). There is no solid research proving that topical zinc or copper can stop or reverse sagging skin due to elastin damage.

Step 2 in this set is the **Rejuvenating Day Moisturizer with SPF 30** (*1 fl. oz.*). Not surprisingly, this in-part avobenzone sunscreen is a lightweight moisturizer that provides broad-spectrum sun protection and helpful antioxidants. It is worth noting that the Rejuvenating Day Moisturizer leaves a lingering shiny finish that exaggerates any oily areas. Of course, the daytime moisturizer provides sun protection, which is a critical part of keeping skin looking young and healthy and protecting elastin, but other than feeling very silky and despite containing some intriguing ingredients, it isn't going to improve sagging skin or get you anywhere close to what Aveeno describes as "dramatic results." This duo isn't a face-lift for under $40!

Despite the letdown, there is one ingredient in the Rejuvenating Day Moisturizer SPF 30 that deserves further discussion, and that's dill extract. There is one study indicating that on human skin samples and on "dermal equivalents" (which is not the same as intact human skin), dill extract has a strong promotional effect on elastogenesis. Elastogenesis is a fancy way of saying it helps make elastin. The study demonstrated that dill stimulates key enzymes in fake skin that trigger elastin production, although no mention was made of dill being able to repair damaged elastin. We also don't know if dill absorbs into real skin to have a similar impact. Instead, all we know is that dill seems to have this effect on isolated skin cells responsible for elastin production (Sources: naturaldatabase.com; and *Experimental Dermatology*, August 2006, pages 574-581). It is doubtful that the tiny amount of dill extract in this product will lift skin in any manner, but it may turn out to be a promising ingredient.

☺ AVERAGE $$$ **Ageless Vitality Elasticity Recharging System, Eye** (*$42.99*). This two-part system make claims similar to Aveeno's Ageless Vitality Elasticity Recharging System, Day SPF 30 above, only this pairing includes an eye cream instead of a moisturizer with sunscreen. Please refer to the review above for an explanation of the elasticity-recharging claims.

As for the **Revitalizing Eye Cream** (0.33 ounce), it's a beautifully silky formula whose spackle-like texture helps temporarily fill in superficial lines. Examining the eye cream and serum (labeled "**Biomineral Concentrate**") together, both formulas lack a range of ingredients research has proven are beneficial for aging skin. Sadly, this duo isn't the big breakthrough it's made out to be. In all likelihood, you will have better results with a well-formulated moisturizer or serum (it doesn't have to be labeled "eye cream")—any of those rated Best in this book will suffice and are worth considering over this set.

☺ AVERAGE $$$ **Ageless Vitality Elasticity Recharging System, Night** (*$42.99*). This system is nearly identical to Aveeno's Ageless Vitality Elasticity Recharging System, Day SPF 30, except the moisturizer in this duo (**Night Activating Cream**) does not contain sunscreen. The moisturizer has a light, yet emollient texture suitable for dry skin. Otherwise, the same comments about the merits of this system and the claims attached to it apply.

☹ POOR **Positively Radiant Tinted Moisturizer SPF 30** (*$14.99 for 2.5 fl. oz.*). Although this tinted moisturizer is available in workable colors for fair to medium skin tones, it does not contain the UVA-protecting ingredients of titanium dioxide, zinc oxide, avobenzone (also known as butyl methoxydibenzoylmethane), ecamsule, or Tinosorb and is not recommended. It is also doubtful that this contains enough soy to discourage skin discolorations, but without question the insufficient UVA protection will encourage more of what you don't want to see in the mirror: wrinkles and brown spots.

AVEENO SUN CARE

☺ GOOD **Continuous Protection Sunblock Lotion SPF 30, for Face** *($10.49 for 3 fl. oz.)* doesn't contain any ingredients that make it better suited for use on the face and in fact is similar to some of the "body" sunscreens Aveeno sells. Many manufacturers of facial sunscreens today are responding to current research that indicates a complementary and positive effect when antioxidants are included in sunscreens. That includes Aveeno, because this product features vitamins A and E as well as soybean seed extract. As for the "continuous protection" claim in the name, it's misleading. No sunscreen provides continuous protection because all of them must be reapplied at regular intervals to maintain sun protection when you're spending hours outdoors.

☺ GOOD **Continuous Protection Sunblock Lotion SPF 55** *($10.49 for 4 fl. oz.)* is similar to the Continuous Protection Sunblock Lotion SPF 30 above, except this product contains a higher amount of active ingredients necessary to achieve its SPF rating. This provides excellent broad-spectrum protection, and it includes antioxidants.

☺ GOOD **Continuous Protection Sunblock Lotion SPF 55, for Baby** *($10.49 for 4 fl. oz.)* distinguishes itself from the Continuous Protection Sunblock Lotion SPF 55 in name and with the inclusion of anti-irritant oat flour. A sunscreen with this many active ingredients is ill-advised for babies, whose skin is not developed enough to tolerate them. Babies under six months of age should be shielded from sunlight rather than treated with sunscreens of any kind; beyond six months, the best sunscreen actives for a baby's skin are titanium dioxide and/or zinc oxide (Source: cancercare.ns.ca/media/documents/sunexposurebrochurefinal.pdf). This is worth considering by adults.

☺ GOOD **Hydrosport Sunblock Spray SPF 50** *($10.99 for 5 fl. oz.)* is Aveeno's version of sister company Neutrogena's Wet Skin Sunblock Spray SPF 50. The formulas are nearly identical, but for Aveeno's addition of a fragrant plant extract, so the same review applies. The chief selling point of this spray-on sunscreen is that you can apply it to wet skin—no need to towel-dry first. The technology Aveeno uses allows the sunscreen ingredients to cling to wet skin without dripping off, which means that even when you're soaked or perspiring heavily, you'll get reliable sun protection. The problem? Like many spray-on sunscreens, the formula contains a high amount of alcohol. The active ingredients provide broad-spectrum sun protection (and include stabilized avobenzone for critical UVA protection), but the alcohol puts your skin at risk for dryness and irritation that hurts healthy collagen production. However, if the convenience helps you reapply sunscreen after two hours when you're outside doing sports or playing in the water, then go for it—getting sunscreen on is the most important thing!

☺ GOOD **Natural Protection Mineral Block Face Stick SPF 50** *($9.99 for 0.5 fl. oz.).* This fragrance-free sunscreen stick can be used on babies or adults. Its gentle formula provides broad-spectrum sun protection with titanium dioxide and zinc oxide. The twist-up stick texture is expectedly thick and difficult to apply to large areas because it doesn't blend readily. Products like this are best for spot-application to the areas more prone to sunburn (tops of ears and feet, bridge of nose, along the hairline). Once blended, the wax-based formula stays put without leaving a telltale white cast. This sunscreen is suitable for use when extra sun protection is needed, regardless of your age. It is best for normal to dry or sensitive skin that's not prone to breakouts. The tiny amount of anti-irritant oat kernel extract isn't enough to calm skin, but this sunscreen stick is very gentle on its own.

☺ GOOD **Natural Protection Mineral Block Sunscreen Lotion, SPF 30** *($10.99 for 3 fl. oz.).* The name for this sunscreen may make you think it's an all-natural product, but that's not the case. Although the active ingredients titanium dioxide and zinc oxide are naturally sourced, what's needed to make these ingredients useful in sunscreens is anything but natural! That's not bad (no question this sunscreen is an effective option), it just makes the name misleading. Besides, the formula contains a mix of natural and synthetic ingredients, just like the majority of sunscreens on the market. This sunscreen has a lightweight, silky texture that leaves a slightly white cast and a somewhat drying matte finish. Those with normal to oily skin that's also sensitive will do best with this fragrance-free sunscreen. Aveeno included some notable anti-irritants to help calm sensitive skin, although the amounts of each are lower than what we'd like to see, thus keeping this sunscreen from earning our top rating.

☹ POOR **Continuous Protection Sunblock Lotion SPF 70, for Face** *($10.99 for 3 fl. oz.)* contains avobenzone for sufficient UVA protection, but it has an SPF rating that, while accurate, may make you think that you can apply this once and be outdoors all day without a care (of course, the "continuous protection" name doesn't help, either). Although this sunscreen contains some good antioxidants and an anti-irritant, it also contains a preservative (methylisothiazolinone) that is not recommended for use in leave-on products due to its sensitizing potential (Source: *Contact Dermatitis*, October 2006, pages 227–229). Without this problematic preservative, this could have been a good sunscreen for normal to oily skin.

☹ POOR **Continuous Protection Sunblock Lotion SPF 85** *($11.99 for 4 ounces)* is very similar to Aveeno's Continuous Protection Sunblock Lotion SPF 70, for Face above, and the same review applies.

☹ POOR **Continuous Protection Sunblock Lotion SPF 100+ Face** *($11.99 for 3 fl. oz.)*. If you're applying sunscreen liberally as directed, then SPF ratings above 50 are overkill. Keep in mind that the SPF number is not about the quality of the sunscreen, but the length of time it protects. In this case, there simply isn't that much daylight in any part of the world to warrant such extreme protection. However, because most of us under-apply sunscreen, higher SPF ratings can be potentially helpful. For example, if you're applying half the recommended amount of a sunscreen rated SPF 100, you could still potentially be getting SPF 50, which is great. However, there's another issue to consider, too: The high amount of active ingredients required to reach this kind of stratospheric SPF rating puts your skin at greater risk of irritation, even if you're not applying it liberally. For best results when you need sun protection for a longer period of time, we urge you to stick with sunscreens rated SPF 25 to 45 and be sure to apply liberally each and every time. Aside from this product's high SPF rating and the inclusion of avobenzone for critical UVA (think anti-aging) protection, the formula has problems. It is water-resistant, but it lacks a beneficial amount of antioxidants; the formula contains far more fragrance than beneficial ingredients. Also disappointing is the inclusion of the sensitizing preservative methylisothiazolinone, which is generally not recommended for use in leave-on products. When you consider the high amount of sunscreen actives along with the irritation potential from this preservative, it doesn't add up to a day of fun in the sun!

☹ POOR **Continuous Protection Sunblock Spray SPF 70** *($10.99 for 5 fl. oz.)* provides broad-spectrum protection and includes the maximum amount of avobenzone for impressive UVA protection, all in a convenient spray that works from any angle (mothers trying to apply sunscreen to squirming children will love that feature). However, the amount of alcohol is significant, which makes this a tough sunscreen to recommend due to its drying, irritating potential. The alcohol-free spray-on sunscreens from Kinesys (not reviewed in this book or on CosmeticsCop.com), Coppertone Water Babies, or Paula's Choice provide ample sun protection and include ingredients that help rather than harm skin.

AVEENO LIP CARE

☹ POOR **Essential Moisture Lip Conditioner SPF 15** (*$3.79 for 0.15 fl. oz.*) does not contain the UVA-protecting ingredients of titanium dioxide, zinc oxide, avobenzone, Tinosorb, or Mexoryl SX. Aveeno clearly recognizes the importance of UVA protection or they wouldn't be using avobenzone in their Continuous Protection sunscreens.

AVON

Strengths: Consistent UVA protection from almost all the products with sunscreen; a few state-of-the-art moisturizers (some with sunscreen) at near-bargain prices; a selection of formidable concealers, powders, blushes, lipsticks, and lip glosses; fantastic pressed-powder bronzer; the company provides complete ingredient lists on its website and offers some of the most helpful Customer Service associates in the industry.

Weaknesses: The Clearskin products are mostly irritating and poor choices for anyone battling blemishes; the Anew Clinical lineup won't make you cancel that upcoming appointment for whatever cosmetic corrective procedure you've booked; an overreliance on jar packaging diminishes the antioxidants found in many Avon moisturizers; endless, unnecessarily repetitive moisturizers with exaggerated, outlandish claims; several of the foundations look decidedly unnatural or have SPF ratings that are too low; average eyeshadows and pencils; mostly average to disappointing mascaras.

For more information and reviews of the latest Avon products, visit CosmeticsCop.com.

AVON CLEANSERS

☺ GOOD $$$ **Anew Ultimate Age Repair Cream Cleanser** (*$14 for 4.2 fl. oz.*). The big claim for this cleanser is that it hydrates for hours without leaving a greasy residue. If it worked in this manner, then Avon would have to admit that women with dry skin wouldn't need any of their moisturizers; after all, if you've already hydrated your skin with your cleanser, why would you use a moisturizer? But, of course, that's not the case, and Avon isn't really selling this cleanser as a stand-alone option for aging skin; there are other products you're supposed to buy. What about the Pro-Sirtuin Technology Avon mentions? Sirtuins are proteins in skin that work to regulate and control certain cellular interactions and events, which is why they're often referred to as information regulators. Their anti-aging connection has to do with how they regulate aging. It is believed that if certain sirtuins can be modified to work against the mechanisms of aging, then the results might be visible on skin (think fewer wrinkles, less sagging, and greater resiliency). There is no research showing you can manipulate sirtuins in skin in any way as claimed. Yes, sirtuins are being researched for ways to control age-related degenerative diseases, but that research is in its infancy. Of course, that never stops cosmetics companies from making nonexistent research look real. What does seem promising is that topical application of specific sirtuins derived from yeast and the red grape component resveratrol (Avon doesn't use either source) seem to have a protective effect on skin in the presence of oxidative and ultraviolet light stress (think pollution, sun damage, and the air we breathe). Having said all that, the only thing you're getting with this product is a standard, emollient cleansing lotion for normal to dry skin that's not prone to breakouts. Most will find this works very well to remove makeup, but also will find it necessary to use a washcloth, as it does leave a residue.

☺ AVERAGE $$$ **Anew Platinum Cleanser** (*$16 for 4.2 fl. oz.*) has a rich texture as claimed, but its main detergent cleansing agent (TEA-lauryl sulfate) is too drying for all but very oily skin. It does have a few novel ingredients, but in a cleanser they are just rinsed down the drain.

☹ POOR **Anew Rejuvenate Revitalizing 2-in-1 Gel Cleanser** *($12 for 4.2 fl. oz.)* claims to be inspired by professional facials and is supposedly capable of reducing wrinkles, signs of fatigue, and other signs of aging while tightening pores. If you think it can accomplish any of these goals, think again! This is nothing more than a standard water-soluble gel cleanser for normal to oily skin. We suppose it approximates a facial in the sense that your face is cleansed, but the formula doesn't perform extractions or change skin in any way other than to remove surface oil, dirt, and makeup; that's nice, but not impressive. The only impressive things about this formula are the terms Avon uses to describe its effectiveness—Exfo-Smoothing Complex, MiniExtraction Technology, and RevitaFresh Technology—which are nothing more than marketing terms the ingredient manufacturer created out of thin air. They are meaningless when it comes to helping your skin. Avon added the irritant menthyl lactate (a form of menthol) so that you think something special is happening when you feel your skin tingle, but it isn't. In fact, when your skin tingles, you know it's being irritated, which is damaging to skin. None of the minerals or plant extracts in this cleanser will affect a wrinkle or pore anywhere on your face (even if they could, they are rinsed down the drain anyway), though the irritation this cleanser causes can lead to collagen breakdown and increased oil production at the base of the pore.

☹ POOR **Anew Reversalist Renewal Foaming Cleanser** *($13 for 4.2 fl. oz.).* This relatively expensive cleanser (more than $3 per ounce) produces copious foam, but the gentleness of its main ingredients are undermined by a high concentration of alkaline potassium hydroxide (that's lye). This cleanser is too drying for all skin types, and is not recommended. As for the claim of 80% wrinkle reversal from this product, it's 100% bogus.

☹ POOR **Clearskin Blackhead Eliminating Daily Cleanser** *($5.49 for 4.2 fl. oz.).* This water-soluble cleanser is medicated with 2% salicylic acid, but the high pH and the brief contact with skin means it won't provide much, if any, exfoliating benefit. Unfortunately, this isn't worth considering as an inexpensive cleanser either because the formula includes sodium C14-16 olefin sulfonate, a detergent cleansing agent that's too drying and irritating for all skin types. Whether acne is a concern or not, gentle cleansing is a must for all skin types and conditions. The scrub beads in here do provide some exfoliation, which is nice, but they would be far better in a less drying formula.

☹ POOR **Clearskin Blemish Clearing Foaming Cleanser** *($5.49 for 4.2 fl. oz.)* is similar to Avon's Clearskin Blackhead Eliminating Daily Cleanser above and the same comments apply. In addition, this cleanser contains the irritating menthol derivative menthyl lactate. Please see the Appendix to learn why irritants like this are bad news for oily, breakout-prone skin.

☹ POOR **Clearskin Pore Penetrating Gel Cleanser** *($6.49 for 4.2 fl. oz.).* This fragranced, water-soluble cleanser is an overall problem for those struggling with acne. Although it contains some helpful, gentle ingredients, it also contains a couple of problematic irritants that do not make it worth considering over lots of other cleansers for normal to oily skin. Please see the Appendix to learn how problematic ingredients impact acne-prone skin.

AVON EYE-MAKEUP REMOVERS

☺ AVERAGE **Makeup Remover Wipes with Mineral Complex** *($8 for 24 wipes).* The "mineral complex" in this makeup remover's name may entice you, but none of the minerals in these wipes offer special benefits for your skin. These cleansing cloths work decently to remove makeup (although waterproof makeup formulas are a bit too stubborn for this makeup remover), but it is best not to use this around your eyes because it contains a form of radish root that can cause irritation. In addition, any makeup remover meant for use around the eyes should omit fragrance—which these cloths contain. Fragrance, whether synthetic or from plant extracts, can be irritating.

☺ AVERAGE **Moisture Effective Eye Makeup Remover Lotion** *($4 for 2 fl. oz.)* is a very basic, but effective, water- and oil–based makeup remover. It is fragrance-free and OK to use around the eyes, though it is best used prior to washing with your regular cleanser.

AVON TONERS

☹ POOR **Clearskin Blackhead Eliminating Daily Astringent** *($4.49 for 8.4 fl. oz.)*. Like most toners (astringent is another name for toner) designed for acne-prone skin, this one only makes matters worse by subjecting your skin to a potentially damaging amount of alcohol. Although it does contain some intriguing ingredients and is medicated with 2% salicylic acid (BHA) to exfoliate skin, there are better exfoliating toners. Please see the Appendix to learn why alcohol is a problem for all skin types.

☹ POOR **Clearskin Professional Clarifying Toner Pads** *($12 for 45 pads)*. If these products are the professional way to manage acne, why is Avon still selling their regular Clearskin products? The company must not have much faith in them, or why create a second set of anti-acne products with the professional angle? As it turns out, although the Clearskin Professional products contain some novel, potentially helpful ingredients, they have the same problem as the regular Clearskin line: Too many products with alcohol, which actually makes acne worse, not better. These pads list alcohol as the second ingredient, which makes them too drying and irritating for all skin types.

AVON EXFOLIANTS & SCRUBS

☺ GOOD **$$$ Anew Clinical Luminosity Pro Brightening Serum** *($54 for 1 fl. oz.)* is a very expensive, but effective, AHA product from Avon. Although there is absolutely nothing clinical about this product, it does contain approximately 4% glycolic acid formulated at a pH of 4, so it will exfoliate skin, and that's good news. This has a serum texture that's suitable for all skin types, although because it contains fragrance, it is not the best for sensitive skin, despite the relatively low amount of AHA it contains. As for Avon's claims that this is an "injectable-grade skin brightener"… get real! First, there are no injectable fillers that brighten skin. Brightening skin is a cosmetic term, not a reason to get a dermal filler. A dermal filler helps with deep wrinkles, hollowed contours, and loss of facial volume, among other signs of aging, but not brightening. Avon does go on to state that the results are not comparable to such procedures, but then why start out with a lie and then have to correct it? You can expect a smoother texture, more even skin tone, and healthy collagen stimulation from this product—the same benefits that are available from other AHA products that cost far less and that actually provide a higher, more effective amount of AHA.

☺ AVERAGE **Anew Genics Treatment Cream** *($38 for 1 fl. oz.)* claims it stimulates the activity of skin's "youth gene" for skin that looks up to 10 years younger. The premise is intriguing, but what isn't mentioned is there are thousands of genes responsible for how skin looks, how it repairs itself, and how it ages and wrinkles. Certain genes stimulate normal collagen production; others stimulate fibroblasts to generate collagen, reduce inflammation, repair skin's surface, and on and on. In other words, there isn't one youth gene. Avon doesn't identify which gene is the youth gene their product is supposed to stimulate, but assuming their YouthGen Technology has any effect on genes (which it doesn't, and that's a good thing; you don't want cosmetics screwing around with your genes), that's but one factor of turning back the clock on your face. Besides, skin care is never as simple as one product (which Avon would agree to because they have dozens of products). Daily sun protection; gentle, nonirritating products containing the right ingredients (such as lots of antioxidants); and regular use of a well-formulated exfoliant play far more pivotal roles. Not surprisingly, the fine print on Avon's gene-stimulating claim was done in a lab on skin cells, not measured on intact skin. What works in a controlled lab setting may not prove to work as well (or at all) on intact skin, not to mention that without the actual test results, we don't even know what this product actually did to the cells (did the cells even have genes present?). What this product really does is exfoliate skin. It contains approximately 5% of the AHA glycolic acid formulated at a pH of 3.8, a range that permits exfoliation to occur. This fragranced AHA moisturizer is best for normal to dry skin. It contains some intriguing plant extracts and peptides, but these anti-aging ingredients won't remain stable during use because Anew Genics Treatment Cream is packaged in a jar. Please see the Appendix to learn why jar packaging is a problem. The bottom line: This is an effective AHA moisturizer to consider, but its packaging and amount of fragrance makes it less compelling than those on our Best AHA Exfoliants list.

☺ AVERAGE **Anew Platinum Night Tourmaline Emulsion** (*$38 for 1.7 fl. oz.*). Avon boasts that this moisturizer provides a 580% instant moisture boost, but if that's true, it's a problem. "Moisture" almost always refers to some amount of water combined with other ingredients that keep the water in skin's uppermost layers. But skin taking on too much water is a bad thing! When skin takes on too much water, the substances that hold skin cells together become engorged and impaired, leading to a damaged barrier. Think of what your fingers look like after soaking in a bath, even if the bathwater has bath oil added. Most likely the claim is inflated but what about the tourmaline polypeptide complex? Can it protect your skin's collagen? Possibly, but there's no solid research to support the claim, not to mention the peptides won't remain stable for long because this product is packaged in a clear jar. That leaves you with a purple-tinted cream imbued with glitter (why the glitter?) whose main ingredient of interest is the AHA glycolic acid. How much glycolic acid this contains isn't revealed, but it's most likely between 3-5%, and the pH of 3.6 ensures it will function as an exfoliant. Although this is an option as an AHA exfoliant for normal to oily skin, it isn't among the best. The fragrance is intense and lingers, which puts skin at greater risk of irritation, and the jar packaging means the plant extracts this contains (which convey antioxidant benefits) won't be effective for long. As for the tourmaline and other minerals in this product, there is no substantiated research proving they do anything for skin. Tourmaline is said to increase the electric properties of skin, but what does that mean? Is it good or bad? We don't know, and the companies selling products with tourmaline offer little more than marketing-speak for an explanation.

☺ AVERAGE **Anew Rejuvenate Night Revitalizing Cream** (*$30 for 1.7 fl. oz.*) promises results similar to a "professional anti-aging facial." What a ridiculous claim! First, what exactly is an anti-aging facial? To us, it's a vague description that defies comparison, but it does sound impressive. What is certain is that it doesn't work anything like peels or microdermabrasion, and when it comes to traditional facials, well, they don't work to prevent aging either. This product ends up being a lightweight moisturizing cream containing Avon's AHA alternative (thiodipropionic acid) along with salicylic acid. Although this blend has the potential to be effective for exfoliation (hardly unique to this product), the cream's pH of 4.4 is too high to ensure exfoliation will occur. Mica is included for a shiny finish, but this product is ultimately too emollient to make pores look smaller for long, despite the claim. It does contain some great ingredients for normal to dry skin, but many of them will begin to deteriorate once the jar packaging is opened. Whether you choose to waste your money on an anti-aging facial (whatever that means) or this product, either way you won't end up with younger-looking, refined skin.

☺ AVERAGE **Anew Rejuvenate Night Sapphire Emulsion** *($30 for 1.7 fl. oz.)*. The "sapphire" portion of this product's name has nothing to do with the gemstone, but everything to do with this lotion's blue tint, from synthetic dye ingredients, and its blue sparkles, which are characteristics of makeup, not skin-care products. It looks pretty, but it doesn't help your skin! The same is true for the overpowering fragrance—whether synthetic or natural, fragrance is not skin care. Getting past the color and shine, this product is meant to reduce pores but it doesn't offer much benefit in that regard. This contains approximately 4-5% of the AHA glycolic acid, and the pH of 3.6 allows it to function as an exfoliant. This product also has an initially thick, spackle-like gel texture, which may minimize the appearance of pores, but that is a cosmetic benefit, not something you need when you're going to bed. Adding to this product's woes is the jar packaging, which is a problem for keeping the ingredients stable once it is opened. Please see the Appendix for further details on jar packaging.

☺ AVERAGE **Anew Reversalist Night Renewal Cream** *($32 for 1.7 fl. oz.)* is just another well-formulated AHA product. It contains a blend of glycolic acid and Avon's patented AHA thiodipropionic acid, most likely at a 3–5% concentration, although Avon wouldn't reveal the exact percentage to us. These ingredients are pH-sensitive, and the pH of 3.6 permits exfoliation to occur. As for the claims, they're mostly accurate in terms of what daily use of any decent AHA product does for skin. With ongoing use, you can expect a pH-correct AHA product to renew skin, refine its texture, reduce signs of sun damage (including the look of wrinkles), and enhance collagen production for firmer skin (Sources: *International Journal of Cosmetic Science*, June 2008, pages 175–182; *Phytotherapy Research*, November 2006, pages 921–934; *Journal of Cosmetic Dermatology*, September 2006, pages 246–253; *Aesthetic and Plastic Surgery*, May-June 2006, pages 356–362; and *Journal of Dermatology*, January 2006, pages 16–22). Avon blended their AHAs in a silky base, which also helps enhance skin's texture and the perception of smoothness. So why isn't this rated higher? Jar packaging. Although that won't impact the effectiveness of the AHAs, it will affect the antioxidant plant ingredients Avon included. Please see the Appendix for further details on jar packaging.

☺ AVERAGE **Anew Reversalist Night Sterling Emulsion** *($32 for 1.7 fl. oz.)* is similar to Avon's Anew Rejuvenate Night Sapphire Emulsion above, but this version makes no claims of erasing pores; instead, the claims are all about firming skin and reactivating its youthful structure. Given that this is basically an AHA exfoliant, the claims aren't as far-fetched as they come across because to some extent that is what any well-formulated AHA (usually glycolic acid or lactic acid) or BHA (salicylic acid) exfoliant can do. This product contains approximately 4–5% glycolic acid (AHA), and the pH of 3.8 allows it to function as an exfoliant (the efficacy of AHAs is pH dependent). That's great news and definitely conveys an anti-aging benefit, but this product also contains a great deal of wafting synthetic fragrance, which can cause irritation. Plus, it comes in jar packaging, which means the beneficial ingredients (antioxidants and peptides) won't remain stable once it is opened. The product also contains glitter; yes, glitter. Shine and fragrance have nothing to do with good skin care, and as such this product looks better in its packaging than it does on your face!

☺ AVERAGE **Anew Ultimate Night Gold Emulsion** *($34 for 1.7 fl. oz.)* is an effective AHA moisturizer with a gel-like texture. It contains approximately 5% glycolic acid and Avon's own AHA ingredient—thiodipropionic acid and trioxaundecanedioic acid. The very fragrant formula is infused with particles of gold shine, no doubt in an effort to reinforce the product's name, not really to provide a precious benefit to skin. Despite the gel texture, this can leave oily skin feeling too slick and greasy. It is best for normal to dry skin. Pay no mind to Avon's claims that their Pro-Sirtuin TX Technology stimulates this special class of proteins. (Sirtuins are types of proteins involved in metabolism, cell growth cycle, and DNA repair.) As far as Avon's formula goes, there is no research proving any of the peptides or other ingredients in this product, or in any product, have an effect on sirtuins in your skin. Even if they could, Avon's choice of clear jar packaging won't keep the ingredients stable once the product is opened.

☺ AVERAGE $$$ **Anew Clinical Advanced Retexturizing Peel** *($25 for 30 pads)* are supposed to be akin to a 35% AHA peel, but don't count on it. The water-based pads contain about 10% ammonium glycolate with glycolic acid, at a pH of 4, so exfoliation will occur. However, alcohol is the fourth ingredient listed, and that increases the potential for irritation. Although effective (just not to the extent of a physician-administered AHA peel), there are better, less expensive AHA products available.

☹ POOR **Anew Clinical Resurfacing Expert Smoothing Fluid** *($38 for 1 fl. oz.)*. First, this AHA exfoliant is not formulated with "professional-grade" ingredients. It is formulated with standard cosmetic ingredients Avon uses in many of their other products that are not sold with any sort of "professional" claims. This exfoliant is supposed to be almost as effective as microdermabrasion, but here's the thing: other than making skin feel smooth, microdermabrasion isn't all that amazing. Comparing what's possible from a well-formulated AHA exfoliant (which this isn't, but more on that in a moment) to microdermabrasion is like comparing what's possible on an iPad to a desktop computer from the early 1990s! Although this contains an impressive amount (likely 10%) of AHA glycolic acid, it's second ingredient is alcohol, which makes it a problem for all skin types. Alcohol causes free-radical damage, hurts healthy collagen production, and impairs skin's ability to heal. The tiny amount of moisture-binding agents Avon added to this exfoliant are little consolation for the damaging effects from the alcohol. Companies such as Alpha Hydrox, Paula's Choice, and NeoStrata offer much better exfoliants that don't put your skin at risk for needless irritation.

☹ POOR **Clearskin Pore Penetrating Invigorating Scrub** *($6.49 for 2.5 fl. oz.)*. There is every reason to believe this problematic scrub will not only make your acne worse, but also confuse your skin due to its blend of oil with alcohol and other drying, irritating ingredients. It is not recommended. Please see the Appendix for details on why irritation is bad for your skin.

☹ POOR **Clearskin Professional Deep Pore Cleansing Scrub** *($12 for 4.2 fl. oz.)* won't reduce oily skin for long—if anything, the irritants in this scrub will stimulate oil production directly in the pore, clearly something that oily skin doesn't need more of. The salicylic acid in this scrub is wasted because it will be rinsed from skin before it has a chance to work (and if acne is your concern, 0.5% salicylic acid likely won't be enough to make a difference). None of this is professional!

AVON MOISTURIZERS (DAYTIME & NIGHTTIME), EYE CREAMS, & SERUMS

☺ GOOD **Clearskin Professional Oil Free Lotion SPF 15** *($16 for 2.5 fl. oz.)*. This daytime moisturizer with an in-part avobenzone sunscreen is designed not only to protect skin from sun damage, but also to help reduce acne. It contains glycolic and salicylic acids to combat acne, although the amounts are too low for either to exert much benefit, so this isn't a 2-in-1 sunscreen/exfoliant product (in addition, the pH of 4.4 is too high for exfoliation to occur). The zinc derivative in this product deserves a bit of explanation because there is a growing body of research demonstrating zinc's second-tier role in minimizing acne. The research deals primarily with oral consumption of pure zinc, which is different than the type Avon uses in this product. However, there have been some intriguing in vitro studies as well that show zinc's role as an anti-inflammatory agent when applied to cultured skin cells. One study compared the effects of topical application of zinc acetate with the effects of common disinfectants such as benzoyl peroxide and topical antibiotics. The zinc acetate didn't win out as the superior choice, but it held its own by comparison (Sources: *Seminars in Cutaneous Medicine and Surgery*, September 2008, pages 170–176; *European Journal of Dermatology*, November-December 2007, pages 492–496; *Journal of the European Academy of Dermatology and Venereology*, March 2007, pages 311–319; and *The Journal of Dermatological Treatment*, 2006, pages 205–210). Given the potential helpfulness of the zinc, this product's relatively lightweight texture suitable for normal to oily skin, and the inclusion of some potentially helpful cell-communicating ingredients, this is worth considering. It does contain fragrance.

☺ GOOD **Solutions a.m. Total Radiance Day Lotion SPF 15** *($13 for 4 fl. oz.)*. This daytime moisturizer with an in-part avobenzone sunscreen came close to earning a Best Product rating, but lost our highest honor due to the inclusion of potentially problematic plant extracts. Among the not-wanted extracts are *Aframomum melegueta* (grains of paradise) and fennel. Both plants contain volatile constituents that can be skin-irritants (Source: naturaldatabase. com), although neither is present in this product in a large amount, which is why it is still worth considering. This is best for normal to slightly dry or slightly oily skin, and the formula contains a broad assortment of antioxidants, skin-identical ingredients, and even some cell-communicating ingredients, all packaged to ensure stability.

☺ GOOD $$$ **Anew Ultimate Day Age Repair Cream SPF 25** *($34 for 1.7 fl. oz.)*. This daytime moisturizer with AHAs has a lot going for it and is definitely a product to consider if you want to combine an in-part avobenzone sunscreen with the exfoliating power of AHAs. This silky, slightly thick cream for normal to dry skin contains a blend of glycolic acid and ammonium glycolate at approximately a 3% concentration and has a pH of 3.6. It is light enough to work well under makeup, too. The downside is the jar packaging, which won't keep the antioxidants and peptides this contains stable during use. You can ignore Avon's claims that this product stimulates youth proteins and restores natural volume to aging skin—this isn't surgery in a jar and there is no such thing as "youth proteins" (there aren't old proteins either). Natural volume in the face is about muscle tone and fat deposits; this product will not do anything to increase or change those aspects of your face. What this will do is provide broad-spectrum sun protection and exfoliation, a combination that is traditionally difficult to pull off because sunscreens require a higher pH to remain stable in emulsions, while AHAs work best at lower pH levels. Somehow Avon has succeeded (NeoStrata also sells sunscreens with AHAs), and that, plus how silky-smooth this feels on skin, are compelling reasons to give this daytime moisturizer an audition.

☹ AVERAGE **Anew Platinum Day Cream SPF 25** *($38 for 1.7 fl. oz.)* contains platinum, which cannot "restore youthful cell shape" as Avon claims, though this fragranced daytime moisturizer will provide reliable broad-spectrum sun protection. Avobenzone is on hand for critical UVA (think anti-aging) protection and this has a lightweight, silky cream texture. Beyond sunscreen, this contains surprisingly little in terms of beneficial anti-aging ingredients. The plant extracts will not remain stable because this is packaged in a jar, which is the least preferred type of container to ensure product stability once it has been opened. For the money, your skin deserves better.

☺ AVERAGE **Anew Platinum Night Cream** *($38 for 1.7 fl. oz.)* was created for women age 60 and older, playing up the mistaken notion that age is a skin type. Of course, many women in their 60s and beyond are dealing with the issues this serum claims to fix; namely, deep lines, sagging along the jaw line and neck, and a loss of youthful contours, but so are women in their 40s and 50s. Avon's solution for tackling these varied issues is to use patented technology said to boost the production of paxillin. Paxillin is a type of protein involved in cell signaling pathways in skin. Essentially, it serves as a "docking protein," which means it recruits and helps utilize cellular substances (such as enzymes) that otherwise would not know how to reach their target cells. When the correct connections occur, paxillin helps regulate how cells move about and function. What does this have to do with sagging skin? When the correct connections occur, paxillin can potentially tell a cell (cell communication) to help make better cells. What does this have to do with sagging skin? Paxillin may improve skin's structural support. Avon is banking that all it takes to lift sagging skin back into place is to stimulate more paxillin in your skin (Sources: nature.com/onc/journal/v20/n44/full/1204786a.html; and *Critical Reviews in Oncogenesis*, volume 8, issue 4, 1997, pages 343–358). What's missing from Avon's theory is that there are myriad other proteins and substances involved in cell communication as well, and there is no research proving that paxillin is the one capable of lifting skin. Even if paxillin could somehow shore up skin, which would be a real leap of physiology, stimulating more of it or any other protein in skin doesn't address the numerous factors (sun damage, gravity, fat pad shifting, bone loss, estrogen depletion, muscle laxity, and on and on) that cause skin to sag and lose its youthful contours. It just isn't possible for skin-care products, regardless of their ingredients, to lift sagging skin back to where it once was. Again, even if that were possible, where would the excess skin go? Sagging skin is about excess—lax skin that starts falling—it has little to do with support. Sagging is one area of skin aging where the cosmetics industry does not have a great solution. As for the formula itself, it's actually an effective (meaning pH-correct) AHA exfoliant in a thick cream base for dry skin. Although Avon wouldn't reveal the percentage of the AHA glycolic acid in this product, it's most likely in the 5–8% range, which is great, but again we're just making an educated guess. The problem, though, is that the AHA is the only exciting aspect of the formula, unless you like exotic plant extracts with no established skin-care benefit. Even if those plant extracts were effective, the jar packaging means the beneficial ingredients won't remain stable once it is opened. See the Appendix for further info on why jar packaging is a problem.

☺ AVERAGE **Anew Reversalist Day Renewal Cream SPF 25** *($32 for 1.7 fl. oz.)* isn't one of Avon's better daytime moisturizers with sunscreen (avobenzone is included for reliable UVA protection). It has a lightweight, silky texture and contains some good natural and synthetic antioxidants, but the jar packaging will render them less effective, not to mention the hygiene issue of sticking your fingers into the jar every day. Avon's Activinol Technology cannot reverse wrinkles, and there's no proof to the contrary. Besides, if this technology is so wonderful for wrinkles, why doesn't Avon include it in all their other antiwrinkle products? If you're curious about Activinol, it is a blend of two plant ingredients they claim will boost production of a molecule in skin known as activin. Activin is a naturally occurring growth factor that helps repair skin and control cellular division. Like most good things in skin, its production slows down as we accumulate more sun damage over the years. The thing to keep in mind about this type of claim is that activin is but one compound that helps skin regulate and repair itself; there are hundreds of others that work in harmony as well. So, to think that boosting production of only one of them is all that's needed is not true. Moreover, neither plant extract Avon includes has any research proving that it boosts activin's role in skin repair. Interestingly, animal studies on wounded skin have shown that when activin production is boosted too much, the result is poor wound-healing and excessive scarring. When it is selectively activated, the wounds healed normally (Source: *Laboratory Investigation*, February 2009, pages 131–141). Based on those facts, if Avon's product can manipulate activin levels in your skin, it may not be a good thing (and, of course, wrinkles aren't the same as wounds).

☺ AVERAGE **Anew Rejuvenate Day Revitalizing Cream SPF 25** *($30 for 1.7 fl. oz.).* You're asked to believe that this daytime moisturizer with an in-part avobenzone sunscreen is akin to getting a professional facial every time it's applied. Talk about an overstatement! This product cannot perform extractions as claimed; just the notion of that is ludicrous—are blackheads and blemishes just going to fall off after applying this product? As for the exfoliating claim, although this contains salicylic acid, the amount is less than 1% and this product's pH isn't within the required range for exfoliation to occur. The only hackneyed claim for this product that makes some sense is Avon's Revitafresh Technology. This is said to "reinforce cell bonds and help make skin look more even and smoother." Yes, that sounds impressive, but in reality most well-formulated moisturizers and serums can make the same claim because they contain ingredients that help reinforce skin's barrier and, as a result, make skin look even and smoother. This contains several ingredients that make skin look beautifully smooth, including silicone, polymers, and a film-forming agent. They're hardly unique to this product, however, and it's disappointing that Avon included fennel extract because this plant (and a few others in this product) contain volatile components that cause irritation. What really makes this product a waste of your money is the jar packaging, which allows the air-sensitive ingredients to break down. If you decide to give this fragranced daytime moisturizer a go, it is best for normal to oily skin.

☺ AVERAGE $$$ **Anew Clinical Lift & Firm Pro Serum** *($54 for 1 fl. oz.).* The claims for this product are confusing. On the one hand, they make it sound stupendous, but then the next comment, in essence, says, no, it really doesn't do what we just told you it can do. Here's an example: First, Avon says this serum contains "injectable grade ingredients" for "dramatic lifting power," which makes it sound as if it will work like dermal injections, procedures performed by doctors to plump out wrinkles. But then Avon goes on to state that this product will not give you the results you get by having these ingredient injected into your skin. Which is it? The truth is the latter; there is absolutely nothing in this product that will provide anything even remotely like what you get from injected dermal fillers. Even when skin-care products contain the same ingredients used in some dermal fillers (hyaluronic acid, for one), these ingredients cannot reach the same level of skin that dermal fillers can. What you're getting is a silky but exceptionally basic AHA serum that contains approximately 5% glycolic acid formulated at a pH that allows it to work as an exfoliant. AHAs have multiple benefits for skin, but no cosmetic ingredient can lift sagging skin, and definitely not "from every angle," as Avon states. No skin-care product can. This serum contains a film-forming agent (PVP, most often seen in hair gels and hairsprays) that can make your skin feel tighter—but feeling tighter isn't the same as actually making it tighter or lifting it.

☺ AVERAGE $$$ **Anew Platinum Eye & Lip Cream** *($36 for 0.5 fl. oz.)* is a fragrance-free moisturizer that claims to be special for the lips and eyes, but isn't. In fact, other than containing a small amount of some unusual ingredients, this is an average moisturizer masquerading as a specialty product. Avon boasts of their Paxillium Technology for this product, but all of their Anew Platinum products contain a blend of some ingredients they indirectly refer to as

Paxillium Technology (discussed in the review above for Avon's Anew Platinum Night Cream), which doesn't really set this one apart from the other Platinum products. Second, this product contains a mix of emollient ingredients that help moisturize, along with some absorbent (and potentially drying) ingredients (e.g., cornstarch and boron nitride) that ideally aren't the best in a product meant to hydrate skin and make it look less wrinkled. Even if Paxillium Technology were the answer for aging skin around the eyes or lips, this product is packaged in a jar, so won't keep the ingredients stable after opening. See the Appendix for further details on why jar packaging is a problem.

☺ AVERAGE $$$ **Anew Rejuvenate 24 Hour Eye Moisturizer SPF 25 Day/Night Cream** *($28 for 0.66 fl. oz.)*. This two-part product provides an eye-area moisturizer with sunscreen for daytime, **A.M. Eye Cream**, and a no-sunscreen eye cream for nighttime use, **P.M. Eye Cream**. Sounds convenient, and the dual-sided jar packaging is clever, but cleverness and convenience don't always add up to good skin care, which is the case with this product. Aside from the jar packaging (see the Appendix for details), the main problem is the directions for the A.M. Eye Cream, which contains synthetic sunscreen active ingredients, state that you should apply this to your eyelid. Doing that is not a good idea, because it's very likely that the sunscreen ingredients will migrate into your eye and cause irritation (and if you perspire while wearing this as directed, eye contact is guaranteed). For the eyelid area, titanium dioxide and zinc oxide are the only two active sunscreen ingredients you should use because they won't cause burning or irritation. If the eye area weren't the issue (though given the name and price, that is how most women will use it), it does include avobenzone for UVA protection and is formulated in a lightly emollient, silky base. The main plant extract, *Tinospora cordifolia*, has research showing it has immune-stimulating effects when taken orally, and it also is an antioxidant (Sources: *Journal of Ethnopharmacology*, June 1999, pages 277–281; and *International Immunopharmacology*, December 2004, pages 1645–1659). However, there is no research demonstrating the effectiveness of this plant when applied topically. Plus, stimulating the immune system can't affect dark circles or reduce puffiness, which is what this eye cream claims to do. The P.M. Eye Cream is similar to but silkier than the A.M. Eye Cream and, as mentioned, does not contain sunscreen. Both products contain several antioxidants and retinol, but these ingredients are wasted due to the jar packaging, which allows them to degrade. This duo can help make slightly dry skin anywhere on the face look better, but the sunscreen portion should not be applied as close to the eye as Avon recommends.

☺ AVERAGE $$$ **Anew Reversalist Illuminating Eye System** *($30 for 0.59 fl. oz.)*. With all of the eye creams and serums Avon sells, it's shocking any of us still have any eye-area problems to complain about. After all, if they worked as claimed, wrinkles, sagging skin, dark circles, and puffiness would be distant memories. Of course, that's not the case, but it doesn't stop Avon from continuing to churn out more eye-area products with ever-more-tempting claims. This time around it's about treating very dark under-eye circles while dramatically reversing wrinkles. In order to accomplish this, Avon provides two products in one jar package (hint: the jar packaging isn't good news for the formula or for daily hygiene). The **Eye Cream** is a silky moisturizer containing a synthetic antioxidant (thiodopropionic acid) that Avon uses in several products. Several antioxidant plant extracts are also included, but none of them are proven to do a thing for wrinkles or dark circles. What's more, any potency these

🌹 Highly fragranced products smell good, but won't help your skin! See the Appendix for details.

ingredients may have will be steadily decreased because of jar packaging. At best, the Eye Cream will smooth superficial lines and improve skin's texture—something almost any moisturizer will do. Part 2 of this product is the use-when-needed **Veil**. This is little more than a thick, silicone-enhanced moisturizer whose spackle-like texture assists the Eye Cream with temporarily filling in superficial lines around the eye. It has a brightening effect on dark circles due to the cosmetic pigments it contains; however, this effect isn't as convincing as using a good concealer for dark circles. This "illuminating" system ends up being an OK option for all skin types, but is pricey for what you get. Please see the Appendix to find out why, in truth, you don't need special products for the eye area.

☺ AVERAGE $$$ **Anew Reversalist Renewal Serum** *($44 for 1 fl. oz.)* comes in truly odd packaging, resembling something most women would be embarrassed to admit they own. (One glance at the packaging will give you a clear idea of what we mean; who knows what Avon was thinking when they made this decision?) Packaging choice aside, what we have here is a highly fragranced serum containing approximately 3% glycolic acid along with Avon's patented AHA, thiodipropionic acid. As an AHA product, the pH is just above the level needed for maximum effectiveness. Avon claims that their Activinol Technology helps reignite skin's repair process and improves wrinkles. It is well known that as we age our skin's natural repair mechanisms become faulty, largely due to cumulative sun damage and years of using products that contain irritating ingredients, plus genetic factors that are beyond our control. The two plant extracts that make up this Activinol complex have some reliable research concerning their antioxidant and anti-cancer abilities, but nothing that proves they can reactivate any element of skin's repair process, and certainly not any more so than hundreds of other plant extracts with the exact same properties (Sources: *Journal of Cellular and Molecular Medicine*, January 2009, ePublication; *Natural Medicines*, July 2008, pages 300–307; and *Acta Poloniae Pharmaceutica*, July-August 2009, pages 423–428). Of course, this serum also is supposed to tighten skin and provide a 100% improvement in discolorations. Such a vague claim is intended to give you the impression that all your skin discolorations will be gone, but the claim doesn't say 100% of what; even a teeny improvement could be a 100% improvement, depending on what you're basing that on. Claims aside, there is nothing in this product that offers much in the way of improvement in skin discolorations. It doesn't contain sunscreen, and the small amount of AHA isn't all that helpful for cell turnover. Also, there are no ingredients in this product that can bring about a dramatic reduction in discolorations. The tightness claim is 100% bogus, although your skin may feel temporarily tighter due to the powdery, dry finish you get from many of the ingredients, but that is hardly moisturizing for normal to dry skin. This contains cosmetic pigments that add shine to skin, but shine isn't skin care. Using Anew Reversalist Renewal Serum isn't nearly as effective as using a pH-correct AHA product with a serum or moisturizer loaded with antioxidants and cell-communicating ingredients that do improve wrinkles.

☺ AVERAGE $$$ **Anew Ultimate Contouring Eye System** *($32 for 0.59 fl. oz.)* offers yet another duo claiming to prevent the skin around your eyes from aging. As you may well suspect, nothing about this two-part product has the power to "reshape, repair, and recontour" your eye area—this isn't an eye-lift in a jar, and neither formula should be packaged in a jar in the first place (see the Appendix to find out why jar packaging is a problem)! One part of the dual-sided jar contains **Concentrated Elixir**. This nonaqueous moisturizer has an emollient silkiness and contains enough silicone and wax to serve as a temporary spackle for lines around the eyes. How long the effect lasts depends on how expressive you are and on what else you apply to the eye area (e.g., foundation, concealer). Concentrated Elixir contains the plant oil from *Perilla ocymoides*. Although this oil is a great source of fatty acids for skin and has been shown to have an anti-inflammatory effect when consumed, it is also known to cause contact dermatitis. This is attributed to two constituents present in the oil: 1-perillaldehyde and peril-lalcohol (Source: naturaldatabase.com). Avon would've done better to include a non-problematic oil, such as evening primrose or borage. The Elixir also contains several ingredients that will quickly lose their potency thanks to the jar packaging. This includes a form of retinol mixed with liquid silicone (retinoxytrimethylsilane), which is really disappointing. The second part of the product is labeled **Intensive Repair Cream**. It is neither intensive nor reparative in the least because it contains nothing more than water, slip agents, gel-based thickener, preservatives, and iron oxides for color, all-in-all a formula that would have been considered antiquated even 20 years ago. Taken together, Anew Ultimate Contouring Eye System is a mediocre system with the additional misfortune of being stuck in a jar.

☺ AVERAGE **$$$ Anew Ultimate Elixir Premium** (*$59 for 1 fl. oz.*) is supposed to retighten and lift skin's structure on the face and neck, all thanks to Avon's Pro-Sirtuin Technology. Sirtuins are discussed in the review above for Avon's Anew Ultimate Age Repair Cream Cleanser. At best this research is in its infancy and there is no evidence that it is possible or even safe. Getting beyond the sirtuin story (and there's no reason to believe any ingredient in this serum will have the claimed effect), it is very disappointing that there's alcohol in this product. The amount likely is too low to cause much harm, but it's listed before several state-of-the-art ingredients, which doesn't make this a serum to contact your Avon salesperson about. When you really examine the formula, the name for this product is downright embarrassing. It isn't "ultimate" or "premium" in any way, save for the deluxe packaging! The only way it can possibly defy the effects of gravity on your face is if you apply it while hanging upside down from a trapeze.

☺ AVERAGE **$$$ Anew Ultimate Night Age Repair Cream** (*$34 for 1.7 fl. oz.*) is a good AHA moisturizer for those with normal to slightly dry skin who prefer a creamy texture. The blend of ammonium glycolate and glycolic acid seems to be present in an efficacious amount, and the pH of 3.6 permits exfoliation. Avon also includes a smaller amount of antioxidants and plant-based water-binding agents, but the jar packaging won't keep them stable once this product is in use. Still, this has merit if you're looking for a well-formulated AHA product.

☹ POOR **Anew Clinical ThermaFirm Face Lifting Cream** (*$32 for 1 fl. oz.*). In case the name of this product wasn't obvious enough, it's designed as an alternative to Thermage treatments. Thermage is a cosmetic corrective procedure that uses radiofrequency energy to heat skin, causing a controlled, nonablative wound that stimulates new collagen production. It is a viable option for tightening skin and smoothing the appearance of wrinkles, and the results continue to improve as more is learned about how to perform the procedure to get the best outcome. Does Avon's alternative even come close to mimicking the effect of Thermage? Not in the least. This is a surprisingly lackluster formula for a cream advertised as having "potent ingredients." Avon refers to this as their "most advanced and powerful facial lifting product ever." Well, it isn't, at least not from any published research, or any research Avon is willing to part with, and not in comparison to other products Avon sells. At best, this is a decent moisturizer for someone with normal to slightly dry skin, but the menthol derivative (menthyl lactate, used in a small amount to create the impression that the product is doing something) isn't the best for any skin type. In fact, the irritation this can cause (and other irritants like fennel don't help, either) can hurt skin's healing process and ability to produce healthy collagen.

☹ POOR **Anew Platinum Serum** *($64 for 1 fl. oz.).* As Avon's most expensive serum, you may be expecting this to be Avon's best, just because it costs the most. This type of "expensive-must-mean-better" logic is one many consumers use when shopping for cosmetics—don't believe it! It isn't true, but it's easy to fall into the trap. The absolute truth is that in the world of makeup and skin care, expensive does not mean better. Anew Platinum Serum was created for women age 60 and older, but age isn't a skin type, so the designation is silly. Of course, many women in their 60s and beyond are dealing with the issues this serum claims to fix; namely, deep lines, sagging along the jaw line and neck, and a loss of youthful contours. However, women in their 30s, 40s, and 50s are all struggling with these as well; again, age is not a skin type. Avon's solution for tackling these varied issues is to use their patented technology, which they claim boosts the production of paxillin. Please refer to the review for Avon's Anew Platinum Night Cream above for details on paxillin. As for this product's formula, it is truly disappointing and overpriced. You're getting mostly water, slip agents, silicone, alcohol, and dry-finish solvents that create a silky texture. Truly state-of-the-art, proven anti-aging ingredients are missing, and the amount of alcohol, while not prodigious, is potentially enough to cause free-radical damage that leads to collagen breakdown, which is the opposite of what you want if your skin-care goal is anti-aging. Based on the price, unproven claims, and lack of a bona fide advantage for women concerned with sagging skin, this serum is not worth your time or money.

☹ POOR **Anew Rejuvenate Flash Facial Revitalizing Concentrate** *($40 for 1 fl. oz.).* Avon claims this water-based serum works like thousands of "micro-extractions to help visibly shrink pores," along with a host of other attributes all designed to provide smooth, poreless skin. Never mind that we need our pores for health, but the claim is supposed to make someone with visible pores feel assured this is the product that will finally clean out and close the gaping appearance of blackheads and open pores. But all this does is provide light hydration, while temporarily filling in pores. Skin appears smoother and may feel tighter due to the amount of film-forming agents (think hairspray) this contains, but pore size itself isn't affected; it hasn't and can't change one little bit from applying this product. Flash Revitalizing Concentrate contains shiny coloring agents claimed to blur imperfections, but adding sheen to skin doesn't blur anything, it just makes skin look shiny. And again, shine isn't the same as using ingredients known to improve the shape of a pore. Nothing in here actually hides pores—they will still be in plain sight and you certainly won't be able to forgo foundation or concealer. Particularly troubling is that this serum contains the irritating menthol derivative menthyl lactate. The cooling sensation this provides may make you think the serum is working, and it is—just not the way you hoped. The irritation from menthyl lactate can lead to collagen breakdown and stimulate oil production at the base of the pore, making pores appear larger than they really are (Sources: *Inflammation Research*, December 2008, pages 558–563; *Archives of Dermatologic Research*, July 2008, pages 311–316; *Skin Pharmacology and Physiology*, June 2008, pages 124–135 and November-December 2000, pages 358–371; *Journal of Investigative Dermatology*, April 2008, pages 15–19; *Journal of Cosmetic Dermatology*, March 2008, pages 78–82; *Mechanisms of Ageing and Development*, January 2007, pages 92–105; and *Medical Electron Microscopy*, March 2001, pages 29–40). Although this serum contains an impressive roster of antioxidants, some skin-identical ingredients, and a cell-communicating ingredient, none of these work like micro-extractions to rid pores of oil or of a buildup of dead skin cells that lead to blackheads. Most of the claims are as gimmicky as it gets, particularly the one concerning your skin looking dramatically younger in two weeks.

AVON SUN CARE

☺ GOOD $$$ **Anew Solar Advance Sunscreen Face Lotion SPF 45** *($34 for 2.6 fl. oz.)* provides critical UVA protection with avobenzone, and comes in a silky, lightweight lotion formula that contains a decent blend of antioxidants. Some of the plant extracts are fragrant, which isn't the best, but the amounts are small enough that it's not likely to be a problem. This sunscreen also contains additional fragrance. This isn't the most advanced sunscreen around, but it's a good option for those with normal to oily skin that's prone to breakouts.

☹ POOR **Anew Solar Advance Sunscreen Body Lotion SPF 30** *($34 for 5 fl. oz.)* makes several missteps, and just doesn't make the grade. The base formula contains a high amount of barium sulfate, a mineral compound cited frequently as a skin-irritant (Sources: *British Journal of Dermatology*, September 2004, pages 557–564; and *Handbook of Cosmetic and Personal Care Additives*, Second Edition, volume 1, Synapse Information Resources, Inc., 2002, page 907). Considering that the synthetic sunscreen actives in this product can cause irritation for some people, it doesn't make sense to add high amounts of any known irritant because doing so increases the risk of a reaction. As such, this isn't a sunscreen we can recommend.

AVON LIP CARE

☺ GOOD **Care Deeply with Aloe Lip Balm** *($0.99 for 0.15 fl. oz.)* is a standard, effective petrolatum-based lip balm that does its job of making dry, chapped lips feel better. For less than one dollar, that's not such a bad deal!

☹ POOR **Beyond Color Plumping Lip Conditioner SPF 15 with Double the Retinol** *($8 for 0.13 fl. oz.)*. Despite its impressive name, there is no reason to consider this lip balm. Given the lack of UVA-protecting ingredients, this certainly isn't all that anti-aging. As for the retinol, doubled or not, there is barely any of it in here; there is more fragrance than retinol. Besides, what does double the amount mean anyway? What is being doubled? You can double zero, but you still have zero. Plus, retinol in any amount isn't going to plump lips, not even a little. The double disappointment—(1) insufficient sunscreen and (2) minimal presence of state-of-the-art ingredients plus packaging that won't keep them stable—makes this a lip product to avoid.

☹ POOR **Moisture Therapy Intensive Moisturizing Lip Treatment SPF 15** *($0.99 for 0.15 fl. oz.)* is not a good choice for daytime wear if your goal is sun protection for the lips. That's because the active ingredients do not provide sufficient UVA protection. Just as with facial or body sunscreens, you want to make sure one or more of these ingredients are listed as active: avobenzone, titanium dioxide, zinc oxide, Mexoryl SX (ecamsule), or Tinosorb.

AVON SPECIALTY SKIN-CARE PRODUCTS

☺ GOOD **Clearskin Professional Acne Mark Treatment** *($12 for 1.7 fl. oz.)*. Acne marks are a concern for many. Although a breakout may go away in a matter of days (or sooner with proper treatment), the pink, red, or brown marks they leave behind may linger for months. When you have lots of these on your face, you understandably want to take action, but can this Clearskin product help? The tube packaging is outfitted with a roller ball applicator that dispenses a thin layer of a lightweight BHA (salicylic acid) exfoliant. Salicylic acid (present here in a 2% concentration) can help fade acne marks by reducing inflammation and also enhancing cell turnover. The catch is that in order for it to be effective, it needs to be formulated within a narrow pH range—and this product is! That means it is a very good, effective BHA exfoliant to use on red marks or all over your face. The texture is best for normal to oily or combination skin. Drawbacks include the somewhat sticky finish (though it's tolerable) and the inclusion of fragrance. Thankfully the amount of fragrance is low but in any amount, fragrance isn't skin care. Also disappointing is the lack of anti-irritants or antioxidants to help skin heal and become healthier. However, this is still worth considering because an effective exfoliant that can help fade red marks. Note that the inclusion of glycolic acid is likely too low to have an exfoliating action, but that's fine because the amount of salicylic acid does the job.

☺ AVERAGE **Clearskin Professional Clear Pore Thermal Mask** *($12 for 2.5 fl. oz.)* causes a warming sensation when it's mixed with water (or applied to damp skin), but that's merely a chemical reaction, it has no benefit for skin. It may feel pleasant, but it won't help acne, nor can it clear pores of the debris that's clogging them. Gimmicky products like this aren't anti-acne skin care, but they can be fun if you like that sort of thing.

☺ AVERAGE **Solutions Vibes Power Cleanser** *($15)*. This hand-held, battery-powered device is meant to be used with Avon's disposable Solutions Vibe Cleansing Pads (included with the device and also sold separately). When powered on, the device vibrates and supposedly makes the textured cleansing pads work better at removing dirt and excess oil by increasing the pressure and scrubbing action. Although the pads themselves are fine, the device is more gim-micky than useful, plus it's easy to get carried away and overdo the scrubbing part, damaging your skin's barrier and leading to dryness, flaking, and irritation.

☹ POOR **Anew Rejuvenate Mineral Facial Rinse-Off Treatment** *($25 for 1.7 fl. oz.)* is nothing more than a poorly formulated clay mask masquerading as a specialty product meant to leave skin looking smooth and poreless. The amount of alcohol it contains is potentially drying and irritating, not to mention that it causes free-radical damage and stimulates oil production at the base of the pore. None of the fermented minerals in this mask can shrink pores, but the absorbent nature of the clay can remove oil from the top portion of the pore, making it ap-pear smaller for a short while, similar to hundreds of other masks, many without the irritating ingredients this version contains. Avon also included their AHA alternative thiodipropionic acid and the BHA salicylic acid, but they are present in amounts too small for exfoliation, not to mention that the pH of this mask is not within the range needed for exfoliation to occur.

☹ POOR **Clearskin Blackhead Eliminating Deep Treatment Mask** *($5.49 for 2.5 fl. oz.)* contains the irritating menthol derivative menthyl lactate. Without it, this would be a very good option for those with oily, acne-prone skin. This mask is medicated with anti-acne ingredient salicylic acid, but the product's pH keeps it from working as an exfoliant—another strike. By the way, this mask won't eliminate blackheads. If it did, why is Avon selling so many other products claiming to do the same thing? The truth is blackheads can be hard to eliminate, and it takes persistent use of the right products, rather than occasional use of a mask, to do it.

☹ POOR **Clearskin Blemish Clearing Acne Pads** *($4.49 for 30 pads)*. Sigh… Here's yet another anti-acne product whose formula is based around alcohol. The 1% salicylic acid plus inclusion of AHAs is great, and the pH of the pads is within range for exfoliation to occur, but the alcohol's negative impact trumps all of that and makes this a problem for skin. See the Appendix to learn why alcohol is a problem for all skin types.

☹ POOR **Clearskin Blemish Clearing Spot Treatment** *($5.49 for 0.5 fl. oz.)*. Despite a 2% concentration of salicylic acid formulated at an effective pH for exfoliation to occur, this spot treatment contains too much alcohol to recommend. See the Appendix to learn why alcohol is a problem for all skin types. Unless your acne is occasional and minor in nature, spot treating tends to just cause you to chase blemishes all over your face—as soon as one area heals, more show up elsewhere, and the chase continues.

⊗ POOR **Clearskin Professional Acne Treatment System** *($32)*. Avon heavily promotes this trio of anti-acne products as an even better version of the popular infomercial brand ProActiv. You can go ahead and read this entire review for the details if you like, or you can stop right now, because we assure you that this system is not as effective as ProActiv. The reasons, you ask? (1) the formulas include needless irritants and (2) they do not include a topical disinfectant to fight the bacteria that contribute to acne. Avon claims their exclusive zinc hexapeptide-11 ingredient warrants their superior difference because it helps control surface oil. That's not much of a claim when you consider how many other cosmetic ingredients have the same action, such as kaolin, certain silicone polymers, talc, and aluminum starch to name a few. If it can work in some other manner, there is no published research proving that to be true, so consumers just have to take Avon's word for it and the ingredient manufacturer (and we all know how trustworthy cosmetics companies can be about their claims—not to mention, this isn't the first product Avon has claimed would clear up your acne, clearly the ones that came before didn't work so well). Avon makes a great fuss of the fact that this ingredient is exclusive to their formula, but exclusivity doesn't equate to exclusive results. Their oil claim is not unique and their ingredient not the only apple in the barrel. Interestingly, however, there is a growing body of research demonstrating zinc's second-tier role in minimizing acne. The research deals primarily with the oral consumption of zinc, but there have been some intriguing in vitro studies as well that show zinc's role as an anti-inflammatory agent when applied to cultured skin cells (Sources: *Seminars in Cutaneous Medicine and Surgery*, September 2008, pages 170–176; *European Journal of Dermatology*, November-December 2007, pages 492–496; *Journal of the European Academy of Dermatology and Venereology*, March 2007, pages 311–319; and *The Journal of Dermatological Treatment*, 2006, pages 205–210). However, none of these studies examined what role zinc hexapeptide-11 may have in mitigating acne, reducing inflammation, or affecting oil production. There are three products in this kit: a cleanser/scrub, pre-soaked medicated pads, and a salicylic acid (BHA) lotion. The **Deep Pore Cleansing Scrub** contains a tiny amount of the abrasive agent polyethylene mixed with water, clay, detergent cleansing agent, and alcohol. It features 0.5% salicylic acid as an active ingredient, but this small amount and the fact that the product is rinsed from the skin before it can have a benefit assures minimal to no efficacy. In addition, the scrub also contains menthol, which is irritating, and the formula isn't the easiest to rinse from skin, so we're not off to a good start. Step 2 involves swabbing your skin with **Clarifying Toner Pads**. Avon again disappoints with an alcohol-laden formula and irritating cinnamon bark extract. Alcohol causes free-radical damage, inflammation, and hurts the skin's healing process. What a shame, because there are some state-of-the-art ingredients in this product. The last step is to apply the **Daily Correcting Lotion**, which contains 0.5% salicylic acid, just like the pads in step 2. As a leave-on BHA product this almost has merit for skin. The small amount of salicylic acid isn't necessarily ideal, but the serious cause for concern is the amount of alcohol in this lotion. All told, there is little reason to try this kit. What Avon claims makes it unique isn't proven, and even if it worked as claimed, at best you'd enjoy less oily skin (temporarily) at the expense of causing lots of irritation and doing little to kill acne-causing bacteria. ProActiv and any other cosmetics company making effective, yet gentle, anti-acne products have nothing to worry about with this problematic trio from Avon.

⊗ POOR **Clearskin Professional Daily Correcting Lotion** *($16 for 2 fl. oz.)*. Here's a prime example of why Clearskin Professional is a joke: Many of the regular Clearskin products from Avon contain an effective amount of salicylic acid (BHA), yet the Professional version contains 0.5%, an amount that won't do much for those with persistent, stubborn acne. How is that professional? It isn't, nor is the inclusion of an irritating amount of alcohol along with cinnamon bark extract, which can increase oil production, further clogging pores. There are some intriguing ingredients in this BHA lotion, but they're saddled with the problematic ingredients destined to make acne and oily skin worse. For better results and a slam-dunk formula you can rely on, consider the anti-acne products from Paula's Choice CLEAR line instead.

⊗ POOR **Clearskin Professional Invisible Blemish Treatment** (*$12 for 0.5 fl. oz.*). This anti-acne product with 2% salicylic acid isn't worth considering and is about as far from a professional solution to acne as you can get. With alcohol as the second ingredient, this is a problem for all skin types. You may notice some initial benefit, but because alcohol can stimulate oil production at the base of your pores, you're essentially setting your skin up for more blemishes. What a shame, because without the alcohol (and, to a lesser extent, the witch hazel), this would've been a slam-dunk for acne-prone skin. The formula contains some very good anti-irritants and its pH permits the salicylic acid to exfoliate, but your skin doesn't deserve or need to suffer from the alcohol it contains.

AVON FOUNDATIONS & PRIMERS

✓☺ BEST **Smooth Minerals Pressed Foundation** (*$11*) is an outstanding medium-to-full coverage pressed-powder foundation for all skin types. The texture is creamy and smooth, if a bit dry, yet the effect is incredibly skin-like, leaving a luminous, non-chalky glow without shimmer (with the exception of those in the Deep shade range, which have noticeable shine). The "mineral" designation is silly, but many women have been brainwashed into thinking "mineral" powders are better for them, so everyone in the cosmetics industry slaps the word "mineral" on their products. Regardless of the name, it goes on beautifully, without exaggerating lines or caking around blemishes. The shades are equally impressive, with workable options for both fair and medium-to-dark skin tones. Nutmeg proved to be an especially lovely neutral shade for dark skin tones, while Spice was a bit too orange. Rather than gunk up your brushes, this foundation applies better with a sponge, but a brush can work if you desire more sheer coverage. Though it lacks an SPF rating, Smooth Minerals applies well over moisturizer with sunscreen, and there's enough titanium dioxide and other sunscreen ingredients in the formula that it wouldn't be a surprise if Avon announces later on that this does indeed provide some sun protection.

☺ GOOD **Ideal Flawless Invisible Coverage Liquid Foundation SPF 15** (*$11*). This liquid foundation with sunscreen has a wonderfully light, yet lush texture that feels substantial, but not heavy on normal, dry, or very dry skin. The texture is very blendable, but because it's highly pigmented, it doesn't sheer out easily (which means finding the perfect shade is essential). As it sets, the foundation meshes with skin and sets to a soft matte finish with a hint of luminosity. The overall effect is medium to full coverage that looks surprisingly natural, and it lasts through the day. The inclusion of titanium dioxide means that broad-spectrum sunscreen is assured, and the pump bottle is a nice touch! So why did this otherwise stellar foundation not earn our top rating? The inclusion of an irritating form of alcohol could spell trouble for your skin. Though the amount isn't huge, there are plenty of foundations that don't include any irritants, so the question becomes why consider this over those that present no risk of irritating your skin? Shades run from fair to dark, but the deepest shades—Earth, Dark Cocoa, and Rich Espresso—do not have an SPF rating, which is disappointing. These shades also have a thinner texture and a slight sheen to their finish.

☺ GOOD **Ideal Shade Cream-to-Powder Foundation SPF 15** (*$10*) claims to contain essential true-tone pigments to match any skin tone, but that doesn't explain why several shades of this cream-to-powder makeup don't resemble real skin tones in the least. Cover Girl and L'Oreal did much better with their foundations, for which they make similar claims. More creamy than powdery, this compact foundation from Avon applies smoothly and blends easily—you can quickly achieve sheer, uniform coverage. The finish hints at being powdery, but any oily areas will be showing shine before you know it. This is a potential winner for those with normal to dry skin, and it's great that the sunscreen is in-part titanium dioxide. Many of the shades are impressive; the ones to avoid due to overtones of pink, peach, or orange include Light Ivory, Cream Beige, Medium Beige, Soft Honey, and Nutmeg.

☺ AVERAGE **Anew Beauty Age-Transforming Foundation SPF 15** *($16)* is a beauty first! This silky liquid foundation not only provides an in-part titanium dioxide sunscreen, but contains approximately 3% glycolic acid at a pH of 3.4, which permits exfoliation. It blends smoothly and offers light to medium coverage with a satin finish that feels moist. So why didn't this innovative foundation receive our highest rating? Because, for all its positive traits, it looks very much like a layer of makeup sitting on top of your skin. The formula settles easily into lines, large pores, and facial crevices, and trying to soften this effect noticeably diminishes the coverage it provides. If you decide the benefit of sun protection and AHA exfoliation is worth the trade-off, there are some suitably neutral colors among the shades.

☺ AVERAGE **ExtraLasting Cream-to-Powder Foundation SPF 15** *($12)*. For a foundation claiming 18-hour wear, this one's overall staying power is sparse at best. The coverage is light initially (and can be built up to medium with blending and layering), but within a few hours the color begins to fade and appear splotchy. One claim it does live up to is water resistance, and though the color may fade, it does stay put; we know that sounds odd, but that's exactly what happens. Cream-to-powder foundations are typically great for normal to combination skin types because of their dry, powdery finish, but this version with built-in broad-spectrum sunscreens contains emollient ingredients that leave a slightly greasy satin finish that will make any oiliness look and feel worse. The formula and finish make it best suited for dry skin. The range of fair to dark shades is impressive, but they're not one-for-one matches of the other ExtraLasting formulas that have the same shade names, which makes it confusing to coordinate shades if you use more than one formula. Speaking of shades, note that the darker shades—Earth, Dark Cocoa, and Rich Espresso—are not SPF-rated and have a slightly slicker texture and a more dewy finish.

☺ AVERAGE **MagiX Face Perfector SPF 20** *($10)* does not contain active ingredients capable of protecting skin from the full range of UVA light, so its use as a sunscreen is not recommended. As a primer for those with oily skin, it is capable of creating a very smooth, matte surface for makeup while keeping excess oil in check for a period of time (the length of time depends on how oily your skin is and what skin-care products you use). The silicone-heavy formula has a silky, dry finish, but cannot "perfect" skin better than many other primers or, better yet, silicone-enhanced serums loaded with antioxidants. Despite this product's merit as a primer, it doesn't deserve better than an average rating because of its deficient sunscreen.

☹ POOR **MagiX Cashmere Finish Liquid Foundation SPF 10** *($11)*. This medium to full coverage, long-wearing liquid foundation had a lot of promise, but ultimately disappoints in nearly every way. The mousse-like texture is easy to apply and blend, and it sets to a flattering matte finish, but in two of the three full-size tubes tested, the product had separated, and even vigorous shaking couldn't restore it to its original "cashmere" texture. As delighted as we were to see that Avon included titanium dioxide for broad-spectrum sunscreen protection, the SPF 10 doesn't meet the minimum SPF 15 that is recommended by almost every medical board in the world. The strong fragrance didn't help matters, either. The final straw was the shades: Almost all are too pink, orange, or ash.

☹ POOR **Smooth Minerals Foundation** *($12)* is definitely smoother and less dry than Avon's previous loose-powder mineral makeup, but it has its own set of problems. The main issue is that the formula isn't easy to blend. It quickly grabs to any moist areas of skin, and that affects how the color looks. The result is uneven, with the slightly moist areas getting moderate coverage and the drier areas getting sheer, spotty coverage. This finishes to a satiny glow, but still feels dry. Those with dry skin or dry areas will feel their skin getting progressively drier after several hours of wear, while those with oily skin will likely find it pools in large pores and looks blotchy. No mineral makeup is worth this much compromise. Most of the shades are too peach, orange, copper, or rose to come close to resembling real skin tones, so it's back to the drawing board, Avon!

AVON CONCEALERS

☺ GOOD **Anew Beauty Age-Transforming Concealer SPF 15** *($10)* provides the benefits of an illuminating concealer, an in-part titanium dioxide sunscreen, and glycolic acid in one concealer. The pH of 3.6 allows the glycolic acid (present at about 3%) to exfoliate, but such exfoliation isn't needed for the immdiate under-eye area, which is precisely where this concealer is likely to be applied. The click-pen applicator dispenses the product onto a brush, and although initially too slippery, it sets quickly to a matte (in feel) finish that has a soft shimmer. Coverage is moderate; this hides minor redness and dark circles, but requires layering for more pronounced flaws. Six shades are available: Natural Golden is slightly peach, but may work for some medium skin tones; Natural Deep turns slightly ash due to the amount of titanium dioxide it contains; Natural Medium is too pinky-peach and best avoided. Based on the formula, this will make skin smoother and protect it from sun damage—just be cautious about using it too close to the eye due to the acidic pH.

☺ GOOD **Ideal Shade Concealer Stick** *($6)* has a thick texture with minimal slip, so initial application is tricky. It is best applied in small dots that you blend together with a concealer brush or clean fingertip. The fact that this concealer has minimal movement impedes blending a bit, but ends up being advantageous because it stays in place and is prone to only minor creasing into lines. This provides excellent coverage, so unless you have a very dark spot or extreme redness you'll be pleased with the results. Almost all the shades are recommended. Be careful with the slightly peach Light Medium and avoid the orange-y Dark shade. Fair, Light, and Neutral are the best of the bunch. Two more comments: The waxes and thickening agents make this concealer a poor choice for use on blemishes. Also, this contains ethylhexyl methoxycinnamate, a sunscreen ingredient that may cause irritation when used around the eye. If you notice any stinging or burning when you use this concealer under your eyes, it may very well be due to this ingredient.

AVON POWDERS

✓☺ BEST **ExtraLasting Pressed Powder SPF 15** *($11)* is everything you could want in a powder: shine control, broad-spectrum sun protection, soft matte finish, and a finely milled texture that's easily picked up with a brush and doesn't appear cakey on skin. Truly impressive, as is Avon's shade range, which runs from translucent all the way to shades for dark skin tones (though Fawn, Mocha, and Toffee have no SPF rating, which is puzzling). This formula will work for all skin types, except dry to very dry.

✓☺ BEST **Ideal Shade Loose Powder** *($9)*. This talc- and mica-based powder is said to contain light-adjusting pigments so your skin looks its best in any light. The goal is to "glow without the glare," but we've never seen any powder look glaring on anyone's skin, although they can look shiny. Just to be clear, cosmetic pigments used in powders (such as iron oxides) have nothing to do with shine—that's where the mica (a pearlescent mineral pigment) comes into play. The good news is that this loose powder does add a glow without adding noticeable "glaring" shine. You won't see an adjustment taking place as you go from indoor to outdoor lighting as claimed (other than what light does to shiny particles on the face normally); rather, this powder looks fantastic on skin regardless of the lighting. It has a beautifully silky texture and seamless application; its overall effect and formula are best for those with normal to dry skin. All the shades are great, including the two offered for darker skin tones.

AVON BLUSHES

☺ GOOD **Smooth Minerals Blush** *($10)*. Loose powder is not the best for applying blush, even if you're a fan of mineral makeup. Avon's version has a smooth yet noticeably dry texture that must be applied very sheer or it tends to deposit unevenly, making skin look blotchy instead of softly blushed with color. The shine is of the sparkling variety and it clings decently. Although we suspect most women who want powder blush will prefer pressed instead of loose, this is a viable option for shiny cheeks.

☺ GOOD **True Color Blush** *($8)* has a smooth, dry texture and soft, non-powdery application. The palette offers enough enticing options to make this a worthwhile option, but bear in mind that every shade has at least a slight shine. Rose Lustre and Golden Glow Light/Medium have the most shine, though the latter is an acceptable shimmer powder for evening. Earthen Rose is a great tan color for contouring.

AVON EYESHADOWS

☺ GOOD **Jillian Dempsey Professional Perfect Eyes Kit** *($9)*. Cleverly designed, this eyeshadow palette opens to reveal shadow pans segmented into distinct eye area shapes (crease, brow bone, eyeliner, etc.) that make creating an eyeshadow design quite easy—if not foolproof. The texture of the powder shadows is pleasantly smooth, with a vibrant, shimmery finish that blends easily and doesn't flake. The only element of the kit that's lacking is the powder liner, which doesn't deliver rich enough color whether applied wet or dry. The overall pan size is generous, making this a real value if you find one of the four kits to your liking.

☺ AVERAGE **Extralasting Powder Eyeshadow** *($9)* is a loose-powder eyeshadow that comes with a pointed sponge-tip applicator. Why these products keep showing up is anyone's guess—a pressed-powder eyeshadow is so much easier to work with. Although this isn't all that messy to use and the formula sets almost immediately and then doesn't move, you're still left with a stripe of intense shine that may temporarily blind anyone who catches your gaze (OK, we're exaggerating, but you get the idea). The sponge-tip applicator hurts more than it helps; however, even if you shake some powder out and attempt to apply it with an eyeshadow brush, it grabs on skin right away and won't move, which you might at first think is a good thing, but only if a stripe of glitter is what you are looking for. With all of these drawbacks, does it really matter how long this lasts?

☹ POOR **True Color Eyeshadow Quad** *($9)* has a smooth texture but not the best application. Every shade in these quads is shiny (and the shine tends to flake), making for an overall eye design that's shine overload, not to mention that most of the color combinations are unworkable or predominantly blue, green, or purple.

AVON EYE & BROW LINERS

☺ GOOD **Glimmersticks Brow Definer** *($7)* has been improved and now this automatic, retractable brow pencil is a strong contender for enhancing brows. Its four colors (including a good option for blonde brows) go on smoothly and evenly, each with a soft powder finish that lasts.

☺ GOOD **Glimmersticks Waterproof Eye Liner** *($7)* applies easily and the retractable pencil doesn't require sharpening, which is always a plus. These glide so well you'll need to be extra careful to not over-apply, and each slightly to moderately shiny shade sets to a fairly immovable finish. True to the name, this is a waterproof formula, though it does come off with a water-soluble cleanser.

☺ GOOD **SuperShock Eye Liner** *($7)*. This waterproof, smudge-proof, and all-around budge-proof gel eyeliner will absolutely stay put once it sets. The gel texture is smooth, but applies somewhat sheer and on the dry side, which means you'll need patience, precision, and a good eyeliner brush to dramatically define the eye. All four shades are infused with metallic shimmer, and it comes off easily with a good makeup remover.

☺ AVERAGE **Big Color Eye Pencil** *($7)* is a standard chunky pencil with a smooth, silicone-enhanced application and a soft, slightly creamy finish. Every color is quite shiny and most are pastel, but if that's your thing these do hold up reasonably well.

☺ AVERAGE **ExtraLasting Eye Liner** *($9)*. This inkwell-style liquid liner applies smoothly and sets to a semi-gloss finish. Avon claims it stays put for up to 12 hours, but we noticed smudging around the corners of the eye by lunch, and by the end of the day the color had started to fade. That's a shame because the wet formula creates quite dramatic emphasis along the lashline, largely due to the flexible felt-tip applicator.

☺ AVERAGE **Ultra Luxury Brow Liner** *($6)* is an ordinary brow pencil that has a typical dry texture, but it is easier to apply than most. The price is right, and this is one to consider if you prefer brow pencil to powder and don't mind routine sharpening.

☺ AVERAGE **Ultra Luxury Eye Liner** *($6)* has an attractive price for a standard pencil that applies easily and offers a smooth, dry finish. This is still prone to mild smearing as the day wears on.

☹ POOR **Glimmersticks Eye Liner** *($7)* is an automatic, retractable pencil with a texture that's too creamy to last for long, particularly as eyeliner. If you prefer pencils, there are better ones available in this price range from Revlon, L'Oreal, and others.

AVON LIP COLOR & LIPLINERS

✓☺ BEST **Glazewear Liquid Lip Color/Glazewear Metallics Lip Gloss** *($6)* is a very good, medium-coverage lip gloss that has a slick application and a non-sticky, glossy finish. The color range is extensive and gorgeous, owing to this product's deserved popularity. Avon occasionally rotates in Glazewear Metallics Lip Gloss, which differs little from original Glazewear save for its metallic finish.

☺ GOOD **Extralasting Lipstick** *($9)*. This silky, lightweight lipstick is supposed to be transfer-resistant, but it isn't. Even once it sets to a slight matte finish it comes off easily—on cups, significant others, napkins, forks, spoons, and anything else your lips touch. The good news is that the color intensity is so strong that it takes several hours for the color to fade to the

---

point where a touch-up is necessary (though all bets are off if you try to get through an entire meal with this intact). The only other point worth mentioning (other than Avon's impressive, versatile shade selection) is that this isn't the most comfortable lipstick unless you're used to the somewhat dry feel of matte and other transfer-resistant lipsticks. That's not a deal-breaker, but know beforehand that this isn't going to feel lush and creamy for long.

☺ GOOD **Glimmersticks Lipliner** *($7)*. If it weren't for this automatic, retractable lipliner's somewhat tacky finish, it would be among the best for smooth application and ability to keep lipstick from feathering into lines around the mouth. As is, it's recommended for those willing to tolerate the finish, though that becomes less of an issue when paired with a lipstick.

☺ GOOD **Lip Stain Marker** *($9)* is packaged just like a felt-tip marker, which makes application as easy as using a pen, although the applicator may be too small for those with ample lips. While the formula doesn't grab onto dry skin or travel around on lips (a big complaint with many liquid stains), the trade-off is that this one doesn't feel great on your lips. Although its sticky texture and dry feel may be hard to get used to, the transfer-resistant color stays true for hours and fades evenly. The four shades look quite different on lips than they appear on the packaging.

☺ GOOD **Ultra Color Rich Lipstick** *($7)* is a traditional creamy lipstick with a large selection of full-coverage colors, most with a satin finish.

☹ AVERAGE **Satin Satisfaction Lip Color SPF 15** *($8)* delivers smooth, rich color that looks and feels fabulous on lips. The pop of color along with the creamy texture make it extra unfortunate that the sunscreen portion does not supply adequate UVA (think anti-aging) sun-protecting ingredients. What's the point of using an SPF-rated lip product if you're leaving your lips vulnerable to sun damage? See the Appendix to find out why the right UVA-protecting ingredients matter.

☹ AVERAGE **Smooth Minerals Lip Gloss SPF 15** *($9)* omits adequate UVA protection necessary for anti-aging benefits. This is otherwise outstanding. Packaged in a tube with a wand applicator is an exceptionally smooth, non-sticky gloss with lots of reflective flecks of shimmer that don't feel gritty as the moisture wears away. There are plenty of shades available, but all contain shimmer and go on quite sheer.

☹ AVERAGE **SuperShock Liquid Lip Shine SPF 15** *($8)*. The only thing all that shocking about this otherwise ordinary lip gloss with sunscreen is that it lacks adequate UVA-protecting ingredients to shield your lips from the sun's most aging rays. Your lips deserve sufficient broad-spectrum sun protection, but this SPF-rated product falls short. Note that the oversize applicator makes it tricky to apply, especially if you have a small mouth or thin lips. See the Appendix to find out which UVA-protecting ingredients you should look for.

☹ AVERAGE **Ultra Color Rich Moisture Seduction Lipstick SPF 15** *($8)* claims to deliver a 500% boost in moisture, and indeed, its moisturizing ingredients make your lips feel soft and hydrated, but also a little greasy. Although greasy, this lipstick feels lightweight and delivers a good stain, even if it does bleed slightly into lines around the mouth—a typical problem for even slightly greasy lipsticks. The 500% boost in moisture claim is meaningless; 500% moisture can be overkill and actually cause your lips to become drier. Keeping water-balance in lips is a good thing, which almost any lipstick or gloss can do. Even if this were a perfect lipstick, its sunscreen doesn't provide sufficient UVA (think anti-aging) protection, which makes this one to skip. See the Appendix to find out which UVA-protecting ingredients you should look for.

☹ AVERAGE **Ultra Luxury Lipliner** *($6)* has a great price for a standard pencil that isn't too dry or too creamy for precise application. The fact that it needs sharpening prevents it from earning a Good rating.

AVON MASCARAS

☺ GOOD **ExtraLasting Mascara** *($9)*. Those seeking length and definition will likely love this waterproof mascara's effect. The tapered rubber bristles on the slender brush separate and perfectly coat each lash from root to tip, resulting in fringed and fluttery lashes. A second coat (applied before the first one dries) amplifies the effect. What's not to love, you ask? The "extralasting" claim. Indeed, this mascara won't flake, smudge, smear, or run, but trouble comes at the end of the day—we needed several applications of makeup remover and a good amount of elbow grease to remove all traces.

☺ GOOD **Super Curlacious Mascara** *($9)*. Curling lashes is what this mascara is supposed to do, and it does so quite well. Mind you, your lashes won't be as precisely curled as if you had used an eyelash curler, but this goes on smoothly and leaves lashes noticeably fringed and uplifted. Length and thickness are respectable and this doesn't clump. Removal is easy with just a water-soluble cleanser. The only drawback, and it's minor, is that this tends to make lashes feel stiffer than many other mascaras.

☺ GOOD **Supershock Mascara** *($9)* is described as Avon's boldest mascara, one that's capable of delivering twelve times your lash's normal volume in a single step. Let's get real here: This is an impressive mascara, but building lashes to "larger than life proportions" is not in its bag of tricks. The large applicator has a brush that contains many tiny, thin bristles that stand up straight. A few coats produces lots of length, but building thickness (volume) is difficult. This is worth considering if you're looking for clump-free length and reliable wear with easy removal. But if you want to spend less and get more bang for your buck, Cover Girl's Lash Blast Mascara trounces this because it allows you to build on the results without messing up a careful application.

☹ AVERAGE **Super Extend Mascara** *($9)* claims to visibly lengthen top lashes by 55%, which is true, but the same could be said for any number of lengthening mascaras. Although this applies easily and evenly, the formula causes the top and bottom lashes to stick together slightly, which is not only uncomfortable, but also unsightly. There are far too many excellent and affordable mascaras on the market to have to tolerate anything less than great.

☹ AVERAGE **SuperShock Max Mascara** *($9)* claims "shocking results" in one sweep, and indeed, you can achieve impressive volume and thickness with a single swipe of its robust brush. However, the instant thickness can look goopy if you don't take extra care to comb through your lashes, and don't add too much more mascara or the goopiness will quickly overtake your lashes, no matter how much you comb through them. All this work may be for naught, though, because this mascara flakes within a few hours. Initially, the results are impressive, but a truly great mascara stays on your lashes, not your skin, through the day.

☹ AVERAGE **Wash-Off Waterproof Mascara** *($6.50)* is oddly named, because you don't expect a mascara to wash off, right? This one does, though as with most waterproof mascaras, you'll need more than a water-soluble cleanser to remove it completely. The real question is why anyone would bother with this lackluster mascara. It provides some length without clumps or smears, but no thickness. That's not terrible, but far better waterproof mascaras are available for the same amount of money at the drugstore.

AVON MARK

Strengths: Mostly good foundations; incredible powders; great inexpensive eyeshadow; good shimmer products; good cleansers; outstanding daytime moisturizer with SPF 30; some worthwhile moisturizers.

Weaknesses: Some of the makeup brushes fail to impress even a little bit; the products for oily and acne-prone skin are mostly unimpressive and needlessly irritating.

For more information and reviews of the latest Avon Mark products, visit CosmeticsCop.com.

AVON MARK CLEANSERS

☺ GOOD **Calming Effect Comforting Milk Cleanser** *($9 for 6.7 fl. oz.)* is a very good, inexpensive water-soluble cleanser for all skin types except for very oily. It contains some notable soothing agents, though their effect in a cleanser won't add up to much given how quickly it is either removed or rinsed from skin. A strong point is this takes off makeup without drying skin. It contains fragrance in the form of vanilla and banana fruit extracts, but those have little to no risk of causing irritation.

☺ GOOD **That's Deep Purifying Gel Cleanser** *($9 for 6.7 fl. oz.)*. Although this doesn't clean deeper than any other water-soluble cleanser, it is a good option for normal to oily skin. Makeup comes off easily and skin is left soft and refreshed. This contains fragrance in the form of black currant and orange flower.

☹ POOR **Help Wanted Anti-Acne Exfoliating Cleanser Apple/Cinnamon** *($10 for 5 fl. oz.)* is a very fragrant cleanser that contains many problematic ingredients acne-prone skin doesn't need. Chief among them are the fragrant plant extracts (is this potpourri or a cleanser?) that include cinnamon, apply, rosemary, and peppermint. This also contains a skin-confusing mix of ingredients that add up to a cleanser that's difficult to move over wet skin and also tricky to rinse. The amount of salicylic acid (an anti-acne superstar) is too low to be of much benefit, not to mention it will be rinsed before it really has a chance to work.

AVON MARK SCRUB

☹ POOR **Berry Grand Super Exfoliating Beads** *($9 for 0.8 fl. oz.)*. This tiny product contains a blend of dry ingredients you mix with water and use as a face scrub. Although that's the intention, the ingredients (while natural) make for an abrasive way to polish your skin. Rice powder is OK, but the corn cob meal and apricot seed powder can be too rough when they're not in a base to cushion them (water alone doesn't cut it). If you prefer a scrub, there are better options to consider. Ultimately, exfoliating with a well-formulated AHA or BHA product is a far better way to go for all skin types, including teens and young adults.

AVON MARK MOISTURIZERS (DAYTIME & NIGHTTIME) & EYE CREAMS

✓☺ BEST **For Goodness Face Antioxidant Skin Moisturizing Lotion SPF 30** *($18 for 1.7 fl. oz.)*. What a great name and, thankfully, it is also a great sunscreen with the actives including in-part avobenzone (for UVA protection) in a lightweight moisturizing base. All in all, it is a very good daytime moisturizer for normal to oily skin. The airless jar packaging helps keep the many antioxidants and plant extracts in here stable during use, and it also contains a cell-communicating ingredient. Some of the plant extracts are fragrant, but their antioxidant ability offsets this minor setback.

☺ GOOD **Light Bright Lighten & Depuff Eye Gel** *($8 for 0.17 fl. oz.)* contains over a dozen plant extracts, none of which are capable of reducing puffy eyes or dark circles. The main plant extract is lotus, and Avon maintains this reduces the look of tired eyes. Don't count on it: the research on lotus doing anything of the sort is conspicuously absent. Some of the plant extracts are there for fragrance, while others have anti-irritant ability or function as antioxidants. All told, this is a good lightweight moisturizer for slightly dry skin anywhere on the face—just don't count on any of the eye-area claims to actually come true.

☺ GOOD **See Things Clearly Brightening Moisturizer** *($18 for 1.7 fl. oz.)* is a very good shimmery finish moisturizer (the shimmer provides the brightening effect) for normal to slightly dry or slightly oily skin. It contains an impressive amount of antioxidants and cell-communicating ingredients along with a tiny amount of water-binding agents. Some of the plant extracts are potentially irritating, but this is likely offset by the nonirritating plant extracts that precede them. The airless jar packaging will help keep the antioxidant ingredients stable during use.

☹ AVERAGE **Need a Shrink? Pore Minimizer Lotion** *($8 for 0.17 fl. oz.)*. The clever name doesn't reflect a clever product. While it would be nice if this could make pores smaller, at best the absorbent ingredients that comprise the bulk of the formula will help keep excess oil in check for a short period of time. Keeping skin matte can help pores look smaller (pores look larger and more apparent when they're engorged with oil), but that in and of itself doesn't actually reduce their size. Like it or not, pore size is genetically determined and no skin-care product has a permanent effect on reducing their size. This is merely an OK lightweight moisturizer for oily skin, but several of the plant extracts are potentially irritating.

☹ POOR **Calm & Composed Super-Soothing Moisturizer** *($18 for 1.7 fl. oz.)*. To soothe and calm sensitive, reddened skin that's also dry, you first need a product that doesn't contain any irritants. Avon missed the mark on that essential detail because this product contains fragrance which, in any form, synthetic or natural, is irritating. Irritating already-sensitive skin can lead to a host of problems, the least of which is ongoing redness, but irritation also hurts skin's healing process and damages healthy collagen production, making it all but impossible for sensitive skin to really improve.

☹ POOR **Matte Chance Mattifying Lotion** *($18 for 1.7 fl. oz.)* lists alcohol as the second ingredient, which negates the worthwhile ingredients in this serum-type product and makes it too irritating and drying for all skin types. Clinique, Paula's Choice, and Smashbox offer much better products to help keep skin matte without the "chance" of irritation.

AVON MARK SPECIALTY SKIN-CARE PRODUCTS

☹ POOR **Back Me Up Anti-Acne Back Treatment Liquid Spray Apple/Cinnamon** *($10 for 4 fl. oz.)*. This spray-on BHA (salicylic acid) product is a great idea for treating acne, whether on the back or anywhere else from the neck down. Though applying creams and lotions to the back is difficult as a solo task, acne on the back should not be left untreated. The problem is that this BHA mist is a terrible way to go about improving acne. While the 2% salicylic acid content and the effective pH are strong points, the base formula contains alcohol and witch hazel, not to mention cinnamon bark. All three of these ingredients, especially the alcohol, are damaging to skin (see the Appendix for further details). Avon Mark also added so much fragrance to this product that it seems more like Febreze® for your back instead of an acne treatment. Keep in mind that fragrance is not skin care.

☹ POOR **Blemish Banisher Anti-Acne Treatment Pads Apple/Cinnamon** *($12 for 50 pads)* are a mixed bag of good and bad ingredients. The good part is the blend of 1% salicylic acid with a decent amount of glycolic acid that could be helpful for exfoliation, even though the salicylic acid would be completely effective on its own from a treatment point of view. When it comes to acne, glycolic acid isn't all that effective because it can't penetrate through the oil in the pore and it doesn't remove dead skin cells from the surface of the skin as well as salicylic acid. The bad news is that the pH of these pads doesn't allow the salicylic acid to function as an exfoliant, plus the formula contains several irritants, including peppermint, cinnamon, and rosemary, and a lot of alcohol. Irritants of any kind, especially alcohol, can stimulate oil production at the base of your pores, hurt the skin's healing process, and cause collagen to break down. All of this adds up to a headache for your skin, making it more red and inflamed—given that acne is red enough on its own, why add fuel to the fire? The apple cinnamon should be for your oatmeal in the morning, not part of your skin-care routine.

☹ POOR **Break Out Plan Anti-Acne Gel Lotion Apple/Cinnamon** *($18 for 1.7 fl. oz.)* is bad skin care. The apple cinnamon is better for you on oatmeal in the morning than it is for your skin. This product does contain a 1.5% concentration of salicylic acid, which is helpful for acne, but the pH of the lotion is too high for the salicylic acid to function very well as an exfoliant. What is really a breakout waiting to happen is the amount of alcohol, peppermint, cinnamon, and rosemary. These ingredients are seriously irritating and irritation hurts the skin's ability to heal, stimulates oil production at the base of your pores, and causes collagen to break down, all of which make acne worse, not better. The amount of redness and inflammation that accompanies these ingredients also will make acne look redder than it already is.

☹ POOR **Get Clearance Anti-Acne Blemish Treatment Gel** *($8 for 0.17 fl. oz.)*. Despite containing 2% salicylic acid, this ends up being another irritating anti-acne product due to the excessive and unnecessary amount of alcohol it contains. It is not recommended.

☹ POOR **Get Treatment Anti-Acne Overnight Fix Apple/Cinnamon** *($12 for 0.84 fl. oz.)* disappoints due to the amount of alcohol it contains. Alcohol is a bad ingredient for all skin types, as we explain in the Appendix. In addition to the alcohol, this also contains several fragrant irritants, making this anti-acne product even less impressive. It is medicated with 1.7% salicylic acid, a proven acne fighter, and the pH is within range of it to work, but the irritants mentioned above makes this a poor option to consider.

AVON MARK LIP CARE

☺ GOOD **Kiss Dry Goodbye Lip Smoother** *($8 for 0.17 fl. oz.)*. This emollient lip balm takes brilliant care of dry, chapped lips. Note: This is flavored with the artificial sweetener saccharin, a bit shocking given how out-of-date an ingredient that is, but you shouldn't be licking your lips anyway, so if you can avoid doing that the saccharin isn't much of a problem.

AVON MARK FOUNDATIONS & PRIMERS

☺ GOOD **Get A Tint Tinted Moisturizer Lotion SPF 15** *($12)* has a lotion-like consistency and provides titanium dioxide for sufficient UVA protection. Best for normal to slightly dry or slightly oily skin, it slips on evenly and blends readily to a sheer, moist finish. The colors tend toward being peach, with the most obvious being Honey/Golden. Avoid that shade. The others are acceptable but do not include options for fair or very dark skin tones.

☺ GOOD **Primed For Perfection Face Primer** *($10 for 0.4 fl. oz.)* is a standard but good foundation primer that, like most others of its ilk, contains silicones for a silky-smooth finish. It's nice that Avon includes some antioxidants, too, as many primers leave these important ingredients out. The formula also includes some dry-finish, mattifying ingredients to help absorb excess oil, making this best for normal to oily skin. Although the absorbent finish is a boon for oily skin, the inclusion of the shiny mineral pigment mica may not make those with oily skin happy; given that oily skin is already shiny, you certainly don't want to add more shine to your face.

AVON MARK CONCEALERS

✓☺ BEST **Get Bright Hook Up Highlighter** *($6.50)*. Accurately described as a pearly liquid highlighter, this lightweight fluid is easy to blend and adds just the right amount of subtle glow to skin. It is ideal for highlighting under the eyes, on the brow bone, or on top of cheekbones. The flesh-toned shades correspond to various skin tones, from fair to tan. All of these are sheer and can be used with or without foundation. Consider this inexpensive shine done right, especially if you've used more expensive highlighters, such as those from Giorgio Armani.

☺ AVERAGE **Save the Day Anti-Acne Concealer Stick** *($9)*. Covering a blemish is tricky: You want enough coverage to conceal redness, but not in a formula that will make matters worse. That's exactly the dilemma with this twist-up stick concealer: It offers nearly full coverage, but the formula is not recommended for use on acne- or blemish-prone skin because of its potential to clog pores and aggravate existing acne. That said, this blendable, matte-finish concealer is a good option for dealing with redness or discoloration from post-acne red marks for those who break out only occasionally. However, it's not for under-eye discolorations because the formula contains the anti-acne ingredient salicylic acid, which can be a problem for use so close to the eye. The bottom line: This concealer is not going to clear acne or make it heal faster, but the coverage and formula still has merit for discolorations if one of the shades proves a good match for your skin tone. This concealer's limitations keep it from earning a higher rating.

☹ POOR **Good Riddance Hook Up Concealer** *($6.50)* is a mini pencil concealer that needs routine sharpening, so expect its lifespan to be brief and usage more time-consuming than any other type of concealer. Actually, you can expect brief results, too, thanks to this concealer's thick, oil–based texture. It covers well and the shades are workable (Light/Medium is slightly peach), but it tends to crease mercilessly and fade within an hour. This simply isn't worth considering over several other concealers.

AVON MARK BLUSHES & BRONZER

✓☺ BEST **Bronze Pro Bronzing Powder** *($10)*. This incredibly smooth pressed-powder bronzer comes in a sturdy black plastic compact, complete with a half-moon natural-hair brush, which doesn't work as well as a big powder brush, but it's far better than a puff. The talc-based powder goes on evenly and can be easily layered to create a truly convincing tan because none of the three shades are too orange, red, or sparkly. In fact, Avon describes this product as being "lightly shimmery," but aside from a lovely glow, there's no detectable shimmer at all, making this an outstanding, affordable bronzing option worthy of our highest rating!

✓☺ BEST **Good Glowing Mosaic Blush** *($8)*. This pressed-powder blush has an almost creamy feel and a very smooth, even application that enlivens skin with soft to moderate shimmer (depending on how much you brush on). The mosaic pattern unites a range of complementary colors that come off as one shade on skin, so consider the design more of an aesthetic feature rather than a practical advantage. This inexpensive blush is recommended for anyone looking for glow-y cheeks and soft color.

✓☺ BEST **Just Pinched Instant Blush Tint** *($8)*. Fans of sheer cream blush, take note: This is an excellent option. The creamy formula isn't too slick, so blending can be more precise, yet the finish maintains a satin-like creaminess that makes this blush best for dry skin. It is not recommended for those prone to blemishes (powder blush is preferred). All the shades are attractive but their sheerness makes them preferred for fair to medium skin tones. This works well to create that soft, translucent color, but don't expect it to last all day without a touch-up.

☺ GOOD **Cheekblossom Cheek Color Tint** *($6.50)*. This silicone-based gel blush is supposed to react with your skin's chemistry to change color, but it ends up turning the same soft pink shade on anyone (think of mood lipsticks from the 60s, exact same concept). Those with darker skin will find the color barely registers even if you apply a lot of it. It has a silky, nearly weightless finish laced with subtle sparkles and is ultimately best for those with fair to light skin.

AVON MARK EYESHADOWS & EYE PRIMERS

☺ GOOD **I-Mark Custom Pick Eyeshadow** *($6)* wins points for its ultra-smooth texture that feels almost creamy and applies evenly without flaking. Since this makeup collection was designed to appeal to teens, it explains why almost half the shades are purple or pink. Still, there are some worthwhile, easy-to-work-with shades, plus the brighter-looking shades go on sheerer than they appear in the pan. Every shade has some amount of shine, but that shouldn't be a problem for teens and most young women prefer shiny eyeshadows anyway.

☹ POOR **Please Hold Eye Primer** *($8)* ends up missing the mark completely. The initial smooth, non-greasy texture seemed very promising, as did the easy blending on lids, but within an hour of wear we saw creasing and no enhanced staying power or richness of color in the eyeshadow. Even more disappointing was that this primer had the strange tendency to turn the lighter shadows orange. A liquid concealer with a matte finish is a great option to use as an eyeshadow primer.

AVON MARK EYE & BROW LINERS

✓☺ BEST **Keep It Going Longwear Eyeliner & Shadow** *($11)* has a creamy gel texture that can be used as an eyeliner and/or eyeshadow. The smudge- and flake-resistant formula glides on smoothly and easily before setting to a long-wearing finish. There are two shades, each housed in a cleverly designed compact featuring a tightly sealed protective cover so the formula won't dry out. The colors go on with dramatic intensity, and some have a metallic finish, but not all duos offered look good together (or even alone). For example, a metallic green and fuchsia combination is more futuristic and colorful than classic and understated, but if you want a bright, somewhat shocking eye design these colors get the job done. If you find a color pairing that suits you, this is an excellent eyeliner/eyeshadow option that delivers long-lasting results.

☺ GOOD **Get in Line Hook Up Waterproof Eyeliner** *($6.50)* must be shaken before use to distribute the cosmetic pigments. Once that's done, the firm brush makes it easy to draw an even line of soft color. This liquid eyeliner sets quickly to a subtle metallic finish, and is waterproof as claimed. Whether it wears for 10 hours depends on what else you've applied around your eyes and if you have oily eyelids. This doesn't hold up nearly as well as the numerous gel eyeliners available.

☺ GOOD **On the Edge Hook Up Liquid Eyeliner** *($6.50)* has a lot going for it! The long, thin brush isn't as precise as others that are shorter and have a pointed tip, but it works well to apply an even line of color (and the color doesn't peter out before you cover the entire lash line). The formula dries quickly and, once set, is generally impervious to smudging or flaking.

☺ GOOD **$$$ Brow Factor Hook Up Clear Brow Gel** *($6)* does a very good job of holding unruly brows in place without making them look or feel stiff. The spoolie brush is dense enough to get between even the thickest brows. While this product performs well, it's also overpriced: You get a very tiny amount of product (0.08 fl. oz.) in this specialty hook-up component (which is meant to "hook up" with another Avon Mark product of your choice on the other end of it).

☺ AVERAGE **What a Line Felt Tip Eyeliner** *($10)* is a very standard pen-style, felt-tip liquid eyeliner, but because the formula is on the dry side, it doesn't go on smoothly or evenly and the dry finish means it doesn't have the depth of color one would expect from a great liquid liner.

☺ AVERAGE **$$$ No Place to Run Longwear Eyeliner** *($9)* is a standard eyeliner pencil that can be blended before it quickly sets to a smudge-proof matte finish. True to claim, the stay-put formula is resistant to sweat, oil, and water, just like almost all eyeliner pencils. The shade selection is a mixture of classic and colorful options. If you don't mind routine sharpening this is a decent option; we would rate it higher if routine sharpening weren't part of the deal.

AVON MARK LIP COLORS

☺ GOOD **Gloss Gorgeous Stay On Lip Stain** *($11)*. Addressing the drying nature of lip stains, this click-pen version has an emollient gloss-like base that delivers equal amounts of moisture and tint. As the moisture and shine wear away, the tint remains, making this a very good, not to mention unique, lip stain option. The eight shades all appear brighter on the packaging than the color they deposit on lips, with Bella proving to be a very versatile red. One note: This does contain "aroma/flavor," which produces a fleeting tingle, although it pales in comparison to the intensity associated with poorly rated lip-plumping products.

☺ GOOD **Glow Baby Glow Luxe Hook Up Lip Gloss** *($6.50)* works fine as a lightweight, shimmery lip gloss. It comes in a tube with a brush applicator, and can be "hooked up" with other Mark products (concealer, mascara, nail polish) if desired. This gloss has a slick, non-sticky feel and imparts subtle color and lots of shine. A similar version called **Glow Baby Glow Hook Up Lip Gloss** *($6.50)* is also available. These shades have minimal to no shimmer and feature a sponge-tip applicator.

☺ GOOD **Lipclick Full Color Lipstick** *($11)* claims that it provides full coverage and has staying power. It does have a decent stain and it can stay in place for a few hours. The finish is slick, but not greasy, and it feels creamy and very lightweight on lips. The 12 shades include an impressive range of options for every skin tone, and none include shimmer. Wondering about the product's cute name? It's because the magnetic tube clicks shut after each application!

☺ AVERAGE **Juice Gems Squeeze On Lip Gloss with Real Fruit** *($7.50)* contains fruit extracts, which aren't the same as real fruit. That's a good thing, because real fruit wouldn't last long in a cosmetic. This is a standard, sheer, sticky lip gloss that has a potent fragrance (and, strangely, it isn't the least bit reminiscent of fruit).

☺ AVERAGE **Lipclick SPF 15 Color Shine Lipstick** *($11)*. Even though this lipstick goes on smoothly and imparts sheer color with a shiny finish and soft shimmer, it doesn't have the active ingredients necessary to ensure broad-spectrum sun protection. Please see the Appendix for details on the active sunscreen ingredients to look for when shopping for SPF-rated products.

☺ AVERAGE **Pro Gloss Hook Up Plumping Lip Shine** *($6.50)*. This thick, slightly sticky lip gloss plumps lips temporarily by irritating them with cinnamon bark extract. You'll feel the tingly, warming sensation almost instantly, but that's not the best experience to put your lips through, especially on a daily basis. Although this is not nearly as irritating as many "plumping" glosses, it is still best reserved for only occasional use. The range of shades is great and all impart translucent color via the handy brush applicator.

AVON MARK MASCARA

☺ AVERAGE **Scanda-Lash Hook Up Mascara** *($6.50)* has a great name but doesn't exactly perform scandalously. Its strength is that it doesn't clump and with some effort it does go the distance, but for thickening and impressive length, you'll have to turn to other mascaras.

AVON MARK FACE & BODY ILLUMINATORS

☺ GOOD **Touch & Glow Shimmer Cream Cubes All Over Face Palette** *($16)*. These individual cubes of pressed powder come in a small but workable range of shades for use on cheeks and eyes, and it's readily apparent which shades work best on each area—there are colors here that shouldn't go anywhere near your eyes unless you want to look like your allergies are in overdrive. The soft "baked" texture is prone to crumbling, so be sure to purchase this with one of the refillable compacts Mark offers. Color payoff is good and application with a brush is smooth. Indeed, these practically blend themselves. The shine is a subtle to moderate glow depending on how liberally you apply, and it stays in place well.

☺ AVERAGE **Glowdacious Illuminating Powder** *($13)*. This pressed-powder compact means to combine bronzer and highlighter into one product, but the result is too shiny for any sort of practical use. The flecks of shimmer in the bronzer flake, leaving behind a blaring, frosted sheen. With the three shades housed around one another in graduating rings, it's impossible to really control how much of each shade you get on your brush, and so it's impossible to control the degree of shine or color, which makes this far more trouble to apply than it's worth.

AVON MARK BRUSHES

The brushes from Avon Mark include some very good, inexpensive options. Full reviews of each are posted on CosmeticsCop.com, but in summation, here's how they rate:

✓☺ BEST **All Over Eye Shadow Brush** *($8)* and **Concealer Brush** *($7)*. ☺ GOOD brushes include Mark's **Angled Contour Face Brush** *($10)*, **Blush + Bronzer Brush** *($8)*, and **Powder Brush** *($10)*. ☺ AVERAGE brushes include the **Angled Contour Eyeshadow Brush** *($8)*, **Eye Shadow Brush** *($7)*, **Flat Eyeliner Brush** *($7)*, and **Foundation Brush** *($8)*.

☺ AVERAGE **Go with the Pro Mini Brush Kit** *($16)*. These tiny brushes aren't what any professional makeup artist would turn to, but it's not a bad set to have on hand for secondary, on-the-go use. None of the brushes are that soft, but they work OK for touch-ups. You get a brush for powder, concealer, lipstick/gloss, eyeliner, and one for eyeshadow. The lip brush works better to apply eyeliner, while the eyeliner brush works best to apply lipstick, at least by practical standards. While not a professional-caliber set, it's an option to keep in your office drawer or weekend travel bag where space is limited.

BARE ESCENTUALS

Strengths: Good makeup removers; a couple of well-formulated loose powders with SPF; some nice eyeshadows and impressive mascaras; great "100% natural" lip gloss and lipliner; several elegant brush options; not too expensive.

Weaknesses: Mineral makeup has its share of pros and cons and isn't for everyone; several of the loose powder products with shine have a grainy feel and cling poorly; some of the skin care contains problematic ingredients.

For more information and reviews of the latest Bare Escentuals products, visit CosmeticsCop.com.

BARE ESCENTUALS CLEANSERS

☹ POOR **bareMinerals Purifying Facial Cleanser with RareMinerals ActiveSoil Complex** *($20 for 6 fl. oz.)* is strategically named to make you believe the cleansing benefit is coming from the RareMinerals ActiveSoil Complex, but it isn't. First, there is no such thing as "ActiveSoil"; it is merely a marketing term to make dirt sound fancy. Second, the ingredient label lists "soil minerals," which means there is no way to know what is rare (if anything) about the dirt in this product or what you're actually putting on your face. Just because it's a mineral doesn't mean it contains something rare—minerals can contain sulfur, lead, chlorides—how rare does that sound? And last, the ingredients in this product that actually are responsible for cleansing your face are standard detergent cleansing agents. That's just fine, but this cleanser also contains several fragrant plant extracts and two forms of irritating lavender oil. These ingredients stand a good chance of causing needless irritation, and irritation is the last thing your skin needs (see the Appendix for details on why irritation and lavender oil is bad for your skin).

☹ POOR **bareMinerals Deep Cleansing Foam with RareMinerals ActiveSoil Complex** *($20 for 4.2 fl. oz.)* makes the same "RareMinerals" claim as the cleanser above, and the same comments apply here, too. The ingredients in this cleanser that actually are responsible for cleansing your face are similar to the cleansing agents found in soap, and they are potentially too drying and irritating for any skin type. This cleanser also contains an unusually high amount of alcohol, and the lavender oil causes further problems. Frankly, the only rare thing about this cleanser is that it is one of the worst ones we've reviewed in quite some time! See the Appendix for details on why irritation and lavender oil are so bad for your skin.

☹ POOR **bareMinerals Exfoliating Treatment Cleanser with RareMinerals ActiveSoil Complex** *($26 for 2.5 fl. oz.)* is a clay-based cleanser that is not only difficult to use (clay isn't the most elegant ingredient on which to base a cleanser), but also contains several fragrant oils capable of causing irritation. The "100% pure RareMinerals ActiveSoil Complex" offers no special benefit for anyone's skin. Between the problematic ingredients and the abrasive nature of this cleanser, it isn't a treatment we'd suggest you try, especially if having clean skin that isn't dry or tight is your goal. Please see the Appendix for details on why irritation is bad for your skin.

BARE ESCENTUALS EYE-MAKEUP REMOVERS

☺ GOOD **On The Spot Eye Makeup Remover** *($5 for 24 swabs)* provides a very gentle eye-makeup remover inside the hollow center of a cotton swab. Snapping the swab at the indicated point feeds the fluid onto the cotton tip, making for quick, convenient application. This isn't the most economical way to remove makeup, and the formula is too mild for stubborn or waterproof makeup, but it's an option.

☺ GOOD **bareEyes Eye Makeup Remover** *($14 for 4 fl. oz.)* is a standard, fragrance-free, silicone-based eye-makeup remover that does the job, and quickly, too! This is excellent for removing all types of makeup, including long-wearing and waterproof formulas.

BARE ESCENTUALS EXFOLIANTS

☹ POOR **bareVitamins Skin Rev-er Upper** *($21 for 2.3 fl. oz.)* used to rate as a very good 1% BHA (salicylic acid) product with a pH of 3.5 to ensure exfoliation will occur. It seems the company changed the formula, and not for the better. This contains several plant extracts that are a distinct problem for skin, with the biggest offender being arnica. This also contains St. John's Wort, listed by its Latin name of *Hypericum perforatum*. Applied topically, this plant contains several components that are toxic in the presence of sunlight (Sources: *Planta Medica*, February 2002, pages 171–173; and *International Journal of Biochemistry and Cell Biology*, March 2002, pages 221–241). What a shame, because this is no longer a BHA product we can recommend, and there are so few options! Paula's Choice is among the only companies that offer a range of truly effective, fragrance-free BHA exfoliants for all skin types.

BARE ESCENTUALS MOISTURIZERS, EYE CREAMS, & SERUMS

☹ POOR **Active Cell Renewal Night Serum** *($50 for 1 fl. oz.)* is water-based serum that contains some good water-binding ingredients to help hydrate normal to slightly dry skin, but in terms of anti-aging ingredients with solid research behind them, it falls short. There is nothing special about the soil minerals in this serum. More of a fancy way to describe dirt, soil minerals most likely cannot penetrate skin as the molecular structure of the minerals is simply too large. But even if they could penetrate, what good would that do? Minerals require enzymes and other substances in the body in order to work—just adding them to a serum isn't going to bring skin to its "ideal renewed state." The chief problem with this serum is the inclusion of lavender oil and, to a lesser extent, orange extract and fragrance ingredients known to cause irritation. Please see the Appendix to learn why lavender oil is a problem for all skin types.

☹ POOR **bareMinerals Firming Eye Treatment** *($28 for 0.5 fl. oz.)* contains some intriguing ingredients, but none of them are targeted exclusively to the needs of the eye area or capable of reducing puffiness. The RareMinerals ActiveSoil Complex is merely a fancy way to describe what amounts to mineral-rich dirt, which offers no special benefits for skin. And, given that the label merely states "soil minerals," you have no idea what you're actually putting on your face. Just because it's a mineral doesn't mean it contains something rare—minerals can contain sulfur, lead, chlorides—how rare does that sound? What's most problematic about this eye cream is the inclusion of fragrant ylang-ylang oil (listed by its Latin name *Canaga odorata*) and other fragrance ingredients. These ingredients can promote irritation that hurts skin's healing process and its ability to look and act younger, and they're even more of a problem when used close to the eyes. This eye cream contains a blend of shiny pigments that may make dark circles appear less obvious, but the effect is strictly cosmetic. Please see the Appendix to learn why you don't need a separate eye cream for the eye area.

☹ POOR **Purely Nourishing Cream with RareMinerals ActiveSoil Complex: Dry Skin** *($28 for 1.7 fl. oz.)* is touted as an emollient moisturizer for dry skin powered by Bare Escentual's RareMinerals ActiveSoil Complex, but it isn't. ActiveSoil is just a fancy term for, well, dirt. Minerals, from the soil or anywhere else, cannot increase skin's firmness or elasticity, or offer any sort of anti-aging benefit. If cosmetics companies are to be believed, it seems there's nothing a blend of minerals cannot do! Minerals aside, this moisturizer ends up being surprisingly basic. All of the intriguing ingredients are listed after the preservative (phenoxyethanol) and so don't amount to much. What does amount to a problem for all skin types is the lavender oil in this moisturizer. See the Appendix to learn why lavender oil is a problem for all skin types.

☹ POOR **Purely Nourishing Moisturizer with RareMinerals ActiveSoil Complex: Combination Skin** *($28 for 1.7 fl. oz.)*. It's been said that it only takes one bad apple to spoil the bunch, and with this moisturizer, the "bad apple" is lavender oil. This fragrant oil may appeal to your nose, but it's a problem for your skin. What a shame, because this moisturizer is loaded with beneficial ingredients, including some very good antioxidants and anti-irritants. As for the RareMinerals ActiveSoil Complex, that's essentially a fancy way to describe dirt, and no matter the source, minerals don't offer special benefits for your skin. See the Appendix to learn more about why lavender oil is a problem for all skin types.

☹ POOR **Renew & Hydrate Eye Cream** *($32 for 0.5 fl. oz.)* contains some great ingredients, yet none of them are special or unique for the eye area, and that includes the allegedly miraculous "soil minerals." More of a fancy way to describe dirt, soil minerals most likely cannot penetrate skin as the molecular structure of the minerals is simply too large. But even if they could penetrate, what good would that do? Minerals require enzymes and other substances in the body in order to work—just adding them to an eye cream isn't going to make your wrinkles, dark circles, or puffiness retreat. Considering how much Bare Escentuals hypes their soil minerals, it's interesting to note they haven't pointed to any research proving why this complex is so amazing. Instead, we get consumer use studies of the products, yet this type of information is rarely helpful, despite seeming so. This eye cream makes two errors that cannot be overlooked. The first is jar packaging. The other issue that truly puts your skin at risk is the inclusion of lavender oil. Please see the Appendix to learn more about why lavender oil and jar packaging are problems—and why, in truth, you don't need an eye cream.

BARE ESCENTUALS SUN CARE

☺ GOOD **$$$ bareMinerals SPF 30 Natural Sunscreen** *($28)* is a loose powder with a sunscreen that's pure titanium dioxide. Housed in a cylindrical component affixed with a soft, decently shaped applicator brush, you shake powder from the base so it feeds through the bottom of the brush, and then apply it to your face. The powder has a soft, sheer texture and minimal shine (much less shine than other powders from Bare Escentuals). This is a great way to add to the sun protection you're already getting from your daytime moisturizer or foundation with sunscreen, plus it helps blot excess shine. Three shades are available, and while all are workable, the Tan shade works best as bronzing powder (strategically applied to cheeks and temples) rather than as all-over face powder. The titanium dioxide is micronized so it doesn't leave a thick, pasty appearance on skin.

BARE ESCENTUALS LIP CARE

☺ GOOD **$$$ bareMinerals Lip Rev-er Upper** *($16 for 0.06 fl. oz.)* is a stick lip balm based on macadamia nut oil. It applies smoothly and the amount of film-forming agent (it's the second ingredient) has some ability to keep lipstick in place, though it's not foolproof. This isn't the best for very dry or chapped lips, but is worth testing if you want something lighter to wear under lipstick.

BARE ESCENTUALS SPECIALTY PRODUCTS

☺ GOOD **$$$ i.d. Shine Control Sheets** *($8 for 30 sheets)* are standard, non-powdered oil-blotting papers housed in a slim, matchbook-style holder that's perfectly portable. Although they work well (and quickly) to absorb excess oil, they're pricey considering the number of sheets you get. Still, if the price doesn't bother you, these work as well as most other blotting papers to temper excess shine.

☹ POOR **bareMinerals Blemish Therapy** *($18 for 0.03 fl. oz.)* is not recommended for several reasons: its active ingredient of 3% sulfur, while antibacterial, is way too drying and irritating for skin; the absorbent minerals will only exacerbate the dryness from the sulfur; and the retinol and niacinamide will be useless because of the unfortunate choice of jar packaging and the high pH of the sulfur. It is also interesting to note that products with a pH over 8 can increase the amount of acne-causing bacteria in skin. Last, this contains several fragrance ingredients known to cause irritation. In short, this is a big mistake if your goal is reducing blemishes and the red marks they leave.

BARE ESCENTUALS FOUNDATIONS & PRIMERS

☺ GOOD **bareVitamins Prime Time Foundation Primer** *($22 for 1 fl. oz.)* is a standard, silicone-based, waterless primer. Like others cut from the same cloth, it makes skin feel very silky and can improve foundation application. It's not a must-have if you're already using a silicone-enhanced moisturizer or serum pre-makeup.

☺ AVERAGE **bareMinerals Foundation SPF 15** *($26)* is the loose-powder foundation that put Bare Escentuals on the map and it is the backbone of their makeup line. This talc-free, mica-based powder has a soft, almost creamy texture and an undeniably shiny finish (not a good look for someone with oily skin). The titanium dioxide and bismuth oxychloride lend this powder its opacity, medium to full coverage, and slightly thick finish. The formula includes broad-spectrum sun protection, but because most women won't apply this liberally enough, it is best paired with another form of SPF. This foundation can be tricky to blend, and is best applied with a powder brush. The best options shade-wise are for fair to light skin, though there are a few exceptions. In fact, there are plenty of shades for women of color, but the high amount of titanium dioxide causes them to look or turn ashy on darker skin.

☺ AVERAGE **$$$ bareMinerals Matte Foundation SPF 15** *($28)* is a loose-powder foundation with a very soft texture and smooth application. The formula provides broad-spectrum sun protection, which is imperative for an anti-aging benefit. Just be sure to pair it with another form of SPF to ensure full sun protection (most women won't apply this liberally enough to achieve that). You can expect medium to almost full coverage. Despite the name, this foundation doesn't have a truly matte finish; you still get a soft, non-sparkling glow that someone with very oily skin won't appreciate. The silica base coupled with calcium silicate and the mineral sunscreen agents can make this feel quite dry, so it's not the best for dry skin. What Bare Escentuals did well is the closure for this loose-powder makeup. The sifter can be completely sealed so powder doesn't spill all over the place, although you'll still get some residual powder in the cap and on the sifter with each use, but the mess is minor when compared with the mess of many other loose powders. Where this foundation takes a sharp nosedive is in its shades. Most of the light colors are fine, but all the darker shades have a strong ashen finish that can make dark skin tones look drab and gray.

☹ POOR **Prime Time Oil Control Foundation Primer** *($22 for 1 fl. oz.)* contains witch hazel extract as the main ingredient, which is a needless form of irritation and a problem for all skin types. This primer sets to a slightly matte finish, but the same can be achieved with nonirritating products. See the Appendix to learn how irritation makes oily skin worse.

☹ POOR **Prime Time Brightening Foundation Primer** *($22)* is a fluid, silky foundation primer with a thin texture that blends well and leaves a soft glowing finish that brightens your complexion. The problem? No matter how long you wait, this primer never really sets, so your skin is left feeling slick and almost greasy. Because this primer never sets, it's tricky to apply foundation evenly over it without the makeup looking streaky or uneven.

BARE ESCENTUALS CONCEALER

☺ GOOD **$$$ bareMinerals SPF 20 Concealer** *($18)* is a loose powder concealer whose texture doesn't offer as much coverage as you would get with a liquid or cream concealer. However, if powder is the way you want to go, this is a decent option, as long as you don't use it for the under-eye area, because if you have any wrinkles around the eye area, powder will make them more obvious. The range includes neutral shades for light to dark skin, and it offers broad-spectrum, mineral-based sun protection for added anti-aging benefit. The colors go on too sheer to conceal more noticeable discolorations, but they do color match nicely with the bareMinerals powder foundations.

✹ Sunscreens must provide reliable UVA (anti-aging) protection. See the Appendix for details.

BARE ESCENTUALS POWDERS

☺ GOOD $$$ **bareMinerals Mineral Veil SPF 25** *($20)* is a sheer loose powder that is great for two reasons: It boosts the sun protection your moisturizer or foundation with sunscreen provides, and absorbs excess oil. You also can use it alone for sun protection, but you have to apply it liberally and that can look thick and exacerbate dryness. It has a sheer, dry texture and a lasting matte finish on skin. The shades apply translucent, so this will be workable for all skin tones.

☺ GOOD $$$ **bareMinerals Natural Light Face Lifting Duo** *($19)* is housed in a tiny component that includes a closable sifter. Inside the component are two loose powders designed to highlight skin. The sifter mechanism can be set so that both shades of powder dispense at the same time, or you can use them individually. It's a thoughtful packaging touch and the closable sifter also helps minimize mess. Each powder has a sheer, gossamer texture that highlights skin, leaving a soft, subtle glow. Whether you use the pale yellow or pale peach shade (or both), this powder brightens without adding sparkles to skin, and it doesn't feel heavy or look dry. Although highlighting with a pressed powder is easier and neater than using loose powder, if loose is your preference this is a very good option, especially for those with fair to medium skin tones. One more comment: This powder, even when artfully applied, won't lift skin or even make it look lifted. It will highlight and brighten, but sagging skin won't suddenly appear firmed up.

☺ GOOD $$$ **bareMinerals Radiance** *($19)*. "Radiance" describes this loose powder perfectly as it has a sheer, shimmery finish that works well for highlighting. The light, silky-soft powder texture adheres to skin with no signs of flaking. The shades are mostly pale versions of rose, peach, cream, and bronze, and can be layered over your powder blush for added luminescence. Just be aware that the shiny finish can emphasize wrinkles and make oily skin appear oilier.

☺ GOOD $$$ **Mineral Veil** *($20)* is a talc-free loose powder with a softer and much lighter consistency than the bareMinerals Foundation SPF 15, and it applies matte. The shades are sheer and have a dry finish that's best for someone with normal to oily skin.

☹ AVERAGE $$$ **bareMinerals READY SPF 15 Touch Up Veil** *($22)* is a touch-up pressed powder with a lightweight feel and reliable, mineral-based broad-spectrum sun protection. The Translucent shade goes on very sheer and is an easy way to add sun protection throughout the day (just be aware that it does leave a slight white cast on the skin). The Tinted shade could be used for medium-tan skin tones or as a sheer bronzer. The reason this is not rated higher is because it contains fragrant ylang-ylang oil (listed by its Latin name *Canaga odorata*). Most powders with sunscreen omit fragrant irritants, so this option is less desirable.

☹ AVERAGE $$$ **Hydrating Mineral Veil** *($20)*. Don't be misled by the name of this loose powder. Although water is the second ingredient, it contains plenty of absorbents, including the main ingredient, silica. This fact doesn't make Mineral Veil the least bit hydrating, but hey, at least silica is a mineral. This powder has a notable dry, slightly thick texture upon application but it quickly lightens, leaving skin feeling very dry and looking very matte. On skin the application looks iridescent, with an almost metallic shade of pink—so this isn't something you want to swirl all over your face during the day or even at night, unless you want a very shiny, somewhat other-worldly complexion. Because of its absorbency and finish, this powder is best for normal to very oily skin; however, as mentioned, you must be willing to tolerate a lot of iridescence, which almost always makes oily skin look oilier. Plus, the hydrating claims are ludicrous; this is a drying powder—there is nothing moisturizing about it, despite it containing some moisturizing lipids from rice. They simply cannot hydrate skin when paired with high amounts of absorbent ingredients.

☹ POOR **bareMinerals Redness Remedy** *($27)* is a yellow-toned loose powder that is touted as being able to "reduce facial redness on contact and over time." It fails on both counts. First, this powder is too sheer to counteract redness; you'd have to cake it on to see any sort of camouflaging, not to mention that the yellow color isn't going to work on all skin tones without adding a jaundiced appearance over the areas that aren't red. (This assumes it worked over redness, which isn't what we found.) Second, you are not going to see any anti-redness benefit from this powder over time. Although the formula contains some very good anti-irritants, such as licorice and chamomile, the jar packaging won't keep air out, thus allowing these oxygen-sensitive ingredients to start breaking down once it is opened. Bare Escentuals claims that the Redness Remedy is "powered by [their] ActiveSoil Complex," which is listed as "soil minerals" on the ingredient list. In essence, they are claiming to sell fancy dirt, though "soil minerals" is a recognized ingredient term by U.S. regulatory standards. There are supposed to be 72 minerals in this soil, but they don't tell you what the 72 minerals are or what else the soil contains. (Lead and cadmium are minerals present in soil and they're natural, too, but you wouldn't want them in abundance on your skin.) Soil also contains a large amount of sand, which has no benefit for skin. Think about this—an acre of soil may contain 900 pounds of earthworms, 2,400 pounds of fungi, 1,500 pounds of bacteria, 133 pounds of protozoa, and 890 pounds of arthropods and algae. It turns out "virgin soil" isn't really as "pure" as the marketing claims make it sound. All in all, this is a complete dud!

☹ POOR **Pure Transformation Night Treatment** *($60)* comes in four shades, including a Clear option that still imparts some color, and most of them provide enough coverage to camouflage minor flaws and redness, so you will perceive that your skin looks better. The recommendation to wear this at night is just shocking to us. Be forewarned that sleeping with this product on your face will result in makeup stains on your pillowcase, and leaving this stuff on overnight would most likely be drying and irritating. Minerals on the skin, even plain talc or chalk or soil of any kind, aren't soothing in the least and need to be washed off, not worn to bed, and this product is no exception.

Getting back to the mineral claims, is there anything to them? Does this "pure mineral concentrate" hold the secret to revitalized, youthful skin? Regardless of the purity of the soil, minerals cannot be absorbed by skin (their molecules are just too big), so any effect would be entirely superficial. Moreover, while there hasn't been much research on topical application of minerals, we do know that whether they are applied topically or ingested, minerals depend on other factors (most notably coenzymes) to work, and even when that happens the benefits aren't all that exciting (Sources: *Cosmeceuticals*, Elsner & Maiback, 2000, pages 29–30; and *International Journal of Cosmetic Science*, 1997, page 105). There is no substantiated research proving that minerals, whether concentrated or not, exfoliate skin or have any effect on pore size. Any perceived reduction in pore size from using this product is solely from its reflective quality and natural opacity, the same as any other powder foundation. It can work to temporarily fill in large pores, but when it's washed off any potential benefit is washed away at the same time.

You may be wondering about the vitamin C (ascorbic acid) in this product. According to the chemists we spoke with, ascorbic acid tends to remain stable in an anhydrous (waterless) product, which this powder certainly qualifies as. How much of the vitamin C reaches the skin is a question, however, along with whether this uses an effective amount.

Cause for concern must be expressed due to the amount of barium sulfate present. This natural mineral compound can be poisonous if ingested and is noted for the way it frequently causes skin reactions. This same ingredient is consumed orally before having certain types of X-rays taken; it is believed that barium sulfate's low solubility and the body's ability to excrete it both help promote its negligible bioavailability. Still, it's not the best ingredient to see so prominently in a skin-care product designed to be used every night.

BARE ESCENTUALS BLUSHES & BRONZER

☺ GOOD $$$ **Faux Tan Matte** *($19)* is a loose bronzing powder that's packaged in a standard clear jar with a closable sifter. Loose bronzing powder is inherently messier to use than pressed or liquid bronzers, but if loose is your preference, Faux Tan Matte has some good qualities, and the closable sifter helps keep the mess to a minimum. The texture is smooth, but somewhat dry, so it's best to apply this sparingly with a large, fluffy powder brush. This bronzer has a matte finish.

☹ AVERAGE $$$ **bareMinerals All Over Face Color** *($19)* is in the blush category because most of the shades are suitable as blush, not colors you'd want to dust all over the face. This is another loose powder with a shiny finish that will emphasize large pores and wrinkles. The shine doesn't flake all over the place, which is great, but it's intense enough to make oily skin look oilier. You may also want to consider this shiny loose powder for highlighting, as several of the shades are pale and sheer, though they still impart a strong shimmer finish.

☺ AVERAGE $$$ **bareMinerals Blush** *($19)* has the same basic texture as the loose foundation above, and the comments about its being messy and hard to control apply here, too. There are several beautiful shades to choose from, some of which have a matte finish, and the application is soft and relatively even once you've mastered how much loose color to pick up on your brush for best results.

BARE ESCENTUALS EYESHADOWS & EYE PRIMERS

☺ GOOD $$$ **bareMinerals High Shine Eyecolor** *($16)* is a surprisingly good loose-powder eyeshadow. With all of the pressed-powder eyeshadows available, normally we wouldn't recommend the mess that the loose format typically entails, but Bare Escentuals has solved this problem with their ingenious packaging. Essentially, the deeply pigmented loose-powder shadow is picked up by a chunky but pointed sponge-tip applicator that "wipes" the excess powder before you've completely removed the applicator. The excess powder falls back into the container, not all over your counter. It also helps that this powder has excellent cling and yet is fairly easy to blend (although difficult to soften). Again, this isn't a dusty, flake-prone powder, and that's really impressive. The shades have rich color payoff, and most have a strong metallic sheen that is not recommended if you have pronounced wrinkles in the eye area because it will draw more attention to them. Despite the intensity of the shine, most of the shades are beautiful!

☺ GOOD $$$ **bareMinerals READY Eyeshadow** *($20-$40)*. Pressed-powder eyeshadow is a first for bareMinerals, and we're probably not the only ones wondering what took them so long. This version has a silky powder texture that blends on easily and doesn't have any of the problems of loose-powder eyeshadows. A bevy of shimmer and matte-finish shades are available, too. The shadows are sold in sets of 2, 4, or 8, and these groupings explain the step-up in pricing for each, with the duos costing $20, and so on. While not all the color combinations go well together, there are some attractive shades to consider for either classic or trendy eye designs.

☺ GOOD **$$$ Prime Time Primer Shadow** *($18)* is an eyeshadow primer that comes in a range of eyeshadow colors, so in essence it's a double-duty product that functions as a long-wearing cream-to-powder eyeshadow. The initially thick, slightly creamy texture feels silky and blends readily. It has a good amount of slip without being slick, so you can better control color placement. This sets to a matte (in feel) powder finish, but each shade leaves a metallic sheen laced with light-catching shimmer. High shine is the look you get, but at least these don't crease or fade easily, although some fading is apparent after several hours of wear. Once set, these become smudge-proof and hold up beautifully if your eye area gets wet.

☺ AVERAGE **bareMinerals Eyecolor** *($13)* has a silky, lightweight loose-powder texture that applies and blends well. Most of the shades go on softer than they look, and some appear matte in the container, but their noticeable shine is revealed on application. Speaking of shine, it runs the gamut here, from a "you're glowing" to a "you're blinding me" finish. This is still a messy way to apply eyeshadow, and the shiniest shades don't cling as well as they should. Watch out for the "Glimmer" shades, which have a grainier texture than the others.

☺ AVERAGE **$$$ bareMinerals Prime Time Eyelid Primer** *($18)* is a good, though not must-have, eyeshadow primer. It has a silky texture that blends easily and sets to a soft powder-like finish that makes eyeshadow application easier. Products like this work, but you can save money (and space in your makeup bag) by simply prepping your eyelids with a matte-finish concealer or foundation, which work just as well.

☺ AVERAGE **$$$ Well Rested SPF 20 Eye Brightener** *($18)* is marketed as an "eye brightener" for dark circles beneath the eyes, but this loose powder fails to impress. Although the texture is smooth and the coverage adequate, the singular yellow-toned shade isn't going to work on everyone (especially for darker skin tones) and won't make dark circles disappear. The one saving grace is that it contains reliable broad-spectrum sun protection for added anti-aging benefit, but there just really isn't anything special about this product that a well-formulated powder couldn't do.

BARE ESCENTUALS EYE & BROW LINERS

☺ GOOD **bareMinerals Big & Bright Eyeliner** *($14)* is an automatic, retractable eye pencil whose wax-based formula glides across your lash line and imparts soft color with a slightly creamy finish. The thicker texture makes drawing a thin line difficult, while the creamier finish doesn't have impressive staying power. On balance, this pencil and its range of attractive, sultry shades is best for creating smoky eyes, which means you apply the pencil and then smudge the line before it smudges on its own.

☺ GOOD **$$$ bareMinerals Brow Finishing Gel** *($14)* is a very standard, but good, colorless brow gel that's easy to apply. The conical brush isn't anything special, but it does the job of grooming stray brow hairs without creating a gummy mess. Once set, this feels almost weightless and it doesn't leave a trace of stickiness.

☺ GOOD **$$$ Buxom Lashliner** *($16)*. This gel eyeliner tried to distinguish itself from the pack with its claims of also being a thickening and conditioning lash treatment. The claims are carefully worded to avoid actually stating that it will increase lash growth or the amount of lashes you have; indirectly, however, that's the message the consumer will get. It's a message you should ignore, because if you don't, you're wasting your money. There isn't anything in this product that can affect lash growth and the tiny amount of natural ingredients doesn't make this better than any other gel eyeliner. Rather, simply applying eyeliner (any eyeliner) close to the base of the eyelashes will make it appear as if you have lashes that are thicker and fuller.

Mascara completes the illusion, but in the end, no lash growth or conditioning is taking place with this product. As a gel eyeliner, the whipped-cream texture applies almost effortlessly and sets quickly to a long-wearing matte finish. This eyeliner isn't rated better because its soft texture makes application consistently tricky; you have to be extra careful you don't pick up too much on your brush each time, because you'll make a mess and it will chip and flake.

☺ GOOD $$$ **Buxom Pen & Ink Long-Last Eyeliner** ($20) is a liquid eyeliner with a unique, flat-head felt tip that allows you to draw on either a thick or thin (though not super thin) line. It takes a little practice to master the applicator, but once you get the hang of it, the results are a nice, even line of dramatic color.

☺ AVERAGE **bareMinerals Liner Shadow** ($13) would indeed work as eyeliner, and these intensely pigmented loose powders function wet or dry. The shades are imbued with shine, some featuring a metallic or glittery finish (and yes, the glitter flakes). This is a messy way to line your eyes, but if you're willing to tolerate that and have a smooth, wrinkle-free eyelid and lower lash line, go for it.

☺ AVERAGE $$$ **Buxom Insider Eyeliner** ($14) is an automatic, retractable pencil available in classic or trendy shades, ranging from purple to pearl to black. It claims to be gentle enough to line even the inner rim of the eyes, but the formula doesn't bear that out. Lining the inner rim of the eye with this pencil is a problem due to the formula's extreme creaminess. You could wait for hours for this to set and you'd still be waiting. All things considered, there are many far better eyeliner options to consider before this one.

☹ POOR **bareMinerals Brow Color** ($11) isn't the way to go if you want to add color and definition to your brows. The loose texture makes it difficult to apply in a controlled manner and results in quite a mess, with powder spilling onto the eyelid and under-brow area. Despite an extensive color selection, including an option for redheads, there's no way we can recommend this given that there are superior, mess-free brow powders that are pressed, not loose, which unquestionably makes them easier to work with.

BARE ESCENTUALS LIP COLOR & LIPLINERS

☺ GOOD **bareMinerals 100% Natural Lipgloss** ($15) comes close to being all-natural, but it isn't, at least not in terms of ingredients. Perhaps they were referring to the way this will look on your lips, but most consumers think "100% natural" means they are getting a "better-for-you formula." You aren't. Still, you may want to consider this moderately thick, oil–based gloss. It has a stickier finish than glosses rated Best, but the colors are sheer and versatile enough to work with most lipsticks. The brush applicator works well and isn't prone to splaying.

☺ GOOD **bareMinerals 100% Natural Lipliner** ($11) is an automatic, retractable lip pencil with a smooth but greasy application due to its plant oil–based formula. Application is swift, but the line doesn't last long and it will bleed into any lines around the mouth. If that's not a concern for you and you want a lipliner whose ingredients are truly 100% natural, give this an audition. The shade range is small, but it's filled with can't-go-wrong colors.

☺ AVERAGE $$$ **bareMinerals Pretty Amazing Lipcolor** ($16) is outfitted with an angled sponge-tip applicator that's supposed to "hug your lips" like a race car driver's car hugs the racetrack, but it's not nearly so precise. It's not the applicator's fault as much as it is this liquid lipstick's thick formula, which makes it tricky to apply evenly without going outside the boundaries of your mouth. On the plus side, the colors are richly pigmented and last for hours, but the formula somehow manages to transfer to everything your lips touch. Despite the fact that this comes off on everything (and bleeds into lines around the mouth), the color leaves a stain so your lips don't look "undone" after that first cup of coffee.

☹ POOR **bareMinerals 100% Natural Lipcolor** *($15)* does indeed contain nothing but natural ingredients. But don't take that to mean this emollient cream lipstick is better than others. If anything, quite the opposite is true: The third ingredient in this lipstick is barium sulfate, a natural mineral compound that can be poisonous if ingested and that is noted for the way it frequently causes skin reactions. This same ingredient is consumed orally before having certain types of X-rays taken; it is believed that barium sulfate's low solubility and the body's ability to excrete it both help promote its negligible bioavailability. Still, it's not the best ingredient to see so prominently in a lipstick. Also unfortunate is that each opaque, highly pigmented shade also contains lavender oil, which can cause skin-cell death even when used in low amounts. This lipstick is a great example of a natural product not being as advantageous as a product with a mix of natural and synthetic ingredients.

☹ POOR **Buxom Big & Healthy Lip Cream Lip Polish** *($18)* is a creamy lip gloss that comes in vibrant shades of pink, purple, peach, and red, with a moisturizing, smooth texture. Unfortunately, the formula contains irritating fragrance and the menthol derivative menthone glycerin acetyl, which, with continued use, can make lips chapped and dry. The same comments and rating applies to the company's **Buxom Big & Healthy Lip Polish** *($18)*.

☹ POOR **Buxom Big & Healthy Lip Stick** *($18)* is merely an automatic, nonretractable lip crayon claiming to be a 3-in-1 product (lipliner, lipstick, and lip plumper), but it barely does even one of these right. Used as a lipliner, it sufficiently prevents feathering, but it needs to be manually sharpened into a tip that's fine enough to do so. As a lipstick, it has a semi-matte finish and staying power, but the formula is so dry that it drags across lips, preventing smooth application. To top it all off, Bare Escentuals opted to include the irritant menthone glycerin acetal to trigger some lip plumping (meaning it causes irritation, which is never good for lips), but it only causes a telltale tingle and a minimal, temporary plumping effect. Although the shade range is impressive with numerous attractive options, this multitasking formula simply fails to deliver.

☹ POOR **Buxom Big & Healthy Lip Tarnish** *($18)* is a creamy lip color in pencil form that could have been a delightful product, but instead Bare Escentuals loaded it with irritating fragrance and menthone glycerin acetyl, which, with continued use, can make lips chapped and dry. The built-in sharpener, non-sticky silky-smooth texture, and pretty colors are great, but all in all, it's just not worth the damage to your lips!

BARE ESCENTUALS MASCARAS

✓☺ BEST **$$$ bareMinerals Flawless Definition Curl & Lengthen Mascara** *($18)* doesn't quite deliver maximum curl, but it does leave lashes perfectly lengthened with a soft, upswept fringe, and not a clump in sight. This is quite impressive from the get-go and it wears without a hitch.

✓☺ BEST **$$$ bareMinerals Flawless Definition Volumizing Mascara** *($18)* is a wonderful mascara that allows you to build equal parts length, definition, and thickness with just a few strokes. Clumping doesn't happen and successive coats further define lashes without making them look spiked or overdone.

☺ GOOD **bareMinerals Magic Wand Brushless Mascara** *($15)* doesn't have a brush, so the name is accurate. Instead, you get a stick with grooves that grab and coat the lashes, providing dramatic length in the process. It can go on heavy and wetter than usual, which sticks lashes together rather than creating a separated, fringed look. Still, the results are impressive if you're looking for lengthening mascara.

☺ GOOD $$$ **bareMinerals Flawless Definition Waterproof Mascara** *($18)* is a strongly waterproof mascara (you'll have no problem swimming with this on your lashes) that excels at lengthening and, despite some minor clumps, separates lashes beautifully. Thickness is minimal so this isn't the waterproof mascara to buy if you want lots of oomph. Otherwise, this holds up well and requires an oil- or silicone-based makeup remover when you're ready to go back to natural.

☺ AVERAGE $$$ **bareMinerals Flawless Definition Mascara** *($18)* has an application that's wetter than usual and can lead to smearing. This darkens lashes considerably and provides ample length, while allowing you to build slight thickness. After it sets, minor flaking during wear is apparent, which doesn't bode well considering the number of mascaras that don't flake.

☺ AVERAGE $$$ **bareMinerals Lash Builder** *($15)* is a standard lash primer, meaning its formula closely matches that of a regular mascara, minus the pigment that gives mascara its lash-darkening color. This doesn't do anything you cannot achieve with an outstanding mascara. If you're using a mascara that doesn't add much thickness, applying Lash Builder first helps add bulk to lashes for more volume and drama, but that still doesn't make it an essential product.

☹ POOR **Buxom Amplified Lash Mascara** *($22)* comes with a unique, twist-up wand that allows you to adjust the brush length and the bristle density. While that may pique your curiosity, the brush is actually harder to control than most due to its large size and cut-straight shape. Your lashes may look thicker, but at the expense of being clumped together, which is never sexy. Couple that with the fact that it flakes and smudges as the day wears on and you'll see that the only thing amplified about this mascara is the mess it creates.

BARE ESCENTUALS BRUSHES

☺ GOOD **Bare Escentuals Brushes** *($10-$30)* are impressive, with almost as many options as makeup artist-driven lines such as M.A.C. Unfortunately, many of them use hair that isn't as soft as it could be, or they aren't shaped as well as others. Among the best options are the **Precision Liner Brush** *($12)*; **Soft Focus Liner** and **Soft Focus Shadow** brushes *($22)*; **Blending Brush** *($18)*; **Flawless Application Face Brush** *($22)*; **Eye Defining Brush** *($16)*; **Tapered Shadow Brush** *($14)*; **Wet/Dry Shadow Brush** *($18)*; **Eyeliner Brush** *($12)*; **Crease Defining Brush** *($18)* and **bareMinerals Refillable Buffing Brush** *($29.50)*.

The brushes not worth your time or money include **bareMinerals Brow Brush** *($12)*, **bareMinerals Maximum Coverage Concealer Brush** *($20)*, **Flathead Shadow Brush** *($15)*, **Heavenly Liner Blending Brush** *($14)*, **Full Coverage Kabuki Brush** *($28)*, and the **Lash Comb** *($10)*.

BEAUTICONTROL

Strengths: The Cell Block-C products include stabilized vitamin C; several well-formulated moisturizers; decent AHA and scrub products; excellent retinol products; several good cleansers plus an exceptional makeup remover; Lip Apeel; very good lip balm with sunscreen; good self-tanner; some great foundations (including one with full coverage); very good powder blush and eyeshadow trios; excellent liquid eyeliner and lip gloss.

Weaknesses: Most of the body-care products contain irritating ingredients, as do several others throughout the line; jar packaging; most of the toners contain problematic ingredients that can hurt skin; limited options for sunscreens, although what's available provides sufficient

UVA protection; the Skinlogics Sensitive skin-care line contains ingredients that are problematic for those with sensitive skin; mostly problematic concealers; limited to poor foundation, concealer, and powder shades for women of color.

For more information and reviews of the latest BeautiControl products, visit CosmeticsCop.com.

BEAUTICONTROL CLEANSERS

☺ GOOD **$$$ Skinlogics Clear Deep Cleansing Gel** *($20 for 6.7 fl. oz.)* is an OK water-soluble option for normal to oily skin. It would be better without the fragrant plant extracts, but they're not present in a high amount. This works well to remove makeup and rinses cleanly.

☺ GOOD **$$$ Skinlogics Platinum Plus Nourishing Creme Cleanser** *($21 for 6.7 fl. oz.)* is a gentle water-soluble foaming cleanser that contains emollients helpful for normal to dry skin. This cleanser also contains several antioxidants and skin-identical substances, most of which won't remain on skin after rinsing. This contains fragrance in the form of methyldihydrojasmonate.

☺ AVERAGE **$$$ BC Spa Facial Purifying Cleansing Lotion** *($24 for 6.7 fl. oz.)* has a milky texture that's best for normal to slightly dry or slightly oily skin and is a pricey water-soluble cleanser. It does remove makeup, but it's a problem for use around the eyes because it contains fragrant plant extracts, which can cause irritation.

☺ AVERAGE **$$$ Skinlogics Sensitive Gentle Cleansing Lotion** *($20 for 6.7 fl. oz.)*. This water-soluble cleansing gel contains too many ingredients that are ill advised for all skin types, but especially for sensitive skin. Geranium, lavender, lime, and orange may smell delicious, but all of them spell trouble for skin in a delicate state.

☹ POOR **BC Spa Facial Purifying Cleansing Gel** *($24 for 6.7 fl. oz.)* is a poor choice for all except those with oily skin because its main detergent cleansing agent (sodium C14-16 olefin sulfonate) is drying. Most disappointing is the inclusion of fragrant plants that cause irritation and are a distinct problem for use around the eyes. The irritating plant extracts and drying cleansing agent make this cleanser impossible to recommend.

☹ POOR **Skinlogics Cleansing Gel** *($18 for 6.7 fl. oz.)* contains several fragrant citrus and other plant extracts (plus jasmine oil) that can be irritating. It would definitely be a problem for use around the eyes, and as a cleanser you'll probably use this around the eyes to help remove makeup.

BEAUTICONTROL EYE-MAKEUP REMOVERS

✓☺ BEST **Skinlogics Lash and Lid Bath** *($12 for 4 fl. oz.)* is a very good, exceptionally gentle cleanser that BeautiControl positions as an eye-makeup remover. It works well for that purpose, and it's fragrance-free. This is similar to removing your eye makeup with Johnson & Johnson's Baby Shampoo, which means you can expect it to perform gently, but it is incapable of removing long-wearing eyeliner or waterproof mascara. If you don't routinely wear that type of eye makeup, this is worth purchasing.

BEAUTICONTROL TONERS

✓☺ BEST **$$$ Skinlogics Platinum Plus Relaxing Tonic** *($23 for 6.7 fl. oz.)* sells itself as more than just a toner, and it is! Although this has a lingering floral scent some may find unappealing, there's no denying this milky toner is a state-of-the-art formulation for normal to very dry skin. It is loaded with water-binding agents, antioxidants (including nonfragrant plant oils), and ingredients that help reinforce skin's protective barrier. The label does not list fragrance, but the product does contain fragrance ingredients, which it would be better off without.

☺ AVERAGE $$$ **BC Spa Facial Regenerating Tonic with PHAs** *($24 for 6.7 fl. oz.)* is an alcohol-free toner that contains polyhydroxy acids (PHA), such as gluconolactone, which are often used as alternatives to AHAs. The theory is that PHAs are gentler on the skin, but research hasn't shown that to be the case, at least not to a significant degree. Just like AHAs, PHAs require an acidic pH of 3-4 to be effective, but the pH of this toner is too high for the PHAs to exfoliate. Also unfortunate is that this toner contains a high amount of the plant irritants arnica and comfrey (the latter listed by its Latin name *Symphytum officinale*). What a shame, because BeautiControl also included a nice mix of beneficial ingredients—the kind you should be seeking when shopping for a well-formulated toner. As is, the plant irritants can hurt your skin's healing process and impair healthy collagen production.

☺ AVERAGE $$$ **Skinlogics Tonic** *($18 for 6.7 fl. oz.)* is a basic toner containing mostly water and slip agents that make skin feel silky, but it isn't as impressive as it could've been.

☹ POOR **Skinlogics Clear Blemish Control Tonic** *($20 for 6.7 fl. oz.)* is an irritating anti-acne toner in several ways. Its pH of 2 is extremely acidic, which negates the benefits of the salicylic acid. Coupled with the low pH, it is an alcohol-based formula that also contains witch hazel, which adds more fuel to the fire. Please see the Appendix to learn why alcohol is a problem for all skin types, and why irritation makes oily skin worse.

☹ POOR **Skinlogics Gold Tonic** *($18 for 6.7 fl. oz.)* has grapefruit extract high up on the ingredient list, so the potential for irritation makes this a tonic to overlook, particularly for sensitive skin. It can't reduce the appearance of puffiness as claimed.

☹ POOR **Skinlogics Herbal Hydrating Mist** *($12 for 6.7 fl. oz.)* is a very basic toner containing a problematic amount of irritating ivy and arnica extracts. In addition, the tiny amount of nonirritating plant extracts present offers minimal benefit to skin, making this a toner to ignore.

☹ POOR **Skinlogics Sensitive Rinse & Restore Tonic** *($20 for 6.7 fl. oz.)* is far from a logical choice for sensitive skin. This in-some-ways-promising toner containing a significant amount of mugwort extract (listed by its Latin name *Artemisia vulgaris*), a plant whose volatile components, including camphor, are too irritating for all skin types (Source: naturaldatabase. com). Mugwort has no known benefit for skin, either—nor do the other problematic plants in this toner.

BEAUTICONTROL EXFOLIANTS & SCRUBS

☺ GOOD $$$ **Skinlogics Thermal Facial Scrub** *($20 for 2.6 fl. oz.)* warms when mixed with water, making it just another scrub whose novelty is a simple chemical reaction that's also present in less expensive scrubs from drugstore lines. The bottom line is that it's not necessary for good skin care. The warming reaction, which begins quite intensely and then subsides, may feel good, but it has zero impact on clogged pores or cleansing skin. This type of product can be a problem for anyone with sensitive skin, especially those with rosacea. However, it's a good scrub for someone with normal to oily skin, whether or not you think the warming (thermal) effect is neat.

☺ AVERAGE $$$ **BC Spa Resurface Microderm Abrasion for Face** *($56 for 2.5 fl. oz.)* is an absurdly overpriced scrub, but is a decent option for all skin types except oily or blemish-prone because the oils and thickeners it contains aren't good for that skin type. It includes alumina as the abrasive agent, similar to what's used in microdermabrasion treatments. However, massaging this over the skin with your hands isn't the same thing as an in-office microderm-abrasion session. To that end, BeautiControl sells the **BC Spa Microderm Abrasion Facial**

Buffer ($14), a battery-powered hand-held device equipped with a rotating facial brush that does help to create an impact similar to that of the real deal. The device has two speeds and the brush head is composed of synthetic bristles. Used with this scrub, it produces more thorough results than just using your fingers. However, it's easy to get carried away with this device, and coupled with the scrub particles (which are overly abrasive), you may get more irritation than benefit. For that reason, it's best to use this scrub without the device (you can try the Facial Buffer with your favorite cleanser).

☺ AVERAGE $$$ **BC Spa Resurface Multi-Acid Resurfacing Peel** *($50 for 30 pads)* contains approximately 10% glycolic acid (AHA) at a pH of 4.1. For an AHA product, a slightly lower pH value around 3.5 would have been a lot better. Although this also contains other AHA ingredients—lactic acid, lactobionic acid, and gluconolactone—they don't make up much of the total content, which further reduces the possibility of exfoliation (i.e., "resurfacing"). The pads are meant to be swiped over skin, you leave the residue on for 10–20 minutes, and then rinse. You'll definitely want to rinse because these pads leave a sticky film on skin that interferes with the application of other products. This doesn't come close to having anything to do with a professional peel from a doctor or aesthetician. Note that for a lot less money you can purchase well-formulated AHA products from Alpha Hydrox, Neutrogena, or Paula's Choice.

☹ POOR **BC Spa Facial Exfoliating Polish** *($20 for 2.6 fl. oz.)* has a gentle cleansing base and contains rounded jojoba beads to polish your skin without excess abrasiveness. However, BeautiControl added a mix of fragrant plant extracts that irritate skin.

☹ POOR **BC Spa Facial Regenerating Tonic with AHAs** *($24 for 6.7 fl. oz.)* contains glycolic acid, an AHA exfoliant. Exfoliating skin with an AHA- or BHA (salicylic acid)-based product is great for your skin because they build collagen, smooth the skin's surface, lessen the appearance of wrinkles, and reduce skin discolorations. AHAs and BHA can function only within a specific pH range, and this product meets that standard. The problem is the amount of witch hazel (listed by its Latin name *Hammamelis virginiana*) along with other irritants such as alcohol and fragrant plant extracts. See the Appendix to learn why irritation is bad for all skin types.

BEAUTICONTROL MOISTURIZERS (DAYTIME, NIGHTTIME), EYE CREAMS, & SERUMS

✓☺ BEST **BC Spa Facial Defend & Restore Moisture Creme SPF 20** *($32 for 2.6 fl. oz.)* is a fragrance-free daytime moisturizer with a pure titanium dioxide sunscreen, which provides gentle, broad-spectrum protection in a creamy, antioxidant-rich base that's excellent for normal, dry, or sensitive skin.

✓☺ BEST **BC Spa Facial Defend & Restore Moisture Lotion SPF 20** *($32 for 2.6 fl. oz.)* is a daytime moisturizer with sunscreen nearly identical to BeautiControl's BC Spa Facial Defend & Restore Moisture Creme SPF 20 above. Other than a texture that's slightly less creamy, the same review applies.

✓☺ BEST **Cell Block-C New Cell Protection SPF 20** *($30 for 1 fl. oz.)* is a remarkable mineral sunscreen (titanium dioxide is the sole active ingredient) for normal to dry or sensitive skin. It is fragrance-free and loaded with antioxidants and cell-communicating ingredients, and the packaging will keep these sensitive ingredients stable during use. The only sour note is the price. It may discourage liberal application, which is essential for achieving the sun protection your skin needs daily (though this is still less expensive than many department store offerings).

✓☺ BEST $$$ **Cell Block-C P.M. Cell Protection** *($40 for 1 fl. oz.)* is an impressive, silky-textured moisturizer for normal to dry skin, and for once the claims of strengthening skin and enhancing its repair process are accurate. That's because the numerous antioxidants, lightweight emollients, and cell-communicating peptides are capable of helping skin help itself when it's exposed to damaging elements (except sunlight, so you'll still need sunscreen). This contains fragrance in the form of citronellyl methylcrotonate.

✓☺ BEST $$$ **Regeneration Overnight Retinol Recovery Eye Capsules** ($38 for 30 capsules) are fragrance-free silicone-based capsules and an excellent way to treat skin to the benefits of stabilized retinol. Each capsule contains enough serum to cover skin around both eyes with little excess, so you're not wasting product. However, you should apply the contents of these capsules all over the face, as the face and eye area need the same beneficial ingredients. Further praise is warranted because the formula contains antioxidant green tea and the anti-irritant bisabolol. This product is suitable for all skin types.

✓☺ BEST $$$ **Regeneration Overnight Retinol Recovery Serum** ($46 for 1 fl. oz.) is a silky, lightweight serum with retinol, an ingredient that helps improve skin by changing the way new skin cells are produced. The packaging will keep the light- and air-sensitive retinol stable, which is a must. This fragrance-free serum also treats skin to a host of other beneficial ingredients, including antioxidants and several water-binding agents. It is recommended for all skin types, although those with sensitive skin may find the retinol too irritating.

✓☺ BEST $$$ **Regeneration Platinum Plus Face Serum** ($65 for 1 fl. oz.) is another one of BeautiControl's "breakthrough" products, so it's natural (at least for us) to wonder why so many are needed. If just one of them worked to deliver breakthrough results, then what is this one for? Does that mean the other ones don't really work? This serum doesn't hold any special secrets to address the needs of women aged 50+ or any age for that matter, and it won't reduce sagging skin—no skin-care product can do that (see the Appendix to find out why). What it does have going for it is a lightweight lotion texture that's loaded with several beneficial ingredients for skin of any age, and that's why it earns a Best Product rating. This is best for normal to slightly dry skin; it contains fragrance in the form of citronellyl methylcrotonate.

✓☺ BEST $$$ **Regeneration Tight, Firm & Fill Eye Firming Serum** ($44 for 0.46 fl. oz.) is a lightweight, water-based eye gel that helps smooth and plump skin, including superficial wrinkles, thanks to its blend of hydrating glycerin, peptides, and some good repairing agents, including hyaluronic acid. It is fragrance-free and also contains some lesser-known antioxidants. This is suitable for all skin types, but please keep your expectations realistic because this won't tighten or fill in wrinkles; it's not even remotely equivalent to the results you get from dermal fillers.

☺ AVERAGE $$$ **BC Spa Resurface Daily Resurfacing Serum** ($40 for 1 fl. oz.) is a very good, wonderfully silky serum that competes favorably with costlier serums BeautiControl sells. It contains a good assortment of antioxidants, cell-communicating peptides, and repairing ingredients, which is why it's a shame to mention the one significant drawback: the problematic preservative methylisothiazolinone. This preservative is typically not advised for use in leave-on products due to its sensitizing potential (Source: *Contact Dermatitis*, November 2011, pages 276–285). The amount is low, but it's still cause for concern and keeps this otherwise outstanding serum from earning our top rating. Note: The enzymes this contains are not known to exfoliate skin or improve age spots, not to mention the enzymes are likely not active in this serum due to their inherent instability. This serum contains a citrus ingredient for fragrance.

⊘ Think "hypoallergenic" means safe for sensitive skin? See the Appendix to find out the truth.

☺ AVERAGE $$$ **BC Spa Solutions Radical Hydration Concentrate** ($30 for 0.5 fl. oz.) is radical in name only, unless you consider a blend of plant oils plus vitamins and fragrant plants a revolution for skin care (just to be clear, they're not). Since this simple moisturizer for dry skin is mostly just safflower and soybean oil, you could purchase either at your grocery store and mix a drop or two with your regular moisturizer for those times when you need more hydration.

☺ AVERAGE $$$ **Regeneration Tight Firm & Fill Extreme Tri-Peptide Complex** ($95 for 1 fl. oz.). What's particularly upsetting about this serum is how similar it is to others BeautiControl (and other brands) sell, yet this option costs more than twice as much! For the extra money you're not getting an exponentially better serum, despite the fact that this one has an overall great formula. The silky, water-based texture contains a good amount of vitamin C (the form used is tetrahexyldecyl ascorbate) and a nice range of antioxidant plant extracts, including some that double as anti-irritants. Peptides are on hand as well, though these cannot "turn back time in as little as 30 minutes." The name for this serum sounds exactly what many struggling with signs of aging want, but the truth is that no skin-care product or specific skin-care ingredient can tighten sagging skin or fill wrinkles in an "extreme" manner. This product is not Botox or dermal fillers in a bottle! See the Appendix to learn why products like this don't help sagging skin. We opted to downgrade this serum's overall good formula because it contains the preservative methylisothiazolinone. This ingredient is generally not recommended for use in leave-on products due to its sensitizing potential (Source: *Contact Dermatitis*, November 2011, pages 276–285).

☺ GOOD $$$ **Cell Block-C Intensive Multivitamin Face Serum** ($42 for 30 capsules) comes packaged in single-use capsules, which is a good way to preserve the efficacy of the anti-oxidant vitamins it contains. The nonaqueous, silicone-based formula feels incredibly silky and is suitable for all skin types except sensitive (due to the ascorbic acid). Overall, although the formula is good, it's not as impressive as Elizabeth Arden's Ceramide Gold capsules or Paula's Choice RESIST Super Antioxidant Concentrate Serum.

☺ AVERAGE **Skinlogics Moisturizer** ($20 for 3.5 fl. oz.) has a rich, silky texture that feels wonderful on dry skin. The price is a bargain for what you get, too, and this works great under makeup. The downside is that it contains a skin-confusing blend of beneficial and problematic ingredients. Overall, the skin-helpful ingredients outweigh the skin-detrimental ones, but really why bother with a product that is fighting itself instead of just focusing on helping your skin? One more comment: Despite the claim, this does contain ingredients capable of clogging pores, making it not a great choice if you're struggling with blemishes.

☺ AVERAGE $$$ **Regeneration Tight, Firm & Fill Face Cream** ($52 for 1 fl. oz.) is said to make skin tighter immediately, but doesn't contain any ingredients capable of doing that. Even if it did, the effect would likely be irritating and assuredly only temporary (think minutes, not hours). Although this moisturizer for normal to dry skin contains several peptides, the jar packaging BeautiControl chose isn't likely to keep them stable during use. As for the "hyaluronic filling spheres" they claim are in this product—don't count on them performing in any way like the dermal filler products that contain hyaluronic acid. Because this product is applied topically and not injected under the wrinkle, the plumping/line-filling effect isn't even a close comparison (though repairing agents like sodium hyaluronate can temporarily plump dry skin).

☺ AVERAGE $$$ **Skinlogics Platinum Plus Renewing Night Creme** ($31 for 1.4 fl. oz.) ends up being one of the disappointing BeautiControl moisturizers, but not because the formula is lacking. What separates this from their outstanding options is the choice of jar packaging, which won't keep the antioxidants in it stable during use. Without the boost these ingredients provide, this is relegated to the status of a standard emollient moisturizer for normal to dry skin. Although the label does not list fragrance, the product does contain fragrance ingredients. One more comment: absolutely nothing about this formula is unique to skin over the age of 50.

☹ POOR **BC Spa Facial Defend & Restore Night Creme** (*$38 for 1 fl. oz.*) is a creamy moisturizer that contains plentiful amounts of great ingredients for dry skin—antioxidants and other anti-aging ingredients—but most of them won't remain potent thanks to the jar packaging. Please see the Appendix to learn why packaging is a problem. This is rated poorly because it contains a couple of plant extracts known to be irritating.

☹ POOR **BC Spa Facial Restructuring Eye Creme** (*$35 for 0.5 fl. oz.*) contains many excellent ingredients. Even though you don't need an eye cream (see the Appendix to find out why), if you're intent on buying an extra product called eye cream, it actually should contain many of the excellent ingredients this one does. Unfortunately, this also contains a few ingredients that shouldn't be applied to any part of your face or eyes. Another strike against it is the jar packaging, because all the great ingredients won't remain stable once you open the jar and let air in.

☹ POOR **BC Spa Solutions Under Eye Dark Circle & Puffiness Solution** (*$30 for 0.25 fl. oz.*) leaves no question as to what problems this eye gel is supposed to treat. Given that dark circles and puffy eyes are a major concern for many women, the cosmetics industry offers thousands of products claiming to do what BeautiControl claims for their product. Is this finally the solution you've been looking for? Of course not. There isn't one ingredient in here that is going to rid your eyes of puffiness or dark circles. Caffeine is a major ingredient, and it shows up in many eye-area products claiming to minimize puffiness. Although caffeine may help alleviate mild puffiness due to its constricting effect, it also can be an irritant when used in high amounts, so it's not something you want to apply to your eye area on a daily basis. Perhaps more important, caffeine has zero effect on age-related puffiness, which is what occurs when the fat pads beneath the skin shift and slip out of place. Even if caffeine were the answer, you have to wonder why all those mornings drinking coffee didn't help. If you are still curious to see if caffeine is an ingredient that works like this, why not just take the leftover coffee in your coffee pot and apply it to your eye area? Of course you don't really want to do that because it would be irritating, but you get the point. We can concede to using this product occasionally because it does contain some intriguing anti-aging ingredients, but it also contains other ingredients that have potentially negative impacts on skin. For example, arnica and *Cupressus sempervirens* (Italian cypress) are skin-irritants and neither is helpful for reducing dark circles, puffiness, or bags under the eyes. How anything in this product is supposed to "flush out fluid" that can occur under the eye isn't explained, most likely because BeautiControl knows this product can't really do that. Actually, all you have to do is stand up and start walking around and fluid buildup, around your eye or anywhere else in your body, will begin to go away. But fluid retention has little to do with puffy-looking eyes, that's about fat pads and muscle laxity, something that no skin-care or cosmetic product can affect. Don't be misled: This isn't a spa solution to common under-eye concerns of any kind.

☹ POOR **Platinum Regeneration Rejuvenating Eye Treatment** (*$42 for 6 pairs*) is sold with the promise of giving you younger-looking eyes in 30 minutes by using the pre-treated eye patches. The mundane formula is mostly water, glycerin, film-forming agent (think hairspray), and a small amount of red algae and peony extract, although the latter two have no research showing they are beneficial for the eye area or for skin anywhere else on the body. Glycerin is a good skin-care ingredient, but it's about as basic as you can get. You'll find these patches make the skin around the eyes look smoother and feel a bit tighter, but the effect is temporary and potentially irritating, because a product with a film-forming agent listed second on the ingredient list is not skin care. This also contains alcoxa, an ingredient that has constricting effects on skin and can be irritating, which is harmful to skin, not helpful.

☹ POOR **Regeneration Tight, Firm & Fill Firming Neck Serum** *($40 for 1 fl. oz.).* Regrettably, the claims for this neck serum are as over-the-top as it gets and this product can't make good on any of them. Before we discuss the claims a bit more, it is worth noting that this serum contains plenty of state-of-the-art ingredients. Yet even the most special anti-aging ingredients cannot undo the effects of gravity and age-related sagging that eventually shows up on the neck and face. It just isn't possible! As for reducing fat or fluid accumulation in that area, there is nothing you can put on topically to get rid of fat. (Our thighs would be thrilled if that were possible!) In terms of fluid retention, reducing your salt intake and standing up and walking around is the best way to reduce fluid buildup. But, fluid retention has nothing to do with skin sagging anywhere on your body. With all the beneficial ingredients in this serum, why the Poor rating? Because BeautiControl added several irritating fragrant plant extracts and citrus oil, and irritation is never good for your skin. Irritating ingredients cause collagen to break down and that's not a good thing from any skin-care viewpoint.

☹ POOR **Skinlogics Clear Oil Control Moisturizer** *($22 for 3.4 fl. oz.)* is a gel-textured moisturizer whose claims go far beyond what its ingredients can actually do. Forget about the claims of controlling oil production or detoxifying the skin because there are no botanicals that can do that, and toxins have nothing to do with acne. This moisturizer goes on silky, but has a slightly tacky finish that doesn't do much to keep skin matte. The amount of citrus extracts is a concern and has no benefit for any skin type; some of the other plant extracts aren't the best, either. It's a shame that there are more potentially troublesome ingredients than beneficial ones.

☹ POOR **Skinlogics Sensitive Hydra-Calm Moisturizer** *($22 for 3.5 fl. oz.)* is said to reduce the appearance of redness, according to the claims, due to the arnica extract in this lightweight moisturizer. We don't know where the proof is for that, because arnica is a known irritant and the amount of it in this product is bound to be troublesome for all skin types. The arnica's negative impact is intensified with the inclusion of other plant irritants as well, while the anti-irritants are unfortunately a lot less prominent (so their effectiveness is negligible). Whoever was in charge of formulating this moisturizer seemingly has no idea what sensitive skin needs to provide barrier protection and reduce inflammation.

BEAUTICONTROL LIP & SMILE CARE

✓☺ BEST **Skinlogics Lip Balm SPF 20** *($12 for 0.06 fl. oz.)* is a very good lip balm with an in-part avobenzone sunscreen. It contains effective emollients and leaves a soft gloss finish. The only misstep is the inclusion of orange oil, but the amount is so small as to be inconsequential.

✓☺ BEST **$$$ Lip Apeel** *($22 for 1.25 fl. oz.)* is a two-part product (peel and balm) that helps the user manually peel dry skin off the lips and then places a thick, glossy balm on them afterward. The peel contains waxes and silicates that can indeed rub off dead skin as you massage the lips. The balm is well formulated, but would be even better without the orange oil. Still, this cleverly packaged product is a very good way to keep lips smooth, flake-free, and moisturized.

✓☺ BEST **$$$ Platinum Regeneration Age Defying Lip Treatment** *($23.50 for 0.09 fl. oz)* is a very well-formulated tinted lip balm if you can look past the overhyped anti-aging claims. The oil–based formula comes in stick form, and its slim component is great for traveling and on-the-go use. It contains ingredients capable of preventing moisture loss and chapped lips, and includes a nice range of beneficial ingredients such as antioxidants and skin-repairing substances. Those extras don't necessarily justify this product's cost, but at least you're getting more than a standard lip balm for your money. This lip product has a slightly sweet scent and flavor.

☹ POOR **Regeneration Tight, Firm & Fill Extreme Lip Treatment** *($26 for 0.9 fl. oz.)* is a surprisingly standard, overpriced lip balm with a thick, waxy texture. Although it contains an impressive range of antioxidants and even includes some peptides, they cannot plump lips or stop signs of aging on lips or around the mouth. What's most disappointing is the inclusion of peppermint (listed by its Latin name of *Mentha piperita*). Peppermint causes irritation that damages healthy collagen production and impairs lip's ability to heal. Its cooling, tingling sensation may make you think this lip treatment is working, and it is, but just not in the way you're hoping!

BEAUTICONTROL SPECIALTY SKIN-CARE PRODUCTS

✓☺ BEST **Cell Block-C Intensive Brightening Elixir** *($30 for 1 fl. oz.)* is a lightweight moisturizer that claims to reduce hyperpigmentation. The various forms of vitamin C in this product may have some impact on discolorations, but the amount is likely not enough to fade discolorations with the same proficiency as hydroquinone or arbutin (Sources: *Dermatologic Therapy*, September-October 2007, pages 308–313; and *International Journal of Dermatology*, August 2004, pages 604–607). Still, even if only minimal fading of discolorations occurs, this elixir has a lot going for it in terms of providing an antioxidant boost to normal to slightly dry skin. Moreover, the opaque tube packaging helps keep the vitamin C and other antioxidants stable during use. This contains fragrance in the form of citronellyl methylcrotonate.

✓☺ BEST **Skinlogics Platinum Plus Brightening Day Creme** *($26 for 3.5 fl. oz.)* claims to lighten age spots (which are really sun-damage spots that can occur at any age); this product is better positioned as a well-formulated moisturizer for normal to dry skin. It contains a very good mix of emollients, cell-communicating ingredients, several antioxidants, and beneficial plant extracts. The alpha-arbutin in this product may have some impact on brown skin discolorations, but we suspect the amount isn't enough to net what most consumers would consider significant improvement. Still, this is definitely worth a try if you need a great moisturizer and want to see if an alternative to hydroquinone may help lighten sun-induced discolorations. This contains fragrance in the form of various fragrance ingredients, though the amounts are likely too small to cause irritation.

✓☺ BEST $$$ **Regeneration Tight, Firm & Fill Dermal Filling Moisture Masque** *($40 for 5 fl. oz.)* will keep you from the dermatologist's office, or so the marketing geniuses at BeautiControl obviously want you to believe. They lead you to believe that this mask replaces what dermatologists do when they inject dermal fillers into lines. The concept is as funny as buying a skin-care product suggesting that it is the same as a heart transplant. Why see a dermatologist for fillers when all you need is this mask? In reality, no skin-care product can even vaguely mimic what real dermal fillers do for skin, any more than a skin-care product can mimic heart surgery. Now that we're done discussing the absurdity of the claims, the good news is that this is a truly well-formulated moisturizing mask that's a very good, though needlessly expensive, option for dry skin. Again, this won't fill in wrinkles or restore lost volume (think sunken cheeks) to an aging face, but if dryness is your concern and you want a mask, this is one to strongly consider. For less money and an equally impressive formula, consider Paula's Choice Skin Recovery Hydrating Treatment Mask.

✓☺ BEST $$$ **Regeneration Tight, Firm & Fill Extreme Wrinkle Concentrate** *($40 for 0.04 fl. oz.)* is a fragrance-free wrinkle filler packaged in a pen-style component with a built-in synthetic brush applicator. The idea and claim is to "paint" the product over visible, deep wrinkles, and the formula helps "fill" them, thanks to the peptides. First, peptides don't have any filling effect on wrinkles. Theoretically, they are great cell-communicating ingredients that may stimulate collagen production, but regardless of the peptide concentration used, they don't have a magical, instant filling effect on wrinkles. What helps this product temporarily fill wrinkles is its spackle-like texture. The effect isn't as pronounced as the claims would have you believe, but products like this can make a subtle difference. What's more, this wrinkle filler also provides your skin with stabilized vitamin C along with other antioxidants and skin-repairing ingredients. All of those can help improve the appearance of wrinkles, especially if you're diligent about daily sun protection. Note: This product's rating is for its overall formula, not because it works as claimed to mitigate deep wrinkles.

☹ POOR **BC Spa Detoxifying Clay Masque** *($36 for 5.7 fl. oz.)*. Your skin isn't harboring toxins that this mask must expunge; in fact, no one at BeautiControl could name any specific toxins this mask eliminates. On the other hand, what you might define as toxic are the irritating ingredients this mask contains, such as the numerous fragrant plant extracts. BeautiControl included absorbent clay and silt, which are great for oily skin, but not when they're accompanied by irritants capable of triggering more oil production at the base of your pores. This is not the type of mask you should be using if your goal is healthier, less oily, or less sensitive skin.

☹ POOR **Skinlogics Clear Purifying Scrub/Masque** *($20 for 5 fl. oz.)* is well intentioned, but the company made a major misstep by including drying, irritating sulfur in this clay scrub/mask hybrid. It also contains some plant extracts with irritant potential, but they're less of a concern relative to the amount of sulfur. See the Appendix to learn why irritation is a big problem for oily skin.

☹ POOR **Skinlogics Clear Spot Treatment Duo** *($18 for 0.5 fl. oz.)* is a clever two-sided product combining a topical disinfectant with benzoyl peroxide on one end and a BHA (salicylic acid) gel on the other. Although the pH of the 2% BHA **Gel** is low enough for exfoliation to occur, it's lower than usual (pH 2.6) which makes it too irritating for skin. That, coupled with the alcohol base, makes this portion of the product too irritating to recommend for blemishes or oily skin. Irritation increases oil production in the pore and alcohol causes free-radical damage. The **Clearing Lotion with Benzoyl Peroxide** portion is fine, but there are several less expensive products that contain the same amount of this active ingredient.

BEAUTICONTROL FOUNDATION & PRIMERS

✓☺ BEST **BC Color Tinted Moisturizer SPF 15** *($22)* is for those with normal to dry skin who prefer the sheerness of tinted moisturizers and also want reliable broad-spectrum sun protection. Although the shade range is limited to those with medium to tan skin tones (the Light shade is too dark for those with fair to light skin), it has a creamy, smooth texture that blends readily and sets to a satin finish. Skin is left protected with a soft, healthy glow. The formula includes numerous antioxidants along with some notable skin-identical ingredients, making this a tinted moisturizer that provides more than just sheer color and sun protection. Well done, BeautiControl!

✓☺ BEST **Secret AGEnt Undercover Makeup** *($18)* is an excellent option for those needing a full coverage foundation. Although it doesn't look natural on skin, no foundation with this amount of coverage does; that's the trade-off for the amount of camouflage you get. This feels silky and sets to a long-wearing matte finish that doesn't look too powdery or flat. Perhaps the best news is that the shades are mostly exemplary. The only ones to avoid due to obvious overtones of peach or pink include Y-4, P-2, P-3, and P-4. Shade P-5 is also not recommended due to a strong copper tone. There are plenty of neutral options for those with fair to medium skin tones, and P-6 is great for dark skin tones.

☺ GOOD **Secret AGEnt Color Primer** *($12)* is a clear silicone-based primer that makes skin feel supremely silky. It is fragrance-free and compatible with most liquid or powder foundations. The texture allows for smoothing and minor "filling" of superficial wrinkles or large pores, but as with most products like this, the effect is fleeting.

☺ GOOD **$$$ Perfecting Creme to Powder Finish** *($18)* is a traditional cream-to-powder makeup that looks beautiful on skin but is very difficult to pick up with a sponge or your fingers. Just swiping your finger across the top barely picks up any product, and with a sponge you almost have to dig in to pick up enough makeup for what amounts to light coverage with a natural satin finish best for normal to dry skin that's not prone to breakouts. Almost all of the shades are very good, and present options for fair to dark skin tones. The ones to avoid due to overtones of peach or orange include P-3, N-4, and P-5. Although this missed being rated a Best Product, it is definitely worth exploring if you prefer this type of foundation.

BEAUTICONTROL CONCEALERS

☺ GOOD **$$$ Regeneration Tight, Firm & Fill Concealer** *($16)* is a satin-finish liquid concealer providing plenty of coverage, but it doesn't blend as easily as it should for smooth natural-looking concealing. Although its finish helps smooth out fine lines, it has the potential to eventually settle into deeper lines if you don't set it with a powder. This comes in three neutral shades and is best for normal to dry skin.

☹ POOR **Platinum Regeneration Age-Defying Concealer** *($20 for 0.9 fl. oz.)* is an oil–based, creamy stick concealer with a colorless moisture core that has an uneven application that requires more blending than usual. Once blended, this provides spotty coverage. The finish remains greasy, so this fades and settles into lines around the eyes (or mouth) quickly. Don't bother!

BEAUTICONTROL POWDERS

☺ GOOD **$$$ Perfecting Wet/Dry Finish Foundation** *($22)* is a talc-based pressed-powder foundation with a smooth texture that's drier than it is silky. Used wet or dry, it provides light to medium coverage and a soft matte finish that is best for normal to slightly dry skin. The formula isn't absorbent enough to handle combination skin with oily areas and definitely not skin that's oily all over. This looks better on skin when used with a damp sponge rather than applying it dry. The shades are mostly excellent, particularly those in the Y and N range. BeautiControl only falters with the peach-tinged P-3 and ash P-5 and Y-5.

☺ AVERAGE **$$$ Secret AGEnt Mineral Makeup SPF 15** *($26)*. This loose-powder foundation has a dry texture but smooth application that sets to a matte finish laced with sparkles. It appears slightly waxen on skin and provides medium to nearly full coverage if you brush on several coats. The shade range is mostly impressive, though keep in mind that the high amount of titanium dioxide and zinc oxide contribute to this foundation's ashen finish on skin. This is less apparent in the lighter shades (Neutral Light and Pin Light are great for fair skin), but the darker shades suffer. These shades are not recommended: Neutral Dark, Pink Dark, and Yellow Dark. This fragrance-free foundation is best for normal to oily skin.

BEAUTICONTROL BLUSH & BRONZER

✓☺ BEST **$$$ BC Color Mineral Blush** *($16)* is terrific! You get two complementary colors in one pan without a divider, so it's best to swirl your brush over both and apply the blush as one color. Application is smooth and the color payoff is impressive. All the shades are matte except Tawny, which has a moderate shimmer most will find too much for professional daytime makeup.

☺ AVERAGE **$$$ Secret Agent Tri-color Bronzing Powder** *($16)* includes a striped design of tan, a mid-tone color, and a pale shade for highlighting. The colors all go on as one when this is applied with a standard powder brush, so the design is more for visual appeal in the compact than expert results on your face. The powder has a smooth but flyaway, dusty texture and slightly grainy finish with sparkles that cling poorly. For the money, this isn't one of the better bronzing powders available.

BEAUTICONTROL EYESHADOWS & EYE PRIMERS

☺ GOOD **BC Color Intense Mineral Shadow Trio** *($20)* provides one matte and two shiny shades per compact. The shiny shades include a color with moderate shimmer and one with a stronger, metallic sheen. Each has a smooth, slightly dry texture and a color deposit that's uneven enough to require careful blending. The included dual-sided applicator just makes a mess of things and is best discarded; use full-size, professional eyeshadow brushes for best results. Although the majority of each trio plays up the shine, the good news is that it won't flake unless you really overdo application.

☺ GOOD **$$$ BC Color Mineral Shadow Trio** *($18)*. All the color sets in these trios are well coordinated. Each includes a light, medium, and dark shade, with the darkest shade in each being deep enough to double as eyeliner. The texture is smooth and dry (be sure to knock excess shadow from your brush to prevent fallout) and application is soft and even. Every trio has at least one shiny shade, but the shine isn't glaring and most users will likely appreciate the effect. The best trios are Sedona, Au Natural, Wisteria Lane, and Sandstone. The minerals in this eyeshadow formula are the same ones used industrywide in powder eyeshadows.

BEAUTICONTROL EYE & BROW LINERS

✓☺ BEST **Liquid Eye Liner** *($12)* is one of the best liquid eyeliners available. The felt tip-style applicator allows for a precise, thin line and the formula dispenses evenly and dries quickly. Once set, this won't budge until you take it off, so you're in for a day of worry-free wear. Classic black and dark brown shades are available, along with a navy hue that's an attractive alternative to black.

☺ GOOD **BC Color Eye Perfecting Pencil** *($12)* is not quite perfect, but pretty close! This fine-tip eyeliner pencil is conveniently retractable and comes in an array of muted but interesting shades, like Amethyst and Jade, which can play up your eye color without looking clownish. While it applies smoothly, it's not very blendable, which can be an issue if you like to smudge or soften your line. Each shade has a satin finish and lasts through the day.

☺ GOOD **$$$ Brow Kit** *($18)* provides two matte, pressed brow powders in a thin compact, plus a clear brow wax for a non-sticky finishing touch. The powders apply well and enhance the brows nicely, though toss the included brush, which is too stiff and scratchy. Having two colors to work with isn't a must, but for those who want to customize, these tone-on-tone shades work well together.

BEAUTICONTROL LIP COLOR & LIPLINERS

✓☺ BEST **BC Color Lip Perfecting Pencil** *($12)* is an outstanding retractable, fine-tip pencil that deposits rich, matte color and keeps creeping lipstick at bay—we love it! The shade range includes versatile colors that complement a wide array of lipsticks, whether you prefer nude, plum, or pink tones.

✓☺ BEST **Lip Gloss** *($16)* is a home run. The texture is light yet moisturizing, and the finish is completely non-sticky. Almost all the shades are infused with some degree of shimmer; each goes on softer than it looks. This is highly recommended unless you prefer tenacious, syrupy glosses.

☺ GOOD **BC Color Mineral Lip Color** *($14)* has the word "minerals" in the title, but they account for only a small portion of this cream lipstick's formula and if you're thinking the minerals make this a more natural lipstick, think again: one of the main ingredients is (the very synthetic) polyester! Not to worry though, because it contributes to this lipstick's smooth texture and cling. This provides a soft gloss finish and comes in an attractive range of shades that includes bright and softer tones. All the colors leave enough of a stain to help this lipstick last until lunch.

☺ GOOD **$$$ Clear Lip Gloss** *($11)* is a basic, but good, clear lip gloss whose only drawback is its too-thin texture. The shiny effect doesn't last long, though this isn't the least bit sticky and, being colorless, is compatible with any lip color.

☹ AVERAGE **Platinum Regeneration Age-Defying Lip Color** *($20)* is an expensive lipstick that gets its anti-aging chops from a tiny amount of peptide plus claims that after several weeks lips are softer and smoother, which would be true after using any lipstick that's as slick and oily as this one. This will quickly travel into lines around the mouth and the glossy, slippery finish is fleeting. A true age-defying lipstick would contain sunscreen, something this formula lacks.

BEAUTICONTROL MASCARAS

✓☺ BEST **SpectacuLash Mascara** *($10)* lengthens lashes without a single clump, smear, or flake to impede the results. You won't get much thickness (the law of diminishing returns applies here), but lashes are left beautifully long and softly fringed.

✓☺ BEST **$$$ SpectacuLash Thickening Primer and Maximum Length Mascara** *($20)* is a dual-sided mascara that includes a colorless lash primer and regular mascara. With the **Thickening Primer** applied first, noticeable bulk is added to lashes. When followed with the **SpectacuLash Maximum Length Mascara**, the result is impressive, at least compared to applying the Maximum Length Mascara (which goes on a bit too wet) alone. With the primer, you get more thickness and greater oomph, and the results look great. Although this is recommended, you should know that Maybelline and L'Oreal sell similar (in some instances better) versions of this product for less money.

☺ GOOD **SpectacuLash Maximum Volume Mascara** *($10)* isn't as wondrous as the name implies. You get noticeable thickness and reasonably long lashes with greater depth. This doesn't wow in the thickness department, but it's still a good mascara to consider.

☹ POOR **SpectacuLash Waterproof Mascara** *($10)* is waterproof, but that's its only redeeming quality. Considering the wealth of excellent waterproof mascaras, there's no reason to consider this one. It goes on too wet, smears in a blink, and clumps after only a few strokes with the brush.

BENEFIT

Strengths: One of the few cosmetics lines that tries to bring fun back to skin care, but succeeds more with their makeup; nice SPF 15 powder foundation; well-deserved reputation for liquid blush; several excellent powder blushes and a good bronzer; good brow-enhancing options; beautiful lip colors; excellent shimmer products.

Weaknesses: Clever names and product descriptions are much more interesting than product contents; skin care lacks impressive formulas and contains fragrance; cream concealers fall short; average mascaras.

For more information and reviews of the latest Benefit products, visit CosmeticsCop.com.

BENEFIT CLEANSER

☺ AVERAGE **$$$ Foamingly Clean Facial Wash** *($21 for 4.5 fl. oz.)* is a foaming, truly ordinary cleanser that's a mixed bag of pros and cons because it contains gentle and drying cleansing agents along with fragrance ingredients that aren't helpful for use around the eyes. This is an OK option for oily skin and it removes makeup easily, but it cleanses almost too thoroughly, putting your skin at risk of feeling tight and dry, and those feelings aren't part of a healthy skin-care routine for any skin type—gentle cleansing is critical for everyone.

BENEFIT EYE-MAKEUP REMOVER

☺ GOOD **$$$ Remove It Makeup Remover** *($21 for 6 fl. oz.)* is a standard, but effective, makeup remover that uses detergent cleansing agents and slip agents rather than oils or silicone to remove makeup. The fragrance-free formula is gentle and suitable for use around the eyes, but it's expensive for what you get.

BENEFIT TONERS

☹ AVERAGE **$$$ Moisture Prep Toning Lotion** *($29 for 6 fl. oz.)* is an overpriced toner that is not worth considering, even if you have money to burn. It is over-fragranced and the third ingredient is alcohol, which causes dryness, free-radical damage, and irritation that hurts healthy collagen production. Granted, the amount of alcohol is likely low enough to pose minimal risk, but why take chances when there are great toners that completely omit irritants?

☹ AVERAGE **$$$ Ultra Radiance Facial Re-Hydrating Mist** *($26 for 4.5 fl. oz.)* is an OK moisturizing toner for normal to dry skin, but the amount of fragrance should give you pause; fragrance isn't skin care. Companies such as Paula's Choice offer superior toner formulas that nix the fragrance in favor of lots of beneficial ingredients. If Benefit had done the same, this would be highly recommended; as is, this toner remains average at best.

BENEFIT SCRUB

☹ AVERAGE **$$$ Refined Finish Facial Polish** *($22 for 4.5 fl. oz.)* is an expensive, utterly ordinary facial scrub that contains standard, rounded polyethylene beads to polish skin to a smooth finish. The clay (kaolin) in this scrub offers little benefit, but it does make it a bit more difficult to rinse than many other scrubs. Ultimately, this isn't anything special; for the money, it doesn't beat exfoliating with a well-formulated AHA (alpha hydroxy acid) or BHA (beta hydroxy acid) exfoliant. If you decide to try this, it's best for combination to oily skin.

BENEFIT MOISTURIZERS (DAYTIME &NIGHTTIME), EYE CREAMS, & SERUMS

☹ AVERAGE **$$$ Total Moisture Facial Cream** *($38 for 1.7 fl. oz.)* is a heavy-duty, thick-textured moisturizer for dry to very dry skin. We'd love to be able to recommend this very emollient facial moisturizer because there just aren't many of these around, but this relatively pricey formula ends up disappointing. It just doesn't offer dry skin the range of ingredients it needs to significantly help it be repaired and look radiant. Instead of a range of anti-aging ingredients, the formula contains standard emollients and thickening agents, with more fragrance and preservatives than state-of-the-art ingredients. Plus, the tiny amount of antioxidants won't remain potent for long due to the clear jar packaging. Please see the Appendix for details on why jar packaging is a problem.

☺ AVERAGE **Triple Performing Facial Emulsion SPF 15** *($28 for 1.7 fl. oz.)*. Doesn't the name of this product sound like it does it all? Well, it doesn't—at least not if your expectations are to take the best possible care of your skin. Although it's great that this provides broad-spectrum sun protection (avobenzone is on hand for critical UVA screening), the lightweight lotion formula doesn't deliver a dose of the ingredients that all skin types need to look healthier and act younger.

☹ POOR **It's Potent! Eye Cream** *($32 for 0.5 fl. oz.)* claims to fade dark circles and smooth fine lines, but its formula is truly disappointing and can't deliver. Of course, no one needs an eye cream (check out the Appendix to find out why), but if you're intent on using one, this isn't the one to consider. The main problem with this cleverly named product is the amount of film-forming agent. As the second ingredient, it can make skin feel smoother and temporarily tighter, but it also puts your skin at risk of irritation. Irritation around the eyes makes wrinkles, sagging, and dark circles worse, not better! Maybe that's what Benefit means by "It's Potent!"?

The rest of the formula fails to impress; there's more preservative and alcohol than state-of-the-art anti-aging ingredients, including the peptides that are supposed to improve dark circles. Adding to the formulary woes is the fact that this eye cream is packaged in a jar, which won't keep any of the potentially helpful ingredients stable.

BENEFIT LIP CARE

☹ POOR **Benetint Lip Balm SPF 15** *($20)* has a smooth texture that moisturizes without feeling sticky, and it comes in a sheer, cherry-red shade that flatters most skin tones. In terms of sun protection, it's disappointing that the formula lacks UVA-protecting ingredients (titanium dioxide, zinc oxide, avobenzone, ecamsule, Tinosorb, or Mexoryl SX), so your lips will remain vulnerable to the sun's aging rays. Also disappointing is the inclusion of fragrance ingredients known to cause irritation. These strikes make this lip balm with sunscreen difficult to recommend.

☹ POOR **Lip Plump** *($22)* supposedly smoothes and builds the contour of the lips, but is really just a lightweight, flesh-toned concealer that minimally fills in lip lines and takes too long to set. Interestingly, the Benefit staff we spoke with about Lip Plump didn't speak highly of it, either.

BENEFIT SPECIALTY SKIN-CARE PRODUCTS

☺ AVERAGE **$$$ The POREfessional** *($29 for 0.75 fl. oz.)* bills itself as a "pro balm" to make pores disappear and give your face a smoother appearance and matte finish. You're directed to apply POREfessional after a moisturizer, and reapply as needed to absorb oil and minimize pores as they "come out of hiding." The moisturizer step is a potential mistake because if you have enlarged pores and oily skin, applying most traditional moisturizers will almost certainly exaggerate both issues. If you have oily skin and large pores with dry, flaky patches, you want to use a lightweight, gel-type moisturizer for smoothing without a creamy or slick finish. Looking at the ingredients, POREfessional is almost entirely silicone blends and film-forming agents, with a token amount of vitamin E. Like similar silicone-based mattifiers, POREfessional goes on dry, silky and initially shine-free. However, the fragrance is nothing short of intense, and it made reapplication (a necessity if you have oily skin, because this won't hold back shine for long) a challenge because you definitely don't want to be inhaling this all day. This mattifier's ability to minimize pores is overstated at best, and the benefit of the beautifully smooth, matte feel upon application won't surpass the powerfully strong fragrance (it really lingers). You can find similar silicone-based products that deliver on their claims and are fragrance-free, including Paula's Choice Shine Stopper Instant Matte Finish.

BENEFIT FOUNDATIONS

✓ ☺ BEST $$$ "Hello Flawless" Oxygen Wow Liquid Foundation SPF 25 *($34)*. Thankfully, this fragrance-free liquid foundation with an in-part titanium dioxide sunscreen has several "wow" factors that have nothing to do with oxygen. Using products that increase the skin's oxygen level (which the claims for this imply) is a bad thing, because oxygen causes free-radical damage, inside and outside our bodies—and cumulative free-radical damage is a leading causative factor of aging. The whole concept of using antioxidants is all about reducing the oxidative damage caused by oxygen and other types of free radicals. Oxygen claim aside, this foundation has a slightly moist but silky texture that feels light and is easy to blend. You'll get light coverage and a soft, natural-looking matte finish that's best for normal to oily or combination skin. The shade range is best for light to medium skin tones; there are no colors for fair or very dark skin, and the darkest shade ("I'm So Glamber" Amber) has an orange overtone that won't work for most dark skin. Both "Cheers to Me" Champagne and "I'm So Money" Honey are slightly peach but still worth testing. All told, save for those shade missteps, Benefit has produced an excellent foundation with reliable broad-spectrum sunscreen.

☺ GOOD $$$ "Hello Flawless!" SPF 15 *($34)* is a pressed-powder foundation that includes an in-part titanium dioxide sunscreen, so it does double duty and makes an excellent adjunct to your liquid foundation with sunscreen. It has a smooth, dry texture. Applied with a brush (but don't use the one included in the compact; it's awkward and applies powder unevenly), you get sheer coverage; applied with a sponge, you get medium coverage and a soft matte finish that looks quite natural. If you're using this to beef up the sun protection your foundation or moisturizer provides, it's best applied with a sponge, and you can use a brush to dust off any excess powder. The shade range includes options for light to medium skin tones. The synthetic sunscreen actives may be a problem for use around the eyes, so use caution and don't apply to the eye area if there are signs of irritation.

☺ GOOD $$$ Play Sticks *($34)* is one of the few foundation sticks left and remains a very good choice. It must be blended quickly because it dries to a powder finish almost immediately, and the finish does have longevity. Coverage can go from light to medium and the drier finish makes this suitable for normal to slightly oily skin only; it won't hold up as the day goes by for those with very oily skin.

☺ GOOD $$$ Some Kind-A-Gorgeous *($29)* is meant to be a sheer foundation that "evens skin tone without the look or feel of makeup." Although this is indeed lightweight thanks to its silicone-enhanced cream-to-powder texture, it isn't translucent enough to work on all skin tones. The shades offered are best for fair to medium skin tones, with the exception of the darkest shade which has unflattering orange undertones. This provides minimal coverage with a satin matte finish.

☹ POOR You Rebel SPF 15 *($30 for 1.7 fl. oz.)* does not include the ingredients needed to shield your skin from the sun's entire range of damaging UVA rays, which is essential for anti-aging benefits. See the Appendix to find out which active ingredients an SPF-rated product should contain.

☹ POOR You Rebel Lite SPF 15 *($30 for 1.7 fl. oz.)* does not improve on Benefit's original You Rebel SPF 15, mostly because this version's sunscreen does not provide sufficient UVA protection. The creamy-smooth texture is great for those with normal to dry skin who prefer sheer coverage and a moist finish, but the sunscreen issue is a big one, and doesn't make this a practical three-in-one product to consider.

BENEFIT CONCEALERS

☹ AVERAGE **$$$ Boi-ing** *($19)* is a cream-to-powder concealer (which leans toward being creamier) and provides almost complete coverage. It blends on easily and layers well if you need to camouflage very dark circles, but won't last through the day unless it's set with powder, which can make the under-eye area look dry and cakey. Among the three shades, only Medium is too peach to strongly consider.

☺ AVERAGE **$$$ Erase Paste** *($26)* is a creamy concealer in a pot that is almost too creamy for its own good! You'll certainly achieve considerable coverage that can be layered for more camouflage, but doing so requires careful blending and makes this already crease-prone formula more apt to do so. Benefit offers three shades, all of which have potential, though they're not the most neutral around.

☺ AVERAGE **$$$ Powderflage Powder Concealer** *($28)*. This product's name is a big-time misrepresentation because it does not provide any camouflage and it doesn't work like a concealer. It's a pale pink loose powder infused with small particles of pearlescent shimmer. Used on its own, it's way too sheer to provide meaningful coverage and it can make the under-eye area look too white.

☹ POOR **Eye Bright** *($20)* is a pale pink, slightly greasy pencil meant to be used on the dark inner corners of the eyes. It is completely unnecessary because any neutral-shade concealer can do the same without the unflattering pink tint.

BENEFIT POWDERS

☺ GOOD **$$$ Get Even Pressed Powder** *($30)* is a talc-based pressed powder that goes on sheer and blends smoothly for a polished, not powdered, look. Coverage is minimal and ideal for mid-day touch-ups. The shade range is limited, but because this powder goes on sheer it can work for a range of skin tones.

☺ GOOD **$$$ Matterial Girl Matte Finish Setting Powder** *($24)* is a talc-based loose powder with a silky, slightly creamy texture that belies its absorbent finish. It does a good job of setting makeup and keeping breakthrough shine in check, but the results don't last as long as those of powders that omit the shiny and slightly emollient ingredients this contains. The single shade goes on semi-translucent and is best for fair to medium skin tones.

BENEFIT BLUSHES & BRONZER

✓☺ BEST **$$$ Benetint** *($29)* has become a beauty classic, though it's not for everyone. This simple, rose-tinted, liquid cheek color only looks good on flawless, smooth skin because it has a tendency to seep into pores and indentations. It can be used as a lip stain, and is relatively long-lasting in that capacity. If you prefer liquid blush, this is deservedly one of the best.

✓☺ BEST **$$$ Cha Cha Tint** *($29)* has an opaque, lotion-like texture that is easier to work with than Benetint. This fragrance-free, liquidy cheek color sets quickly, so blending must be swift, but it offers a bit more playtime than Benetint, so you're less likely to make a mistake. Cha Cha Tint imparts a soft, sheer peachy pink coloration that looks fresh and attractive—and it lasts! It doesn't leave a shimmering finish, instead making cheeks look lit-from-within. The formula is suitable for all skin types—and it won't magnify the appearance of large pores like Benetint (and other liquid or gel blushes) can.

☺ GOOD **$$$ CORALista** *($28)* is a shimmery, coral pink powder that adds a healthy glow to your cheeks. The shimmer is subtle and CORALista will look great on many skin tones. Brushing on a sheer layer wakes up and adds a soft color to your skin. Lighter skin tones can use this as a blush, whereas darker skin tones will find it works best as a highlighter. The included brush is too small for proper application and the powder does have a faint peach scent to it, but neither of these factors should keep you from giving CORALista a try.

☺ GOOD **$$$ Dandelion** *($28)* is positioned as a highlighting powder but works best as a pale pink blush. It has a very soft gold undertone and a sheer amount of shine. This has a nice, smooth texture and the pressed powder is finely milled, so application is even, if a bit sheer. Color-wise, Dandelion is best for those with fair to light skin tones who want a touch of shine.

☺ GOOD **$$$ Dallas** *($28)* promises an "outdoor glow for the indoor gal" and it delivers this via shine that leaves skin with a healthy glow. The nude pink shade has a soft tan undertone and is a Benefit favorite because it is foolproof for many skin tones, whether you live in Dallas or elsewhere!

☺ GOOD **$$$ Hervana** *($28)* is a pressed-powder blush named after its supposed "heavenly flush." Like Benefit's other powder blushes, this comes in a box and, in this instance, there are four shades that are swirled together for pinkish, iridescent color. The lightweight, silky powder texture blends well and offers a slightly radiant glow, but the color goes on so light and sheer that you'll likely have to do some layering to see any color, and those with darker skin tones won't see much color no matter how much layering they do.

☺ GOOD **$$$ Hoola** *($28)* is a pricey, but excellent, bronzing powder. If you don't mind parting with this much moola, you'll find that Hoola has a smooth texture, minimally shiny finish, and a believable tan color that is very flattering on fair to medium skin.

☹ AVERAGE **$$$ Bella Bamba** *($28)* is a pressed-powder blush with shine packaged in a large, colorful cardboard container. Regrettably, the texture is an odd mix of creamy and crumbly. Despite that, if you're careful and use a full-size blush brush, application is even and you get translucent pink color with a soft golden shimmer that makes cheeks almost look wet. This fragranced blush is more novelty than must-have, but some may like it.

☹ AVERAGE **$$$ Posietint** *($29)* is sold as a liquid blush and cheek stain. It imparts a translucent flush of warm pink that stays put. The trouble (and major drawback) is with application: this sets to a stain almost immediately, so blending must be lightning-fast because it doesn't budge easily once set. For that reason, using this as a sheer cheek tint is difficult. However, using it as a long-wearing lip stain is an option, assuming you like the color. The brush applicator works well on lips, but its size means extra caution if lips are small.

☹ AVERAGE **$$$ Thrrrob** *($28)* is the least impressive of Benefit's "House of Powders." Thrrrob has a reasonably smooth yet dry texture and sheer application, imparting a pale, cotton candy–pink shade with a touch of silvery shine. It doesn't impart the rush of color the description mentions; actually, it takes a lot of product to build noticeable color.

BENEFIT EYESHADOWS & EYE PRIMERS

☺ GOOD **$$$ Creaseless Cream Eyeshadow/Liner** *($19)* has a silky-smooth, cream texture with a shiny finish. It blends evenly and goes on sheer, but can be layered to build more color intensity if desired. The color range is extensive and beautiful. Despite its creamy texture, this eyeshadow isn't likely to crease for those with normal to dry skin. Those with oily eyelids may

🍸 Did you know alcohol in skin-care products is a big problem? See the Appendix to learn more.

experience some creasing by the end of the day, but likely not much more than they normally would with a powder eyeshadow. Note: Due to this product's texture, it is best to apply it with an eyeshadow brush made of synthetic (rather than natural) hair.

☺ GOOD **$$$ Velvet Eyeshadow** *($18)* has a very smooth, powder texture and sheer application that imparts proportionately more shimmer than color. Even the darker shades apply quite sheer, and building intensity takes some effort. This eyeshadow blends readily and the shine clings well, but it's only for those who want minimal color and moderate shimmer.

☹ POOR **Stay Don't Stray** *($26)* is sold as a primer for use under concealer and eyeshadow. That sounds intriguing, but because the liquidy cream texture is prone to creasing itself, it ultimately makes matters worse. Packaging-wise, you have to deal with a dispenser that pumps out way too much product, so you end up wasting a lot. The single shade is OK, but one shade never works for everyone (think about one-size-fits-all pantyhose, those didn't work either).

BENEFIT EYE & BROW LINERS

☺ GOOD **$$$ BADgal Liner Waterproof** *($20)* applies smoothly and wears well through the day. The smudger tip on the opposite end of the pencil is useful for softening and blending the liner once applied. The color will begin to fade after 12 hours or a sweaty workout, but it won't wear off completely. In fact, you'll definitely need an eye-makeup remover to take this off completely!

☺ GOOD **$$$ Brow Zings** *($30)* is housed in a compact with two coordinated brow colors (in a creamy wax and powder cake) along with two tiny but functional brushes and a mini pair of tweezers. It's true that brushes this size are no match for those of standard length, but for travel or purse, what's included here is workable and not scratchy or flimsy. The non-greasy, wax-based color is good for tinting and grooming unruly brows, while the powder is for softer accenting or less dramatic shading. There are shades for light, medium, and dark brows.

☺ GOOD **$$$ Magic Ink Liquid Jet-Black Eyeliner** *($20)* does the trick. The finely tapered brush allows for smooth, defined application and the dramatic color won't flake or smudge. Those who like bold and dramatic eyeliner will love this!

☺ GOOD **$$$ Speed Brow** *($16)* works well as a sheer brow tint (available in one shade), while helping to groom and keep stray hairs in place. Speed Brow dries quickly and the brush is small enough to allow for precision grooming of thin or sparse brows.

☺ AVERAGE **$$$ Instant Brow Pencil** *($20)* delivers quick, smooth application and excellent shades (best for light brown to brunette brows). The pencil has a soft tip, so requires light pressure or short, feathering strokes through brow hairs for best results. We wish the finish didn't remain tacky on brows because it can feel and look a bit gummy, which may be why Benefit included a spoolie brush at the opposite end of this pencil to smooth out the problem application.

☹ POOR **BADgal Kohl Pencil** *($20)* is a standard chunky pencil that is creamy enough to consistently smear and fade. It may seem impressive that it is heralded by major fashion magazines, but remember, such publications applaud many products that are mediocre to poor, or just plain irritating.

BENEFIT LIP COLOR & LIPLINERS

☺ GOOD **$$$ Full-Finish Lipstick** *($18)* implies full coverage, but that's not what you get with this creamy-smooth lipstick. The shade range is attractive and each leaves a decent, doesn't-fade stain as it wears, but layering any color only adds up to moderate coverage and a soft gloss finish. This is a good cream lipstick to consider; it just has a misleading name.

☺ GOOD **$$$ Pocket Pal** *($20)* is a dual-sided wand that features a vial of Benetint liquid on one end and a clear lip gloss on the other. You brush the Benetint on lips, allow it to dry, and then top it with the lip gloss (which is necessary because Benetint on its own does not moisturize lips). If you like the way Benetint colors your lips and want a glossy finish, this is recommended!

☺ GOOD **$$$ Silky-Finish Lipstick** *($18)* glides on velvety smooth and is exceptionally moisturizing. The shades, some of which have shimmer, are attractive and impart a cream-gloss finish that's a bit on the slick side. The slightly glossy finish means this lipstick can bleed into lines around the mouth, but if that isn't an issue for you, then this is a beautiful option.

☺ GOOD **$$$ Ultra Shines Lip Shine** *($18)* is a sparkling gloss that glimmers in an array of vibrant colors. The texture is pleasantly smooth and coats lips with shine, minus the sticky feeling that many glosses leave.

BENEFIT MASCARAS

☺ GOOD **$$$ They're Real! Mascara** *($22)*. Benefit would have you believe that this mascara can deliver results as impressive as false eyelashes, but that just isn't so. Nonetheless, this mascara does lengthen lashes and increase thickness with multiple coats. Despite claims to the contrary, it doesn't curl lashes any better than regular mascara. The brush is on the larger side, which makes it a little difficult to use, but the bristles are well engineered to give lashes more definition without clumping.

☺ AVERAGE **$$$ BADgal Lash Mascara** *($19)*. From the box to the oversized brush, everything about this mascara is big except the results. It does apply cleanly and evenly, with no clumps in sight, but after much effort for moderate length and minimal thickness, BADgal Lash Mascara is a disappointment.

☺ AVERAGE **$$$ BADgal Waterproof Mascara** *($19)*. "Bad" mascara would be a more appropriate name for this lackluster mascara that does little more than add some pigment to the lashes. It doesn't lengthen, thicken, or curl lashes at all. The only good thing to say is it doesn't smudge and it is waterproof, as the name indicates.

BENEFIT FACE & BODY ILLUMINATORS

✓☺ BEST **$$$ 10** *($28)* tempts you to "be a perfect 10," and although it takes more than this cosmetic to go from bland to glam, without question you'll be pleased with the wonderfully silky texture and smooth application. This pressed shimmer powder is housed in a large cardboard box and includes a pale pink and sheer bronze shade with no divider in between. The concept is to bronze and highlight, but this is best for highlighting by adding soft touches of shine because the bronze shade is so sheer. The shine clings well and is glow-y without being too show-y, making for an attractive, though pricey, evening look.

☺ GOOD **$$$ Girl Meets Pearl** *($30)* is a face illuminator that offers a hint of glimmer and has a silky liquid texture. Its peachy pink hue is laced with subtle shimmer that leaves a pearlescent sheen, although the effect is quite subtle. The twist-up applicator allows you to pat the product directly on your skin, or you can use your fingertips for more precision and control. We recommend testing this product before purchasing to see if the illuminating effect shows up on your skin as much as you'd like; if so, this is a great option for those desiring a soft, luminous glow.

☺ GOOD **$$$ High Beam** *($26)* comes in a nail polish bottle and is applied to the face with a brush (or you can use a sponge or your fingers). It is a silvery pink shimmer lotion that dries to a matte (in feel) finish, leaving the shine behind.

☺ GOOD **$$$ Moon Beam** *($26)* is identical to High Beam except that it imparts golden-apricot color instead of pink. Both products tend to stay put and are much easier to control than shimmer powders with their minimal ability to cling.

☺ GOOD **$$$ One Hot Minute** *($30)* is a sheer, shiny loose powder with a talc-based formula that promises to make your skin look "sexy in seconds." Sexy-looking skin doesn't require shine (we'd argue that healthy, smooth skin is far more alluring), but this powder has a beautifully smooth texture that blends and adheres well. The shiny effect is of the sparkling variety rather than the shimmering variety, and it's workable for daytime if you want to add shine to your routine. The sole shade is accurately described as rose-gold, which is not a one-size-fits-all match.

☺ GOOD **$$$ Sugarbomb** *($28)* combines four triangles of different powders—in shimmery shades of pink, peach, and plum—meant to be swirled to create a sheer, rosy powder that can be used to highlight or as blush, depending on your skin tone. The shine is stronger than the color payoff, but the sheerness is due in part to how finely milled the pressed powder is.

☺ GOOD **$$$ Sun Beam** *($26)* is a liquid highlighter with a golden-bronze shimmering finish. It's housed in what looks like a large bottle of nail polish and can be applied with the included brush, but is easiest blended on with your fingers. Sun Beam blends on evenly and dries down to allow the shine to stay put.

☺ GOOD **$$$ "That Gal" Brightening Face Primer** *($29)* is a highlighting lotion whose pale pink shimmer adds a soft glow and moist feel to skin. Benefit is selling this as a primer, which means they intend for it to be applied all over the face. That's an option, but only if you have normal to dry skin and want forehead-to-chin shimmer. The click dispenser on top of the glue stick–like package takes some getting used to and can dispense too much product if you're not careful.

☹ AVERAGE **$$$ Ooh La Lift** *($22)* feels like an "instant eye lift!"—or so Benefit would like you to believe. This is just a pale pink liquid highlighter with a smooth texture and a slight shine. There is absolutely nothing in it to support the "depuffing and firming" claims, though using this under the eyes to banish dark areas will make puffiness less apparent.

☹ AVERAGE **$$$ Watt's Up! Soft Focus Highlighter For Face** *($30)* is a creamy highlighter stick with a velvety texture that blends well into skin, especially with the sponge blending tool that's affixed to the opposite end. It offers a luminous shimmering sheen with peach and champagne undertones. The downside is that the color and the beautiful glow rub off easily, leaving you to wonder why you bothered, especially given the cost!

BENEFIT BRUSHES

✓☺ BEST **$$$ Foundation Brush** *($24)* is a great option if you prefer to apply foundation with a brush! Its soft, synthetic hair allows for smooth blending. The brush is large enough to cover large areas quickly, but the slightly contoured tip allows for more control where you need it.

☺ GOOD **$$$ Hard Angle / Definer Brush** *($20)* works well if you want to apply a powder brow product or eyeshadow. The synthetic brush hairs are thin-textured, dense, and firm, but not "hard," as the name implies, or scratchy. The brush has just enough give to smoothly apply brow powders for a natural yet defined look.

☹ AVERAGE **$$$ Concealer Brush** *($22)* is intended to be used with cream concealers, but it's so wide that it's difficult to use for small blemishes or spot treatments. On the other hand, Concealer Brush has soft yet dense brush hairs that are suitable for applying concealer to larger areas.

☺ AVERAGE **$$$ The Talent Brush** *($18)* is touted as offering a "precision tip" for lining eyes, while the flat side of the brush is supposed to be used for shading and contouring. Although the synthetic brush hairs are soft to the touch and have enough density to apply eyeshadow, in terms of contouring, there are better brushes. The tip of the brush is not fine enough to allow for the tight control you need for eyelining, so that leaves you with a mediocre eyeshadow brush.

BENEFIT SPECIALTY MAKEUP PRODUCTS

☹ POOR **Prrrowl Iridescent Mascara Topcoat & Shimmering Lip Gloss** *($28)* is not recommended for anyone, not even on Halloween. There is no reason to waste your money on this poor performer! The iridescent mascara top coat imparts a layer of blue glitter that tends to cake up on lashes and, simply put, looks ridiculous. The shimmering lip gloss isn't much better, as it imparts an iridescent peachy pink hue with specks of light blue glitter.

BIOTHERM (SKIN CARE ONLY)

Strengths: Sunscreens now include the right UVA-protecting ingredients; some good cleansers and makeup removers.

Weaknesses: Redundancy, especially within the moisturizer category where there are far too many products whose differences are more tied to name and claims than formula; overuse of alcohol in the moisturizers (the drying kind, not benign fatty alcohols such as cetyl or stearyl); jar packaging; bland toners; ineffective AHA, BHA, and skin-lightening products; overly fragrant products make this brand a poor choice for those with rosacea or sensitive skin.

Note: Biotherm's claims and advertised ingredients would lead you to believe their products are all about natural formulations, and that is absolutely not the case. These products are steeped in synthetics, some that are great for skin, but also some that are definitely problematic.

For more information and reviews of the latest Biotherm products, visit CosmeticsCop.com.

BIOTHERM CLEANSERS

☺ GOOD **Biosource Softening Cleansing Milk, for Dry Skin** *($19 for 6.7 fl. oz.)* is a good cleansing lotion for normal to dry skin and it rinses well without the aid of a washcloth (though you may still need one to reach stubborn makeup at the hairline or around the eyes). This cleanser contains fragrance, which isn't the best to use around the eyes.

☺ AVERAGE **Biosource Biosensitive Dermo-Neutral Cleanser Gentle Milk** *($19 for 6.7 fl. oz.)* has a fluid texture and does not contain detergent cleansing agents (which means it can be gentler on skin), but the inclusion of coriander oil is a misstep that doesn't make this cleanser a safe bet for someone with sensitive skin. It's an OK option for normal to dry skin.

☺ AVERAGE **$$$ Biosource Clarifying Cleansing Milk** *($19 for 7 fl. oz.)* is a lightweight cleansing milk whose exceptionally basic formula is OK for normal to slightly dry skin, but for the money, this is nothing special. If anything, the amount of fragrance and the fragrance ingredients it contains put skin at risk for irritation. A fragrance-free cleansing milk, such as those from Boots, Clinique, or Paula's Choice RESIST, is preferred because omitting fragrance is a gentler way to go for your face and for cleansing around your eyes.

☺ AVERAGE **$$$ Biosource Softening Exfoliating Cleansing Gel for Dry Skin** *($19 for 5 fl. oz)* is a cleansing gel with scrub granules that could not be more basic and is ill-suited for dry skin. It's overpriced for what you get and contains enough fragrance to put skin at risk of irritation. See the Appendix for details on the problems daily use of highly fragranced products can cause.

☺ AVERAGE **$$$ Biosource Tonifying Exfoliating Cleansing Gel With Thermal Plankton Cellular Water for Normal and Combination Skin** *($19 for 5 fl. oz)* is a cleansing gel with scrub granules and could not be more basic. It's overpriced for what you get and contains enough fragrance to put skin at risk of irritation. See the Appendix for details on the problems daily use of highly fragranced products can cause.

☹ POOR **White D-Tox Brightening Micro-Scrub Cleanser** *($38 for 4.2 fl. oz.)* contains a small amount of jojoba beads for a mild scrub action. It is supposed to fight skin pigmentation (discoloration) issues, but dark spots cannot be scrubbed away. You need to treat dark spots with leave-on products and proven ingredients like vitamin C, hydroquinone, or niacinamide (among others); purchasing a special (and expensive) cleanser to improve dark spots isn't the answer. And, of course, fighting dark spots is a losing battle if you're not diligent (if not neurotic) about daily use of a sunscreen rated SPF 15 or greater (and greater is better). In terms of using this as a cleanser, the formula contains soap-like ingredients, which make it too drying and irritating for all skin types. Of particular concern is the amount of potassium hydroxide (that's lye), an alkaline ingredient that is very drying. Adding to this problem is a high amount of fragrance and fragrance ingredients known to cause irritation. See the Appendix for details on why irritation is bad for everyone's skin.

BIOTHERM EYE-MAKEUP REMOVERS

☺ GOOD **$$$ Biocils Make-up Removal Gel, for Sensitive Eyes** *($17.50 for 4.2 fl. oz.)* is a very good, fragrance-free eye-makeup remover that is adept at removing most types of water-soluble eye makeup (meaning it won't remove waterproof mascara); it may be used before or after cleansing.

☺ GOOD **$$$ Biosource Total and Instant Cleansing Micellar Water all Makeup Face & Eyes** *($19 for 4 fl. oz.)* has only one drawback and that is the inclusion of fragrance, which makes this ill-advised for sensitive skin; plus, using fragranced products to remove eye makeup isn't the best idea due to the risk of getting the fragrance in your eyes. Still, this works swiftly to remove all types of makeup, including waterproof formulas.

☹ POOR **Biosource Hydra-Mineral Lotion Softening Water** *($19 for 4 fl. oz.)* has a basic and somewhat problematic formula and it's just not a good option for skin. What makes it less than desirable is the inclusion of alcohol. As the fourth ingredient, it may not be present in a huge amount, but its inclusion should give you pause: Why tempt irritation when so many makeup removers do not contain any irritating ingredients? Moreover, this remover doesn't work as well as those that contain silicones or have more emollient ingredients that break down makeup, allowing it to be more easily washed away. Last, the inclusion of fragrance makes this a poor choice for sensitive skin and using fragranced products so close to the eye itself (as you'd likely do with a makeup remover) isn't the best idea.

BIOTHERM TONERS

☹ POOR **Biosource Hydra-Mineral Lotion Toning Water** *($19 for 4 fl. oz.)* lists alcohol as its second ingredient, which means it isn't hydrating, it's irritating. See the Appendix to learn why alcohol is a problem for all skin types.

☹ POOR **Biosource Instant Hydration Softening Lotion with Thermal Plankton Cellular Water for Dry Skin** *($19 for 6.76 fl. oz)* contains "thermal plankton cellular water" but you can forget about having benefit for dry skin because this toner contains enough alcohol to put skin at risk of dryness and irritation. Even without the alcohol, this toner is a boring formula that contains too much fragrance and not nearly enough of the kind of ingredients that dry skin needs to be hydrated and healthier. It's not that this toner lacks good ingredients, it's just that there are too many problematic ingredients to make it worth using—and the good ingredients could've been replaced by even better ingredients, which is what you should expect considering this toner's price!

☹ POOR **Biosource Instant Hydration Toning Lotion with Thermal Plankton Cellular Water** *($19 for 6.76 fl. oz.)* is nearly identical to Biotherm's Biosource Instant Hydration Softening Lotion with Thermal Plankton above, and the same comments apply.

☹ POOR **White D-Tox Translu-Cell Clarifying Renovating Lotion** *($38 for 6.7 fl. oz.)* lists alcohol as the second ingredient, making it too drying and irritating for all skin types. See the Appendix for details on the problems alcohol causes for all skin types. As for using this to fight skin discolorations, it contains a couple of plant extracts with minimal research (none on human skin, it was done on plants and animals) on their ability to improve dark spots, but even if the research was plentiful and solid, it doesn't excuse the inclusion of alcohol. Perhaps most disappointing is that although this toner contains ingredients that exfoliate skin (which can be a critical step for improving discolorations), the product's pH allows it to function as an exfoliant, and it contains the AHA ingredient glycolic acid as well, but the amount is too low for it to function as an exfoliant.

BIOTHERM EXFOLIANT

☺ AVERAGE **$$$ Skin.Ergetic Signs of Fatigue Repairing Concentrate** *($58 for 1.7 fl. oz.)* has a serum-like texture and contains salicylic acid (also known as BHA) formulated at a pH to allow exfoliation to occur. Unfortunately, the amount of salicylic acid is less than 0.5%, so it's not present in an amount that can truly benefit your skin. Also, this product contains a potentially troublesome amount of skin-damaging alcohol along with fragrance ingredients known to cause irritation. Those are not helpful for skin that's showing signs of fatigue or for improving signs of aging ("fatigue" actually has nothing to do with aging; tired skin needs sleep and exercise, not anything a skin-care product can provide). See the Appendix to learn why irritation is so bad for all skin types.

BIOTHERM MOISTURIZERS (DAYTIME & NIGHTTIME), EYE CREAMS, & SERUMS

☺ AVERAGE **$$$ Age Fitness Elastic Re-Elastifying Anti-Ageing Care, Dry Skin** *($64 for 1 fl. oz.)* could have been a great product for dry skin to fight aging, but it falls short from every angle. It can't build elastin as the name implies because it is almost impossible to regenerate elastin, and this formula definitely won't do it. While this does have a rich, silky texture it contains more alcohol, fragrance, and preservatives than beneficial ingredients. What it should contain is an abundant amount of the anti-aging ingredients all skin types need to look and act younger. See the Appendix for details on the problems that alcohol and fragrance in skin-care products cause.

☺ AVERAGE **$$$ Age Fitness Nuit Power 2 Recharging & Renewing Night Treatment, Normal/Combination Skin** *($65 for 1.7 fl. oz.)* is a basic, silky moisturizer for normal to slightly dry skin. Although this contains some very good olive-based antioxidants plus a cell-communicating ingredient, those substances won't remain stable because this moisturizer is packaged in a jar. Also, the formula contains more alcohol than anti-aging ingredients, and alcohol is pro-aging. This product falls short of keeping skin fit (if by "fitness" Biotherm means healthier, younger-looking skin).

☺ AVERAGE $$$ **Age Fitness Power 2 Active Smoothing Care, Dry Skin** *($60 for 1.7 fl. oz.)* is a rich, emollient moisturizer best for dry skin. Although it contains olive-derived antioxidant ingredients as claimed, they will not be able to provide anti-aging benefits because this product is packaged in a jar, which won't keep these important ingredients stable after the container is opened. Please see the Appendix to learn why jar packaging is a problem. In better packaging, this would be worth considering, although you don't need to spend this much to get a well-formulated moisturizer. This moisturizer will feel good over dry skin, but given that its anti-aging benefits will be squandered due to the jar packaging, it comes down to a "why bother?"

☺ AVERAGE $$$ **Aquasource 24h Deep Hydration Replenishing Balm, Very Dry Skin** *($36 for 1.7 fl. oz.)* leaves much to be desired, especially if you're concerned about mitigating signs of aging. The thick-textured moisturizer may feel good over dry to very dry skin and contains some helpful antioxidants, the fact that it's packaged in a jar means these critical ingredients won't remain stable after it is opened (see the Appendix for further details). In terms of this providing "deep hydration," it won't go any deeper than lots of other moisturizers, including many that treat dry skin to a better range of ingredients proven to make a positive difference.

☺ AVERAGE $$$ **Aquasource 24h Deep Hydration Replenishing Cream, Dry Skin** *($45 for 4.5 fl. oz.)* contains some helpful ingredients for dry skin, but it also contains a potentially problematic amount of alcohol, which causes free-radical damage. Also, like many Biotherm moisturizers, it is heavily fragranced. Neither alcohol nor fragrance are good for anyone's skin; see the Appendix to find out why. In terms of this providing "deep hydration," it won't go any deeper than lots of other moisturizers, including many that treat dry skin to a better range of ingredients proven to make a positive difference.

☺ AVERAGE $$$ **Aquasource Biosensitive Riche Dermo-Stabilising Hydrator for Dry to Very Dry Skin** *($45 for 1.7 fl. oz.)* is an OK moisturizer for normal to dry skin. It contains mostly water, glycerin, silicone, thickener, Vaseline, more thickeners, sunscreen agent, plant oils, and a tiny amount of vitamin E.

☺ AVERAGE $$$ **Biofirm Lift Firming Anti-Wrinkle Filling Cream - Face & Neck for Dry Skin** *($65 for 1.7 fl. oz.)* is one of the more emollient moisturizers Biothem offers, but its lifting and firming ability is an impossibility. The claims make it sounds like a re-sculpting face-lift awaits, but the most you can count on is smoother, softer skin and improved appearance of wrinkles over dry areas (something almost every moisturizer can do). The jar packaging renders the antioxidant vitamin E ineffective shortly after the product is open.

☺ AVERAGE $$$ **Biofirm Lift Firming Anti-Wrinkle Filling Cream - Face & Neck Normal/Combination Skin** *($65 for 1.7 fl. oz.)* is a basic option for its intended skin type, but won't lift skin a centimeter or provide a firming benefit. See the Appendix to find out why the jar packaging this comes in is a problem.

☹ AVERAGE $$$ **Biofirm Lift Firming Anti-Wrinkle Micro-filling Cream for Eyes** *($52 for 0.5 fl. oz.)* contains mostly water, silicone, slip agent, thickeners, alcohol, absorbents, more thickener, and vitamin E. Lesser amounts of several plant oils and some antioxidants are also included, but the jar packaging won't keep their best traits stable once the product is open. This product won't firm skin and its caffeine content cannot reduce puffy eyes. All in all, this is a dated formula, though it works as a basic moisturizer for slightly dry skin, so it's a little like using a washboard instead of a washing machine to clean your clothes. See the Appendix to find out why, in truth, you don't need an eye cream.

☺ AVERAGE $$$ **Hydra D-Tox Bio-Defensis Hydra-Detoxifying Gel for Under-eye Bags & Dark Circles** *($40 for 0.5 fl. oz.)* contains an extract from the anti-inflammatory herb *Terminalia sericea*, but neither this nor the other plant ingredients have a proven ability to reduce most cases of puffy eyes or dark circles. At best, this water- and silicone-based gel hydrates while providing a soothing benefit. It is fragrance-free, but see the Appendix to find out why, in truth, you don't need an eye cream.

☺ AVERAGE $$$ **Multi Recharge SPF 15 Daily Protective Energetic Moisturizer** *($49 for 1 fl. oz.)* is a daytime moisturizer with sunscreen that contains Mexoryl SX for reliable UVA protection, although we're skeptical that the amount Biotherm included will be enough, so this is recommended for sun protection with some reservations. The texture is a lightweight cream that's best for normal to slightly dry skin, and although the formula contains some helpful antioxidants and nonfragrant plant oils, the jar packaging won't keep these important ingredients stable during use (see the Appendix for details on the problems jar packaging presents).

☺ AVERAGE $$$ **Multi Recharge Yeux Energetic Eye Care** *($40 for 0.5 fl. oz.)* is an exceptionally basic eye cream that cannot erase signs of fatigue as claimed. You may be surprised to learn you don't need an eye cream (see the Appendix to find out why), but if you want to use one anyway, it should have a better formula that treats your eye area to proven anti-aging ingredients. Like many eye creams, this contains cosmetic pigments (mica and titanium dioxide) for a subtle brightening effect. That effect is makeup, however, not skin care, and although it can be attractive it holds no special benefit for the eye area—plenty of facial moisturizers have these brightening pigments, too.

☺ AVERAGE $$$ **Nutrisource Highly Nurturing Rich Cream** *($50 for 1.7 fl. oz.)* is a very emollient moisturizer for dry to very dry skin. It's not much for antioxidants, but even if it were chock-full, the jar packaging would undermine them. This contains a potentially irritating amount of coriander oil, so proceed with caution, since coriander can cause contact dermatitis and may have mutagenic properties (Source: *Handbook of Cosmetic and Personal Care Additives*, Second Edition, Volume 1, 2002). All told, this isn't worth strong condsideration.

☺ AVERAGE $$$ **Rides Repair Nuit Pur Silicium Intensive Wrinkle Reducer Ultra-Revitalizing Night Cream, Dry Skin** *($70 for 1.7 fl. oz.)* contains some great ingredients! Sadly, because of the jar packaging, many won't remain stable because repeated exposure to light and air destroys these ingredients. See the Appendix for further details on jar packaging. As for this product's antiwrinkle ("rides" is French for "wrinkles") ability, it doesn't have any edge over most other emollient moisturizers, including many that cost less and are in stable packaging. If anything, this formula contains some dated ingredients (cornstarch and wax?) and is short on giving your skin the range of beneficial ingredients (like antioxidants) it needs to look and act younger.

☺ AVERAGE $$$ **Rides Repair Nuit Pur Silicium Intensive Wrinkle Reducer Ultra-Revitalizing Night Cream, Normal/Combination Skin** *($70 for 1.7 fl. oz.)* is similar to Biotherm's Rides Repair Nuit Pur Silicium Intensive Wrinkle Reducer Ultra-Revitalizing Night Cream, Dry Skin above, and the same review applies.

☺ AVERAGE $$$ **Rides Repair Pur Silicium Intensive Wrinkle Reducer Ultra-Regenerating & Smoothing, Dry Skin** *($65 for 1.7 fl. oz.)* has an emollient texture that makes dry skin feel better, but its overall formula isn't what current research shows that skin needs to improve and resist signs of aging. Normally we'd comment on the problem jar packaging presents by causing light- and air-sensitive ingredients to break down, but there are so few of those types of ingredients in here it's not worth further discussion; it just doesn't contain anything of importance for skin. As for this product's antiwrinkle ("rides" is French for "wrinkles") ability, this doesn't have any edge over most other emollient moisturizers, including many that cost less.

☺ AVERAGE $$$ **Rides Repair Pur Silicium Intensive Wrinkle Reducer Ultra-Regenerating & Smoothing, Normal/Combination Skin** *($65 for 1.7 fl. oz.)* is similar to Biotherm's Rides Repair Pur Silicium Intensive Wrinkle Reducer Ultra-Regenerating & Smoothing, Dry Skin above, and the same comments apply.

☺ AVERAGE $$$ **Skin.Ergetic Non-Stop Anti-Fatigue Moisturizer with Fruit & Vegetable Fractions Cream Gel** *($49 for 1.7 fl. oz.)* contains fractions (extracts) of fruits and vegetables that function as antioxidants, but most of them aren't present in amounts your skin will notice—even if they were, the poor choice of jar packaging means they won't remain stable for long. See the Appendix to find out why jar packaging for products like this is always a bad idea. The goal of this moisturizer for normal to combination skin is to reduce signs of "fatigue" before they become signs of aging, but one doesn't cause the other. Yes, we tend to look "older" when we're fatigued, but most signs of aging come from cumulative sun exposure, smoking, an unhealthy diet, menopause, genetics, and gravity; it has nothing to do with being fatigued. Being fatigued simply exaggerates what's already there, but that's not the same as fatigue causing signs of aging; getting a good night's sleep and exercise is what you need to combat fatigue, not this product.

☺ AVERAGE $$$ **Skin.Ergetic Non-Stop Anti-Fatigue Moisturizer with Fruit & Vegetable Fractions Rich Cream** *($49 for 1.7 fl. oz.)* is nearly identical to Biotherm's Skin.Ergetic Non-Stop Anti-Fatigue Moisturizer with Fruit & Vegetable Fractions Cream Gel, save for its thicker texture. Otherwise, the same review applies.

☺ AVERAGE $$$ **Skin Vivo Nuit Overnight Reversive Anti-Aging Care** *($75 for 1.7 fl. oz.)* is an expensive moisturizer that has anti-aging aspirations; however, its formula cannot deliver, mostly because it comes up short on beneficial ingredients and the amount of alcohol it contains is potential cause for concern. Moreover, the almost nonexistent amount of antioxidants present won't remain stable during use because this moisturizer is packaged in a jar (see the Appendix for further details); plus, modern-day, proven anti-aging ingredients are absent. In short, this formula is largely incapable of repairing skin from a day's worth of environmental aggressors that "accelerate the aging process."

☺ AVERAGE $$$ **Skin Vivo Uniformity Renovating Anti-Age Moisturizer SPF 15** *($70 for 1.7 fl. oz.)* is a daytime moisturizer with sunscreen that contains a good mix of actives that provide broad-spectrum protection. Stabilized avobenzone and Mexoryl SX are on hand for reliable UVA (think anti-aging) protection. Although sun protection is assured, the base formula is mostly lacking in state-of-the-art, anti-aging ingredients. It has a silky, lightweight texture suitable for normal to combination skin, but the amount of vitamin-based antioxidants is paltry, and they won't remain stable once this jar-packaged product is opened (see the Appendix for details on jar packaging). You'll see a subtle brightening/radiance-boosting effect thanks to the mineral pigments this contains, but that alone isn't worth the price of admission. Even adding in the broad-spectrum sun protection, this daytime moisturizer is a tough sell.

☺ AVERAGE $$$ **Skin Vivo Yeux Anti-Aging Eye Gel** *($50 for 0.33 fl. oz.)* Biotherm's claims go on and on about reversing aging and rejuvenating skin through the vital impulse of your genes, all supposedly backed up by "in vivo science" and patents. If that's really the case, we couldn't find the research Biotherm did to prove their assertions, and they weren't willing to share it with us. What's certain is that the formula is far from extraordinary, and you don't need a special product for the eye area anyway (see the Appendix to learn why). As for patents: A patent has nothing to do with efficacy. A patent is obtained without any proof that what you're patenting actually works. The "patented" claim always sounds impressive to unsuspecting consumers, which is why lots of companies use it, but it isn't proof of anything except acknowledgment that you have laid claim to the use of an ingredient or ingredients for a specific purpose. This eye-area gel has a silky texture that's slightly spackle-like, so it can, to a minor extent, temporarily fill in superficial lines around the eye. How long the effect lasts depends on how expressive you are and what products you apply over it, but no one is going to mistake you for being even one year, let alone ten years, younger simply because you applied this product around your eyes. It contains a tiny amount of emollient shea butter and the mineral pigment mica for shine, but shine isn't skin care—and it's far removed from Biotherm's talk of "gene's vital impulses"! Speaking of genes: Our skin has plenty of them working in a carefully orchestrated manner to handle the formation, movement, and shedding of skin cells. As skin becomes damaged (mostly due to sun exposure), gene function can become faulty and eventually cause the process to malfunction, in turn causing a host of problems, from deep wrinkles to leathery texture. Using products with ingredients that protect skin and help repair some of the damage should allow these genes to begin functioning in a normal, healthier manner—but products like this aren't the answer because they don't contain the types of ingredients all skin types need to look and act younger.

☺ AVERAGE $$$ **White D-Tox Bright Cell Intense Brightening Cream** *($72 for 1.7 fl. oz.)* has a lightweight texture suitable for normal to slightly dry skin, but its jar packaging misses the mark for keeping the one significant brown spot–improving ingredient this contains stable during use. This product contains ascorbyl glucoside, a form of vitamin C that shows up in many products claiming to correct dark spots. There's some good research behind this ingredient's efficacy, but like all forms of vitamin C, it degrades and loses effectiveness when routinely exposed to light and air—which is exactly what happens when you opt for jar packaging (see the Appendix for further details). Biotherm claims they use three active ingredients to fight against pigmentation changes, but that really isn't the case. Only the form of vitamin C mentioned above has published research proving its worth for lightening discolorations. There is some information about *Palmaria palmata*, a type of algae, playing a role in controlling the pathway that causes melanin (skin pigment) formation, but there's so little to go on it's mostly speculation that this would work on intact skin; plus, concentration protocols have not been established and this product contains only a minute amount. What this product does have is a shockingly ordinary formula that makes its price that much harder to accept. As with most Biotherm products, it contains fragrance ingredients known to cause irritation, and it lacks the state-of-the-art anti-aging ingredients all skin types need to look and act younger.

☹ POOR **Age Fitness Power 2 Yeux Smoothing Relaxing Eye Care** *($50 for 0.5 fl. oz.)* contains a great range of beneficial ingredients for skin anywhere on the face, not just the eye area. Nothing in here is unique for the eye area, and in fact you don't need an eye cream (see the Appendix to learn why), which this formula proves in no uncertain terms; you just get charged twice as much for a virtually identical face cream. This has a lightweight yet hydrating texture that contains several antioxidants, and the opaque bottle packaging will keep them stable during use. Biotherm included small amounts of helpful skin-repairing and cell-communicating ingredients, too, and these provide further anti-aging benefits. Unfortunately, an overall impressive formula is sidetracked by the inclusion of fragrant coriander oil. This fragrant plant oil is known to cause contact dermatitis and also to make skin more sun-sensitive due to its chief fragrant component, linalool. Skin anywhere on the face does not need irritating ingredients, but when these ingredients are applied close to the eye, they become even more of a problem; plus applying fragrant irritants around the eye can make dark circles look worse.

☹ POOR **Age Fitness Re-Elastifying Anti-Ageing Care, Normal and Combination Skin** ($64 for 1 fl. oz.) is said to combine an anti-aging moisturizer and serum in one, but if that's the case Biotherm should stop selling the serums they offer. Separate from that notion, the formula is a big disappointment. It could have been a great product for combination skin to fight aging, but it falls short from every angle. It can't build elastin as the name implies because it is almost impossible to regenerate elastin, and this formula definitely won't do it. This lightweight moisturizer contains far more alcohol, fragrance, and preservative than it does the anti-aging ingredients all skin types need to look and act younger. With alcohol as the second ingredient, this ends up being more pro-aging than anything else because alcohol causes free-radical damage, which is just the opposite of what you need from a skin-care product! It is also highly fragranced, which isn't helpful for anyone's skin. Please see the Appendix for details on the problems that alcohol and fragrance cause.

☹ POOR **Aquasource 24h Deep Hydration Replenishing Gel, Normal/Combination Skin** ($45 for 0.5 fl. oz.) is said to provide deep hydration for 24 hours, but with alcohol as the fourth ingredient, it ends up being more problematic than helpful, and is bound to make combination skin worse. This lightweight moisturizer contains more alcohol than the kind of anti-aging ingredients all skin types need to look and act younger. It also contains several fragrance ingredients (albeit in small amounts) known to be irritating, which isn't helpful for anyone's skin. Please see the Appendix for details on the problems that alcohol and fragrance cause. This also is not recommended because it contains the irritating menthol derivative menthoxypropanediol. The tingle you experience upon application may feel refreshing, but it's your skin telling you it is being irritated.

☹ POOR **Aquasource Biosensitive Dermo-Stabilising Hydrator for Normal/Combination Skin** ($45 for 1.7 fl. oz.) won't reduce shine in oily areas but is a good moisturizer for its intended skin type. Unfortunately, it contains a problematic amount of skin-irritant coriander oil, which makes it a problem for anyone's skin. Coriander can cause contact dermatitis and make skin more sun-sensitive (Source: naturaldatabase.com).

☹ POOR **Aquasource Biosensitive Fragile Eye Contour Hydra-Soothing** ($40 for 0.5 fl. oz.) contains some good moisturizing agents, but nothing you won't find in numerous facial moisturizers, proving once again that eye creams are an unnecessary addition to your skin-care routine. This one is an especially bad option because it contains coriander oil, a fragrant oil known to cause contact dermatitis and make skin more sun-sensitive (Source: naturaldatabase.com).

☹ POOR **Aquasource Nuit High Density Hydrating Jelly** ($48 for 1 fl. oz.) is a fragranced, artificially colored gel-like moisturizer that lists alcohol as its second ingredient, which makes it a problem for all skin types. Alcohol isn't the least bit hydrating and, because it generates free-radical damage, it works against the anti-aging ingredients this lightweight moisturizer contains. See the Appendix for further details on the problems that alcohol causes. In addition to the alcohol, it contains numerous fragrance ingredients, which may please your nose, but won't make your skin happy because whether the fragrance is natural or synthetic, it causes irritation. You can ignore the claims of this being enriched with thermal plankton water, etc., etc. That sounds natural and spa-like, but water is water (skin can't really tell the difference) and considering the missteps this product makes, the called-out extras are not worth getting excited about.

Lavender oil smells great, but fragrance isn't skin care! Find out why in the Appendix.

⊗ POOR **Aquasource Skin Perfection 24h Moisturizer High Definition Perfecting Care, All Skin Types** *($48 for 1 fl. oz.)* is not appropriate for anyone's skin because it lists alcohol as the third ingredient. Alcohol isn't hydrating or skin-perfecting; rather, it causes free-radical damage. This also contains the irritating menthol derivative menthoxypropanediol. The tingle you experience upon application may feel refreshing, but it's your skin telling you it is being irritated, and that's not a good thing (see the Appendix to learn why irritation is a problem for all skin types). In addition to this lightweight moisturizer containing more alcohol than the kind of anti-aging ingredients all skin types need to look and act younger, it also contains several fragrance ingredients known to be irritating, which isn't helpful for anyone's skin.

⊗ POOR **Aquasource Superserum Intensely Moisturizing Oligo-Thermal Concentrate** *($46 for 0.5 fl. oz.)* lists alcohol as the third ingredient and plenty of fragrance ingredients, so it's far from being "super" and has limited appeal as a moisturizer. It also contains the irritating menthol derivative menthoxypropanediol, whose strong tingle is your skin telling you it's being irritated. See the Appendix for details on why alcohol, fragrance, and irritating ingredients are a problem for all skin types. If the formula weren't bad enough, the claims are over the top! The story is that Biotherm's biologists captured thousands of liters of thermal spring water, said to be a rich source of minerals—but, in a skin-care product the minerals are removed as part of the necessary purification process all water goes thorough before being mixed into a cosmetic formula. Then they combined this allegedly special water with pink sea salt from millions of years ago. There is no research showing any of this is good for skin; the story doesn't even make sense. The entire concept is ridiculous because minerals in water don't penetrate skin (their molecular structure is too large) and salt is drying (think of how your skin feels after you've been swimming in the ocean or how much salt hurts if you get it in an open wound). Regardless of the story, and regardless of the source of the water and salt, there is no research proving they can "insulate skin from environmental harm." If anything, the combination of salt water and alcohol impairs skin's barrier function, leaving its surface wide open to environmental damage. And it's certain this combination cannot protect skin from sunlight, which is its biggest environmental threat. Ultimately, this serum is a poor choice for all skin types. Although it contains some beneficial ingredients, they're intermixed with problematic ingredients, and your skin deserves only the good ingredients, preferably without hokey claims.

⊗ POOR **Hydra-Detox Bio-Defensis Detoxifying Moisturizer Rosy Glow Active Protection** *($49 for 1.7 fl. oz.)* is not only incapable of detoxifying your skin (skin does not eliminate toxins; the liver and kidneys take care of that), but also, with alcohol as the second ingredient, you're getting a strong hit of irritation, which is toxic for skin. The irritation causes dryness and hurts your skin's ability to heal and produce healthy collagen—none of which is "ultra-moisturizing" as claimed! This has a silky, lightweight texture, but so do many other moisturizers that cost less yet provide superior formulas without all of the skin-detox nonsense.

⊗ POOR **Rides Repair Yeux Pur Silicium Intensive Wrinkle Reducer Eye Contour** *($51 for 0.5 fl. oz.)*. This fragrance-free eye cream's instant smoothing effect is due to the silky silicone it contains, an ingredient that's not unique to Biotherm (indeed, almost any eye cream with an elegant, silky texture contains one or more silicones). If you're wondering about the first part of this eye cream's name, "rides" is French for "wrinkles," but in many ways this product is antiwrinkle in name only. Although the formula contains some skin-smoothing emollients and an impressive amount of vitamin E (tocopheryl acetate), its jar packaging won't keep the key ingredients stable during use. See the Appendix for details on why jar packaging is a problem. Ultimately, this eye cream is just further proof of why you don't need a separate product for the eye area; this contains nothing that is special for the eye area and, in fact, is merely an all-around ordinary product.

☹ POOR **Skin.Ergetic Overnight High Recovery Moisturizer with Tea & Seed Fractions** *($49 for 1.7 fl. oz.)* is an emollient moisturizer that contains fractions (extracts) of fruits and vegetables that function as antioxidants, but the poor choice of jar packaging means they won't remain stable for long, so your skin cannot reap their benefits. See the Appendix to find out why jar packaging for products like this is always a bad idea. This fragranced moisturizer's overall formula and unfortunate packaging are a problem for everyone's skin. This contains citrus oils and higher amounts of fragrance ingredients known to cause irritation, which hurt the skin's ability to heal and repair itself.

☹ POOR **Skin Vivo Reversive Anti-Aging Care Cream Gel for Normal/Combination Skin** *($70 for 1.7 fl. oz.)* is an expensive moisturizer that has anti-aging aspirations which this formula cannot deliver, mostly because it's dated and because it contains the irritating menthol derivative menthoxypropanediol. Irritants like this keep products from being anti-aging, and for those with oily skin, the irritation can stimulate more oil production at the base of the pores. See the Appendix for further details on why irritation is a problem for all skin types. Although this formula contains a small amount of antioxidants, they will not remain stable once this product is opened, all thanks to jar packaging. In short, this formula is incapable of repairing skin from environmental aggressors that "accelerate the aging process." At best, this meets the basic needs of normal to dry skin, but does so with an overly fragranced formula that can cause further problems.

☹ POOR **Skin Vivo Reversive Anti-Aging Serum** *($80 for 1.7 fl. oz.)* promises 10 years of youth after four weeks of use, but we wouldn't start counting down just yet! With alcohol as the second ingredient, there is more risk than benefit. Alcohol causes dryness and free-radical damage, and hinders your skin's ability to heal and produce healthy collagen—the exact opposite of what any product labeled "anti-aging" should do! The silicones this contains make skin feel silky, but you can get that benefit from numerous serums that don't contain alcohol. The teeny-tiny amount of antioxidants this contains will be of little help, and the salicylic acid cannot exfoliate owing to its low amount and to the fact that the pH of this serum is not within the range for exfoliation to occur. Add to this a smattering of fragrance ingredients known to cause irritation and you have a serum that no one should be using.

☹ POOR **Source Therapie 7 Skin Perfection Catalyzing Serum** *($64 for 1.7 fl. oz.)* contains a mix of beneficial and problematic ingredients. Despite its tempting, science-themed name, in many ways the formula cannot compete with today's best serums. Not only is this mostly lacking in state-of-the-art anti-aging ingredients, but also it contains a potentially problematic amount of skin-damaging alcohol and the menthol derivative menthoxypropanediol. The tingle you'll feel when you apply this serum isn't proof it's doing something good; rather, it's proof your skin is being irritated (see the Appendix to learn why irritation is bad for all skin types). Although this contains a handful of good ingredients, including sodium hyaluronate and antioxidant vitamin E (tocopheryl acetate), they're not unique to this serum—and when you add in the irritation from the bad ingredients mentioned above plus the fragrance ingredients, you have a serum that's not worth your time or money.

BIOTHERM LIP & SMILE CARE

☹ POOR **Beurre De Levres Replumping and Smoothing Lip Balm** *($36 for 0.43 fl. oz.)* has an outrageous price, and you will think so too when you realize it's mostly mineral oil and waxes. Are they kidding? Although these ingredients can help moisturize dry lips and protect them from chapping, they're not as elegant as several other ingredients found in less expensive lip balms, and definitely not any better than just using Vaseline. Even if the price doesn't raise an eyebrow, you need to know that the formula contains fragrant coriander oil, which is known to be sensitizing and to cause contact dermatitis, not to mention making lips more sun-sensitive (Source: naturaldatabase.com). The irritation coriander causes may lead to minor, temporary lip plumping, but the trade-off from daily application is more problems with chapping and, over time, damaged production of healthy collagen, which leads to thinner lips.

BIOTHERM SPECIALTY SKIN-CARE PRODUCTS

☺ AVERAGE **$$$ Hydra D-Tox Hydra-Detoxifying Mask** *($39 for 75 ml)* won't oxygenate skin any more than drinking a lot of coffee will make you sleepy, but it's an OK, basic moisturizing mask for normal to slightly dry skin.

☺ AVERAGE **$$$ White D-Tox Translu-Cell Intense Brightening Cream** *($82 for 1 fl. oz.)* should be loaded with ingredients proven to fight dark spots and uneven skin tone, especially with this price. Unfortunately, the formula will be of minimal use in addressing this concern because the lightening ingredients it contains have minimal research proving their efficacy. So, in all likelihood, your discolorations won't improve much, if at all, with this product, especially if you don't use a well-formulated sunscreen, which is the most important product to improve skin discolorations. This contains a small amount of *Palmaria palmata,* a type of algae believed to play a role in controlling the pathway that causes melanin (skin pigment) formation, but there's so little to go on it's mostly speculation that this would work on intact skin. Moreover, concentration protocols have not been established, so we don't know how much is needed to improve discolorations. Also present is the pomegranate-derived antioxidant ellagic acid, which has some research explaining how it works to affect melanin production. However, the studies on this ingredient were done on mushrooms and mice, not on human skin, and the main conclusion was that oral consumption helped more than topical application (Sources: *Bioscience, Biotechnology and Biochemistry*, volume 69, 2005, pages 2368–2373; and *International Journal of Cosmetic Science*, August 2000, pages 291–303). Ironically, this product contains the fragrance ingredient limonene (along with other fragrance ingredients known to cause irritation), which is known to cause skin discolorations when skin is exposed to sunlight. Limonene certainly is not the ingredient you want to see in any skin-care product, especially if your concern is lightening dark spots! Granted, it's present in a low amount, but really it shouldn't be here at all.

☹ POOR **Aquasource Non-Stop Emergency Hydration Mask** *($35 for 2.5 fl. oz.)* will likely conjure up wonderful spa images, but this mask's formula for normal to dry skin isn't as helpful as it could be, and the missteps make it not worth considering. This contains some good moisturizing plant oils and shea butter plus silicones for a silky feel, and the amount of vitamin E is greater than what Biotherm products typically have. That's great, as is the inclusion of some helpful skin-repairing ingredients. Things go wrong because this mask also contains the irritating menthol derivative menthoxypropanediol, as well as fragrance ingredients known to be irritating. Your skin doesn't need to suffer any bad ingredients to get good ones, as there are plenty of moisturizing masks that give your skin only helpful ingredients. See the Appendix to learn why irritation and fragrance are a problem for all skin types.

☹ POOR **Skin Vivo Uniformity Anti-Dark Spots Reversive Concentrate** *($49 for 0.5 fl. oz.)* contains far too many problematic ingredients to earn a recommendation. Things start off badly with alcohol as the second ingredient (which causes free-radical damage and other problems), and the only skin-lightening ingredient (ascorbyl glucoside, a form of vitamin C) of note is likely present in an amount too low for it to improve dark spots. Even if the vitamin C content were greater, the alcohol is a deal-breaker (see the Appendix to find out why). Adding to the problem with alcohol is the inclusion of several fragrance ingredients known to cause irritation; it's almost a "who's who" of every problematic fragrance ingredient known! The formula contains some mineral pigments (mica and titanium dioxide) for shine and a subtle brightening effect, but this visual trick is strictly cosmetic; it cannot improve dark spots. Last, the amount of salicylic acid is likely too low for it to function as an exfoliant—and even if it were present at a 1% concentration, this product's pH is too high for exfoliation to occur.

BOBBI BROWN

Strengths: A good cleanser and eye-makeup removers; a few stably packaged products loaded with advanced ingredients to keep skin in top shape; one of the best neutral shade ranges for foundation; foundation options for all skin types and preferences; very good blush and eyeshadows (powder and cream), including several matte shades; the pressed and loose sheer powders excel; the Gel Eyeliner and Shimmer Brick are impressive; mostly excellent brushes.

Weaknesses: As with most Lauder-owned companies, the well-formulated moisturizers are hindered by jar packaging, which compromises the effectiveness of light- and air-sensitive ingredients; several otherwise effective products marred by irritating fragrant oils or fragrance ingredients; concealers are a mixed bag; mostly unappealing lip glosses, and none of those with sunscreen provide sufficient UVA protection.

For more information and reviews of the latest Bobbi Brown products, visit CosmeticsCop.com.

BOBBI BROWN CLEANSERS

☺ GOOD **$$$ Lathering Tube Soap** *($26 for 4.2 fl. oz.)* is a standard foaming cleanser that uses the soap-derivative potassium myristate as the main cleansing agent, which can be drying and sensitizing for some skin types. However, this cleanser also contains a battery of nonirritating plant oils for extra cushioning while cleansing. There are minute amounts of lavender, jasmine, and grapefruit for fragrance, but likely not enough to be problematic. Though pricey, this is still a decent cleansing option for normal to slightly dry skin.

☺ AVERAGE **$$$ Hydrating Rich Cleanser** *($26 for 4.2 fl oz.)* is a thick-textured cleanser that contains some good ingredients for dry skin, but the chief emollient in use is not the easiest to rinse, so expect to need a washcloth for complete removal. Getting every trace of this cleansing cream off skin is mandatory because the formula contains a couple of fragrant plant oils (lavender and rose), plus other fragrance ingredients known to cause irritation. Dry skin already has a compromised surface, so adding an irritating ingredient to the mix isn't going to help it improve, not to mention fragrant irritants can hinder healthy collagen production and cause sensitized reactions. The amount of fragrance isn't that high, but no question this would be better without the scent. As is, this is an OK though overpriced cleanser for dry to very dry skin.

☹ POOR **Brightening Gentle Cream Cleanser** *($30 for 3.3 fl. oz.)* is an expensive foaming cleanser that is water-soluble, but contains some drying cleansing agents and enough potassium hydroxide (also known as lye) to leave skin feeling tight, as if cleansed by standard bar soap. The formula also contains fragrant orange oil and fragrance ingredients that can cause irritation, especially if used around the eyes. None of this adds up to gentle!

☹ POOR **Extra Balm Rinse** *($58 for 7.3 fl. oz.)* is a very rich, luxurious cleansing balm for dry to very dry skin, but the olive oil prevents it from rinsing well without the aid of a washcloth. That's not a big deal, but the amount of the fragrant component limonene in this product is. Limonene is a volatile compound found in most citrus fruits, and its topical application causes contact dermatitis (Source: naturaldatabase.com).

BOBBI BROWN EYE-MAKEUP REMOVERS

✓☺ BEST **$$$ Instant Long-Wear Makeup Remover** *($24 for 3.4 fl. oz.)* is a standard, but very good, dual-phase makeup remover. The blend of solvent and silicones quickly removes all types of makeup, including waterproof mascara and lip stains. What makes this product a cut above many similar options is its lack of fragrance and any other ingredients problematic for use around the eyes. It is recommended for all skin types.

☺ GOOD **$$$ Eye Makeup Remover** *($24 for 3.4 fl. oz.)* is a very standard, detergent-based eye-makeup remover that contains fragrant rose water and soothing cornflower extract. It works well, but so do many similar removers that cost much less than this one and omit the fragrance.

BOBBI BROWN TONERS

☺ AVERAGE **$$$ Hydrating Face Tonic** *($28 for 6.7 fl. oz.)* ends up not being as well formulated a toner as it could have been. The disappointing ingredients—lavender, orange, and palmarosa—are a problem for all skin types. These fragrant plant extracts have no established benefit for skin, yet each is capable of causing irritation that damages collagen and hurts the skin's ability to heal. It's doubtful that the amounts and forms included in this toner will be a problem, but they shouldn't be in here at all. Without question, your skin could have benefited from the range of antioxidants and hydrating agents included in this toner, along with the smaller amounts of skin-repairing ingredients, but the irritating ingredients are hard to ignore.

☹ POOR **Brightening Hydrating Lotion** *($52 for 6.7 fl. oz.)* is a toner that contains some helpful ingredients for skin, including vitamin C. However, something that's not helpful is the potentially problematic amount of fragrant bitter orange oil. Also known as neroli, this plant oil can make skin more sun-sensitive, especially fair skin. As with many fragrant oils, it contains chemical components capable of causing irritation (Source: naturaldatabase.com).

BOBBI BROWN SCRUB

☺ GOOD **$$$ Buffing Grains for Face** *($42 for 0.99 fl. oz.)* are made to sound special because you can add these loose grains to any cleanser to create a custom scrub. The novelty may be fun, but this concoction is simply polyethylene beads (plastic beads) with adzuki bean powder and tiny amounts of plant oils, plus a detergent cleansing agent that is activated by water. Polyethylene is used in most topical scrub products; you don't need to spend this much money for its benefit. While a viable option if you don't mind shelling out the money for this, a soft washcloth works just as well (if not better) than a scrub.

BOBBI BROWN MOISTURIZERS (DAYTIME & NIGHTTIME), EYE CREAMS, & SERUMS

✓☺ BEST **$$$ Intensive Skin Supplement** *($67 for 1 fl. oz.)* has some impressive ingredients and a lightweight, water-based serum texture built around slip agents and silicones. The amounts of vitamin C and mulberry root extract are probably not enough to have an effect on melanin production, but between them, the other antioxidants, and a cell-communicating ingredient, this is a well-formulated product that can be used by all skin types.

☺ GOOD $$$ **Brightening Advanced Serum** *($105 for 1.6 fl. oz.)* contains some beneficial antioxidants all skin types need to look and act younger, but it's not worth the investment. Bobbi Brown is owned by Estee Lauder, and Lauder's namesake line as well as sister company Clinique offer similar yet better serums for less money. This is a good, but overpriced, serum that's suitable for normal to slightly dry or oily skin.

☺ GOOD $$$ **Brightening SPF 50 UV Protective Face Base** *($38 for 1.7 fl. oz.)* is a very good daytime moisturizer with sunscreen for normal to dry skin, and it's not packaged in a jar! UVA protection is provided by avobenzone, and the emollient base formula contains an impressive mix of antioxidants to boost the sunscreen's efficacy. The mineral pigment mica is on hand for its cosmetic brightening effect, but in terms of ingredients that can affect hyperpigmentation, this treats your skin to only small amounts of ingredients capable of lightening discolorations. Despite this, the sunscreen element of this product will help keep new discolorations at bay, while also providing several helpful ingredients that dry skin needs to look and feel better.

☺ AVERAGE $$$ **Extra Eye Repair Cream** *($68 for 0.5 fl. oz.)* contains a brilliant assortment of ingredients for dry to very dry skin anywhere on the face. Unfortunately, it's packaged in a jar so the potency of several state-of-the-art ingredients will be diminished during use. Of course, regardless of how dry the skin around your eyes may be, you don't need a special product labeled "eye cream" to find relief. Refer to the Appendix to learn more about jar packaging and why you don't need an eye cream.

☺ AVERAGE $$$ **Hydrating Eye Cream** *($46 for 0.5 fl. oz.)* definitely contains ingredients that can hydrate skin around the eyes or elsewhere on the face, but it's an overall lackluster formula whose antioxidant vitamins are compromised by jar packaging. This eye cream is fragrance-free, but see the Appendix to find out why you don't need an eye cream.

☺ AVERAGE $$$ **Hydrating Intense Night Cream** *($60 for 1.7 fl oz.)* has a wonderfully creamy, cushiony texture that feels great on dry skin. Its formula is front-loaded with substantial emollients to prevent moisture loss and make dry skin feel comfortable, and numerous antioxidant plant oils are included. While all of that is excellent, what's not so good is the jar packaging. See the Appendix to find out why jar packaging is a bad idea. What's even more disappointing is the inclusion of fragrant oils known to cause irritation. These may smell great, but fragrance isn't skin care and, in fact, skin does better without fragrance. This also contains the fragrance ingredient methyldihydrojasmonate, putting skin at further risk of irritation. See the Appendix to learn why daily use of over-fragranced products is a problem.

☺ AVERAGE $$$ **Oil Control Lotion SPF 15** *($48 for 1.7 fl. oz.)*. Other than having a soft matte finish that someone with oily skin will appreciate, this daytime moisturizer with an in-part avobenzone sunscreen cannot control oil. Oil production is controlled by hormones, and as such is not affected by what you apply topically to your skin (although certain ingredients can absorb excess oil, but that's not the same as controlling oil production). So, with its matte finish and reliable sunscreen, why isn't this a slam-dunk for normal to oily skin? Because the amounts of lavender extract and irritating geranium oil surpass the amounts of several state-of-the-art ingredients. For what this product costs, you should expect more of the good stuff and little to none of the bad.

☹ POOR **Extra Eye Balm** *($68 for 0.45 fl. oz.)* is an extremely emollient, rich moisturizer that would have been a slam-dunk for those with dry skin (and an imposing skin-care budget) if it did not include appreciable levels of potent irritants like mint oil, orange oil, and galbanum oil, among others. None of these ingredients should go anywhere near the eye. What a shame, because aside from those irritants this is an exceptionally well-formulated product. See the Appendix to learn how irritants hurt your skin's ability to look and act younger.

☹ POOR **Extra Face Oil** *($62 for 1 fl. oz.)* contains some highly effective oils for dry to very dry skin, including olive, sesame, and jojoba. Not willing to leave well enough alone, this product also contains the irritants neroli, patchouli, lavender, and sandalwood, along with problematic fragrant components such as geraniol and linalool. Using plain olive oil would be preferred to this well-intentioned, but faulty, product.

☹ POOR **Extra Repair Moisturizing Balm** *($90 for 1.7 fl. oz.)* ends up being a very expensive way to supply skin with Vaseline and silicone, the main ingredients (next to water) in this rich balm. The antioxidant plant oils are rendered ineffective by this product's jar packaging, and the geranium oil, while smelling nice, can cause skin irritation (Sources: *Contact Dermatitis*, June 2001, pages 344–346; and *Journal of Applied Microbiology*, February 2000, pages 308–316). Choosing plain Vaseline not only costs considerably less, but also spares your skin an irritant response that can damage healthy collagen production. In better packaging and without the fragrant plants, this would be a good, rich moisturizer for those with very dry skin.

☹ POOR **Extra Repair Moisturizing Balm SPF 25** *($90 for 1.7 fl. oz.)* has avobenzone for UVA protection, but contains irritating bitter orange, grapefruit, and geranium oils, all of which cause irritation, plus the citrus oils are photosensitizing (Source: naturaldatabase.com). What are those ingredients doing in a product whose intention is to protect skin while outdoors? And even if it didn't include these problem ingredients, how liberally are you going to apply a sunscreen with a price like this? See the Appendix to learn why jar packaging is a bad idea.

☹ POOR **Extra Repair Serum** *($105 for 1 fl. oz.)* contains good ingredients for skin (though nothing exciting or worthy of this price tag), but their beneficial effects are counteracted by the inclusion of several fragrant plant oils, most of which cause irritation, which in turn hurts your skin's ability to look and act younger, and they're not repairing in the least! See the Appendix for details on why irritation is bad for your skin.

☹ POOR **Extra Soothing Balm** *($58 for 0.5 fl. oz.)* contains triglycerides, waxes, emollients, and plant oils that can protect and restore dry skin to a healthier-looking and smoother-feeling state. What's not the least bit soothing is the inclusion of ginger root and bitter orange oils. Both can be irritating to skin and they keep this product from being a worthwhile purchase (Source: naturaldatabase.com).

☹ POOR **Hydrating Face Cream** *($52 for 1.7 fl. oz.)* is a fragrant moisturizer that contains a blend of helpful and irritating ingredients. The problematic ingredients include coriander oil, jasmine, rosemary, and lavender. All of these can prompt irritation that hurts skin's healing process and hinders healthy collagen production. The jar packaging is also a problem; see the Appendix to find out why—and please avoid this moisturizer.

☹ POOR **Hydrating Gel Cream** *($52 for 1.7 fl. oz.)*. Although this moisturizer for normal to dry skin has a silky, gel-cream texture that feels light but still moisturizes well, the inclusion of several fragrant irritants makes it impossible to recommend. Also disappointing is the fact that this is packaged in a jar. Please see the Appendix to learn why this type of packaging is a problem and why irritation is bad for everyone's skin.

☹ POOR **Protective Face Lotion SPF 15** *($48 for 1.7 fl. oz.)* wins points for its in-part titanium dioxide sunscreen and a silky lotion base laced with soothing chamomile, several antioxidants, and cell-communicating ingredients. The problem is the inclusion of fragrance ingredients linalool, limonene, and cinnamyl alcohol, the latter of which is a known skin sensitizer and inappropriate for use in a product meant to protect skin from sun damage (Source:

Chemical Research in Toxicology, March 2004, pages 301–310). It's interesting that cinammyl alcohol and its aldehyde form are part of a standard fragrance mix used by dermatologists to determine whether a patient is suffering allergic contact dermatitis from fragrance (Source: dermatologytimes.com/dermatologytimes/article/articleDetail.jsp?id=396332).

BOBBI BROWN LIP CARE

☹ POOR **Lip Balm SPF 15** *($19 for 0.5 fl. oz.)* lacks the UVA-protecting ingredients of titanium dioxide, zinc oxide, avobenzone, Tinosorb, or Mexoryl SX, and is not recommended.

BOBBI BROWN FOUNDATIONS

✓☺ BEST **$$$ Oil-Free Even Finish Compact Foundation** *($42)* is a silicone-based, creamy compact makeup that applies and blends beautifully. This has a natural, slightly moist finish that isn't really powdery—it actually leaves skin with a soft glow that only those with oily skin will want to avoid. It provides light to medium coverage, but if you layer it you can net nearly full coverage, a feature that also makes it an option for use as concealer. Several beautiful shades are available.

✓☺ BEST **$$$ SPF 15 Tinted Moisturizer** *($40 for 1.7 fl. oz.)* has an in-part titanium dioxide–based sunscreen, and the silicone-based formula has a light but noticeably moist feel on the skin. The colors are exceptional and include options for porcelain to dark skin tones. This is an outstanding tinted moisturizer for normal to slightly dry skin. As expected, coverage is sheer and even. The tiny amount of fragrance ingredients is not cause for concern, though without question the formula would be better off without them.

✓☺ BEST **$$$ Skin Foundation Mineral Makeup SPF 15** *($38)* is a loose-powder foundation that goes on sheer so it looks natural, but it has enough coverage to even out your skin tone without looking chalky. The finely milled texture is super fluffy and light; as a result, it can get a little messy when transferring the product from the brush to your face, but, once applied, the result is an effortlessly smooth finish, weightless feel, and broad-spectrum sun protection all rolled into one. Keep in mind that we don't recommend relying on any SPF-rated loose powder as your sole source of sun protection because it is unlikely that anyone will apply it liberally enough to achieve optimal sun protection (a light dusting will not protect you from the sun's damaging rays). It is best to use an SPF 15 powder in conjunction with a moisturizer or foundation rated SPF 15 or greater.

☺ GOOD **$$$ Foundation Stick** *($41)* was the debut foundation from Bobbi Brown, and it's interesting (and worthwhile) to note that the shade range has improved considerably over the years. Initially, the small lineup was very yellow, though it was clear Brown was heading in the right direction—there wasn't a pink or rose-toned shade to be found. Today's array mostly of mostly neutral shades runs the gamut from fair to very dark, with just a few missteps along the way. Texture-wise, this remains creamy, is surprisingly easy to blend, and provides medium coverage that can be sheered if desired. We disagree with the company's "for all skin types except very oily" claim, because this is not the type of foundation someone with blemishes should use, nor does it have a matte quality to please someone with an oily T-zone. It is best for normal to dry skin.

☺ GOOD **$$$ Luminous Moisturizing Foundation** *($46)* has an elegant, fluid texture with just enough slip to make blending over normal to dry skin a pleasure. This does indeed have a luminous, satin-like finish, casting a healthy glow on skin. Coverage goes from light to medium and, as usual, almost all the shades are flawlessly neutral. We wouldn't label this foundation "super-moisturizing" as the company does, but it will hydrate. Just don't expect it to firm or lift the skin as the showcase ingredient with that alleged benefit (acetyl hexapeptide-3) is barely present and doesn't work in that manner anyway. The only thing keeping this from earning a Best Product rating is the inclusion of lavender extract, which lends a noticeable lavender fragrance to this otherwise top-notch foundation.

☺ GOOD $$$ **Skin Foundation SPF 15** *($46)* is a very good option for fans of tinted moisturizer looking for a bit more coverage and who still want the convenience of an all-in-one product. Skin Foundation SPF 15 provides sheer to medium coverage and broad-spectrum sun protection, though at 1% titanium dioxide, the UVA protection is not as impressive as many others with a higher concentration. The creamy texture blends easily, drying down to a satin finish that leaves the skin with a natural-looking yet polished finish. As is the case with most Bobbi Brown foundations, the shades tend to be golden in tone, and there are some very good options for light to dark skin tones with just a few shades to avoid. This foundation will work for all skin types.

☺ GOOD $$$ **SPF 15 Tinted Moisturizer Oil-Free** *($40)* is a fragrance-free tinted moisturizer with an in-part titanium dioxide sunscreen and a lightweight, slightly creamy texture that applies smoothly and blends evenly. The only real negatives are the price and the rather low amount of titanium dioxide, a crucial ingredient for UVA protection. Nonetheless, it still provides soft color, weightless hydration, and sheer coverage with a natural matte finish. As a bonus, this contains cell-communicating ingredients and antioxidants for extra benefits, and the packaging Brown chose will keep these delicate ingredients stable. Best for normal to oily or combination skin, this comes in a range of mostly neutral shades for fair to dark (but not very dark) skin tones.

☹ AVERAGE $$$ **Illuminating Finish Powder Compact Foundation SPF 12** *($42)*. If this talc-based powder foundation were rated SPF 15 or greater, it would easily rate a Best Product. As is, and because SPF 15 is the minimum level recommended for daily protection by medical boards all over the world, we cannot rate this as highly as we'd like. If you're still curious or if you're willing to apply this over a daytime moisturizer with sunscreen or a pressed powder with sunscreen (again, rated at least SPF 15 or higher), then here's what you need to know: The texture is superbly smooth and it applies beautifully. Few powder foundations have such an amazingly natural, skin-like matte finish. Skin looks fresh and polished, never dry or dull. Despite the name, this isn't illuminating, but the matte finish is sheer and attractive. Coverage is also sheer, but you can layer for slightly more camouflage. The formula is best for those with normal to oily skin. As for the shades, the range is extensive, with options for fair to tan skin tones and, with a couple of exceptions, soft and neutral. Getting back to the sunscreen, we're impressed that it's in-part titanium dioxide. Actually, considering the amount of titanium dioxide and the addition of a second sunscreen active, we're surprised this didn't meet the benchmark SPF 15.

☹ AVERAGE $$$ **Moisture Rich Foundation SPF 15** *($46 for 1 fl. oz.)* has a wonderfully soft, fluid-but-creamy texture that blends beautifully and dries to a natural, soft glow finish. Coverage is in the light to medium range and the shades are almost impeccable with just a few exceptions. African-American skin tones are well-served here, as are those with skin in the very fair range. Lamentably, the sunscreen is without sufficient UVA-protecting ingredients, which means this must be paired with another product that provides that critical protection. How shortsighted—because this is otherwise a formidable foundation for someone with normal to dry skin.

☺ AVERAGE $$$ **Natural Finish Long Lasting Foundation SPF 15** *($46)* was designed for those with oily skin who don't want to spend their day powdering to tone down excess shine. It succeeds with that purpose thanks to its soft, weightless matte finish and absorbent formula. Regrettably, some of the absorbent benefit is from the amount of alcohol this silky liquid foundation contains, and alcohol is never good for anyone's skin type. Between that and the low amount of titanium dioxide, this foundation becomes less desirable, especially for someone with oily skin seeking to use foundation as their sole source of facial sunscreen. This does blend on beautifully and provides light to medium coverage that manages to look impressively natural. As usual for Brown, her shade range is mostly top notch. There are ample shades for fair to light skin tones and a couple of good shades for dark skin tones, too. The medium to tan shades suffer a bit from overtones of yellow, orange, copper, or red. Given the pros and cons, it didn't earn a better rating, but it is still worth a test drive if you're curious how it could perform for you.

☹ POOR **Extra Repair Foundation SPF 25** *($56)*. Unfortunately, the main extra you're getting from this rich, creamy foundation for dry skin is an extra dose of irritation. The formula provides broad-spectrum sun protection that includes avobenzone for UVA (anti-aging) screening, but it also contains several fragrant plant oils and extracts. Combined with the active ingredients this foundation contains, you most likely will be getting a good amount of irritation, which will not repair skin. Irritation can cause collagen breakdown and impair your skin's ability to heal. Without the fragrant irritants, this would be a very good foundation for dry skin. It has a smooth texture, hydrates without feeling greasy, and leaves a soft, dewy finish while providing light to medium coverage. The shade range is admirable and includes excellent options for fair to dark skin tones. Some of the medium to deep shades are too orange, gold, or copper, but it's not worth describing the specific shades because, regardless of color, this pricey foundation is impossible to recommend. Bobbi Brown offers better foundations with sunscreen that spare your skin the needless irritation.

☹ POOR **Extra SPF 25 Tinted Moisturizing Balm** *($52 for 1 fl. oz.)* includes an in-part avobenzone sunscreen. But for this greasy tinted moisturizer, that benefit is negated by the many fragrant oils, all of which are irritating to skin and counteract the anti-irritants present in the formula. Without them, this would have been a good option for those with very dry skin, and all the shades are impeccably neutral. What a shame!

BOBBI BROWN CONCEALERS

☺ AVERAGE $$$ **Creamy Concealer** *($22)* is truly creamy with a thick texture and moist finish. Even when set with powder (which this absolutely needs), it can settle into lines around the eye and also magnifies large pores. It doesn't help that the shade range is hit or miss, with some neutral shades nestled alongside strong peach, pink, or gold tones. This concealer's only ace is the great coverage it provides. Note: This product is also sold in Brown's **Creamy Concealer Kit** *($32)*, which also includes a loose powder to set the concealer.

☺ AVERAGE $$$ **Face Touch Up Stick** *($23)* has a creamy texture and medium coverage that make it easy to use, blend, and layer, but those are attributes that several other, less expensive concealers also have. If you're eager to try this concealer anyway, shop carefully; some of the shades are very orange.

☹ POOR **Brightening Spot Treatment Corrector SPF 25** *($35)* is a resounding dud. Not only is the price exorbitant, but also the sunscreen's paltry amount of titanium dioxide (less than 1%) isn't what you want to see in a concealer meant to minimize discolorations.

The texture is dry and difficult to blend and the silicone wand applicator doesn't help matters. Dabbing this on trouble spots provides nearly complete camouflage, but because most of the shades are terrible, you're just trading one problem for another. Even worse, once this sets, the clay-like matte finish is immovable—any blending mistakes cannot be softened, so you have to start all over. This concealer is sold as "Bobbi's secret," but as it turns out, it's a secret she should've kept to herself.

☹ POOR **Corrector** *($22)* has the same texture, application, and level of coverage as Bobbi Brown's Creamy Concealer, but this version is meant for those with very dark circles. The shades are almost all strongly peach or pink, but the logic from Brown is that such hues cancel the purple tinge dark circles have. They do cancel it, but the effect is not nearly as flattering or neutral as it is from a neutral- to yellow-toned concealer. If anything, using a noticeably pink or peach-toned concealer over purple skin discolorations just replaces one discoloration with another.

☹ POOR **Tinted Eye Brightener** *($38)* has a weightless, liquid formula that blends on incredibly smooth and offers light coverage for minor imperfections. The pen applicator is convenient and easy to use, dispensing just the right amount of product. So why the Poor rating? Once it goes on, the matte finish settles unevenly on skin, drawing attention to wrinkles and fine lines. To make matters worse, several of the shades are unflattering peach tones (no one has peach-colored skin). To brighten as claimed, you'll need to select a shade lighter than your natural skin color, and considering all the peachy shades and the wrinkle-emphasizing finish, this product is so not worth it!

BOBBI BROWN POWDERS

✓☺ BEST **$$$ Sheer Finish Loose Powder** *($35)* is a talc-based powder that has a light, silky texture and smooth, slightly dry finish thanks to the cornstarch it contains. It feels weightless and looks very natural, yet makes skin look polished. Among the shades there are several flattering options for fair to dark skin, but watch out for those with a slightly peach undertone or stark white color.

✓☺ BEST **$$$ Sheer Finish Pressed Powder** *($34)* is talc-based with a silky, lightweight texture and beautiful finish. There are flattering shades for fair to dark skin except for a couple of shades that are slightly peach or stark white.

BOBBI BROWN BLUSHES & BRONZER

☺ GOOD **$$$ Blush** *($24)* is a pressed powder blush that features gorgeous colors that apply and blend evenly with a smooth matte finish (a few shades have a negligible amount of shine). This blush deposits stronger color, so if you want a sheer look, apply sparingly.

☺ GOOD **$$$ Bronzing Powder** *($35)* shows Brown knows what she's doing when it comes to creating believable tan shades. All the shades are attractive and convincing, each possessing a smooth application and soft finish with a tiny amount of visible shine. Those with fair skin should apply this sparingly and build as needed—a little goes a long way. This is preferred to Brown's **Illuminating Bronzing Powder** *($35)*, whose colors are a mixed bag and whose shiny finish looks uneven.

☺ GOOD **$$$ Shimmer Blush** *($24)* is a beautiful shiny powder blush. The color selection is small but what's available is good, especially if you prefer vibrant pastel tones. As for the shine, it's a blend of low-glow shimmer with crystalline sparkles, which tend to flake slightly. The silky, suede-like texture is wonderful and what you should expect from a powder blush at this price point.

BOBBI BROWN EYESHADOWS

✓☺ BEST $$$ **Long-Wear Cream Shadow** *($24)* is a silky, cream-to-powder eyeshadow that is highly recommended. Application is surprisingly easy, but you better be fast because the formula sets quickly. It also doesn't have as much initial movement as powder eyeshadows, which can make blending difficult, but with practice (and a good, synthetic hair eyeshadow brush) it can be done. In terms of long wear, this passes with flying colors and absolutely refuses to crease—though you may notice slight fading at the end of the day. Many of the shades impart shimmer, but the shine level is mostly subtle to moderate.

✓☺ BEST $$$ **Metallic Long-Wear Cream Shadow** *($24)*. Other than offering a metallic shimmer finish, these fragrance-free cream eyeshadows are identical to Brown's regular collection of Long-Wear Cream Shadow above, and the same review applies.

☺ GOOD $$$ **Eye Shadow** *($21)* has a silky, smooth-blending texture and most of the colors are beautifully matte (those that aren't true matte have a very soft, nonintrusive shine). There are some great choices for darker skin tones, and many of these shades would work well for lining the eyes or defining the eyebrows. The lighter shades apply sheerer than the medium to deep shades, which isn't necessarily advantageous, but can make blending colors a bit easier.

☺ GOOD $$$ **Metallic Eye Shadow** *($21)* is a powder eyeshadow with a smooth, almost creamy texture that is a pleasure to apply. Considering the amount of metallic shine, the effect is still flattering and doesn't overwhelm the face. The shine is a mix of finely milled shimmer with large particles of shine; the larger particles exhibit average cling, so expect some flaking unless you apply this sheer. Brown offers many attractive shades and the pigmentation in each is strong. You can also use these wet for an intensified effect or as eyeliner.

☺ GOOD $$$ **Shimmer Wash Eye Shadow** *($21)* is how Brown chose to separate her matte Eye Shadows from the obviously shiny powder ones. These have the same smooth texture and even application, except every shade has a non-flaky shimmer finish. There are shine-enhancing options for all skin tones.

BOBBI BROWN EYE & BROW LINERS

✓☺ BEST $$$ **Long-Wear Gel Eyeliner** *($22)* is a cream-gel eyeliner that is applied with a brush. It goes on like a liquid liner, and quickly sets to a long-wearing, budge-proof finish. It's truly an extraordinary product for lining the eyes, especially for anyone who finds powders or pencils fade or smear by the end of the day (or sooner). Brown's selection of shades often sees high-shine options rotated in seasonally, but the core assortment of blacks, charcoal brown, and steely grays are perfect.

☺ GOOD $$$ **Brow Pencil** *($20)* requires routine sharpening, and admittedly, we're not big fans of that. It's an inconvenience compared to twist-up pencils, and it ends up wasting product. That said, we were pleasantly surprised: Despite the fact that this pencil needs sharpening, it applies beautifully and is ideal for softly filling in and shaping brows. The texture is dry without being too hard or waxy, and it has a silky powder finish that doesn't flake or smear. Best of all are the shades, which include natural-looking options for blonde to brunette brows, but no good colors for redheads. If you prefer brow pencils to powders or gels and don't mind routine sharpening, this is worth a look, assuming the price doesn't bother you.

BOBBI BROWN LIP COLOR & LIPLINERS

☺ GOOD $$$ **Creamy Lip Color** *($23)* feels more greasy than creamy, but some women may indeed prefer this super-emollient lipstick with a glossy finish. The texture isn't slick or overtly slippery, but the oils will definitely cause color to migrate into lines around the mouth. This is not as pigmented as Brown's regular Lip Color, and as such doesn't last as long. Still, there are some gorgeous colors to consider.

☺ GOOD $$$ **Lip Color** *($23)* is a traditional cream lipstick with nice opaque coverage and great colors, including less conventional but still attractive options. Regardless of depth, the shades have minimal stain, so don't expect long wear.

☺ AVERAGE $$$ **Brightening Lip Gloss** *($23)* has a thick, syrupy texture that ends up being quite sticky, and also tenacious. The brightening part comes from the noticeable shimmer in each shade of this sheer gloss.

☺ AVERAGE $$$ **Lip Gloss** *($23)* is an extremely overpriced, standard, thick, sticky gloss. The same comments apply to Brown's **Shimmer Lip Gloss** ($23).

☺ AVERAGE $$$ **Lip Liner** *($20)* is a standard creamy lip pencil that features a smooth application and beautiful shade range, but the pencil has limited longevity compared to many others, including those that need sharpening, as this does.

☺ AVERAGE $$$ **Rich Lip Color SPF 12** *($23)* fails to provide sufficient UVA protection. What a shame considering everything else about it is flawless. We love the elegant, smooth cream texture that moisturizes without feeling slick or immediately moving into lines around the mouth. If only the SPF rating was higher and included the right UVA-protecting ingredients (see the Appendix for details).

☺ AVERAGE $$$ **Treatment Lip Shine SPF 15** *($23)* is a slim lipstick offered in a stunning array of colors, many of which are infused with soft shimmer or finish with a metallic sheen. The texture is smooth, silky, and hydrating, although this has enough movement to easily slip into lines around the mouth. As for it being a treatment—don't count on it. The sunscreen doesn't provide sufficient UVA protection because it doesn't contain titanium dioxide, zinc oxide, avobenzone, ecamsule, Mexoryl SX, or Tinosorb, and those are the only ingredients that cover the UVA spectrum. Also, the formula contains the same thickeners and emollient oils found in classic creamy lipsticks, and the packaging doesn't keep the few specialty ingredients (antioxidants) in here stable, so you're not really getting anything special for your money. If this lipstick with sunscreen offered better broad-spectrum sun protection, it would easily earn a higher rating. As is, it's not worth your time or money.

☹ POOR **High Shimmer Lip Gloss** *($23)* does indeed contain an astronomical amount of shimmer with an ultra-glittery, reflective finish. In fact, it's so glittery that you can feel the grainy, unpleasant finish the glitter leaves behind as the gloss wears off. What's more problematic is the amount of peppermint, which causes a stinging sensation on application. That tingling means this gloss is irritating your lips.

☹ POOR **Rich Color Lip Gloss** *($23)* imparts rich, nearly opaque color as the name states, and the finish is a flattering soft gloss. What a shame this gloss is hampered by the inclusion of irritating peppermint oil. The tingle it causes upon application is your lips telling you they're being irritated, and it's the reason this gloss isn't recommended.

BOBBI BROWN MASCARAS

✓☺ BEST $$$ **No Smudge Mascara** *($24)* really doesn't smudge but its performance goes beyond that. You'll enjoy how quickly this mascara lengthens lashes without clumping, and

Wondering why that product claiming to lift sagging skin didn't work? See the Appendix!

it provides more thickness than most waterproof mascaras. It stays on all day whether you're swimming or getting caught in the rain, and doesn't make lashes feel dry or brittle. Removing it requires more than a water-soluble cleanser, but that's par for the course. This is one to try if you prefer shopping for mascara at the department store.

☺ GOOD $$$ **Everything Mascara** *($24)* is a great all-purpose mascara, but it doesn't excel in any particular area. Moderate length and thickness are both present in equal proportion, so if you're looking to build amazingly long or dramatically thick lashes, this mascara won't bring you "everything." However, it does nicely separate lashes, doesn't clump or smear, and leaves lashes feeling soft rather than stiff or brittle.

☺ GOOD $$$ **Extreme Party Mascara** *($24)* applies cleanly and provides good length with appreciable thickness. You won't have to worry about clumps and it comes off easily with a water-soluble cleanser. The only drawback is the price: For what this costs, the results should be spectacular—that's what would make for a good party.

☹ AVERAGE $$$ **Lash Glamour Extreme Lengthening Mascara** *($24)* is only glamorous if your definition of the word as it pertains to mascara is "minimal length and no thickness after much effort." This mascara is best for a natural look, and it applies cleanly without flaking.

BOBBI BROWN FACE ILLUMINATORS

☺ GOOD $$$ **Shimmer Brick Compact** *($39)* includes five individual shades of powder (which resemble stacked bricks, hence the name), and all of them are viable options for adding a soft shine to the skin. The powder applies well, despite the fact that it feels drier than most, but the shine tends to migrate and dissipate after a few hours of wear. If the colors appeal to you, go for it—just don't expect the shimmer effect to go the distance.

☹ AVERAGE $$$ **Highlighter Pen** *($32)* is housed in a pen-style applicator outfitted with a built-in synthetic brush. This liquid highlighter (as a reminder, highlighter is applied over concealer or used alone to brighten naturally dark, shadowed areas) has a fluid texture and decidedly moist finish. Brown claims the effect is dewy, and she's right, but this also adds quite a bit of shine. Using this around wrinkled eyes isn't recommended because the shine will only magnify the wrinkles. The moist finish also has a tendency to crease into lines unless set with powder, but doing that somewhat defeats the purpose of using a highlighter.

BOBBI BROWN BRUSHES

☺ $$$ **Bobbi Brown Brushes** *($25-$60)* are quite nice, with well-tapered edges and dense bristles, though the prices are on the high side. There are some to carefully consider, and some to ignore altogether. The best, most useful brushes are the **Ultra Fine Eyeliner Brush** *($25)*, **Eye Shadow Brush** *($28)*, **Eye Contour Brush** *($28)*, **Eye Smudge Brush** *($28)*, **Foundation Brush** *($35)*, **Concealer Brush** *($25)*, **Touch Up Brush** *($28)*, and **Retractable Lip Brush** *($25)*.

BOOTS

Strengths: Inexpensive; the Expert skin-care line offers many outstanding options for sensitive skin; some great cleansers, including a few without fragrance; all sunscreens provide sufficient UVA protection; a smoothing, soothing lip balm; the only mass-market makeup line with testers for almost every product; mostly impressive foundation shades; very good powders and powder blush; great sheer lipstick; a handful of good mascaras.

Weaknesses: Abundance of ordinary formulas; Botanics line products contain few botanical ingredients; Time Dimensions line lacks sunscreen and provides more shine than proven anti-aging formulas for skin; repetitive formulas and a penchant for including the good stuff in amounts too small to be all that helpful; majority of products are surprisingly average; no effective AHA or BHA products; no products to help battle blemishes or lighten skin discolorations; jar packaging; foundations are more expensive than the competition, but do not best them; mostly disappointing eyeshadows; average to poor eye, brow, and lip pencils; inferior makeup brushes; superfluous or just plain unattractive specialty products.

For more information and reviews of the latest Boots products, visit CosmeticsCop.com.

BOOTS CLEANSERS

✓☺ BEST **Beautifully Balanced Purifying Cleanser, for Oily/Combination Skin** *($7.99 for 6.6 fl. oz.)* is a slightly fluid, fragrance-free, water-soluble cleanser that is suitable for its intended skin type. The smaller amount of detergent cleansing agent doesn't allow for complete removal of makeup, but this is an option as a morning cleanser or for those who wear minimal makeup.

✓☺ BEST **Expert Anti-Blemish Cleansing Foam** *($5.29 for 5 fl. oz.)* is a basic, but very good, water-soluble cleanser for all skin types. It is fragrance-free and works well to remove excess oil and makeup. There isn't anything about this cleanser that makes it preferred for blemish-prone skin, but it's not a cleanser those dealing with blemishes shouldn't consider, either.

✓☺ BEST **Expert Sensitive Cleansing & Toning Wipes** *($4.49 for 30 wipes)* are steeped in a mild cleansing solution that's fragrance-free and ideal for dry, sensitive skin—including those dealing with rosacea (though the rubbing of facial cloths on skin can exacerbate rosacea symptoms, so use caution). These cloths remove most types of makeup (eye makeup is trickier, especially waterproof formulas) and are a great on-the-go solution for using while traveling or to remove makeup before exercising.

✓☺ BEST **Expert Sensitive Gentle Cleansing Lotion** *($4.49 for 6.7 fl. oz.)* is a very standard but exceptionally gentle detergent-free cleansing lotion for dry, sensitive skin. Most will find a washcloth is necessary for complete removal. This works beautifully to take off makeup, including waterproof formulas, without drying or stripping skin. Although the formula is essentially a liquid cold cream, this deserves a high rating due to its value for sensitive, easily irritated skin. The price is great, too!

✓☺ BEST **Expert Sensitive Gentle Cleansing Wash** *($4.49 for 5 fl. oz.)* is a gentle, very basic formula that is a good option for sensitive skin whether it's oily or dry. The formula is so mild that it isn't much for makeup removal, but is fine for those who wear minimal makeup or for use as your morning cleanser. It is fragrance- and colorant-free.

✓☺ BEST **Soft & Soothed Gentle Cleanser, for Normal/Dry Skin** *($7.99 for 6.6 fl. oz.)* is a good detergent-free cleansing lotion for its intended skin types. The fragrance-free formula is very gentle, yet removes makeup easily (though you may need a washcloth to avoid leaving a residue of mineral oil).

☺ GOOD **Complexion Refining Deep Clean Mousse** *($8.99 for 5 fl. oz.)* is a basic but good water-soluble cleanser for all skin types except very oily.

☺ GOOD **Skin Brightening Deep Clean Gel** *($6.99 for 5 fl. oz.)* is a very good water-soluble cleanser for normal to oily skin. It removes makeup and won't leave skin feeling stripped.

☹ AVERAGE **Age Defense Cleansing Balm** *($9.99 for 6.7 fl. oz.)* doesn't offer much defense against aging. If anything, the citrus extracts it contains can cause irritation—the kind that increases rather than reduces signs of aging. Plus, the citrus extract and the sugarcane extract do not function as AHAs, despite the claim on the packaging that they can exfoliate skin—even if they could function like that, in a cleanser they are just rinsed down the drain.

This removes all types of makeup, but it doesn't rinse easily without the aid of a washcloth. It's an OK option for normal to dry skin, but should not be used around the eyes because it contains fragrant plant extracts.

☺ AVERAGE **Radiance Boosting Hot Cloth Cleanser** *($9.99 for 6.7 fl. oz.)* is a standard, fragranced cream cleanser for dry skin that comes with its own "washcloth" made of muslin (a sheer, woven cotton fabric). Although it's nice that Boots supplies a washcloth with their cleanser, the cloth's thin texture means it doesn't hold up as well as a standard cotton washcloth, although some may prefer the feel of muslin. Note that the "hot" part of the name refers to the temperature of the water you're supposed to use during cleansing; the formula itself doesn't warm as it's used. However, you should never use hot water to cleanse your skin because it is a strong source of irritation, hurting the skin's surface and impairing healing; warm to lukewarm water is preferred, especially for dry skin.

☺ AVERAGE **Skin Brightening Cleanser** *($6.99 for 8.4 fl. oz.)* won't brighten skin, but it can be a good cleansing lotion for normal to very dry skin. The mineral oil doesn't rinse easily without the aid of a washcloth.

☹ POOR **Cleansing Milk Geranium** *($7.99 for 5 fl. oz.)* would be an OK, albeit greasy, option for dry skin, but it contains too many irritating fragrant oils and fragrance ingredients to earn even a slight recommendation

☹ POOR **Cold Cream Rose** *($7.99 for 1.69 fl. oz.)* is a very antiquated cold cream formula that is not preferred to the classic version from Ponds. Because cold cream–style cleansers do not rinse easily from skin, you're leaving the problematic ingredients right where they're not needed. And the jar packaging is a completely unhygienic way to get almost any skin-care product on your face or body.

BOOTS EYE-MAKEUP REMOVERS

✓☺ BEST **Organic Face Nourishing Eye Makeup Remover** *($6.99 for 2.5 fl. oz.)*. Those looking for a makeup remover that's as close to natural as possible may wish to consider this product. The oil–based formula is noticeably greasy (and best used prior to washing your face), but it removes all types of makeup with minimal effort. It is fragrance-free, which makes it ideal for sensitive skin. This product's value for sensitive skin (it only contains six ingredients) is why it earned a Best Product rating.

☺ AVERAGE **Cleanse & Care Eye Make-Up Remover** *($7.99 for 3.3 fl. oz.)* is a silicone-in-water dual-phase makeup remover that works well to take off all types of makeup. This is labeled as suitable for even the most sensitive skin, but the preservative 2-bromo-2-nitropropanc-1,3-diol can be problematic (Source: *Handbook of Cosmetic and Personal Care Additives*, 2nd Edition, volume 1, Synapse Information Resources, 2002). Almay and Neutrogena sell the same type of makeup remover with gentler preservatives.

☺ AVERAGE **Expert Sensitive Gentle Eye Makeup Removal Lotion** *($5.49 for 6.7 fl. oz.)* is a basic, oil–based eye-makeup remover anyone can use. The formula is quite greasy and requires a separate cleanser to avoid a residue, but it works fine to remove all types of eye makeup. It is fragrance-free.

☺ AVERAGE **Expert Sensitive Gentle Eye Makeup Removal Pads** *($5.49 for 60 pads)* are soaked in an oily base that works to remove makeup (including waterproof formulas), but not without leaving a greasy film that must be washed off. The simple formula is fragrance- and preservative-free (the lack of water means preservatives aren't essential). This is similar to using plain mineral oil on a cotton pad, except it costs a lot more.

BOOTS TONERS

☺ AVERAGE **Complexion Refining Toner** *($7.99 for 5 fl. oz.)* is a water-based toner that contains two kinds of clay, which allows it to have a matte finish. The amount of castor oil is small, making this an OK option for normal to oily skin. This also contains rosemary leaf extract which poses a slight risk of irritation but again, the amount is likely too small for it to cause problems.

☺ AVERAGE **Expert Sensitive Gentle Refreshing Toner** *($3.99 for 6.7 fl. oz.)* is an exceptionally basic, gentle toner whose fragrance-free formula is suitable for all skin types, including sensitive skin. It woud be rated higher if it contained a selection of skin-identical ingredients and at least one antioxidant of note.

☺ AVERAGE **Soft & Soothed Gentle Toner, for Normal/Dry Skin** *($7.99 for 6.6 fl. oz.)* provides skin with a tiny amount of soothing agents, but is otherwise a lackluster fragrance-free formula that merely helps remove the last traces of makeup and leaves normal to dry skin soft.

☹ POOR **Expert Anti-Blemish Toner** *($4.29 for 6.7 fl. oz.)* isn't expert at anything except perhaps causing needless irritation and excess free-radical damage due to the amount of alcohol it contains. Willowbark extract isn't much of a weapon against blemishes, and definitely not in an irritating toner like this.

☹ POOR **Organic Face Rosewater Toner** *($7.99 for 5 fl. oz.)* is little more than eau de cologne disguised as skin care. Water, alcohol, and rose oil do not add up to good skin care any more than a martini flavored with a liqueur adds up to a balanced diet.

☹ POOR **Skin Brightening Toner** *($6.99 for 8.4 fl. oz.)* contains enough alcohol to be irritating, and the plant extract horsetail has constricting (not oil-reducing) properties that are not helpful for skin. The citrus and sugar cane extracts are supposed to be natural alternatives to the AHA glycolic acid, but they do not work in the same manner. But by far the biggest concern is the amount of alcohol. See the Appendix to learn why alcohol is a problem for all skin types.

BOOTS EXFOLIANTS & SCRUBS

✓☺ BEST **Expert Sensitive Gentle Smoothing Scrub** *($5.49 for 3.3 fl. oz.)* is a simply formulated but very gentle fragrance-free scrub. It is suitable for all skin types, including sensitive (assuming your sensitive skin can tolerate a gentle scrub). The sheer, gel-like formula rinses cleanly and doesn't contain extraneous ingredients skin doesn't need. Well done!

☺ GOOD **Time Dimensions Clarifying Facial Exfoliator** *($9.99 for 5 fl. oz.)* is a good fragrance-free scrub for dry to very dry skin. The water- and mineral oil–based formula contains a small amount of silica beads and pumice for a gentle polishing, but this doesn't rinse as well as water-soluble scrubs.

☺ GOOD **Total Renewal Micro-Dermabrasion Exfoliator** *($14.99 for 2.5 fl. oz.)* has alumina as its abrasive ingredient and, as such, this scrub can be grittier and potentially too abrasive unless used with great care. This does rinse easily.

☺ AVERAGE **Expert Anti-Blemish 2-in-1 Scrub and Mask** *($5.79 for 3.3 fl. oz.)* is an OK option for normal to dry skin. Polyethylene is the scrub agent, and it's buffered by the oil so there's less chance of overdoing it. The oil makes this scrub more difficult to rinse than most others. It is a poor choice for blemish-prone skin for two reasons: willow bark has minimal blemish-busting activity (and even less in a product that's rinsed from skin) and acne cannot be scrubbed away. In fact, scrubbing active acne lesions can cause further redness and risk spreading acne-causing bacteria to areas of the face that may not have breakouts.

The Reviews B

☹ POOR **Advanced Renewal Anti-Ageing Glycolic Peel Kit** *($24.99)*. The **Gentle Glycolic Peel** part of this kit contains an unspecified amount of the AHA glycolic acid. The company wouldn't reveal the percentage when we called, but it is likely between 5% and 10%. That's promising for effective exfoliation, but the bad news is that it also contains alcohol, which is anything but gentle! Alcohol is a major ingredient in this product, and the dryness, irritation, and free radical damage it causes are not the path to smoother, healthier skin. What a shame, because the pH of the Peel is within range for exfoliation to occur. Part two of this kit is the **Soft Neutralizing Pads**, which are just water with slip agents and a tiny amount of anti-irritants. A post-peel product like this isn't needed because you can use plain tap water to neutralize (i.e., stop the action of) an AHA peel. In the end, your skin will be much happier if you use a well-formulated AHA gel or lotion that doesn't assault your skin with a needless irritant and that doesn't need to be rinsed off.

BOOTS MOISTURIZERS (DAYTIME & NIGHTTIME), EYE CREAMS, & SERUMS

☺ GOOD **Expert Sensitive Hydrating Serum** *($7.49 for 1.69 fl. oz.)*. Although labeled a serum, this product's formula is much closer to a moisturizer. It contains some good, though standard, slip agents and emollients and is also fragrance-free. It's an unquestionably safe option for those with dry, sensitive skin and/or rosacea. It works quite well under makeup, though be sure your foundation contains sunscreen and is rated SPF 15 or greater.

☺ GOOD **Expert Sensitive Light Moisturizing Lotion** *($5.99 for 6.7 fl. oz.)*. You can completely ignore the oily skin claims for this moisturizer. This isn't a product anyone with oily skin should be using because the oil and triglyceride it contains will contribute to making skin even oilier. This is a basic, bare-bones moisturizer for normal to dry skin that's sensitive or affected by rosacea. Its merit for sensitive skin is why it is rated above average. All other skin types should be using something else because this formula completely lacks beneficial extras.

☺ GOOD **Expert Sensitive Restoring Night Treatment** *($6.99 for 1.69 fl. oz.)* is a bland, very basic fragrance-free moisturizer that is only recommended if you have dry skin that's prone to sensitivity or you're struggling with rosacea and need a basic moisturizer to help keep skin smooth.

☺ GOOD **Intensive Wrinkle Reduction Serum** *($14.99 for 1 fl. oz.)* has a beautifully silky silicone-enhanced texture but sadly, most of the intriguing ingredients (including vitamin A and the peptides) are listed after the preservative. That means skin isn't going to see much benefit other than the general smoothing and softening the core ingredients in this serum provide. This does contain an impressive amount of stabilized vitamin C, so it may be worth considering if you're curious to see what C can do for you, but skin care isn't as simple as one great ingredient. This fragrance-free serum is suitable for all skin types.

☺ GOOD **Radiance Renewal Night Serum** *($13.99 for 1 fl. oz.)* is a very good, ultra-light moisturizer for normal to oily skin. It contains bilberry extract as the main antioxidant, and it has anti-inflammatory benefits. The citrus extracts and sugarcane do not function as AHAs, but do contribute to this serum's water-binding properties. However, the citrus is potentially irritating, and that keeps this serum from earning a Best Product rating.

☺ AVERAGE **Advanced Hydration Day Cream SPF 12** *($14.99 for 1.69 fl. oz.)* provides sufficient UVA protection via its in-part avobenzone sunscreen, but the SPF rating is disappointing because you cannot use this as your only source of daily sun protection. Another letdown is that this day cream for normal to dry skin contains just a dusting of several state-of-the-art ingredients, including ceramides and phytosphingosine.

☺ AVERAGE **Advanced Hydration Day Fluid** *($14.99 for 1 fl. oz.)* is an OK (not advanced) moisturizing lotion for normal to slightly dry or slightly oily skin. It lacks antioxidants, and the amounts of skin-identical ingredients found in healthy skin are in very short supply.

☺ AVERAGE **Advanced Hydration Night Cream** *($15.99 for 1.69 fl. oz.)* is a standard lightweight moisturizer for normal to slightly dry skin. Jar packaging is irrelevant because this does not contain any air- or light-sensitive ingredients. The truly elegant ingredients round out the ingredient list, but that's not where you want to see them, especially in a moisturizer labeled "advanced."

☺ AVERAGE **Botanics Soothing & Calming Eye Base** *($8.99 for 0.25 fl. oz.)* contains a tiny amount of soothing licorice extract, but is otherwise a bland blend of thickeners, mineral oil, aluminum starch, and several waxes. The iron oxide pigments provide a bit of sheer color and coverage, but we wouldn't choose this over a great liquid or cream concealer.

☺ AVERAGE **Calm Skin Redness-Relief Gel** *($19.99 for 1 fl. oz.)* is better described as a moisturizer than a gel because the thickeners and emollients it contains don't combine to create a gel texture or finish. It's a fairly average product that achieves some silkiness from the silicones. Regrettably the anti-irritants it contains, which could help squelch redness, are present in such negligible amounts they are pretty much useless; ditto for the range of skin-identical ingredients. It's good that this product is fragrance-free, but it is not a good choice if your goal is combating persistent redness.

☺ AVERAGE **Expert Anti-Redness Serum** *($7.99 for 0.84 fl. oz.)*. There are some great ingredients in this serum that all skin types can benefit from, including ceramides and anti-irritants. Unfortunately, most of them are present in paltry amounts your skin won't notice. That leaves you with a moisturizer (it's definitely more of a moisturizer formula than a serum) that's an OK emollient option for normal to dry skin not prone to blemishes. It is fragrance-free.

☺ AVERAGE **Expert Sensitive Anti-Blemish Serum** *($7.99 for 1 fl. oz.)* contains willow bark but this plant is not considered an effective anti-acne ingredient, though it has anti-inflammatory properties. There is no research proving willow bark is helpful for those with oily skin, either. Consider this a very basic serum whose few interesting ingredients are present in amounts too small to matter.

☺ AVERAGE **Expert Sensitive Hydrating Eye Cream** *($6.99 for 0.67 fl. oz.)* is a very basic emollient eye cream for day use. It can be used anywhere on the face, though it's fragrance-free, gentle formula is a plus for use near the sensitive eye area. Expect this to moisturize skin, but that's all. The formula doesn't contain a single state-of-the-art ingredient.

☺ AVERAGE **Expert Sensitive Hydrating Moisturizer** *($4.99 for 1.6 fl. oz.)*. There isn't anything "expert" about this moisturizer except the name. It's a gentle, fragrance-free formula that's suitable for sensitive or rosacea-affected skin, but doesn't offer skin any beneficial extras such as antioxidants or cell-communicating ingredients. This is only recommended if you have dry, sensitive skin that does better with less. The choice of jar packaging is not of great concern for this moisturizer due to its basic formula (though there's still the hygiene issue from dipping your finger in a jar each day).

☺ AVERAGE **Expert Shine Control Lotion** *($5.99 for 3.38 fl. oz.)*. This lightweight moisturizer's oil-control claims are a joke. The second ingredient is a thickening agent that is incapable of keeping skin matte for eight minutes, let alone eight hours as claimed! At best, this is an OK fragrance-free moisturizer for slightly dry skin. The amount of alcohol is potentially cause for concern.

☺ AVERAGE **Intensive Nourishing Serum** *($14.99 for 1 fl. oz.).* Labeling this a serum is not accurate because texture- and formula-wise, it is best described as a traditional moisturizer for normal to dry skin not prone to breakouts. Skin will get some antioxidant benefit from the olive oil it contains, but the amount of vitamin C is unimpressive and not enough to be part of the company's so called "brightening complex" that this is supposed to contain. This isn't a bad moisturizer for the money, but it doesn't live up to the claims on the label and is outpaced by many other well-formulated products for about the same cost.

☺ AVERAGE **Instant Radiance Beauty Balm** *($15.99 for 1 fl. oz.)* adds radiance from the shiny mineral pigment mica and the slightly greasy finish it leaves on skin, and that's it. Keep in mind, shine isn't skin care, and the formula lacks the advanced beneficial ingredients, such as antioxidants, your skin needs to repair itself and to look and act younger. There are lots of products that provide shine plus those beneficial ingredients, so no need to settle for less.

☺ AVERAGE **Lifting & Firming Eye Cream** *($19.99 for 0.5 fl. oz.)* provides moisture to slightly dry skin and has a silky texture, but that's the extent of this eye cream's abilities. See the Appendix to learn why, in truth, you don't need an eye cream (and definitely not one like this).

☺ AVERAGE **Lifting & Firming Night Cream** *($19.99 for 1.69 fl. oz.)* is nearly identical to the Lifting & Firming Eye Cream above, except this is more emollient for dry skin. Otherwise, the same review applies—and this Night Cream can be used around the eyes.

☺ AVERAGE **Moisture Quench Day Cream, For Normal/Dry Skin** *($12.99 for 1.69 fl. oz.)* fails to impress because the majority of its formula is ho-hum, and the good stuff that shows up at the end of the ingredient list is too little, too late. There are several superior formulas for dry skin available elsewhere.

☺ AVERAGE **Moisture Quench Day Fluid, For Normal/Dry Skin** *($12.99 for 3.3 fl. oz.)* is the Lotion version of the Moisture Quench formula above, and the same review applies.

☺ AVERAGE **Moisture Quench Night Cream, for Normal/Dry Skin** *($12.99 for 1.69 fl. oz.)* is a standard emollient moisturizer for dry to very dry skin. Someone with normal skin will likely find this too rich. And someone shopping for a brilliantly formulated moisturizer not packaged in a jar will be disappointed (see the Appendix to learn why jar packaging is a problem).

☺ AVERAGE **Moisturising Eye Cream** *($13.99 for 0.84 fl. oz.)* is a very basic moisturizer for normal to dry skin anywhere on the face. The amount of mica leaves a noticeable shine on skin. Grape seed oil is a great antioxidant, but the jar packaging won't let it maintain its potency during use. See the Appendix to learn why jar packaging is a problem, and why you don't need an eye cream.

☺ AVERAGE **Night Moisture Cream** *($13.99 for 1.69 fl. oz.)* is an OK lightweight moisturizer for normal to slightly dry skin. The amount of grape seed oil is impressive, but the jar packaging won't keep its antioxidant elements stable during use. See the Appendix to learn why jar packaging is a problem.

☺ AVERAGE **Nourishing Night Cream** *($14.99 for 1.69 fl. oz.)* is a good, basic emollient moisturizer for dry skin. Although it can definitely improve signs of dryness and make skin feel comfortable, the antioxidant ability of the plant oils and extracts will be diminished due to jar packaging. See the Appendix to learn why jar packaging is a problem.

☺ AVERAGE **Organic Face Moisturising Eye Cream** *($14.99 for 0.5 fl. oz.)* is a basic emollient moisturizer suitable for dry skin anywhere on the face. It is fragrance-free and contains several natural ingredients that will benefit skin. This would earn a higher rating if it contained a more interesting mix of ingredients. As is, there are better moisturizers to consider. Remember, you don't need a special moisturizer labeled "eye cream" (see the Appendix to find out why).

☺ AVERAGE **Organic Face Super Balm** *($8.99 for 3.2 fl. oz.)* is a good choice for treating very dry skin anywhere on the body, but it is best for stubborn dry areas like heels, cuticles, and elbows. Simple isn't bad for skin, but the jar packaging won't keep the air-sensitive natural ingredients in this product stable.

☺ AVERAGE **Protect & Perfect Beauty Serum** *($19.99 for 1 fl. oz.)* reigns above every other Boots product in terms of reader curiosity due to reports this serum is comparable to tretinoin, the active ingredient in Retin-A and Renova. The research was carried out by scientists at the University of Manchester, with the conclusion that this Boots serum was just as effective at stimulating collagen production as tretinoin, yet costs considerably less. That sounds great until you learn that Boots paid for the research, which means they had a vested interest in making sure the study made their product look great. Also, because the study was done "blind" instead of double-blind, the researchers knew who was getting which treatment. This type of study isn't as reliable as double-blind studies because, especially when money is at stake, there is a natural bias toward making sure the product in question comes out in the best possible light. Comparing a product to tretinoin in a short period of time is just absurd. Tretinoin works over time (there's abundant research about that); it initially makes the skin worse due to the irritation it can cause, such that over time there is no way to know what the results would have been.

Protect & Perfect Beauty Serum is silicone-based and contains a small amount of vitamin C as sodium ascorbyl phosphate (which research has shown is not as effective as ascorbic acid, though it is more stable). A nearly insignificant amount of vitamin A (as retinyl palmitate, not retinol as claimed) and other antioxidants hardly makes this an anti-aging product worth any amount of frenzy. Its vitamin C content and other attributes are not even worth mild enthusiasm when you consider that several companies offer serums that are infinitely more state-of-the-art. And if you're looking for peptides (or hope that the ones used in this Boots serum will spell certain doom for your wrinkles), this isn't the product that will flood your skin with them. In fact, there are more preservatives than peptides in this fragrance-free serum. Despite out dispelling the hype this product generated (and remember, it all began with funding from Boots, and no one else has reproduced the results from their "study"), it can be a good serum-type moisturizer for all skin types, and the silicones make skin feel wonderfully silky.

This product comes in translucent glass packaging that will compromise the stability of the vitamin C and vitamin A unless this is constantly kept away from light.

By the way, there is plenty of substantiated, published research indicating that topically applied vitamin C can stimulate collagen production, but so can a lot of other ingredients (for example any sunscreen comes to mind), but you would need more vitamin C than what is in this Boots serum (Sources: *Journal of Cosmetic Dermatology*, June 2006, pages 150–156; *Pharmaceutical Development and Technology*, November 2006, pages 255–261; *Dermatologic Surgery*, July 2005, pages 814–817; and *Experimental Dermatology*, June 2003, pages 237–244).

Keep in mind that one skin-care ingredient is never enough for skin, just like one type of food (like broccoli) doesn't make for a healthy diet. It is the combination of healthy substances that is truly the best for skin; there isn't one miracle ingredient to be found anywhere.

And by the way, even Boots doesn't believe their own claims or they wouldn't be selling dozens of products making the same promises about getting rid of wrinkles. If the one they launched works, what are all the others for?

☺ AVERAGE **Protect & Perfect Day Cream SPF 15** *($19.99 for 1.69 fl. oz.)* doesn't list active ingredients and, therefore, it cannot be relied on for adequate sun protection. This con-

The Reviews B

tains several sunscreen ingredients, but a product sold in the United States must follow FDA regulations for over-the-counter drug products, and Boots isn't doing that. However, even if they modify the labeling so that it follows regulations, this jar-packaged moisturizer will be a resounding disappointment for anyone hoping there is truth behind its claims of being a fantastic moisturizer for younger-looking skin. Any of the daytime moisturizers with sunscreen from Olay or Paula's Choice are preferred to this.

☺ AVERAGE **Protect & Perfect Eye Cream** (*$19.99 for 0.5 fl. oz.*) doesn't contain exceptional levels of any state-of-the-art ingredients and it does not have any ability to chase dark circles and puffiness away. Puffy eyes and dark circles do not have a skin-care solution, unless they are the result of using poorly formulated products around your eyes and actually are causing the puffiness and darkness, in which case you could stop using them. This cream contains a smattering of peptides and some antioxidants, but even combined, the amount is likely too small to make much difference for eye-area skin, plus none of them have any research showing they can improve problems around the eyes. See the Appendix to find out why, in truth, you don't need an eye cream.

☺ AVERAGE **Protect & Perfect Intense Beauty Serum** (*$22.99 for 1 fl. oz.*). Boots lauded this product based on the results of a 12-month study they performed. The results were that 70% of the "volunteers" using this product showed a "marked improvement" in the appearance of their sun-damaged skin. That's hardly surprising, given that this serum contains some ingredients that can help sun-damaged skin look better, just like countless other serums and moisturizers. Regardless, the study claim is bogus because this so-called study wasn't published or peer-reviewed. We don't know if it was done double-blind, if the effect of the Boots serum was compared with the effect of other products, or even if the participants were using other products at the same time. For example, if they were using sunscreen during the test period that would have had far more impact than this serum as far as the results go. As is, this "study" is meaningless and poses more questions than answers, but it does make for great marketing headlines.

In short, there is no real evidence that this is the serum everyone with sun-damaged skin needs. Based on the ingredient list, this isn't anything special for anyone's skin. It's remarkably similar to Boots Protect & Perfect Beauty Serum—the very same one that caused a frenzy because it was said to work as well as tretinoin without the irritation. If that serum (which the company still sells) is so remarkable, why do they need another version with a nearly identical formula? The logical answer is that they want to continue the marketing hype of its progenitor and sell more product using this thinly veiled pseudo-science. Don't fall for it; this serum pales in comparison to many others, including several from Olay and Neutrogena. The only intense thing about it is the name, not what it does for aging skin.

Note that this serum is sold in Canada as No7 Refine & Rewind Beauty Serum.

☺ AVERAGE **Protect & Perfect Night Cream** (*$19.99 for 1.69 fl. oz.*). How important does Boots consider the Protect & Perfect complex in this moisturizer? Not very, or even slightly. If they did, the key anti-aging ingredients would amount to more than a mere dusting. As is, your skin is getting more fragrance and preservative than antioxidant vitamins and peptides. Moreover, those ingredients won't remain potent for long due to the jar packaging. See the Appendix to learn why jar packaging is a problem.

☺ AVERAGE **Rebalancing Day Gel, for Oily/Combination Skin** (*$12.99 for 1.69 fl. oz.*) will not revitalize skin with green tea and seaweed because those ingredients are barely present. This is merely a boring gel moisturizer that's suitable for its intended skin types. It's nice that fragrance was omitted, but why weren't more beneficial ingredients added?

☺ AVERAGE **Rebalancing Night Fluid, for Oily/Combination Skin** *($12.99 for 3.3 fl. oz.)* is a skin-confusing mix of slip agent, silicone, zinc oxide, emollients, clay, talc, and wax. It's too light and absorbent for dry skin, yet too potentially troublesome for oily skin or oily areas. We suppose it's OK for normal skin, but overall it's an unimpressive formula.

☺ AVERAGE **Time Dimensions Brightening Facial Balm** *($16.99 for 1 fl. oz.)* is a fluid moisturizer whose silicone content will make all skin types feel silky while the mica imparts a noticeable shine, but shine isn't skin care. The amount of antioxidants and peptides is disappointing, and certainly doesn't make this a top choice for improving skin of any age.

☺ AVERAGE **Time Dimensions Intensive Restoring Treatment** *($18.99 for 1 fl. oz.)* is neither intensive nor restorative. This is a simple, light-textured lotion with a lot of mica for a shiny finish. Vitamin A and peptides are supposed to be major players here, but their presence amounts to a non-speaking, walk-on part in a movie, not the "top billing" your skin needs to look and feel its best.

☺ AVERAGE **Time Dimensions Nourishing Eye Cream** *($18.99 for 0.5 fl. oz.)* is a below-standard lightweight moisturizer for slightly dry skin anywhere on the face. The mica leaves a soft shine finish, but this has nothing to do with boosting collagen or elastin, or reducing fine lines or puffiness in the eye area. See the Appendix to learn why, in truth, you don't need an eye cream.

☺ AVERAGE **Time Dimensions Rejuvenating Day Moisturiser** *($16.99 for 1.69 fl. oz.)* is a thicker version of the Time Dimensions Nourishing Eye Cream above, except this version doesn't contain mica. Otherwise, the same basic comments apply.

☺ AVERAGE **Time Dimensions Restoring Night Moisturiser** *($17.99 for 1.69 fl. oz.)* contains a teeny-tiny amount of antioxidants and peptides, features jar packaging, and is otherwise very similar to the Time Dimensions Rejuvenating Day Moisturiser. Skip it.

☺ AVERAGE **Time Dimensions Softening Line Smoother** *($15.99 for 0.5 fl. oz.)* is merely a blend of silicones and slip agents whose texture is meant to serve as a sort of spackle for superficial lines and wrinkles. It works marginally well, but how long the effect lasts depends on how much you move your face. This is an option for those who want to try such a product but don't want a shiny or sparkling finish.

☺ AVERAGE **Time Resisting Day Cream SPF 12** *($19.99 for 1.69 fl. oz.)* deserves credit for its in-part avobenzone sunscreen, but the base formula for normal to slightly dry skin offers little of substance for skin, not to mention the SPF 12 is below the minimum standard SPF 15 recommendation. The mica provides a soft shine finish and, while Boots talks up this sunscreen's antioxidant complex, the amount of antioxidants is likely too small for skin to gain any benefit.

☺ AVERAGE **Time Resisting Night Cream** *($19.99 for 1.69 fl. oz.)* does not contain retinol as claimed (retinyl palmitate is not the same thing), and ends up being another plain emollient moisturizer for normal to dry skin. It is far less elegant than the moisturizer options from many other drugstore lines, including Olay, Paula's Choice RESIST, and Neutrogena.

☺ AVERAGE **Triple Action Day Moisture Cream SPF 15** *($12.99 for 1.69 fl. oz.)* is a standard, but good, daytime moisturizer with sunscreen for normal to slightly dry skin. UVA protection is provided by avobenzone and this contains a couple of antioxidants. It's nothing special, but the price is reasonable and this would work well under makeup.

☺ AVERAGE **Ultimate Lift Eye Gel** *($13.99 for 0.5 fl. oz.)* is so basic and boring that the name is embarrassing. This won't lift skin in the least; it's just water, slip agents, plant extract, film-forming agent, and preservatives. See the Appendix to learn why you don't need a special product for the eye area, gel or otherwise.

☹ POOR **Expert Anti-Blemish Night Moisturizer** *($4.99 for 1.69 fl. oz.)* lists alcohol as the second ingredient. That's not a helpful or "expert" ingredient for any skin type, blemishes or not. Definitely a product to leave on the shelf!

☹ POOR **Expert Shine Control Instant Matte** *($5.99 for 0.5 fl. oz.)* lists alcohol as the second ingredient. It is not recommended due to the dryness and irritation this much alcohol causes. Alcohol can de-grease the skin, but the oil will be back in no time and likely worse than before.

☹ POOR **Rebalancing Day Fluid SPF 15, Oily/Combination** *($12.99 for 3.3 fl. oz.)* does not list any active sunscreen ingredients, so you can't know exactly the protection you are getting. It does contain sunscreen ingredients capable of providing broad-spectrum sun protection, but the lightweight lotion formula contains a potentially skin-damaging amount of alcohol. The formula also lacks antioxidants and other skin-repairing ingredients that all skin types need every day. Please see the Appendix for details on why alcohol can be a problem in skin-care products. Bottom line: This product isn't poised to rebalance anything, and may make your oily areas worse due to the amount of alcohol.

☹ POOR **Time Resisting Day & Night Eye Care** *($19.99 for 0.66 fl. oz.)*. Housed in one dual-chamber pump bottle are a cream and gel for the eye area. The **Eye Cream** *(0.33 ounce)* differs little from most of the Boots' facial moisturizers, which means it is an unexciting formula whose few intriguing ingredients are listed after the preservative, so they're not going to be of much help given the paltry amount. The **Eye Gel** *(0.33 ounce)* has a lighter texture than the Cream, but otherwise doesn't wow, either, although each of the products has a pleasant enough texture. Because the Eye Gel contains the irritating menthol derivative menthyl PCA, it isn't recommended. See the Appendix to learn why irritation is a problem for everyone's skin.

BOOTS LIP CARE

✓☺ BEST **Botanics Organic Lip Balm** *($6.99 for 0.33 fl. oz.)* is a very good emollient (and notably greasy) lip balm that is 100% natural. The shea butter-based formula is fragrance- and colorant-free, and doesn't contain any irritants, which is great. The greasy nature of this balm makes it best for use at night because it makes a mess, whether paired with lipstick or by itself, something you wouldn't want during the day.

☺ AVERAGE **Lip Salve Rose & Geranium** *($6.99 for 0.5 fl. oz.)*. There is much to praise about this lip balm because it has what it takes to protect lips from chapping and to prevent moisture loss. Unfortunately, Boots couldn't resist adding fragrant oils (rose and geranium) that are not helpful for anyone's lips. Applying these fragrant oils to lips isn't as bad as slathering them all over your face, but there are better lip balms to consider, including those from The Body Shop and Paula's Choice.

☺ AVERAGE **Protect & Perfect Lip Care** *($7.99 for 0.33 fl. oz.)* contains ingredients to help moisturize lips and make them feel silky, but the complex referred to in this product's claims won't do anything to repair signs of aging around the mouth. This is a decent, waxy, lanolin- and Vaseline-based, lightweight lip moisturizer, but that's about it.

☹ POOR **Time Dimensions Instant Lip Plumper** *($9.99 for 0.27 fl. oz.)* is perhaps the most irritating lip plumper being sold today. Most such products contain one or two irritants that cause lips to swell slightly by virtue of irritation. Boots uses menthol (a lot of it), spearmint oil, eugenol, clove oil, pepper extract, methyl eugenol, and cinnamon. All we can say, besides "buyer beware," is "Ouch!" And Boots calls this product a "special treat"!

✎ Buying skin-care products packaged in jars? See the Appendix to learn why that's a bad idea.

Boots Specialty Skin-Care Products

☺ GOOD **Conditioning Clay Mask** *($8.99 for 4.2 fl. oz.)* is a very standard but good clay mask that is an option for oily to very oily skin. It is fragrance-free and the sole plant extract, burdock root, has soothing properties.

☺ GOOD **Expert Scar Care Serum** *($7.99 for 1.6 fl. oz.)* doesn't contain any ingredients capable of eliminating scars. However, massaging this over scars or skin anywhere on the body will result in a silky softness that can improve skin's appearance. Any scar reduction seen from the use of this product (such as color or length of scar) is purely coincidental. In many cases, skin continues to remodel and heal after a scar forms. That means the scar will continue to improve with time, regardless of what you use. Keeping scars protected from sunlight and treating skin with a well-formulated serum or moisturizer (this product doesn't quite meet that standard) will go a long way toward encouraging the most productive healing and best-looking outcome.

☺ GOOD **Expert Shine Control Papers** *($4.49 for 50 sheets)* are imbued with chalk (calcium carbonate), which has absorbent properties and will leave a fresh matte finish. You may find you don't need to follow with powder after using these blotting papers.

☹ AVERAGE **Expert Anti-Blemish Serum** *($7.99 for 1 fl. oz.)* doesn't contain a single ingredient that has a shred of published research showing it can be helpful for reducing acne breakouts.

☹ AVERAGE **Intensive Line Filler** *($17.99 for 0.67 fl. oz.)* is packaged in a tube and has a slightly thick texture that includes mineral pigments (what the company refers to as "light-diffusing particles"), but shine isn't skin care. This is an OK option to temporarily fill in and smooth superficial wrinkles and enlarged pores, but there are better products for this purpose, including those from BeautiControl's Regeneration Tight line. The amount of peptides in Intensive Line Filler is inconsequential for skin.

☹ AVERAGE **Intensive Moisture Face Mask** *($19.99 for 3.3 fl. oz.)* is an exceptionally standard moisturizing mask for dry to very dry skin. What you get for your money isn't worth the cost, but this will cover the basics in terms of making dry skin feel smoother and more comfortable.

☹ POOR **Complexion Refining Clay Mask** *($8.99 for 1.69 fl. oz.)* is a below-standard clay mask due to the amount of irritating isopropyl alcohol. It cannot draw out "even the most deep-rooted impurities"—you won't see a marvelously clear complexion after use, and your skin may feel uncomfortably dry.

☹ POOR **Expert Anti-Blemish Concealer Duo** *($5.99 for 0.32 fl. oz.)* features an anti-acne fluid on one end and a concealer on the other. The **Blemish Lotion** is loaded with alcohol and will be of precious little help against acne; the **Concealer** has a thick, occlusive texture that is no match for today's best concealers. We guarantee your acne will not improve or be convincingly hidden if you choose to try this product.

Boots Foundations & Primers

✓☺ BEST **Intelligent Balance Mousse Foundation** *($13.99)* is an outstanding, feather-light mousse foundation for normal to very oily skin. The sponge-like texture blends seamlessly over skin, leaving a smooth matte finish without a hint of flatness. The powdery silicones (which comprise the bulk of this nonaqueous formula) do a good job of keeping excess shine in check, although this foundation's finish can magnify dry areas, so be sure to prep your skin beforehand. You'll enjoy sheer to light coverage that holds up surprisingly well throughout the day, except for very oily areas, which will require some blotting and perhaps a powder touch-up or two. The only drawback (well, aside from there being no shades for dark skin tones) is the jar packaging, which isn't the most sanitary way to use makeup. One other comment about the jar packaging: Once you're about half way through this foundation, the relatively narrow opening makes it more difficult to get product out. All of the shades are very good, and finish lighter than they appear, but Target offers testers for the Boots makeup, so seeing if one of the shades will work for you is convenient.

✓ ☺ BEST **Soft & Sheer Tinted Moisturiser SPF 15** *($11.99 for 1.69 fl. oz.)* is a great find for those with normal to dry skin! Titanium dioxide is partially responsible for UVA protection, while the creamy-smooth texture applies and blends beautifully, providing sheer coverage and a fresh, moist finish. All three shades are recommended.

✓ ☺ BEST **Stay Perfect Foundation SPF 15** *($13.99)* makes reference to the skin-strengthening ceramides it contains, but the amount of them in this silky liquid foundation is barely a dusting. Although this isn't skin care disguised as makeup, it contains an in-part titanium dioxide sunscreen, feels nearly weightless, and sets to a smooth matte finish. Sheer to light coverage is obtainable and the overall formula is best for normal to very oily skin. There are ten mostly great, neutral shades.

☺ GOOD **Lifting and Firming Foundation SPF 15** *($14.99 for 1 fl. oz.)* gets its sun protection partly from titanium dioxide, though it would be better if a higher percentage were included (1.6% is low). This is otherwise a very silky liquid foundation for those with normal to oily skin seeking medium coverage and a non-powdery matte finish. Seven of the eight shades are recommended; Truffle is too peach for its intended range of skin tones. Do we need to state that this won't lift or firm skin in the least?

☺ GOOD **Stay Perfect Foundation Compact SPF 15** *($15.99 for 0.24 fl. oz.)* is a traditional cream-to-powder makeup with an in-part titanium dioxide sunscreen. The creamy texture sets quickly to a powder finish. This is best for normal to slightly oily skin not prone to blemishes, and provides light to medium coverage. Each of the four shades is soft and neutral, though options for fair and dark skin tones are lacking. The crescent-shaped sponge accompanying this foundation is almost useless; a full-size circular sponge works much better.

☺ GOOD **True Identity Foundation** *($12.49 for 1.3 fl. oz.)* is an amazing foundation—if you need barely any coverage. The silicone- and talc-based formula feels silky, provides a real-skin finish, and has a hint of color. It is best for normal to oily skin, and all the shades are great (but again, this is not one to pick if you need coverage beyond what strategically placed concealer provides).

☹ AVERAGE **Complexion Refining Foundation** *($11.99 for 0.84 fl. oz.)* begins slightly creamy, but sets to a nearly weightless matte finish suitable for normal to oily skin. Coverage goes from sheer to light, and each of the eight shades is a winner (there are options for fair skin, too). The only drawback is the inclusion of volatile fragrant components, which can cause irritation.

☹ AVERAGE **Mineral Perfection Foundation** *($13.99)*. Boots' contribution to the glut of mineral makeup doesn't bring anything new to the table, unless you happen to believe that ruby, amethyst, and sapphire powders are great for skin (they're not); even if they were, the trace amounts in this product translate into a nothing for skin. Aside from the gimmick, this loose-powder foundation has a silky texture that's nearly weightless. It provides sheer to almost medium coverage and leaves a sparkling shine finish. Boots includes a brush with a stubby handle but full-size head, and it's much better than the applicators that accompany several other mineral makeups on the market. The one drawback to this otherwise very good powder is the colors, each of which goes on darker than it looks and errs on the peach side rather than being neutral. There are no shades suitable for fair to light skin tones. Avoid Buff and note that all shades of this foundation can easily appear streaky if not carefully blended.

BOOTS CONCEALERS

☺ GOOD **Complexion Refining Concealer Stick** *($9.99)* is a find for those who prefer lipstick-style concealers and are not using them to cover blemishes (because the ingredients that keep this in stick form can contribute to clogged pores). It blends very well, leaves a satin-smooth finish, and poses just a slight risk of creasing into lines around the eye. Only two shades are available, one of which (Sweet Ginger) will be too peach for some, so this is recommended only if you have light skin.

☻ AVERAGE **Radiant Glow Concealer** *($12.99)* functions best as a highlighter because it brightens shadowed areas, but provides minimal coverage. The finish feels matte but has a slight shine to it, which works to a subtle extent to reflect light away from dark areas. You push a button at the bottom of the pen-style component, and the product is fed onto a built-in synthetic brush. There are better versions of this product from Estee Lauder (Ideal Light) and Yves Saint Laurent (Touche Eclat Radiant Touch), but both cost twice as much.

☹ POOR **Quick Cover Blemish Stick** *($9.99)* lists its first ingredient as chalk and, as expected, looks chalky on skin. This lipstick-style concealer contains wax-like ingredients that are not recommended for use on blemishes, though it does provide sufficient coverage. Still, each of the four shades tends toward pink and peach tones, and overall this has more strikes than positives.

BOOTS POWDERS

✓☺ BEST **Perfect Light Loose Powder** *($11.99)* has a feather-light texture and seamless, dry finish. The aluminum starch- and talc-based formula is excellent for normal to oily skin because it absorbs well without looking chalky or thick. Although Boots advertises four shades on their website, the Target stores we visited consistently sold only two, both of which are sheer and recommended. Bonus points are deserved because the packaging for this loose powder works great to minimize mess. Also available and equally recommended is **Perfect Light Portable Loose Powder** *($12.99)*.

☹ POOR **Botanics Lighter Than Air Loose Powder** *($12.99)* has an accurate name, but although the feel is weightless, the finish is unnaturally dry and lends a flat, overly powdered appearance to skin, even when applied sheer. Moreover, this powder has a strong scent and contains volatile fragrance ingredients. Why consider this when there are so many great powders without this one's drawbacks?

☹ POOR **Perfect Light Pressed Powder** *($11.99)* has a texture that feels waxy and dry at the same time. That not only makes application with a brush difficult (the powder doesn't pick up easily), but also creates a heavy appearance on skin. The finish is made even more obvious because each of the shades has a slight pink or peach tone.

BOOTS BLUSHES

✓☺ BEST **Cheek Tint** *($9.99)*. In a word, this cream-to-powder blush's performance is impressive. Packaged in a generously sized compact, the color goes on sheer, but can be built up easily if a more dramatic look is desired. Once this sets, the color's intensity fades a bit, but that helps to create a very natural-looking blush that lasts and lasts. Application is hassle-free, because this contains just the right amount of slip along with having an ample play time during blending, which is about as easy as it gets. Though it doesn't exaggerate pores to the extent of some cream-to-powder blushes, this product does contain multiple ingredients that can clog pores and is not recommended for blemish-prone skin. Of the three shades, all are lovely and universally flattering, with Maple Silk being a noteworthy choice for medium to dark skin tones.

The Reviews B

☺ GOOD **Botanics Cheek Colour** *($8.99)* isn't the silkiest powder blush, but it's a definite option for those who prefer soft colors that apply sheer, build well, and impart subtle shine.

☺ GOOD **Natural Blush Cheek Colour** *($8.99)* isn't the silkiest powder blush around, but is a definite option for those who prefer soft colors that apply sheer, build well (if more color is desired), and come in a selection of very good matte shades.

☺ AVERAGE **Mineral Perfection Blush** *($9.99)*. Applied with a better brush than what's included, this goes on evenly and imparts a soft wash of color. The two shades are best for fair to light skin tones, and each has enough shine to make them too much for daytime wear, but they're fine for evening glamour. Keep in mind that this can be a messy way to apply blush—and that the minerals in this blush show up in most powder blushes not labeled "mineral."

BOOTS EYESHADOW & EYE PRIMERS

☺ GOOD **Botanics Eye Colour** *($3.99-$6.99)* has a smooth, silky texture. Application is effortless, and the color, though sheer, is buildable and really lasts, but you may see minor flaking from the shades with flecks of shine. The shade selection includes some almost matte nude and brown tones (which go on more vibrant than the shimmer shades) alongside shiny blues and greens that are best left alone. This comes in singles and duos.

☺ AVERAGE **Mineral Perfection Eye Shadow Palette** *($8.99)* is mica-based eyeshadow and, because mica is a mineral, the name is apropos, yet the formula is nothing unique or different when compared with hundreds of other eyeshadows. Although the powder eyeshadows in these sets have a smooth texture, their waxy nature disrupts color pickup on the brush, so application doesn't go past sheer; even the darker colors barely register on skin. Still, these can work for a soft eyeshadow design and the Rose and Topaz trios are decent. Avoid the too colorful Breeze and Heather trios unless you're looking for a blatant and very noticeable effect that's far from a classic eye design.

☺ AVERAGE **Stay Perfect Eye Mousse** *($7.99)* has a light-as-mousse texture but so much slip that controlled blending becomes an issue. Once set, these tend to last with minimal creasing, though because the shine is intense they're not for wrinkled skin. Only a tiny dab is needed, and again, blending must be done carefully or this will slide all over the eye area.

☺ AVERAGE **Stay Perfect Eye Shadow Single** *($5.99)* has a smooth but dry texture that applies better than expected but can be tricky to blend with other colors (it doesn't have much movement). The range of colors allows for some good pairings, but each has strong shine, so these aren't for women with wrinkles or sagging around the eyes.

☹ POOR **Stay Perfect Smoothing & Brightening Eye Base** *($6.99)* is a pink-tinted cream meant to function as an anchor so eyeshadow lasts longer. The thick, creamy formula does just the opposite: your eyeshadow won't make it to lunch without fading, creasing, or smearing, and the pink color is obvious enough to interfere with any eyeshadow color used over it. Stay away from this product if you want your eye makeup to stay perfect!

BOOTS EYE & BROW LINERS

☺ GOOD **Lash & Brow Perfector** *($7.99)* is a clear mascara that works best as a lightweight brow gel. Although application is wetter than most, this does not feel sticky or stiff once it dries, yet it holds brows neatly in place. Used as mascara, you'll get a smidgen of emphasis, but that's it.

☺ AVERAGE **Amazing Eyes Pencil** *($6.99)* needs sharpening, but other than that this is quite good, and preferred to the Botanics Eye Definer below. It glides on swiftly, deposits strong color (which is what you want for eye lining) that can be softened with the built-in sponge tip, and stays in place. The only issue is minor fading, which will be a deal-breaker only for those with oily eyelids.

☺ AVERAGE **Botanics Eye Definer** *($5.99)* is a very standard eye pencil that needs routine sharpening and is available in classic colors. This applies easily and feels almost powdery but is still slightly prone to smudging.

☺ AVERAGE **Cream Eye Liner** *($7.99)* applies smoothly and evenly, but the colors don't go on as rich as you might expect and tend to fade throughout the day. The included brush is OK if you're in a pinch, but you're better off using a higher-quality eyeliner brush. Overall this is a so-so option for eyeliner.

☺ AVERAGE **Liquid Eye Liner** *($8.99)* comes in inkwell packaging and features a thin, flexible brush that works well; if only the color deposit weren't so sheer. The sheerness means successive layers are needed to build color, which increases the chance of smearing. This dries quickly, but will fade before long, so overall it doesn't compare favorably with liquid liners from L'Oreal and Almay, to name just two.

☹ POOR **Beautiful Brows Pencil** *($6.99)* won't create beautiful brows unless your definition of that includes flaking color and matted brow hairs from this substandard pencil's waxy texture and finish. This is one of the worst brow pencils we've ever come across. Great colors, though.

BOOTS LIP COLOR & LIPLINERS

✓☺ BEST **Botanics Lip Gloss** *($7.99)* earns its rating because it has a superior smooth texture, moisturizes lips without feeling goopy, isn't sticky, and provides a beautiful selection of sheer to moderate colors, each with a sexy gloss finish and subtle shimmer.

✓☺ BEST **Sheer Temptation Lipstick** *($9.99)* feels rich and emollient, and while the colors look quite bold in the tube, each goes on sheer, as the name states. This has a glossy finish yet isn't too slippery, and the colors are great. If you want sheer lip color, what more could you ask for?

☺ GOOD **High Shine Lip Gloss** *($7.99)* is a traditional sheer lip gloss applied with a sponge tip attached to a wand. It feels smooth and is non-sticky, and has a soft but glossy finish.

☺ GOOD **Lip Glace** *($9.99)* comes in a tube and is a standard, thick lip gloss with a slightly sticky finish and wet, glossy shine. Some of the colors go on sheer, while others go on more intense and imbue lips with sparkles.

☺ GOOD **Mineral Perfection Lipstick** *($9.99)*. Minerals play a minor role in this lipstick, other than the mica that gives almost every shade in this small collection a slight shimmer. This is otherwise a very standard, lightweight cream lipstick with a smooth, slick finish. It will travel into lines around the mouth, but if that's not an issue for you, this is a viable lipstick. The color deposit is moderate.

☺ GOOD **Moisture Drench Lipstick** *($9.99)* is a standard, but good, cream lipstick. Each of the attractive colors provides moderate coverage and a soft, moisturizing finish. Several shades provide a dimensional shimmer, which can create the illusion of fuller lips.

☺ GOOD **Stay Perfect Lip Lacquer** *($9.99)* is a two-part product that includes a lip paint and a clear top coat to ensure a glossy finish and comfortable wear (the lip paint used by itself makes lips feel dry). Although this version doesn't have the same impressive longevity as long-wearing lip paints from Cover Girl or Maybelline, we were pleasantly surprised that not once in several hours of wear did we feel compelled to apply more top coat. Perhaps we should have, as this might have "protected" the color from fading so much; but at least when that occurred, it did so evenly rather than peeling or flaking off. All in all, this is worth a look despite the fact that it does not keep color looking perfect for eight hours, as claimed.

☺ GOOD **Stay Perfect Lipstick** *($9.99)* has a lightweight texture and smooth, creamy finish that remains a bit slick, so this will migrate into lines around the mouth. If that is not a concern, this is definitely worth auditioning.

☹ AVERAGE **Botanics Lip Liner** *($6.99)* applies easily but tends to smear and travel into lines around the mouth. This needs-sharpening pencil works best when applied all over lips and blended with a gloss for a soft, stained effect.

☹ AVERAGE **Wild Volume Lipstick** *($9.99)* goes on slick, but also provides a decent stain that lasts a bit longer than the time it takes for the moisture to wear away (which doesn't take long). The big deal about this lipstick is the volume, which Boots attributes to the inclusion of pea and senna extracts, but it's more likely due to whatever irritant creates the tingling sensation. As a rule, any distinct tingling from a lip product is a sign of irritation and with continued use can cause dry, chapped lips. All told, there is nothing particularly special about this lipstick, except that it's only available in various shades of red and brown.

☹ POOR **Line & Define Lip Pencil** *($6.99)* is a decent automatic, retractable lip pencil that applies easily. Unfortunately, the finish feels (and stays) tacky, and the colors, while initially rich, fade too quickly.

BOOTS MASCARAS

✓☺ BEST **Exceptional Definition Nutrient Enriched Mascara** *($7.99)*. The unique design of this mascara's rubber-bristled brush allows it to work to your advantage, at least if what you expect from mascara is clean, clump-free, perfectly defined lashes. The bristle alignment features various rows of different lengths, so you get smooth length and enough thickness to satisfy unless you're looking for major volume. This leaves lashes looking beautifully fringed and defined but never too "show-y," and removes easily with a water-soluble cleanser.

☺ GOOD **Botanics Volumising Mascara** *($6.99)* ranks as the best non-waterproof mascara from Boots. You'll enjoy equal parts length and thickness without clumps or smearing, resulting in moderately dramatic, beautifully separated lashes.

☺ GOOD **Extreme Length Mascara** *($7.99)*. This mascara's thin, rubber-bristled brush delivers defined lashes and smooth length, and allows you to easily coat difficult-to-reach lashes. Despite the name, we wouldn't say the length is "extreme," but lashes do look slightly emphasized. The formula is smudge-free, flake-free, and leaves lashes softly fringed.

☺ GOOD **Lash 360°** *($7.99)*. This mascara's odd brush is its only point of difference. Unfortunately, the variable bristles, which are thicker and shorter in the center of the brush and longer on the ends, don't translate into unique lash effect. You'll find this allows for ample length and slight thickness without clumps, along with great lash separation, just like many other recommended mascaras. It leaves lashes soft and is easy to remove with a water-soluble cleanser. That's nice, but this wasn't a necessary addition to the already-crowded lineup of mascaras from Boots.

☺ GOOD **Maximum Volume Waterproof Mascara** *($7.99)* is minimally waterproof (your eyes getting misty won't cause this to budge, but don't go into the pool with the expectation this will stay put). It is otherwise a very good lengthening and thickening mascara that builds well without getting too dramatic, and it doesn't clump. Removing this takes just a water-soluble cleanser.

☺ GOOD **Stay Perfect Mascara** *($7.99)* is a very good, understated mascara, one that's nearly impossible to overdo. The traditional bristle brush applicator deposits just the right amount of mascara and the formula is dry enough that lashes feel light, but not stiff. With a couple of coats, there's adequate lengthening and thickening, with an enviable amount of separation too boot—especially surprising considering how densely packed the bristles are.

☺ GOOD **Super Sensitive Mascara** *($7.99)* has fewer ingredients than most mascaras, although that's not a guarantee that someone with sensitive eyes won't have a problem (and the bulk of this formula consists of ingredients found in most mascaras). Still, this has a very clean application that lets you build impressive length and some thickness with zero clumps. As a bonus, it leaves lashes very soft and doesn't flake.

☺ AVERAGE **Botanics Lash Defining Mascara** *($6.99)* winds up being merely average and is an option only if you want to barely enhance your lashes because you're 99% satisfied with the way they look minus mascara.

☺ AVERAGE **Maximum Volume Mascara** *($7.99)* is below average if you were banking on the name translating into copiously thick lashes. This does little to enhance lashes in any respect, but is OK if you want a minimalist look.

☹ POOR **Botanics Waterproof Mascara** *($6.99)* is not recommended at any price unless you want minimal length, sparse definition, and no thickness regardless of how many coats you apply. It is waterproof and comes off with a water-soluble cleanser, but so what?

☹ POOR **Extravagant Lashes Mascara** *($7.99).* Picture this: A mascara brush with a series of large angular ridges (rather than bristles) that wrap around its squared applicator head. What you have just envisioned is possibly the weirdest, least attractive or effective mascara we've ever experienced. Not only is it strange to look at, but its performance is a joke. It's impossible to apply without clumping lashes together (square angles don't take to lashes too well—imagine that!). Even a comb-through revealed nothing impressive, let alone "extravagant." What Boots was thinking when they designed this we may never know, but this is definitely a mascara we'll remember, if only for its bizarreness!

BOOTS FACE & BODY ILLUMINATORS

☺ GOOD **Botanics Shimmer Pearls** *($12.99)* are identical to the Sun Kissed Bronze Shimmer Pearls reviewed below, except there are more pink and peach beads, so the result is a soft blush color that applies sheer and leaves a subtle shine.

☺ GOOD **Bronze Shimmer Pearls** *($11.99)* are multicolored powder beads packaged in a jar. You swirl a brush over the beads and apply a sheer layer of powder, which creates a peachy tan color and provides a radiant finish. Although gimmicky, this is a good way to perk up a sallow complexion and add a soft, non-sparkling shine.

☺ GOOD **High Lights Illuminating Lotion** *($12.99 for 1 fl. oz.)* is a standard lightweight shimmer lotion that applies easily and sets to a matte (in feel) finish that stays put. The shine is moderate and not sparkling or glittery, making it a good choice for evening makeup. The pale, opalescent pink color works best on fair to light skin tones.

BOSCIA (SKIN CARE ONLY)

Strengths: All the sunscreens provide sufficient UVA protection; the packaging for many products not only keeps the plant-based and antioxidant ingredients stable but also helps minimize these preservative-free products' exposure to bacteria and organisms, that can cause unhealthy changes; some good cleansers and moisturizers.

Weaknesses: Expensive considering the smaller-than-average sizes; several products are marred by the inclusion of irritating ingredients; no effective options for managing acne; no options for lightening skin discolorations.

For more information and reviews of the latest Boscia products, visit CosmeticsCop.com.

BOSCIA CLEANSERS

☺ GOOD $$$ **Clear Complexion Cleanser with Botanical Blast** *($26 for 5 fl. oz.)* is a standard but good water-soluble cleanser suitable for all skin types except very oily. The fact that this is preservative-free likely necessitates a small size (so you use it up quickly), but it makes for an expensive cleanser that is only worth considering if you know you're sensitive to preservatives (even when they're in rinse-off products).

☺ GOOD $$$ **Purifying Cleansing Gel** *($26 for 5 fl. oz.)* can work for most skin types except very dry. All in all, it is nearly identical to Boscia's Clear Complexion Cleanser with Botanical Blast above, so the same comments apply.

☺ AVERAGE $$$ **Detoxifying Black Cleanser** *($28 for 5 fl. oz.)*. This thick cleanser is said to dissolve pore-clogging impurities, but it isn't impurities (such as dirt or pollution) that clog pores. It's dead skin cells and natural cellular debris mixing with your skin's oil. None of that is "toxic" either, and in fact this cleanser cannot detoxify skin. Within the human body, the liver and kidneys do the detox work, not skin. Your skin doesn't have toxins that need to be removed by a special cleanser, nor do you need to pay this much for a good cleanser. This ends up being a cleanser that's somewhat difficult to use due to its texture and it contains a fragrant plant oil known to cause irritation. If you decide to try this (the black coloration comes from charcoal powder), it's an OK option for normal to oily skin. Note: This cleanser warms when mixed with water, but the warming sensation is more tactile than a skin-care benefit. The warmth won't soften impurities or oil any better than simply washing with lukewarm water.

☺ AVERAGE $$$ **Soothing Cleansing Cream** *($26 for 5 fl. oz.)*. This thin-textured, detergent-free cleansing cream is an OK option for normal to dry skin not prone to breakouts. It does not rinse well without the aid of a washcloth, but does remove makeup efficiently.

☹ POOR **Makeup-Breakup Cool Cleansing Oil** *($26 for 5 fl. oz.)*. This waterless, emollient cleansing oil contains eucalyptus oil and menthol to create a cooling effect. Unfortunately, this effect has nothing to do with cleansing or makeup removal. In this product, it has everything to do with causing irritation, especially if you use it to remove eye makeup.

BOSCIA TONERS

☺ AVERAGE $$$ **Clear Complexion Tonic with Botanical Blast** *($24 for 5 fl. oz.)*. This spray-on toner is based around lavender flower water, which, while not as problematic as pure lavender oil, isn't skin care—it's eau de cologne. Of course, lavender oil is in this toner as well, though likely not in an amount that's troublesome for skin. The water-binding agents and anti-irritants are helpful for all skin types, though the rosemary and gardenia extracts aren't ideal. *Phellodendron amurense* bark has anti-inflammatory activity when applied to skin, but we can't tell if Boscia included enough of it to be soothing. Even if they did, the lavender water and oil likely cancel out its effect.

☹ POOR **Balancing Facial Tonic** *($24 for 5 fl. oz.)*. Lavender flower water comprises the bulk of this toner, making it an eau de cologne, not skin care. There also is lavender oil in here, and in any form, that's not soothing, balancing, or an essential ingredient for skin. In fact, lavender can cause cell death, and its fragrant components are irritating (Source: *Cell Proliferation*, June 2004, pages 221–229). The anti-irritants in this toner can be helpful for skin, but would be more beneficial if the lavender didn't get in their way.

BOSCIA MOISTURIZERS (DAYTIME & NIGHTTIME), EYE CREAMS, & SERUMS

✓☺ BEST $$$ **Restorative Day Moisture Cream SPF 15** *($48 for 1 fl. oz.)*. This daytime moisturizer with an in-part avobenzone sunscreen is packaged in an airless jar to preserve the efficacy of the plant ingredients and antioxidants it contains. Its silky, slightly thick texture is best for normal to dry skin. Best of all, the fragrance-free formula contains an impressive blend of skin-identical ingredients, emollients, cell-communicating ingredients, and soothing plant extracts. An intriguing ingredient in this product that deserves further comment is magnolia bark extract. It seems that magnolia bark contains several chemical constituents that have a cortisone-like effect. In theory, this should help calm skin and reduce signs of sensitivity, though bear in mind that the active ingredients in this daytime moisturizer with sunscreen preclude its recommendation for those with sensitive skin (titanium dioxide and zinc oxide are the preferred active ingredients for this skin type). The research on magnolia bark related to ingestion rather than topical application, but theoretically its soothing benefits should be applicable to your skin, too.

✓☺ BEST $$$ **Restorative Night Moisture Cream** *($48 for 1 fl. oz.)* is a rich cream that's best for dry, sensitive skin that's not prone to breakouts. It contains several proven emollients and some notable plant extracts, and the airless jar packaging will help keep these important ingredients stable during use. Also on board are cell-communicating ingredients and some good water-binding agents, along with an impresive amount of antioxidant rose hip oil (listed by its Latin name of *Rosa centifolia* flower, though the form Boscia chose isn't all that potent). Still, this fragrance-free moisturizer is a boon for those with sensitive skin that's uncomfortably dry. See the review of the Restorative Day Moisture Cream SPF 15 above for comments on the magnolia bark ingredient the Night Moisture Cream also contains.

☺ GOOD **Oil-Free Daily Hydration SPF 15** *($36 for 1.4 fl. oz.)* is a very good lightweight daytime moisturizer. Those with normal to oily skin will appreciate the soft matte finish, while the in-part avobenzone sunscreen shields skin from UVA rays. Several anti-irritants are included, some of which also have antioxidant ability. This product is also fragrance-free and, like all Boscia products, does not contain preservatives.

☺ GOOD **Oil-Free Nightly Hydration** *($36 for 1.4 fl. oz.)*. This lightweight, fragrance-free moisturizer is said to contain "oil-moderating botanicals," but the plant extracts it includes do not have this benefit, although they do offer antioxidant and anti-inflammatory benefits, and that's great. Perhaps what Boscia was trying to convey is that by treating skin gently and reducing inflammation, you potentially can reduce the oiliness of your skin. That logic has merit because we know from research that treating oily skin with harsh, irritating ingredients stimulates more oil production, so treating it gently won't make matters worse; in that sense, Bosica has a point. Interestingly, some of the plant extracts in this moisturizer do have anti-bacterial properties. Despite this, none of them have solid research proving their antibacterial action works against acne-causing bacteria, so relying on this to fight acne would be a mistake. The ingredient oleanolic acid is a fatty acid found in some plants. There is one study showing that this fatty acid has some antibacterial action against acne-causing (and other types of) bacteria, but it did not perform as well as other plant substances such as usnic acid (Source: *Phytomedicine*, August 2007, pages 508–516), which isn't in this product. Still, you may get some anti-acne benefit from this moisturizer, and its light lotion texture doesn't feel greasy. On balance, this is a very good option for normal to oily or combination skin prone to blemishes.

☺ GOOD **Vital Daily Moisture SPF 15** *($36 for 1.4 fl. oz.)*. With a few deletions and more bells and whistles, this in-part avobenzone sunscreen would be an excellent daytime moisturizer for normal to dry skin. It contains some very good anti-irritants and olive oil, a good emollient and antioxidant. Unfortunately, it loses points by adding fragrant jasmine oil and rosemary extract. The rosemary extract is less of a concern, but jasmine oil is a known skin irritant (Source: *Journal of Investigative Dermatology*, December 1987, pages 540–546). Although the small amount of jasmine oil is unlikely to be problematic, this would still be better off (and rated higher) without it.

☺ GOOD $$$ **Enlivening Amino-AG Eye Treatment** *($38 for 0.5 fl. oz.)*. This silky, light-weight moisturizer contains a selection of effective ingredients for slightly dry skin anywhere on the face. The inclusion of rosemary oil in a product meant for use around the eyes is not wise, as it can be an irritant, although the amount this contains is not likely to be a problem. Mid-priced for an eye cream, this is one of the better options from Boscia, but, truth be told, you don't need an eye cream (see the Appendix to find out why).

☺ GOOD $$$ **Recharging Night Moisture** *($44 for 1.4 fl. oz.)*. Boscia highlights the oriental botanicals in their description of this product, but it's the blend of glycerin, silicones, and plant oils that treat normal to dry skin to a respectable complement of what it needs to look and feel its best.

☺ GOOD $$$ **Restorative Amino-3P Firming Treatment** *($48 for 1 fl. oz.)*. Those with dry to very dry skin, take note: Despite being labeled "firming treatment," this is actually an oil-rich moisturizer that is a great option if persistent dryness is a problem. The texture isn't greasy, and some with very dry skin may still find this doesn't supply enough moisturizer, but it's certainly worth a try. Olive oil is antioxidant-rich but Boscia includes other plant-based antioxidants (and some good anti-irritants), too. This moisturizer would earn our top rating if it did not contain fragrant rosemary extract in the amount it does. It also contains other fragrant plants that make it a tough sell for those with sensitive, reddened skin.

☺ GOOD $$$ **Restorative Eye Treatment for Under-Eye Bags** *($48 for 0.5 fl. oz.)*. This eye cream may state it's for under-eye bags, but the formula cannot do a thing to change this type of puffiness, which is almost always related to fat pads shifting underneath the eye area, leading to loose skin that pouches and won't go away no matter what products you use. The truth (and we wish this wasn't the case) is that most cases of under-eye bags can only be treated via cosmetic surgery. Searching for and spending untold dollars on eye creams claiming to help will only waste your time and money—money that would be better spent on a surgical procedure that really works. If under-eye bags are not your concern, this is a well-formulated eye cream for dry skin. You may be surprised to learn that you don't need a special product for the eye area, whether labeled eye cream or something else. Refer to the Appendix to learn more!

☺ GOOD $$$ **Skin Refining Treatment** *($48 for 1 fl. oz.)*. This water-based serum contains enough silicone to have the requisite silky finish. Unfortunately, other than some good water-binding agents, there's not much else to talk about. Antioxidants are in short supply, and despite everything this serum brags about not containing, it doesn't feature an impressive roster of key ingredients to make it competitive with today's best serums.

☹ AVERAGE $$$ **Intensive Eye Treatment** *($48 for 0.68 fl. oz.)*. Boscia claims the rice bran oil in this water- and silicone-based moisturizer can have a lifting effect on skin—nothing could be further from the truth. No plant oil of any kind can lift sagging skin, any more than a cupcake would be useful as a doorstop! This product has good moisturizing ability and contains several plant-based antioxidants, but the ivy extract makes it too irritating to use around the eyes. And the brightening effect isn't all that intensive; it's merely a cosmetic effect that results from the shine. This is not a terrible moisturizer; the texture and formulary are nice, but there isn't anything in it that's unique for the eye area or for any other part of the face. All in all, it's just okay, and your skin deserves better than just okay.

☺ AVERAGE $$$ **Restorative Night Treatment** *($48 for 1 fl. oz.)*. This lightweight moisturizer for normal to slightly dry or slightly oily skin would be a much better "treatment" if it contained a broader mix of skin-repairing ingredients, antioxidants, and some cell-communicating ingredients. It will hydrate without heaviness, but the amount of fragrant bitter orange is cause for concern (though it's better that Boscia used the diluted water form than pure bitter orange oil). On balance, this isn't one of the better anti-aging moisturizers around.

☹ POOR **Antioxidant Recovery Treatment C** *($48 for 1 fl. oz.)* contains a form of vitamin C, which has mounting research pertaining to its efficacy against brown spots, but it also contains senseless irritants, including peppermint, anise, and orange oils. What a shame! Also cause for concern is the amount of potassium hydroxide (lye) this product contains.

☹ POOR **Clear Complexion Moisturizer with Botanical Blast** *($36 for 1.4 fl. oz.)* does not contain any ingredients capable of clearing breakouts. The only ingredient that's even related to this claim is willow bark extract. Willow bark contains salicin, a substance that, when taken orally, is converted by the digestive process into salicylic acid (BHA, a staple anti-acne ingredient). The biological processes of converting willow bark to salicylic acid and then into salicin is complex, requiring enzymes and other chemical reactions, and skin cannot do to willow bark what the digestive tract can. Further, salicin, much like salicylic acid, is stable only under acidic conditions, and this product isn't acidic. Adding to the limitations is that the amount of willow bark in this product is too small for it to be effective, even if it could be converted into salicylic acid. Willow bark may indeed have some anti-inflammatory benefits for skin because, in its natural form, it appears to retain more of its aspirin-like composition, but there are lots of anti-inflammatory ingredients that can benefit skin; willow bark is hardly the only one. This product also contains other antioxidant extracts, which is helpful; unfortunately, it also contains fragrant oils, all of which are capable of causing irritation—the very kind of irritation that triggers more oil production at the base of pores, potentially leading to more breakouts (and bigger pores).

☹ POOR **Clear Complexion Treatment with Botanical Blast** *($35 for 1 fl. oz.)*. Talk about a misguided product with faulty claims! Although this does have a lightweight gel texture as described, not a single ingredient in this moisturizer can control oil, clear breakouts, or prevent further breakouts. The combination of orange, lavender, fennel, and clove leaf oils will only serve to irritate and inflame skin, and that's not a "gentle and effective" way to keep breakouts at bay.

BOSCIA SPECIALTY SKIN-CARE PRODUCTS

✓☺ BEST **Fresh Blotting Linens** *($10 for 100 sheets)*. These standard oil-blotting papers are composed of a natural fiber created from the abaca leaf, a plant that resembles bananas. They absorb excess oil without depositing powder or fragrance on your skin. They are also fragrance-free, which is why they deserve our top rating, not to mention the abaca leaf is a sustainable resource, making these blotting papers a good "green" option.

☺ GOOD **California Orange Blotting Linens** *($10 for 100 sheets)*. Composed of abaca leaf fibers, these papers absorb excess oil while depositing fragrance on skin in the form of orange extract. Absorbing oil is one thing, but it does not need to be accompanied by something to perfume your skin, which explains why almost all other oil-blotting papers omit this additive. Still, these can soak up excess shine for those with oily skin. Also available are **Green Tea**, **Vanilla**, **Lavender**, **Peppermint**, and **Rose Blotting Linens** ($10 for 100 sheets). The Rose, Peppermint, and Lavender versions are not recommended due to their strong fragrance.

☺ AVERAGE $$$ **Clear Complexion Mask with Botanical Blast** *($30 for 2.8 fl. oz.)* contains a skin-confusing mix of helpful and irritating plant extracts, although at least the scales are tipped in favor of the good plant extracts. However, your skin will still be confused and that can lead to problems. Also bound to confuse oily skin is the blend of absorbent clay with a high amount of emollient waxes, including beeswax (think candles). The wax content makes this mask difficult to rinse and can lead to more clogged pores. All in all, this isn't "the perfect addition" to your anti-acne routine. It's a mask your skin will do better without.

☺ AVERAGE $$$ **No Pores No Shine T-Zone Treatment** *($36 for 1 fl. oz.)*. This mattifier contains some very good dry-finish silicones and polymers that work to absorb excess oil to keep skin shine-free. The formula also contains some beneficial extras (such as antioxidants and repairing ingredients) not typically seen in mattifiers or oil-absorbing primers. With such positive comments you may wonder why this didn't rate higher. In a word, irritation. For reasons unknown to us, Boscia added the irritating menthol derivative menthyl lactate to this otherwise great formula. The amount isn't much, but its presence takes what could've been a top option and knocks it down to potentially problematic. The cooling sensation this ingredient provides isn't a skin-care benefit; it's your skin telling you it is being irritated. If you decide to try this, you should know that the irritation from menthyl lactate can stimulate nerve endings at the base of the pore, leading to your oily skin becoming worse.

☹ POOR **Clarifying Detox Mask** *($25 for 2.8 fl. oz.)*. This below-standard, basic clay mask contains rosemary, peppermint, lavender, and eucalyptus oils, which is way too many irritating ingredients for one product. None of these can detoxify skin in any manner. Strangely enough, several anti-irritants precede these problem ingredients on the list, but their effect is minimal given the long list of problematic plant extracts.

☹ POOR **Luminizing Black Mask** *($34 for 2.8 fl. oz.)*. Using this peel-off mask exposes your skin to a drying, irritating amount of polyvinyl alcohol (a hairspray ingredient, listed second), witch hazel water (which is part alcohol), pine bark, and fragrant rosemary oil. We mean, really, what a pathetic group of ingredients for any skin type. As for the toxins that this allegedly pulls from your skin, no one at Boscia could tell us what those toxins are or why the ingredients they included were "toxic" on their own. The soothing agents this mask contains are too little, too late; they can't make up for the irritation caused by the other ingredients.

☹ POOR **Pore Purifying Black Strips** *($15 for 6 strips)* are essentially an expensive version of what the Biore brand has been selling at the drugstore for years. The same concept applies: You apply an adhesive strip that's cut to fit across your nose, leave it on for several minutes, then peel it off. The strip is supposed to remove excess oil along with blackheads and other pore-clogging debris. Unfortunately, they address only part of the problem, and do so in an irritating manner, which ends up making matters worse. The strong adhesive helps pull out the top portion of blackheads and it leaves your skin feeling smooth, but it can also be very irritating. These strips require firm pressure to adhere to skin, and removing them can be tricky. If the adhesive weren't bad enough, Boscia added the potent irritants menthol, alcohol, and witch hazel. All three of these ingredients cause irritation that hurts skin's healing process, damages healthy collagen production, and triggers more oil production at the base of the pore. The reason pore strips are a bad option for blackheads is that they remove only the uppermost portion (the part you can see) without remedying what's going on inside the pore lining, where the blackhead begins. For stubborn blackheads, a well-formulated BHA (beta hydroxy acid, active ingredient salicylic acid) and a handheld tool known as a comedone extractor are much better options because they work in combination to get to the "root" of the problem. You'll find our top picks for BHA Exfoliants at the end of this book.

BURT'S BEES (SKIN CARE ONLY)

Strengths: Budget-priced (it's always a letdown when you pay too much for lackluster to ineffective products); good lip gloss; complete ingredient lists for every product are available on the company's website; one of the few lines that actually adheres to its all-natural marketing (though the results aren't always best for skin).

Weaknesses: Pervasive use of irritating ingredients, all of which have documentation proving their problematic nature for skin (and lips); average to poor sunscreens; no effective anti-blemish products; poor selection of cleansers; antioxidants sullied by reliance on jar packaging.

For more information and reviews of the latest Burt's Bees products, visit CosmeticsCop.com.

BURT'S BEES CLEANSERS

☺ GOOD **Natural Acne Solutions Purifying Gel Cleanser** *($10 for 5 fl. oz.)* is a very good water-soluble cleanser for all skin types. The detergent cleansing agents are quite gentle and so are not especially adept at removing makeup, but those who wear minimal to no makeup won't find this to be an issue. The active ingredient is 1% salicylic acid, but its blemish-busting effect is limited when it's in a product that's quickly rinsed from skin. The salicylic acid isn't derived from willow bark as claimed, so this product shouldn't be construed as a natural alternative to other anti-acne cleansers. Willow bark contains salicin, a chemical that can be converted via enzymes into salicylic acid when ingested, but not when applied topically (Source: naturaldatabase.com).

☺ GOOD **Radiance Daily Cleanser** *($10 for 6 fl. oz.)* is a very good, mild cleansing lotion suitable for dry skin not prone to blemishes. Although the detergent cleansing agent isn't great for removing makeup, the sunflower emollient picks up the slack. The formula contains a small amount of jojoba beads for exfoliation, but you may still want to use a washcloth for a more thorough "scrub" and to avoid a residue. The fruit acid complex referred to in the claims is a collection of citrus and sugar extracts that do not function like AHAs.

☹ AVERAGE **Sensitive Facial Cleanser** *($10 for 6 fl. oz.)*. Other than tiny amounts of alcohol and witch hazel extracts (neither of which is suitable for any skin type, let alone sensitive skin), this is a very good, very rich cleanser for dry to very dry skin. Its water- and oil–based formula removes makeup, but between the oil and wax content, this does not rinse easily so have a damp washcloth ready or you will be left with a residue. This creamy cleanser contains several soothing plant extracts and eschews the fragrant plants often used in Burt's Bees other products—a nice change of pace!

☹ POOR **Soap Bark & Chamomile Deep Cleansing Cream** *($8 for 6 fl. oz.)* contains several problematic ingredients for skin, especially for use around the eyes, and is not recommended.

BURT'S BEES TONERS

☹ POOR **Garden Tomato Toner** *($12 for 8 fl. oz.)* lists alcohol as the second ingredient, which makes this toner too drying and irritating for all skin types. Alcohol also causes free-radical damage and collagen breakdown, which goes against what the antioxidants in this toner do to benefit your skin. This also contains citrus peel oils that contain irritating components that cause further damage. Ouch!

☹ POOR **Natural Acne Solutions Clarifying Toner** *($10 for 5 fl. oz.)* contains many natural ingredients, some good ones and some bad ones. Chief among the bad ingredients is

☞ Did you know you don't need an eye cream? It's true! See the Appendix to find out why.

alcohol. Alcohol shows up in many anti-acne products, and it's never welcome; see the Appendix to find out why. Although this toner is medicated with anti-acne superstar salicylic acid, the pH of the product is too high for it to function as an exfoliant. Even if the pH were within the proper range, the amount of alcohol remains a problem, as does the needlessly high amount of fragrance.

☹ POOR **Rosewater & Glycerin Toner** *($12 for 8 fl. oz.)* lists alcohol as the second ingredient, which makes this toner too drying and irritating for all skin types. See the Appendix for further details on why alcohol is a problem for all skin types.

BURT'S BEES SCRUBS

☹ POOR **Citrus Facial Scrub** *($8 for 2 fl. oz.)* is an inelegant scrub whose abrasive agents are composed of nutshells whose uneven shape can cause tiny tears in the skin during use (in contrast, perfectly rounded polyethylene beads polish skin without this effect). Although the nutshells aren't the best, they don't make this product a poor contender. What does are the nutmeg and clove powders, which only serve to provide fragrance and irritate skin.

☹ POOR **Natural Acne Solutions Pore Refining Scrub** *($10 for 4 fl. oz.)* is a mess on several counts. The main issue is that it contains several plant oils that are inappropriate for anyone struggling with blemishes. Secondary issues include the thick, creamy texture and the fact that it doesn't rinse without leaving a waxy film on skin (it really feels awful over oily areas). The active ingredient is salicylic acid, but it has minimal chance of being helpful due to this scrub's brief contact with skin (not to mention it has all those oils to work through before it can touch your skin). From any direction, this is a serious problem for blemish-prone skin.

☹ POOR **Peach & Willowbark Deep Pore Scrub** *($8 for 4 fl. oz.)* contains an appreciable amount of sodium borate. Also known as borax, this ingredient has a drying effect on skin due to its alkaline pH. It is fine in small amounts, but that's not the case here, making this a scrub to avoid.

BURT'S BEES MOISTURIZERS (DAYTIME & NIGHTTIME), EYE CREAMS, & SERUMS

☺ GOOD **Sensitive Daily Moisturizing Cream** *($15 for 1.8 fl. oz.)* contains mostly natural ingredients, and given that this fragrance-free moisturizer is meant for those with sensitive skin, we're glad Burt's Bees left out the problematic plant extracts and fragrant oils. Instead, skin is treated to a thick-textured cream rich in nonfragrant plant oil and a rather high amount of zinc oxide. In addition to functioning as a sunscreen (though this product does not have an SPF rating), zinc oxide also functions as a skin protectant (it's the active ingredient in most diaper rash creams because of the strong barrier properties it has). That can be helpful for sensitive skin, but the drawback is zinc oxide can feel too heavy and occlusive—and there are other soothing, protective ingredients that help sensitive skin. Still, if you have sensitive, dry skin you'll likely find the texture of this product acceptable. The plant extracts this contains function as antioxidants and some have research pertaining to their anti-inflammatory properties, so ultimately this is worth considering and a welcome change of pace from most of the other Burt's Bees moisturizers.

☺ GOOD **Sensitive Eye Cream** *($15 for 0.5 fl. oz.)* is very similar to Burt's Bees Sensitive Daily Moisturizing Cream above, and there's no reason that cannot be applied around the eyes, too. If anything, the Moisturizing Cream is the better choice because it contains a much lower amount of denatured alcohol than the Eye Cream. Granted, in both products the amount is likely too low to be cause for concern, but why include it at all, especially in a product meant for use around the eyes? This cannot help with puffiness at all; in fact, its heavier texture may worsen the appearance of puffy eyes (if your puffiness comes from fluid retention, in which case heavier products can pull the distended skin).

☺ AVERAGE **Beeswax & Royal Jelly Eye Creme** *($15 for 0.25 fl. oz)* contains a tiny amount of royal bee jelly (in powder form), but this ingredient, despite tempting folklore, has no established benefit for skin. It can cause contact dermatitis, though the amount of it in this product likely negates that possibility (Source: naturaldatabase.com). This is otherwise a boring formula and in truth you don't need an eye cream (see the Appendix to learn why).

☺ AVERAGE **Beeswax Moisturizing Day Creme** *($15 for 2 fl. oz)* is described as a light-weight formula, but it contains too much oil to make that claim a reality. This is a good, basic moisturizer for dry skin but definitely lacks state-of-the-art ingredients. The jar packaging won't keep key ingredients stable and has other issues, too, all described in the Appendix.

☺ AVERAGE **Beeswax Moisturizing Night Creme** *($15 for 1 fl. oz.)* is primarily plant oil, water, wax, and aloe. It serves its purpose for dry skin, but also leaves skin wanting more.

☺ AVERAGE **Naturally Ageless Intensive Repairing Serum** *($25 for 0.45 fl. oz.)* consists of a blend of oils, most of which are helpful for dry to very dry skin, but dry skin and wrinkles are not associated so the ageless claim is unwarranted. It is also mislabeled as a serum; it's really more an oil mix and the oils in this product are easily replaced by those available in any health food store, and then you won't have to risk irritation from the fragrant oils this product contains.

☺ AVERAGE **Naturally Ageless Line Diminishing Day Lotion** *($25 for 2 fl. oz.)* is an unsuitable choice for daytime unless your foundation contains a sunscreen rated SPF 15 or higher and you apply it evenly to your face. This moisturizer is an average option for normal to dry skin. The amount of antioxidant-rich pomegranate (supposedly "packed" into this formula) is less than the amount of denatured alcohol, which causes free-radical damage, dryness, and irritation. For the money, this is a disappointing formula and far from what a state-of-the-art anti-aging moisturizer should be.

☺ AVERAGE **Naturally Ageless Line Smoothing Eye Creme** *($25 for 0.5 fl. oz.)* is an emollient moisturizer for dry skin, but one that's not advised for use around the eyes because the amount of alcohol it contains can be potentially irritating and drying. The formula overall is boring, lacking state-of-the-art ingredients, and the jar packaging won't keep the minimal amount of antioxidants in this product stable. See the Appendix to learn why you don't need an eye cream.

☺ AVERAGE **Naturally Ageless Skin Hydrating Night Creme** *($25 for 2 fl. oz.)* wastes its few antioxidants because of the poor choice of jar packaging, which won't keep them stable. Otherwise, it's a basic, emollient moisturizer for normal to dry skin not prone to blemishes. The fact that it includes more denatured alcohol than it does state-of-the-art ingredients is disappointing at any price, and nothing about this fragranced moisturizer is skin-firming.

☹ POOR **Natural Acne Solutions Daily Moisturizing Lotion** *($18 for 2 fl. oz.)* is a light-weight lotion that has an odor reminiscent of chlorine and citronella, so we're not off to a good start if your olfactory sense is especially acute. It's also a letdown that the main ingredient is sunflower oil, which someone with blemish-prone skin does not need—yet the company claims this product controls oil! How? By adding more? That's like telling an obese person they'll slim down by consuming more calories and not exercising! The theory that oily skin is producing too much oil because it needs more has no basis in fact. Skin makes oil because of androgens (male hormones). Adding to the misinformation is the fact that this contains 1% salicylic acid as its active ingredient, a decidedly unnatural ingredient (so much for a natural solution for acne), but the pH of 5 prevents it from exfoliating skin or from affecting the bacteria that cause acne. Last, this has an unappealing waxy, tacky finish on skin that is far from representative of how today's best moisturizers (those with and without salicylic acid) feel.

☹ POOR **Radiance Day Creme** *($18 for 2 fl. oz.)* is not suitable for daytime because it doesn't contain a sunscreen. Yes, you can apply this and follow with a foundation rated SPF 15 or greater, but the greasy base isn't the best for makeup application, even if skin is very dry. Some of the plant extracts in this product are irritating and serve no pleasant purpose other than adding fragrance; unfortunately, fragrance isn't a skin-care benefit. See the Appendix for further details about daily use of highly fragranced products.

☺ AVERAGE **Radiance Day Lotion SPF 15** *($18 for 2 fl. oz.)* is a mineral sunscreen that contains an effective blend of titanium dioxide and zinc oxide for broad-spectrum sun protection. The creamy, borderline greasy base formula is recommended only for dry skin not prone to blemishes. Royal jelly doesn't have miraculous benefits for skin, so just ignore the claims for this ingredient. It would be better for you if Burt's Bees had included some potent antioxidants, but this is really just an average moisturizer with sunscreen. By the way, this isn't an all-natural product, although it's fairly close if you want to stretch your definition of what constitutes natural.

☹ POOR **Radiance Eye Creme** *($18 for 0.5 fl. oz.)* is nearly identical to Burt's Bees Radiance Day Creme above, proving once again that eye cream formulas rarely differ from facial moisturizers.

☹ POOR **Radiance Night Creme** *($18 for 2 fl. oz.)* is a very basic emollient moisturizer for dry skin. It contains mostly natural ingredients, but several of the plants have irritant potential for skin and the amount of fragrance is much higher than it should be (ideally, fragrance-free is best for your skin).

☹ POOR **Radiance Serum with Royal Jelly** *($18 for 0.45 fl. oz.)* is practically all about royal jelly. We have no idea why royal jelly still gets the occasional promotion in skin-care products, but it does, despite there being no research showing it has special benefit for skin (but, then, that has never stopped the cosmetics industry before). We suspect Burt's Bees includes royal jelly because of its association with the "bees" in the company name, and because it is naturally secreted by honeybees and used for nourishment. But, none of that has anything to do with good skin care, just good marketing. Even if royal jelly were a proven nutritional powerhouse for skin, you shouldn't ignore the fact that this serum contains a potentially irritating amount of alcohol; in fact, there's more alcohol present than the played-up royal jelly! This serum isn't worth your time or money. Please see the Appendix for details on why the irritation alcohol causes is a problem for all skin types.

BURT'S BEES LIP CARE

☺ GOOD **Replenishing Lip Balm With Pomegranate Oil** *($3 for 0.15 fl. oz.)* has pomegranate oil, which is great, and contributes to making this a good lip balm capable of taking care of chapped lips.

☺ GOOD **Tinted Lip Balm** *($7 for 0.15 fl. oz.)* is a twist-up lip balm that comes in floral-inspired shades (like Rose, Tiger Lily, and Hibiscus) with a soft tint, light scent, and lots of moisture. There's an abundance of emollient oil ingredients included that will make lips feel soft, smooth, and moisturized. Although the flower-derived fragrant plant waxes pose a slight risk of irritation, this is nevertheless a very good formula that gives lips a splash of soft color.

☺ AVERAGE **Honey Lip Balm** *($3 for 0.15 fl. oz.)* is a wax-based flavored lip balm that can do an OK job of preventing moisture loss and helping with chapped lips. The fact that it's flavored isn't the best because anything that tempts you to lick your lips (which flavor does) means the lip balm won't last as long as it should, so you'll be reapplying more often than with an unflavored balm.

☺ AVERAGE **Nourishing Lip Balm with Mango Butter** *($3 for 0.15 fl. oz.)*. There's one potential concern in this emollient, plant oil–based lip balm and that's the amount of fragrance. It's listed as aroma, a clever way to confuse the customer about what they are really buying. Your lips have no more use for fragrance than your skin, so ideally a fragrance-free lip balm is best. This will help heal chapped lips and prevent moisture loss, but its fruity scent and flavor isn't the best. If anything, the flavor may encourage you to lick your lips, which will wear away the balm and can lead to more dryness and chapping.

☺ AVERAGE **Rejuvenating Lip Balm with Acai Berry** *($3 for 0.15 fl. oz.)* is nearly identical to the Burt's Bees Nourishing Lip Balm with Mango Butter reviewed above, save for a change in smell and flavor. As such, the same review applies.

☺ AVERAGE **Sun Protecting Lip Balm with Passionfruit SPF 8** *($4 for 0.15 fl. oz.)* contains a pure titanium dioxide sunscreen, but its SPF rating is far below the standard SPF 15 recommended by medical boards around the world. That's a shame because the emollient formula is otherwise excellent for keeping dry, chapped lips in kissably soft shape, although the amount of flavor it contains may encourage excess lip-licking, which isn't the best.

☹ POOR **Beeswax Lip Balm Tin** *($3 for 0.3 fl. oz.)* is the company's most popular product, but it isn't one we'd recommend because it contains irritating peppermint oil.

☹ POOR **Beeswax Lip Balm Tube** *($3 for 0.15 fl. oz.)* is identical to the Beeswax Lip Balm Tin, and the same review applies.

☹ POOR **Lip Shimmers** *($5)* are sheer, glossy lipsticks that apply well but irritate lips with a potent mix of peppermint and rosemary oils. Your lips deserve better than irritation!

☹ POOR **Medicated Lip Balm** *($4 for 0.15 fl. oz.)* is not the least bit soothing as general skin care for your lips. It does contain some very good emollient oils and waxes to protect against chapped lips, but it also contains several potent irritants that can make chapping and dryness worse. Camphor, menthol, and clove oil are present, and there is some marginal research, and we mean really minor research, showing a potential to heal herpes cold sores (menthol and camphor) or reduce the discomfort (clove oil). However, it would be wiser to apply only the pure essential oil over the area, including tea tree oil, which this product doesn't contain, for an alternative treatment than to irritate your entire lip area on a daily basis with these ingredients, which have no benefit for lips that don't have cold sore breakouts. Keep in mind that none of these ingredients can prevent a herpes breakout.

☹ POOR **Res-Q Lip Balm SPF 15** *($4 for 0.15 fl. oz.)* includes a pure titanium dioxide sunscreen to provide reliable broad-spectrum protection. It also has a smooth, plant oil and wax base that helps keep lips smooth and protected against chapping. All of that is great, which is why it's disappointing to see that this balm also contains fragrant lavandin oil. A hybrid of lavender oil, lavandin contains many of the fragrance ingredients that make pure lavender oil a problem for skin and lips. See the Appendix to learn why lavender oil and its derivatives should be avoided.

☹ POOR **Ultra Conditioning Lip Balm with Kokum Butter** *($4 for 0.15 fl oz.)* could've been a top-notch lip balm for uncomfortably dry, chapped lips, but the fragrant oils are potent irritants and this also contains fragrance ingredients known to cause irritation, making this a lip balm to avoid.

BURT'S BEES SPECIALTY SKIN-CARE PRODUCTS

☺ GOOD **Natural Acne Solutions Maximum Strength Spot Treatment Cream** *($13 for 0.5 fl. oz.)* is an intriguing anti-acne product to consider! The lightweight cream contains a good blend of anti-inflammatory plant extracts and its only potentially problematic ingredient is a tiny amount of witch hazel extract. The helpful, redness-reducing ingredients are in abundance, though it's a shame this contains fragrance and a couple of fragrance ingredients known to be irritating. Although this isn't preferred to anti-acne products medicated with benzoyl peroxide or salicylic acid (willow bark is not the same as salicylic acid, and does not work the same when applied topically), it is a worthwhile option to consider. At the very least, it should help fade red marks and provides a slight antibacterial punch due to the glucose oxidase and lactoperoxidase ingredients it contains.

☹ POOR **Natural Acne Solutions Targeted Spot Treatment** *($10 for 0.26 fl. oz.)* may contain several natural ingredients, but many of them are nothing more than an assault on skin that's already reddened and inflamed from acne. The main ingredient is alcohol, which not only is irritating, but also stimulates oil production at the base of your pores. (How ironic that it is indeed natural, but once again, natural as a skin-care category doesn't tell you anything about whether or not a product has benefit for your skin.) If that weren't bad enough, you're also getting a potent dose of lemon peel oil and lesser, but still problematic, amounts of other irritating plants, including eucalyptus.

CAUDALIE PARIS (SKIN CARE ONLY)

Strengths: Good cleansers; an excellent scrub for dry skin; air-tight packaging; a good lip balm and moisturizing mask; one truly state-of-the-art moisturizer for dry skin.

Weaknesses: Expensive; mundane to irritating serums, moisturizers, and eye creams; limited sun protection options; no AHA or BHA products; no products to lighten skin discolorations; several products contain irritating plant extracts.

For more information and reviews of the latest Caudalie products, visit CosmeticsCop.com.

CAUDALIE PARIS CLEANSERS & MAKEUP REMOVER

☺ GOOD **$$$ Gentle Cleanser Face And Eyes, For Normal To Dry Skin** *($26 for 6.7 fl. oz.)* would be better classified as "gentle" if it didn't contain fragrance, but it is still an effective, detergent-free cleansing lotion for normal to dry skin not prone to blemishes. It will remove makeup and rinses fairly well, though you may find you need a washcloth for complete removal. This cleanser does not protect your skin from free radicals—that is impossible. Even to come close to achieving that, you'd have to be in an environment without oxygen, which would mean you couldn't breathe, and that wouldn't be good! There isn't any product anywhere that can stop free-radical damage; at best we can only reduce the impact.

☺ GOOD **$$$ Instant Foaming Cleanser** *($26 for 5 fl. oz)* is a standard water-soluble cleansing gel suitable for its intended skin type. The price is out of line for what you get, but it works well and won't leave your skin feeling tight or dry. This does contain fragrance.

☺ AVERAGE **$$$ Cleansing Water Face And Eyes, For All Skin Types** *($14 for 3.4 fl. oz.)* is a fragrance-free liquid makeup remover that contains enough oil to leave a slightly greasy finish (so this is best used before you cleanse your face). It works to remove just about any type of makeup, though most will find a silicone-enhanced formula superior at removing waterproof formulas. Caudalie's claim about "micelle" water being able to capture dirt like tiny magnets is true, but that is true of any detergent-based makeup remover. Micelle technology is simply one way of explaining how a detergent cleansing agent combines with water and interacts with oils to clean any surface, including skin. That technology is not by any means unique to this product. Lastly, this is not preferred to any of the fragrance-free makeup removers because anything you use so close to the eye itself should not contain fragrance.

CAUDALIE PARIS TONERS

☺ AVERAGE $$$ **Grape Water, for All Skin Types** (*$8 for 1.7 fl. oz*) is an incredibly simple toner that contains only grape water. You might as well mist your skin with pure grape juice, because at least that isn't diluted, and it certainly costs less than this. Either way, it takes more than grapes to give your skin what it needs to look its best.

☺ AVERAGE $$$ **Toning Lotion** (*$26 for 6.7 fl. oz.*) is an OK toner for normal to dry skin. Caudalie maintains this toner contains a high concentration of what they refer to as "Vinolevure," an ingredient said to be extracted from yeast. This contains a form of beta-glucan, an antioxidant that can be derived from yeast, but is hardly unique to this product or the only thing skin needs to improve itself.

☹ POOR **Beauty Elixir, for All Skin Types** (*$46 for 3.4 fl. oz.*) lists alcohol as the second ingredient, making it too drying and irritating for all skin types; plus alcohol causes free-radical damage and cell death. Even if this were alcohol-free, it contains several irritating plant oils that will leave your skin less than beautiful.

CAUDALIE PARIS SCRUB

☺ GOOD $$$ **Gentle Buffing Cream** (*$35 for 2 fl. oz.*) is an excellent scrub for normal to very dry skin not prone to blemishes. It would be gentler (and better for sensitive skin) without the fragrance and fragrance ingredients such as geraniol, but in terms of abrasiveness and ingredients that cushion skin as you scrub, this is quite mild.

CAUDALIE PARIS MOISTURIZERS (DAYTIME & NIGHTTIME), EYE CREAMS, & SERUMS

☺ GOOD $$$ **Vinoperfect Day Perfecting Cream SPF 15** (*$68 for 1 fl. oz.*) provides UVA protection with an in-part avobenzone sunscreen, and is formulated in a lightweight cream base ideal for normal to dry skin. (Someone with oily skin will find this too heavy, so the "all skin types" designation should be ignored.) This contains a smattering of antioxidants and interesting water-binding agents, but is not rated a Best Product because most of the really intriguing ingredients are listed after the fragrance.

☺ GOOD $$$ **Vinosource Anti-Wrinkle Nourishing Cream** (*$50 for 1.3 fl. oz.*) impresses with its lightweight yet creamy texture and antioxidant-rich formula, and it contains other helpful ingredients for dry skin, including borage oil, olive esters, and glycerin. Although not quite on par with today's best moisturizers, it is one of the better formulas from Caudalie and, like all their moisturizers, the opaque tube packaging will help keep the antioxidants stable during use.

☺ GOOD $$$ **Vinosource Intense Moisture Rescue Cream** (*$38 for 1.3 fl. oz.*) is an excellent though pricey moisturizer for dry to very dry skin. It contains a good range of emollients along with antioxidants, plus some cell-communicating ingredients. The only drawback, beyond the price, is that this contains a rather high amount of fragrance plus sensitizing fragrant components that are present in many other Caudalie moisturizers. The amount of the fragrance ingredients (such as limonene) isn't high, but their inclusion plus the amount of generic "fragrance" keeps this moisturizer from earning our top rating. In the end, this has a

The Reviews C

good range of ingredients to help skin look and act younger, assuming you're protecting your skin every day with a well-formulated sunscreen rated SPF 15 or greater.

☺ AVERAGE $$$ **Fresh Complexion Tinted Moisturizer** *($39 for 1 fl. oz.)* is a lightweight, fluid tinted moisturizer suitable for normal to slightly dry skin. Both of the shades are too peachy pink and each imparts shine from mica (which is why it is not recommended for oily areas, unless you want to look extra shiny). The formula will leave your skin wanting more; it really is boring, and highly fragranced as well so it's less desirable than better tinted moisturizers from Aveda, Bobbi Brown, and Neutrogena (and their options include the added benefit of a broad-spectrum sunscreen).

☺ AVERAGE $$$ **Premier Cru The Creme** *($150 for 1.7 fl. oz.)* is supposed to create "unparalleled age-fighting power," yet if that's true, Caudalie should own up to the fact that none of their other antiwrinkle products are as good and stop selling them. Of course, they won't do that, and consumers will continue to be puzzled by this brand's many repetitive options claiming to leave their face line-free. As it turns out, this product, whose name is similar to Lauder's Creme de la Mer, shouldn't be at the top of anyone's premier list of anti-aging moisturizers, or any moisturizer for that matter. It's a fairly standard blend of water, thickeners, slip agent, and plant oils. Grape, olive, and sesame oils have antioxidant ability, but they show up in lots of other products sold at more realistic prices and with far better formulations. Several of the more enticing ingredients are present in amounts too small for skin to notice, including the peptides. For what Caudalie is charging, those ingredients should be front and center, not relegated to mere dustings. At best, this is an overly fragranced moisturizer for normal to dry skin. It cannot, we repeat, cannot, fill wrinkles, lift skin, or reduce discolorations. Lots of other companies offer moisturizers whose formulas come a lot closer to achieving anti-aging results than this does.

☺ AVERAGE $$$ **Premier Cru The Eye Cream** *($95 for 0.5 fl. oz.)* is Premier Cru The Creme facial moisturizer's eye-cream counterpart, even though you don't need an eye cream (see the Appendix to find out why). Although beautifully packaged, this eye cream isn't worth its price. You'll get some hydration, but you're also getting a lot more shine (from the mineral pigment mica) than you are state-of-the-art anti-aging ingredients, and shine is not skin care. This is just an OK option for normal to dry skin, but at this price, you should be getting an outstanding product. The fact that this eye cream contains fragrance isn't good. Fragrance isn't skin care and can be especially problematic in products to be used in the eye area.

☺ AVERAGE $$$ **Pulpe Vitaminee 1st Wrinkle Cream** *($58 for 1.03 fl. oz.)* cannot prevent sagging as claimed. The multiple factors that cause skin to sag (i.e., sun damage, bone loss, gravity, loss of estrogen, fat pads shifting beneath the skin, and so on) cannot be addressed by any skin care product. We wish that weren't the case, but it's the absolute truth. Sagging can be addressed only with cosmetic corrective and/or surgical procedures. Knowing that this product cannot halt sagging, is there any other reason to consider it? For the money, no; however, it is a good emollient moisturizer that can address the needs of those with dry skin. It does not have a matte finish as claimed and, in fact, contains very little to help keep skin matte. What this moisturizer is missing is a greater range of antioxidants along with skin-repairing and cell-communicating ingredients. You'll find better moisturizers with those types of ingredients listed in our Best Products chapter.

☺ AVERAGE $$$ **Pulpe Vitaminee 1st Wrinkle Fluid** *($58 for 1.3 fl. oz.)* is a light, thin-textured moisturizer for normal to oily skin. Contrary to claim, this is not "remarkably effective" at reducing sagging skin; in fact, it cannot affect sagging in the least. Skin-care products cannot affect the physiological reasons behind sagging skin, plus this contains no sun protection. On balance, this expensive moisturizer contains little of anti-aging interest and its fragrance ingredients pose a risk of irritation.

☺ AVERAGE $$$ **Pulpe Vitaminee 1st Wrinkle Serum** *($62 for 1 fl. oz)* is supposed to reverse the first signs of aging. If it could do that, Caudalie wouldn't need to sell so many other antiwrinkle/firming products making the exact same claim, but of course they do. This serum contains some intriguing ingredients for skin, but none of them are capable of reversing aging. What's most disappointing is that many of the intriguing ingredients are listed after the preservatives, so they don't count for much. This is an average, overpriced serum for normal to dry skin.

☺ AVERAGE $$$ **Pulpe Vitaminee Eye and Lip Cream** *($49 for 0.5 fl. oz.)* is a fairly standard fragrance-free moisturizer whether applied around your eyes or on your lips. Its only exciting aspect is a high amount of antioxidant vitamin E (listed as tocopheryl acetate, which is not the most exciting form of this ingredient). That's nice, but it doesn't make this product worth the price, not to mention that you don't need a separate eye cream (see the Appendix to find out why). Overall, this is an ordinary formula with not much to offer skin anywhere on the face, especially not for the price tag.

☺ AVERAGE $$$ **Vinexpert Anti-Ageing Serum Eyes And Lips, For Skin Lacking Vitality** *($70 for 0.5 fl. oz.)* is terribly overpriced and is actually a nearly do-nothing water-based serum for normal to slightly oily skin. The amount of witch hazel is potentially irritating, and all the intriguing ingredients are listed after the preservative. Nothing in this serum can diminish puffiness or dark circles, either. See the Appendix to learn why, in truth, you don't need a special product for the eye area.

☺ AVERAGE $$$ **Vinexpert Firming Serum** *($79 for 1 fl. oz.)* has a barely discernible tightening effect on skin; however, the effect is only temporary, and strictly cosmetic. This is otherwise an embarrassingly overpriced water-based serum whose bitter orange and rose flower water can cause irritation. Very few ingredients beneficial for skin are included, but at least this serum is not a total waste of money.

☺ AVERAGE $$$ **Vinexpert Night Infusion Cream** *($68 for 1 fl. oz.)* is a lightweight cream moisturizer for normal to dry skin, but its regenerating action is limited unless you believe that grape seed oil is the only antioxidant to seek. It's a worthwhile ingredient for skin, but its effect in this product is likely offset by the amount of fragrance and the potentially irritating fragrant components it contains.

☺ AVERAGE $$$ **Vinexpert Radiance Day Fluid SPF 10** *($68 for 1 fl. oz.)* is an OK daytime moisturizer with sunscreen for normal to oily skin, but it's overpriced for what you get, and the SPF rating is disappointing. SPF 15 is the minimum recommended by most major medical and dermatologic organizations, so even though this product provides UVA protection with the active sunscreen ingredient avobenzone, its low SPF rating means you must pair it with another product that contains sunscreen. The lotion-textured base formula isn't very exciting. Several antioxidants are included, but Caudalie added larger amounts of fragrance and mica (for shine) than it did many of these essential ingredients. That's not what you want to see for a product that costs this much, especially when you consider that the more you spend on a facial moisturizer with sunscreen, the less likely you are to apply it liberally (which is essential for getting the amount of sun protection stated on the label).

☺ AVERAGE $$$ **Vinexpert Riche Radiance Day Cream SPF 10** *($68 for 1 fl. oz.)* is similar to Caudalie's Vinexpert Radiance Day Fluid SPF 10, save for it's richer, almost greasy, texture. Otherwise, the same comments apply.

The Reviews C

☺ AVERAGE $$$ **Vinoperfect Cell Renewal Night Cream** *($68 for 1 fl. oz.)* claims to work overnight at diminishing dark spots and tightening pores, yet the ingredients in this cream show up in almost all of Caudalie's other moisturizers, which seems to mean that they do all those other things, too, right? Wrong! This standard, overpriced moisturizer for normal to dry skin contains nothing that can fade the faintest freckle, nor can it tighten pores (triglycerides and shea butter are not what pores need if they are clogged or engorged with too much oil). The tartaric and malic acids are present in amounts too low for them to function as AHAs, and the pH of 4.4 wouldn't permit exfoliation anyway.

☺ AVERAGE $$$ **Vinoperfect Complexion Correcting Radiance Serum** *($79 for 1 fl. oz.)* has such an average formulation that the price just seems to be in bad taste. The small amount of grape extract means that this product likely has minimal antioxidant ability—and what about skin-identical substances, cell-communicating ingredients, or an anti-irritant or two? All of those are hallmarks of state-of-the-art serums, which this product certainly is not.

☺ AVERAGE $$$ **Vinoperfect Day Perfecting Fluid SPF 15 PA++** *($68 for 1 fl. oz.)* is a good, though needlessly expensive, daytime moisturizer with sunscreen for normal to dry skin. Important UVA (think anti-aging) protection is provided by stabilized avobenzone, and the formula has an impressive amount of antioxidant-rich grape seed oil. The problem with a daytime moisturizer being so expensive is that you're less likely to apply it liberally each morning, which means you won't be getting the stated level of sun protection. In terms of Caudalie's skin transformation claims, the dewy finish this leaves will help revive radiance, and the act of protecting your skin from further sun damage will help fade the dark spots that formed due to sun damage (because the dark spots are not constantly being exposed to the UV light that caused them). Although all that's great, these traits are common to any well-formulated sunscreen for normal to dry skin—you don't need to spend in this range to obtain these anti-aging benefits.

☺ AVERAGE $$$ **Vinopure Matte Finish Fluid, For Combination Skin** *($49 for 1.3 fl. oz.)* contains a frustrating combination of beneficial and irritating ingredients for its intended skin type. The sage leaf water doesn't get this off to a great start because sage can be a skin irritant. This is an OK moisturizing fluid with some good antioxidants, but it absolutely cannot regulate oil production. Its texture and finish is soft matte, and it works well under makeup; however, the matte feel doesn't have any effect on what's happening in your skin's oil glands.

☺ AVERAGE $$$ **Vinosource Quenching Sorbet-Creme** *($40 for 1.3 fl. oz.)* is a fairly standard moisturizer for dry skin. Despite claims of an "ultra-natural formula," there are plenty of synthetic ingredients on board. The blend of natural and synthetic ingredients is mostly good, but the amount of fragrance is cause for concern, especially when you consider that Caudalie recommends this moisturizer for ultra-sensitive skin. Regardless of skin type, fragrance isn't skin care! Also disappointing is that there is more fragrance and alcohol in this moisturizer than soothing ingredients and antioxidants. See the Appendix to find out why alcohol and a high amount of fragrance are skin-care problems, not benefits.

☹ POOR **Pulpe Vitaminee Regenerating Concentrate** *($44 for 0.5 fl. oz.)* is based around the antioxidant-rich grape seed extract, but this serum-style product ends up being a major source of irritation for all skin types. It contains several fragrant oils that have questionable, if any, benefit for your skin, but research has made it clear that each can cause irritation (Source: naturaldatabase.com). Of particular concern is the lavender oil. It may smell great, but the oil causes numerous problems for skin, all discussed in the Appendix.

☹ POOR **Vinosource Moisturizing Concentrate, For Dry Skin** *($44 for 0.5 fl. oz.)* contains rosewood and palmarosa oils along with other fragrant irritants such as eugenol, limonene, and citral. None of these are suitable for dry skin; you'd be better off applying pure grape seed or jojoba oil to treat dry skin instead of wasting your money on this product.

CAUDALIE PARIS SUN CARE

☺ GOOD **$$$ Teint Divin Self Tanner Face** *($39 for 1 fl. oz.)* is a very good self-tanner for dry to very dry skin, but the price is just silly. It contains dihydroxyacetone to turn skin tan, the same ingredient that's present in almost every self-tanner sold today, from L'Oreal to Neutrogena and Coppertone, and for a fraction of the price—just take a look at how tiny this container is! This is a good self-tanner, but absolutely not worth the extra money.

CAUDALIE PARIS LIP CARE

☺ GOOD **$$$ Lip Conditioner** *($12 for 0.14 fl. oz.)* is a standard, mineral oil– and wax-based lip balm that contains a nice array of emollients to help lips feel smooth, soft, and comfortable, but labeling this "antioxidant-rich" is definitely an exaggeration.

CAUDALIE PARIS SPECIALTY SKIN-CARE PRODUCTS

☺ GOOD **$$$ Vinoperfect Enzymatic Peel Mask** *($40 for 1.3 fl. oz.)* This fragranced moisturizing mask for normal to dry skin claims to peel skin along with tighten pores and reduce oily skin. Looking at the ingredient list, there's no way these results are possible. The formula contains mostly water, glycerin, emollient thickener, plant oils, and lots more thickeners and emollients, none of which have an exfoliating (peeling) or pore-reducing effect. If anything, applying a heavy-duty mask like this to areas with enlarged pores will only make them appear larger! All this mask can realistically do is leave your skin feeling smooth and soft. The emollient ingredients it contains are great for dry to very dry skin, which is why this is rated well. If you're willing to disregard all the claims, this can be a good moisturizing mask.

The claim of Caudalie's "Viniferine" (from grapes) being 62 times as effective as vitamin C is not supported by published research. It's just a marketing claim because Caudalie is all about grapes, often to the exclusion of other beneficial antioxidants. Even if it was as great as they say, so what? There are many antioxidants available, so comparing one to another isn't really helpful. Why not acknowledge both are great and include them (plus others) in one product?

☺ AVERAGE **$$$ Vinosource Moisturizing Cream-Mask Face and Eyes, for Dry Skin** *($40 for 1.6 fl. oz.)* is a glycerin-rich mask for dry skin, and supplies an impressive amount of antioxidant grape seed oil, which makes this a decent, though needlessly pricey, option.

☹ POOR **Vinopure Purifying Mask, for Combination Skin** *($35 for 1.6 fl. oz.)* is a standard clay mask wrapped up in one of the longest ingredient lists you're likely to see. The odd mix of absorbents and emollient, oily, or wax-based thickeners is bound to be confusing for your skin. Contrary to the claim, this mask cannot regulate oil production, something that is controlled by hormones and not affected by products like this. Moreover, the bergamot, lavender, clary, and sandalwood oils are all irritating for any skin type. See the Appendix to learn why irritation is a big problem for oily skin.

CERAVE (SKIN CARE ONLY)

Strengths: Affordable, gentle, and fragrance-free; excellent body moisturizers (reviewed on CosmeticsCop.com) and facial cleansers; daytime moisturizer provides broad-spectrum sun protection.

Weaknesses: Hydrating Cleanser does not remove makeup well on its own; formulas are effective but don't go the extra mile to supply dry skin with a wider complement of beneficial ingredients.

For more information and reviews of the latest CeraVe products, visit CosmeticsCop.com.

CERAVE CLEANSERS

✓☺ BEST **Foaming Facial Cleanser** *($11.99 for 12 fl. oz.)* is a gentle, water-soluble cleanser that's best for normal to oily skin and ranks among the top cleansers available at any price. The formula produces a slight lather, removes makeup easily, and rinses without a hint of residue. The inclusion of skin-identical ingredients is a nice touch, although these state-of-the-art ingredients are best when included in products meant to be left on the skin. Foaming Facial Cleanser is an excellent option for those with oily, sensitive skin, too, including those struggling with rosacea. An added bonus is that the built-in pump dispenser is easy to use.

✓☺ BEST **Hydrating Cleanser** *($11.40 for 12 fl. oz.)* deserves serious consideration by anyone with normal to dry skin that's also sensitive, including those dealing with rosacea. It is an exceptionally gentle, soothing cleanser that contains several ingredients that mimic the structure and function of healthy skin. These are a good, but not essential, addition to a cleanser (ideally, they are ingredients that should be left on your skin). But when you're dealing with an impaired barrier, which is a hallmark of consistent dryness, every little beneficial extra helps. This cleanser is fragrance-free; its only drawback is its limited ability to remove makeup unless used with a washcloth.

CERAVE MOISTURIZERS (DAYTIME & NIGHTTIME)

✓☺ BEST **Facial Moisturizing Lotion PM** *($13.99 for 3 fl. oz.)* is a very good option for normal to dry skin. In addition to numerous skin-identical ingredients, it contains a generous amount of the cell-communicating ingredient niacinamide, which offers multiple benefits. Its lightweight cream texture provides substantial moisture. This fragrance-free moisturizer is highly recommended for sensitive or rosacea-affected skin, hence the high rating. The only formulary drawback is the lack of antioxidants, but you can remedy that by applying an antioxidant-rich serum under or over this product.

☺ GOOD **Facial Moisturizing Lotion AM SPF 30** *($13.99 for 3 fl. oz.)* includes an in-part zinc oxide sunscreen for reliable UVA protection in a formula with a lightweight lotion texture that feels elegant and wears well under makeup. Other than the sunscreen, the star ingredient in this daytime moisturizer is the cell-communicating ingredient niacinamide. This fragrance-free product also contains an impressive mix of skin-identical ingredients. The only thing holding it back from a higher rating is the lack of antioxidants; it is well established that adding antioxidants to sunscreens not only boosts the effectiveness of the sunscreen, but also boosts your skin's ability to fight the free-radical damage sun exposure causes. This is still worth strong consideration for its overall formula and affordability, but it doesn't quite qualify as a best option. It's best for normal to slightly dry or slightly oily skin.

CERAVE SPECIALTY SKIN-CARE PRODUCTS

☺ GOOD **SA Renewing Lotion** *($15.95 for 8 fl. oz.)*. This fragrance-free body lotion from CeraVe is said to exfoliate skin, and to that end it contains the BHA salicylic acid. Although

---

🔥 Irritating ingredients are a problem for all skin types. Find out why in the Appendix.

salicylic acid is an exfoliating superstar, its effectiveness in that regard depends on the product's pH, which is where this product falls down a bit. After several tests, we determined that the pH of SA Renewing Lotion is 4.5, which is beyond the ideal range (pH 3–4) that salicylic acid needs to function optimally as an exfoliant. With a pH of 4.5, you'll likely get some efficacy against breakouts and chicken skin (keratosis pilaris), but not as much as you would from a BHA body lotion with a lower pH. This product also contains the AHA derivative ammonium lactate, but again the higher pH keeps this from working as well as it could. What about using this as a regular body lotion? Its silky, slightly emollient formula contains some very good ingredients for normal to dry skin, and it is absolutely worth considering for all-over smoothing and hydration without a greasy feel. Like CeraVe's other body lotions (reviewed on CosmeticsCop.com), it contains a good mix of skin-repairing ingredients, but is short on antioxidants.

CETAPHIL (SKIN CARE ONLY)

Strengths: Inexpensive; mostly fragrance-free products; affordable and widely available; offers complete ingredient lists on its website; the sunscreens offer sufficient UVA protection.

Weaknesses: No anti-acne products; no state-of-the-art moisturizers; the original Gentle Skin Cleanser is a dated formula that isn't nearly as elegant or efficacious as many other water-soluble cleansers (despite its near-constant mention in fashion magazines as a best cleanser).

For more information and reviews of the latest Cetaphil products, visit CosmeticsCop.com.

CETAPHIL CLEANSERS

☺ GOOD **Daily Facial Cleanser for Normal to Oily Skin** _($8.49 for 8 fl. oz.)_ is a standard, detergent-based cleanser that can work for most skin types except for dry to very dry skin. It removes makeup nicely, far better than the original Cetaphil Gentle Skin Cleanser, and doesn't irritate the eyes or dry out the skin. It does contain fragrance, which seems a misguided idea from this company.

☺ GOOD **Dermacontrol Oil Control Foam Wash** _($11.99 for 8 fl. oz.)_ is a good, lightly fragranced cleanser for normal to oily or combination skin. Cleanser such as this (and there are many) are great for acne-prone skin because they don't over-cleanse but instead remove excess oil and rinse without leaving a residue. This contains zinc gluconate, an ingredient that has been studied in comparison to antibiotics for managing acne. The research on this ingredient was done with oral supplements, not topical application via a cleanser, so it's a stretch to state it applies here, too. However, zinc gluconate has anti-inflammatory activity that can be helpful for reducing redness from acne, though it would be best used in a leave-on product (Sources: _Archives of Dermatological Research_, December 2011, pages 707–713; _Journal of Investigative Dermatology_, January 2011, pages 59–66; _European Journal of Dermatology_, May-June 2005, pages 152–155; and _Dermatology_, Volume 203, 2001, pages 135–140). In terms of the "oil control" portion of the name, this cleanser cannot control oil beyond simply washing it from the surface of skin, just as any well-formulated cleanser like this can do.

☺ AVERAGE **Gentle Cleansing Bar** _($4.79 for 4.5 fl. oz.)_ is similar to Dove's original Beauty Bar and is a soap-free bar cleanser. It's an OK option for use from the neck down, but the sodium tallowate and sodium palm kernelate may clog pores and exacerbate breakouts.

☺ AVERAGE **Gentle Skin Cleanser** _($7.99 for 8 fl. oz)_ is a cleanser we have recommended for years, but no more. In many ways the formula has become dated and is now a poor representation of the best of the best when it comes to facial cleansers. Part of what led us to this reconsideration (well, beyond the wealth of beautifully formulated water-soluble cleansers) is the amount of sodium lauryl sulfate in this so-called "gentle" cleanser. Although the amount is likely 1% or less of the product's contents, there are many other cleansers available that don't use this potentially problematic ingredient and that are far better for skin. There is little reason to consider this over dozens of other options plus this cleanser is not adept at removing makeup.

☹ POOR **Antibacterial Gentle Cleansing Bar** *($4.79 for 4.5 fl. oz.)* is a standard bar cleanser with the antibacterial active ingredient triclosan. There isn't a lot of research demonstrating triclosan's effectiveness against acne-causing bacteria, but it has the potential to be a good first line of defense when acne is the concern. However, in a bar cleanser like this, the ingredients holding the cleanser in bar form won't reduce acne and may make it worse. It is not preferred to Cetaphil's water-soluble cleansers.

CETAPHIL MOISTURIZERS (DAYTIME & NIGHTTIME)

☺ GOOD **Daily Facial Moisturizer SPF 15** *($13.99 for 4 fl. oz.)* is a good, avobenzone-based sunscreen in a standard moisturizing base that is OK for someone with normal to dry skin. The product is fragrance-free; adding antioxidants and a broader array of ingredients that mimic the structure and function of healthy skin would make this good daytime moisturizer superior.

☺ GOOD **Daily Facial Moisturizer SPF 50** *($13.99 for 1.7 fl. oz.)* contains an in-part titanium dioxide sunscreen for reliable UVA protection. However, we take issue with their claim that the UV filters chosen are an "optimum blend" because that isn't the case. The blend is fine, but the combination of actives isn't unique to this product, nor is it the only one to provide such a high level of sun protection. Another questionable claim is that this is nonirritating. If titanium dioxide were the only active, we would agree with the claim, but that's not the case. It's disingenuous to state that your sunscreen is nonirritating when it contains sunscreen actives that people can (and sometimes do) react to. That's the reality, though it doesn't mean such sunscreens should be avoided (many people can tolerate any sunscreen active); just be aware there is the potential for a skin reaction. Although this is recommended for those with normal to dry skin, it absolutely isn't non-greasy as claimed. Also, the amount of titanium dioxide lends a slight white cast that cannot be blended away (though it's much less noticeable than that of many other mineral sunscreens). It's disappointing that antioxidants were given short shrift. A token amount of vitamin E is all that's included, which won't help this product compete with others at the drugstore that offer a range of potent antioxidants. Still, this deserves a Good rating for its sun protection ability, for its acceptable aesthetics, and because it is fragrance-free.

☺ GOOD **Dermacontrol Oil Control Moisturizer SPF 30** *($16.99 for 4 fl. oz.)* is a fragrance-free daytime moisturizer with sunscreen that's said to be a 3-in-1 option for oily skin because it hydrates, protects, and controls shine. It ends up doing two of the three decently well, though on balance the formula isn't all that exciting. The blend of absorbent and film-forming agents in this moisturizer prevent it from being hydrating, though it does have a lightweight texture and absorbent, soft matte finish those with oily skin will appreciate. It protects with an in-part avobenzone sunscreen, so critical UVA (think anti-aging) protection is assured. That's excellent because oily skin needs daily sun protection, too! What this is missing, at least in meaningful amounts, are antioxidants and ingredients to reduce redness and calm acne-prone skin. Cetaphil included tiny amounts of vitamin E, a component of soothing licorice, anti-irritant allantoin, and zinc gluconate, but that's about it and we're concerned it's too little to make much difference. The zinc gluconate addition is interesting because of the research linking it to improving acne (at least when consumed orally) and for reducing inflammation by regulating the inflammatory process in skin that leads to acne (Sources: *Archives of Dermatological Research*, December 2011, pages 707–713; *Journal of Investigative Dermatology*, January 2011, pages 59–66; *European Journal of Dermatology*, May-June 2005, pages 152–155; and *Dermatology*, Volume 203, 2001, pages 135–140). Cetaphil's Dermacontrol Oil Control Foam Wash contains this ingredient, too, but based on the research it is a better bet in a leave-on rather than a rinse-off product. This potentially helpful option for oily, acne-prone skin is worth a try; we only wish it had a better range and greater amounts of the kind of ingredients all skin types need to look and act younger and healthier. To that end, Olay and Paula's Choice have formulas for oily skin that are more well-rounded while still being lightweight and providing broad-spectrum sun protection.

CHANEL

Strengths: Sleek and occasionally elegant packaging; almost all the sunscreens contain avobenzone for UVA protection; a handful of good cleansers and topical scrubs; some good foundations with sunscreen; some very good concealers; several good mascaras; a sheer lipstick with sunscreen that includes avobenzone; all the powder eyeshadows have superb textures; some elegant shimmer liquids.

Weaknesses: Expensive, with an emphasis on style over substance; overreliance on jar packaging; antioxidants in most products amount to a mere dusting; no products to effectively address sun- or hormone-induced skin discolorations; mediocre to poor eye pencils and brow-enhancing options; extremely limited options for eyeshadows if you want a matte finish.

For more information and reviews of the latest Chanel products, visit CosmeticsCop.com.

CHANEL CLEANSERS

☺ GOOD **$$$ Gel Purete Rinse-Off Foaming Gel Cleanser** *($45 for 5 fl. oz)* is an efficient water-soluble cleanser for normal to oily skin, which is the good news. The bad news: The price is positively ridiculous. Paying this much for something you can get at the drugstore for less than ten dollars (and the same size container) is ludicrous, and advised only if you steadfastly refuse to cleanse your face with anything but a Chanel product.

☺ GOOD **$$$ Lait Confort Creamy Cleansing Milk** *($45 for 5 fl. oz.)* is a standard, insanely overpriced, detergent-free cleansing lotion suitable for dry to very dry skin that's not prone to breakouts. It removes makeup easily and feels silky, but likely will require a washcloth to ensure you're not leaving residue behind. Tulip extract isn't capable of removing pollutants from skin, and lily extract isn't hydrating. Even if those plants had such properties, the amount of them in this product is minuscule.

☹ AVERAGE **$$$ Mousse Confort Rinse-Off Foaming Cleanser** *($45 for 5 fl. oz.)* is a standard, exceptionally overpriced cleanser that can be too drying for most skin types. The potassium-based cleansing agents aren't as prevalent as they are in some other foaming cleansers, which makes this a slightly gentler option, but it would be important to keep this away from the eye area. It does remove makeup and rinses cleanly, but that is hardly unique or worth this amount of money.

☹ AVERAGE **$$$ Mousse Douceur Rinse-Off Foaming Mousse Cleanser** *($45 for 5 fl. oz.)* is a cleanser for normal to oily skin which produces copious amounts of mousse-like foam, but the potassium-based ingredients responsible for creating all the foam can be needlessly drying for skin. This removes makeup easily and rinses cleanly, but there are gentler foaming cleansers to consider.

☺ AVERAGE **$$$ Mousse Exfoliante Purete Rinse Off Exfoliating Cleansing Foam Purity + Anti-Pollution** *($45 for 5 fl. oz.)* is a basic, ridiculously overpriced cleansing scrub whose potassium-based, soap-like cleansing agents can be too drying for all but oily skin, and even then you would want to be careful because too much cleansing action can damage skin's barrier, and that isn't good. Chanel includes a mix of polyethylene (plastic) spheres and jojoba beads for a mild scrub action and, as usual, includes a fairly strong amount of fragrance.

☹ POOR **Le Blanc Fresh Brightening Foam Cleanser** *($60 for 5 fl. oz.)*. This needlessly expensive foaming cleanser rinses cleanly and removes makeup well, but it contains soap-like cleansing agents that make it too drying for all skin types. The majority of this cleanser is cleansing agents, so it tends to clean too well, which is part of what leaves your skin feeling tight—and, of course, none of this has a positive effect on skin discolorations. In fact, when discolorations are the concern, you don't need a special cleanser to lighten them, because these spots cannot be washed away (if only it were that easy!), and the type of ingredients that can impact skin color need to be left on, not washed off. Although this contains a tiny amount of licorice root extract (an ingredient known to help improve discolorations), its benefit is rinsed down the drain before it can improve your skin. Plus, there's more fragrance than licorice root in this cleanser, and fragrance isn't skin care.

CHANEL EYE-MAKEUP REMOVERS

☺ GOOD **$$$ Demaquillant Yeux Intense Gentle Biphase Eye Makeup Remover** *($32 for 3.4 fl. oz.)* is a standard, but good, water- and silicone-based makeup remover. It makes short work of long-wearing makeup, including waterproof mascara, but so do similar removers from Neutrogena, Almay, Maybelline New York, and Paula's Choice.

CHANEL TONERS

☺ AVERAGE **$$$ Lotion Confort Silky Soothing Toner** *($45 for 6.8 fl. oz.)* lends a silky texture and smooth finish for normal to dry skin. However, the formula doesn't make it worth the inflated price. Several of the intriguing ingredients are listed after the preservative, and there's no proof anywhere that tulip extract combats pollutants or that lily extract hydrates skin as Chanel claims. Furthermore, what pollutants are they referring to that require a special ingredient anyway, especially tulips?

☹ POOR **Le Blanc Brightening Moisture Lotion** *($67.50 for 5 fl. oz.)*. With alcohol as the second ingredient and almost no helpful ingredients for skin, this is a problem product any way you look at it. The alcohol causes dryness and free-radical damage, among other negatives (see the Appendix for further details), and the lack of antioxidants and skin-repairing ingredients is shameful. What about the pearl protein and licorice extract? Can they help lighten brown spots? It's a "no" for the pearl protein (listed as hydrolyzed conchiolin protein). As for the licorice: Two forms are included—dipotassium glycyrrhetinate and licorice root extract—and there's some research showing how they work to correct discolorations, but they're not worth considering in a product like this, which overloads your skin with alcohol and fragrance. There are lots of products using forms of licorice extract to improve skin discolorations, among other beneficial ingredients that cost less and are far better formulated.

☹ POOR **Lotion Douceur Gentle Hydrating Toner** *($45 for 6.8 fl. oz.)* is laden with alcohol and "gentle" and "hydrating" are not the words we'd choose to describe this toner. It is a problem for all skin types because alcohol causes dryness, irritation, and free-radical damage—everything that a smart skin-care routine is designed to avoid.

⊗ POOR **Lotion Purete Fresh Mattifying Toner** *($45 for 6.8 fl. oz.)* contains some intriguing ingredients for skin, including unique water-binding agents. However, the beneficial ingredients are trumped by the amount of skin-damaging alcohol Chanel included. Alcohol can degrease the skin and leave it temporarily matte, but the resulting irritation stimulates skin's oil glands to produce more oil, so in almost no time oily skin is back and worse than before.

CHANEL MOISTURIZERS (DAYTIME & NIGHTTIME), EYE CREAMS, & SERUMS

☺ AVERAGE $$$ **Hydramax + Active Creme, Active Moisture Cream** *($72 for 1.7 fl. oz.)* is a decent moisturizer for normal to dry skin, but vitamin E is the only significant antioxidant and elegant skin-identical ingredients are absent, so you're not getting your money's worth. The few intriguing ingredients are listed well after the preservatives and fragrance, making them inconsequential.

☺ AVERAGE $$$ **Hydramax + Active Serum Active Moisture Boost** *($82 for 1 fl. oz.)* features a "powerful formula" that "performs at the source of dehydration," according to Chanel, but somehow the ad copy didn't mention that this product contains a high amount of alcohol (it's the third ingredient). When alcohol is listed before such skin-identical ingredients as glycerin and sodium PCA, it means your dry skin won't get the moisture boost it deserves. This product does contain a strong, lingering fragrance. See the Appendix to learn why alcohol and high amounts of fragrance are bad for everyone's skin.

☹ AVERAGE $$$ **Sublimage Essential Regenerating Cream (Texture Supreme)** *($375 for 1.7 fl. oz.)*. Although Chanel sells numerous antiwrinkle, skin-firming products, this one is the ultimate, according to their marketing copy, which of course explains why the price is so completely out of synch with reality, even though the formula is far from state-of-the-art. Just as with their other Sublimage products, you're supposed to believe that vanilla fruit oil and Chanel's special fractionation process is the key to vanquishing everything that keeps skin from looking youthful. (Fractionation is strictly a chemical process, not a miracle of any kind, and certainly not unique to Chanel.) Admittedly, this emollient moisturizer for dry skin has a rich, elegant texture that feels great, but almost all the ingredients creating that texture are as standard as it gets. Perhaps most frustrating is that the effectiveness of the few antioxidants and plant extracts that are included will be compromised due to the jar packaging, which won't keep them stable for very long. For what Chanel is charging, you should expect the most airtight packaging available (along with an attractive pair of gold earrings). Enough said, other than that, there are no words fit for print to describe what a tremendous waste of money this moisturizer is.

☺ AVERAGE $$$ **Sublimage Essential Regenerating Cream (Texture Universelle)** *($375 for 1.7 fl. oz.)* is a very emollient moisturizer for dry to very dry skin. It contains several ingredients that make dry skin feel smoother and softer, but so do hundreds of other moisturizers that wouldn't dare charge this much. The air-sensitive ingredients in this product (antioxidants and the vanilla) will become almost instantly useless once you open it, thanks to the unwise choice of jar packaging. Putting your faith and dollars in this product won't bring you any closer to a wrinkle-free face—and personally we'd rather devote these funds to new shoes or a night at the theater or an investment toward a face-lift.

☺ AVERAGE $$$ **Sublimage Eye Essential Regenerating Eye Cream** *($200 for 0.5 fl. oz.)* doesn't carry the same sticker shock as Chanel's other Sublimage products, but is still outrageously priced for what amounts to a standard emollient moisturizer for dry skin anywhere on the face. It contains mostly water, glycerin, emollient thickening agents, canola oil, film-forming agent, wax, more film-forming agent, a cell-communicating ingredient, silicone, preservatives,

The Reviews C

and a tiny amount of vanilla oil and antioxidants (which are rendered ineffective due to jar packaging). You don't have to spend even one-third this much to get a good moisturizer, and in this case, unless you believe the claims, why would you? See the Appendix to learn why, in truth, you don't need an eye cream.

☺ AVERAGE $$$ **Sublimage Serum Essential Regenerating Concentrate** *($425 for 1 fl. oz)* is an underwhelming, truly ordinary, serum. It's merely a blend of standard ingredients, beginning with water (you'd think for $400 they would eliminate the least expensive ingredient in any cosmetic product) and including what Chanel deems the star attraction, vanilla. $400 for a tiny amount of vanilla! Unbelievable! Apparently, this serum gets immediate must-have status because of the precious vanilla water and vanilla oil it contains. It should be noted, however, that the vanilla oil is listed after the preservative, while the vanilla water (vanilla tea) is more prominent—again, for the money, Chanel shouldn't be diluting the alleged good stuff. Is there any reason to believe vanilla in any form can regenerate skin and provide "unprecedented results" for wrinkles? Not according to any published research. In fact, some forms of vanilla can cause contact dermatitis and skin sensitivity, and as you might expect, that would become only more likely in a product that contains concentrated amounts of it, as this serum claims. The lack of supporting evidence for vanilla makes this serum a ludicrous investment—nothing else it contains is unique and you're getting no special benefit for the money.

☺ AVERAGE $$$ **Ultra Correction Lift Lifting Firming Day Cream SPF 15** *($150 for 1.7 fl. oz.)* contains an in-part avobenzone sunscreen and follows the same pattern as many other Chanel products: Showcase a star ingredient, in this case something called elemi PFA, attach an anti-aging claim to it, then include just a dusting of it in the formula and don't bother to mention that there's no research anywhere proving it lifts skin. But wait, there's less: They not only include a mere dusting of their allegedly superior ingredient (elemi PFA), but also package the product in a jar so that if it did have any potency, it will be diminished once the product is opened. Add a lot of fragrance to those disappointments and this doesn't shape up to be a brilliant choice for anyone's skin, regardless of age or amount of sagging.

☺ AVERAGE $$$ **Ultra Correction Lift Lifting Firming Day Fluid SPF 15** *($150 for 1.7 fl. oz.)* is the lotion version of Chanel's Ultra Correction Lift Lifting Firming Day Cream SPF 15, above, and the same review applies.

☺ AVERAGE $$$ **Ultra Correction Lift Total Eye Lift** *($85 for 0.5 fl. oz.)* supposedly stimulates the production of tensin, a protein in skin that specific cells create as part of skin's repair process, particularly when it is wounded. Of course, wrinkles aren't the same as wounds, and there's no research proving that stimulating tensin production in skin has a lifting effect once skin begins to sag or pooch; sagging isn't a wound either. As is typical for the cosmetics industry, Chanel has chosen to focus on one element of skin repair to the exclusion of many other factors that cause skin to look older. Even if you could fix this one aspect of aging, it wouldn't address the hundreds of processes that negatively affect skin daily. Addressing one small aspect of "aging" won't change skin. Analyzing the ingredient label makes it clear there is nothing distinctive in this eye moisturizer. The formula is mostly water, slip agents, film-forming agent, silicone, and emollients. Several intriguing ingredients are present, but in amounts so small that your skin is unlikely to notice, not to mention that their potency will be short-lived due to the jar packaging. In the end, this product is neither lifting nor correcting, and isn't remotely useful for the eye area. See the Appendix to learn why, in truth, you don't need an eye cream.

☺ AVERAGE $$$ **Ultra Correction Lift Ultra Lifting Firming Night Cream** *($165 for 1.7 fl. oz.)* has an emollient texture that will feel great on dry skin. However, the price is absurd for what amounts to a completely ordinary, ho-hum formulation. Aside from a pathetic amount of state-of-the-art ingredients, the little it does contain won't remain stable due to the jar packaging. Chanel includes more fragrance than intriguing plants and peptides, and for what they're charging those ingredients should be up front and center. None of the ingredients in this moisturizer can stimulate building blocks in skin so it becomes lifted and firmer. See the Appendix to learn why fragrance and jar packaging won't help your skin.

☺ AVERAGE $$$ **Ultra Correction Line Repair Anti-Wrinkle Comfort Day Cream SPF 15** *($125 for 1.7 fl. oz.)* will give you reliable broad-spectrum protection if you apply this daytime moisturizer with sunscreen liberally, but chances are, given what it costs, you're not going to be slathering this on your face and neck every morning. Not applying a sunscreen liberally is a recipe for more wrinkles because skimping on sunscreen is almost as bad as going without it. That said, given the mundane, out-of-date base formula, this moisturizer is absurdly overpriced. It isn't capable of repairing lines or significantly improving the appearance of aging skin, other than the sun protection it provides, which is something you can get from dozens of far less expensive sunscreens. The blend of thickeners with glycerin and film-forming agent will make dry skin look and feel smoother and hydrated, but so can any $10 moisturizer. However, state-of-the-art ingredients with research showing they can repair skin are in short supply. Another problem is the jar packaging, which means the beneficial ingredients won't remain stable after the jar is opened. See the Appendix for details on the other issues jar packaging presents.

☺ AVERAGE $$$ **Ultra Correction Line Repair Anti-Wrinkle Day Fluid SPF 15** *($125 for 1.7 fl. oz.)* has an unimpressive base formula and the antiwrinkle action of this daytime moisturizer comes from its in-part avobenzone sunscreen. It has a lightweight, silky lotion texture those with normal to oily skin will enjoy, but there's far more fragrance than state-of-the-art ingredients that your skin needs, and that you should expect, if not demand, at this price. There is no logical reason to purchase this product because you can get even better formulas with sunscreen from Olay, Neutrogena, and Paula's Choice without breaking the bank.

☺ AVERAGE $$$ **Ultra Correction Line Repair Anti-Wrinkle Eye Cream** *($85 for 0.5 fl. oz.)* has a silky, slightly creamy texture that feels nice but that's the only good thing about this product. Just like any moisturizer (it doesn't have to be labeled "eye cream"), this will soften the appearance of wrinkles. Sadly, other than a pleasant texture, Chanel didn't add any state-of-the-art ingredients that would've given this standard eye cream far more real antiwrinkle properties. As such, this isn't much for treating wrinkles, although it is fragrance-free as claimed. See the Appendix to learn why, in truth, you don't need an eye cream.

☺ AVERAGE $$$ **Ultra Correction Line Repair Anti-Wrinkle Night Cream** *($135 for 1.7 fl. oz.)* contains many emollient ingredients needed by those with dry skin, which is nice, but for this amount of money your skin deserves a whole lot more. Even more disappointing is that the problems far outweigh the benefits, making this an expensive mistake. The biggest problem is the jar packaging, which means the beneficial ingredients won't remain stable once it is opened. In this formula the most intriguing ingredients—those that actually may have some antiwrinkle action—are present only in the tiniest amounts possible. You're getting a lot of fragrance, but fragrance isn't the least bit anti-aging.

☺ AVERAGE $$$ **UV Essentiel Multi Protection Daily UV Care SPF 50** *($52 for 1 fl. oz.)* contains an in-part zinc oxide sunscreen and that's the good news about this daytime moisturizer. Unfortunately, you don't get anything else for what amounts to little more than a mundane, overpriced sunscreen. The denatured alcohol that's included is an exceedingly irritating and skin-damaging ingredient, and it's especially a concern because it's listed before

The Reviews C

any of the intriguing ingredients. This daytime moisturizer has a light, fluid texture and soft matte finish those with normal to oily skin will appreciate, but other than the sun protection, it offers there is nothing of significance to extol. See the Appendix to learn more about the problems alcohol presents.

☹ POOR **Hydramax+Active Active Moisture Gel Cream** *($72 for 1.7 fl. oz.)* is marketed exclusively for those with normal skin. Regardless of skin type, this product is not recommended due to the amount of skin-damaging alcohol. Alcohol causes free-radical damage, irritation, and dryness, none of which are good for skin. Estee Lauder, Clinique, and Paula's Choice offer much better lightweight moisturizers.

☹ POOR **Le Blanc Brightening Concentrate** *($195 for 1.7 fl. oz.)*. This is said to be the most concentrated of Chanel's Le Blanc products, which claim to lighten dark spots. The claims mention an ingredient known as TXC along with pearl protein as what's responsible for improving skin tone. The pearl protein has no research showing it can do anything for skin, but what about the TXC? Chanel claims it's "the first active brightening ingredient registered in Japan as a quasi-drug by a Western company," which merits some explanation. Japan's cosmetics regulatory system has a category known as "quasi-drugs." Essentially, this is their way of regulating cosmetic ingredients, such as retinol and vitamin C, that go beyond the basic benefits of other ingredients that give skin-care products their texture and stability, which can be significant, but the Japanese government has chosen a select few for some unknown reason. Among the cosmetics regulated in Japan as quasi-drugs are "effective essences that contain whitening components," which applies to this Chanel product due to its TXC ingredient. So why does the Japanese cosmetics regulatory board think TXC improves skin color? We have no idea.

The technical name for TXC is cetyl tranexamate HCL; there is no published research proving this ingredient is the one to use for lightening brown spots. Because concentration protocols haven't been established for this ingredient, we don't even know how much is needed to get results for brown spots (and this product contains only a teeny-tiny amount of TXC, despite the claims of being "concentrated"). Perhaps the Japanese government knows something about TXC the rest of the world doesn't, but that information is not available. Either way, this is a lot of money to spend to find out if it's worth the price tag, especially considering there are other formulations that are supported by research as being effective for skin discolorations. Even if the TXC ingredient was a proven option for dark spots, Le Blanc Brightening Concentrate's overall formula is a big disappointment! Alcohol is listed as the second ingredient, which means your skin will experience dryness and free-radical damage along with other problems (see the Appendix for details). This skin-lightening product contains a form of vitamin C (ascorbyl glucoside) that has some solid research pertaining to improving discolorations, but the amount of alcohol in this product makes it not worth considering. You can find this form of vitamin C and others in superior products that cost a lot less.

☹ POOR **Le Blanc Brightening Moisturizing Cream** *($130 for 1.7 fl. oz.)* is part of Chanel's collection of products claiming to lighten dark spots. The claims mention an ingredient known as TXC along with pearl protein as having "intensifying dark spot correction" properties. See our comments about these ingredients plus the vitamin C in the review of Le Blanc Brightening Concentrate above. What is most disappointing about this formula is that alcohol is listed as the second ingredient, which means your skin will experience dryness and free-radical damage along with other problems. It's also packaged in a jar, which hurts the stability and effectiveness of key ingredients (see the Appendix for details).

☹ POOR **Purete Ideale Serum Intense Refining Skin Complex** *($75 for 1 fl. oz.)* gets its matte finish from silicone and alcohol, but the amount of alcohol here, along with witch hazel, makes this water-based serum too drying and irritating for all skin types. Alcohol won't balance oil production because oil production is controlled by hormones, and topically applied products like these have no effect on what's happening hormonally.

☹ POOR **Sublimage Essential Regenerating Fluid** *($295 for 1.7 fl. oz.)* is a poorly formulated, overly expensive serum. The marketing geniuses call this "the ultimate in anti-aging luxury," but if this is truly their ultimate, then why are they selling so many other antiwrinkle products that make similar boasts? This lightweight moisturizer for normal to oily skin joins the other wildly overpriced Sublimage products, except that this one has an even more mediocre formula than the others. With alcohol as the third ingredient, this moisturizer is not antiwrinkle in the least. If anything, the alcohol is pro-wrinkle because the irritation it causes leads to collagen breakdown and inflammation. The ingredients that follow the alcohol on the list are pathetically commonplace and inexpensive to include in a product, which makes the price of this moisturizer a joke—a joke on the consumer that isn't funny in the least.

☹ POOR **Sublimage Essential Revitalizing Concentrate** *($425 for 1 fl. oz.)*. "Shockingly bad" isn't strong enough to describe this serum's formula. Although it contains a handful of good ingredients (mostly water-binding agents), the second ingredient is alcohol. That means that for over $400 you're getting a serum that stands a good chance of making your skin look and act older, not younger. See the Appendix to learn about the problems alcohol causes for all skin types, and why it's about as far from anti-aging as you can get. Chanel's spin on this serum is that it contains a rare plant ingredient sourced from the Himalayas (it's never sourced from, say, the suburbs of Chicago) that is said to detoxify cells so skin can be born again. Sigh. The message is that our skin cells harbor toxins that lead to signs of aging, and if these toxins are not removed (by a rare, purified plant, of course), then youthful skin isn't possible. It isn't true. Skin cells do not harbor toxins that keep you from looking younger. Toxins from food, air pollution, and the like are filtered from the body by the liver and kidneys, not the skin. And even if skin cells were harboring toxins that needed to be removed, there's no research proving the plant extracts in this serum can do anything of the sort.

☹ POOR **Ultra Correction Lift Intensive Lifting Concentrate** *($165 for 1 fl. oz.)* is a classic example of why expensive doesn't mean better. Despite the Chanel name and the gorgeous sleek packaging, this serum is mostly water and alcohol. Can you believe that?! For what this costs, it should be overflowing with proven anti-aging ingredients to build collagen and firm skin. Sadly, it's not; in fact, the amount of alcohol in this serum poses significant problems for all skin types. Please see the Appendix for details on why alcohol in this amount is something you should avoid. The claims are enticing, but in truth this serum cannot lift skin, not even a fraction of a millimeter. Chanel maintains that this serum contains an ingredient known to stimulate tensin, a protein in skin. Tensin is one of the proteins that make up fibroblasts, which are substances in skin that generate collagen. Despite the claim, skin is far more complex than one protein, and the alcohol will kill off fibroblasts, not increase them. The extract from the plant *Canarium luzonicum* is the ingredient Chanel refers to in their claims, calling it elemi PFA, but there is no research proving what effect, if any, this ingredient has on tensin in skin (or any facet of skin, for that matter). If Chanel has research proving tensin is wonderful, they're not sharing it. Plus, if this ingredient is so beneficial, you have to wonder why they're not including it in many of their other anti-aging products that also claim to lift skin. Even if this ingredient were proven effective, Chanel includes only a dusting of it. Fragrance, it seems, is more important, even though the research is clear that fragrance is a problem for keeping skin in top shape.

☹ POOR **Ultra Correction Lift Sculpting Firming Concentrate** *($165 for 1 fl. oz.)* wouldn't be worth it even if it were free! This water-based serum lists alcohol as the second ingredient, which means it will cause dryness, irritation, and free-radical damage. Of course, it cannot lift or sculpt an aging face in any way, shape, or form—unless you count the tightening effect from the film-forming agents (think hairspray for your face) as a remarkable benefit. It isn't, and the effect is strictly cosmetic. Even fragrance is listed before anything of real benefit for skin. Overall, this is a poorly formulated product you should just ignore. See the review for Chanel's Ultra Correction Lift Intensive Lifting Concentrate above for a discussion of the elemi PFA that's said to be so miraculous.

☹ POOR **Ultra Correction Line Repair Intensive Anti-Wrinkle Concentrate** *($135 for 1 fl. oz.)* is a shockingly ordinary, overpriced, water-based serum incapable of repairing lines or having even a modest antiwrinkle action, and it doesn't even provide much hydration. Instead it assaults your skin with a lot of alcohol, fragrance, and alumina. Meanwhile, the potentially helpful ingredients are barely present, which is insulting for what Chanel is charging for this poorly formulated serum. This contains cosmetic pigments that subtly brighten skin, but you can achieve that with countless products costing a lot less than this does! Two words: Don't bother.

CHANEL LIP CARE

☺ GOOD **$$$ Hydramax + Active Lip Care** *($45 for 0.3 fl. oz.)* is a very emollient, intensely moisturizing lip balm whose buttery texture will feel great. It contains a good mix of fatty acids, waxes, and plant oil along with Chanel's customary dose of fragrance and a fragrant plant extract or two. Dry lips will benefit from this balm, but the price should give you serious pause. You're not getting much extra for your money though this still deserves a Good rating for its overall formula. For the record, Paula's Choice Lip & Body Treatment Balm is worth considering over this, and has a much more realistic price.

☹ POOR **Ultra Correction Lift Plumping Anti Wrinkle Lips and Contour** *($85 for 0.5 fl. oz.)* is so basic and boring that the price is a stinging insult. Both the allegedly special ingredients and the truly intriguing ingredients are present in the smallest amounts you can imagine, and for what Chanel is charging, these ingredients should be front and center. The big deal about this lip balm is that it stimulates the production of tensin, a protein in skin that specific cells produce as part of skin's repair process, particularly when it is wounded. Of course, wrinkles aren't the same as wounds, and there's no research proving that stimulating tensin production in skin has a lifting or firming effect on skin anywhere on the face (or body, for that matter). This lip balm is a monumental waste of time and money, unless you think coating lips with plastic, talc, and wax is the pinnacle of anti-aging therapy.

CHANEL SPECIALTY SKIN-CARE PRODUCTS

☺ GOOD **$$$ Masque Destressant Purete Purifying Cream Mask** *($50 for 2.5 fl. oz.)* is a basic clay mask for normal to oily skin (those with very oily skin would want something more absorbent). The thickening agents (including beeswax) may be problematic for blemish-prone skin, but this does the job in terms of absorbing surface oils without overdrying skin.

☹ POOR **Hydra+Active Active Moisture Mask** *($50 for 2.5 fl. oz.)* is a moisturizing mask for dry skin that contains some good emollients to improve dryness, but it also contains methyl lactate, a potent skin irritant, and more alcohol than beneficial ingredients. This adds up to a poor choice for any skin type. See the Appendix to learn why irritation is a problem for all skin types.

CHANEL FOUNDATIONS & PRIMERS

✓☺ BEST $$$ **Mat Lumiere Long Lasting Luminous Matte Fluid Makeup SPF 15** *($54)* presents a new breed of matte-finish makeup; the only cons are how fleeting the matte-finish can be to over oily areas. Otherwise, this fluid's ultra-smooth foundation is a pleasure to blend. It provides medium to almost full coverage and leaves skin looking what is best described as luminous matte. That means this isn't as reflective or moist-feeling as foundations with a satin finish, but it also isn't powdery matte like most traditional oil-free liquid foundations. This is definitely a consideration for those with normal to slightly oily or slightly dry skin, and its sunscreen is pure titanium dioxide, which is excellent. Among the range of shades are several beautiful options. Ivory is great for fair skin. The shade to avoid due to peach overtones is Naturel. Ginger and Honey are slightly peach, but may work for some medium to tan skin tones.

☺ GOOD $$$ **Lift Lumiere Firming and Smoothing Fluid Makeup SPF 15** *($65)* is described as being more than a foundation; Chanel wants you to know they have created "the consummate skin-caring makeup." That sounds great, but the ingredient list doesn't support the boast. In terms of texture, this has a beautifully silky feel and includes a broad-spectrum sunscreen with an in-part titanium dioxide base, but that's only a start when it comes to ultimate skin-caring makeup. Where are the antioxidants and cell-communicating ingredients? How about some anti-irritants or skin-identical ingredients like ceramides or hyaluronic acid? They're not here, save for a teeny-tiny amount of plant oil and plant extracts with antioxidant ability. That doesn't add up to being worth $65. Even though this is a long way off from being skin-caring makeup, you can count on reliable sun protection, supremely smooth application, and an attractive satin matte finish suitable for normal to slightly dry or slightly oily skin. Coverage begins at medium and can be built to nearly full camouflage, although doing so produces a heavier look that is not easily softened. The majority of shades are neutral and ideal for fair to medium skin tones. Avoid the following shades because they are too pink, orange, or rose to look convincing: Natural Beige, Naturel, and Tawny. One more point: It goes without saying that this foundation won't firm skin in any noticeable way, though it definitely creates the illusion of smooth, even-toned skin.

☺ AVERAGE $$$ **Le Blanc de Chanel Sheer Illuminating Base** *($45)* is a lightweight foundation primer-type product that is basically talc suspended in a moisturizing base. It adds a whitish glow to skin (mica adds some shine), but this is an awfully expensive way to net this ordinary cosmetic effect!

☺ AVERAGE $$$ **Perfection Lumiere Long-Wear Flawless Fluid Makeup SPF 10** *($55)* has a fluid, initially creamy texture that feels amazingly weightless but also provides light, smoothing hydration. It sets to a soft matte finish that works best for normal to combination skin; those with dry skin will find this doesn't provide enough moisture. The formula is exceptionally easy to blend, but make sure you blend thoroughly or it will crease into lines and large pores. Light to medium coverage is possible, and on balance this looks surprisingly natural, while masking minor imperfections. This foundation offers Chanel's most expansive shade range, and there are some excellent colors for light to dark skin tones. Given the number of shades and Chanel's uneven reputation for producing neutral colors, there are several to watch out for: Beige 060 is slightly peach but worth considering; Ambre 104 is noticeably copper, while Ambre 134 will be too red for many dark complexions; Ambre 154 is a gorgeous color for ebony skin; Beige Ambre 054 and 064 suffer from orange overtones; Beige Rose 042 is slightly rose; and Beige Rose 052 is so peachy it looks more like blush than foundation. We wish the sunscreen were rated SPF 15; SPF 10 is below the minimum standard recommended by medical boards around the world. Still, the sole active ingredient is titanium dioxide, so this does provide broad-spectrum protection. But, for best antiwrinkle results, you'll want to pair this with a moisturizer rated SPF 15 or greater. Beyond the letdown of the low SPF rating, this foundation has a fragrance that lingers. Many foundations are fragrance-free, and that's best for your skin (despite the sensory appeal of fragranced products).

☺ AVERAGE $$$ **Teint Innocence Compact Naturally Luminous Compact Makeup SPF 10** ($57) is disappointing because it does not contain the UVA-protecting ingredients of titanium dioxide, zinc oxide, avobenzone, ecamsule, or Tinosorb. Of course, the SPF rating is too low for sufficient daytime protection, so opting to use this requires another product rated SPF 15 or greater. What's sad about the sunscreen deficiency is that this is otherwise a top-notch, cream-to-powder foundation. It blends over skin impeccably and provides medium coverage that perfects without looking artificial. The moist, slightly thick finish is best for normal to dry skin not prone to blemishes. Almost all the shades are neutral, with the best ones being those designed for fair to medium skin tones. Soft Bisque is slightly peach, but may work for some skin tones. This would have earned a Good rating if it had the right UVA-protecting ingredients and was rated SPF 15 or greater.

☺ AVERAGE $$$ **Vitalumiere Aqua Ultra-Light Skin Perfecting Makeup SPF 15** ($45), which contains an in-part titanium dioxide sunscreen, is described by Chanel as "next-generation makeup." It has some very good attributes to support that claim, but there are also formulary drawbacks. It contains alcohol and a strong fragrance, and both are a problem for all skin types (see the Appendix for details).

☺ AVERAGE $$$ **Vitalumiere Moisture-Rich Radiance Fluid Makeup SPF 15** ($55). It is truly disappointing to not be able to give this liquid foundation with sunscreen a better rating. It has so many wonderful attributes, but the sunscreen does not provide sufficient UVA protection, which is odd since most of Chanel's SPF-rated products get this right. Because of this, you shouldn't rely on this foundation as your sole source of sun protection. If you have normal to dry skin and are willing to pair this with a well-formulated sunscreen, here's what you can expect—a fluid, slightly creamy texture that blends impeccably and sets to an attractive, sheer satin finish. Coverage is in the sheer to light range, and this beautifully enlivens skin without looking artificial. The colors are gorgeous and mostly neutral, with options for fair to tan skin. The only shade to consider carefully is the slightly peach Beige 3.0.

☻ POOR **Hydramax + Active Serum Active Moisture Tinted Lotion SPF 15** ($62 for 1.35 fl. oz.) should be an amazing tinted moisturizer in every respect for the price Chanel is charging. As is, the sunscreen leaves skin vulnerable to UVA damage because it does not contain the active ingredients of titanium dioxide, zinc oxide, avobenzone, Mexoryl SX (ecamsule), or Tinosorb. Adding to that serious problem is the base formula, which is as basic as it gets and is overly fragranced to boot. The texture is creamy and the finish soft and radiant from each of the three very sheer shades, but come on! Stila, Bobbi Brown, Estee Lauder, Shiseido, and many other brands offer far better tinted moisturizers that don't leave your skin vulnerable to UVA damage (and treat it to at least a smattering of state-of-the-art ingredients).

CHANEL CONCEALERS

✓☺ BEST **$$$ Correcteur Perfection Long Lasting Concealer** *($40)* has a gorgeously smooth, lightweight texture that blends easily and doesn't crease into lines or magnify their appearance. It has a soft, satin matte finish that lasts and won't make the under-eye area look dry or cakey. Among the mostly excellent neutral shades, be careful with Beige Petale; it is too peach for some medium skin tones. One more note: This concealer contains fragrance; that's not a deal-breaker, but the formula would be better without it.

☺ AVERAGE **$$$ Lift Lumiere Concealer Smoothing and Rejuvenating Eye Contour Concealer** *($46)* is a well-intentioned but poorly conceived concealer. First, a concealer is intended, as the name implies, to provide appreciable coverage—this one doesn't. Second, a concealer should be easy to blend (which this is) and stay in place once it has set—this one doesn't. This begins creamy and stays that way, so it begins creasing into lines and fading in short order and that continues throughout the day. You can set the concealer with pressed powder, but that doesn't help because the powder tends to stick to this emollient concealer, leading to skin that looks matte on top but "crinkled" underneath. Another sour note is the packaging. Although generously sized, the pump bottle dispenses way too much product even when you're being extra careful, so a lot gets wasted (and at this price, wasting even a drop of concealer isn't the goal). It conceals minor flaws reasonably well, but there are dozens of other concealers that out-perform this and its three mediocre shades.

CHANEL POWDERS

✓☺ BEST **$$$ Poudre Universelle Libre Natural Finish Loose Powder** *($52)* has an extremely fine, sifted texture and a soft matte finish that looks beautiful on skin. It is talc-based and comes in four very good, sheer colors. Do you need to spend this much money for a superior loose powder? No, but if you're swayed by Chanel, this won't disappoint.

☺ GOOD **$$$ Poudre Universelle Compact Natural Finish Pressed Powder** *($45)* has a finely milled texture and a sheer, dry finish. This talc-based powder comes in five good shades, suitable for fair to light skin.

☺ AVERAGE **$$$ Poudre Douce Soft Pressed Powder** *($50)* is a silky, slightly dry-textured, talc-based powder that imparts sheer color and a soft shine finish. Only two shades are available, but the color deposit is so minimal that it makes them versatile for fair to medium skin tones, assuming you don't mind the shiny finish. The included compact-sized brush is better than most, but that doesn't completely justify the price of this powder.

CHANEL BLUSH & BRONZERS

☺ GOOD **$$$ Joues Contraste Powder Blush** *($43)* is a winning pressed-powder blush. The texture and application are suede-smooth, with plenty of pigmentation, so a little goes a long way. Every shade has at least a soft shine, and the following shades have a sparkling shine that's a bit too much for daytime wear: Mocha, Orchid Rose, and Tempting Beige. The brush provided is terribly small and the wrong shape for applying a soft wash of color to cheeks.

☺ GOOD **$$$ Soleil Tan de Chanel Bronzing Makeup Base** *($48)* is best used as a sheer bronzing cream for cheeks and other key areas of the face, such as temples or the eye contour. We wouldn't take Chanel's advice and apply this balm-like bronzing base all over your face because the color change is noticeable enough that you'd need to apply it to your neck and

The Reviews C

hands, too, and that's never a good idea for day-to-day makeup. The soft golden tan color works best for light to medium skin tones, and it has a satin powder finish that looks great.

☺ GOOD $$$ **Soleil Tan de Chanel Moisturizing Bronzing Powder** *($50)* is a dry (not moisturizing) powder blush that is almost a bit too powdery for seamless application. Each shade has enough pigment so it's best to start with a sheer application, and you can layer from there. Among the shades, the most attractive and versatile are Desert Bronze and Terre Ambre, each of which has a subtle sparkling shine. It nearly goes without saying that there are equally good and better bronzing powders at the drugstore.

CHANEL EYESHADOWS & EYE PRIMERS

☺ GOOD $$$ **Illusion D'Ombre Long Wear Luminous Eyeshadow** *($36)* is a cream-to-powder eyeshadow brimming with sparkly shimmer, but it has a unique spongy, mousse-like texture that blends on smoothly and can be applied sheer or layered for a more dramatic look. Even after hours of wear, there's no creasing or fading—and it's easily removed with a gentle cleanser or makeup remover. The only drawback is a limited shade selection (only six shades) and the screw-top packaging will cause this cream shadow to dry out if the cap isn't screwed on tightly after each use.

☺ GOOD $$$ **Les 4 Ombres De Chanel Quadra Eyeshadow** *($58)* has an enviably silky, utterly blendable texture and wonderfully even application. It is a pleasure to work with these powder shadows, but working with the colors is another story! In most of these quads, many of the shades are intensely shiny. Either that, or the selected shades are too contrasting to create an attractive, enhancing eye design. Without such intense shine, these would easily merit a Best Product rating. For an equally impressive texture and application with less obvious shine, consider Dior's 5-Colour Eyeshadow.

☺ GOOD $$$ **Ombre Essentielle Soft Touch Eyeshadow** *($28.50)* consists of single eyeshadows accurately described as a creamy-feeling powder, and they apply beautifully—though they are best applied in sheer layers to avoid flaking. You'll find these are pigment-rich, blend smoothly, and their intensity lasts through the day.

☻ AVERAGE $$$ **Ombres Contraste Duo, Eyeshadow Duo** *($42)*. This complementary eyeshadow duo comes as a set: one dark shade with a matte finish and one lighter variation of the same shade with a shimmer finish. Although not bad, this eyeshadow is surprisingly standard for its price.

CHANEL EYE & BROW LINERS

☺ GOOD $$$ **Stylo Yeux Waterproof Long-Lasting Eyeliner Waterproof** *($30)* is indeed waterproof. In fact, this automatic, retractable pencil is nearly budge-proof; it takes considerable effort to remove. However, it applies easily and it lasts; its creamy texture and finish belie its longevity; and it is best for creating a moderately thick, rather than thin, line.

☻ AVERAGE $$$ **Crayon Sourcils Sculpting Eyebrow Pencil** *($29)* is a needs-sharpening pencil with a texture and application that's a step above most brow pencils, and it includes a brush to comb through brows. This goes on softly; has a dry, smooth finish; and would have been rated a Best Product if sharpening weren't required. If you decide to try this, the Taupe shade is great for blondes (but not platinum or very light blonde brows).

☻ AVERAGE $$$ **Ecriture De Chanel Automatic Liquid Eyeliner** *($34)* is packaged in a click-pen applicator with a decent, flexible brush. Problems arise when too much liquid liner is dispensed (which happens fairly often), so you wind up wasting a lot of product. It applies a bit too wet, so don't blink or it will smear, though dry time remains fast. Once set, this wears well but you have to be OK with the fact that each shade has a shiny finish. Given the price and the difficult-to-avoid dispensing of excess product, this is one to consider with caution

☺ AVERAGE $$$ **Le Crayon Khol Intense Eye Pencil** *($28)* is a standard pencil whose creamy texture has a soft powder finish, the colors are quite soft, meaning you need several applications before you get what most consider an intense line.

☺ AVERAGE $$$ **Le Crayon Yeux Precision Eye Definer** *($29)* is a very expensive, utterly standard pencil that has a soft texture, a slightly dry finish, and an angled sponge tip for blending. Nothing is extraordinary here except the price, and it isn't justified by the performance.

CHANEL LIP COLOR AND LIPLINERS

✓☺ BEST $$$ **Rouge Allure Laque Luminous Satin Lip Colour** *($32)* is expensive. And, yes, you can find similar options at the drugstore (Maybelline New York Color Sensational Lip Gloss comes to mind). However, if you're keen on Chanel, this opaque lip gloss with its dazzling lacquered finish is highly recommended. It has a thin yet emollient texture that imparts rich color, whether you prefer bold reds or muted pinks. It isn't sticky and it applies evenly with its angled sponge-tip applicator.

✓☺ BEST $$$ **Rouge Coco Hydrating Creme Lip Colour** *($32.50)* is another cream lipstick by Chanel. Did they really need another? The salesperson assured me this was better than their others, which begs the question of why they're still selling lipsticks that aren't as good, but we weren't in the mood to debate this point while at the counter. The "better" portion is said to be a richer color payoff, which this rich, emollient lipstick definitely has. It's beautifully creamy without being greasy or too slick, and the shade range offers something for everyone. Unlike many of Chanel's other lipsticks and glosses, Rouge Coco has minimal fragrance.

☺ GOOD $$$ **Aqua Crayon Lip Colour Stick** *($26)* is an automatic, nonretractable lip pencil that applies well and has good pigmentation to ensure long wear. It's not as creamy as it used to be, and so is a better (though needlessly pricey) option than it once was.

☺ GOOD $$$ **Rouge Allure Extrait De Gloss, Pure Shine Intense Colour Long Wear Lip** *($32)* is a creamy lip gloss that makes lips feel velvety smooth, while imparting a semi-opaque color in a variety of flattering shades.

☺ GOOD $$$ **Rouge Allure Luminous Satin Lip Color** *($32.50)* promises alluring color and sensational comfort, and it does deliver—but so do many other creamy lipsticks that cost much less than this one. The semi-opaque, shimmer-infused shades slip over lips and feel comfortably light, but the slight amount of stain doesn't promote longevity, so frequent touch-ups are necessary.

☺ GOOD $$$ **Rouge Coco Shine Hydrating Sheer Lipshine** *($32.50)* is a sheer lipstick that glides on beautifully and leaves a subtle wash of color along with a shiny finish and plenty of shimmer. This is far less pigmented and creamy than the original Rouge Coco lipstick, but the shade selection is just as lovely. What this lipstick lacks in staying power, it makes up for in feel—it's never greasy, grainy, or sticky.

☺ GOOD $$$ **Rouge Double Intensite Ultra Wear Lip Colour** *($34)* mirrors the same concept introduced by Max Factor and then Cover Girl (i.e., a lip color that dries to a matte, unmovable finish, accompanied by a clear gloss that doesn't disturb the color to create a comfortable finish). This is a formidable option for those looking for long-wearing lip color. The shade selection is smaller than those of competing brands, but each shade is quite attractive, with colors that are complementary to light and dark skin tones (the dark shades are very dark, so test them before purchasing). It does wear well throughout the day (and night), but as with similar products, it requires regular reapplication of the glossy top coat to keep lips from feeling dry and chapped.

CHANEL MASCARAS

✓☺ BEST $$$ **Inimitable Waterproof Mascara** *($30)* impresses in every respect, which it should at this price! The rubber-bristled, spiky-looking brush quickly thickens and lengthens lashes for outstanding definition without clumps. It wears without flaking or smearing, and is very waterproof (you will need an oil- or silicone-based remover when it's time to take this off).

☺ GOOD $$$ **Inimitable Mascara Multi-Dimensionnel** *($30)* allows you to achieve length and thickness in nearly equal measures, but neither is extraordinary and there are some clumps along the way (which can be brushed through without incident). This wears all day without a flake or smear, and keeps lashes remarkably soft and with a slight curl. Note: Based on the brush style and rubber bristles, you should know that similar results are obtainable from Cover Girl's Lash Blast or Lash Blast Length Mascara.

☹ AVERAGE $$$ **Inimitable Intense Mascara Multi-Dimensionel Sophistique Volume Length Curl Separation** *($30)* has a too-heavy application from the first coat. Subsequent coats applied in an effort to smooth lashes from a blatant over-deposit of mascara doesn't help, so you will need a separate lash brush or comb handy. Chanel's promise of no clumps or spiky lashes doesn't come true, which is precisely why you need the lash comb! With effort, you can achieve dramatic, defined lashes that have a lush, voluminous appearance, but why go through the extra work and pay Chanel's exorbitant price when several drugstore mascaras produce dramatic results without hassles?

CHANEL FACE & BODY ILLUMINATORS

✓☺ BEST $$$ **Eclat Lumiere Highlighter Face Pen** *($40)* is a beautiful highlighter housed in a click-pen component with a built-in synthetic brush applicator. Whether you choose the golden or beige rose shade (which isn't rose at all), you'll get a soft, slightly creamy texture that's a pleasure to blend and sets to a soft matte finish complete with a subtle glow. The finish is ideal for highlighting around the eyes, down the bridge of the nose, or the top of the cheekbones. This is thicker and easier to control than Yves Saint Laurent's popular Radiant Touch product.

☺ GOOD $$$ **Base Lumiere Illuminating Makeup Base** *($42)* works to promote smooth skin and leaves a silky feel that isn't the least bit heavy. Sold as a foundation primer, it does facilitate application of makeup, but so do many other lightweight, silicone-based gels and serums. So, while the effect is nice, you don't necessarily need another step in your routine to achieve results.

CHANEL BRUSHES

✓☺ BEST $$$ All Chanel's **Eyeshadow Brushes** *($28–$38)* are worth considering if you don't mind the expense. The **#25 Large Eyeshadow Brush** ($38) is flat, wide, and well-shaped to apply a powder eyeshadow to the entire eyelid area with ease. Less impressive but still worth considering for those with money to burn is the **#27 Angled Eyeshadow Brush** ($32). Also available are the **Face/Cheek Brushes** ($32–$65), but they're not quite as elegant as we were hoping. The **#6 Powder Brush**, which costs over $60, isn't worth it though there's no denying its soft and works well to deposit powder. The **#4 Blush Brush** ($54) is merely average and also not worth its price. The **#2 Angled Powder Brush** ($60) is worth considering for blush or contouring, while the excellent, sumptuously soft **#8 Touch-Up Brush** ($45) is great for touch-ups or buffing powder into skin.

CLARINS

Strengths: Broad selection of effective, broad-spectrum sunscreens; some good self-tanning products; some good cleansers and gentle topical scrubs; a great foundation primer; superb foundations and powders; very good powder blush; wonderfully creamy lipsticks; great lip glosses and mascaras.

Weaknesses: Overpriced; pervasive reliance on jar packaging; most products have more fragrance than beneficial plant extracts; poor toners; an overabundance of average moisturizers; no effective products for lightening discolorations or treating acne; no effective AHA or BHA products; disappointing eye pencils; average eyeshadows and makeup brushes.

For more information and reviews of the latest Clarins products, visit CosmeticsCop.com.

CLARINS CLEANSERS

☺ GOOD $$$ **Gentle Foaming Cleanser With Shea Butter** *($21 for 4.4 fl. oz.)*. By no means is this a bad cleanser, but the fragrance and preservatives it contains shouldn't be in a product meant for sensitive skin. Best for normal to dry skin, this water-soluble foaming cleanser has a lotion-like texture that removes makeup well, if you can stand the amount of fragrance (which sensitive skin definitely should not risk). Another issue is the price, which is significantly higher than that of any cleanser we recommend from the drugstore. You're not getting extra benefits with this Clarins cleanser, other than the prestige and French flair the brand espouses.

☺ GOOD $$$ **One-Step Gentle Exfoliating Cleanser with Orange Extract** *($35 for 4.4 fl. oz.)* is a standard, but good, water-soluble cleanser that contains gentle detergent cleansing agents. Plant cellulose provides a mild exfoliating effect, and is fine for occasional use by all skin types—just use caution and avoid massaging this over blemishes. Clarins claims this cleanser purifies and smoothes the skin with natural botanicals, but their presence is sparse and mainly provides an orange-tinged fragrance. Actually, the ratio of synthetic to natural ingredients in this product is 5:1, which pretty much nullifies any credibility for the botanical claim.

☺ GOOD $$$ **Water Comfort One-Step Cleanser, for Normal to Dry Skin** *($32.50 for 6.8 fl. oz.)* is a water- and solvent-based cleanser that contains gentle cleansing agents and, aside from fragrance, no problematic ingredients. That's a positive step since this product is meant to be a convenient cleanser that does not require rinsing. It is an option for normal to slightly dry skin, but is not adept at removing long-wearing or waterproof makeup.

☹ AVERAGE $$$ **Extra-Comfort Cleansing Cream with Shea Butter, for Dry or Sensitized Skin** *($44 for 6.8 fl. oz.)* is a rich, cold cream–style cleanser for dry to very dry skin. It is not recommended for sensitized skin due to its fragrance and the presence of fragrant components. This requires use of a washcloth for complete removal.

☹ POOR **Cleansing Milk with Alpine Herbs, for Dry or Normal Skin** *($29.50 for 7 fl. oz.)* is a basic cleansing lotion that rinses decently but contains some problematic plant extracts, including arnica, St. John's wort, and Melissa (balm mint), along with fragrant components that are irritating for skin, including eugenol and linalool. This is not recommended for any skin type.

☹ POOR **Cleansing Milk with Gentian, for Combination/Oily Skin** *($30 for 7 fl. oz.)* contains a lot of sage extract, way too much fragrance, and lesser but still potentially problematic amounts of fragrant components, including eugenol. This is not recommended because even without the irritants, it is way too emollient for its intended skin type.

☹ POOR **Gentle Beauty Soap** *($15 for 5.3 fl. oz.)* is certified organic, but that doesn't change the fact that this is classic soap—the same kind that's drying and irritating to your skin, not to mention the residue it leaves behind. For your money (way too much money for such an ordinary product that is easily replaced at the drugstore for $2, but you shouldn't do that to your face at any cost), you're getting mostly drying soap ingredients with water and fragrance.

☹ POOR **Gentle Foaming Cleanser for Combination or Oily Skin** *($21 for 4.4 fl. oz.).* The amount of potassium hydroxide in this cleanser is cause for concern and disqualifies it as a gentle formula. The potassium hydroxide, combined with some of the other main ingredients, makes this closer to a drying soap than to a gentle water-soluble cleanser. All the intriguing plant extracts are wasted in a cleanser because they are just rinsed down the drain, and the fragrance is so potent this product ends up being far more problematic than dozens of others. All told, this is a terrible cleanser and the tight dry feeling it leaves on skin is not good skin care for anyone.

☹ POOR **Gentle Foaming Cleanser for Normal or Combination Skin** *($20 for 4.4 fl. oz.)* is nearly identical to the Gentle Foaming Cleanser for Combination or Oily Skin above, and the same review applies.

☹ POOR **Pure Melt Cleansing Gel, for All Skin Types** *($32.50 for 3.9 fl. oz.)* is supposed to veil skin in gentleness, but if that's the case, why did Clarins choose the preservatives methylchloroisothiazolinone and methylisothiazolinone for this residue-leaving, emollient, oily cleanser? Both preservatives are known for their sensitizing potential, and are not the best choice for a cleanser whose oil and emollient ingredients remain on your skin even after rinsing. This will remove any kind of makeup easily, but the ingredients Clarins used to do that are incredibly commonplace. Two far better versions of this product are Clinique's Take the Day Off Cleansing Milk or Take the Day Off Cleansing Balm, and both cost less than this Clarins gel.

CLARINS EYE-MAKEUP REMOVERS

☺ GOOD $$$ **Instant Eye Make-Up Remover** *($26.50 for 4.32 fl. oz.)* is a standard, silicone-in-water, dual-phase fluid that works very well to remove stubborn makeup and waterproof mascara. The rose flower water is primarily fragrance, and doesn't make this preferred to less expensive silicone-based removers from Almay or Neutrogena, among others.

☹ AVERAGE $$$ **Gentle Eye Make-Up Remover Lotion** *($26.50 for 4.32 fl. oz.)* is an exceptionally standard, water-based makeup remover that contains a lot of fragrant rose water along with soothing cornflower water. The rose water isn't the best for use around the eyes, making this not preferred to less costly options that omit fragrant additives.

CLARINS TONERS

☹ AVERAGE $$$ **Extra-Comfort Toning Lotion, for Dry or Sensitized Skin** *($21 for 6.8 fl. oz.)* is a fairly basic toner, but it does contain some decent ingredients for dry skin. The problem is that the really beneficial ingredients are listed after the preservative and the fragrant ingredients, so there's little chance this will be what sensitized skin needs.

☹ AVERAGE $$$ **Super Restorative Wake-Up Lotion** *($40 for 4.2 fl. oz.)* is highly fragranced and if you like to wake up by applying a highly fragranced toner on your skin, this is one way to do it. Unfortunately, fragrance isn't skin care (synthetic fragrance is high up on the ingredient list) and this toner for slightly dry skin offers too few beneficial ingredients to make it even a consideration for your skin. The price is just galling when you consider that the formula undermines everything a well-formulated toner should be doing to improve your skin.

☹ AVERAGE $$$ **Toning Lotion with Camomile, for Dry or Normal Skin** *($20 for 6.8 fl. oz.)* is an OK toner for normal to dry skin, but does not distinguish itself from several less expensive options. It contains some good skin-identical ingredients, but leaving the fragrant components on the skin after daily use isn't the best idea (see the Appendix for more details).

☹ POOR **Toning Lotion with Iris, for Combination or Oily Skin** *($30 for 6.8 fl. oz.)* contains more fragrance than beneficial ingredients and also contains a lesser but still worrisome amount of iris root extract. None of this is about "promoting well being" for skin, but it is likely to leave those with combination skin more confused. The amount of fragrance in this product is just over the top, and it also contains several fragrance ingredients known to cause irritation. Consider this a perfect example of how Clarins uses fragrance under the mistaken notion that it's skin care—and see the Appendix to find out how daily use of highly fragrant products hurts your skin.

CLARINS EXFOLIANTS & SCRUBS

☺ GOOD $$$ **Bright Plus HP Gentle Brightening Exfoliator** *($30 for 1.7 fl. oz.)* has the properties of a cleanser, topical scrub, and clay mask all in one product, with the clay and its absorbency being the dominant quality. This is an interesting option for someone with normal to oily skin, but is best used in the morning because this much clay isn't going to help remove makeup. Nothing in this product will reduce the appearance or occurrence of dark spots.

☺ GOOD $$$ **Gentle Refiner Exfoliating Cream with Microbeads** *($30 for 50 ml)* is a standard, but good (and, it must be said, way overpriced) scrub for normal to slightly dry or slightly oily skin. Cellulose fiber is the abrasive agent, and it's definitely a better alternative to, say, ground-up walnut shells. As is the case with most Clarins skin-care products, this is highly fragranced. However, it rinses fairly well so the fragrance isn't going to linger on your skin.

☺ AVERAGE $$$ **Gentle Peeling Smooth Away Cream** *($30 for 50 ml)* is an absurdly expensive, antiquated formula for what is little more than a creamy scrub, whose waxy texture helps eliminate dry, flaky skin by rubbing it over the skin for a minute or two. You apply this thick, scrub-like product to dry skin and then remove it by smearing it over the skin. The rubbing action causes the paraffin wax it contains (the second ingredient) to ball up on your skin, taking dead, dry skin with it as you rinse, which isn't an easy task because wax is difficult to get off the skin. This is an OK but outdated way to attain smoother skin, and the rubbing action isn't good for skin. A standard, water-soluble scrub or, better yet, a well-formulated AHA or BHA product is a much better way to go—and the AHA or BHA products offer numerous other benefits that no scrub can match. If you decide to try this, it is best for normal to dry skin not prone to breakouts.

☹ POOR **Bright Plus HP Gentle Renewing Brightening Peel** *($38 for 4.2 fl. oz.)* is a fluid exfoliant that contains the AHA glycolic acid, although the amount is less than 2%. That's not necessarily bad news because the formula also contains other AHAs, tartaric acid, plus the BHA ingredient salicylic acid. The problem is that the pH of 4.1 is borderline for exfoliation to occur. Even if the overall AHA and BHA content were greater, this product lists skin-damaging alcohol as the second ingredient, and it is highly fragrant. Both of these issues keep us from recommending this product because of the problems these ingredients cause for skin. Please see the Appendix to learn why alcohol and fragrance are not the least bit beneficial for your skin.

CLARINS MOISTURIZERS (DAYTIME & NIGHTTIME), EYE CREAMS, & SERUMS

☺ GOOD $$$ **Gentle Day Cream, for Sensitive Skin** *($60 for 1.7 fl. oz.)* isn't more gentle than most Clarins moisturizers and the fact that it contains fragrance shows they're not taking the needs of truly sensitive skin seriously. Still, this can be a good moisturizer for normal to dry skin not prone to blemishes, and most of the plant extracts are soothing and anti-inflammatory, which is a nice change of pace.

The Reviews C

☺ GOOD $$$ **Gentle Night Cream** *($70 for 1.7 fl. oz.)* is nearly identical to the Gentle Day Cream, for Sensitive Skin above, and its higher price isn't justified. Either option is best for normal to dry skin not prone to blemishes.

☺ AVERAGE $$$ **Advanced Extra-Firming Day Lotion SPF 15, for All Skin Types** *($78.50 for 1.7 fl. oz.)* doesn't disappoint with its in part avobenzone sunscreen and silky, lightweight lotion base. However, for the money, this supplies skin with almost no extras beyond basic sun protection, and any firming benefit would have to be accidental, because none of the ingredients in this daytime moisturizer have that effect. It is best for normal to slightly oily or slightly dry skin.

☺ AVERAGE $$$ **Advanced Extra-Firming Eye Contour Cream** *($60 for 0.7 fl. oz.)*. If this is Clarins' idea of an advanced formula, then we assume their chemists are still using textbooks dating back at least a decade or two. Far from being a "revolutionary nighttime treatment," this water-based moisturizer has a temporary tightening effect on skin, thanks to the amount of absorbent rice starch it contains and a significant amount of film-forming agent. (Neither of these ingredients is beneficial or helpful for dry skin.) The truly beneficial ingredients are few and far between, including tiny amounts of the plant extracts Clarins always boasts about, but that isn't unique to this product. For an absurd amount of money, you're getting mostly water, thickener, glycerin, rice starch, slip agent, film-forming agent, preservatives, and vitamin E. Not very exciting, and in no way should this be considered a state-of-the-art anti-aging moisturizer for the eyes or elsewhere. See the Appendix to learn why, in truth, you don't need an eye cream.

☺ AVERAGE $$$ **Advanced Extra-Firming Eye Contour Serum** *($60 for 0.7 fl. oz.)* makes the same claims and has the same nonadvanced formulary issues as the Advanced Extra-Firming Eye Contour Cream above, except this has a serum texture and omits the rice starch. It still has enough film-forming agent to produce a temporary tightening effect on skin, and the silica lends a drier finish, but this type of effect can eventually make the eye area look dry and more wrinkled. This product does not contain anything that can lift or regenerate skin.

☺ AVERAGE $$$ **Advanced Extra-Firming Neck Cream** *($82 for 1.7 fl. oz.)* claims to be the ultimate firming neck treatment, but that's about as true as saying Ivory soap is the ultimate cleanser. This product contains mostly water, silicone, thickeners, slip agent, preservative, and fragrance. None of it is firming, but it will make dry skin look and feel smoother. That's probably not what you were expecting for $82, but it's the truth. And it must be said that you don't need a special cream for skin on your neck. A well-formulated facial moisturizer can and should be applied to your neck, too.

☺ AVERAGE $$$ **Beauty Flash Balm** *($45 for 1.7 fl. oz.)* is an extremely average moisturizer that contains absorbent rice starch, which can be problematic for dry skin.

☺ AVERAGE $$$ **Bright Plus HP Intensive Brightening Smoothing Serum** *($69 for 1.06 fl. oz.)* is a surprisingly good serum from Clarins, although that's not much of an accolade considering the mostly lackluster anti-aging products they sell. This silky serum contains a good amount of vitamin C, but the form of vitamin C is not the form that has considerable research behind it showing it to be effective for discolorations. Still, it has *some* research and this serum contains a teeny-tiny amount of other plant extracts that may have a disruptive effect on melanin synthesis. (That's what leads to the brown discolorations you see on your skin.) Overall this serum ends up being a mixed bag. The amount of fragrance and the presence of numerous fragrance ingredients known to irritate skin are causes for concern. Some of the other ingredients may be helpful for discolorations, but there are much better options, and many of those cost far less.

☺ AVERAGE **$$$ Bright Plus HP Repairing Brightening Night Cream** *($65 for 1.7 fl. oz.)* doesn't contain much to be excited about, other than a good amount of ascorbyl glucoside (a form of vitamin C). It is overpriced for what amounts to a stunningly basic, ordinary formula, especially when you consider that the vitamin C won't remain effective for very long after the product is opened, thanks to the jar packaging. See the Appendix for details on why jar packaging is a problem. All you're getting for a lot of money is an average emollient moisturizer for dry skin. The plant extracts and "white flowers" it contains cannot provide protection against dark spots.

☺ AVERAGE **$$$ Extra-Firming Day Cream, Special for Dry Skin** *($78.50 for 1.7 fl. oz.)* is an overall mundane formula with an undeserved price. The emollients will make dry skin feel better, but the fragrance is cause for concern (see the Appendix for details) and this isn't firming, extra or otherwise, in the least.

☺ AVERAGE **$$$ Extra-Firming Night Cream, Special for Dry Skin** *($86 for 1.7 fl. oz.)* contains a smattering of plants, but is primarily a water- and mineral oil–based moisturizer joined by several thickeners, glycerin, shea butter, and peanut oil. It will take good care of dry to very dry skin, but it won't make it firmer. It's interesting that although some Clarins products contain mineral oil, we have dealt with several salespeople from this line who love to speak of the alleged evils of this ingredient, ignoring (or oblivious to) the fact that Clarins uses it. Just to be clear, mineral oil is not harmful or suffocating to skin in the least and it doesn't deserve its reputation as a problematic ingredient.

☺ AVERAGE **$$$ HydraQuench Cream, for Normal to Dry Skin** *($49.50 for 1.7 fl. oz.)* claims to satisfy the needs of everyone who has normal to dry skin, regardless of temperature variations or climate. Yet this boring moisturizer definitely leaves your skin wanting more beneficial ingredients. It certainly isn't a barometer for skin exposed to varying temperatures or climate shifts; if that were true, the same could be said for countless other moisturizers because the ingredients Clarins used to create this product are at best described as commonplace. In addition, the jar packaging won't keep the smattering of antioxidants stable during use, and you have to tolerate a lot of fragrance, a trait seen throughout the Clarins line. Regarding the claim that this moisturizer is able to address all the needs of normal to dry skin: No way! What about the need for sunscreen, stable packaging, and state-of-the-art ingredients that help create and maintain healthier skin? All of that is missing here; it's only the claims and sales pitch that could make you think you're getting more—more than you really are.

☺ AVERAGE **$$$ HydraQuench Intensive Serum Bi-Phase, for Dehydrated Skin** *($58 for 1 fl. oz.)* is a water-based serum that contains some good emollients and water-binding agents, along with a type of Peruvian nut oil whose fatty acid content is helpful for normal to dry skin. We wouldn't consider this a slam-dunk solution for dehydrated skin in unforgiving climates, but it's a decent, albeit ordinary, serum-type moisturizer for normal to slightly dry skin (assuming you pair it with a sunscreen or foundation with sunscreen for daytime use).

☺ AVERAGE **$$$ HydraQuench Lotion SPF 15, for Normal to Combination Skin or Hot Climates** *($49.50 for 1.7 fl. oz.)* contains avobenzone to provide sufficient UVA protection, and comes in a lightweight base with an odd mix of absorbents (aluminum starch) and emollients (shea butter). It is likely to leave those who have normal to dry skin wanting more moisture and those with normal to oily or combination skin feeling it is too heavy. Although this contains some helpful ingredients to reinforce healthy skin, it isn't nearly as advanced as the best daytime moisturizers from the Lauder companies, Paula's Choice, or Olay.

☺ AVERAGE $$$ **HydraQuench Rich Cream, for Very Dry Skin or Cold Climates** (*$49.50 for 1.7 fl. oz.*) is simply a more emollient version of Clarins' HydraQuench Cream, for Normal to Dry Skin. Adding mineral oil and shea butter does make this better for dry to very dry skin, and the emollients can indeed help protect your skin when subjected to cold weather. However, that benefit isn't by any means unique to this product, which is actually a pretty ordinary moisturizer even with their list of plant extracts (with unproven benefits), which cannot help skin defend itself from climate changes. The claim is based on the fact that the plants can survive dramatic climatic extremes, and Clarins wants you to believe that extracts from these plants can transfer that benefit to your skin. Just because a plant can survive under extreme climatic conditions in its native environment doesn't mean the mechanisms that allow it to do so are transferable to your skin, especially when you consider that the plants are harvested and processed and then teeny amounts of them are added to a cosmetic product. As with almost all of the HydraQuench products, this is highly fragranced.

☺ AVERAGE $$$ **Multi-Active Day Early Wrinkle Correcting Lotion SPF 15** (*$56 for 1.4 fl. oz.*) is a "wrinkle control" product from Clarins that at least makes more sense than the others they've launched for daytime use because it provides broad-spectrum sunscreen protection. The lightweight base formula has a lotion texture and is short on significant anti-aging ingredients for skin, but it's much better than the other Multi-Active Day products from Clarins. This is an OK option for normal to slightly dry skin; mica provides a shiny finish.

☺ AVERAGE $$$ **Super Restorative Day Cream** (*$114 for 1.7 fl. oz.*) is another fairly standard moisturizer from Clarins with the usual assortment of wow-factor claims, including smoothing wrinkles, helping skin feel "lifted," and restoring a youthful appearance. If you have dry, dehydrated skin, any moisturizer can make skin look younger and feel smoother, so where are the state-of-the-art ingredients to justify the hefty expense? There are barely enough to mention. To make matters worse, this isn't the best choice for daytime because it lacks a sunscreen, and there is no recommendation on the label to make sure you use sunscreen in addition to this product. Given such an ordinary emollient moisturizer, your money is best saved for some other splurge.

☺ AVERAGE $$$ **Super Restorative Day Cream SPF 20** (*$114 for 1.7 fl. oz.*) has an in-part titanium dioxide sunscreen, but that's the only positive element of this vastly overpriced, overhyped moisturizer. Nothing about it is a restorative treatment for aging skin, and some of the fragrant components can be a problem on skin that's exposed to sunlight.

☺ AVERAGE $$$ **Super Restorative Decollete and Neck Concentrate** (*$105 for 1.7 fl. oz.*) purports to reduce visible signs of aging on the neck and chest because of the "high-performing plant extracts" it contains. The plant extracts must be able to exert stellar performance at minuscule concentrations, however, because that's all you're getting in this wolf-in-sheep's-clothing moisturizer disguised as a specialty treatment. Plenty of emollients and skin-silkening agents are on hand to make normal to dry skin look and feel better, but none of the plants can affect pigmentation (age spots from sun damage) or restore the elegant, feminine qualities to an aged-looking decolletage. If anything, the volatile fragrant components in here can cause irritation (see the Appendix for details), and possibly make the chest and neck look blotchy and red. Besides, there is no research anywhere proving the neck and chest need special products. A well-formulated facial moisturizer can and should be applied to these areas, too.

☺ AVERAGE $$$ **Super Restorative Night Wear** (*$122 for 1.7 fl. oz.*) is nearly identical in emollient feel and performance to the Super Restorative Day Cream above, and the same basic comments apply.

☺ AVERAGE $$$ **Super Restorative Serum** *($132 for 1 fl. oz.)* is a classic case of a product's name, price, and marketing agenda not adding up to what's inside the bottle, which, for all intents and purposes, is just another thin-textured moisturizer (it really doesn't have a standard serum look or feel; in fact, the finish is a bit tacky, not silky). The Clarins sales staff would no doubt blanch at that statement, as most of the counter personnel we spoke to treated this product as if it were the fountain of youth, yet they clearly must be entranced by their company's assertions, because nothing in this product can firm, lift, restore, or tone the skin. This product contains mostly water, slip agents, thickeners, emollient, silicone, film-forming agent, water-binding agent, fragrance (lots of fragrance), several plant extracts (all present in minute amounts), caffeine, preservatives, and coloring agents. Clarins tends to favor exotic-sounding plants over state-of-the-art skin-care ingredients such as proven antioxidants or anti-irritants. Although that is undeniably enticing to some consumers, it doesn't help skin and it often causes irritation. There is no reason to consider this product an anti-aging treatment. If you're shopping for serums or moisturizers at the department store and want a selection of modern, elegant formulas, your skin and pocketbook would be better off exploring the options from Estee Lauder, Peter Thomas Roth, DDF, or Clinique before just about anything Clarins offers.

☺ AVERAGE $$$ **Super Restorative Total Eye Concentrate** *($82 for 0.53 fl. oz.)* promises to banish all manner of under-eye skin complaints, from puffiness to crow's feet. Yet all it can do is moisturize the skin, and at most temporarily reduce the appearance of wrinkles. It contains mostly water, silicone, glycerin, thickeners, emollient, preservative, plant extracts, and the tiniest amount of peptides you're likely to find in a skin-care product. Nothing in this eye cream will protect skin from pollution, a claim Clarins is fond of making for many of their moisturizers and specialty items. See the Appendix to find out why, in truth, you don't need an eye cream.

☺ AVERAGE $$$ **UV Plus HP Day Screen High Protection SPF 40** *($38 for 1.7 fl. oz.)* is highly fragranced and for a product line that's all about plants, there's very little of them here. On the plus side, this all-titanium dioxide sunscreen assures broad-spectrum sun protection and the silicones promote a silky finish, but beyond that there isn't much to get excited about. Those with normal to oily skin who, for some reason, want to overspend on a moisturizer with sunscreen will do best with this lightweight product. The numerous fragrance ingredients make this a bad choice for those with sensitive skin, despite the sunscreen active being very gentle. Those with dry skin will find this provides minimal hydration. One more thing: This cannot protect skin from all types of environmental pollution, as claimed; not only is that impossible (this isn't an invisible shield between your skin and the environment), but Clarins included such a tiny amount of antioxidants that the claim becomes all the more laughable. This product is about lightweight, mineral-based sun protection, period. Tinted options are available as well, for those with light to medium skin tones.

☺ AVERAGE $$$ **Vital Light Day Illuminating Anti-Ageing Comfort Cream** *($85 for 1.7 fl. oz.)* has a creamy texture those with dry skin will appreciate, but the overall formula leaves much to be desired; it's hardly the pinnacle of anti-aging, or a "vital breakthrough." Does this restore a youthful glow? Yes, but not in any meaningful way. Rather, this ordinary, overpriced, underwhelming formula with standard emollients contains a shiny pigment to add a bit of glow to the skin. Hardly worth $85 by any standard, except to cosmetics companies who overcharge for their products. The shine this provides can make your skin look lit-from-within, but so can lots of other products that add shine to your face, from powders to primers and shine enhancers, but you don't have to spend nearly this much for that effect. As for the tiny amount of exotic plant extracts Clarins brags about as having special powers for skin, they don't, but it doesn't matter because none of them will remain stable once this jar-packaged product is opened. The same goes for the antioxidants (plant extracts and antioxidants deteriorate in the presence of air), so all you're paying for is shine, basic emollients, and a lot of fragrance.

☺ AVERAGE $$$ **Vital Light Day SPF 15 Illuminating Anti-Ageing Cream-All Skin Types** *($85 for 1.7 fl. oz.)* contains stabilized avobenzone for critical UVA (think anti-aging) protection. What a shame it's so expensive and that the jar packaging won't keep the antioxidants it contains stable during use. Please see the Appendix for further details on the problems jar packaging presents. This has a lightweight creamy texture that makes skin look smooth, while the amount of film-forming agent (polymethyl methacrylate) it contains can make skin feel a bit tighter (but keep in mind that feeling tighter isn't the same as sagging skin actually becoming tighter). The amount of alcohol is potential cause for concern, as is the fact that this product contains far more fragrance than state-of-the-art anti-aging ingredients. The formula doesn't contain anything known to reawaken skin's luminosity, but keeping it protected from further sun damage will definitely result in better-looking (and acting) skin.

☺ AVERAGE $$$ **Vital Light Night Revitalizing Anti-Ageing Comfort Cream** *($85 for 1.7 fl. oz.)* is a pink-tinted moisturizer that is another basic, overpriced formula for dry skin. The main ingredients help dry skin look and feel better, but they are commonplace and definitely don't justify the cost. None of the ingredients in this moisturizer can boost micro-circulation as claimed, although admittedly, the very act of applying skin-care products stimulates circulation because you're massaging them into or over your skin. So really, the claim isn't a big deal and doesn't provide any special benefit. As with most products from Clarins, this contains more fragrance and preservatives than antioxidants. Also, the plant extracts that provide the antioxidant benefits won't remain potent for long thanks to the jar packaging, which allows them to break down. See the Appendix for further details on the problems jar packaging presents.

☺ AVERAGE $$$ **Vital Light Serum** *($85 for 1 fl. oz.)* isn't worth its price tag. The strongly fragranced formula contains mostly water, slip agents, film-forming agent, and preservative. It also contains the novel skin-lightening ingredient hexylresorcinol (discussed in detail below) which Clarins maintains is four times as effective as 2% hydroquinone, the reigning gold standard skin-lightening ingredient in over-the-counter and prescription products. There is no published, substantiated research to support that claim, but the resorcinol portion of this ingredient is capable of causing dryness and irritation. Not surprisingly, Clarins offers no research to support their claim for hexylresorcinol. Ironically, hexylresorcinol is a synthetic ingredient. Clarins makes a big deal about how many natural ingredients they use, yet this so-called breakthrough product is built around a synthetic. That's not bad; it just makes Clarins "natural" positioning all the more misleading. Hexylresorcinol is a preservative and antiseptic with a pale yellow color and somewhat heavy texture. It has a strong odor, which is likely why Clarins added fragrance and fragrant plant extracts to this skin lightener. High amounts of this ingredient can burn skin, but that's true of many ingredients when used in high amounts. In this product, Clarins is likely using around 1%, so the risk of burning is practically zero. This ingredient is believed to have efficacy similar to hydroquinone because, like hydroquinone, it plays a role in melanin (skin pigment) production. In contrast, though, hydroquinone (and other alternatives, such as vitamin C) have mounds of research and a history of safe use supporting their use, while hexylresorcinol is the new kid on the block—and consumers are left to take the cosmetics company's

---

🖋 Exposing oily skin to irritating ingredients makes it worse! See the Appendix to learn more.

word for its efficacy. One of the plant ingredients in this serum is *Atractylodes lancea* root. There is one in vitro study showing this plant inhibits melanin production, but it wasn't compared to known skin-lightening actives, so it's a mystery as to how well this plant works compared to other lightening ingredients (Source: *Biological and Pharmaceutical Bulletin*, April 2007, pages 719–723). Another plant ingredient, *Cochlearia officinalis*, is a natural source of fragrance ingredients and mustard oil, a known irritant (naturaldatabase.com). This would be a much better option had Clarins chosen plants that are proven effective without exposing skin to volatile fragrance ingredients whose irritation can lead to collagen breakdown. For certain, this product is nearly a do-nothing for wrinkles and it absolutely cannot lift skin. Many skin-care products claim they can firm and lift skin, but none of them work, at least not to the extent claimed. A face-lift-in-a-bottle isn't possible, but with the right mix of products, you will see firmer skin that has a more lifted appearance—and that's exciting! In order to gain these youthful benefits, you must protect skin from any and all sun damage every day, use an AHA (glycolic acid or lactic acid) or BHA (salicylic acid) exfoliant, and use products that have a wide range of antioxidants and skin-repairing ingredients. This combination of products (remember, one product doesn't do it all) has extensive research showing how they can significantly improve many of the signs of aging such as firming skin, reducing wrinkles and brown spots, and eliminating dullness.

☺ AVERAGE $$$ **Younger Longer Balm** *($99 for 1.7 fl. oz.)* has a great, succinct name. No question as to what this product is supposed to do! Clarins goes off the deep end with claims for this product, especially with their statement that it "maintains proper functioning of skin nerve endings." What we apply to our skin can indeed affect nerves in our skin—just touching your skin affects the nerve endings, but "proper functioning"? Our question is: How do your nerve endings behave improperly? By reacting? If anything, the nerve endings in skin may be adversely affected by the amount of fragrance in this moisturizer for normal to dry skin. For the money, you're not getting anything special; all of the intriguing ingredients are listed after the fragrance, as is typical of Clarins. All in all, this product is really disappointing, at least if you're expecting protection from free radicals and a reduction in broken capillaries. For less money, you'd be wise to consider any of the non-jar-packaged moisturizers from Clinique or Estee Lauder.

☹ POOR **Bright Plus HP Brightening Hydrating Day Lotion SPF 20** *($60 for 1.7 fl. oz.)* provides broad-spectrum sun protection that includes avobenzone for critical UVA screening, but the highly fragranced base formula contains far too much alcohol to be labeled "hydrating." The alcohol causes free-radical damage, collagen breakdown, and impairment of skin's healing process. This isn't the way to look younger, especially given the number of daytime moisturizers with sunscreen that nourish and restore rather than hurt skin.

☹ POOR **Contouring Facial Lift** *($70 for 1.7 fl. oz.)* lists alcohol as the second ingredient, and that makes this serum too irritating for all skin types. Nothing in this product will minimize signs of slackened skin.

☹ POOR **Extra-Firming Day Wrinkle Lift Cream, for All Skin Types** *($80 for 1.7 fl. oz.)* is a very boring, exceedingly overpriced concoction of water, emollients, glycerin, slip agents, cornstarch, preservative, and fragrance. It is not suitable as a day cream because it doesn't contain sunscreen. The amount of plant extracts (none of which have a firming effect) is so small as to be nearly inconsequential for skin. This is too emollient for all skin types; it is best for normal to dry skin not prone to breakouts. But even if you have normal to dry skin, think twice before purchasing this highly fragranced moisturizer. See the Appendix to find out why the jar packaging this comes in is bad news.

☹ POOR **Extra-Firming Night Rejuvenating Cream, For All Skin Types** *($86 for 1.7 fl. oz.)* has a formula similar to, but more boring than, that of the Extra-Firming Day Wrinkle Lift Cream, for All Skin Types, and absolutely not worth the price.

☹ POOR **Extra-Firming Tightening Lift Botanical Serum** *($80 for 1 fl. oz.)* is another firming, tightening product. Do you ever wonder how anyone successfully shops the Clarins line given all the extra-firming, lifting, sculpting, and antiwrinkle products they offer? How do the salespeople make sense of it all!? Luckily you're reading this review, so you'll be forewarned before you present your credit card for this below-average, way-overpriced product. The firming and tightening sensation you get from this water-based serum comes from tapioca starch, an ingredient you can buy at the grocery store for pennies per use. The rest of this product is mostly slip agents, anti-irritant, gel-based thickener, pH adjuster, and fragrance. The amount of peptide is so small it's a joke, and that minuscule amount pales in comparison to the amount in other products with peptides (if that's what you're after), including Olay Regenerist and Olay Definity. Moreover, Clarins included pepper extract (listed as *Capsicum annuum* fruit), a needless irritant that interferes with the soothing action of the oat kernel extract, essentially canceling it out.

☹ POOR **HydraQuench Cooling Cream-Gel, for Normal to Combination Skin or Hot Climates** *($49 for 1.7 fl. oz.)* lists alcohol as the second ingredient. That certainly explains the cooling effect of this "anti-heatwave" gel (clearly this line is aimed at menopausal women or women afraid global warming is hurting their skin), but it also makes this too drying and irritating for all skin types, regardless of the climate. Plus the effect is transient at best, lasting only a few seconds, and then it's gone. There is no reason to subject your skin to this misguided, overly fragranced product.

☹ POOR **HydraQuench Cream SPF 15** *($49.50 for 1.7 fl. oz.)* is a daytime moisturizer sunscreen lacking the UVA-protecting ingredients of titanium dioxide, zinc oxide, avobenzone (also known as butyl methoxydibenzoylmethane), ecamsule, or Tinosorb and is not recommended. The base formula is definitely moisturizing, but the jar packaging won't keep the good, though air-sensitive, ingredients stable once it's opened. See the Appendix for further details on why jar packaging is a problem.

☹ POOR **Multi-Active Day Early Correction Wrinkle Cream, All Skin Types** *($56 for 1.7 fl. oz.)* is a bland, overpriced moisturizer that doesn't contain sunscreen. The wrinkle-control claims this product makes are nothing more than a bad joke for your skin, however, we doubt you'll be laughing. There is nothing about this formula that's preferred for younger skin not yet showing signs of aging. This is just a moisturizer and a highly fragranced one at that (there is more fragrance in this product than beneficial skin-care ingredients), and the jar packaging won't keep the small amount of good plant extracts stable after opening. This also contains the preservative methylisothiazolinone, which is known to be sensitizing. Given the preservative, the fragrance ingredients, and the lack of sunscreen, what you have is a very misguided product that won't prevent wrinkles, but will cause irritation.

☹ POOR **Multi-Active Day Early Correction Wrinkle Cream, Dry Skin** *($56 for 1.7 fl. oz.)* is more emollient than, but otherwise very similar to, the Clarins Multi-Active Day Early Correction Wrinkle Cream, All Skin Types above, and the same review applies.

☹ POOR **Multi-Active Skin Renewal Serum** *($63 for 1.04 fl. oz.)* is another, boring, poorly formulated product from Clarins. If there's a unique flower out there, Clarins will find it and build a product (often a product line) around it, regardless of research to support its benefit, or lack thereof, for your skin. This serum has a silky texture but contains considerably more fragrance than state-of-the-art ingredients. Talk about a disappointment! Where are the skin-identical and cell-communicating ingredients? What about antioxidants that don't have irritancy potential (Clarins includes lemon extract in this serum)? This serum isn't capable of rejuvenating skin, nor is it gentle as claimed. Not only is the amount of fragrance potent, but also this contains several fragrance ingredients known to cause irritation. Clarins also included the preservative methylisothiazolinone, which is contraindicated for use in leave-on products due to its sensitizing potential (Sources: *Actas-dermosifiliograficas*, January-February 2009, pages 53–60; *Contact Dermatitis*, October 2005, pages 226–233; *Regulatory Toxicology and Pharmacology*, December 2003, pages 269–290; and *American Journal of Contact Dermatitis*, June 2000, pages 115–118). This serum has the potential to be multi-irritating, rather than multi-active for younger-looking skin!

☹ POOR **Truly Matte Pore Minimizing Serum** *($49 for 1 fl. oz.)* leaves skin with a soft matte finish, but the amount of alcohol here means this isn't the best for any skin type. None of the plant extracts in this serum have any effect on pores. Even if they did, the amount of each is minuscule when compared with the amount of fragrance. Clinique's Pore Minimizer products are much better than this, or you can consider the options from Paula's Choice.

☹ POOR **Truly Matte Ultra-Matte Rebalancing Lotion** *($40 for 1.7 fl. oz.)* lists alcohol as the second ingredient, which means this won't rebalance anything. The alcohol will irritate skin and generate more oil production at the base of your pores, which is exactly what those struggling with oily skin don't need. This product also contains a significant amount of fragrance; the most helpful ingredient, green tea, is listed last. See the Appendix to learn why irritation and fragrance are problems for all skin types.

CLARINS SUN CARE

☺ GOOD **After Sun Moisturizer with Self Tanning Action** *($32 for 5 fl. oz.)* is sold to prolong and enrich a natural tan, a choice that is infuriating from a company with so many products that claim to forestall aging and wrinkles, because getting a tan from the sun is what causes the wrinkles in the first place. (Well, perhaps that's job security for Clarins?) Despite the lack of ethics involved in encouraging tanning, this is a good self-tanning lotion that contains dihydroxyacetone (DHA) and a small amount of erythrulose, an ingredient similar to DHA that develops color at a slower rate.

☺ GOOD **Liquid Bronze Self Tanning, for Face and Decollete** *($34 for 4.2 fl. oz.)* is a very silky self-tanning lotion that can be used anywhere on the body. It turns skin tan with DHA and a lesser amount of the self-tanning ingredient erythrulose.

☺ GOOD **Self Tanning Instant Gel** *($34 for 4.4 fl. oz.)* contains DHA to turn skin tan, along with a tiny amount of erythrulose, all in a silky lotion base that doesn't feel thick or greasy. Clarins states there's no need to wait before dressing once this is applied, but we'd play it safe and wait at least 30 minutes to avoid streaks and stained clothing.

☺ GOOD **Self Tanning Milk SPF 6** *($34 for 4.4 fl. oz.)* has an in-part avobenzone sunscreen, but the SPF rating makes it too low for daytime protection. Given that most people don't apply self-tanner daily, formulating one with a sunscreen is an odd choice. This product is recommended as a standard, creamy self-tanner, though its tanning ingredient, dihydroxy-acetone, is found in many self-tanning products that cost less than this.

☺ GOOD **Sunscreen Care Milk Lotion Spray SPF 20, Moderate Protection** *($32 for 5.2 fl. oz.)* leaves skin wanting more in terms of antioxidants (fragrance got higher priority but fragrance isn't skin care). However, this is easy and convenient to apply plus it includes 3%

stabilized avobenzone for UVA protection. The water-resistant formula is suitable for oily to very oily or breakout-prone skin. Sunscreens like this may be applied to face or body (but don't spray directly on your face or it may get in your eyes). Note that inclusion of several fragrance ingredients in this sunscreen makes it less desirable. These fragrance ingredients increase the likelihood of a reaction from the active ingredients this product contains.

☺ GOOD $$$ **Radiance-Plus Self Tanning Cream-Gel** *($54 for 1.7 fl. oz.)* is a lightweight, silicone-enhanced moisturizer with a lesser amount of the self-tanning ingredient DHA and the slower-acting self-tanning ingredient erythrulose. The reduced amount of self-tanning "actives" means less color, so this can be a good option for fair skin tones or for times when you want a hint of sunless tan rather than that "day at the beach" look. The texture of this fragranced self-tanner is best for normal to oily or breakout-prone skin.

☺ GOOD $$$ **Sunscreen Care Cream SPF 30, High Protection** *($32 for 4.4 fl. oz.)* has too many synthetic active ingredients and too much fragrance to make it a safe bet for sensitive skin, but it does include titanium dioxide for sufficient UVA protection. This water-resistant sunscreen has a silky-smooth finish that doesn't feel too thick, and is best for normal to slightly dry or slightly oily skin.

☹ AVERAGE $$$ **Delectable Self-Tanning Mousse with Mirabelle Oil, SPF 15** *($42 for 4.1 fl. oz.)* is a good, though needlessly expensive, self-tanner that includes an in-part avobenzone sunscreen. Most self-tanners use the same ingredient, DHA, to change the color of surface skin cells. So, regardless of the price tag or the product line, the products do the exact same thing. Combining self-tanners with sunscreen isn't helpful and can be problematic because the two are diametrically opposed in terms of how they are supposed to be applied. For sunscreen to provide enough protection, you must apply it liberally. When it comes to self-tanners, however, liberal application can result in uneven absorption causing streaking, a darker color than you want, and a patchwork appearance. That said, this self-tanner is an option for normal to slightly oily skin. The plant oil and extracts it contains (plus some antioxidants) won't remain potent for long due to the jar packaging, although in a self-tanner they aren't of much help anyway. In a sunscreen, however, they would be great, but you just can't count on them in this product.

☹ AVERAGE $$$ **Delicious Self Tanning Cream** *($42 for 3.9 fl. oz.)* could not be a more basic self-tanning lotion if it tried, and labeling this as having "skin-nourishing benefits" is like labeling M&Ms as health food. Like most self-tanners, this turns skin color with DHA. A secondary self-tanning agent (erythrulose) is in here as well, so your color will continue to develop after the initial tan appears within hours. That's nice, but many other self-tanners offer this perk, and few dare to charge as much as Clarins. If you want a self-tanner from Clarins, they offer several options more elegant than this.

☹ AVERAGE $$$ **Sunscreen Care Cream SPF 20, Moderate Protection** *($37.50 for 6.8 fl. oz.)* is a broad-spectrum sunscreen said to ensure an even, long-lasting tan, which is an unethical claim for any cosmetics company to make, especially one with as many anti-aging products as Clarins. Although this has a lightweight, silky texture and contains titanium dioxide for reliable UVA (think anti-aging) protection, the formula contains more fragrance than beneficial extras like antioxidants. This also contains several fragrance ingredients known to cause irritation, which isn't a step in the right direction. Between the claims that encourage tanning and the problematic extras, this isn't a sunscreen worth your time or money.

☹ AVERAGE $$$ **Sunscreen Care Milk-Lotion Spray SPF 50+** *($32 for 5.3 fl. oz.)* is a spray-on sunscreen lotion providing broad-spectrum sun protection that includes stabilized avobenzone for sufficient UVA protection. What's disappointing is the price, which may discourage the liberal application necessary to reach the stated SPF rating, and the fact that Clarins added more fragrance than beneficial antioxidants. Fragrance is a hallmark of most of their products, but fragrance is not skin-caring in the least. And, with the amount of active ingredients in this sunscreen, the fragrance increases the likelihood you'll have a sensitized reaction from the sun. Please see the Appendix for details on why high amounts of fragrance are a problem for all skin types.

☺ AVERAGE **$$$ Sunscreen Care Milk-Lotion Spray SPF 50+, Very High Protection** *($32 for 5.3 fl. oz.)* is a spray-on sunscreen lotion with a light texture that's suitable for normal to slightly dry or slightly oily skin. It provides broad-spectrum protection and includes stabilized avobenzone for critical UVA (think anti-aging) protection. Although sun protection is assured and the application method is convenient, it's disappointing that this sunscreen contains far more fragrance than beneficial extras such as antioxidants.

☺ AVERAGE **$$$ Sun Wrinkle Control Cream for Face SPF 50+, Very High Protection** *($30 for 2.5 fl. oz.)* claims to provide sun protection and reduce sun-induced skin aging; it also "promotes a more even tan"! Make no mistake, any amount of color from the sun is your skin telling you it has been damaged and this damage leads to wrinkles and potentially skin cancer. Using sunscreen to protect your skin and getting a tan is the wrong approach; it's sort of like taking vitamin supplements in the hopes that it will reduce the risks associated with smoking cigarettes—it doesn't! Despite the disingenuous tanning claim, this sunscreen provides great broad-spectrum protection and includes stabilized avobenzone for critical UVA (think anti-aging) protection. The lotion formula is best for normal to dry skin, but the lack of protective antioxidants is disappointing. This sunscreen contains a high amount of fragrance as well as fragrance ingredients known to cause irritation. Because the sunscreen actives themselves will be sensitizing for some people, it's best to use fragrance-free sunscreens to ensure your skin gets the protection it needs without excess irritation.

☹ POOR **Intense Bronze Self Tanning Tint for Face and Decollete** *($34 for 4.2 fl. oz.)* has a thin, almost liquid consistency, and the amount of alcohol is a potential problem. Alcohol causes dryness, irritation, and free-radical damage, and it's best to avoid skin-care products where it is the main ingredient. Given the vast number of self-tanners (including others from Clarins) that are alcohol-free, it doesn't make sense to overspend on this one and risk irritation.

☹ POOR **Sunscreen Care Oil Free Lotion Spray SPF 15, Moderate Protection** *($32 for 5.1 fl. oz.)* is a spray-on sunscreen and is oil-free as claimed, but it also contains skin-damaging alcohol and an unusually high amount of fragrance. Both are problematic for all skin types, especially when they are the main ingredients in a product. See the Appendix for further details. It's great that this sunscreen spray provides broad-spectrum protection (including avobenzone for critical UVA screening), but the base formula definitely leaves your skin wanting more to protect from aging.

CLARINS LIP CARE

☺ GOOD **$$$ Moisture Replenishing Lip Balm** *($24 for 0.5 fl. oz.)* is a mineral oil–based lip balm that contains an effective blend of emollient thickeners and helpful plant extracts. It's a pricey way to care for dry, chapped lips, but will do the job if you decide to splurge. The amount of peptide is so small as to be inconsequential.

☺ AVERAGE **$$$ Extra-Firming Lip & Contour Balm** *($37.50 for 0.45 fl. oz.)* contains cosmetic pigments to reflect light away from lips, which can (cosmetically) make them appear fuller. This lip balm will reduce chapping and dryness, but it cannot make lips appear any fuller or younger-looking than any other lip balm or Vaseline for that matter. The simple act of moisturizing lips with any helpful ingredient will make them look younger and fuller (moist lips look fuller than dry, cracked lips); however, any shimmering lip gloss has the same effect. In short, we can't discredit this product for being ineffective on dry lips, but we encourage you to ignore the anti-aging claims and realize you don't have to spend anywhere near this amount of money to have smooth, soft lips.

☺ AVERAGE $$$ **Extra-Firming Lip & Contour Gentle Exfoliator** (*$28 for 0.6 fl. oz.*) is a lip scrub, which blends mineral oil (a non-plant ingredient Clarins uses way more often than they like to admit, and their counter personnel continually admonish it as a terrible ingredient), and sugar, which does indeed work as a gentle exfoliant. Of course, part of the gentleness depends on the user not applying too much pressure, but if you take care, the result is flake-free, smoothed lips. You can create this product at home by blending any nonfragrant oil with a small amount of sugar. Mix until a paste is formed, and gently massage this over your lips, then rinse with warm water. You can also use a soft baby's toothbrush to gently exfoliate dry, flaky skin from lips. By the way, regardless of the method, exfoliating lips isn't going to make them firmer, "extra plump" or otherwise.

CLARINS SPECIALTY SKIN-CARE PRODUCTS

☺ AVERAGE $$$ **Bright Plus HP Intensive Brightening Mask** (*$32.50 for 2.24 fl. oz.*) has a brightening effect which is simply cosmetic; there is nothing intensive about it. According to Clarins, 97% of women who used this mask reported more luminous skin. That sounds impressive, but it's what we don't know about this statistic that matters. How many women tried the mask? Who were they? Were they paid to test the product or do they work for Clarins? What was done to their skin beforehand? If it was stripped with alcohol and then this moisturizing mask was applied, of course it's going to make skin look luminous—but so would several other products. And just because skin appears more luminous doesn't mean the ingredients that got it to look that way are beneficial. Adding shimmery sparkles to the product can make skin luminous, but they serve no skin-care benefit. In the case of this mask, the packaging is supposed to make you think you're getting potent, individually packaged "doses" of a special treatment, but you're not. The brightening effect comes from titanium dioxide, while the rice starch and clay promote a matte finish (an odd trait for a moisturizing mask, and one that likely will confuse dry or oily skin). The tiny amounts of plants (a common characteristic of Clarins products) have minimal impact on skin. This mask contains a lot of fragrance and also includes several fragrance ingredients that are potential irritants. See the Appendix to learn why irritation and excess fragrance are detrimental for everyone's skin.

☺ AVERAGE $$$ **HydraQuench Cream-Mask** (*$35 for 2.5 fl. oz.*) is an OK moisturizing mask for dry skin, but considering the price and the small container, this product is a waste of money. It's mostly a blend of water with glycerin, silicone, and thickeners, which are hardly unique and not at all specialized for the needs of those with dry, dehydrated skin. It also contains far more fragrance than intriguing ingredients for skin, which furthers the disappointment factor.

☺ AVERAGE $$$ **Instant Smooth Line Correcting Concentrate** (*$32.50 for 0.9 fl. oz.*) is a wrinkle filler housed in a pen-style component with a smooth, angled applicator. Turning the base of the component dispenses product onto the tip, and from there you smooth it over wrinkles. Does it work? To some extent, yes, but as with all wrinkle fillers the effect is temporary, and how long it lasts depends on how much you apply and how expressive you are. The formula contains a blend of silicone ingredients whose texture has a slight, spackle-like effect on lines. It's very similar to Clarins Instant Smooth Perfecting Touch, which provides the same effect, but you get a lot more product for your money. Both products contain mineral pigments that leave a soft shiny finish. Compared with Instant Smooth Perfecting Touch, the Line Correcting Concentrate contains a tiny amount of antioxidant vitamin E and a skin-repairing ceramide, but not enough to make a significant difference. It's also fragrance-free, which makes it great for use around the eyes, but skin anywhere on the face will benefit from fragrance-free products because fragrance isn't skin care, something Clarins ignores in almost all their other products.

☺ AVERAGE $$$ **Super Restorative Replenishing Comfort Mask** *($62 for 2.5 fl. oz.)* contains some great emollients and plant oils that are capable of replenishing skin and restoring a smooth appearance to the face for dry to very dry skin. The claim of removing dead skin cells is tied to the glycolic acid in this product, but the amount is too small (and the pH too high) for it to function as an exfoliant. This mask contains more fragrance than beneficial ingredients; although they may please your olfactory sense, fragrance is not skin care. This mask also contains the preservative methylisothiazolinone, which is known to be sensitizing, but because this mask is intended to be rinsed off, it's not likely to be a problem. Still, this isn't worth the time or expense.

☺ AVERAGE $$$ **Truly Matte Pure & Radiant Mask** *($29 for 1.7 fl. oz.)* contains more moisturizing ingredients than absorbents, which may leave combination to oily skin confused rather than purified. This mask is best for normal to slightly dry skin, but for the money it's a rather superfluous product. Contrary to claim, the thickening agents this mask contains can clog pores.

☹ POOR **Bright Plus HP Intensive Brightening Botanical System with Snow Lotus** *($155 for 1.2 fl. oz.)* is a beautifully packaged product and packaging plays a huge role in how consumers perceive products. In fact, in many instances, the packaging has far more draw and effect than what's inside. In this case, however, the packaging is not only a lure but also truly deceiving because it makes this vastly overpriced kit seem like a specialized treatment. The goal of this two-step system is to "brighten tired-looking skin" and restore "a luminous and healthy-looking glow in just 3 weeks." How is this supposed to be accomplished? Step 1 involves applying **Age Control Concentrate**. A cursory look at the ingredient list reveals what a joke the name of this product is. It's mostly water and alcohol, the latter of which is age-promoting, not reversing. Other than tiny amounts of vitamins C and E, there is nothing positive about this product. It contains a large amount of fragrance and is laced with fragrance ingredients known to cause irritation. What a slap in the face to women looking to take the absolute best care of their skin, regardless of cost! Step 2 is the **Brightening Concentrate**, a bland yet silky moisturizer that contains a tiny amount of vitamin C, most certainly not enough to affect skin discolorations. Again, the amount of fragrance is cause for concern, as is the inclusion of several fragrance ingredients known to be irritating. Used separately or alone, there is no reason to believe either of these products will do much more than make skin feel smoother while inciting inflammation and irritation: two things that lead to increased signs of aging. And who wants to pay good money for that?

☹ POOR **Bright Plus HP On-The-Spot Brightening Corrector** *($35 for 0.34 fl. oz.)* lists alcohol as the second ingredient and that makes this product too irritating and drying for all skin types. In addition, none of the ingredients can fade sun or age spots, and the pH of the product is too high for the tiny amount of salicylic acid it contains to function as an exfoliant.

⊗ POOR **Truly Matte Blemish Control** *($23 for 0.34 fl. oz.)* has a roll-on applicator that may seem convenient, but this product contains too much alcohol and too little of anything capable of minimizing blemishes. The antibacterial agent triclosan is likely somewhat effective, but the irritants that precede it aren't a good trade-off. Wintergreen and volatile fragrant components make this even more troublesome for inflamed, reddened skin. See the Appendix to learn why irritating ingredients make oily, blemish-prone skin worse.

CLARINS FOUNDATIONS & PRIMERS

☺ GOOD **$$$ Instant Light Complexion Perfector** *($33)* is a unique primer that feels weightless and leaves skin silky-smooth. The uniqueness comes from the subtle opalescent shine of this fluid product. You'll get a low-glow shine that enhances the complexion by making it look luminous without obvious sparkles. The matte (in feel) finish provides an excellent base to apply foundation over, and this works well to optically minimize darkness in shadowed areas (although a good concealer or other highlighters can do so, too). The only drawback is the inclusion of a small amount of fragrance ingredients known to cause irritation. Their inclusion isn't a deal-breaker, but keeps this from earning our top rating.

☺ GOOD **$$$ Everlasting Foundation SPF 15** *($36)* is a concentrated liquid foundation including titanium dioxide as the sole active ingredient. That's great for gentle sun protection, although I'm concerned that the amount (2%) is barely enough to achieve the SPF rating on the label. Still, when an SPF and active ingredients are listed, it's reasonable to assume that Clarins did due diligence in terms of FDA-required sunscreen tests—at least we hope so. This has a supremely silky texture with decent slip, so blending isn't difficult. It goes on nearly opaque, and is tricky to soften to less than medium to full coverage, so if you're looking for sheer coverage, this is not the foundation for you. The powdery matte finish is definitely long-wearing, but 15 hours as claimed is pushing matters, especially if you have oily skin. This is assuredly a foundation to test before purchasing because not everyone with oily skin will like the amount of coverage and the finish. Where Clarins really excels is their shade selection: There's not a bad one in the bunch and there are plenty of options for fair to light skin tones. The darkest shade isn't all that dark, but Clarins foundations don't typically cater to women with dark skin tones. As for the claims of "triple protection against free radicals," don't count on it. The sunscreen provides protection from free-radical damage from the sun, but the tiny amount of one antioxidant (green tea) in this foundation isn't going to provide much, if any, protection from anything.

☺ GOOD **$$$ Extra-Firming Foundation SPF 15** *($42.50)* contains only a dusting of ingredients capable of firming skin, extra or otherwise, but of course the sunscreen helps prevent further signs of aging. Although the name is misleading, it doesn't stop this noticeably fragranced foundation from being a good choice for someone with normal to dry skin. Its texture and application are creamy-smooth, setting to a soft matte finish that remains slightly moist to the touch, which provides a healthy glow. You can attain medium to full coverage, and this is easy to blend evenly. The range of shades has some impressively neutral options for fair to tan skin tones, including #114, which is the darkest color (but not very dark). Be careful with shade #11 (Toffee), which is slightly peach, and #113 (Chestnut), which has a slight orange cast that won't work for most medium to tan skin tones.

☺ GOOD **$$$ Instant Smooth Foundation** *($38)* is a soft-textured whipped mousse foundation that goes on creamy and transforms almost instantly to a silky, weightless matte finish that gives skin an attractive dimensional quality. Coverage is sheer to modestly medium, meaning this isn't for anyone with a noticeably uneven skin tone or dark discolorations. The silicone-heavy formula is best for normal to slightly dry or slightly oily skin. Those with oily skin will see shine in short order (the formula contains vegetable oil), while those with dry skin won't really get the moisture Clarins promises; but this does go on smooth. Almost all the shades are worth considering by those with fair to slightly tan skin tones. Avoid 05, which is too peach. Shades 0 and 1.5 are remarkably neutral. Note: As with many Clarins products, this has a strong fragrance. Those looking for a similar foundation for a lot less money should consider Maybelline New York's Dream Matte Mousse Foundation or Cover Girl's TruBlend Whipped Foundation.

☺ GOOD $$$ **Super Restorative Foundation SPF 15** *($60)*. Taken on its own merits as a foundation with an in-part titanium dioxide sunscreen, this is a beautifully done option for normal to dry skin. The initially creamy texture becomes lighter (in feel) as you blend, and it sets to a gorgeous satin matte finish that enlivens skin rather than making it look like a layer of makeup intended to mask it. You'll get medium coverage that's ideal for evening out your skin tone and reducing minor flaws. All in all, this is excellent—and there isn't a bad shade in the bunch. Now, to the over-the-top claims that are likely the reason some women may be willing to spend this much money on a foundation, even when there are perfectly beautiful foundations available for less than half the price. Clarins wants you to believe you can fight aging and wrinkling with this foundation, but the only anti-aging element in this foundation is its sunscreen, which is the same for any well-formulated foundation with sunscreen. This makeup isn't restorative on any level other than sunscreen, and it doesn't contain any ingredients capable of lifting skin. It also is not a specialized formula for those over the age of 50. Such a ridiculous notion won't go away, but please don't shop for skin-care or makeup products based on the number of candles on your birthday cake—age is not a skin type. Such claims rarely lead you to the products you really need, especially if you're in your 50s and still struggling with breakouts, oily skin, rosacea, blackheads, whiteheads, or overly sensitive skin. Clarins included a lot of fragrance, which keeps this from earning a Best Product rating, and the allegedly "super-restorative" plant extracts are but a dusting, so you're left with the unsung heroes of today's best foundations: silicones and silicone polymers. These are what create the silky, unbelievably smooth textures and finishes that, when combined with modern pigment technology, result in foundations that look more skin-like than ever.

☺ GOOD $$$ **Super Restorative Tinted Cream SPF 20** *($79)* is way too overpriced! While this has some strong points, the price is just a joke and easily replaced by other less expensive options. Pricing aside, this creamy tinted moisturizer with a pure titanium dioxide sunscreen has a beautiful smooth texture that feels luxurious and enlivens dull skin with sheer, luminescent color. Each of the four shades has a peach to orange cast, but the sheerness makes it a non-issue except for the darkest shade (05 Tea). The formula sets to a satin matte finish that remains slightly moist to the touch. As for the claims, all I can say is they are as inflated as Goldie Hawn's lips in *The First Wives Club* (remember that scene? It's one of our favorites)! In order to justify the expense of what amounts to a good tinted moisturizer with sunscreen, Clarins claims this replenishes and lifts the complexion. The only skin-lifting you'll see is if you do a handstand while applying this (thus causing sagging facial skin to go in the opposite direction) and its replenishment ability is not reflected in a state-of-the-art formula. Consisting mostly of water, several silicones, salt, and fragrance, this is minimally replenishing (though the silicones add their special silkiness, which enhances application). All the intriguing ingredients are present in the tiniest amounts, so calling this super restorative is not accurate. For less money and a better formula, check out the tinted moisturizers from Bobbi Brown, Neutrogena, or Paula's Choice.

☺ AVERAGE $$$ **Everlasting Compact Foundation SPF 15** *($36)* has a pure titanium dioxide sunscreen. Although that's great, as a general rule we don't recommend relying on any powder with sunscreen for your daily sun protection. It's not that they don't protect from sun damage—it's that most women are unlikely to apply the necessary amount to reach the level of sun protection stated on the label. For best results, powders with sunscreen should be applied over your daytime moisturizer or foundation with sunscreen. This has a sheer, dry texture that doesn't blend as readily as the best powder foundations. Its powdery matte finish is best for oily skin, though the finish tends to magnify wrinkles and even the slightest hint of dry or flaky skin. Coverage is in the light to medium range. The shade range caters to those with light to slightly tan skin tones. Cream, Sand, Wheat, and Honey are particularly good shades, though with any of the colors you'll be putting up with a powder foundation that doesn't look as smooth and natural as others. As for Clarins's claims that this foundation lasts for 15 hours once applied, don't bet on it. Although it will hold up quite well over oily areas, you will need to touch-up because this doesn't control shine from morning until evening.

☺ AVERAGE $$$ **Instant Smooth Perfecting Touch** *($32.50 for 0.5 fl. oz.)* calls itself "the modern, magic makeup base" and has "innovative line-filling technology" that claims to do all sorts of astounding things for skin. Reading the description, you might be curious how you ever got away with wearing makeup before this jar of wonder arrived. As it turns out, this is nothing more than a multiple silicone primer whose spackle-like texture and silky finish does work (temporarily) to fill in superficial wrinkles and large pores. How long the effect lasts depends on your skin type and, in the case of wrinkles, how expressive you are. The pale pink color adds a subtle luminous quality to skin, but that's camouflaged if you follow it with foundation. It's an option for a silky-feeling pre-makeup moisturizer, but not as impressive as silicone-based serums loaded with antioxidants and other skin-beneficial ingredients (and Clarins did not include any).

☺ AVERAGE $$$ **Skin Illusion SPF 10 Natural Radiance Foundation** *($36)* is a beautiful liquid foundation. We wish this didn't have a couple of major drawbacks that keep it from getting a higher rating. The first problem is the low SPF rating; SPF 15 is the recommended minimum rating by medical boards and organizations all over the world, and many consider even higher SPF ratings to be better. The second problem is that this contains a potentially problematic amount of skin-damaging alcohol. Alcohol causes free-radical damage, irritation, dryness, and collagen breakdown. Broad-spectrum sun protection is provided by titanium dioxide in this easy-to-blend foundation, but again, SPF 10 isn't enough. If you decide to pair this with a moisturizer rated SPF 15 or greater, it leaves a soft, dewy finish that provides light coverage and is best for normal to slightly dry skin. Clarins typically does well with their foundation shades, and this follows suit—almost all the colors (which are best for fair to medium skin tones) are soft and neutral. Wheat is slightly peach, but workable, but Chestnut is best avoided due to its orange overtone. The darkest shade (Cappuccino) is best for tan, not dark, skin tones.

☹ POOR **HydraQuench Tinted Moisturizer SPF 6** *($44)* is a tinted moisturizer with sunscreen that has several issues making it less desirable than many other options in this category. To begin, the SPF rating is below the minimum SPF 15 recommendation from medical boards worldwide—this isn't a wise choice as your sole source of daily sun protection (although the active ingredient is a good one). Next, the formula is highly fragrant and contains several fragrance ingredients known to cause irritation. Please see the Appendix to learn why this is a problem. This has a smooth, creamy texture suitable for normal to dry skin and it sets to a radiant satin finish with sheer coverage, yet the shades tend to be unusually peach, so even though this goes on sheer the peachy tone isn't the most natural look on the skin tones the shades work best for (which would be light to medium). In terms of hydration, this isn't a very exciting or state-of-the-art formula. It contains more mica (a shiny mineral pigment) than intriguing ingredients, and again, the wafting fragrance is a problem for all skin types, making this a tinted moisturizer to avoid.

CLARINS CONCEALERS

☺ GOOD $$$ **Concealer Stick** *($25)* is packaged like traditional lipstick. It applies smoothly, but its creaminess borders on greasy. Although that may sound like a problem, this ends up having a slight powder finish that's only minimally prone to creasing into lines around the eye. Best for dry skin and not recommended for use on blemishes; this comes in three workable shades.

☺ GOOD $$$ **Instant Light Brush-On Perfector** *($30)* is a fragrance-free liquid highlighter packaged in a click pen–style component that includes a built-in synthetic brush applicator. What's dispensed is a soft, initially creamy liquid that applies smoothly and more sheer than you might expect. Best for highlighting rather than concealing, this sets to a satin finish that has a slight tendency to crease into lines around the eyes. The creasing isn't a deal-breaker, however, because this works quite well over your regular concealer, and a light dusting of powder makes the minor creasing almost a non-issue. Clarins offers three shades: a pale, flesh-toned soft pink, neutral ivory, and nude beige. They are best for fair to light-medium skin tones or you can mix it with your regular concealer to add a subtle brightening effect while camouflaging dark areas.

CLARINS POWDERS

✓☺ BEST $$$ **Loose Powder** *($35)* comes in a generous container and has a silky, feather-light texture and a sheer, dry application that looks beautiful and feels weightless on the skin. The two sheer shades are good, each with a satin finish—meaning this is best for those with normal to dry skin who want to avoid a true matte finish.

☺ GOOD $$$ **Powder Compact** *($30)* has a very silky, ultrafine texture and a dry, non-powdery finish. The talc-based formula comes in three sheer shades appropriate for fair to light skin.

CLARINS BLUSHES & BRONZER

✓☺ BEST $$$ **Multi-Blush** *($28.50)* is an excellent option for cream-to-powder blush. The formula is very easy to blend, and all but one of the colors are beautiful. Avoid Tender Raspberry because it's intensely fuchsia and not easy to soften to a more flattering tone.

☺ GOOD $$$ **Blush Prodige Illuminating Cheek Color** *($28.50)* is a great pressed-powder blush that offers four complementary shades in one compact. Each compact holds a large "square" of blush surrounded by three small "rectangles" of blush, which you can mix with your brush and apply as one uniform color or apply separately, although we don't advise doing so because the results will look striped or contrived. The manner in which this blush is presented is visually appealing, but separating the tone-on-tone shades isn't necessary for great results. This powder blush has a smooth texture that applies softly and builds well if you desire more intensity. The shade in each compact offer matte and shiny finishes, but the shine is subtle and doesn't hold up well. The shade range works best for fair to medium skin tones, which is true for most makeup from Clarins.

☺ GOOD **$$$ Bronzing Powder Compact** *($36)* is a standard, really overpriced, pressed bronzing powder with the requisite smooth yet dry texture and shiny (not overly so) finish. All the shades apply sheer and can be difficult to build should you want more color. Morning Sun is OK for fair skin, but applies as a peachy blush rather than a true bronze or tan color.

CLARINS EYESHADOWS & EYE PRIMERS

☺ GOOD **$$$ Instant Light Eye Perfecting Base** *($24.50)* comes packaged in a click-pen applicator with a built-in synthetic brush tip. Housed inside is a smooth liquid concealer that blends well, evening out the appearance of skin on the eyelid or under-eye area. This has a crease-free matte finish that adds a touch of shine to skin, though not distractingly so. Both shades are good, but they are best for fair to light skin tones. Although this is an impressive product, it is superfluous if you're already using an excellent concealer in the eye area.

☹ AVERAGE **$$$ Colour Quartet for Eyes** *($40)*. The compact for these eyeshadow quads is gorgeous; too bad the color combinations (most of which are pastel-oriented) aren't. Each powder eyeshadow in the sets has a smooth, dry texture that deposits color somewhat unevenly and with some minor flaking. Every shade is also shiny, so we're talking maximum spotlight on less-than-taut or wrinkled eye-area skin.

CLARINS EYE & BROW LINERS

☹ AVERAGE **$$$ Eyebrow Pencil** *($23)* is an utterly standard brow pencil that requires routine sharpening. It has a firm, dry texture that demands a bit of pressure to deposit color. The powdery finish won't smear and it isn't prone to fast fading, but the price is really out of line for what you get.

☹ AVERAGE **$$$ Waterproof Eyeliner Pencil** *($23)* has a tenacity that can survive swimming and tears, so it is waterproof—but you have to tolerate sharpening it, and a finish that remains tacky to the touch. It's an OK occasional-use option, but there are smoother, silicone-based eye pencils that are also waterproof, even though they may not advertise that fact.

☹ POOR **Eye Liner Pencil** *($23)* is a standard pencil with substandard attributes. This soft-textured pencil glides on but is too creamy for it not to smudge and smear, though the built-in sponge-tip applicator facilitates smudging and smearing if you use it.

CLARINS LIP COLOR & LIPLINERS

✓☺ BEST **$$$ Joli Rouge** *($24.50)*. "Joli" is a French word that means attractive, and this luscious cream lipstick certainly is. Exceptionally moisturizing, smooth, and pigment-rich, the colors glide on easily and leave a beautiful cream finish that doesn't veer toward being too glossy or slick. Be careful because this is creamy enough to bleed into lines around the mouth, but if that (and this lipstick's price tag) isn't an issue for you, it is one of the best cream lipstick options at the department store.

✓☺ BEST **$$$ Rouge Prodige True Colour & Shine Lipstick** *($24.50)* leaves lips feeling velvety smooth with its creamy texture and hint of shine. There are plenty of flattering colors from which to choose, including shades of nude, pink, coral, mauve, and red, all of which offer good color saturation. While Clarins claims that this lipstick delivers long-lasting color, we wouldn't put Rouge Prodige Lipstick in the same category as other top-rated long-lasting lipsticks, but it does have the potential to stay put through your first cup of morning coffee. All factors considered, if the price doesn't hold you back, this lipstick is worth a try!

☺ GOOD **$$$ Gloss Appeal** *($21)* is a lip gloss whose deep, bold colors may look imposing at first glance, but that actually go on watercolor sheer. The slightly thick texture feels balm-like but isn't sticky, and leaves an attractive gloss finish with a blend of gold and silver shimmer.

☺ GOOD **$$$ Instant Light Lip Perfector** *($21)* is simply a shimmering lip gloss available in three sheer shades (pastel rose, apricot, and beige). It has a smooth, non-sticky texture and a sheer, glossy finish. Clarins suggests using this under lipstick, but that only leads to a messy application that takes more time to neaten than just applying gloss after lipstick.

☹ AVERAGE **$$$ Joli Rouge Perfect Shine Sheer Lipstick** *($24.50)* is a very sheer, glossy lipstick with the distinction of maintaining a glossy look without being too slick or slippery. Instead, you get an emollient texture that offers a soft wash of translucent color. The color fades within an hour, but that's the nature of most sheer, glossy lipsticks. The main drawback is that each shade is imbued with glitter particles that, while not garish, feel grainy as this lipstick's finish wears off. You can get better results with the sheer, glittery lipsticks from Wet n' Wild for less than $4.

☹ AVERAGE **$$$ Lip Definer** *($23)* is a standard pencil that has an easy-to-apply texture, but it needs sharpening and doesn't hold a candle to many other automatic lip pencils.

CLARINS MASCARAS

✓☺ BEST **$$$ Wonder Perfect Mascara** *($24)* is a mascara that builds notable volume and length, and adds an attractive fringed curl to lashes. You'll notice some minor clumping, but given how quickly this produces great results, that's a negligible trade-off. Besides, the clumping is easily combed through because the brush is so adept at separating and defining every lash. This counts as perfect mascara if its best attributes are on your ideal mascara checklist!

☺ GOOD **$$$ Wonder Volume Mascara** *($24)* provides substantial lash enhancement without being too dramatic, and the formula wears well without making lashes feel brittle.

☹ AVERAGE **$$$ Double Fix Mascara Waterproofing Seal** *($22)* is sold as a waterproofing top coat for use with non-waterproof mascaras. It works, but applying this over mascara isn't always flattering because—depending on which mascara you're wearing—it either clumps lashes together, makes them look spiky, or creates a wet look that may not be to your liking. Why bother with this (and the extra expense) when there are dozens of excellent waterproof mascaras available?

☹ AVERAGE **$$$ Eye Definition Mascara** *($24)* is advertised as an ultra-voluminous mascara with intense color. The volume comes at the expense of some clumping, which isn't ideal, but they really do deliver on the deeply pigmented, jet-black color. The tip of the applicator brush has a smaller/thinner portion designed for hard-to-reach lashes, but it ends up making the application even clumpier. In terms of length, you won't notice much improvement.

☹ AVERAGE **$$$ Wonder Length Mascara** *($24)* works well to make lashes longer, though not without a slightly uneven application and not with the same extensive elongation as several superior drugstore mascaras. The real wonder is how Clarins gets women to spend this much on an average mascara! Those who prefer the style of brush offered by Clarins should consider Maybelline New York Lash Discovery Mascara instead.

☹ POOR **Instant Definition Mascara** *($24)* has a unique brush whose tip contains narrowly spaced, short bristles for added emphasis along the lash line and outer fringe of lashes.

The Reviews C

Applied very carefully to avoid a mess (a too-casual application can quickly backfire because this deposits a lot of mascara), this lets you build dramatically thick, long lashes that just keep getting bigger with each stroke of the brush. Despite a heavy application, the brush prohibits clumping; however, the formula remains creamy and as such this mascara is prone to smearing and smudging throughout the day. It also breaks down and runs with the slightest hint of water, so getting misty-eyed leads to swift mascara meltdown.

CLARINS BRUSHES

☺ AVERAGE **$$$ Clarins Brushes** *($18.50–$34)* are decent, but they pale in comparison to what most makeup artistry lines sell for the same amount of money. The hair quality isn't up to par, nor are the brush shapes as elegantly functional as they could be, all of which makes this small brush collection one to consider carefully, if at all. **The Brush** *($20)* is meant as a take-along powder applicator, but since it isn't retractable you're looking at a messy makeup bag or purse after a few uses.

CLARINS SPECIALTY MAKEUP PRODUCTS

☹ POOR **Fix' Make-Up Refreshing Mist** *($26 for 1 fl. oz.)* is designed as a spray-on mist to set your makeup, this product does little more than make skin feel damp and slightly sticky. It contains nothing that enhances (or could possibly enhance) makeup wear; in fact, overdoing this can lead to makeup meltdown or streaking, plus this contains fragrance ingredients and fragrant plant extracts capable of causing irritation. The finish leaves a lingering stickiness, too, and the formula doesn't provide a skin-care benefit. Whoever thought this overpriced, gimmicky product was a good idea needs to go back to the drawing board!

CLARISONIC (SKIN CARE ONLY)

Strengths: Cleans skin well, but not as well as the claims state.

Weaknesses: Very expensive; system provides only minuscule amounts of cleanser (though you can use this with any cleanser).

For more information and reviews of the latest Clarisonic products, visit CosmeticsCop.com.

CLARISONIC CLEANSERS

☺ GOOD **$$$ Refreshing Gel Cleanser** *($25 for 6 fl. oz.)* is a good, though overpriced, water-soluble cleanser for normal to oily or combination skin. It isn't necessary to use this or any other Clarisonic cleanser with the Clarisonic brush, but this gentle formula is an option if you don't mind overspending. It foams slightly, removes makeup, and rinses without leaving a residue. This does contain fragrance.

☺ AVERAGE **$$$ Nourishing Care Cleanser** *($25 for 6 fl. oz.)* is more emollient than Clarisonic's other cleansers, and the amount of oils it contains impedes rinsing (not to mention that using this with the Clarisonic brush can push the plant oils farther into the pores, potentially causing blemishes). This contains a small amount of *Cymbopogon schoenanthus* oil, a plant also known as camel grass and that is related to lemongrass, but there is no information pertaining to its benefit or risk for skin. Still, as a fragrant plant oil it can irritate skin, and there are plenty of cleansers that treat skin gently without exposing it to fragrance.

☹ POOR **Gentle Hydro Cleanser** *($25 for 6 fl. oz.)* contains gentle cleansing agents that remove makeup without drying skin, but where this cleanser really goes astray is by including several fragrant oils. Lemon, lime, bergamot, and orange all cause irritation and are a problem for use around the eyes. Using this cleanser with the Clarisonic brush means these irritants are pushed deeper into your pores, where their problematic effects are magnified. Any gentle, water-soluble (and, ideally, fragrance-free) cleanser can be used with the Clarisonic brush, so this overpriced entry can be ignored.

CLARISONIC MOISTURIZERS (DAYTIME & NIGHTTIME), EYE CREAMS, & SERUMS

☺ GOOD $$$ **Opal Anti-Aging Sea Serum** (*$65 for 1.7 fl. oz.*) is a water-based serum sold with the Clarisonic Opal, a device designed to "infuse" anti-aging ingredients deeper into skin around the eyes via sonic vibrations. The Opal system is reviewed below, but for those so inclined, the accompanying serum may be purchased separately. Although pricey, this certainly isn't the most expensive serum around and it contains several beneficial ingredients (though none of them are unique or special for the eye area). Chief among them is willowherb, a great anti-irritant. This also contains elastin, which is a good water-binding agent but it cannot fuse with or replenish elastin fibers in your skin (elastin is what gives skin its ability to bounce back when stretched). This serum is primarily about soothing agents and doesn't contain much in the way of proven antioxidants. In that sense, it isn't as well-rounded as the best serums, but is still worth considering if you have normal to slightly dry skin. This isn't a slam-dunk for sensitive skin because it contains ginger root extract, a potential irritant, especially if used around the eyes. The amount is likely too low to be cause for concern, but its presence precludes a recommendation for sensitive or rosacea-affected skin.

☺ AVERAGE $$$ **Renewal Serum** (*$75 for 1 fl. oz.*) is a mixed bag of pros and cons. The pros include the inclusion of a cell-communicating peptide and some good antioxidants and repairing ingredients. The cons are the fact that this is a water-based serum (for the money, you should expect a more substantial base than plain water), it contains a lot of film-forming agent (think hairspray-type of ingredients), and it includes fragrant plant oils, which can be irritating. For the money, there are many other serums whose formulas outpace this one and that don't subject your skin to fragrant irritants. See the Appendix to learn why irritation is a problem for all skin types.

CLARISONIC SPECIALTY SKIN-CARE PRODUCTS

☺ GOOD $$$ **Clarisonic Skin Care System** (*$195*) is a battery-powered, rechargeable oscillating brush designed for your face. You are supposed to use this device for one minute, which the company claims "Leaves skin feeling and looking smoother" and "Deeply cleanses and clarifies the skin." The system is also supposed to remove six times more makeup than just using a cleanser. Why should you spend this much money on a rotating brush to clean your skin? Well, the makers of Clarisonic have a rather official-looking study showing that it reduces oil on the skin. Their study looked at 30 adults with oily skin. During one visit, each participant had one side of their forehead manually cleansed and the other half was cleansed with the Clarisonic brush and cleanser. The results? The amount of "surface sebum remaining after cleansing with the Clarisonic was found to be significantly less than that remaining after cleansing manually." We wouldn't hang our hats on this trivial research. Comparing the brush to just regular washing isn't much of a comparison—what about comparing the Clarisonic to manual cleansing with a cleanser other than the Clarisonic version? Perhaps their cleanser isn't adequate for removing oil without using their brush. What would have been more relevant would have been to compare the Clarisonic to manual cleansing with a washcloth. We suspect that the washcloth would have proven just as effective and, to say the least, far less expensive.

The Reviews C

Such a comparison was done at a later date, and published in the February 2005 issue of the peer-reviewed journal, *Cosmetic Dermatology*. The dermatologist who authored the report stated that the Clarisonic cleaned best because it removed the most makeup compared to standard cleansers, a scrub, and a face cloth. Aside from the fact that Clarisonic paid for the study (there have been no independent studies), what wasn't mentioned was the brand names of the cleansers used, or what the results would have been had the participants used a makeup remover before cleansing. The Clarisonic website lists other studies to support their claims and efficacy, but all of them were conducted by the team behind these products. In that sense, they're simply not as reliable as third-party, double-blind, substantiated research. Bottom line: We're not saying that Clarisonic's brush is not a good way to clean skin. What we are saying is that it is not the only nor is it the best way to clean skin or remove makeup. Without question, it is needlessly expensive and not something anyone should go into debt for out of concern their skin is not getting clean enough. Besides, if you want to see what all the fuss is about, you can check out the similar cleansing brush system from Olay's Pro-X brand (this retails for around $30). The only other published piece of information about Clarisonic simply described how the sonic cleansing worked to provide consistent results and help loosen debris trapped in pores due to the oscillating brush head. Sounds promising, but the piece was written by Pacific Bioscience Laboratories, the company that, you guessed it, sells Clarisonic (Source: *Journal of Cosmetic Dermatology*, June 2006, pages 181–183). This brush will certainly help clean skin (and for that reason it deserves a Good rating), but it won't reduce wrinkles, pore size, or blemishes—at least not to a degree where you'll be glad you splurged on the system. The basic system includes two brush heads (for normal and sensitive skin); a Delicate brush head is available for separate purchase (all brush heads cost $25 apiece). The Delicate brush is recommended for very sensitive skin; however, regardless of brush head chosen, use caution if you're attempting to use Clarisonic and have rosacea or sensitive skin.

Note: If you decide to use this or any other cleansing brush on your skin, please be gentle. Overzealous usage can lead to inflammation that can hurt your skin's healing process. Pay attention to how your skin responds and discontinue (or reduce the frequency of) use if you see signs of irritation.

☺ AVERAGE $$$ **Clarisonic Opal Sonic Infusion System** *($185)* consists of a battery-powered, handheld device you use with the accompanying Anti-Aging Sea Serum (reviewed above) to sonically infuse antiwrinkle ingredients into skin around the eyes. Specifically, this device is meant to target crow's feet around the eyes. Consumer reviews for this product are mixed, with many women reporting no change and others swearing they see a difference. Here's an account from a Paula's Choice staff member who volunteered to put this device through its paces (the tester was using this system to reduce wrinkles around the eyes): "The system itself is compact and cleverly designed (think of a flat egg with a silver 'crack' across the middle) with the serum stored in the top part of the egg and the bottom portion of the egg containing the sonic applicator. Following the instructions, I pressed a button on the side which dispensed a pre-measured pea-sized amount of serum on the applicator. I switched the applicator on, which started the vibrating motion and pressed it against the crow's feet area of my face, rotating the applicator in a circular motion. The feeling was a bit odd; for those of you who have used a Sonicare toothbrush it was the same strange tickling feeling except on your skin—not in your mouth! After 30 seconds the applicator beeped and shut off, automatically. Once it was ready to go again, I repeated the steps around my other eye. After 60 seconds, as promised, I was done! Easy enough! I closely examined the skin around my eye area. Nothing had changed—I looked exactly the same just a little greasy due to the residual serum (which by the way is very nice, goes on smoothly and absorbs quickly. Next morning I found myself in the bathroom using the Opal Sonic Infusion as instructed. Before I started, I was surprised to see that the fine lines and wrinkles around my eyes actually looked better! I couldn't believe it! With great enthusiasm I applied the serum with the special powered applicator again. But my enthusiasm was short-lived when I noticed later in the day my fine lines and wrinkles were as before. I stuck to the plan and used the Opal Sonic Infusion that night. Once again, I saw the same impressive results the next morning. This pattern continued for several weeks—elation in the morning, disappointment by the end of the day. I wondered how this could be. Why do my crow's feet look better in the morning, yet go back to their normal state in the evening even though I use the Clarisonic Opal in the morning and evening? I came up with a theory as to why I was experiencing daily ecstasy and agony over my crow's feet: Was the constant vibrating of the Clarisonic applicator slightly irritating my skin, causing it to swell, thus making my wrinkles look less pronounced? By the end of the day the inflammation calmed down, which would explain why 8-10 hours later my crow's feet returned to their normal state. If my theory was true, could the inflammation the Opal Sonic Infusion was potentially causing eventually result in my crow's feet getting worse over time? Eventually, I stopped using the product but my attention was still completely focused on my eye area. Day one, two and three: no change; however, on day four I did see a change. My eye area looked worse. I didn't see more crow's feet but those I have looked deeper and more pronounced. Nothing got better after 3 months of using this system every day—the wrinkles got worse."

Your experience may differ, but we suspect that the staffer's theory is correct, and that the improvement one may see from this system is due to inflammation from the vibration and pressure applied while using Clarisonic Opal. We cannot enthusiastically recommend this device, and without question it's quite an investment. In the end, most will find greater results putting their money toward cosmetic dermatology procedures such as Botox or dermal fillers artfully injected around the eyes. These are not long-term solutions and they need to be repeated, but the results, when done correctly, will be much more impressive than this underwhelming system.

CLEAN & CLEAR (SKIN CARE ONLY)

Strengths: Inexpensive; an excellent 10% benzoyl peroxide product; some very good cleansers.

Weaknesses: The majority of products contain irritating fragrant extracts, alcohol, menthol, menthyl lactate, or other problematic ingredients; below-average moisturizers; poor choices for anyone struggling with breakouts and blackheads.

For more information and reviews of the latest Clean & Clear products, visit CosmeticsCop.com.

CLEAN & CLEAR CLEANSERS

✓☺ BEST **Daily Pore Cleanser, Oil-Free** *($5.49 for 5.5 fl. oz.)* is a very good, water-soluble cleanser/scrub hybrid for oily to very oily skin. It removes makeup easily and rinses cleanly. This is definitely one of Clean & Clear's better cleansers!

✓☺ BEST **Foaming Facial Cleanser, Sensitive Skin** *($5.29 for 8 fl. oz.)* is not only Clean & Clear's best cleanser, thanks to its gentle yet very effective water-soluble formula, but is also one of the best beauty buys at the drugstore. It would be even better without fragrance, but that's a minor concern. This cleanser removes makeup easily and is suitable for all skin types except very dry.

☺ GOOD **Finishes Oil-Free Pore Perfecting Cleanser** *($1.99 for 8 fl. oz.)* is a standard, gentle cleanser that works best for normal to oily or combination skin. This cost-effective formula removes excess oil without leaving skin dry, and is also adept at removing most types of makeup, although waterproof or long-wearing formulas likely will require a separate remover.

☺ GOOD **Foaming Facial Cleanser, Oil Free** *($5.29 for 8 fl. oz.)* is recommended if you prefer a water-soluble cleanser with copious foaming action. The foam has no cleansing ability, but the impression it gives is one some consumers prefer, and in the case of this product is not irritating or drying. The antibacterial agent triclosan is listed as an active ingredient, and although its contact with skin will be brief, it can be a helpful start to the process of reducing acne-causing bacteria.

☺ GOOD **Makeup Dissolving Facial Cleansing Wipes, Oil-Free** *($5.99 for 25 wipes)* are a great way to remove makeup and refresh skin. They're particularly useful for travel because they almost always make it through airport security in your carry-on luggage. They are capable of removing long-wearing or waterproof formulas, though wipes aren't the best method for gently removing mascara. A liquid makeup remover applied with a cotton pad or swab gives you greater control and less pulling.

☹ POOR **Advantage 3-in-1 Foaming Acne Wash** *($8.49 for 8 fl. oz.)* is medicated with 2% salicylic acid, but this proven anti-acne ingredient is of little use in a cleanser because it is rinsed from the skin before it has a chance to work. Although this cleanser avoids menthol-type ingredients, its main cleansing agent is sodium C14-16 olefin sulfonate, which makes it too drying for all skin types.

☹ POOR **Advantage 3-in-1 Exfoliating Cleanser** *($6.99 for 5 fl. oz.)* is an all-around mess of a formula that's all but guaranteed to make acne and redness from breakouts worse. It's medicated with 5% benzoyl peroxide, the gold standard ingredient for killing acne-causing bacteria; however, in a cleanser that's rinsed from the skin, its impact will be minor at best. The formula contains a drying detergent cleansing agent (sodium C14-16 olefin sulfonate) along with fragrance, and the potent irritant menthol. Please see the Appendix to learn why irritation is a problem for all skin types. The scrub ingredient is polyethylene, which is great; however, acne cannot be scrubbed away, and the fact that this contains mineral oil along with petrolatum (that's Vaseline) makes it difficult to rinse, plus it can leave your skin feeling greasy. See what we mean by an all-around mess?

☹ POOR **Continuous Control Acne Cleanser** *($5.99 for 5 fl. oz.)* contains 10% benzoyl peroxide, but this topical disinfectant is of little use to skin because it is quickly rinsed off. The menthol in this unusually creamy cleanser makes it too irritating for all skin types.

☹ POOR **Deep Action Cream Cleanser, Sensitive Skin, Oil-Free** *($5.99 for 6.5 fl. oz.)* contains menthol and is not recommended for any skin type. Without it, this would be an appropriate cleanser for sensitive skin.

☹ POOR **Makeup Dissolving Foaming Cleanser, Oil-Free** *($5.99 for 6 fl. oz.)* definitely has a strong foaming action, but its main detergent cleansing agent (sodium C14-16 olefin sulfonate) makes it too drying and irritating for all skin types. Clean & Clear offers gentler yet still effective cleansers, as do its sister companies Neutrogena and Aveeno (all owned by Johnson & Johnson).

☹ POOR **Morning Burst Detoxifying Facial Cleanser** *($5.99 for 8 fl. oz.)* has contradictory claims: On the one hand, it's supposed to oxygenate skin to remove impurities, but on the other hand it contains antioxidant-filled beads that burst as you cleanse (antioxidants work against oxygen to prevent it from damaging cells, clearly Clean & Clear assumes their consumers wouldn't notice this incongruity). As it turns out, this isn't an oxygenating experience for skin, and that's a good thing. The bad part of this very basic cleanser is the inclusion of irritating menthyl lactate (a form of menthol).

☹ POOR **Morning Burst Facial Cleanser** *($6.49 for 8 fl. oz.)* is a below-standard, water-soluble cleanser that "wakes you up" with an irritating dose of menthol and the menthol derivative menthyl lactate, which leaves your face tingling after rinsing. Without those trouble-makers and an assortment of irritating plants, this would've been a great cleanser for oily skin.

☹ POOR **Morning Burst Skin Brightening Facial Cleanser, Oil-Free** *($5.99 for 8 fl. oz.)* is similar to the Morning Burst Facial Cleanser above, and the same review applies.

☹ POOR **Morning Burst Shine Control Facial Cleanser** *($6.49 for 8 fl. oz.)* contains menthol and menthyl lactate along with irritating citrus extracts, and is not recommended. The irritating ingredients this contains can make oily skin worse (see the Appendix for details).

CLEAN & CLEAR TONERS

☹ POOR **Deep Cleaning Astringent** *($3.99 for 8 fl. oz.)* contains 2% salicylic acid, but the pH is too high for it to function as an exfoliant. Even with its pH in the correct range, the amount of alcohol in this anti-acne toner makes it a problem for all skin types.

☹ POOR **Deep Cleaning Astringent, Sensitive Skin** *($3.99 for 8 fl. oz.)* contains enough alcohol to make it problematic, while the amount of salicylic acid (plus this toner's pH) isn't going to be helpful for those struggling with breakouts. This is absolutely not for sensitive skin!

CLEAN & CLEAR EXFOLIANTS & SCRUBS

☹ POOR **Blackhead Eraser Scrub** *($5.99 for 5 fl. oz.).* The touted ACELERA Complex in this scrub is supposed to help deliver the 2% salicylic acid it contains "deep to the pores." In a scrub, that isn't possible with any formula because it is rinsed from the skin before it can do much. Salicylic acid is far better at helping to treat acne when it's in a leave-on product. When properly formulated in leave-on products, salicylic acid can penetrate into the pore lining, where blockages occur, which is a major reason why it can be so helpful for those struggling with blackheads. In a rinse-off product like this, however, it's basically wasted. In the end, despite the superior-sounding claims, this scrub isn't recommended, for the above reasons and because it contains the irritating menthol derivative menthyl lactate, which is irritating, and irritation stimulates more oil production at the base of your pores (see the Appendix for details).

☹ POOR **Deep Action Exfoliating Scrub, Oil-Free** *($4.99 for 5 fl. oz.)* contains the irritating ingredient menthol, so this cleanser-scrub hybrid is not recommended. Without it, Clean & Clear would have had a very good scrub for normal to oily skin.

☹ POOR **Morning Burst Detoxifying Facial Scrub** *($5.99 for 5 fl. oz.)* cannot oxygenate skin (which is good, because adding oxygen to skin causes free-radical damage), but it will irritate it thanks to the inclusion of the menthol derivative menthyl lactate. This is not a wise way to get your morning skin-care routine off to a good start.

☹ POOR **Morning Burst Facial Scrub** *($5.49 for 5 fl. oz.)* is similar to the Morning Burst Detoxifying Facial Scrub above, and the same review applies.

☹ POOR **Morning Burst In-Shower Facial** *($5.99 for 4 fl. oz.)* isn't close to approximating what occurs during a facial, at least not one performed by a competent aesthetician. The amount of fragrance makes it irritating, and to make matters worse, this also contains the irritant menthol and several problematic plant extracts. See the Appendix to learn why irritation is bad for everyone's skin.

☹ POOR **Morning Burst Shine Control Facial Scrub** *($5.99 for 5 fl. oz.).* has the same problem as the Morning Burst Detoxifying Facial Scrub above, and the same review applies.

CLEAN & CLEAR MOISTURIZERS (DAYTIME & NIGHTTIME)

☺ AVERAGE **Advantage Acne Control Moisturizer Oil-Free** *($7.49 for 4 fl. oz.)* is an OK lightweight moisturizer for normal to oily skin. The 0.5% concentration of salicylic acid isn't that helpful for blemishes, and it's not effective in this product given that its pH is above 4. The cinnamon and cedar bark extracts pose a risk of irritation.

☺ AVERAGE **Finishes Pore Perfecting Moisturizer SPF 15** *($7.49 for 1.7 fl. oz.)* includes avobenzone for reliable UVA protection. That's the good news. The bad news is that the base formula includes several fragrant citrus extracts that can cause irritation. The "minerals" touted in this product as being able to diffuse the appearance of pores are those that show up in hundreds of other products. The thing is, these minerals (including mica) add shine to skin, and shine isn't going to make large pores less noticeable; instead, it has the opposite effect! When you have oily skin, more shine is not the goal.

☹ POOR **Morning Glow Moisturizer SPF 15, Oil-Free** *($6.79 for 4 fl. oz.)* contains a form of menthol that can cause skin to tingle (not glow) with irritation, and that is unquestionably a problem. Without it, this in-part avobenzone sunscreen would have been highly recommended as a basic, lightweight, affordable sunscreen for normal to slightly oily skin.

CLEAN & CLEAR SPECIALTY SKIN-CARE PRODUCTS

✓☺ BEST **Persa-Gel 10, Maximum Strength** *($5.99 for 1 fl. oz.)* remains a very potent, fragrance-free topical disinfectant for blemishes. It contains 10% benzoyl peroxide, the maximum amount approved for over-the-counter sales. Although this amount can be drying and potentially irritating, this is an option for stubborn cases of acne. If you haven't used a benzoyl peroxide product in the past, start with a 2.5% or 5% strength rather than jumping to the maximum strength—you may find the lower strengths work great!

☺ GOOD **Oil-Absorbing Sheets** *($5.79 for 50 fl. oz.)* are an interesting twist on the standard oil-absorbing papers. These are more like soft plastic sheets with a slight rubbery feel. They work well enough, but it takes several of them to make a difference, just as it does with any of the more standard oil-absorbing papers.

☹ POOR **Advantage Acne Control Kit** *($19.99)* is supposed to make fighting acne as easy as 1-2-3, but each of the products in this misguided kit has its share of problems. The **Advantage Acne Control Cleanser** contains 10% benzoyl peroxide, a concentration that can be quite drying, although it won't have time to work because it is rinsed quickly from your skin. A larger problem is the drying detergent cleansing agent sodium C14-16 olefin sulfonate along with menthol, neither of which helps combat blemishes, and which just add irritation and inflammation to skin. Step 2 is the **Advantage Acne Control Moisturizer**, which is reviewed on its own above. Last is the **Advantage Fast Clearing Spot Treatment**, which contains 2% salicylic acid, but also enough alcohol to cause irritation, and that problem is not reduced by the inclusion of cinnamon and cedar bark extracts. In short, there is little reason to expect relief from acne with this kit, and every reason to expect irritated, reddened skin. See the Appendix to learn why irritation is the last thing oily, breakout-prone skin needs.

☹ POOR **Advantage Acne Spot Treatment** *($6.99 for 0.75 fl. oz.)* is a 2% salicylic acid gel with a pH of 3.2, so it can exfoliate the skin's surface and inside the pore lining. That's great, but the alcohol base is problematic, especially when combined with the cinnamon and cedar bark extracts here. You would fare better (a lot better) with the BHA products from Paula's Choice.

☹ POOR **Advantage Mark Treatment** *($6.49)*. Red marks from past acne breakouts are a common problem, but this product is not a good solution. It does contain 2% salicylic acid (BHA) along with the AHA ingredient glycolic acid, and the formula's pH allows exfoliation to occur (and regular exfoliation helps these red marks fade faster). Unfortunately, the base formula contains alcohol and witch hazel, both of which cause significant irritation, which makes red marks worse. Please see the Appendix for details on why irritation is a problem for all skin types, and a real negative for those struggling with breakouts.

CLINIQUE

Strengths: Extensive selection of state-of-the-art moisturizers and serums loaded with ingredients that research has shown are of great benefit to skin; excellent sunscreens; several Redness Solutions products excel; an outstanding benzoyl peroxide product; good selection of self-tanning products; some very good cleansers and eye-makeup removers; some unique mattifying products; a large and impressive selection of foundations, many with reliable sun protection (and shades for darker skin tones), good concealers, some remarkable mascaras, great eyeshadows, loose powder, most of the blush products, some brilliant lipsticks and lip gloss, gel eyeliner, priced lower than most competing department-store lines yet they often offer better (certainly less fragrant) products.

Weaknesses: The three-step skin-care routine because of the bar soaps and irritant-laden clarifying lotions; jar packaging downgrades several otherwise top-notch moisturizers; incomplete routines for those prone to acne; skin-lightening products with either unproven or insufficient levels of lightening agents; the pressed-powder bronzer and brow pencil disappoint; lip plumper; one truly awful mascara.

For more information and reviews of the latest Clinique products, visit CosmeticsCop.com.

CLINIQUE CLEANSERS

✓☺ BEST **Liquid Facial Soap Extra Mild** *($16 for 6.7 fl. oz.)* is not necessarily water-soluble due to its oil content, but it is an excellent option for someone with dry to very dry skin. A true lotion cleanser, it does not contain any detergent cleansing agents, and so is actually a smart choice for someone with sensitive or easily irritated skin (and infinitely better for skin than any of Clinique's bar soaps). The oil content helps dissolve makeup, including mascara, but you'll need a washcloth for complete removal. One nice touch is the anti-irritants, although they are not as beneficial here as they are in leave-on products.

✓☺ BEST **$$$ Comforting Cream Cleanser** *($19.50 for 5 fl. oz)* is an excellent, lotion-type cleanser for normal to dry skin that is close to being water-soluble, but still requires the use of a washcloth for complete removal. This would be an option for normal to dry or sensitive skin, and it is truly fragrance and irritant-free.

✓☺ BEST **$$$ Redness Solutions Soothing Cleanser** *($21.50 for 5 fl. oz.)* is an emollient cleansing lotion that is a fantastic option for those with dry, sensitive skin because it lacks detergent cleansing agents. The emollients and silicone are what remove makeup, though they can impede rinsing and might make it necessary to use a washcloth. This cleanser contains several anti-irritants that are beneficial for all skin types, and because the formula doesn't rinse easily, some of the soothing agents will be left on skin, which is good. The claim that this can make skin smoother with mild exfoliation is inaccurate; there are no exfoliating ingredients in this fragrance-free cleanser. Overall, this should prove a helpful option for those with rosacea and/or dry skin.

✓☺ BEST **$$$ Take The Day Off Cleansing Balm** *($27.50 for 3.8 fl. oz.)* is a modern-day version of a classic cleansing cream. It contains emollients and plant oil to dissolve makeup, and is capable of removing stubborn or waterproof formulas. This is best for dry to very dry skin or sensitive skin not prone to breakouts.

✓☺ BEST **$$$ Take The Day Off Cleansing Milk** *($26 for 6.7 fl. oz.)* is a oilly, light weight cleansing lotion whose solvent dissolves makeup quickly and easily. This doesn't rinse completely without the aid of a washcloth, but is nevertheless a very gentle option for those with normal to dry, sensitive skin. It is fragrance-free. This would be a prime choice for someone with dry skin and rosacea.

☺ GOOD **Wash-Away Gel Cleanser** *($19.50 for 5 fl. oz.)* is a very good, fragrance-free cleanser for oily skin. It feels refreshing, produces a gel-based lather, and rinses without a hint of residue. This also works to remove makeup, though if you wear waterproof mascara you will likely need a separate makeup remover.

☹ AVERAGE **$$$ Liquid Facial Soap Mild Formula** *($16 for 6.7 fl. oz.)* is a fairly basic cleanser that runs the risk of being drying for most skin types because it contains so much salt (sodium chloride). Sodium chloride is present in lots of skin-care products due to its many helpful functions. But, generally, you don't want to see it so high up on the ingredient list because, well, it's salt, and salt is drying (think how your skin feels after a day in the ocean or if you get salt in a cut).

☹ POOR **Acne Solutions Cleansing Bar for Face and Body** *($14 for 5.2 fl. oz)* contains 2% salicylic acid, which is good for acne but useless in a rinse-off product. Beyond that, this bar soap is a poor choice for all skin types, blemishes or not as it may be irritating and drying to skin.

☹ POOR **Acne Solutions Cleansing Foam** *($18.50 for 4.2 fl. oz.)* would have been an excellent liquid-to-foam cleanser for normal to oily skin, but the peppermint is a problem and salicylic acid's benefit in a cleanser is minimal at best because it is rinsed from skin before it can penetrate into the pore lining. This cleanser does contain some very good (and some unique) water-binding agents, but again, their impact on skin won't be great and the peppermint remains a problem.

☹ POOR **Facial Soap Extra Mild** *($12 for 5.2 ounce bar)* may be mild, but it's still standard bar soap and as such can be needlessly drying and irritating to skin. If you prefer bar cleansers, Dove's original Beauty Bar is actually a better, less expensive formulation.

☹ POOR **Facial Soap Mild** *($12 for 5.2 ounce bar)* is a less emollient version of the Facial Soap Extra Mild above, and the same review applies.

☹ POOR **Facial Soap Oily** *($12 for 5.2 ounce bar)* contains a high amount of menthol and sodium borate, both of which are irritating to skin. The irritation from this soap can make oily skin worse (see the Appendix for details).

☹ POOR **Liquid Facial Soap Oily Skin Formula** *($16 for 6.7 fl. oz.)* is similar to the Liquid Facial Soap Mild Formula above, but loses points for the senseless inclusion of menthol. This irritant has no benefit for skin, oily or not. What a shame, because without the menthol this would have been a slam-dunk recommendation for normal to oily skin.

☹ POOR **Rinse-Off Foaming Cleanser** *($19.50 for 5 fl. oz.)* produces copious, creamy foam, but the potassium-based cleansing agents can be drying for most skin types, though they certainly clean well (almost too well, as anyone with dry areas will find them feeling tight and possibly looking flaky from using this cleanser).

CLINIQUE EYE-MAKEUP REMOVERS

✓☺ BEST $$$ **Take The Day Off Makeup Remover for Lids, Lashes & Lips** *($18 for 4.2 fl. oz.)* is a very good, silicone-in-water, dual-phase remover that makes quick work of even the most stubborn foundations, lipsticks, and waterproof mascaras. It is Clinique's most efficient makeup remover and may be used before or after cleansing.

☺ GOOD **Rinse-Off Eye Makeup Solvent** *($17 for 4.2 fl. oz.)* is a basic, no-frills eye-makeup remover that contains mild detergent cleansing agents to dissolve makeup. It does not contain extraneous ingredients that may irritate the eye.

☺ GOOD $$$ **Naturally Gentle Eye Makeup Remover** *($17 for 2.5 fl. oz.)* is indeed gentle, but also oily enough to make it difficult to rinse from the eye area or eyelashes. It is an option, but Clinique's Take the Day Off Makeup Remover for Lids, Lashes & Lips is less messy, easier to rinse, and effectively removes all types of eye makeup.

CLINIQUE TONER

☺ GOOD $$$ **Moisture Surge Face Spray Thirsty Skin Relief** *($21 for 4.2 fl. oz.)* is a very good spray-on, alcohol-free toner. This is a good choice for all skin types, including oily or blemish-prone skin that has minor dry patches.

CLINIQUE EXFOLIANTS & SCRUBS

✓☺ BEST $$$ **Turnaround Concentrate Radiance Renewer, All Skin Types** *($42.50 for 1 fl. oz.)* has claims and a formula that put it in the category of exfoliant, but the formula does more than that, and it's to your skin's benefit. The main exfoliant is the polyhydroxy acid (PHA) lactobionic acid. Functionally similar to AHAs (such as glycolic acid), lactobionic acid's claim to fame is that it is less potentially sensitizing than AHAs, while better at repairing skin's barrier function. There is limited research showing that to be the case, so it isn't a given that lactobionic acid is superior to AHAs or to salicylic acid, a BHA that Clinique includes in other Turnaround products (Sources: *Journal of Cosmetic Dermatology*, March 2010, pages 3–10; and *Cutis*, February 2004, pages 3–13). Still, it can be a good alternative for those who cannot tolerate AHAs, and it is capable of exfoliating skin when formulated within the correct pH range, which is the case for this Turnaround product! Going beyond daily exfoliation, this silky, serum-textured product supplies skin with a wide range of antioxidants and skin-repairing ingredients to improve its texture and fight signs of aging. The fragrance-free formula is suitable for all skin types, including sensitive skin. Some of the plant extracts have intriguing research demonstrating efficacy in lightening sun-induced brown spots, but first and foremost this is an exfoliant, which also supplies skin with a good range of beneficial ingredients. Note: This product contains a small amount of the mineral pigment mica. As such, it leaves a slightly shiny finish that those with oily skin may not like.

☺ GOOD $$$ **7 Day Scrub Cream Rinse-Off Formula** *($18.50 for 3.4 fl. oz.)* rinses decently, but may still require use of a washcloth for complete removal. It also contains polyethylene as the scrub agent, and is an option for normal to slightly dry skin not prone to blemishes.

☺ GOOD **Mild Clarifying Lotion** *($12.50 for 6.7 fl. oz.)* puts all of Clinique's other Clarifying Lotions to shame with its alcohol-free formula that contains 0.5% salicylic acid at an effective pH of 2.9. Although a higher concentration of salicylic acid would be more effective for someone battling blemishes and blackheads, this is a step in the right direction and contains some very good skin-identical ingredients.

☺ AVERAGE $$$ **Turnaround Instant Facial** *($36.50 for 2.5 fl. oz.)* is a water- and silicone-based scrub that contains diatomaceous earth (ground-up porous rock composed of the skeletons of sea creatures) to manually scrub skin. The formula also features salicylic acid, but the pH is too high for it to function as an exfoliant. Even if it worked in this manner, you're not going to gain much benefit from the 5 minutes this product is supposed to be left on skin before rinsing. Not to mention that scrubbing the skin for 5 minutes is just plain excessive, and potentially damaging to the skin. Consider this an expensive face scrub that can be difficult to rinse because of the silicones (though ironically the silicones help buffer skin from the abrasiveness of the diatomaceous earth). The beneficial ingredients Clinique added look good on the label, but antioxidants, anti-irritants, and cell-communicating ingredients are most effective in leave-on products; rinsing them down the drain doesn't help your skin. Turnaround Instant Facial is best for normal to dry or slightly oily skin.

☹ POOR **Acne Solutions Clarifying Lotion** *($14 for 6.7 fl. oz.)* doesn't improve on Clinique's long-standing Clarifying Lotions. This version still contains a lot of alcohol and a lesser but still potentially problematic amount of witch hazel. Without those, it would be an excellent toner for all skin types, though the 1.5% salicylic acid cannot exfoliate due to the pH of the formula.

☹ POOR **Clarifying Lotion 1** *($12.50 for 6.7 fl. oz.)* still lists alcohol as the second ingredient, and that makes this BHA (salicylic acid) product too irritating for all skin types. The alcohol this contains will trigger oil production at the base of your pores, not to mention cause free-radical damage and irritation.

☹ POOR **Clarifying Lotion 2** *($12.50 for 6.7 fl. oz.)* is an alcohol-based BHA exfoliant that contains potent skin-irritants witch hazel and menthol. The Clinique salespeople may claim that the alcohol is "cosmetics-grade," which sounds nice, but doesn't make this product any less irritating. The alcohol this contains will trigger oil production at the base of your pores, making oily or combination skin worse. See the Appendix for further details.

☹ POOR **Clarifying Lotion 3** *($12.50 for 6.7 fl. oz.)* lists alcohol as the second ingredient, and that makes this BHA product too irritating for all skin types. The alcohol this contains will trigger oil production at the base of your pores, not to mention cause free-radical damage and irritation.

☹ POOR **Clarifying Lotion 4** *($12.50 for 6.7 fl. oz.)* lists alcohol as the second ingredient, and that makes this BHA product too irritating for all skin types. The alcohol this contains (and its aroma is unmistakable) will trigger oil production at the base of your pores, not to mention cause free-radical damage and irritation.

☹ POOR **Exfoliating Scrub** *($18.50 for 3.4 fl. oz.)* is Clinique's most abrasive topical scrub and also its most irritating, thanks to menthol. This is a great way to abrade skin's surface, causing barrier disruption that leads to persistent dry, flaky skin or skin that's "dry underneath and oily on top." If that describes your skin and you're using this scrub, please stop.

CLINIQUE MOISTURIZERS (DAYTIME & NIGHTTIME), EYE CREAMS, & SERUMS

✓☺ BEST **City Block Sheer Oil-Free Daily Face Protector SPF 25** *($19 for 1.4 fl. oz.)* protects skin from sun damage with its actives of titanium dioxide and zinc oxide. The lightweight but still moisturizing base is best for normal to dry or sensitive skin, including those dealing with rosacea. Clinique included a very good blend of antioxidants and cell-communicating ingredients, so this is highly recommended for those seeking a gentle sunscreen. It is slightly tinted to offset the whitening effect from the amount of mineral sunscreens it contains.

✓☺ BEST **Redness Solutions Daily Protective Base SPF 15** *($18.50 for 1.35 fl. oz.)* gets the gentle sunscreen right with its pure titanium dioxide and zinc oxide blend. The base formula is similar to that of Clinique's City Block Sheer Oil-Free Daily Face Protector SPF 25 above, which is also suitable for someone with sensitive, reddened skin (and that's why this earns a Best Product rating). Both products contain some very good water-binding agents, skin-identical substances, and antioxidants. However, it is worth nothing that the aforementioned Clinique City Block Sheer offers skin a greater complement of beneficial ingredients. The only advantage of the Redness Solutions is its sheer green tint (if you consider that a plus). When applied to skin, the green tint becomes a pale flesh tone that provides a bit of coverage. If you have superficial, minor redness, you'll notice it is less apparent, but that would be true for any tinted moisturizer, too. Anyone with lingering or persistent redness (such as occurs with rosacea) will want to pair this with a foundation that supplies at least medium coverage. One more thing: The finish of this product is matte, but also somewhat chalky. It can lend a flat appearance to skin that someone not bothered with oiliness may not like.

✓☺ BEST **Sun SPF 30 Face Cream** *($19 for 1.7 fl. oz.)* is among Clinique's sunscreens (in their sun-care line, not in their "regular" facial-care line) that claim to use what the company refers to as SolarSmart technology. This technology is supposed to trigger a repair mechanism in skin to help prevent signs of aging. What they're really referring to are the antioxidants in this sunscreen; the claim is basically just a new way of stating what we've known for some time: that antioxidants added to sunscreens help boost the efficacy of the active ingredients while also helping skin defend itself against sun damage (Sources: *Clinics in Dermatology*, November-December 2008, pages 614–626; and *Photochemistry and Photobiology*, July-August 2006, pages 1016–1023). That doesn't mean Clinique's sun-care products are superior to others that also contain antioxidants, although that could certainly be inferred from the claims they're making. Nevertheless, this is an outstanding sunscreen formula for normal to dry skin. It contains a wide range of antioxidants and cell-communicating ingredients as well as stabilized avobenzone for UVA protection. We disagree with Clinique that this sunscreen is gentle enough for sensitive skin. Without question, the active ingredients it contains can absolutely be sensitizing for all skin types, although that doesn't mean they shouldn't be considered or that they don't have value when it comes to protecting skin from sun damage. Anyone with sensitive, reactive skin should stick with sunscreens whose only active ingredients are titanium dioxide and/or zinc oxide. This sunscreen is fragrance-free and contains mica, a mineral pigment that leaves a slight shimmer on skin. Its formula is a bit tricky to use with makeup, but it works well if you prefer pressed-powder foundations over creams or liquids.

✓☺ BEST **Sun SPF 50 Face Cream** *($19 for 1.7 fl. oz.)* is similar to Clinique's Sun SPF 30 Face Cream above, and the same comments apply. Keep in mind that SPF 50 is probably too much (there aren't that many hours of daylight in most parts of the world), but if you tend to be someone who doesn't apply sunscreen liberally, this will help ensure you get enough sunscreen ingredients on your skin to at least equal an SPF 20 or so depending on how much you apply.

✓☺ BEST **$$$ Super Rescue Antioxidant Night Moisturizer, for Combination Oily to Oily Skin** *($44.50 for 1.7 fl. oz.)* claims that using this will protect your skin from free-radical damage and help make it stronger. It's true that antioxidants applied topically (and consumed as part of a healthy diet) do much to diffuse and reduce free-radical damage, but it isn't physically possible to stop free-radical damage in its entirety. Antioxidants have their place in skin-care products, but they are not an all-out rescue from or an impervious shield against free-radical damage. Super Rescue is suitable for normal to combination skin, but is probably too heavy for oily skin or really oily areas. It contains some great emollients, silicone, slip agents, several antioxidants, Vaseline, cell-communicating ingredients, and soothing plant extracts. The only frustrating element is that half of the really intriguing ingredients are listed after one of the preservatives, which means that they're basically window dressing. However, even without considering the mere dustings of those ingredients, this fragrance-free moisturizer is still antioxidant-packed, and it is recommended for normal to slightly dry or slightly oily skin. What's more, the opaque tube packaging keeps the many light- and air-sensitive ingredients stable during use. All of Clinique's Super Rescue Antioxidant Night Moisturizers are fragrance-free and suitable for sensitive skin.

✓☺ BEST $$$ **Super Rescue Antioxidant Night Moisturizer, for Dry Combination Skin** *($44.50 for 1.7 fl. oz.)* is similar to the Super Rescue Antioxidant Night Moisturizer for Combination to Oily Skin above, except this has a more emollient texture that's best for normal to dry skin. It will feel too heavy on oily areas and is not the best for breakout-prone skin.

✓☺ BEST $$$ **Super Rescue Antioxidant Night Moisturizer, for Very Dry to Dry Skin** *($44.50 for 1.7 fl. oz.)* is the richest of Clinique's three Super Rescue Antioxidant Night Moisturizers, and is appropriate for dry to very dry skin. Interestingly, this version contains greater amounts of antioxidants known for their potent anti-inflammatory effect. That attention to detail can help dry skin repair itself because the less inflammation skin endures, the better able it is to strengthen itself and repair damage. Otherwise, the same comments made above for the Super Rescue Antioxidant Night Moisturizer for Combination to Oily Skin apply here, too.

☺ GOOD **Dramatically Different Moisturizing Gel in Tube** *($13 for 1.7 fl. oz.)* is more a lotion than a gel, but does feel quite light and silky on the skin. It does not contain any oils or heavy thickening agents, and this fragrance-free moisturizer is appropriate for normal to slightly dry or slightly oily skin. The only issue we have with the product is its meager antioxidant content (though it has some great anti-irritants). Most of Clinique's moisturizers are brimming with state-of-the-art ingredients, but this one, though certainly effective for its intended skin types, is plain by comparison—yet dramatically better than their original and still incredibly popular yellow lotion.

☺ GOOD $$$ **Even Better Skin Tone Correcting Lotion Broad Spectrum SPF 20 Combination to Oily Skin** *($44.50 for 1.7 fl. oz.)*. This is a very good, lightweight daytime moisturizer with sunscreen. It is well suited for its intended skin types, and contains stabilized avobenzone for critical UVA (think anti-aging) protection. The silky, fluid texture slips easily over skin, but if you were hoping for an absorbent or matte finish, you're out of luck: this leaves a sheen despite feeling light. If you follow with a matte finish foundation and/or powder, the sheen is a non-issue, and it's great that the formula contains a range of antioxidants, including vitamin C as well as smaller but potentially helpful amounts of repairing ingredients. This contains grapefruit peel extract which poses a slight risk of irritation, but it's certainly not as bad as pure grapefruit peel oil (which is a concentrated source of fragrant irritants skin doesn't need). Although this contains salicylic acid, the pH is markedly out of the range it needs to function as an exfoliant. Even if the pH was within the required range, the amount of salicylic acid present is likely below 0.5%, which isn't enough to exfoliate skin. Still, this fragrance-free Even Better product has a lot going for it, though you don't need to spend in this range for an effective, broad-spectrum moisturizer with sunscreen.

☺ GOOD **$$$ Repairwear Laser Focus Wrinkle & UV Damage Corrector** *($44.50 for 1 fl. oz.)* is just another well-formulated serum that will make your skin (and wrinkles) softer and smoother, just like countless other well-formulated options. Just to make sure you're aware, this doesn't have anything to do with what real lasers can do for skin. Not a single ingredient (or mix of ingredients) in this serum is capable of even vaguely creating the results a dermatologist can provide. By associating this with laser treatments, Clinique has garnered a considerable amount of attention for this Repairwear product. According to the company, after 12 weeks of applying this serum every day, results come close to what's possible from a laser treatment. Of course, Clinique didn't publish their study, so there is no way to know what their purported results mean, if anything. What will grab consumers is the fact that this serum isn't expensive, at least not when compared with its department store competitors (or with laser treatments), and the packaging will keep the ingredients stable. The formula does contain a nice mix of antioxidants, silicones, and a smaller, but still potentially helpful, amount of cell-communicating and skin-identical ingredients. Ironically, for all the hoopla surrounding Repairwear Laser Focus, its formula isn't as impressive as the formulas of Clinique's now-discontinued Repairwear serum or many products from other Estee Lauder–owned lines, including the Lauder brand, whose Perfectionist and Advanced Night Repair Concentrate serums have better formulas for aging skin. According to one of the press releases for Repairwear Laser Focus (which is not a study), it was tested side-by-side with Erbium laser treatments. (An Erbium laser is an ablative laser that removes several layers of the epidermis to improve wrinkles and discolorations.) Subjects applied the serum to one side of their face and had an Erbium laser treatment done on the other. It wasn't specified if the subjects had one or several laser treatments, but given that results were monitored every four weeks, it is highly unlikely the Erbium laser was used each time. Just one treatment with this laser can result in downtime of a week or more as skin heals, but the results can be remarkable, surpassing what any serum can provide. More important, the benefits from any laser treatment take time to show up, and Clinique only measured results at 4, 8, and 12 weeks! And lasers aren't serums or moisturizers! Of course, none of this reality stopped Clinique from stating that results from Repairwear Laser Focus were nearly equivalent to what you can expect to see after a series of three Erbium laser treatments. But again, the details of the study are unavailable, so you're left to put your faith in Clinique and hope for the best. The problem? As most ethical cosmetic dermatologists will tell you, skin-care products cannot and do not have the same effects as laser treatments. Serums like this can improve skin's texture and help stimulate healthy collagen production, but they cannot affect skin the same way lasers do, and there's no research proving otherwise, despite Clinique's press release. Your skin will feel better and your wrinkles will appear softer when you apply this serum, but that's true of any well-formulated serum. For the best of both worlds, a smart approach to anti-aging is to pair a state-of-the-art skin-care routine with the cosmetic corrective procedures that are appropriate for addressing the concerns you have about how your skin is aging. One more comment: There's an ingredient blend in this serum known by the trade name Pinoxide, which is a blend of pinanediol, camphanediol, and butylene glycol. These glycol-type ingredients are categorized as skin-conditioning agents, but there is research—from the ingredient manufacturer and biopharmaceutical company AGI Dermatics—that Pinoxide can reduce dark circles, increase circulation, and strengthen skin's elasticity and collagen production (Source: miinews.com/pdf/sep_oct_07/AGIDerm_Ed_ABG0907v4-082207.pdf). That sounds promising, but there is no independent, peer-reviewed research to support these claims. Besides, lots of ingredients can help stimulate collagen production and help repair sun-damaged skin (to some extent). Pinoxide is not the best, must-have ingredient blend.

☺ AVERAGE **Dramatically Different Moisturizing Lotion** (*$24.50 for 4.2 fl. oz.*) is one of Clinique's flagship products, but it's really just a basic, mundane, out-of-date, yellow-toned moisturizer built around mineral oil and sesame oil. It's an option for dry skin and is fragrance-free, but other than its reasonable price tag, there is nothing especially attractive or beneficial about this product. You can do far better for your skin.

☺ AVERAGE **Pore Refining Solutions Stay-Matte Hydrator Dry Combination to Oily** (*$36 for 1.7 fl. oz.*). This is nearly identical to Clinique's former Pore Minimizer Refining Lotion. This is a water- and silicone-based fluid lotion that also contains a good deal of film-forming agent (which can temporarily make pores look smaller) along with alcohol and the absorbents silica and talc. Clinique claims that, with ongoing use, this product makes pores smaller, but nothing in this formula supports that claim. If anything, daily exposure to the high amount of film-forming agent and alcohol can cause chronic irritation, and that won't strengthen pores in the least. This is best used as a temporary mattifying product, though products like Paula's Choice Shine Stopper Instant Matte Finish or Smashbox's Anti-Shine Foundation are more effective options. And for even better results, you can use a well-formulated BHA exfoliant to further improve pore size and prevent clogging. This contains an ingredient blend known as LipoLight, which is said to diffuse light to "drastically reduce the appearance of skin imperfections." This complex is a blend of the polymer polydodecanamideaminium triazadiphenylethenesulfonate and polyvinyl alcohol, a film-forming ingredient most often found in peel-off masks and hair sprays. The polymer complex gives this product an interesting texture and helps skin appear smoother, but its benefit isn't unusual or special. In any light, your pores will look a bit smaller with this on, but the trade-offs from the problematic ingredients this product contains aren't really worth it—not when there are other products that reduce pore size without irritation.

☹ AVERAGE **Super City Block Oil-Free Daily Face Protector SPF 40** (*$19 for 1.4 fl. oz.*) is a daytime moisturizer with sunscreen, which contains titanium dioxide and zinc oxide for UVA protection along with a couple of synthetic sunscreen actives. Because of the synthetic actives, this is not preferred to Clinique's Super City Block with SPF 25 for those with sensitive skin. On balance, this isn't preferred in general because it contains several fragrant plant extracts including angelica, which is known to cause a phototoxic reaction when skin is exposed to sunlight. Granted, with a product like this you're getting sun protection so the likelihood of a reaction between sunlight and the angelica plant is low, but still, why include it at all? It's not as though it's a superior ingredient or there aren't any other antioxidant plant extracts to consider. This has a sheer, flesh-toned tint and also contains mica for a soft shine finish. The formula is best for normal to slightly dry or slightly oily skin but again, it's a tough sell. Clinique offers better options for daytime sun protection, as do its sister brands Estee Lauder and M.A.C.

☺ AVERAGE **$$$ All About Eyes** (*$29 for 0.5 fl. oz.*) is one of Clinique's most popular items, and its silicone-based formula leaves skin very smooth and silky. It contains some outstanding ingredients to fortify skin and allow it to repair itself, but many of these are compromised by packaging that exposes them to light and air. Clever cosmetic pigment technology changes the way light is reflected off shadowed areas, temporarily improving the appearance of dark circles (sort of like a concealer but without coverage). If only Clinique would get this out of a jar and into an opaque tube, it would be a winner! See the Appendix to learn why jar packaging is a problem and why, despite the positives of All About Eyes, you don't need an eye cream.

☺ AVERAGE **$$$ All About Eyes Rich** (*$29 for 0.5 fl. oz.*) is an emollient version of the All About Eyes, but unlike that product, whose silkiness is largely due to its silicone base, All About Eyes Rich contains several emollients, chiefly shea butter. It is indeed a moisture-rich product and is preferred for dry to very dry skin around the eyes or elsewhere on the face. It cannot diminish dark circles or puffy eyes as claimed. The usual roster of antioxidants, anti-irritants, and ingredients that mimic the structure and function of healthy skin are present, but the antioxidants won't remain potent for long given the jar packaging. See the Appendix for details on the problems jar packaging presents and find out why, in truth, you don't need an eye cream.

☺ AVERAGE $$$ **All About Eyes Serum De-Puffing Eye Massage** (*$26 for 0.5 fl. oz.*). This "serum" is really a water-based, thin-textured gel. It is housed in a cylindrical component and the product is dispensed onto a metal roller-ball applicator. Massaging this serum around the eyes does feel soothing, and the metal ball applicator provides a brief cooling effect. However, most cases of puffy eyes, particularly those related to aging, cannot be massaged away. If only it were that simple, who would bemoan their puffy eyes, right? Like most Clinique facial and eye-area moisturizers or serums, the formula contains an impressive mix of antioxidants, cell-communicating ingredients, and some skin-identical substances. With one exception (explained below) none of them have solid research demonstrating they're the solution for dark circles or under-eye puffiness; however, they certainly have benefit for skin, around the eyes or elsewhere. The exception ingredient in this eye serum is caffeine. When applied topically, caffeine serves as an anti-inflammatory and has a constrictive effect on skin, which may lead to a reduced puffiness, assuming it arises from edema (swelling) and not aging (Sources: *Planta Medica*, October 2008, pages 1548–1559; and naturaldatabase.com). It is disappointing that fragrant tangerine peel extract is included in an amount that's likely to cause irritation. Tangerine peel contains volatile components that can irritate on contact. Although we don't typically comment on our personal experience with a skin-care product, we did experience a stinging reaction from All About Eyes Serum. For this reason, it's a tough product to recommend, especially given that lots of other facial moisturizers (which are fine to use around the eye) contain beneficial ingredients without the risk of irritation.

☺ AVERAGE $$$ **Even Better Skin Tone Correcting Moisturizer SPF 20** (*$44.50 for 1.7 fl. oz.*) has enticing claims but this is just another in-part avobenzone sunscreen, similar to others from Clinique's Superdefense line, right down to the price and the unfortunate use of jar packaging. Interestingly, the Superdefense products offer SPF 25, but in this case the Even Better with SPF 20 is supposed to be the one that provides a "high level" defense! Other than the difference in SPF rating, the main point of difference between Even Better and Superdefense is that Even Better claims to "break apart surface darkening and exfoliate it away." That's an enticing claim, but one that won't come true. The only ingredient in Even Better with proven exfoliating ability is salicylic acid (BHA), which when properly formulated, is a great exfoliant (among other benefits). In this product, however, both the low amount of salicylic acid (less than 1%) and the high pH don't permit it to work as it could. The only research showing that acetyl glucosamine is effective for improving skin discolorations comes from the cosmetics companies using it. That's not terrible but not as balanced as it could be, either. You'll get reliable broad-spectrum sun protection from this moisturizer for normal to slightly dry skin, but that's about it. Keeping skin protected from sunlight will help prevent future discolorations, but that's true for all well-formulated sunscreens. But, back to the jar packaging issue: It's a shame Clinique is still relying on jars. As is the case with most of their moisturizers, those with and without sunscreen, this contains a brilliant array of beneficial ingredients for skin, but many of them won't remain stable due to the jar packaging. See the Appendix for further details on jar packaging.

☺ AVERAGE $$$ **Moisture Surge Extended Thirst Relief** *($36 for 1.7 fl. oz.)* is in jar packaging, which will ensure that the antioxidants this contains won't remain potent after the product is opened. Also, the amount of peptide is rather small, which isn't what most people would consider impressive. Promising to never let skin go thirsty again (which is odd because it takes much more than water to replenish dry skin), this silicone-enhanced moisturizer ends up being an OK option for normal to slightly dry or slightly oily skin, but Clinique definitely sells better moisturizers.

☺ AVERAGE $$$ **Moisture Surge Intense Skin Fortifying Hydrator** *($36 for 1.69 fl. oz.)* doesn't contain a brilliant assortment of ingredients for seriously dry, dehydrated skin. Its texture and fragrance-free formula are best for normal to slightly dry skin or for oily skin struggling with dry patches. As is typical for Clinique, this moisturizer contains several antioxidants, repairing ingredients, and cell-communicating ingredients. Skin needs all of these to repair itself and act younger. The problem? Many of those ingredients are not stable upon repeated exposure to light and air—and this moisturizer is packaged in a jar, so that exposure is guaranteed to happen. See the Appendix for further details on the problems jar packaging presents.

☺ AVERAGE $$$ **Redness Solutions Daily Relief Cream** *($42.50 for 1.7 fl. oz.)* is an impressive soothing moisturizer for dry, reddened skin—but the jar packaging remains an issue. The plethora of antioxidants (Clinique is rarely stingy with such ingredients) is not going to be of much ongoing benefit once the product is opened. This is an overall brilliant moisturizer formula, but any major benefits are lost due to the poor packaging decision. See the Appendix for further details on the issues with jar packaging.

☺ AVERAGE $$$ **Repairwear Day SPF 15 Intensive Cream** *($49.50 for 1.7 fl. oz.)* is an excellent, in-part zinc oxide sunscreen in a moisturizing base that's characteristic of the best moisturizers from Clinique, but it also has jar packaging (see the Appendix to find out why that's a problem). Some of the plant extracts can be problematic, but they are present in small amounts and the beneficial plant extracts and cell-communicating ingredients have them outnumbered. Clinique maintains that Repairwear "helps block and mend the look of lines and wrinkles," though that's true only to the extent that an effective sunscreen, which this product contains, can prevent further skin damage. As well-formulated as this product is, please don't be fooled into thinking it can repair your skin and eliminate wrinkles, or you're bound to be disappointed. The fact that this is described as an intensive cream may make you think it is for very dry skin, but it's actually best for normal to dry skin.

☺ AVERAGE $$$ **Repairwear Day SPF 15 Intensive Cream, Very Dry Skin Formula** *($49.50 for 1.7 fl. oz.)* is a more emollient, dry-to-very-dry-skin-appropriate version of the Repairwear Day SPF 15 Intensive Cream above, and the same comments apply.

☺ AVERAGE $$$ **Repairwear Intensive Eye Cream** *($40 for 0.5 fl. oz.)* has a lot going for it in terms of its plentiful antioxidant content—that's why the choice of jar packaging was a bad one, because these ingredients won't remain potent once the product is opened and used repeatedly. It's a good emollient eye cream for dry skin, but opaque tube packaging would have made it a slam-dunk. See the Appendix to learn why, in truth, you don't need an eye cream.

☺ AVERAGE $$$ **Repairwear Intensive Night Cream** *($49.50 for 1.7 fl. oz.)* is an elegant formulation that covers all the bases when it comes to a modern combination of emollients, skin-identical ingredients, antioxidants, and cell-communicating ingredients—yet the effectiveness of several of those ingredients is compromised due to the jar packaging. This does contain a jasmine oil–derived fragrance in the form of methyldihydrojasmonate, which refutes Clinique's

100% fragrance-free assertion. One more thing: other than not containing sunscreen (essential for daytime) nothing about this moisturizer is special for use at night.

☺ AVERAGE $$$ **Repairwear Intensive Night Cream, Very Dry Skin Formula** (*$49.50 for 1.7 fl. oz.*) is a richer, creamier version of the Repairwear Intensive Night Cream above, and the same basic comments apply.

☺ AVERAGE $$$ **Superdefense SPF 25 Age Defense Moisturizer, for Combination Oily to Oily Skin** (*$44.50 for 1.7 fl. oz.*) contains in-part avobenzone, so the critical UVA portion is covered (and the avobenzone is stabilized by octocrylene, another active sunscreen ingredient). This daytime moisturizer is loaded with antioxidants, water-binding agents, and cell-communicating ingredients. The silky-textured formula is ideal for its intended skin types because it supplies light hydration and skin-beneficial ingredients without potentially problematic thickening agents. Unfortunately, the choice of jar packaging takes this daytime moisturizer from "super" to "average," and that's not what your skin needs. See the Appendix to learn why jar packaging is a problem you shouldn't overlook.

☺ AVERAGE $$$ **Superdefense SPF 25 Age Defense Moisturizer, for Dry Combination Skin** (*$44.50 for 1.7 fl. oz*). The silky-textured lightweight cream formula is suitable for its intended skin types, but those with oily areas will not be pleased with the satin sheen finish. Otherwise, the same comments made above for the Superdefense SPF 25 Age Defense Moisturizer, for Combination Oily to Oily Skin apply here, too.

☺ AVERAGE $$$ **Superdefense SPF 25 Age Defense Moisturizer, for Very Dry to Dry Skin** (*$42.50 for 1.7 fl. oz*) has a cream-textured, substantive formula that is well suited for its intended skin types. Otherwise, the same comments made above for the Superdefense SPF 25 Age Defense Moisturizer, for Combination Oily to Oily Skin apply here, too.

☺ AVERAGE $$$ **Turnaround Overnight Radiance Moisturizer, Very Dry to Combination Oily** (*$44.50 for 1.7 fl. oz.*) is another of Clinique's offerings for various Turnaround products over the years, yet none of them have ever been all that great. This is mostly due to the fact that although salicylic acid is included for exfoliation, the pH is above 4, which means it cannot function as an exfoliant. That wouldn't necessarily be a deal-breaker because this product provides numerous other great ingredients. Unfortunately, the jar packaging won't keep many of them stable once you begin using this, and that includes several antioxidants that would otherwise benefit your skin. See the Appendix for further details on why jar packaging is a problem. Getting back to the exfoliation, you may see some skin-smoothing benefits from the form of urea and acetyl glucosamine they include in this product, but there isn't a lot of research to fall back on, and there are only small amounts anyway. Nothing about this formula is optimized to assist your skin's renewal process at night. Skin is renewing and attempting to repair itself 24 hours a day; there is no research proving that this process somehow ramps up or becomes vastly more efficient during the evening hours. Besides, what would that mean for people who work all night and sleep during the day? Would their skin be less renewed because they're awake during hours most of us sleep? At best, this is an OK moisturizer for normal to dry skin.

☺ AVERAGE $$$ **Youth Surge Night Age Decelerating Night Moisturizer Dry Combination** (*$44.50 for 1.7 fl. oz.*) is just like Clinique's Youth Surge daytime moisturizers with sunscreen. The nighttime version is sold around the concept of sirtuin technology. This technology is said to enhance your skin's ability to repair itself, but is there anything to it? Sirtuins are proteins that are involved in regulating biological processes by controlling the chain of events that cause these processes to occur, which is why they're often referred to as information regulators. The anti-aging connection has to do with their potential to regulate cellular processes responsible for aging. It is believed that if certain sirtuins can be modified to work against the mechanisms of aging that the results might be visible on skin: think fewer wrinkles, less sagging, and greater resiliency. Although there is no research showing that skin-care products can change or manipulate sirtuin production to affect wrinkles in any way, Clinique's advertising for this product subtly suggests otherwise implying that the research about sirtuins and degenerative disease is somehow related to wrinkles. More to the point is what about all of Clinique's other "de-agers" that don't contain sirtuins? Do those not work as well because they lack this technology? What seems promising is that topical application of specific sirtuins derived from yeast and the antioxidant resveratrol (in this case from the root of the plant *Polygonum cuspidatum*) seem to have a protective effect on skin in the presence of oxidative and ultraviolet light stress. However, more research is needed before we'd suggest anyone run out and look for products that increase sirtuin activity in their skin. Plus, we don't know the risks associated with manipulating sirtuins; doing so might have negative side effects. The problem is twofold. First, there is limited research showing how much and what type of sirtuin is needed topically to cause desirable cellular changes that might lead to younger-looking skin. Plus, the bioavailability of a topically applied source of sirtuins is questionable given that we don't know how efficiently they penetrate intact skin. (Testing skin cells in a lab setting with concentrated doses of ingredients that stimulate sirtuins is an entirely different story from using moisturizers on intact skin.) Second, and an even bigger concern, is that whenever normal cellular processes are manipulated, you run the risk of causing a potential overproliferation of cells. In other words, how would the sirtuin-influenced cells know when too much of a good thing becomes a problem? How long is too long to keep skin cells active? You also must consider how much manipulation of biological processes is enough to start a cascading negative chain of events, the consequences of which could be cancer (Sources: *Current Medicinal Chemistry*, 2008, pages 1887–1899; *Journal of Drugs in Dermatology*, June 2007, pages 14–19; and *Nature Reviews: Drug Discovery*, June 2006, pages 493–506). Putting aside the marketing nonsense about sirtuins, this lightweight cream moisturizer for normal to slightly oily or slightly dry skin is loaded with antioxidants, cell-communicating ingredients, and, to a lesser degree, skin-identical (repairing) substances. Unfortunately, the jar packaging won't keep the majority of these state-of-the-art ingredients stable during use. Please see the Appendix to learn more about why jar packaging is a problem.

☺ AVERAGE $$$ **Youth Surge Night Age Decelerating Night Moisturizer, Very Dry to Dry** *($49.50 for 1.7 fl. oz.)* is a more emollient version of Clinique's Youth Surge Night Age Decelerating Night Moisturizer, Dry Combination, and other than its richer texture for dry skin, the same review applies.

☺ AVERAGE $$$ **Youth Surge SPF 15 Age Decelerating Moisturizer, Combination Oily to Oily** *($48.50 for 1.7 fl. oz.)* is said to leverage sirtuin technology to tackle lines and wrinkles. Before we discuss sirtuins and skin, it is worth asking what the company means by "leverage." By stating in their ads that their product is "Leveraging sirtuin technology," they could mean gaining advantage from this technology, paying to use this technology, or, really, whatever they want it to mean. It doesn't say the technology is making a difference and changing the structure of your skin. Look closely at the claims for the Youth Surge products and you'll see that every statement they make is a purely cosmetic claim. "Visible effects" could mean anything—visible effects of what? "Seem to evaporate" doesn't mean that lines and wrinkles will really go away, it could mean that water evaporates, and the word "seems" doesn't mean it is actually happening. "Skin gains strength" is a strange claim that might lead you to believe it will build collagen or skin will appear more taut, but it could really mean just about anything you want it to mean. That's the art of cosmetics ad copy. Please see the review for Youth Surge Night Age Decelerating Night Moisturizer Dry Combination above for a discussion of sirtuins and their use (or lack thereof) for aging skin. This daytime moisturizer with sunscreen includes reliable UVA protection (from titanium dioxide, though a higher percentage would be preferred) and is loaded with antioxidants, cell-communicating ingredients, and, to a lesser degree, skin-identical substances. Unfortunately, jar packaging won't keep the majority of these state-of-the-art ingredients stable during use. Youth Surge's sunscreen is the only "age decelerating" effect you can rely on, but we'd advise you to look for equally impressive formulas in better packaging. If you decide to try this anyway, it's best for normal to dry skin; those with oily skin will find it way too creamy.

☺ AVERAGE $$$ **Youth Surge SPF 15 Age Decelerating Moisturizer, Dry Combination** *($49.50 for 1.7 fl. oz.)* is similar to Clinique's Youth Surge SPF 15 Age Decelerating Moisturizer Combination Oily to Oily above, though this version is preferred for dry skin. Those with combination skin (meaning oily and dry areas) will find this to be too emollient for their oily areas—and sunscreen needs to be applied all over. Otherwise, the same comments and cautions apply.

☺ AVERAGE $$$ **Youth Surge SPF 15 Age Decelerating Moisturizer, Very Dry to Dry** *($49.50 for 1.7 fl. oz.)* is similar to Clinique's Youth Surge SPF 15 Age Decelerating Moisturizer Combination Oily to Oily above, though this version is preferred for normal to dry skin. Those with very dry skin will likely prefer the Youth Surge formula for Dry Combination skin, though please see the comments on sirtuin technology and jar packaging above before handing over your credit card for this moisturizer.

☺ AVERAGE $$$ **Zero Gravity Repairwear Lift Firming Cream, for Combination Oily to Oily Skin** *($56 for 1.7 fl. oz.)* promises an instant firming sensation but a sensation isn't the same as an actual result, and about all this moisturizer will do instantly is make skin feel smoother and softer. That won't help skin stand up to gravity's downward assault, but then again, no skin-care product can do that. As is true for most of Clinique moisturizers, this is loaded with antioxidants, cell-communicating ingredients (including retinol), and ingredients that mimic the structure and function of healthy skin. The problem with this product is twofold: jar packaging won't keep the buzzworthy ingredient stable during use and the inclusion of alcohol (it's the sixth ingredient) prior to any antioxidant is a letdown because alcohol causes free-radical damage (see the Appendix for further details on jar packaging and alcohol). Considering the price and aforementioned detriments, this moisturizer is a tough sell. The mineral pigments in this product lend a soft glow to skin.

☺ AVERAGE $$$ **Zero Gravity Repairwear Lift Firming Cream, for Dry Combination Skin** *($56 for 1.7 fl. oz.)* makes the same claims as the Zero Gravity Repairwear Lift Firming Cream, for Combination Oily to Oily Skin, but omits the alcohol and contains several thickeners to create a creamier texture suitable for normal to dry skin (not combination skin, assuming part of this combination includes oily areas). It's still unfortunate that so many light- and air-sensitive ingredients are prone to breaking down quickly once this jar-packaged moisturizer is opened.

☺ AVERAGE $$$ **Zero Gravity Repairwear Lift Firming Cream, for Very Dry to Dry Skin** *($56 for 1.7 fl. oz.)* has a surprisingly lighter texture than the Zero Gravity Repairwear Lift Firming Cream, for Dry Combination Skin above, despite being labeled for very dry skin.

The glycerin, plant oil, and emollient thickeners are certainly capable of making any degree of dry skin look and feel better, but the state-of-the-art efficacious ingredients (numerous antioxidants and several cell-communicating ingredients, including retinol) won't last for long once this jar-packaged moisturizer is opened.

☹ POOR **Pore Refining Solutions Correcting Serum** *($39.50 for 1 fl. oz.)* has a silky texture and this slightly tinted serum is supposed to clear your pores of the debris that causes them to become enlarged, which in turn, makes magnifying mirrors your skin's worst enemy. Although the formula contains several helpful ingredients (including many antioxidants), the amount of alcohol is cause for concern. Alcohol causes dryness and irritation as well as free-radical damage that hurts your skin's healing process and ability to become healthier. In testing this product we noted a distinct alcohol scent, which is not good news for those hoping this would make their pore problem vanish. See the Appendix to learn why alcohol is especially bad for oily skin. The salicylic acid this contains is present in an amount too low for exfoliation to occur, plus the pH is too high for it to work as an exfoliant (salicylic acid needs a pH range of 3-4 to be effective). In the end, despite Clinique's guarantee of your pores looking 58% smaller, this isn't a great bet for daily use over the long haul.

☹ POOR **Youth Surge Night Age Decelerating Night Moisturizer Combination Oily to Oily** *($49.50 for 1.7 fl. oz.)*. Aside from the marketing nonsense about sirtuins (refer to the review above for Clinique Youth Surge Night Age Decelerating Night Moisturizer Dry Combination), this moisturizer is a step in the wrong direction. Although it contains plenty of beneficial ingredients (including antioxidants, although the jar packaging won't keep them stable), they're trumped by the amount of skin-damaging alcohol. Alcohol is an irritant that causes free-radical damage and collagen breakdown, and hurts skin's ability to heal and repair damage. The lightweight texture of this moisturizer will please those with combination to oily skin, but the amount of alcohol makes it impossible to recommend. See the Appendix for more info on why alcohol and jar packaging are bad news for anti-aging skin care.

CLINIQUE SUN CARE

✓☺ BEST **Sun SPF 15 Face/Body Cream** *($21 for 5 fl. oz.)* is an outstanding sunscreen formula for normal to oily skin. It contains a wide range of antioxidants and cell-communicating ingredients as well as stabilized avobenzone for UVA protection. We disagree with Clinique that this sunscreen is gentle enough for sensitive skin. Without question, the active ingredients it contains can absolutely be sensitizing for all skin types, although that doesn't mean they shouldn't be considered or that they don't have value when it comes to protecting skin from sun damage. Anyone with sensitive, reactive skin should stick with sunscreens whose only active ingredients are titanium dioxide and/or zinc oxide. This sunscreen is fragrance-free and contains mica, a mineral pigment that leaves a slight shimmer on skin.

✓☺ BEST **Sun SPF 30 Body Cream** *($21 for 5 fl. oz.)* is identical to Clinique's Sun SPF 15 Face/Body Cream above, except for a higher concentration of active ingredients needed to reach SPF 30. You can use either one on facial skin, too. This sunscreen is fragrance-free and contains mica, a mineral pigment that leaves a slight shimmer on skin.

✓☺ BEST **Sun SPF 50 Body Cream** *($21 for 5 fl. oz.)* is identical to Clinique's Sun SPF 15 Face Cream above, except for a higher concentration of active ingredients needed to reach SPF 50. You can use either one on facial skin, too. This sunscreen is fragrance-free and contains mica, a mineral pigment that leaves a slight shimmer on skin. Keep in mind that SPF 50 is probably too much (there aren't that many hours of daylight in most parts of the world), but if you tend to be someone who doesn't apply sunscreen liberally, this will help ensure you get enough sunscreen ingredients on your skin to at least equal an SPF 20 or so depending on how much you apply.

☺ GOOD $$$ **Self Sun Body Airbrush Spray** *($21 for 4.2 fl. oz.)* is a fragrance-free, aerosol, spray-on self-tanner that, true to claim, produces a fine mist from any angle. It's a convenient option for covering hard-to-reach areas, but you still need to blend it over your skin to avoid streaks and blotches. Just like almost all self-tanners, this contains the ingredient dihydroxyacetone (DHA) to turn skin tan. It also contains erythrulose, another self-tanning ingredient that works slower than DHA. The combination of these two ingredients can be longer lasting and is worth a test run. The small amount of alcohol in this product is unlikely to cause irritation or dryness, though it does help this self-tanner set quickly.

☺ GOOD $$$ **Self Sun Body Tinted Lotion, Light-Medium** *($21 for 4.2 fl. oz.)* is a very good lightweight self-tanning lotion suitable for all skin types. The Light-Medium designation means there is less of the self-tanning ingredient dihydroxyacetone (DHA) in this product; less DHA means it will turn your skin a deep shade of tan only after a few applications. This particular product is tinted with caramel so you get instant color along with the lasting color that develops after a few hours. Although Clinique's non-acnegenic claim is meaningless (it has no legal definition or requirement), the texture of this product does make it a safer bet for those prone to blemishes. It is fragrance free, too. The mica this contains adds a slight shimmer to skin. Also recommended for a deeper tan is Clinique's **Self Sun Body Tinted Lotion, Medium-Deep** *($21 for 4.2 fl. oz.)*.

☺ GOOD $$$ **Self Sun Face Tinted Lotion** *($20 for 1.7 fl. oz.)* is a great, silky-textured option for all skin types, although there is nothing about this formula that makes it better for the face than the body. You get instant sheer color from the tint this has, and your self-tan color develops within hours thanks to dihydroxyacetone, the same ingredient that shows up in most self-tanning products. This deserves consideration also because it is fragrance-free. The mica this contains adds a slight shimmer to skin.

☺ GOOD $$$ **Sun Advanced Protection SPF 45 Stick** *($19 for 0.21 fl. oz.)* is an emollient, nonaqueous sunscreen stick that provides UVA protection with avobenzone. Although it doesn't contain oils, the wax and emollients that keep this in stick form can certainly contribute to clogged pores. Although the active ingredients in this sun stick are great, we don't advise using it in the eye area unless you know you're not sensitive to the sunscreen agents. Most people should tolerate this well using it on lips, the bridge of the nose, tops of the ears, and other vulnerable areas prone to sun damage due to neglectful application.

☹ POOR **Sun SPF 25 Body Spray** *($21 for 5 fl. oz.)* is a spray-on sunscreen that contains avobenzone for sufficient UVA protection with a base formula of mostly alcohol. This will make the sunscreen too drying and irritating for skin. Alcohol also causes free-radical damage, and for some reason this Clinique sunscreen is woefully short on antioxidants to help offset that damage. Those looking for spray-on sunscreens should consider the better options from Banana Boat and Paula's Choice.

CLINIQUE LIP CARE

☺ GOOD $$$ **All About Lips** *($21.50 for 0.41 fl. oz.)* theoretically smoothes and fills in superficial lip lines and lines around the mouth with silicones and film-former, but test this out before spending the money. Even if it does have an impact, which is merely temporary and quickly undone if you follow with lipstick or gloss (the product's performance largely depends on leaving it undisturbed), it will be convincing only for the most superficial of lines. This also contains salicylic acid, but not in an amount that will exfoliate skin around the mouth—and it is too drying for use on lips.

☺ AVERAGE $$$ **Repairwear Intensive Lip Treatment** *($26 for 0.14 fl. oz.)* functions as a soft spackle for lines on and around the lips. The very thick, lipstick-style balm has several emollients to condition lips, and also contains film-forming agents and waxes that temporarily fill in lines. The addition of peppermint may make you think the product is doing something special, but it's just especially irritating, which isn't great for routine use. Smaller amounts of antioxidants and cell-communicating ingredients are included, but not enough to justify the cost or make this a revolutionary treatment for lip lines.

☹ POOR **Full Potential Lips Plump and Shine** *($17.50)* is said to have a triple-plumping action and promises to keep the plumpness going for hours. The trio of plumping agents include peppermint, capsicum (pepper), and ginger root oils. All of these are irritating for lips, especially if this is a product you intend to use routinely. It's otherwise a standard, slightly thick lip gloss with a sticky finish and an attractive selection of sparkle-infused colors.

☹ POOR **Superbalm Lip Treatment** *($12.50 for 0.25 fl. oz.)* has a lot going for it, but is not recommended over similar lip balms (or even plain Vaseline, which is the main ingredient in Superbalm Lip Treatment) because Clinique added spearmint, grapefruit, and other problematic plants. For better results, check out M.A.C. Lip Conditioner or Paula's Choice Lip & Body Treatment Balm.

CLINIQUE SPECIALTY SKIN-CARE PRODUCTS

✓☺ BEST **Acne Solutions Emergency Gel Lotion** *($15 for 0.5 fl. oz.)* remains an outstanding topical disinfectant for blemish-prone skin with 5% benzoyl peroxide and a good group of anti-inflammatory agents.

✓☺ BEST $$$ **Acne Solutions Oil-Control Cleansing Mask** *($20 for 3.4 fl. oz.)* is a clay mask that lists 1% salicylic acid as its active ingredient. Unfortunately, because clays don't have an acidic pH, the salicylic acid (BHA) won't function as an exfoliant. However, this is still a good, though pricey, oil-absorbing mask that can benefit those struggling with acne (and/or oily skin). It contains soothing plant extracts and is also fragrance-free, which lands it on our short list of the best masks for those with oily, breakout-prone complexions.

☺ GOOD **Acne Solutions Clearing Moisturizer, Oil-Free** *($18.50 for 1.7 fl. oz.)* is one of the most state-of-the-art benzoyl peroxide lotions available today. It contains 2.5% of this topical disinfectant, an excellent amount to apply all over acne-prone skin. The lightweight lotion base feels silky and contains oodles of good-for-skin ingredients, including green tea, acetyl glucosamine, and many soothing plant extracts. The only misstep (one that prevents this product from earning our best rating) is the addition of peppermint extract. The amount is so small as to very likely be a non-issue for skin, but why include it at all when it has no benefit for acne-prone skin?

☺ GOOD $$$ **Even Better Clinical Dark Spot Corrector** *($49.50 for 1 fl. oz.)*. A lot of women struggle with discolorations, so any product claiming to correct this appearance-diminishing issue is going to get attention. Of course, it also helps that Clinique's promotional machine is firing on all cylinders to get the word out that Even Better Clinical Dark Spot Corrector is here and ready to help. The most significant claim being made for Even Better Clinical Dark Spot Corrector is that its efficacy is comparable to prescription products formulated with 4% hydroquinone. As Clinique stated in their press release for Even Better Clinical Dark Spot

Corrector, hydroquinone is the current gold standard treatment for skin discolorations—a fact most cosmetic dermatologists would agree with. Apparently, Clinique has developed a blend of five ingredients they've labeled CL-302 complex. The blend consists of exotic plant extracts (because, of course, a well-known plant such as aloe just isn't that exciting when you're heralding a "breakthrough" product) along with salicylic acid, a form of stabilized vitamin C (ascorbyl glucoside), and a type of black yeast. Clinique maintains their clinical trials validated that their botanical-based complex provided "prescription level results." As expected, Clinique hasn't published their study on this product's alleged efficacy, and it isn't available for public scrutiny. Therefore, we can't know how reliable the results were—we don't even know the protocols of the study. The results sound impressive, but what if Clinique only included results from study participants who had marked improvement? What about the ones whose discolorations didn't improve or, more important, saw greater improvement with hydroquinone? Regardless of the protocol, what we know for certain is that hydroquinone has over 50 years of research attesting to its efficacy and safety. In contrast, the ingredients Clinique chose have a comparably modest track record (Sources: *American Journal of Clinical Dermatology*, July 2006, pages 223–230; *Journal of the American Academy of Dermatology*, May 2006, Supplemental, pages 272–281; *Cutis*, March 2006, pages 177–184; *Journal of Drugs in Dermatology*, September-October 2005, pages 592–597; *Journal of Dermatological Science*, August, 2001, Supplemental, pages 68–75; *Journal of Cosmetic Science*, May-June 1998, pages 208–290; and *Dermatological Surgery*, May 1996, pages 443–447). The form of vitamin C in Even Better Clinical Dark Spot Corrector has minimal (but growing) research demonstrating its efficacy, and earlier studies paired with niacinamide, an ingredient absent from this Clinique lightener (Source: *Skin Research and Technology*, May 2006, pages 105–113). One ingredient in this product deserves further explanation: dimethoxytolyl propylresorcinol. This ingredient, with its chemical-associated name, isn't mentioned in any of the press releases for Even Better Clinical Dark Spot Corrector, well, at least not directly. It turns out it's a chemical compound from the *Dianella ensifolia* plant, which is what Clinique chose to refer to in their marketing information for this product. This ingredient is known to inhibit tyrosinase, which is the enzyme in skin that spurs melanin production. Research has shown that many ingredients inhibit the action of tyrosinase, as this is believed to be a fairly efficient way to control hyperpigmentation. Examples of such ingredients are various types of mushrooms, grape seed, 1-propylmercaptan, and arbutin. To date, there is no conclusive research proving that dimethoxytolyl propylresorcinol is the best one, or that its efficacy is comparable to prescription-strength hydroquinone. That assertion is from Clinique, not from published, peer-reviewed research (and that's what counts for your skin). According to research published in *Drugs of the Future* (volume 33, 2008, pages 945–954), dimethoxytolyl propylresorcinol inhibited pigmentation on reconstituted human skin and animal models. How this ingredient works on reconstituted skin isn't identical to how it will work on intact human skin, but at least it gives researchers some idea of how it works and how it may be used in skincare products. Still, this bit of information isn't a lot to go on. It's an understatement to mention that it pales in comparison to the reams of published research on hydroquinone! Surprisingly, this ingredient was measured not against hydroquinone, but kojic acid—and ingredient with skin-lightening ability but also poor stability. Lots of ingredients can out-perform kojic acid, so it's not that thrilling that dimethoxytolyl propylresorcinol did better in its sole published, comparative test. What about the salicylic acid? Although this BHA ingredient can improve skin cell turnover to help fade discolorations faster, the amount Clinique uses in this product is likely less than 1%, not to mention the pH of 5 prevents it from working as an exfoliant. When all is said and done, there's only a tiny bit of research supporting the lightening claims made for this product. You may experience some good results from this skin lightener, but those with melasma or more widespread hyperpigmentation issues should consider (or stick with) prescription hydroquinone products, along with being neurotic about daily sun protection, which is essential if your goal is reducing discolorations. Even Better Clinical Dark Spot Corrector is suitable for all skin types. Although it's not a slam-dunk for those struggling with discolorations, its blend of antioxidants and skin-identical ingredients warrants a Good rating.

☺ AVERAGE **Acne Solutions Post-Blemish Formula** *($15 for 0.07 fl. oz.)* claims to gently fade the appearance of post-inflammatory hyperpigmentation—those pesky red or brown marks left over for a period of time after a blemish has healed. However, other than the smattering of anti-irritants, nothing in this lightweight lotion (dispensed through a click-pen precision applicator) will hasten the fading of these unsightly marks. That's because the main "ingredient" necessary to fade post-blemish marks is time. The typically red or pink pigmentation you're seeing is a remnant of your skin's healthy immune response to the blemish, and for most skin types and skin colors it tends to linger long after the blemish is gone. The marks will fade, but it can often take 12 months or longer. If you don't have that kind of patience (and who does?), a better option for speeding up the fading of this type of discoloration is to use a topical exfoliant (a pH-effective AHA or BHA product works well) or a tretinoin product (available by prescription). It is also critical that you wear sunscreen daily to prevent more damage that will impede the skin's healing process. Finally, when new blemishes appear, take steps to treat skin gently while using effective blemish-battling products, and, whatever happens, do not pick at them and make scabs—that is a surefire way to damage skin further, resulting in darker and longer-lasting post-inflammatory hyperpigmentation. Bottom line: This Clinique product won't make matters worse, but it won't help things either, and as such is relegated to "why bother?" status.

☹ POOR **Acne Solutions Spot Healing Gel** *($15 for 0.5 fl. oz.)* lists alcohol as the main ingredient, and although it contains 1% salicylic acid, the pH is too high for it to function as an exfoliant, leaving your skin irritated and still blemished. See the Appendix to learn why alcohol is a problem for oily, acne-prone skin.

CLINIQUE FOUNDATIONS

✓☺ BEST **$$$ Almost Powder Makeup SPF 15** *($24)* has a buttery smooth texture that slips on like a second skin and blends to a seamless satin-matte finish with a hint of sparkling shine. This feels incredibly light for a pressed-powder foundation capable of sheer to medium coverage, and you get brilliant sun protection from 13% titanium dioxide (in addition, there's a synthetic sunscreen active, something you don't typically see in a product being sold as mineral makeup). Almost all eight shades are soft and neutral; Deep Honey may be to orange for some skin tones, while Deep is slightly ash, probably due to the amount of titanium dioxide. Deep Golden is best for tan skin tones, which is about as dark as the shade range goes. Whether applied with a sponge for medium coverage or a brush for a sheer look, this is an outstanding powder foundation with sunscreen.

✓☺ BEST **$$$ Even Better Makeup SPF 15** *($26)* claims to make skin look "even better" without makeup. The one thing this beautifully silky liquid foundation has going for it in terms of reducing skin discolorations is its brilliant blend of titanium dioxide and zinc oxide along with a synthetic sunscreen agent. Combined, they provide reliable broad-spectrum protection (assuming you apply this foundation liberally and evenly). As for the other ingredients in this foundation, none of them are known to have a dramatic effect on skin's tone or clarity. However, going back to the sunscreen, it's true that keeping skin protected from sun exposure will enhance its clarity and improve skin tone. That's because you're shielding skin from a major causative source of these complexion detractors. But that capability is hardly unique to this foundation, so the selling point becomes less persuasive. What you'll get with this foundation is a smooth application that blends readily and sets to a soft matte finish that looks very skin-like. It's surprising that something whose finish is so lovely offers fairly significant coverage, especially for minor redness. The only drawback this foundation has is a small amount of grapefruit peel extract. This has the potential to cause irritation, but we doubt the amount used would be much of a problem. Shade-wise, the expansive palette tends to fall to the slightly peach or pink side of neutral. Many of the colors are top-notch, especially for lighter and dark skin tones. The following shades are not recommended due to strong overtones of peach and rose: Porcelain Beige, Cream Caramel, Neutral (which is anything but neutral), Honey, and Beige. There are some good dark tones and the shade range now includes options for very dark skin, too. Even Better Makeup SPF 15 is best for normal to oily skin, and should be suitable for blemish-prone skin unless you know that mineral sunscreen actives make your breakouts worse.

✓☺ BEST $$$ **Perfectly Real Compact Makeup** *($24)* is a talc-based pressed-powder foundation with wow-factor silkiness. It glides over skin and doesn't look the least bit heavy, even when applied with the included sponge. Those with normal to slightly dry or oily skin will enjoy the smooth matte finish and light, buildable coverage. The range of shades is brilliant: Those with fair to medium skin will find neutral option after neutral option. The only potential problem shades are 116 (too yellow) and 120 (slightly peach). Your skin won't look "believably perfect," but will look even and polished. A caveat: Those with melasma or rosacea will likely want more coverage than this foundation provides, but its texture is so light it could be brushed over a medium- to full-coverage liquid foundation without detriment.

✓☺ BEST $$$ **Perfectly Real Makeup** *($24)* is a near-perfect choice for those who want a smooth, lightweight foundation that fulfills its promise of looking as natural as possible. This liquid foundation has a slightly creamy texture that quickly morphs into a soft matte finish once it's blended. Clinique states that Perfectly Real Makeup "feels like nothing at all." It isn't quite that light—you will notice it's there—but your skin will look improved without appearing made-up. It provides sheer to light coverage, so you still need a concealer for red spots or dark circles. The matte finish makes this product preferable for normal to oily skin. It can definitely exaggerate any dry spots, so it's important for your skin to be completely smooth before application. Almost all the shades are gorgeous, neutral options with no strong overtones of peach, pink, ash, or rose. There are options for very light skin, as well as some beautiful darker shades.

✓☺ BEST $$$ **Stay-Matte Oil-Free Makeup** *($23)*. This fragrance-free liquid foundation is oil-free as claimed and contains a beautiful array of silky, lightweight ingredients that won't make oily skin or oily areas feel slick or look greasy. Its soft, slightly fluid cream texture is easy to blend and provides no less than medium coverage from the get-go. This is not the foundation to pick if you want sheer to light coverage, though we suppose you could mix this with a moisturizer to sheer the results. It finish is absorbent, long-wearing, and noticeably matte—any dry areas will be magnified, so be sure to moisturize those spots first. Ideally, this foundation is tailor-made for skin that's oily to very oily all over, as those skin types are most likely to be

The Reviews C

thrilled with how this looks and wears. It does a formidable job keeping excess shine in check, though you may find you need to blot or powder at some point during your day.

The range of shades is extensive, impressive, and mostly warm-toned, so you'll see more yellow to gold tones than pink or rosy tones. The only shade to avoid is Deep Neutral which is strongly peach. Honey is slightly peach but workable, as is Creamwhip. The darkest shades (Spice, Clove, and Amber) are good for dark skin tones though they're quite similar. The shade options for very fair skin are limited, but still worth a look. Those with light to tan skin tones will be happiest with the palette.

☺ GOOD **Supermoisture Makeup** *($24)* is being advertised as a foundation that thinks it's a moisturizer; containing a special time-release technology that places powerful moisturizing agents where and when skin needs them most. We wouldn't count on that, since a makeup doesn't have a radar-like ability to detect dry spots and respond accordingly, while holding back over the oily areas. Still, this creamy liquid foundation is definitely worth considering by those with dry to very dry skin. It has a soft, slightly whipped texture that glides over skin, provides light to medium coverage, and leaves skin visibly hydrated with a soft shimmer glow. Those with very dry skin who want to apply more than the standard amount of foundation will notice increased coverage. The collection of shades is mostly impressive, offering good colors for fair to dark skin tones.

☺ GOOD **$$$ Acne Solutions Liquid Makeup** *($26)* is a very good foundation for those with oily or breakout-prone skin. It's not a reliable choice for treating acne because the amount of salicylic acid is too low to be of much help and the foundation's pH won't permit exfoliation. Even though you'll need to resort to other products to manage acne, this foundation certainly won't make matters worse. It has an unbelievably weightless texture that feels silky and sets quickly to a soft matte finish. You'll see an improved skin tone, and this absolutely doesn't feel like you're wearing makeup. Coverage is in the light to medium range, so you'll need to pair this with a concealer for trouble spots or strong redness. This does a formidable job of keeping oily shine in check, too. Yes, the formula contains a type of alcohol that can be problematic for skin, but the amount is low enough that it won't be all that problematic, although it certainly would have been far better without it. Among the shades to consider carefully are the slightly peach Fresh Beige. The other shades are excellent and best for fair to dark skin tones.

☺ GOOD **$$$ Moisture Sheer Tint SPF 15** *($27)* has a satin-smooth texture and slightly creamy application that sets to a minimally moist finish. This product is aptly named, as it provides sheer, almost nonexistent coverage. Its sunscreen is in-part titanium dioxide, but it's at a level of only 1%, which may be too low to provide sufficient UVA protection for long days outdoors. Three shades are available, and the best among them are Fair and Neutral. The Beige shade is good, but may be too yellow for medium skin tones. This is a good option for someone with normal to slightly dry skin seeking sheer coverage.

☺ GOOD **$$$ Repairwear Laser Focus All-Smooth Makeup SPF 15** *($32.50)*. In no way does this makeup's formula or appearance on skin approximate the improvements possible from laser or light-emitting treatments your dermatologist can provide. It is "laser focus" in name only, although the formula does contain some good skin-repairing ingredients. This liquid foundation with an in-part titanium dioxide sunscreen has a creamy, moist texture that spreads easily, but isn't so slippery that blending is difficult. It sets to a soft, satin finish that feels moist without being greasy. Skin is left looking dewy and you can achieve medium to full coverage, so this works well to camouflage a noticeably uneven skin tone. The main drawbacks include the shades and the fact that, despite claims to the contrary, this foundation, like almost all liquid foundations, tends to emphasize wrinkles more than downplay them. Among the dozen shades, several are slightly to obviously pink, peach, orange, or rose. Shades 01, 1.5, 02, 07, and 08 are the best ones. Consider 03, 04, 05, and 06 carefully, being sure to check the results in natural light or you may have a complexion that looks too rosy. Shades 09 and 11 are also rosy, but their beige tone helps to offset this, at least a bit. Shade 12 is not recommended due to a strong orange overtone. On balance, the shade range has options for fair (but not porcelain-fair) to tan skin tones. This foundation is best for normal to dry skin and suitable for breakout-prone skin, although the moist finish isn't likely to feel great over breakout-prone areas.

☺ GOOD $$$ **Superbalanced Powder Makeup SPF 15** *($34.50)* is the product propelling Clinique into the "mineral makeup" game, too. And it's strictly a marketing gimmick, as mineral makeup is not unique; in fact, most powders are mineral-based. It's great that the sunscreen is pure titanium dioxide and that the jar package includes a sifter that shaves off the solid formed powder as you rotate from its edges. Although that seems clever and allows the user to control how much powder is dispensed, it does little to minimize the mess that is inherent to loose powders. Application-wise, this powder's slightly creamy texture goes on smoothly and provides sheer to medium coverage with a soft matte finish. It is best for normal to slightly dry or slightly oily skin; those with pronounced oily areas will find this isn't absorbent enough, while those with dry areas will find it makes them more noticeable. You may be tempted to try this foundation because it claims to help absorb oil while maintaining skin's moisture balance, but it absolutely cannot do that. The main ingredients are absorbent by nature, and even though Clinique includes some emollient ingredients, they cannot overcome the absorbency of the titanium dioxide, talc, and mica, although the emollients do keep this powder from being as absorbent as it could be, which is why those with oily skin won't be pleased. As for the shades, almost all of them are excellent, but the medium to dark shades (there are no options for very dark skin tones) tend to look slightly chalky unless applied sheer. Natural 6 and Natural 7 suffer a bit from being slightly peach, but are still worth considering.

☺ AVERAGE $$$ **Age Defense BB Cream SPF 30** *($37)* is part of an Asian-inspired trend that has made its way to the United States; but, for the most part, this is one overseas trend you can ignore without feeling as though you're missing out on something great. The concept of blemish balm creams is that they serve as a treatment-based tinted moisturizer to even out skin tone (a blemish in Asia is about skin color, not about breakouts). Most offer sun protection, sheer to light coverage to even out the skin tone, and one or more ingredients to lighten brown discolorations or red marks from acne. Clinique's attempt to capitalize on the BB cream trend doesn't break any new ground; in fact, there are more problems than benefits with this fragrance-free product, especially if you have breakout-prone skin. The texture is thick, creamy, and somewhat opaque. Despite the creaminess, this feels a bit dry as it's applied and sets to a soft matte finish; it doesn't have the elegant slip of today's best foundations. This provides enough coverage to blur minor imperfections (you get more coverage than a standard tinted moisturizer), but only one of the two shades is worthwhile. Shade 01 is a ghostly pink that leaves a distinct white cast on skin; Shade 02 is a soft neutral that's workable for fair to light skin tones. There are no shades for medium to dark skin tones, but that's just as well because this isn't a product worth auditioning. Sun protection is provided by a range of synthetic and mineral actives, so this provides sufficient protection against the sun's aging UVA rays. Unfortunately, the formula lacks ingredients proven to help improve blemishes, whether they are from discolorations or from a breakout. Instead, your skin is treated to some heavy thickening agents and a product that feels slightly heavy and mask-like instead of fresh and "barely there."

The Reviews C

All skin types, blemished or not, would do better with any of the Clinique foundations or tinted moisturizers with sunscreen that we've rated highly.

☺ AVERAGE $$$ **Continuous Coverage SPF 15** *($23)* is a very opaque, full-coverage cream foundation that will certainly not look natural no matter how well you blend. What it will do is provide substantial camouflage for irregular pigmentation or birthmarks. That's what some people need, but we cannot stress enough how the use of foundations such as this should be limited to only areas with prominent discolorations. Applied all over, this can easily look thick and mask-like. The sunscreen active ingredient is all titanium dioxide, and this, coupled with the thick, powdery finish, can lend a chalky look to the skin. The four shades are good (and best for light to medium skin tones), but the pluses and minuses mean that this is definitely a trade-off foundation. It's best for normal to dry skin not prone to breakouts.

☺ AVERAGE $$$ **Redness Solutions Makeup SPF 15** *($26)* is said to be formulated with "probiotic technology [which] helps strengthen the barrier often compromised in redness sufferers." That sounds intriguing, but there is no published research to support the claim that probiotics (which are strains of helpful bacteria) have any benefit when applied topically, or even that they remain stable in a skin-care or makeup formula. Although the probiotics are most likely a bust, this foundation does contain some good anti-inflammatory ingredients that may help reduce redness. What puzzles us is why Clinique decided to include a synthetic sunscreen, octinoxate, in a foundation targeted for sensitive skin?! Mind you, octinoxate is effective and fine for the majority of people, but it carries a higher risk of irritation for those with sensitive skin. The formula would be far better for sensitive, reddened skin if they used zinc oxide and titanium dioxide instead. Beyond the claims, this liquid foundation offers medium coverage to help camouflage redness and blemishes. It sets to a matte finish. Among the shades, avoid Calming Fair, which has pink undertones that emphasize redness, not neutralize it; however, the other shades are flattering, neutral colors in the fair to medium range. Clinique did not create any shades for darker skin tones, perhaps because the darker your skin tone is, the less apparent redness will be.

☺ AVERAGE $$$ **Superbalanced Makeup** *($23)* claims to provide moisture and absorb oil when and where needed—a skin-care dream many women share. However, this ends up doing neither job very well. There is no way a product can differentiate between the oily parts of your face and the dry parts. The absorbent ingredients in it will soak up any oil they come in contact with (including the moisturizing ingredients in this product or in the one you applied to your skin) and the moisturizing ingredients will get deposited over areas you don't want to be moisturized. With Superbalanced Makeup, you get a silicone-in-water liquid that provides light to medium coverage with a smooth, matte-finish foundation that is best for someone with normal to slightly dry or slightly oily skin. Someone with any amount of excess oil would not be happy with the finish or with how it wears during the day. Compared to several other Clinique foundations, the palette of shades isn't as neutral. The following colors are best avoided by most skin tones: Light, Cream Chamois, Ivory, Neutral, and Vanilla. Alabaster and Breeze are the best neutral shades.

☹ POOR **Moisture Surge Tinted Moisturizer SPF 15** *($26)* provides reliable broad-spectrum sun protection (from its in-part titanium dioxide sunscreen) in a slightly creamy base that's best for normal to dry skin. However, because the formula contains the irritating ingredient menthol, it is not recommended (irritation like this is always a problem for skin and best avoided). What a shame, because this tinted moisturizer looks great on your skin.

CLINIQUE CONCEALERS

✓☺ BEST **$$$ All About Eyes Concealer** *($16)* is a state-of-the-art concealer formula thanks to the inclusion of pentapeptides, antioxidants, and elegant skin-identical ingredients. It has a smooth, creamy texture and concentrated pigmentation. A little goes a long way and provides good coverage with minimal slip. The seven shades present mostly true skin-color options, though Light Neutral (the palest shade) is too yellow for most fair skin and Medium Beige is too bright yellow. The others are superb and include options for darker skin. Clinique claims this is recommended for disguising dark circles, and it does indeed work very well for that purpose, without looking thick or cakey.

☺ GOOD **Acne Solutions Clearing Concealer** *($15.50)* is a liquid concealer with 1% salicylic acid as its active ingredient. However, Clinique didn't include any ingredients to establish the acidic pH range that's necessary for salicylic acid to exert its acne-clearing action. Although that's disappointing, this is still a very good concealer for use on oily areas or on acne. It has a fluid texture that offers minimal slip and sets to a long-wearing matte finish while providing sufficient coverage. All the shades are recommended except Corrective Green, which leaves a slightly eerie Wicked Witch of the West tint on the skin.

☺ GOOD **Line Smoothing Concealer** *($15.50)* is a very good liquid concealer with a smooth, even application, the right amount of coverage for most flaws, and a semi-matte finish that leaves a bit of a glow. Of the mostly neutral shades, only Medium Honey (which is bright peach) and Deep Honey (an unattractive ochre hue) should be avoided.

☺ GOOD **$$$ Airbrush Concealer** *($19.50)* is housed in a pen-style applicator; you rotate the base to feed concealer onto the built-in brush tip. It offers a smooth (though too sheer to provide any amount of concealing) application that has an airy, silky texture and sets to a natural matte finish. Two of the three shades are the main issue here, because Fair is too pink and Medium is undeniably peach. Neutral Fair is great. Despite the shade issues, this concealer is so sheer that the misguided colors get toned down. By the way, the finished effect on the skin is not akin to airbrushing a photo, where flaws are eliminated. If anything, even minor flaws will still be visible with this concealer, but, to Clinique's credit, they do describe this as being sheer, so it still deserves a good rating for those looking more for a highlighter/enhancer than for significant coverage.

☹ POOR **Redness Solutions Targeted Corrector** *($19.50)* is a twist-up stick concealer meant to neutralize redness. It does that to some extent, but you most likely won't be impressed with the results because the color goes on too yellow. Essentially, what this does is trade one discoloration problem (redness) for another (sallowness), and the more you blend to soften the yellow cast, the less redness coverage you get. Although this has a smooth, silicone-enhanced texture, its finish tends to magnify the slightest crease and put the spotlight on large pores. Moreover, the formula contains several waxes and thickeners that are a problem for use over acne-prone areas (assuming your redness is from blemishes). Those with sensitive skin should be aware that this color-correcting concealer, which really isn't corrective in the least, contains potentially irritating plant extracts, most notably grapefruit extract. Although not present in a large amount, this needless irritant can hurt your skin's healing process and make redness worse. Interestingly, the magnolia bark extract this contains may have effects on skin similar to the effects of hydrocortisone (Source: naturaldatabase.com). That can help reduce redness, but your skin is still left to deal with the potential irritation from the grapefruit and the tricky yellow cast.

CLINIQUE POWDERS

✓☺ BEST **$$$ Blended Face Powder & Brush** *($21)* is one of the best talc-based loose powders available, and is available in an attractive array of colors. This has a light, supple finish that clings well without caking and doesn't look dry or dull skin's natural glow. Of the shades, use caution with Transparency 2 (pale pink but goes on sheer) and Transparency Bronze (nice color, but too shiny, though it's an option for evening sparkle). The finish this powder leaves is best for normal to dry skin. The Invisible Blend shade goes on translucent but not too white, so it is indeed suitable for most skin tones looking for a powder that tempers shine without adding color. One more point: Toss the brush; it doesn't apply powder well, feels scratchy, and sheds too much.

☺ GOOD **$$$ Redness Solutions Instant Relief Mineral Pressed Powder** *($32.50)*. Clinique maintains this powder reduces redness on contact and it does, but so does any other pressed powder that provides light to medium coverage, and there are lots of those that cost half the price of this one! The formula contains some intriguing ingredients, but none of them have substantial research proving they're a must-have for reddened skin, and they won't remain stable in this kind of packaging anyway. What you can count on is that this powder is unlikely to make red skin worse. It has a refined, silky texture that applies beautifully. The soft matte finish enlivens skin without looking dry or powdery; Clinique even includes a serviceable (if small) brush to sweep this on. Because this is sold as a "specialty" pressed powder, only one shade is available, which obviously limits its appeal. It is a pale yellow color and, therefore, can tone down redness (it's definitely better than mint green). Thankfully, the yellow coloration is soft and doesn't add a strange tone to skin. Despite this plus, the powder is limited to those with fair to light skin tones.

☺ GOOD **$$$ Stay Matte Sheer Pressed Powder Oil-Free** *($21)* is a good, talc-based powder with a slightly dry, powdery, sheer finish. The shades are beautiful and there are some good options for light and dark skin tones.

☺ GOOD **$$$ Superpowder Double Face Powder** *($21)* is a standard, talc-based pressed powder with a smooth, soft texture. It can be used alone or as a regular finishing powder. There are eight very sheer shades, all terrific. Some may find this an acceptable powder foundation, but it is best as a pressed powder that provides light coverage.

☹ AVERAGE **$$$ Redness Solutions Instant Relief Mineral Powder** *($32.50)* purports to "measurably reduce redness on contact," and this claim is somewhat true. The minerals present in this loose powder (mica, bismuth oxychloride) don't make it anything special (nor do they have redness-reducing properties), but this powder's soft yellow color does help reduce the appearance or redness on the face. Nothing in this formulation will actually reduce the redness caused by rosacea; it will simply help to conceal the appearance of redness. If anything, we're concerned that the amount of potentially irritating grapefruit peel extract may make redness worse. Despite that ingredient misstep, this is a good loose powder for use to help even out skin tone and set makeup. As long as you have reasonable expectations, you'll find this a fine option for a loose powder. Toss the small antibacterial brush that's included with this powder. It's too rough to be used on anyone's skin, much less those who are already suffering from sensitivity issues.

CLINIQUE BLUSHES & BRONZERS

✓☺ BEST **$$$ Blushwear Cream Stick** *($21)* is a twist-up, cream-to-powder blush in stick form. This is easy to blend over moist skin and provides a soft wash of color that looks quite natural. Each of the pastel shades has a touch of shine, but the effect is a subtle glow rather than obvious sparkles. Overall, this is an excellent option for those with normal to dry skin who don't wish to use powder blush.

☺ GOOD $$$ **Almost Bronzer SPF 15** *($29.50)*. Titanium dioxide is the active ingredient in this pressed bronzing powder, so it is capable of providing sufficient broad-spectrum protection. The talc-based formula has a smooth, dry texture that applies sheer and leaves a soft shine finish. We wish the colors were better; they appear tan, but they apply peachy, which almost makes this better as blush. The sunscreen element serves as a helpful adjunct to your foundation or moisturizer with sunscreen, but if you use it alone, you'll have to apply way too much over your entire face to get the SPF protection of 15. A brush is included, and although it's not preferred to a full-size powder or blush brush, it's usable.

☺ GOOD $$$ **Blushing Blush Powder Blusher** *($21)* has the smoothest texture and best color deposit of all Clinique's powder blushes, but each shade is laden with shine (on most shades, the shine is metallic-looking rather than a soft shimmer). This powder blush is otherwise very workable and easy to blend, but this much shine is best reserved for nighttime glamour.

☺ AVERAGE $$$ **Quick Blush** *($23.50)* is sold as a powder blush and brush in one, and it is. A tiny disc of pressed-powder blush is housed in the base of the product's cap. You twist the opposite end before opening, which deposits a small amount of color onto the built-in (and surprisingly good) blush brush. The concept is practical and great for on-the-go use, but all the shades go on so sheer you need several applications to get noticeable color. This ends up being an OK option for a very subtle blush effect, but only if you have fair to light skin.

☺ AVERAGE $$$ **Soft Pressed Powder Blusher** *($21)* is decently silky but almost too sheer. Color deposit is minimal and requires successive layers to register on most skin tones (and forget about it showing up at all on dark skin). All the shades are shiny and the shine tends to flake, making this less enticing than the powder blushes from M.A.C., NYX Cosmetics, or Clarins.

☹ POOR **True Bronze Pressed Powder Bronzer** *($25)* has a dry, grainy texture and somewhat spotty, sheer application with shine. It isn't nearly as impressive as it should be, and is not worth considering even though the three tan shades are a balanced mix without too much red or copper.

CLINIQUE EYESHADOWS

✓☺ BEST **Colour Surge Eye Shadow Duo** *($18)* has an ultra-smooth texture and application that is Clinique's best ever. Several sets contain two shiny colors, albeit in mostly workable combinations. The deeper shades apply smoothly and are an option for creating a shiny, smoky, evening eye makeup. There are some blue-toned duos to watch out for, but the odd pairing of purple with pale gold (in the Beach Plum duo) is actually quite attractive. Matte duos are also available, and each has an enviably silky texture and true matte finish. Also recommended is **Colour Surge Eye Shadow Quad** *($25.50)*, which features some attractive groupings, including Teddy Bear, Spicy, and Choco-Latte.

✓☺ BEST **Colour Surge Eye Shadow Soft Shimmer** *($15)* offers a splendid texture and sublimely silky colors that blend beautifully, and although the shine (shimmer) isn't what we consider "soft," the finish is appropriate for daytime makeup if you have unwrinkled eyelids and a smooth under-brow area. The small shade selection is impressive, with only a few pastel tones that you should consider carefully.

☺ GOOD **Colour Surge Eye Shadow Super Shimmer** *($15)* is nearly identical to the Colour Surge Eye Shadow Soft Shimmer, except with more shine. This is best reserved for evening or special occasion makeup.

✓☺ BEST **Colour Surge Eye Shadow Stay Matte** *($15)* leaves a hint of shine in each shade, despite the "matte" in the name of this powder eyeshadow. The shine is light enough to almost be a non-issue, but those shopping for a completely matte option should know that these aren't it. The smooth texture and strong pigmentation (strong for Clinique, as many of their eyeshadows are quite sheer) make for lasting impact. Application is smooth with no flaking, and several of the shades work well for creating the classic smoky eye. Martini is a medium olive-green tone that's muted enough to not be distracting and that works quite well with warm brown or caramel tones.

☺ GOOD **$$$ Colour Surge Eye Shadow Trio** *($22.50)* has a very soft, silky texture and an even, although sheer, application that builds well for a greater "surge" of color. Depending on the trio, the finishes vary from satin matte to soft shine. Totally Neutral and Come Heather are great sets; Ebb and Flow has a greenish shade that's tricky to use, although the color isn't unattractive. The color payoff isn't as noticeable as Clinique's other Colour Surge eyeshadows; perhaps they scaled back for the trios.

☺ GOOD **$$$ Lid Smoothie Antioxidant 8-Hour Eye Colour** *($19.50)* is an impressive cream-to-powder eyeshadow, though not because it offers wonderful skin-care benefits for your eye area. The formula contains a dusting of fruit- and vegetable-based antioxidants and a teeny-tiny amount of peptide, but these won't "coax fine lines into a blanket of smoothness" nor do they make eyelid dropping or sagging look better. An innovative feature of this eyeshadow is its rounded metal-tip applicator. Not only is it contoured to fit the eye area, it remains cool to the touch (as most metals do) and, as a result, this feels cooling when applied but the cooling isn't from irritating ingredients. Lid Smoothie has a slightly thick cream texture that softens as you apply. There's enough slip for even blending without going outside the intended area, and this sets within several seconds. Once set, it tends to stay in place without creasing or fading, though if you have oily eyelids you likely won't experience worry-free wear for as long as 8 hours. Although this eyeshadow's finish is powdery in feel, the look is color with obvious shimmer. The shade range presents some enticing, easy-to-work-with options though the darker shades (Lick-orice, Impromt-Blue, Seventh Heather, and Sassy-fras) go on lighter and sheerer than they appear in the tube.

CLINIQUE EYE & BROW LINERS

✓☺ BEST **Brush-On Cream Liner** *($15)* is a densely pigmented cream-gel eyeliner packaged in a glass jar. The formula applies easily (similar to liquid eyeliner) and sets to a long-wearing finish that won't smear, smudge, or flake even if oily eyelids are a problem. It may seem like a bonus that Clinique included a brush, but unless you want a thick line, you'll want to experiment with fine-tipped options. Among the four shades, Black Honey is shiny and the remainder are classic black, brown, and gray. As with all products of this nature, it must be recapped tightly after each use to prevent the product from drying out.

✓☺ BEST **Instant Lift for Brows** *($15)* is a dual-ended brow pencil and shimmering highlighter designed to define your brows and highlight the skin around them. Of course this has nothing to do with an eye lift, but it does let you create fuller, shapelier brows, with the option to further define them with a hint of shimmer along the brow bone. The brow colors are natural-looking and there are options for blonde to deep brown brows. The highlighter is the same shimmering, light cream shade regardless of which brow color you select.

☺ GOOD **Brow Shaper** *($15)* is a powder brow color that comes in four excellent shades, though now each of them has shine, which is a bit over the top. The texture is slightly heavy, but these blend onto the brow quite well, even though the brush that comes packaged with them is too stiff and scratchy. For the money, a matte, brow-toned eyeshadow would work just as well and could also double as an eyeshadow; Brow Shaper is too heavy for eyeshadow.

☺ GOOD **Superfine Liner for Brows** *($14)* is an automatic, nonretractable, very thin brow pencil that works well to softly accent and fill in brows for those who prefer pencils to powder. It applies without dragging or feeling thick, and has a slightly tacky powder finish that lasts with minimal fading and no smearing. The five shades are excellent, and include options for blondes and redheads.

☺ AVERAGE **Quickliner for Eyes** *($15)* is a standard automatic pencil that provides a smooth, no-tugging application and is very easy to smudge before it sets. Because this stays creamy, its wear-time is compromised and every shade goes on too soft for quick definition.

☹ AVERAGE **$$$ Cream Shaper for Eyes** *($15)* is a very soft-textured eye pencil that goes on creamy and stays creamy, yet (this is the best part) barely smudges. Each shade is infused with shimmer, which should raise a red flag if your eyelids are wrinkled. Otherwise, the glow these pencils provide can be subtly effective. It is best for defining eyes and then smudging the effect for a smoky look, and is not recommended as a lower-lid liner if you have allergies or watery eyes, both of which promote smearing with a creamy pencil like this.

☹ POOR **Brow Keeper** *($15)* is a substandard brow pencil that comes in only two colors. It has a slick texture and slightly creamy, sticky finish that prompts smudging and fading.

CLINIQUE LIP COLOR & LIPLINERS

✓☺ BEST **High Impact Lipstick SPF 15** *($15)* comes with the selling point of having it all, and Clinique is almost right with this cream lipstick. The sunscreen is in-part zinc oxide, so broad-spectrum protection is assured. This also has a beautifully creamy texture that feels neither greasy nor thick. It sets to a soft cream finish and provides medium coverage. Where Clinique went slightly astray, at least in terms of the "have it all" claim, is that the colors aren't full coverage, which compromises their longevity. Most of them have a good stain, but this will wear off the same as most cream lipsticks—it won't maintain a just-applied look for eight hours, even if you avoid lipstick-wrecking activities such as eating and drinking. However, taken as a creamy lipstick with effective sunscreen, there is no question this wins high marks, and the shade range is wonderful. Those who love cool-toned red shades should check out Red-y to Wear!

✓☺ BEST **Long Last Soft Shine Lipstick** *($15)* has a luscious feel and smooth, even application with opaque coverage. It is nicely creamy without being greasy or too glossy. The color selection offers equally impressive pale and deep shades.

✓☺ BEST **Superbalm Moisturizing Gloss** *($15)* comes in a squeeze tube and is an emollient, balm-like lip gloss that moisturizes while imparting sheer, juicy color and a minimally sticky feel. It's a good way to condition lips while adding a hint of color, and some of the shades have a slight shimmer for a glistening effect.

✓☺ BEST **$$$ Vitamin C Smoothie Antioxidant Lip Colour** *($17.50)* is an antioxidant-rich lip color that's housed in a click-style pen with a splay-proof brush applicator. That's great news, not only because it produces superior results, but also because it keeps the antioxidants stable. Consider this a lipstick-lip gloss hybrid because the product imparts creamy, sheer-to-medium color that doesn't feel heavy or sticky in the least, but it does leave a healthy shine and has the kind of staying power you may not expect from something with a glossy finish. The colors are lovely, and the formula impressive, though it would have been better if it contained sunscreen. All told, it's a winner from Clinique!

☺ GOOD **Almost Lipstick** *($15)* is a Clinique classic which includes the shade Black Honey, the company's best-selling lipstick shade. True to claim, it is a flattering color for most skin tones (although it looks imposingly dark in the tube). This remains a smooth, sheer lipstick that provides a soft gloss finish, and the shade selection has gone from a few to several options, including some attractive pink and nude tones, all of which go on sheerer than they look in the tube.

☺ GOOD **Butter Shine Lipstick** *($15)* goes on quite thick and feels considerably more greasy than creamy. It has a glossy finish and comes in an attractive selection of shades seemingly based on best-sellers from Clinique's vast lipstick library—but this will bleed into lines around the mouth almost as soon as you apply it, and its longevity is cut short by the extra-emollient formula. It isn't a bad lipstick by any means, just one to approach with caution if you're prone to lipstick feathering or want long-lasting color.

☺ GOOD **$$$ Chubby Stick Moisturizing Lip Colour Balm** *($16)* is a sheer, thick lipstick-like pencil housed in a twist-up plastic package, so no sharpening is needed! Performance-wise, this applies smoothly with a slick, slightly greasy texture and glossy finish. It quickly moves into lines around the mouth, but if that's not your concern, and you find the novelty of Chubby Stick enticing, it's worth checking out. Almost all the sheer colors are attractive and this also can work as a more substantial lip gloss applied over your regular lipstick.

☹ POOR **Long Last Glosswear SPF 15** *($15)* is one of the most undesirable glosses in recent memory, and it's hard to make an unappealing lip gloss, because most of the ingredients used to create them will make lips feel soft and smooth. Not only does the sunscreen leave lips vulnerable to UVA damage, but the texture is inordinately thick and uncomfortably sticky. This comes close to feeling like you've painted a mix of maple syrup and glue on your lips, and then allowed it to dry. Each sparkle-infused shade (all go on much softer than they look in the tube) provides a vinyl-like shine, but other glosses do that also, and without the unpleasant aesthetics of this. For better results, check out the glosses from Dior, M.A.C., or others from Clinique.

CLINIQUE MASCARAS

✓☺ BEST **High Impact Mascara** *($15)* is simply fantastic and is on our short list of favorite mascaras. If you're looking for mascara that quickly builds substantial length and thickness while defining lashes without clumping, this is a must-try. It wears well throughout the day and is easily removed with a water-soluble cleanser, qualities that make it even more ideal.

✓☺ BEST **Lash Doubling Mascara** *($15)* does a very good job of living up to its name, as this quickly builds lots of length and a fair amount of thickness with ease. The formula sweeps on with no clumps or smearing—each lash is well defined—so unless you're looking for all-out drama, this is an outstanding choice.

☺ GOOD **Lash Power Mascara Long Wearing Formula** *($15)* is a great waterproof mascara that stays on through any precipitation or amount of eye tearing, and is surprisingly easy to remove (it comes off with very warm water, followed by your regular cleanser). Application-wise, the small, pointed brush allows you to reach and elongate every lash, providing clean definition. Thickness and volume are harder to come by because it's a gel-based formula. Those looking for lash separation with length and worry-free long wear are this mascara's target audience, regardless of geographical location!

✍ Lavender oil smells great, but fragrance isn't skin care! Find out why in the Appendix.

☺ AVERAGE **Bottom Lash Mascara** *($10)* is a classic waste of time and money due to its very small brush. Of course this works to apply mascara to your bottom lashes, but so does any regular mascara. It's all about how you hold the brush—you don't need special mascara for your bottom lashes!

☺ AVERAGE **High Impact Curling Mascara** *($15)* is misnamed; it should be called No Impact, No Curl Mascara. This mascara goes on wet and smears easily if you're not careful. It will separate and lengthen lashes, but it doesn't provide much thickness and it has zero curling effect. The curved brush also makes application to the lower lashes needlessly difficult.

☺ AVERAGE **High Lengths Mascara** *($15)* comes with an innovative brush, resembling a thin, elongated claw with three tiny rows of plastic teeth on one side. The shape is meant to mimic the curve of your eyelid, yet it cannot be applied in one swoop from the lash line up without creating a mess. Rather, best results are achieved by combing the end of the brush up through each individual lash. After trying it every which way, this method was the only one that produced an even look with no smudging. That said, and after much effort, even a perfect application can't prevent some smudging by the end of the day.

☺ AVERAGE **Lash Building Primer** *($14)* is nothing to get excited about. This will only impress you if it is used with a mediocre to poor mascara. In that case, you could expect to see increased length and thickness that would not be possible using the inferior mascara alone.

☺ AVERAGE **Naturally Glossy Mascara** *($15)* is a basic mascara that builds some length and minimal thickness, though it leaves lashes feeling dry and stiff due to the film-forming agents and the amount of PVP (an ingredient used in many hairstyling gels) it contains.

☹ POOR **High Definition Lashes Brush Then Comb Mascara** *($15)* is really bad, and that's not something we see too often with mascaras. The dual-sided brush features comblike teeth on one side and standard mascara bristles on the other. You're directed to use the bristled portion first to build thickness, then comb through lashes for length and added drama. Neither side works well, though at least the brush side doesn't leave lashes clumped together and spiky-looking. This is one of the few mascaras that requires more effort to apply and neaten than the results merit.

CLINIQUE FACE & BODY ILLUMINATOR

☺ GOOD **$$$ Up-Lighting Liquid Illuminator** *($25)* is a liquid shimmer lotion whose three sheer shades don't break any new ground for radiant shine. Each applies smoothly and imparts a hint of color and shine that can be layered for more intensity. The shine clings well and the color lasts—though keep in mind the effect of both is subtle.

CLINIQUE BRUSHES

☺ GOOD **The Brush Collection** *($14.50–$34)*. Most of Clinique's brushes are full, well-shaped, and functional for their intended purpose. The prices are similar to most other brushes at the department store. All feature elegant handles that are neither too long nor too short. The best options are the **Blush Brush** ($26.50), **Concealer Brush** ($17.50), **Eye Shadow Brush** ($19.50), **Eye Contour Brush** ($19.50), **Powder Foundation Brush** ($32.50), and **Eye Definer Brush** ($17.50), which is preferred for defining brows rather than eyelining. Adding a unique marketing element to their new brushes is Clinique's assertion that the brush hairs are treated with a long-lasting antibacterial agent to keep them hygienic. That could very well be possible, but it seems Clinique doesn't quite believe it either because they still advise you to clean your brushes monthly for hygienic purposes, and the makeup artists clean the brushes with alcohol after each use. It's also important to keep in mind that the kind of bacteria that grow on brushes aren't the kind associated with breakouts, so the antibacterial claim won't help that aspect of your skin's appearance.

CLINIQUE SPECIALTY MAKEUP PRODUCTS

☺ AVERAGE **$$$ Pore Refining Solutions Instant Perfector** *($18)* is a specialty makeup product claiming to make your pores look smooth and "virtually flawless" with a matte finish that lasts up to 8 hours. Although this has an intriguing, spackle-like texture that temporarily improves the appearance of enlarged pores, its shine control effect fails to impress. At best, the matte finish lasts an hour or so, after which the oil comes roaring back and your pores look as if you hadn't done anything different. You'll be reaching for your blotting papers or powder, which isn't the point of this product. Without question, your first impression of this product will be positive. It feels supremely silky, leaves a weightless, powdery matte finish that initially makes pores appear smaller, and it definitely keeps shine in check. If only the results weren't so short-lived, this would be easy to recommend. It comes in three translucent shades, including Invisible Bright, which has an opalescent pink cast that enlivens skin without adding shine.

COVER GIRL (MAKEUP ONLY)

Strengths: Inexpensive and widely available; a hugely improved selection of foundations, several with reliable sunscreen; good concealers; enviable pressed powders; some fantastic Lash Blast (and other) mascaras; mostly great eyelining options; a vast selection of lip color options, from the long-wearing Outlast to sheer lip glosses to the wholly impressive Lip Perfection lipstick; several great options in the Queen Collection for women of color.

Weaknesses: The older foundations are seriously lacking; the newer Advanced Radiance foundation has great texture but disappointing SPF rating; powder blush and eyeshadows; terrible makeup brushes; all the "Clean" products contain irritating ingredients.

For more information and reviews of the latest Cover Girl products, visit CosmeticsCop.com.

COVER GIRL FOUNDATIONS & PRIMERS

☺ GOOD **Cover Girl & Olay Simply Ageless Serum Primer** *($14.99 for 1 fl. oz.)*. The marriage of Cover Girl and Olay (both brands owned by consumer products juggernaut Procter & Gamble) has generated lots of products, including this serum/primer. Actually, the name "serum primer" is a bit redundant because almost all primers are serums and almost all serums can be primers, but what's in a name anyway; what counts is how this works. Beneficial ingredients are present in this Cover Girl/Olay product, but not to the same extent as in the "regular" serums from Olay and in primers from some other brands. This has the requisite silky texture and enough titanium dioxide to lend a cosmetic brightening effect, along with a rather dry finish, making it best for normal to oily/combination skin. The skin-firming claims are couched in cosmetics language, saying that it "appears" to make skin look firm, although it doesn't really make it firmer. This typical hedge is understandable because the ingredients in here can't firm skin. Surprisingly, the really beneficial ingredients are present in smaller amounts than what Olay includes in their Regenerist serums. This fragrance-free primer works well under makeup, facilitating application by smoothing the skin's texture, and the matte finish helps keep excess shine in check. Oddly, this also contains the sunscreen ingredient ethylhexyl methoxycinnamate, in addition to the titanium dioxide, so you'd think that Cover Girl/Olay would've taken the extra step to determine this product's SPF rating. We asked them about that and their response was that ethylhexyl methoxycinnamate "has emollient properties that strongly influence both how the product feels on application and the product's dry-down profile on skin." The answer doesn't make sense: Why use a sunscreen ingredient that has poor emollient properties in comparison with other emollient ingredients? Without question, ethylhexyl methoxycinnamate can influence a product's texture, but not in a good way. This problem is one of the difficulties in formulating an elegant-feeling sunscreen. This is worth a try, the price is hard to pass up, and if you have normal to oily/combination, you may be truly pleased with the results, but your skin will not be any firmer than it was when you started.

☺ GOOD **Queen Collection Natural Hue Liquid Makeup** *($7.79)* is a standard, but good, lightweight oil-free foundation for normal to oily skin. The shade range is designed for women with dark skin tones. For the most part, the colors are spot-on (though it's a shame there are no testers). Be careful with the orange-tinged Golden Honey and Amber Glow; Rich Mink and True Ebony are gorgeous for very dark skin tones. Regardless of shade, you get sheer to light coverage and a soft matte finish. This must be blended carefully to avoid an uneven appearance.

☺ AVERAGE **Clean Makeup Sensitive Skin** *($6.99)* mercifully omits the sickly sweet scent that is present in the Clean Makeup Normal Skin formula, as well as the irritating extracts. Unfortunately, most of the shades are just too strongly peach, pink, or rose for most skin tones. The only shades worth considering are Ivory, Classic Ivory, and Soft Honey. This has a beautifully lightweight, silky texture that provides light coverage and is easy to blend. The finish is soft matte but again, the shades are mostly awful.

☺ AVERAGE **Cover Girl & Olay Tone Rehab 2-in-1 Foundation Base** *($14.99)* is billed as a 2-in-1 product, the first being a Cover Girl foundation that evens skin tone and the second being an Olay serum that hydrates skin over time. Sounds like a bonus product, but almost any well-formulated foundation will live up to the claim of evening out your skin tone, merely because of the coverage it provides. The Olay serum spirals out along with the foundation, and although the serum does include several beneficial ingredients for skin, it also includes potential skin irritants, including very strong fragrance. Irritation, even if it smells nice, is always a problem for skin (see the Appendix for further details). If you're still interested in giving this a try, you'll find it provides light coverage and leaves a soft matte finish. Its formula is best for normal to dry skin. The 12 shades will suit light to medium/deep skin tones, although the coverage is relatively sheer, which means you have more flexibility with shades if you need it.

☺ AVERAGE **NatureLuxe Liquid Silk Foundation SPF 10** *($11.99)*. Aside from a few natural-sounding ingredients, there is nothing any more natural about NatureLuxe foundation than there is about countless other liquid foundations. What NatureLuxe does offer is built-in broad-spectrum sun protection (albeit a paltry SPF 10, when SPF 15 is the minimum recommended by most medical boards), as well as a decent amount of ingredients with proven benefit for skin, something you don't see very often in other liquid foundations! True to its name, the foundation indeed has a silky texture, but that silkiness doesn't translate into easy application because it sets much too quickly, so you have to blend it on fast. The finish is somewhat powdery and it will stay put, but it has a slight amount of sheen that might be a problem for those with oily skin, which already has enough of its own "sheen." Most of the shades are for fair to medium skin tones, some particularly nice options for fair skin—no surprise, as porcelain-complexioned singer Taylor Swift is the face of NatureLuxe. Finding the right shade will take some experimenting, especially because these shades tend to oxidize (change color) after a few minutes, bringing out noticeable orange and peach undertones. What prevents this from earning a higher rating is the aforementioned low SPF, plus enough fragrance to be not only bothersome, but also a potential irritant (fragrance, whether natural or synthetic, can cause irritation). Cover Girl offers better foundations, or you can check out our Best Foundations list at the end of this book for superior options.

☺ AVERAGE **Queen Collection Natural Hue Compact Foundation** *($9.99)* is a classic cream-to-powder foundation, but in this case, classic isn't a positive thing. Lots of brands offer better cream-to-powder formulas, including Estee Lauder and M.A.C., both lines that offer shades for women of color. Cover Girl's contribution has a waxy yet smooth texture that has OK initial slip but sets almost too quicky to a powdery finish that can appear greasy. What's worse, most of the colors are terrible. They're either too orange, too copper, or too red. The few worthwhile shades include Rich Mink and Warm Caramel. If you opt to try this, it's best for normal to slightly dry skin that's not prone to blemishes.

☹ POOR **Clean Makeup Normal Skin** *($6.99)* is the original Cover Girl foundation (launched in 1961) that hasn't yet been discontinued despite the fact that it has a dated, basic formula that contains clove, menthol, camphor, and eucalyptus, which are extremely irritating for skin, comes in colors that are largely unusable for any skin tone, and has fragrance that is intrusive. This must be selling well, however, or why would they keep it for so many, yet all that means is that there are thousands of women wearing an irritating foundation whose colors haven't kept pace with the vast majority of foundations available, including those from Cover Girl. See the Appendix to learn why the irritating ingredients and fragrance in this makeup are bad for all skin types.

☹ POOR **Cover Girl & Olay Simply Ageless Foundation SPF 22** *($13.99)* is supposed to combine the benefits of Olay Regenerist Serum in a foundation with sunscreen. The claim is that it can stay suspended above wrinkles, covering them evenly without seeping into lines and not clogging pores. Well, don't count on it. The only two redeeming qualities of this foundation are (1) the spokesperson is Ellen DeGeneres (though clearly she's being paid a lot of money for this endorsement, and we doubt that she could possibly believe this product has any merit) and (2) the sponge that's included in the packaging is good for blending. Seriously, that's it, it's all downhill from there. This cream foundation blended with Olay Regenerist serum is all gimmick and hype. The creamy texture is difficult to blend, even with the included sponge, feels greasy on the skin, and sets easily into lines and wrinkles, leaving your face with a heavy and cakey made-up look. If this doesn't clog pores, we don't know what will. Cover Girl & Olay Simply Ageless Foundation SPF 22 isn't recommended for any skin type.

COVER GIRL CONCEALERS

☺ GOOD **Cover Girl & Olay Simply Ageless Concealer** *($11.99)* comes in a generously sized screw-top jar and has the right amount of slip to make blending a breeze. While the shades are mostly neutral (only Medium/Dark has a slightly rose cast), they're suitable mainly for light to medium skin tones. The biggest issue with this concealer is that it tends to slip into creases shortly after application, thereby accentuating wrinkles—probably not what you had in mind, especially given the "ageless" name. A good dusting of powder helps with the slippage problem, but given that this concealer's finish is already quite matte, powdering over it increases the risk of under-eye skin looking and feeling too dry. Olay's contribution to this Cover Girl product comes primarily from the addition of a significant amount of niacinamide, which does indeed give skin an extra boost and is not a light- or air-sensitive ingredient. However, although niacinamide is a great ingredient for skin, it takes more than this B vitamin to make skin look and act younger. This concealer is best for those who do not have prominent wrinkles around the eye.

☺ GOOD **Fresh Complexion Concealer** *($5.29)* is the only Cover Girl liquid concealer to seriously consider. It has a wonderful, lightly creamy texture and a soft application that provides almost too much slip. Although blending this concealer takes a bit more time, the natural matte finish and smooth coverage are worth it. This wouldn't be our top choice if your main concern is great coverage, but those with minor imperfections should check it out. Of the colors, only Natural Beige is too pink to purchase, but be careful with the slightly pink Creamy Beige, too.

☻ AVERAGE **CG Smoothers Concealer** *($7.39)* is a standard, lipstick-style concealer that doesn't go on as greasy as it appears and provides good coverage with minimal creasing. However, four of the six shades are on the peach side, and the coverage is opaque enough for that to be a problem for some skin tones. Neutralizer is OK, but Illuminator is too whitish pink for even very light skin. This concealer is not recommended for use over blemishes or blemish-prone areas.

☹ AVERAGE **Invisible Concealer** *($4.39)* has a formula and mostly poor colors that have caused it to fall out of favor as a recommended concealer. It provides adequate coverage but has a somewhat tacky finish that isn't as elegant as today's best liquid, wand-applicator concealers. Among the five shades, only the darker ones (Honey and Tawny) are workable.

☻ POOR **Cover Girl & Olay Simply Ageless Corrector** *($11.99)* is a creamy yellow concealer that exchanges one skin problem for another. While it is dense and pigmented enough to cover blemishes and dark circles, you then have to work at concealing the corrector. Save yourself the extra step and extra money and opt instead for a concealer that will work all on its own; such options are plentiful, including some from Cover Girl.

COVER GIRL POWDERS

✓☺ BEST **TruBlend Pressed Powder** *($7.79)* continues the remarkable pigment technology introduced with Cover Girl's TruBlend Foundation. This talc-based powder has a silky smooth, slightly thick texture that meshes so well with skin you won't know you're wearing powder. Instead, the skin looks refined and finished rather than pasty or dry, an effect that is flattering on all skin types. Six very good shades are available, and they're versatile enough to work for many skin tones within their respective range. Somehow, the pigments in this powder simply enhance skin without changing its natural color. This is good news, because it means you're not likely to make a mistake choosing a shade—just pick something that looks close to your skin tone and you should be all set (unless skin is very fair or dark, in which case you should turn to the pressed-powder options from L'Oreal or Revlon before Cover Girl TruBlend).

✓☺ BEST **Advanced Radiance Age-Defying Pressed Powder** *($7.79)* has a formula, texture, and finish that are identical to those of the TruBlend Pressed Powder above, so the same basic comments apply. Six shades are available, and there's not a bad one in the bunch.

☺ GOOD **Clean Oil Control Pressed Powder** *($6.99)* is a good, talc-based, affordable pressed powder for normal, combination, or slightly oily skin. The texture is a bit on the dry side, but this is more a matter of preference because it still works to even out skin tone and provide a polished finish without looking dry or cakey. Unfortunately, contrary to the name, what it doesn't do is control oil, at least not any better than dozens of other talc-based pressed powders.

☺ GOOD **Clean Pressed Powder Sensitive Skin** *($6.99)* isn't "cleaner" than any of the other pressed powders in the Cover Girl line. It's a standard, talc-based powder with a smooth application and soft, slightly dry finish suitable for normal to oily skin. The shades are a mixed bag with the light to medium tones faring best (and there are shades for very fair skin). The missteps that should be avoided include Classic Beige, Warm Beige, Creamy Beige, Medium Light, and the borderline-peach Soft Honey.

☺ AVERAGE **Queen Collection Natural Hue Minerals Pressed Powder** *($8.29)* contains mica, a mineral that, along with the talc, gives credibility to this product's name. It has an unusual texture that's smooth yet waxy, and the result is minimal powder deposit and poor shine control. You'll get a sheer satin finish that doesn't look overly powdered, but doesn't do much to enhance skin tone or downplay large pores, either. Oddly, the shade selection doesn't go as dark as the foundations that are part of Cover Girl's Queen Collection. Every color goes on lighter and softer than it appears in the compact, and all except Light Bronze 1 are recommended.

☹ POOR **Clean Pressed Powder for Normal Skin** *($6.99)* is an incredibly fragrant powder that includes eucalyptus oil, clove oil, and camphor, all of which are very irritating even in small amounts. This is, hands down, the most irritating pressed powder at the drugstore and most of the shades are terrible.

COVER GIRL BLUSHES & BRONZER

☺ GOOD **Cover Girl & Olay Simply Ageless Sculpting Blush** *($10.49)* works quite nicely as a blush, coming in four versatile shades that are best suited for light to medium skin tones. Housed in a flat, jar-like package, the product applies a bit greasy, but this allows adequate time for blending (the product's claim of "sculpting" seems a bit of a stretch, especially considering that the tones all hover around pink and peach, colors that aren't used for contouring). Once it sets to a soft powder finish, the results are natural and lasting, although not "ageless," of course!

☺ AVERAGE **Queen Collection Natural Hue Bronzer** *($8.29)* is described as a mineral-enriched formula, and it is. The minerals are talc and mica, and they show up in the majority of bronzing powders sold today. This is a standard bronzing powder that has a smooth, dry texture and soft application (too soft, in fact, for the darker skin tones its intended for). The shades aren't that impressive; only Ebony Bronze is recommended, though this won't register on most dark skin tones.

☹ POOR **Cheekers** *($4.47)* are available in contemporary shades, but have a terribly dry, flaky texture that sweeps on unevenly, creating a blotchy look.

☹ POOR **Classic Color Blush** *($5.49)* is a powder blush that comes in four shades that, although vivid, blend on sheer. These are fairly powdery, and the color intensity is too soft for darker skin tones.

☹ POOR **Instant Cheekbones** *($5.49)* has three colors in one compact—a blush tone, a contour color, and a shiny highlighter. The colors are workable but the formula has a terribly dry, flaky texture that sweeps on unevenly, creating a blotchy look.

COVER GIRL EYESHADOWS

☺ GOOD **Intense ShadowBlast** *($7.99)*. Is an eyeshadow that claims to be long-wearing, water-resistant, and crease-proof too good to be true? The answer is: yes and no. Yes, because this cream eyeshadow lives up to its claims by lasting all day, resisting creasing, and withstanding a moderate amount of moisture (a light mist as opposed to a downpour). No, because the pigmentation is very light and because once it sets, the formula really accentuates wrinkles or even slightly crinkly lids. If that seems like a fair trade-off to you (or if you have perfectly smooth, unlined eyelids), then you'll likely be happy with this eyeshadow. The color selection is limited to six shades, all of which are quite frosty. Note that the bulky sponge-tip applicator is tricky to use at first; try dabbing the product on your lids and then blending out with your fingertips or a soft eyeshadow brush.

☹ POOR **Exact Eyelights Eye Brightening Eyeshadow** *($7.49)* is a collection of four different powder eyeshadow palettes that are designed to "enhance and brighten" your natural eye color, be it blue, brown, green, or hazel. That's an interesting (though tired) concept, but not even one of the four palettes offers workable options that could reasonably complement the corresponding eye color. Instead, Cover Girl included shades that match these eye colors outright, and it's never a good idea to match your eyeshadow to your eye color. Of the four color options, only the palette for brown eyes contains workable shades for any eye color. Consider that moot, however, because the eyeshadow formula is Cover Girl's oldest, and as such has an unpleasantly dry texture and imparts extremely sheer color that flakes away almost as fast as it's applied.

☹ POOR **Eye Enhancers Kit Shadows** *($3.19-$5.49)* come in palettes of one, three or four shades, but have a bit of a nonsense name because one color (or one of anything) does not make a kit. Each shade has a smooth, unusually dry texture that imparts sheer color, but not without some flaking and skipping during application. These apply very sheer—even the black shade goes on almost translucent. Compared to powder eyeshadows from L'Oreal, Sonia Kashuk, and NYX Cosmetics, these aren't worth considering.

☹ POOR **Smoky ShadowBlast** *($8.49)*. Paired into color combinations to easily create a smokey eye effect, this dual-ended cream-to-powder eyeshadow stick is a great idea; unfortunately, the formula doesn't live up to the concept's potential. The colors go on too sheer and too frosty (all shades are heavy on the frost-like shimmer), but there's little color payoff, so the smokey effect is nil. Worse, the colors crease and then fade far too quickly.

COVER GIRL EYE & BROW LINERS

☺ GOOD **Exact Eyelights Eye Brightening Liner** *($6.99)* tries to brighten eye color with shades that just don't work for that purpose. Radiant Sapphire for blue eyes? The best strategy for playing up eye color is to do so with a contrasting color, or better yet, what every model and celebrity has on in fashion magazine after magazine: smokey gray or brown shades, not blue, jade green, purple…. But, if you ignore Cover Girl's recommended pairings, you'll find an automatic, retractable eyeliner, available in some great shade options, that goes on smoothly and has incredible staying power—although for a pencil liner, it sets fast and isn't forgiving if you want to blend it. Of the four options, those with the most baffling names are the best: Vibrant Pearl is a smoky black and Vivid Ruby, a deep brown.

☺ GOOD **Queen Collection Eye Liner** *($4.99)* doesn't require sharpening, but it isn't retractable, so be careful with how much of the tip you expose at once. It has a smooth, creamy application that deposits color evenly, though we expected these to be more pigmented given this pencil is designed for dark skin tones. Once set, the formula stays put and is minimally prone to fading. Avoid the ashen Grey Khaki; the navy Midnight Blue is OK because it's more of a bluish-black.

☺ GOOD **Perfect Point Plus** *($5.79)* is an automatic eye pencil that glides on easily without being greasy, and it maintains a consistent, sharp point. Chestnut is a great shade as an auburn eyeliner, but Midnight Blue is best avoided. Avoid using the smudge tip—it's not well made and can change your eye makeup look from smoky to messy.

☺ AVERAGE **Line Exact Liquid Liner Pen** *($6.99)* offers precision application from a felt-tip style pen that is easier to work with than liquid liners that apply with a long, thin brush. The formula dries quickly, so smearing and smudging are not an issue. The average rating is because this tends to wear unevenly and is prone to fading—so the intense line you begin the day with looks like a shadow of its former self by lunchtime.

☺ AVERAGE **Liquiline Blast Eyeliner Pencil** *($8.79)* features a distinctively shaped rubber tool on the other end that's angled perfectly for smudging out from the lashline. Application is mostly smooth (only a slight amount of drag), and once this sets, it's resistant to smearing and even a tear or two. The vibrant shades range from an ill-advised Green Glow to a rich Violet Voltage. Were it not for the need for routine sharpening, this would've earned a Good rating.

COVER GIRL LIP COLOR & LIPLINERS

✓☺ BEST **Blast Flipstick Blendable Lip Duo** *($7.99)*. This clever lip duo is a genuine bargain because you really get three shades of lipstick in one dual-sided product. How? Each of the 13 duos contains a cream shade and a shimmer shade coordinated to be applied separately or together—the results are impressive and quite fun! Also impressive is how pigmented this lipstick is, delivering vibrant color that lasts for hours with minimal bleeding. The texture is smooth, light, and somewhat dry, so if you like moisturizing lipsticks, you may want to prep with a balm or finish with a gloss. One note about packaging: The small plastic caps on either end of this twist-up tube are prone to coming off if jostled, which puts your makeup bag, purse, or pocket at double the risk for a lipstick disaster.

✓☺ BEST **Lip Perfection Lipstick** *($6.99)* is as close to perfection as you'll find at the drugstore! Between the feather-light feel, semi-matte finish, and incredible staying power, it's a winner for Cover Girl and you.

✓☺ BEST **Outlast All-Day Lipcolor** *($9.29)* features a liquid color you apply to lips (make sure they're clean, dry, and free of any flakes), let set for a moment or two, then apply a glossy top coat for comfortable wear and shine. Outlast wears extraordinarily well. As long as you can commit to regularly applying the moisturizing top coat, you'll be rewarded with feel-good color that lasts through most meals (oily salad dressings or fried foods are this lip color's undoing), and it doesn't come off on cups or people (so go ahead and kiss the ones you love freely).

✓☺ BEST **Queen Collection Lip Gloss** *($5.99)* is a superior lip gloss that is outfitted with a sponge-tip applicator. It applies smoothly; imparts sheer, shimmering color; and hasn't a trace of stickiness. The shade range is well suited to those with darker skin tones, though each color goes on softer than it appears in the package. Consider this a best beauty buy!

☺ GOOD **LipSlicks Lipgloss** *($3.99)* is a basic, emollient, castor oil–based sheer lipstick with some very shiny shades, all in packaging that makes getting it on the lips very tricky for anyone with thin lips.

☺ GOOD **Outlast Double LipShine** *($10.30)* is a sheerer, glossier version of Cover Girl's Outlast Smoothwear All Day Lipcolor. It is not rated as highly as the original Outlast because its promised 10-hour wear time doesn't come close to being true, and it wears unevenly.

☺ GOOD **Outlast Lipstain** *($7.99)* comes packaged like a felt-tip marker. The pointed-tip applicator makes precise application easy, but as with most lip stains the watery color distributes unevenly and will need to be blended with a fingertip or lip brush. Also, the sheer colors apply brighter than they appear on the packaging, so choose carefully. Once this stain sets it wears well on its own and provides a matte base for gloss. If you've been using BeneTint as your lip stain, give Outlast Lipstain a try—you won't be disappointed. Neither will your wallet!

☺ AVERAGE **Lip Perfection Lipliner** *($6.99)* delivers smooth, bold color that lasts, but the need for routine sharpening makes it inconvenient, especially considering the number of twist-up pencils available today that make application effortless every day and all day.

☺ AVERAGE **NatureLuxe Gloss Balm SPF 15** *($5.99)* looks and feels more like a sheer lipstick than a lip gloss or lip balm. It deposits a soft stain of color with a moist finish that wears away after about an hour, leaving behind a soft wash of color. Of the 16 shades, you'll find metallic, frost, and cream finishes, all of which have the same moist texture and sheer color payoff. Anemone looks too bright in the container, but it's actually a cheerful, flattering red. What prevents this otherwise very good product from earning a higher rating is the lack of sufficient UVA-protecting ingredients. See the Appendix to learn which UVA-protecting ingredients should be in any SPF-rated product.

COVER GIRL MASCARAS

✓☺ BEST **Lash Blast Length** *($7.79)* works exactly as claimed, allowing you to build impressively long, perfectly separated lashes. Thickness is minor, but without question this makes lashes really long, and without clumps, smears, or flaking. Removal is easy with a good water-soluble cleanser.

✓☺ BEST **Lash Blast Volume** *($7.79)* has an oversized, rubber-bristled brush that seems imposing at first, but allows you to be surprisingly nimble when defining, lengthening, and slightly thickening your lashes. You're left with a full, dramatic, clump-free sweep of softly fringed lashes that look gorgeous and last all day.

☺ GOOD **Lash Blast 24HR** *($8.99)*. We never recommend anyone wear mascara for 24 hours straight; it's just not a good idea to fall asleep with your makeup on because it causes irritation and makes you look puffy the next morning. But, if you had to, this one would be up to the task. It holds a curl beautifully, adds thickness and length, and each coat looks even more fabulous than the last (with the help of a lash comb). Plus, it does this all without flaking or smudging for, yes, 24 hours (although it depends to some extent on how you sleep). LashBlast 24HR has the same giant rubber brush as the original LashBlast, but its formula is different. What Cover Girl should've made clear is that this formula is waterproof—very waterproof. In fact, it's difficult to remove even with the best eye-makeup remover. While tenacity is clearly this mascara's best point, the fact is that all the tugging on your lashes to remove it is a problem. To avoid premature sagging and wrinkling, it is best to never tug on the skin, especially around the eyes, because it stretches the elastin fibers in your skin and over time they won't bounce back. For regular wear, you want to proceed cautiously with this one.

☺ GOOD **Lash Blast Fusion** *($8.99)*. Marketed attempts to combine the impressive volume of the original Lash Blast with the impressive lengthening of Lash Blast Length to create—you guessed it—their most impressive mascara yet. Does this mascara do it all? Well, almost. The brush is nearly identical to that of Lash Blast Original (orange tube), meaning that it's wide with short, rubber bristles, but the mascara itself is lighter and applies thinly, like Lash Blast Length (in the yellow tube). Unlike Lash Blast Length, however, this isn't a one-coat wonder, although with patience you can come close to creating the separation of the Length version with the fullness of the Original Lash Blast, but you never fully reach the maximum potential of either. So, you end up with lashes that are balanced and beautiful, but lack the full extent of flutter or fullness of their predecessors.

☺ GOOD **Lash Blast Fusion Water Resistant Mascara** *($9.99)* is a good choice for those looking to strike a balance between length and thickness. Your lashes won't get as thick as the original Lash Blast Mascara (orange tube) nor will they be as long as with Lash Blast Length (yellow tube) but many will find the compromise acceptable. This applies smoothly without a clump in sight though can go on a bit unevenly and requires a bit more comb-through than usual (but it's hardly a deal-breaker). The most impressive and unexpected result from this mascara is how well it curls lashes and keeps them upswept! It is definitely worth a look if your lashes need more curl and you don't want to bother with a lash curler. As for being water-resistant, this fits the bill, but so do almost all mascaras not labeled "waterproof." Waterproof formulas tend to stay on when lashes get soaked (think swimming or a shower), whereas water-resistant mascaras are great for minor dampness around the eyes (a light rainfall or when you tear up watching a sad movie). This particular mascara comes off easily with a water-soluble cleanser.

☺ GOOD **Lash Blast Length Water Resistant** *($7.79)* performs just as the regular Lash Blast Length, with the added benefit of being moderately resistant to water. That means it can withstand a couple of tears or a fine mist of rain, but not a downpour or a dip in the pool. Other than that, this mascara works exactly as claimed. This missed a best rating for not being as impervious to water as it should be.

☺ GOOD **Lash Blast Luxe** *($7.99)* comes with a giant rubber-bristled brush that some will love and others will instantly dislike. The differences between Lash Blast Luxe and the original Lash Blast are that the Luxe version is infused with shimmer and it does not enhance thickness the way the original did. The shiny lash effect is very subtle, so aside from the reduced thickness (thickness is what catapulted the original Lash Blast to a Best Product), this mascara is quite similar. The large plastic brush makes it difficult to get an even application on smaller lashes, but once on, Lash Blast Luxe lengthens and separates lashes well with minimal clumping. It doesn't do much for thickness, but it will wear well for hours with no flaking. Removal is easy with a cleanser or an eye-makeup remover.

☺ GOOD **Lash Perfection Volumizing Mascara** *($6.49)* has a retro 1970s look, but its performance (and brush) reminded us of Cover Girl's Lash Blast Fusion (their mascara in the purple tube). Not surprisingly, the performance of Lash Perfection Volumizing Mascara was almost identical to that of Lash Blast Fusion (reviewed above) so the same comments apply.

☺ GOOD **Natureluxe Mousse Mascara** *($8.49)*. The hook with this mascara is that it uses natural waxes instead of "select synthetic polymers" to lengthen and thicken your lashes. Although clearly meant to appeal to women seeking natural makeup, the formula contains the same waxes you see in numerous other mascaras. This contains more natural ingredients than typical mascaras, but not by much, and not enough to make it worth considering over many others. (Plus, synthetic polymers are not bad for your lashes.) Performance-wise, this has a slightly wet application that can be uneven, but the rubber-bristled brush makes it easy to get clean separation. It quickly adds length and decent thickness to lashes. Once set, this wears without flaking or smearing and comes off easily with a water-soluble cleanser.

☺ GOOD **Natureluxe Water Resistant Mascara** *($8.49)* is nearly identical to the Natureluxe Mousse Mascara above, except this holds up better if your eye area gets wet.

☹ AVERAGE **Exact Eyelights Eye Brightening Waterproof Mascara** *($8.49)*. The concept behind this mascara is that you get waterproof protection while adding a brightening shimmer to your lashes. The brightening effect is really subtle, and ends up being a bit annoying because the sparkle particles tend to flake throughout the day. This mascara has a thin, uneven application that takes patience to get what never amounts to more than modest length and no thickness. It's waterproof as stated, but so what? There are lots of waterproof mascaras that handily out-perform this, and you can get the brightening effect from eyeliner or eyeshadow instead.

☹ AVERAGE **Exact Eyelights Mascara** *($8.49)* is supposed to make eyes appear to glisten, and that's because it contains shimmer pigments. Your eyes won't glisten or sparkle with this mascara, but they may become slightly irritated because the shiny particles flake slightly. The other novel feature of this mascara is that its shades are made to correspond with various eye colors. If you notice any difference it will be subtle; for the most part, these are all soft black mascaras lightly tinted with either blue, olive green, copper, or aubergine for a really, really slight effect. As for length and thickness, both are respectable, without a single clump or smear, though not to the same impressive extent as Cover Girl's formidable Lash Blast Mascara.

☺ AVERAGE **Lash Blast Waterproof Volume** *($7.79)* proves that it really is the marriage of a brush and mascara formula that creates a perfect union of beautiful lashes (a problem often discussed among cosmetics chemists who formulate makeup). Cover Girl's original (non-waterproof) version of Lash Blast Mascara is arguably one of their best mascaras (at least if you want gorgeously thick, elongated lashes without a clump in sight). Although the waterproof version has the same spiky, rubber-bristled brush, the results aren't as impressive due to the differences in the formulas. Yes, this is waterproof (and requires an oil- or silicone-based remover when you're ready for it to come off), but it requires a lot more work to get close to "lush, volumized lashes." It out-performs many lackluster waterproof mascaras, but doesn't jump to the head of the class

COVER GIRL BRUSHES

☺ GOOD **Eyeshadow Brush** *($4.49)* isn't the most versatile due to its thickness, and should be flatter and a bit more pointed for better control and blending. This remains an OK option for applying all-over or soft crease color.

☹ POOR **Large Blush Brush** *($4.79)* is a poorly constructed brush that is not recommended because the bristles are too soft and too sparse, making color placement and control an issue.

☹ POOR **Powder Brush** *($5.49)* is cut straight across rather than domed or tapered, a shape that tends to work against the natural contours of the face and makes it easy to over-powder.

DDF - DOCTOR'S DERMATOLOGIC FORMULA (SKIN CARE ONLY)

Strengths: Several good water-soluble cleansers; excellent Photo-Age sunscreens and every DDF sunscreen includes sufficient UVA-protecting ingredients; some truly state-of-the-art moisturizers and serums; a few good AHA and skin-lightening options; a good benzoyl peroxide topical disinfectant.

Weaknesses: Expensive; products designed for sensitive skin tend to contain one or more known problematic ingredients; several irritating products based on alcohol, menthol, or problematic plant extracts; more than a handful of average moisturizers, many in jar packaging.

For more information and reviews of the latest DDF products, visit CosmeticsCop.com.

DDF - DOCTOR'S DERMATOLOGIC FORMULA CLEANSERS

☺ GOOD $$$ **Blemish Foaming Cleanser** *($38 for 6.6 fl. oz.)* is a standard, liquid-to-foam cleanser that contains mostly water, detergent cleansing agents, lather agent, and pH-adjusting agents. Salicylic acid is listed as an active, but its contact with skin is too brief for it to affect blemishes. The token amount of azelaic acid won't impact blemishes even a little. The same can be said for the plant extracts, some soothing and some irritating—but none present in an amount great enough to be a problem or to exert a benefit. This is a good, though pricey, option for normal to oily skin.

☺ GOOD $$$ **Brightening Cleanser** *($38 for 8.5 fl. oz.)* is a detergent-based, water-soluble cleanser for normal to oily skin. It contains the AHA glycolic acid along with a small amount of plant extracts with limited research pertaining to their skin-lightening ability. Although this sounds promising, the AHA and plant extracts need to be left on skin in order to help lighten and "brighten." In a cleanser, they're rinsed down the drain before they have a chance to work, so you're not getting any extra benefits for your money. This deserves a Good rating due to its cleansing and makeup-removing abilities, but note that the amount of glycolic acid can be a problem for use around the eyes.

☺ GOOD $$$ **Non-Drying Gentle Cleanser** *($38 for 8.5 fl. oz.)* is billed as ultra-mild, and for the most part, it is. The detergent cleansing agent is one typically seen in "no more tears" baby shampoos and it is fragrance-free. This is a semi-water-soluble cleanser most suitable for normal to slightly dry skin.

☹ AVERAGE $$$ **Advanced Micro-Exfoliation Cleanser** *($46 for 6 fl. oz.)* isn't anything advanced and is overpriced. Labeling this an advanced cleanser is like calling a typewriter an advanced word processing system. This is mostly a mixture of water, wax, Vaseline, glycerin, and mineral oil, so it is little more than an old-fashioned cold cream base. A basic emollient cleanser that is recommended only for dry to very dry skin, this has a mild scrub action from the rice bran wax it contains, but the emollient base makes it difficult to rinse completely. DDF added some potent antioxidants and cell-communicating ingredients to this product, and because some of it remains on the skin due to the poor rinsability, you may in fact get some benefit from them, but that's a stretch. There are far better ways to get beneficial ingredients to the skin.

☹ AVERAGE $$$ **Salicylic Wash** *($38 for 8.5 fl. oz.)* contains 2% salicylic acid instead of an AHA like glycolic acid. However, both its brief contact with skin and the pH of the base still prevent exfoliation. This is otherwise a very standard, water-soluble cleanser for normal to oily skin. It should be kept away from the eye area.

☹ AVERAGE $$$ **Sensitive Skin Cleansing Gel** *($38 for 8.5 fl. oz.)* is a standard, detergent-based water-soluble cleanser for normal to oily skin. It is not a slam-dunk for sensitive skin (including rosacea) because of the potentially irritating plant extracts and preservatives it contains.

☹ POOR **Glycolic 5% Exfoliating Wash** *($35 for 8.5 fl. oz.)* contains 5% glycolic acid in this detergent-based water-soluble cleanser and is formulated in the correct pH for it to exfoliate, but its contact with skin is too brief for it to provide much benefit because cleansers are rinsed off the skin. Add to that the inclusion of peppermint oil (which does nothing but irritate skin) and this expensive cleanser is one to leave on the shelf.

DDF - DOCTOR'S DERMATOLOGIC FORMULA TONER

☹ POOR **Aloe Toning Complex** *($35 for 8.5 fl. oz.)* contains an amount of comfrey extract that makes it potentially problematic for all skin types. Please refer to the Cosmetic Ingredient Dictionary at CosmeticsCop.com for detailed information on why comfrey is a problem for skin.

DDF - DOCTOR'S DERMATOLOGIC FORMULA EXFOLIANT & SCRUBS

☺ GOOD $$$ **Glycolic 10% Exfoliating Moisturizer** *($52 for 1.7 fl. oz.)* contains 10% glycolic acid at a pH of 3.6, making it an effective exfoliant. The lightweight, silicone-enhanced lotion base is suitable for normal to slightly dry skin. Although it contains some great antioxidants and the packaging will keep them stable, the amount of each is so small as to be almost nonexistent.

☹ AVERAGE $$$ **Glycolic 10% Exfoliating Oil Control Gel** *($52 for 1.7 fl. oz.)* has a pH of 4.1, which limits the effectiveness of the 2% salicylic acid and 10% glycolic acid it contains. Add to that the high amount of alcohol in this formula, and there isn't any other reason to consider this BHA gel.

☹ POOR **Acne Control Treatment Salicylic Acid Acne Medication** *($44 for 1.7 fl. oz.)* should have been a slam-dunk recommendation, but it isn't. This BHA exfoliant designed for acne-prone skin contains 1.5% salicylic acid formulated in a silky lotion base. Alas, the pH of 2.5 is unusually low and bound to be too irritating for all skin types. In addition, the formula includes irritating plants such as witch hazel and ginger root.

☹ POOR **Glycolic 10% Toning Complex** *($40 for 8.5 fl. oz.)* contains alcohol, witch hazel, and menthol, and is not recommended for any skin type. What a shame, because this is otherwise a well-formulated 10% glycolic acid toner.

DDF - DOCTOR'S DERMATOLOGIC FORMULA MOISTURIZERS (DAYTIME & NIGHTTIME), EYE CREAMS, & SERUMS

✓☺ BEST **$$$ Bio-Moisture Eye Serum** *($88 for 0.5 fl. oz.)*. The claims for this eye cream sound scientific, but a quick glance at the formula proves once again why eye creams are an unnecessary extra product when a well-formulated face product will work brilliantly (see the Appendix find out why). More cream than serum, Bio-Moisture Eye Serum contains some great ingredients to fight signs of aging around the eyes. The thing is, those same ingredients are found in great facial moisturizers, which you can (and should) use around your eyes, too! If you choose to try this eye cream (again, it's mislabeled as "serum"), it is best for normal to dry skin. The formula contains enough of the mineral pigment titanium dioxide to have a subtle brightening effect, which can make dark circles less apparent (though a good concealer goes even further).

✓☺ BEST **$$$ Mesojection Antioxidant Moisturizing Serum** *($88 for 0.9 fl. oz.)* is sold as a topical substitute for a procedure known as mesotherapy. This treatment, which according to research is not medically sound, is most commonly used to dissolve fat and improve the appearance of cellulite via injections that contain either homeopathic or pharmaceutical substances. Strangely, there isn't necessarily any consistency in the range of mesotherapy procedures, and the cocktail of ingredients varies from practitioner to practitioner, which makes this treatment very hard to evaluate. The most commonly used substance is phosphatidylcholine, but it also is frequently combined with deoxycholate. A handful of studies have shown that this can successfully reduce fat when injected into the skin, with one study demonstrating this effect for the under-eye area. Theoretically, the reduction of subcutaneous fat may be caused by inflammatory-mediated cell death and resorption. What does any of this have to do with skin? DDF is hoping that the effects associated with the injection of potentially helpful substances will correlate with the effects of topical application of this water-based serum. They state that this product's technology allows for 85% more potent antioxidant activity to be delivered to the deepest layers of the skin's surface (that's really not so deep, since it's still the surface of skin, but it sounds impressive, doesn't it?). But there is no published research to confirm that this antioxidant has any "mesojection" (Who came up with that deceptive term?) impact or any benefit whatsoever. Other than this overblown marketing angle, this contains impressive amounts of several antioxidants in a base that is suitable for normal to dry skin. The amount of salicylic acid is too low for it to be efficacious, although this serum has a pH that would allow it to exfoliate if more were included.

✓☺ BEST **$$$ Pro-Retinol Energizing Moisturizer** *($88 for 1.7 fl. oz.)* presents retinol along with several antioxidants in a slightly emollient lotion base suitable for normal to dry

The Reviews D

---

skin. This well-packaged product contains some beneficial fatty acids and nonvolatile plant oils that go beyond merely moisturizing skin. If you're going to splurge on a moisturizer, this product won't prove to be a letdown (provided you keep your expectations in check about it making you look years younger).

✓☺ BEST $$$ **Protect and Correct UV Moisturizer SPF 15** *($64 for 1.7 fl. oz.)* is an in-part avobenzone sunscreen that makes claims similar to those of Olay's dwindling Definity brand, and the formulation isn't that much different either. That's not surprising given that Olay owner Procter & Gamble is at the helm of DDF, too. Of course, because DDF is a "dermatologist-developed" line sold in upscale stores, the price point is much higher than that of Olay. But the good news is you're getting a well-formulated daytime moisturizer that is suitable for normal to dry skin. The amount of niacinamide along with acetyl glucosamine will likely have a positive impact on skin discolorations, and the formula does include several antioxidants (though only a couple are present in meaningful amounts). The amount of mica in this moisturizer with sunscreen leaves a soft shimmer on skin that, to some extent, can indeed make it look "translucent," but you can get that result from any cosmetic that contains soft shine ingredients.

✓☺ BEST $$$ **Wrinkle Resist Plus Pore Minimizer Moisturizing Serum** *($85 for 1.7 fl. oz.)* is a very good serum that treats skin to smoothing silicone, glycerin, cell-communicating ingredients (niacinamide and peptides), plus notable antioxidants. This pale peach-tinted version from DDF has pigments for a slightly shimmery finish, but in our estimation that doesn't make it worth considering over the considerably less expensive version from Olay (and Olay offers a fragrance-free version in their Regenerist line). Still, if you're loyal to DDF, we can't dispute that this is an impressive formula for normal to slightly dry or slightly oily skin, but then again, so is Olay's.

☺ GOOD $$$ **Amplifying Elixir** *($70 for 1.7 fl. oz.)* is said to boost the results of your skin-care routine by 47%, but that figure is a moving target. What does it really mean, in terms of your skin-care routine? Would someone using bad products with irritating ingredients get a greater increase and someone using brilliantly formulated products see less improvement? Quite possibly, which is why the percentage mentioned is meaningless, especially because we don't know exactly how DDF came to this result. When it comes down to it, this is yet another serum to consider. It contains some good ingredients, but none that make it capable of performing better than any other well-formulated serum. And for what this costs, you should think twice before adding it to your routine, especially if the routine you're using already includes a great serum and/or moisturizer. The fragrance-free formula contains the cell-communicating ingredient niacinamide as a main ingredient, just as many of the serums from Olay do (Olay and DDF are both owned by Procter & Gamble, and their formulas are more similar than most consumers realize). It also contains some novel and potentially helpful antioxidants and immune-modulating plant extracts, all of which may help keep skin healthier and improve its barrier function. Although that's wonderful, this serum is hardly the only product to contain these types of ingredients—and you certainly don't have to spend in this range to get their results. Amplifying Elixir is best for normal to oily skin, but can be used by all skin types. Its water and glycol base lend somewhat of a tacky finish, so this doesn't feel as silky as silicone-based serums, but it still works well under moisturizer.

☺ GOOD $$$ **Erase Eye Gel** *($52 for 0.5 fl. oz.)* is a silky, fragrance-free serum that contains some intriguing ingredients for repairing wrinkles, but nothing that cannot be found in many serums designed for the face, including most sold by Olay Regenerist (and remember,

DDF is owned by the same company that owns Olay). None of the ingredients in this eye serum have research proving they do anything to make dark circles or puffiness better, though the small amount of caffeine may have some impact on minor swelling around the eyes (the kind that's from fluid retention, not from aging). This serum contains mineral pigments to add shine around the eyes, but shine isn't skin care; it's really a makeup effect. To some extent, the shine helps reflect light away from dark circles, but better results can be had from using a good concealer instead. If you decide to try this, it is suitable for all skin types—though see the Appendix to find out why, in truth, you don't need a special product for the eye area.

☺ GOOD $$$ **Restoring Night Serum** *($95 for 0.8 fl. oz.)* is a pricey water-based serum that may have grabbed your attention with its claim of reversing wrinkles by 30%. Who wouldn't be tempted by any product making such a boast? Added to these hope-in-a-bottle marketing shenanigans, DDF uses phrases such as "patented technology" (which is meaningless because patents have nothing to do with efficacy) and "results in 2 weeks" (which is easy to simulate with almost any skin-care product). Supposedly, the patented technology allows elastin, one of skin's supportive elements, to cross link, as it does naturally when we're young and before sun damage occurs. However, unlike collagen, once elastin fibers are damaged, they're most likely irreparable. Also, unlike collagen (which healthy skin loves to make), we have almost all the elastin we ever will have at birth; after that, elastin production decreases significantly. By the time we reach adulthood, elastin production stops almost completely (Source: *Cosmetic Dermatology Principles and Practice*, 2nd Edition, Baumann, Leslie, M.D., McGraw Hill Medical, 2009, pages 9–10). That's just one more reason why sun protection is so important if you want to avoid damaging the elements in your skin that keep it looking young and that cannot easily, if ever, be regenerated. Think of elastin strands as if they were small rubber bands. When a rubber band is fresh and new, it has great bounce-back and resiliency. However, once it is stretched beyond its limits, it either snaps or fails to revert to its original size. Such is the case with damaged elastin fibers in your skin—years of cumulative damage, mostly from environmental sources, cause elastin to lose its ability to snap back into place, resulting in sagging skin and more pronounced wrinkles. However, there is one ingredient in this serum (dill extract) that has the potential to stimulate elastin production, at least with fake skin. There is one study indicating that on human skin samples and on "dermal equivalents" (which is not the same as intact human skin), dill extract had an effect on elastogenesis. Elastogenesis is a fancy way of saying it helped make elastin. The study demonstrated that dill can stimulate key enzymes in fake skin that trigger elastin production, although no mention was made of dill being able to repair damaged elastin (which would be truly exciting) or how much dill was required or whether or not it would work in a cosmetic formula when combined with other ingredients. We also don't know if dill can be absorbed into real skin to have a similar impact. Instead, all we know is that dill seems to have this effect on isolated skin cells responsible for elastin production (Sources: naturaldatabase.com; and *Experimental Dermatology*, August 2006, pages 574–581). Although it is highly doubtful that the amount of dill extract in this product will repair elastin in test tube skin or real skin, there is still the claim about reducing wrinkles by 30% to look at. Understand that percentages indicating improvement are meaningless without the study in hand because there is no way to know how the study was done. If the product was applied after washing and then the face was stripped with alcohol, that could easily account for the improvement, but DDF isn't divulging their study protocol; rather, they're just bragging about the results (sort of like getting an A on a math test but you already had the answers given to you—and everyone knows you cheated).

The Reviews D

Aside from the over-the-top seductive claims, this does contain several beneficial ingredients that can help improve wrinkles and make skin look smoother while reducing inflammation and repairing skin's barrier. All of that is good news; it's just tempered by the fact that DDF's attention-getting, wrinkle-reversing claims won't become reality. Oh, and by the way, DDF is owned by Procter & Gamble, which explains this new formula's similarity to many of Olay's products (also owned by P&G), and those products are a lot less pricey, that's for sure. This fragrance-free serum is suitable for all skin types.

☺ AVERAGE $$$ **Advanced Firming Cream** *($130 for 1.7 fl. oz.)* is indeed an advanced formula for dry skin, we're not going to dispute that. What's not advanced is the jar packaging, which will lead to the light- and air-sensitive ingredients deteriorating shortly after you begin using this moisturizer (see the Appendix for further details). The claim of neutralizing 82% of free radicals is an in vitro claim, not an ongoing effect given skin's continual exposure to the environment. Aside from the claims, this would have gotten a great recommendation if the packaging would help you get the good stuff delivered to your skin.

☺ AVERAGE $$$ **Advanced Moisture Defense UV Cream SPF 15** *($105 for 1.7 fl. oz.)* contains avobenzone for sufficient UVA protection and has a silky base that's loaded with the cell-communicating ingredient niacinamide. The formula also contains several impressive antioxidants, and that's where the jar packaging starts to rain on the parade, because all these state-of-the-art ingredients deteriorate in the presence of air when the package is opened. A great formula is meaningless if it's not in packaging that keeps the most delicate yet effective ingredients stable during use. One more comment: the price of this moisturizer means you'll be less likely to apply it liberally each day—yet that's essential to getting the amount of anti-wrinkle sun protection this provides!

☺ AVERAGE $$$ **Clarifying Hydrator** *($42 for 1.7 fl. oz.)* is another moisturizer from DDF that's strikingly similar to those from Olay's Regenerist line, though Olay costs less and tends to omit the potentially problematic ingredients DDF chose for Clarifying Hydrator. Both Olay and DDF are owned by Procter & Gamble, so the formulary similarities are not surprising; clearly, there's no need to spend more for this product because, although you're getting some great ingredients, there are some troublemakers afoot, too, and so the question is why bother?

☺ AVERAGE $$$ **Wrinkle Relax** *($88 for 0.5 fl. oz.)* is a lightweight, water-based serum that contains an impressive amount of vitamin C (as magnesium ascorbyl phosphate) and not much else of interest, at least not anything present in an amount that would have an astonishing effect on wrinkles or expression lines. The tiny amount of peptide this serum contains has scant research on its ability to reduce wrinkles, though this serum contains enough film-forming agent (think hairspray) to make skin feel temporarily smoother and a bit tighter. Despite these traits, in no way is Wrinkle Relax a viable substitute for the improvements possible from Botox injections or dermal fillers. If anything, for what this costs your money would be better spent on an actual cosmetic procedure!

☹ POOR **Advanced Eye Firming Concentrate** *($88 for 0.5 fl. oz.)* is beautifully formulated, and we would love to give this product a better rating. The caffeine has no special benefit for the eye area, despite the association with waking someone up. However, the jar packaging wastes all the air-sensitive ingredients, including vitamin A and the peptides (see the Appendix to learn more). It is also important to point out that the eye-area claim and the idea it requires a higher price tag is just silly; it doesn't contain any special ingredients exclusively for skin around the eyes. Again, check the Appendix where you'll see why, in truth, you don't need a special product for the eye area—really.

☹ POOR **Weightless Defense Oil-Free Hydrator UV Moisturizer SPF 45** *($52 for 1.7 fl. oz.)* offers significant sun protection and contains avobenzone for protection from the sun's aging rays (UVA radiation), but the amount of alcohol present causes dryness and irritation that leads to free-radical damage and the breakdown of healthy collagen. The alcohol gives this product its lightweight texture and finish, but lots of other ingredients can do that without irritating your skin. See the Appendix for further details on the problems alcohol presents.

DDF - DOCTOR'S DERMATOLOGIC FORMULA SPECIALTY SKIN-CARE PRODUCTS

☺ GOOD **$$$ Benzoyl Peroxide Gel** *($34 for 2 fl. oz.)* is a simply formulated but effective topical disinfectant for blemish-prone skin. The amount of tea tree oil is not enough to function as a disinfectant (it just adds fragrance), but the 5% benzoyl peroxide takes care of that on its own.

☹ POOR **Sulfur Therapeutic Mask** *($40 for 4 fl. oz.)* is a standard clay mask that also contains 10% sulfur. Sulfur is a topical disinfectant that is very irritating and highly alkaline, and can cause problems for skin. See the Appendix to learn how irritation makes oily, breakout-prone skin worse.

DERMA E (SKIN CARE ONLY)

Strengths: Inexpensive considering the formulas; company provides complete ingredient lists on their website; an effective AHA product; tea tree oil–based disinfectants for acne; some good cleansers; well-formulated soothing serum; good masks.

Weaknesses: Jar packaging is rampant for many of the antioxidant-rich products; several boring moisturizers; abrasive scrubs; no BHA options; one skin-lightening product with questionable efficacy; products that contain the controversial ingredient DMAE; several products contain natural ingredients that have not been proven effective for their intended purpose; the anti-aging products with peptides make over-the-top claims not supported by what they contain.

For more information and the latest Derma E reviews, visit CosmeticsCop.com.

DERMA E CLEANSERS

☺ GOOD **Hyaluronic Hydrating Cleanser** *($15.50 for 6 fl. oz.)* is a good, gentle cleanser suitable for all skin types except sensitive. The only concern is the fragrant plants and "Plumeria fragrance" this contains. Fragrance isn't skin care, but at least in a cleanser these ingredients are rinsed from skin before they can cause problems. This cleanser removes most types of makeup (long-wearing or waterproof formulas will require a separate makeup remover) and rinses without leaving a residue. It contains hyaluronic acid as claimed, and this helps keep skin soft during cleansing, but no more so than many other ingredients. Note that this cleanser cannot unclog pores by itself. Cleansers help remove surface oil and debris that contributes to clogging, but for real improvement you need to use a well-formulated BHA (salicylic acid) exfoliant such as those from Paula's Choice.

☺ GOOD **Tea Tree and E Face and Body Wash** *($10.50 for 8 fl. oz.)* is a fairly gentle, water-soluble cleanser that is a good inexpensive option for normal to oily or blemish-prone skin. The amount of tea tree oil adds a medicinal fragrance and warrants caution when using around the eyes. Although tea tree oil has antiseptic and antibacterial properties, its brief contact with skin when included in a cleanser isn't the best way to obtain those benefits because it's just rinsed down the drain before it can have any benefit. Due to the tea tree oil, this should not be used anywhere near the eye area. And if you use this as a body wash, do not apply it on or near the genital area; only use it on breakout-prone areas such as the chest and back, or to wash your feet.

☺ GOOD **Vitamin A Glycolic Cleanser** *($11.50 for 6 fl. oz.)* is similar to the Hyaluronic Hydrating Cleanser above, and the same comments apply, except ideally this one is best for normal to dry skin.

☺ GOOD **Vanilla Bean Cleansing Mousse, Age-Defying Facial Formula** *($15.50 for 6 fl. oz.)*. The botanical ingredients in this cleanser aren't going to optimally nourish skin due to the small amounts included and the fact that this product is quickly rinsed away. What this will do is gently cleanse and remove makeup from normal to dry skin. It rinses without leaving a residue and would be rated a Best if it did not contain fragrant plant extracts that pose a risk of irritation. As for the age-defying portion of the name, that's all it is, just a name. This cleanser holds no special ability over others to make skin look younger or resist wrinkles.

☺ AVERAGE **Anti-Aging Pycnogenol Cleanser, Fragrance Free** *($15.50 for 6 fl. oz.)* would be a much better option if it did not contain a potentially irritating amount of lemon grass extract, which most definitely adds fragrance to this supposedly fragrance-free product. This cleanser's lack of emollients and detergent cleansing agents means that it is not adept at removing makeup, and the antioxidant pycnogenol isn't going to help your skin because it is rinsed away before it can provide any benefit. This is suitable for normal to dry skin.

☺ AVERAGE **DMAE Alpha Lipoic Acid C-Ester Foaming Facial Cleanser** *($15.50 for 6 fl. oz.)*. The amounts of DMAE and alpha lipoic acid in this water-soluble cleanser are too small to affect skin, not to mention that they're rinsed off before they can have any effect. This contains both problematic and soothing plant extracts, so the pros and cons essentially cancel each other out. All told, this is an OK cleanser for normal to oily skin. It would be rated higher and would be better for your skin if it did not contain lemongrass and lavender, both fragrant additives with no established benefit for skin.

☺ AVERAGE **Glycolic Facial Cleanser** *($14.95 for 8 fl. oz.)*. This simply formulated water-soluble cleanser for all skin types would be a much gentler option without the glycolic acid. Plus, it's in a cleanser, so the glycolic acid isn't going to be in contact with your skin long enough for it to provide an exfoliating benefit, and the pH of the product is not low enough for it to function that way. What glycolic acid can do, especially with the amount in this cleanser, is cause eye irritation. Careful application minimizes this risk, but given you're not getting any benefit from the glycolic acid anyway, why bother with a potentially problematic cleanser, especially one like this that doesn't remove makeup all that well?

☺ AVERAGE **Tropical Solutions Facial Cleansing Gel** *($12.50 for 6 fl. oz.)* has the makings of a gentle, water-soluble formula, but we're concerned about the minimal amount of preservatives compared to the high amount of spoilage prone ingredients. Another concern is the unidentified "natural fragrant oils." Not only does this leave consumers in the dark about which oils they're applying to their skin, but this ingredient designation isn't one that's supported by any cosmetics regulatory agency in the world. If a cosmetics company can't get this right, how are consumers supposed to trust other aspects of their formulas? Although this is suitable for normal to dry skin, the formulary concerns are great enough to keep this from earning a better rating.

☹ POOR **Age-Defying Facial Cleanser** *($19.50 for 6 fl. oz.)* costs more than most other cleansers from Derma E, but is the extra money warranted? Not really, because the extra anti-oxidants will be rinsed from skin before they have much chance to work. Although the main ingredients in this water-soluble cleanser are gentle, it contains some irritating plant extracts as well as lavender oil, which is always a problem for skin, even in small amounts (see the Appendix for details). Ultimately, the problematic ingredients in this cleanser don't make it age-defying, but do make it impossible for us to recommend.

☹ POOR **Very Clear Problem Skin Cleanser** (*$15.50 for 6 fl. oz.*). Derma E claims that the natural ingredients in this cleanser are very effective on acne or blemish-prone skin. With the exception of the tea tree oil, that simply isn't true. However, even the tea tree oil has not been shown to be as effective as benzoyl peroxide for fighting acne, and any potential efficacy is just rinsed down the drain in a cleanser. Nourishing skin with plant extracts isn't going to prevent future breakouts because it does nothing to address the causes of breakouts, which are bacteria proliferation combined with excess oil and an inefficient pore lining becoming clogged with oil and dead skin cells. This cleansing lotion is a misguided option for acne-prone skin, and the rosewood oil contains volatile components (chiefly linalool) that can be irritating (Source: naturaldatabase.com). And, of course, it isn't all natural in the least.

DERMA E EYE-MAKEUP REMOVER

☺ GOOD **Eyebright Eye Makeup Remover** (*$12.75 for 4 fl. oz.*) is best described as a gentle, water-soluble cleanser rather than as an eye-makeup remover, even though it works well to remove eye makeup. If you're using one of Derma E's well-rated cleansers, you don't need this product. If not, it's one to consider for all-over use by those with normal to slightly dry or slightly oily skin.

DERMA E TONERS

☺ GOOD **Anti-Aging Pycnogenol Toner, Fragrance Free** (*$15.50 for 6 fl. oz.*) is a very good toner for all skin types, including sensitive. It contains a short but effective list of anti-oxidants and soothing agents, and is indeed fragrance-free. Two things keep this toner from earning a Best rating: The clear bottle packaging, which exposes the product to light and won't keep the light-sensitive ingredients stable, and the omission of repairing and cell-communicating ingredients, which all skin types need to become healthier and act younger. If you decide to try this toner, be sure to store it away from light to preserve the effectiveness of the antioxidants.

☺ AVERAGE **Vanilla Bean Revitalizing Toner, Age-Defying Facial Formula** (*$15.50 for 6 fl. oz.*) contains many beneficial ingredients but also some that are problematic, and these less desirable ingredients aren't present in tiny amounts. As for the vanilla, it has some antioxidant ability for skin, but not in the small amount in this product. If you decide to try this toner, be sure to store the clear plastic bottle away from light to preserve the effectiveness of the antioxidants.

☺ AVERAGE $$$ **Hyaluronic Hydrating Mist** (*$13.50 for 2 fl. oz.*) is a spray-on toner that contains some very good antioxidants and soothing agents. The price is on the high side for the amount of product you get, but we can think of less impressive toners that cost more. Although Derma E included witch hazel extract, it's likely the amount used isn't enough to cause problems for skin (plus the extract isn't as bad for skin as the distillate form). We would've assigned a Good rating to this toner, but it is low on skin-repairing ingredients that should be front-and-center in any toner you consider.

☹ POOR **Age-Defying Balancing Toner** (*$19.50 for 6 fl. oz.*). Talk about a few bad apples spoiling the bunch! This alcohol-free toner is loaded with beneficial ingredients, including some great antioxidants and soothing agents, but it also contains some problematic plants and irritating lavender oil. Lavender oil always a problem for skin, even in small amounts (see the Appendix for details). Other problematic ingredients in this toner include witch hazel and papaya, but it's the lavender oil that makes this a bad choice, especially if you're concerned about reducing signs of aging. What a shame; with a few minor changes this toner would be a brilliant option for all skin types! By the way, despite glycolic acid being the third ingredient, the amount is likely too low to promote exfoliation plus this toner's pH is too high for the glycolic acid to function in this manner.

☹ POOR **DMAE Alpha Lipoic C-Ester Firming Facial Toner** (*$15.50 for 6 fl. oz.*). This toner's DMAE content is negligible, not to mention that DMAE's benefit for skin is controversial (please refer to the Cosmetic Ingredient Dictionary at CosmeticsCop.com for details). Although this toner has some helpful ingredients for skin, it also contains irritants such as witch hazel, lemongrass, and lavender, none of which are firming. (Irritation and firming are not the same thing, and because irritation can deplete skin's collagen content, you get diminishing results over time.) By the way, Derma E likes to claim that their toners can close pores, which absolutely isn't true. Pores do not open and close like window blinds. This is just a sad recurring claim made to attract the attention of women who are endlessly seeking such a benefit. Unfortunately, it remains elusive because there are no cosmetic ingredients that can close pores. What you can do is reduce the size of enlarged pores with ingredients that exfoliate and help normalize pore function. That's not the same as closing pores, because if pores could be closed, skin's surface would quickly dry out and you'd overheat (pores are an integral part of transferring oil to skin's surface and also play a role in regulating body temperature).

☹ POOR **Vitamin A Glycolic Toner** (*$11.50 for 6 fl. oz.*) offers little of value for any skin type but instead puts skin at risk for irritation and collagen breakdown due to the irritants it contains. Witch hazel and papaya extracts are problematic ingredients, while the really beneficial ingredients are present in smaller amounts than these irritants. As for the glycolic acid, the amount in this toner is far too low for it to work as an exfoliant, not to mention the pH is outside the range this ingredients needs to exfoliate skin.

DERMA E EXFOLIANT & SCRUBS

✓☺ BEST **Evenly Radiant Overnight Peel** (*$16.95 for 2 fl. oz.*) is one of the star products in the Derma E line, at least if you're looking for a well-formulated AHA lotion. This peel contains 5% glycolic acid plus lower amounts of the lesser-known AHA ingredients lactic and malic acids, all formulated at an effective pH of 3. This is a recommended exfoliant for normal to dry, sun-damaged skin. It contains a tiny amount of antioxidants and a dry skin–friendly mix of emollients, while the fragrance (from lemon extract) is subtle.

☺ AVERAGE **Fruit Enzyme Facial Scrub** (*$13.95 for 4 fl. oz.*). Despite the fact that this scrub contains some emollient ingredients, the salt-like and cornmeal scrub particles tend to be needlessly abrasive unless you're exceptionally gentle. This scrub is also so fragrant that the scent lingers on your skin long after you rinse it, which isn't a good sign. The claimed enzymatic action of this scrub is nil because including a tiny amount of papaya fruit extract isn't going to give skin an enzyme polish, not to mention that enzymes are difficult to keep stable in cosmetic products in any amount (which is why they are rarely used except by cosmetics companies trying to reinforce their natural claims despite a lack of skin-care benefit). This scrub is an OK option for dry skin if used infrequently and with great care, but that sounds like a real waste of time and money, doesn't it?

☺ AVERAGE **Tropical Solutions Facial Scrub** *($12.50 for 4 fl. oz.)*. The tropical angle of this face scrub is mere marketing rather than formulary excellence. This face scrub contains ground apricot powder as the abrasive agent, and its uneven edges can be too rough unless used with great care. Ironically (at least for those seeking natural skin-care products) synthetic polyethylene beads are the preferred scrub agent. There are other concerns for this product, too: the minimal amount of preservatives compared to the high amount of spoilage-prone ingredients and the unidentified "natural fragrant oils." This ingredient generalization leaves consumers in the dark about which oils they're applying to their skin, not to mention the designation isn't one that's supported by any cosmetics regulatory agency in the world. Although this is suitable for normal to dry skin, the formulary concerns are great enough to keep this from earning a better rating.

☺ AVERAGE **Vitamin A Glycolic Facial Scrub** *($11.50 for 4 fl. oz.)* is similar to the Tropical Solutions Facial Scrub above, and the same comments apply. The amount of glycolic acid is mere window dressing and does not play any role in this scrub's ability to exfoliate skin.

☹ POOR **Microdermabrasion Scrub** *($32.50 for 2 fl. oz.)* is not recommended because it contains several irritating citrus oils that don't bring this anywhere near a "salon-perfect treatment" for your skin. Acne scars cannot be scrubbed away, as this product claims. If anything, the irritation from the citrus oils can encourage oil production at the base of your pores, potentially making acne worse and prolonging the healing process. In so many ways, this scrub is bad news for your skin.

☹ POOR **Very Clear Cleansing Scrub** *($13.95 for 4 fl. oz.)* is meant to bring blemished skin to a clearer state, but what it's most likely to do is confuse your skin and potentially make acne worse. The abrasive agent is apricot seed powder, and it can be quite rough on skin due to the uneven particle size and sharp edges. This scrub also contains thickening agents and plant oils that blemish-prone skin doesn't need, and there are fragrant oils that do nothing but cause irritation, which can stimulate oil production in the pore (see the Appendix for details). None of this will improve acne or lead to new cell growth, which, by the way, has nothing to do with attaining clear skin.

DERMA E MOISTURIZERS (DAYTIME & NIGHTTIME), EYE CREAMS, & SERUMS

☺ GOOD **Hyaluronic Acid Rehydrating Serum** *($29.50 for 2 fl. oz.)* is better described as a lightweight moisturizing lotion rather than as a serum, but it contains vitamin C plus some very good water-binding and repairing ingredients for all skin types. The texture of this makes it preferred for normal to oily skin, and unlike many Derma E products, it contains fragrance rather than fragrant oils. Because the product is in clear bottle packaging, you must store it away from light to preserve the potency of the vitamin C. One more thing: This product contains sodium hyaluronate, which is the salt form of hyaluronic acid. As such, it is not correct to label this product as containing hyaluronic acid. Sodium hyaluronate is a worthwhile water-binding agent for skin, but it is not the same as hyaluronic acid and it does not work in some miraculous fashion for skin; if it did, why doesn't Derma E include this ingredient in all their serums?

☺ AVERAGE **Age-Defying Day Creme** *($39.50 for 2 fl. oz.)*. Billed as Derma E's ultimate antioxidant daily moisturizer, we can't help but wonder why they need so many other moisturizers, too. After all, if this is the "ultimate," what more could you want? Or why not just make the other products better to match this supposedly stellar formula? As it turns out, despite an impressive amount of the antioxidants pcynogenol and astaxanthin, jar packaging allows the potency of these ingredients to degrade shortly after the product is opened (see the Appendix for details). What you're left with is a lightweight moisturizing cream for normal to dry skin not prone to breakouts. It is not recommended for daytime use unless you're willing to pair it with a sunscreen rated SPF 15 or greater. This product has a lingering, pine/herbal scent that means there is enough fragrance in here to make it potentially irritating, and that isn't good news for anyone's skin.

☺ AVERAGE **Anti-Aging Moisturizing Complex SPF 15** *($22.50 for 2 fl. oz.)*. This fragrance-free daytime moisturizer with sunscreen includes in-part zinc oxide for sufficient UVA protection, so the anti-aging portion of the name is apt! It's an OK daytime moisturizer with sunscreen for normal to dry skin not prone to breakouts. The bad news is that jar packaging will render the roster of antioxidants ineffective due to daily exposure to light and air (see the Appendix for details). That's a shame because in better packaging (and with the inclusion of some skin-repairing and cell-communicating ingredients to further help skin act younger) this would be rated higher.

☺ AVERAGE **Ester-C Moisturizing Serum with E Skin Recovery Complex** *($16.95 for 2 fl. oz.)* is a good water-based moisturizer (the texture and formula don't match what most consumers expect from a serum) for normal to slightly dry skin. It contains an impressive roster of proven antioxidants, and little that's extraneous. The antioxidants in this formula have the potential to improve signs of aging, including stimulating collagen production. The average rating is because this serum lacks a good range of skin-repairing and cell-communicating ingredients to provide skin with better anti-aging benefits. Also, the citrus fragrance isn't the best, as all forms of citrus pose a risk of irritation—and that's not the way to obtain younger-looking skin.

☺ AVERAGE **Fruit Smoothee Eye Creme** *($22.50 for 0.5 fl. oz.)* is excellent for dry skin, but using it anywhere on the face, especially around the eyes, may prove problematic. Why? Derma E is fond of using an unknown blend of "natural and fragrant oils," and there are no fragrant oils that do skin any favors (see the Appendix for details). What a shame they didn't leave fragrance of any kind out of this product, because it contains a bevy of helpful ingredients for skin, including several antioxidants. As is, this is a tough sell because you don't know which fragrant oils you're applying. Last, check out the Appendix to find out why, in truth, you don't need an eye cream.

☺ AVERAGE **Fruit Smoothee Moisturizing Creme** *($22.50 for 2 fl. oz.)*. Need proof that facial moisturizers and eye creams rarely differ? This product is a great example. Ingredient-by-ingredient, it is nearly identical to Derma E's Fruit Smoothee Eye Cream above. Of course, because this is for the face, you get four times as much product for the same price. But even if they were different it wouldn't matter, because there is no research showing that eye-area skin needs ingredients that are different from those for use on the face. In this case, due to this product's blatant similarities to the Eye Cream, the same basic review applies.

☺ AVERAGE **Fruit Smoothee Serum** *($22.50 for 1 fl. oz.)* has a texture that's much closer to a standard moisturizing lotion than a serum. It contains some exceptional antioxidants with a proven track record of being helpful for skin. The lightweight texture is ideal for those with normal to slightly dry skin, and the numerous antioxidants play a role in helping to reduce inflammation and protect skin from oxidative damage. Why the Average rating then? For some reason, Derma E lists their fragrance as a blend of unidentified "natural and fragrant oils." As such, you don't know what you're applying to your skin, but without question fragrant oils aren't helping it. Without the fragrant oils, this would have easily earned a higher rating, and the price is great, too.

☺ AVERAGE **Hyaluronic Acid Night Creme** *($29.50 for 2 fl. oz.)*. The bulk of this formula is helpful for dry to very dry skin, which is great. What's not so great is the choice of jar packaging because it allows the unstable antioxidants to degrade shortly after you begin using it (see the Appendix for details). Sodium hyaluronate is the salt form of hyaluronic acid, so despite being a worthwhile ingredient for skin, it is not the same as hyaluronic acid and it does not work in some miraculous fashion for skin. If it did, why doesn't Derma E include it in all their moisturizers?

☺ AVERAGE **Pycnogenol Moisturizing Creme, Fragrance Free** *($29.95 for 2 fl. oz.)*. This fragrance-free moisturizer is a pricey prospect for normal to dry skin when you consider that the potency of the star ingredients will deteriorate due to the jar packaging (see the Appendix for details). With several outstanding antioxidants in this product, this product would've been so much better in an opaque tube, not a jar!

☺ AVERAGE **Pycnogenol Redness Reducing Serum** *($29.95 for 2 fl. oz.)*. This water-based lightweight moisturizer (it really doesn't have a serum texture) includes emollient macadamia nut oil along with synthetic thickening agents, which makes it better for normal to dry skin not prone to blemishes. The blend of anti-irritants and antioxidants this contains are good, but the clear bottle packaging demands careful storage away from light. The amount of arnica extract has the potential to be irritating, which is why, despite some strong positives, this product receives an Average rating.

☺ AVERAGE **Tea Tree & E Antiseptic Creme** *($12.50 for 4 fl. oz.)*. Derma E markets this product as a multipurpose wonder cream for a wide range of skin ailments. The "magic" ingredient, in this case, to handle all these skin woes is tea tree oil. Regrettably, tea tree oil can't live up to even a small part of the claims Derma E puts on the label. Most of what they attribute to tea tree oil is not supported by any published research. What has been proven is that tea tree oil has antimicrobial and some antifungal benefit and that it's an ingredient to consider for acne and a few other skin disorders; but other than that there is no reason to use it (Source: naturaldatabase.com). A bigger reason to leave this product on the shelf is because it is packaged in a jar. This diminishes the potency of the natural ingredients, including the antioxidant vitamins this contains, so any benefit they'd have is steadily decreased each time this product is opened and exposed to air.

☺ AVERAGE **Tropical Solutions Anti-Aging Day Creme** *($19.50 for 2 fl. oz.)*. The tropical angle of this moisturizer is mere marketing rather than formulary excellence. As for being used during the daytime, that's not a wise choice unless you're willing to pair this with a product with sunscreen rated SPF 15 or greater. As a moisturizer, this has an emollient, somewhat inelegant texture that's an OK option for dry skin. The formula contains several antioxidant oils and extracts, but the clear plastic bottle packaging demands storage away from sources of light to preserve the sensitive ingredients. The antioxidants are the only intriguing anti-aging element of this moisturizer. We are concerned about the potentially weak preservative system for a product with so many spoilage-prone ingredients, but this pales in comparison for Derma E's penchant for listing "natural and fragrant oils." This ingredient generalization leaves consumers in the dark about which oils they're applying to their skin, not to mention the designation isn't one that's supported by any cosmetics regulatory agency in the world.

☺ AVERAGE **Tropical Solutions Anti-Aging Eye Creme** *($19.50 for 0.5 fl. oz.)* is nearly identical to Derma E's Tropical Solutions Anti-Aging Day Creme, above except you'll pay the same amount of money for one-fourth as much product. As such, the same comments apply.

☺ AVERAGE **Tropical Solutions Anti-Aging Night Creme** *($19.50 for 2 fl. oz.)* is nearly identical to Derma E's Tropical Solutions Anti-Aging Day Creme above. Unlike the Day Creme, this moisturizer is packaged in a jar. That's bad news for the antioxidants this product contains, as well as bad news for your skin and overall hygiene (think of fingers dipping into a water-based product daily). All told, since the only anti-aging element is the antioxidants and their potency is severely diminished due to jar packaging, there's no compelling reason to consider this relatively inexpensive facial moisturizer.

☺ AVERAGE **Tropical Solutions Facial Moisturizer SPF 15** *($17.50 for 2 fl. oz.)*. This lightweight daytime moisturizer for normal to dry skin contains zinc oxide plus a synthetic sunscreen active for reliable broad-spectrum protection. It has a smooth, creamy texture that blends well, leaving only a faint hint of a white cast and a soft satin finish that doesn't feel thick or greasy. Those are all pros, but this product isn't home free yet: Its pineapple-mango fragrance is knock-your-socks-off strong, and that makes it tough to recommend. That's disappointing because this contains some excellent antioxidant plant oils and other antioxidants such as sta-bilized vitamin C and vitamin E. Fragrance isn't skin care (see the Appendix for details), and its presence in this product shouldn't be overlooked. For the sake of your skin, please experiment with fragrance-free or minimally fragranced options first.

☺ AVERAGE **Tropical Solutions Intensive Serum** *($19.50 for 1 fl. oz.)* is notably similar to the Tropical Solutions Day Creme, Eye Creme, and Night Creme above. All these products share the same antioxidant mix supported by a base that includes glycerin, plant oil, and triglycerides. Those are helpful groups of ingredients for dry skin, but this serum isn't more intensive than any of the other Tropical Solutions products (which is to say, not much). The amount of antioxidants in this serum is impressive, but a well-rounded anti-aging product needs to contain more than just a good mix of antioxidants. More skin-identical substances would be great, and how about a cell-communicating ingredient or two? This contains a pineapple-mango fragrance which may smell nice, but fragrance isn't skin care and products like this are better for your skin without the added scent.

☺ AVERAGE **Vitamin A and Green Tea Creme** *($19.50 for 2 fl. oz.)* sounds truly impressive given all the numbers and potent-sounding ingredients it flaunts on the label, but it's mostly hot air. The claim that retinol is an exfoliant is not true; it's a beneficial cell-communicating ingredient and an antioxidant that helps skin create better, healthier skin cells and increase the amount of skin-support substances. People mistakenly believe it's an exfoliant because it can cause flaking and superficial dry skin, which actually can be a problem if it continues. In fact, this product does not contain retinol. Instead, Derma E includes retinyl palmitate, which is a form of retinol but not the same as pure retinol, which is found in many other products. Even if they had included pure retinol, the choice of jar packaging would render it useless shortly after the product was exposed to light and air. The jar packaging is why this product doesn't deserve better than an Average rating. As for the 20,000 IU (International Units) claim for the vitamin A, that sounds better than it ends up being, and any amount is meaningless anyway because of the poor packaging.

☺ AVERAGE **Vitamin A Retinyl Palmitate Wrinkle Treatment Creme** *($12.50 for 4 fl. oz.)* is an emollient formula for dry skin. It contains retinyl palmitate, as its name tells you, not retinol (they're not the same thing). Although that's not such a letdown, the choice of

---

jar packaging is. Couple the poor choice of packaging (discussed in the Appendix) with the inclusion of unidentified fragrant oils and this is a moisturizer to pass by in favor of numerous other options.

☺ AVERAGE **Vitamin A Retinyl Palmitate Wrinkle Treatment Gel** *($12.50 for 8 fl. oz.)*. This simple, water-based gel moisturizer is ideally for oily skin. It contains a mix of vitamins A and E along with glycerin, a gel-based thickening agent, and preservatives. We suppose it's an OK, affordable option if you're curious to see what these antioxidant vitamins will do for your skin, but neither is going to eliminate dry, aging skin as claimed. If anything, the lack of emollients in this moisturizer will assuredly leave those with dry skin wanting more. Regrettably, Derma-E also included "natural fragrant oils." This ingredient generalization leaves consumers in the dark about which oils they're applying to their skin, not to mention the designation isn't one that's supported by any cosmetics regulatory agency in the world.

☺ AVERAGE **Vitamin E 12,000 IU Creme** *($12.50 for 4 fl. oz.)*. Although 12,000 IU (International Units) of vitamin E sounds like a lot, it ends up being less than 0.28 ounce in total in this 4-ounce product, which doesn't sound as impressive after you take the smoke and mirrors out of the equation. What also is disappointing is that the vitamin E is tocopheryl acetate, which is far less bio-available than several other forms of vitamin E, including alpha tocopheryl or tocotrienols. Another really unimpressive feature is the jar packaging, which will render all the tocopheryl acetate and the other antioxidants ineffective shortly after you begin using it. Consider this yet another Derma E moisturizer to ignore, despite the fact that it contains some great ingredients for dry skin.

☺ AVERAGE $$$ **Age-Defying Eye Creme** *($22.50 for 0.5 fl. oz.)*. There are many helpful ingredients in this light yet emollient eye cream, and it is suitable for dry skin anywhere on the face. The problem is the clear jar packaging, which won't keep the antioxidants stable during use (see the Appendix for details and to learn why you don't need an eye cream). We're also concerned about the amount of witch hazel extract in a product meant for application near the eyes, but the nut oil that precedes it likely mutes its negative impact on skin.

☺ AVERAGE $$$ **Peptides Plus Wrinkle Reverse Eye Creme** *($27.50 for 0.5 fl. oz.)* is similar to but more emollient than Derma E's Peptides Plus Wrinkle Reverse Creme reviewed below, and you get less product for more money. The peptide antiwrinkle claims for this product are over-the-top and completely without proof when it comes to being able to "actually reverse the aging process." No one will be looking decades younger even after months of using this peptide-enhanced moisturizer. Peptides have skin-conditioning benefits and theoretically cell-communicating ability, but how much activity and effect they have on collagen production is unknown. And for certain, peptides don't work like Botox to eliminate wrinkles and expression lines, nor can peptides discourage new wrinkles, especially if you're not applying a well-formulated sunscreen daily, even when the sun isn't shining. Since most eye creams don't contain sunscreen, you're actually doing your skin a disservice by using these types of products during the day. Yes, you can follow with a moisturizer that contains sunscreen, but why not just use that around your eyes instead, and skip the eye cream? We would say this is a good product to try if you're curious to see what peptides can do for your skin, but the jar packaging is a disappointment and it won't keep any of the ingredients stable once the product is opened.

☹ POOR **Age-Defying Night Creme** *($39.50 for 2 fl. oz.)*. Despite an impressive amount of the antioxidants pycnogenol and astaxanthin, jar packaging decreases the potency of these ingredients and the other vitamin-based antioxidants shortly after the product is opened (see the Appendix for details). What you're left with is a lightweight moisturizing cream for normal to dry skin not prone to breakouts. If the packaging issue weren't enough of a disappointment, it's also bad news that this moisturizer contains lavender oil. This fragrant plant oil may smell soothing, but fragrance isn't skin care and in truth lavender has plenty of research proving how bad it is for all skin types, even in small amounts (see the Appendix for details).

☹ POOR **DMAE-Alpha Lipoic-C-Ester Creme** ($22.50 for 2 fl. oz.). A major ingredient in this moisturizer is dimethyl MEA, also known as DMAE. We have written about this controversial ingredient in the past and it is not one we recommend. The latest research has shown that it stunts the growth of fibroblast cells (which contribute to healthy collagen production) and causes cell death, an outcome that other studies have also shown (Source: *Aesthetic Plastic Surgery*, November-December 2007, pages 711–718). (For a detailed explanation of DMAE, please refer to the Cosmetic Ingredient Dictionary at CosmeticsCop.com.) As for the antioxidants in this moisturizer for dry skin, their efficacy is hindered by the jar packaging, which makes this product a waste of time and money, not to mention the potential risks associated with using DMAE.

☹ POOR **DMAE-Alpha Lipoic-C-Ester Serum** ($22.50 for 2 fl. oz.) includes a tiny amount of the ingredient dimethyl MEA, also known as DMAE. Derma E maintains this ingredient is "widely acclaimed," but that certainly isn't reflected in published research. DMAE is a controversial ingredient and one that we do not recommend. Beyond the risk associated with the use of DMAE (mentioned in the review above), there isn't anything in this water-based serum worth getting excited about. The clear bottle packaging won't help keep the antioxidants stable unless you store it away from light, and the amount of alpha lipoic acid is minuscule.

☹ POOR **Hyaluronic Acid Day Creme** ($29.50 for 2 fl. oz.) contains a problematic amount of witch hazel extract, which is mostly alcohol. Added to that is the negative effect of the jar packaging on the antioxidants and this isn't shaping up to be a skin-care product worthy of your money or attention. This contains the salt form of hyaluronic acid (sodium hyaluronate), which is a beneficial ingredient for all skin types, but the amount in this fragranced product doesn't make it a must-try. See the Appendix for details on jar packaging and how irritation hurts your skin.

☹ POOR **Hyaluronic & Pycnogenol Eye Creme, Fragrance Free** ($19.50 for 0.5 fl. oz.). Despite a notable amount of antioxidants, the amount of witch hazel extract, which is mostly alcohol, makes this eye cream impossible to recommend for anyone. See the Appendix for details on all this, and to find out why you don't need an eye cream.

☹ POOR **Peptides Plus Wrinkle Reverse Creme** ($43.50 for 2 fl. oz.) is similar to the Peptides Plus Wrinkle Reverse Eye Creme above, except this contains fragrant ylang-ylang oil, and is not recommended. See the Appendix to find out how daily use of fragrant products damages skin.

☹ POOR **Peptides Plus Wrinkle Reverse Serum** ($43.50 for 2 fl. oz.) is not a true serum, but really a moisturizer. It's similar to the Peptides Plus Wrinkle Reverse Eye Creme above, except this contains fragrant ylang-ylang oil, and is not recommended. See the Appendix to find out how daily use of fragrant products damages skin.

☹ POOR **Pycnogenol Eye Gel, Fragrance Free** ($19.50 for 0.5 fl. oz.). While pycnogenol and green tea are both good antioxidants, witch hazel extract (which is mostly alcohol) is a major ingredient in this eye gel, and trumps the fact that it is otherwise a well-formulated, fragrance-free product. See the Appendix to learn why, in truth, you don't need an eye gel (or cream).

☹ POOR **Skinbiotics Treatment Creme** ($19.95 for 4 fl. oz.). Doesn't the name of this moisturizer make it sound like medicine for your skin? Well, it isn't, at least not the type of medicine that's good for your skin. Derma E took a new approach to marketing this sub-brand by claiming the products help fight bacteria and germs via their antiseptic action. No claims are made for moisturizing skin, fighting wrinkles, etc. Instead, it's all about fighting germs and bacteria. To that end, tea tree and oregano oils are a large part of the formula. Although both are natural and both have potent antibacterial action, oregano oil contains volatile components such as carvacrol and thymol that are irritating to skin. It is these components that earn oregano oil its antibacterial and antifungal stripes, but the risk of irritation is real and not one to ignore (Source: naturaldatabase.com). If you're concerned about bacteria on your skin, such as the kind that can cause acne, there are far better, safer products to consider.

☹ POOR **Skinbiotics Treatment Oil** *($19.95 for 1 fl. oz.)* is similar to the Skinbiotics Treatment Creme above, and the same review applies.

☹ POOR **Very Clear Problem Skin Moisturizer** *($19.50 for 2 fl. oz.)* contains a good amount of tea tree oil, which can have benefit for acne, but not as much benefit as you'd get from benzoyl peroxide and certainly not in such an overly fragrant formula. Adding irritants such as lavender oil and fragrant rosewood oil compromise skin's ability to heal. Lavender and rosewood don't have any proof of efficacy for blemish-prone skin, and nothing in this moisturizer can reduce sebum (oil). Not to worry, however, the tea tree oil won't stay stable long in this jar packaging, so there is no reason to buy this product, because clear skin is not what you'll get for your money. See the Appendix for details on jar packaging, lavender oil, and why irritation makes oily skin worse.

DERMA E LIP CARE

☺ GOOD **Lip Repair Creme** *($14.50 for 0.5 fl. oz.)* is an intriguing lip balm due to its lotion-like texture. It isn't nearly as protective as most emollient- or oil–based lip balms, but it's worth consideration if you find an emollient texture too heavy. This contains oils and more occlusive moisturizing ingredients, but they're a minor part of the formula. Antioxidants are plentiful though antioxidants aren't the slam-dunk answer when lips are dry and chapped. Still, this fragrance-free lip moisturizer has enough strong points to handily deserve its rating.

DERMA E SPECIALTY SKIN-CARE PRODUCTS

✓☺ BEST $$$ **Hyaluronic Hydrating Mask** *($29.50 for 4 fl. oz.)*. Other than the small amount of fragrance this contains, it is a very good, soothing and hydrating mask for dry skin. The formula blends repairing ingredients with beneficial plant extracts, all of which function as antioxidants. This contains hyaluronic acid, too, but a rather small amount given it's a prominent part of this mask's name. Still, this delivers on its claims and will leave parched skin plumped with smoothing moisture while treating it to other beneficial ingredients all skin types need to become healthier and act younger. Although on the pricey side, on balance this is a better formula than many moisturizing masks sold by department store brands. It can be left on skin overnight, and you should definitely do this if your skin is notably dry.

☺ GOOD **Cleansing Enzyme Mask** *($13.95 for 4 fl. oz.)*. This clay mask makes deep cleansing claims based on the fact that it contains sea salt. However, this mask has almost no abrasive action, so you shouldn't consider it if you're looking for a clay mask/scrub product. Salt of any kind isn't deep cleansing, though it can be irritating when it's among the main ingredients. This is a good option for absorbing excess oil and making skin feel smooth, but it cannot detoxify skin. No mask can detoxify skin because skin doesn't have toxins lurking in it that require a product like this to purge them. The myth about removing toxins from skin was developed solely to make you waste your money on useless skin-care products with spectacular claims and ordinary formulations. In terms of enzymes, this contains papaya extract, which can be a source of the enzyme papain. Just because papaya extract is listed doesn't mean what you're getting is papain, so it's anyone's guess as to whether this mask has any enzymatic action. Even if it did, enzymes are unstable ingredients that rely on other factors to exfoliate skin. Without question they are not preferred over exfoliating with a well-formulated AHA or BHA product.

☺ AVERAGE **Skin Lighten** *($24.95 for 2 fl. oz.)*. Derma E's claim that this product is unique has some merit given the formulary, but stating that it's "all natural" is nothing more than a fairy tale, without the happy ending. Since when did stearic acid, phenoxyethanol, and PEG-100 stearate become natural ingredients? They didn't, and they're not, which is why the "all natural" claim from Derma E is a joke. The only ingredient in this thick cream that is capable of lightening skin is licorice root extract. However, the limited research on this ingredient was done in vitro and there are no established concentration protocols for creating skin-care products whose licorice root extract would work to inhibit melanin production (Sources: *Plant Medica*, August 2005, pages 785–787; and *Journal of Agricultural and Food Chemistry*, February 2003, pages 1201–1207). Even if Derma E is including an amount that would be effective, their choice of jar packaging will cause the licorice root extract to become less effective with each use. Jar packaging also hinders the effectiveness of the antioxidants in this skin lightener, and it is not preferred to stably packaged skin lighteners that contain hydroquinone or arbutin as active ingredients.

☺ AVERAGE **Very Clear Spot Blemish Treatment** *($11.50 for 0.5 fl. oz.)* contains the same plant ingredients as all the other products in the Derma E Very Clear lineup, but the results are mixed. Tea tree oil has disinfecting properties similar to the gold standard for acne, benzoyl peroxide. The percentage of tea tree oil is critical to its efficacy, with 5% and up considered effective against acne-causing bacteria. This product appears to meet that percentage requirement and it includes some potent anti-irritants. Unfortunately, it also contains fragrant rosewood oil, an ingredient whose linalool content makes it irritating, and lavender extract isn't a welcome addition. If you're curious to see if tea tree oil will work for your blemish-prone skin, you're better off buying the pure oil and making sure it's housed in a dark bottle to preserve its efficacy.

☹ POOR **Clear Vein Creme Spider Vein/Bruise Solution** *($24.95 for 2 fl. oz.)* is supposed to eliminate unsightly spider veins, broken capillaries, and bruises. Unfortunately, it doesn't contain any ingredients that can eliminate these problems, though some of the plant extracts have research that relates to venous issues. For example, horse chestnut contains aesculin, an ingredient known to decrease the permeability of capillaries and constrict veins, but the information about this effect is based on in vitro studies or intravenous administration, not topical application (Source: naturaldatabase.com). Ironically, another component of horse chestnut can cause increase the risk of bleeding and bruising. Without question, this isn't a "very safe" product as claimed! It's a great example of natural ingredients not being free from risk, just as there are synthetic ingredients that present risks. This product contains other ingredients whose chemical constituents are a problem for skin, such as the tannins in witch hazel and oak bark. In contrast, the rutin ingredient in this product has research indicating it may decrease fragile capillaries and their permeability, but this research was either deemed inconclusive or involved oral, not topical, dosage (Sources: *European Journal of Obstetrics, Gynecology, and Reproductive Biology*, November 2006, pages 3–8; and *The Encyclopedia of Common Natural Ingredients Used in Food, Drugs, and Cosmetics*, 2nd Edition, John Wiley & Sons, 1996). More than anything else, this product isn't any kind of solution and will only disappoint those dealing with the cosmetic concerns large veins and capillaries present. Cosmetic corrective procedures such as lasers or sclerotherapy are much better ways to truly improve these concerns.

☹ POOR **Psorzema Natural Relief Creme** *($19.95 for 4 fl. oz.)*. This specialty moisturizer is said to relieve topical symptoms from the skin disorders psoriasis and eczema. Of course, it's a blend of natural ingredients that are supposed to heal and calm scaly, flaky skin. There are lots of great natural ingredients that can soothe skin and reduce inflammation. Some of them are, in fact, included in this product. However, Derma E also included problematic plant extracts such as neem leaf, which contains sulfur and other irritants (Source: naturaldatabase.com). Neem has anti-inflammatory substances too, but why not use a plant (such as willow herb) that provides this benefit without the risk of irritation? None of the plant extracts in this product, even the exotic ones, have any research pertaining to their ability to improve symptoms of eczema or psoriasis. Some have antifungal properties, but fungus isn't a causative factor in either skin disorder. Also a problem is jar packaging, which won't keep the numerous plant ingredients in this product stable during use (see the Appendix for details). It would be great if this worked as claimed to bring some relief to those struggling with eczema or psoriasis, but the formula doesn't make such relief a reality. Caution: Neem extract, which is the second ingredient in this product, can cause severe poisoning if ingested. If you decide to use this product, it must be carefully stored out of children's reach (we're assuming adults won't try to eat this stuff, but kids certainly might be tempted).

☹ POOR **Scar Gel** *($19.95 for 2 fl. oz.)* is supposed to, surprise, diminish the appearance of scars. It contains the same "active" ingredient used in Mederma, a drugstore product making the same scar-reducing claims. The problem is that this ingredient (onion bulb extract) hasn't been shown to work any better on scars than plain Vaseline and there is no convincing research proving it does much of anything (Sources: *Journal of the American Academy of Dermatology*, December 2009, pages 31–47; and *Dermatologic Surgery*, February 2006, pages 193–197). We are concerned about Derma E's inclusion of lavender fragrance, because lavender oil (which may be part of what creates this product's scent) is known to cause skin-cell death and enhance oxidative damage—two things that discourage healing of scars. Scar Gel won't have any positive effect on stretch marks or burns, either. It's basically an all-talk, no-action product that isn't worth considering.

☹ POOR **Stop Itch Instant Relief Creme** *($19.50 for 2 fl. oz.)* is an anti-itch cream formulated in a moisturizing base. The antioxidant content is impressive, but none of these ingredients will remain stable due to jar packaging (see the Appendix for details). The reason this product works to quell itching is because it contains counter-irritants such as peppermint oil. Counter-irritants are used to induce local inflammation for the purpose of relieving inflammation in deeper or adjacent tissues. In other words, they substitute one kind of inflammation for another, which is never good for skin. Irritation or inflammation, no matter what causes it or how it happens, impairs the skin's immune and healing response (Source: *Skin Pharmacology and Applied Skin Physiology*, November-December 2000, pages 358–371). And although your skin may not show it or doesn't react in an irritated fashion, if you apply irritants to your skin the damage is still taking place and is ongoing, so it adds up over time (Source: *Skin Research and Technology*, November 2001, pages 227–237).

DERMALOGICA (SKIN CARE ONLY)

Strengths: Good eye-makeup remover; a combination AHA/BHA product; a unique lightener product; a couple of commendable moisturizers, one with stabilized Vitamin C.

Weaknesses: Expensive and massively overhyped; almost every category has one or more products that contain irritating ingredients with no established benefit for skin, Clean Start and MediBac lines; poor sunscreens.

For more information and the latest Dermalogica reviews, visit CosmeticsCop.com.

DERMALOGICA CLEANSERS

☺ GOOD $$$ **Tri-Active Cleanse** *($38 for 5.1 fl. oz.)*. This creamy standard, detergent-based, foaming cleanser has lots of potential for those with dry to very dry skin. However, it isn't any more adept at lifting dulling skin cells than any other cleanser; if anything, the emollients in this product impede rinsing, which means more dead skin cells remain than are washed away. The whitening name and brightening claims are meaningless, too, and it's worth noting that this product does not contain enzymes or peptides as claimed. It does contain fragrant ylang-ylang oil, listed by its Latin name *Canaga odorata*. Including ylang-ylang is not great news because fragrant extracts are not skin care, but the amount is likely too low to be problematic. Consider this a worthwhile cleanser for dry skin, but not a specialized brightening product.

☺ AVERAGE $$$ **Essential Cleansing Solution** *($33 for 8.4 fl. oz.)* is a cold cream–style cleanser that is an option for dry to very dry skin, but it's not so enticing owing to the inclusion of a few potentially irritating plant extracts. This removes makeup and rinses fairly well, but you may find you need to use a washcloth to avoid leaving a residue (and the irritating plant extracts) on skin.

☹ POOR **Clean Start Wash Off** *($20 for 6 fl. oz.)* makes impossible claims; no skin-care product can regulate oil production because oil production is primarily a function of androgens, male hormones that everybody has. Any aesthetician who believes the claim needs to go back to Skin Physiology 101. In addition, the main cleansing agent is sodium lauryl sulfate, which poses a high risk of skin irritation. That, plus the inclusion of lavender and orange oils, makes this cleanser too drying and irritating for all skin types.

☹ POOR **Clearing Skin Wash** *($33 for 8.4 fl. oz.)*. This overpriced water-soluble cleanser for acne-prone skin makes the same mistake as most anti-acne products: It contains drying and irritating ingredients that make acne worse instead of better. Of chief concern here is the numerous irritating plant extracts in this product, plus the menthol and camphor. All these can cause your skin extra problems such as redness and increased oil production, because that's what irritating ingredients do to skin. Plus, irritation hurts your skin's healing process (which won't help acne) and hinders healthy collagen production. In addition, the numerous irritants in this cleanser are a distinct problem to use around the eyes. The amount of salicylic acid is wasted in a cleanser, because its brief contact with skin won't be enough to impart a benefit. A leave-on product with salicylic acid is the best way to go if you're struggling with breakouts.

☹ POOR **Dermal Clay Cleanser** *($33 for 8.4 fl. oz.)* is an odd mixture of plant oil, clay, detergent cleansing agents, thickeners, and several irritating plant extracts. This concoction won't help oily or "congested" skin, but could very well make matters worse, mostly because it doesn't rinse well.

☹ POOR **Precleanse** *($35 for 5.1 fl. oz.)* is marketed as an oil that dissolves pore-clogging oil, but is nothing more than a mix of triglyceride with several nonfragrant plant oils. Also included are two forms of lavender and forms of citrus that serve to fragrance the product and irritate skin. For the money, irritant-free jojoba or olive oil is preferred.

☹ POOR **Skin Purifying Wipes** *($18 for 20 wipes)* contain melissa (balm mint), witch hazel, and camphor, all of which are irritating to skin. The amount of salicylic acid isn't sufficient for exfoliation, and the pH wouldn't allow that to happen even if it contained a decent amount.

☹ POOR **Skin Resurfacing Cleanser** *($37 for 5.1 fl. oz.)* is an acidic water-soluble cleanser whose lactic acid content has the ability to exfoliate skin; that is, if you leave it on your skin for at least several minutes. Doing that, however, would only increase the irritation potential of this cleanser, a result of the many fragrant oils, other fragrant components, and the detergent cleansing agents it contains. And getting this cleanser anywhere near your eyes would be a problematic experience! This cleanser is not recommended; you can achieve better results without needless irritation by using a well-formulated AHA exfoliant that contains either lactic or glycolic acid.

☹ POOR **Special Cleansing Gel** *($33 for 8.4 fl. oz.)* contains irritating essential oils of lavender and balm mint (melissa) and is neither recommended nor the least bit special. See the Appendix to learn why daily use of fragrant products is damaging to skin—and something no ethical aesthetician should ever advise.

☹ POOR **Ultracalming Cleanser** *($33 for 8.4 fl. oz.)* contains several problematic fragrant plant extracts known to cause irritation, which prevents this otherwise well formulated cleansing lotion from being ultra-calming or recommended. This also contains some soothing plant extracts, but their benefit will be lost because the irritating ingredients get in the way of this cleanser being even slightly calming. Using this would be a big mistake if you have sensitive or rosacea-affected skin.

DERMALOGICA EYE-MAKEUP REMOVER

☺ GOOD $$$ **Soothing Eye Makeup Remover** *($22 for 4 fl. oz.)* is a standard, but good, detergent-based eye-makeup remover that is free of fragrance and the irritating plant extracts Dermalogica puts in their facial cleansers. Color us surprised!

DERMALOGICA TONERS

☹ POOR **Antioxidant Hydramist** *($37 for 5.1 fl. oz.)* winds up being a very disappointing, poorly formulated toner! The amount of peptides, vitamin C, green tea, and water-binding agents is impressive and somewhat justifies the product's price, but the addition of rosewood, clove, and lemon peel oils is a mistake, as are numerous fragrance ingredients such as eugenol and limonene. These ingredients make this toner too irritating for all skin types and negate any soothing effects the beneficial ingredients might have. By the way, there is no research anywhere showing that the peptides Dermalogica includes in this toner can prevent signs of aging associated with the creation of advanced glycation end-products (AGE).

☹ POOR **Clean Start All Over Clear** *($18 for 4 fl. oz.)* is a spray-on toner that contains the most potent (and irritating) form of witch hazel (the distillate, which is mostly alcohol) as well as fragrant oils that cause irritation. Alcohol also causes free-radical damage, but the irritation stimulates oil production in the pore, which is hardly a control mechanism. Some of the ingredients in this toner are helpful for skin, but not nearly as much as they could be given that they are commingled with irritants.

☹ POOR **Multi-Active Toner** *($32 for 8.4 fl. oz.)* is multi-irritating because it contains lavender, balm mint, pellitory, arnica, and ivy. None of these ingredients are helpful for any skin type. They may please your nose and you may think the scent is refreshing, but what pleases your nose almost never makes your skin happy. We cannot stress enough how irritating this toner is and for what it costs, it's hugely disappointing.

☹ POOR **UltraCalming Mist** *($32 for 6 fl. oz.)*. This spray-on toner is supposed to relieve sensitivity and calm redness, but it contains precious few ingredients proven to do that. In fact, this toner contains a helping of irritating plant extracts, which is the last thing sensitive, reddened skin needs. Instead, sensitive skin needs a gentle, soothing toner, such as those from Paula's Choice RESIST or Skin Recovery lines, and you also can consider any of the toners we recommend in the Best Products chapter at the end of this book.

DERMALOGICA EXFOLIANTS & SCRUBS

☺ AVERAGE $$$ **Skin Prep Scrub** *($32 for 2.5 fl. oz.)* is a detergent-based, water-soluble cleanser that contains cornmeal as the scrub agent. It would probably be better to just use cornmeal from the grocery store if you want a cornmeal scrub, because then at least you wouldn't be applying some of the irritating plant extracts that are present in this product, including arnica, pellitory, and ivy. Although these ingredients are probably present in such small amounts that they don't have much effect on skin, why are they in here at all?

☺ AVERAGE $$$ **Skin Renewal Booster** *($48 for 1 fl. oz.)* is a very expensive, effective, yet ultimately problematic AHA exfoliant. The amount of lactic acid is likely above 5% and that fact coupled with this product's pH of 3.6 ensures exfoliation will occur. Beyond the AHA, this contains a tiny amount of salicylic acid (BHA) but likely not enough for your skin to notice a difference. This is problematic because it contains several fragrant plant extracts known to cause irritation. Combined, they can potentially make oily skin worse by stimulating excess oil production at the base of the pores, not to mention that fragrant plant extracts also stand a good chance of worsening redness. This AHA exfoliant also contains the anti-aging ingredient retinol and, while that may seem convenient, the amount is on the low side and retinol's potential to cause sensitivity is heightened when it is combined with irritating ingredients instead of soothing, skin-fortifying ingredients.

☹ POOR **Clean Start Ready, Set, Scrub** *($21 for 2.5 fl. oz.)*. Skin will be off to an irritating start if you opt to use this scrub/clay mask hybrid product. It contains fragrant plant oils with known cell-damaging properties and irritation potential as well as several forms of menthol, which adds to the irritation. Numerous scrubs out-perform this one without needlessly irritating skin in the process.

☹ POOR **Daily Microfoliant** *($50 for 2.6 fl. oz.)* costs a lot for what amounts to cellulose, magnesium oxide (the exfoliants in this cleansing scrub), detergent cleansing agents, plant extracts, and irritating essential oil of grapefruit peel. There is no reason to choose this over a standard topical scrub, or just using a washcloth with your water-soluble cleanser. The enzyme papain and salicylic acid cannot remain stable in a formula like this because the magnesium oxide throws off the pH, so it won't stay within the acidic range necessary for exfoliation to occur. You will get a granular exfoliation from this scrub, but you'd be better off using a gentler scrub or a damp washcloth with your facial cleanser (and you'll save money, too).

☹ POOR **Daily Resurfacer** *($66 for 0.51 fl. oz.)* is an extremely expensive, somewhat gimmicky way to exfoliate skin, and its exfoliating benefit is dubious. Enclosed in a jar are almost three dozen packets of a liquid solution and a pre-soaked sponge designed to fit on your index finger. You're directed to massage this in circular motions over skin, with no need to rinse. The solution has in its base a bitter-orange extract, which is a fragrant extract and a skin irritant, so things aren't off to a good start. Salicylic acid (BHA) is included, at about a 1% concentration, but the AHAs touted on the label are sugarcane and apple extracts, neither of which are true AHAs that can exfoliate skin, or at least not with any supporting research. Either way, the pH of this solution is too high for exfoliation to occur, so you're left hoping the sponge applicator will be abrasive enough to do the job. (It isn't, but that's a good thing.) Making matters worse, especially because the product remains on the skin, is grapefruit peel oil. This citrus oil can cause contact dermatitis and phototoxic reactions due to its volatile chemical constituents (Source: naturaldatabase.com).

☹ POOR **Gentle Cream Exfoliant** *($36 for 2.5 fl. oz.)* ends up being Dermalogica's idea of gentle, but that includes irritants such as sulfur and lavender oil. Who's formulating these products and marketing them so disingenuously? If the spa or aesthetician you frequent uses or endorses these products, run, don't walk, to the nearest exit and book your facial elsewhere! Note: This scrub's abrasive agent is diatomaceous earth, which is essentially fossilized algae shells. As such, they tend to have a rough, uneven surface that can scratch and tear skin, especially if used zealously.

☹ POOR **Multivitamin Thermafoliant** *($49 for 2.5 fl. oz.)*. Dermalogica has taken an everything-but-the-kitchen-sink approach to exfoliation, and as usual with their products, the results backfire as they make several formulary mistakes. Let's begin by discussing the thermal reaction alluded to in the product's name, which is nothing more than a high school student's science class project. When two of the ingredients in this product, polyethylene glycol and baking soda, are mixed with water, heat is released (you start the reaction when you splash your face with water). The fleeting heat sensation may psychologically feel good, but it isn't doing anything to help your skin (if anything, making your skin too warm can lead to problems). The real exfoliating component of this product consists of abrasive magnesium oxide crystals, which provide manual exfoliation as you massage them over your skin (just like any scrub). This also includes an AHA (lactic acid) and BHA (salicylic acid). Although the latter ingredients are present in a potentially functional amount, the alkaline pH of this product keeps them from exfoliating, not to mention that they are rinsed down the drain before they can have any effect on your skin. Dermalogica included some emollient plant oils to protect your skin during the scrubbing process, but they also added several fragrant oils and fragrance ingredients that do nothing but irritate skin. Rosewood, lemon peel, and clove oils are not what you want to expose your skin to, especially when it is about to be scrubbed. One more point: There is a lot of retinol in this product, but this antiwrinkle ingredient is wasted in a product that you rinse from your skin.

☹ POOR **Powerfoliant2** *($65 for 0.6 fl. oz.)* is nothing more than a gimmicky cleanser that adds AHAs and enzymes to the mix. You combine a small amount of cleansing powder with a liquid mixture that contains lactic acid and you then wash your face with it. Exfoliation will occur, too, but only if you leave it on your skin for several minutes, and that's not a good idea. There are many reasons not to leave this on your skin, including the fact that the product contains irritating grapefruit peel oil and detergent cleansing agents, which are too irritating and compromising to the skin's barrier. Using a separate cleanser and a well-formulated, leave-on AHA product is not only less expensive, but also much better for your skin.

DERMALOGICA MOISTURIZERS (DAYTIME & NIGHTTIME), EYE CREAMS, & SERUMS

✓☺ BEST $$$ **Map-15 Regenerator** *($85 for 0.3 fl. oz.)* ranks as one of the few Dermalogica products that does not assault skin with irritating fragrant oils. That's a plus, and there is every reason (other than the price, that is) to consider this an excellent way to treat your skin to the benefits of stabilized vitamin C. The "Map" in this product's name stands for magnesium ascorbyl phosphate, a form of vitamin C that research has shown to be beneficial for skin (Sources: *Photochemistry and Photobiology*, June 1998, pages 669–675; and *Journal of Pharmaceutical and Biomedical Analysis*, March 1997, pages 795–801). Dermalogica purports to use 15% of this ingredient, which means it can also have skin-lightening ability. The silicone-enhanced, powder-to-lotion texture is unique, and skin is also treated to some good water-binding agents and additional antioxidants, all without a hint of fragrance. This does not contain hyaluronic acid as claimed; rather, it contains the salt form (sodium hyaluronate) of this ingredient. That's fine, but the company shouldn't call out an ingredient that isn't really in the product in its pure form. Map-15 Regenerator is suitable for all skin types, but those with rosacea may not be able to tolerate the amount of vitamin C it contains.

☺ GOOD $$$ **Intensive Moisture Balance** *($40 for 1.7 fl. oz.)* is among the few Dermalogica products we recommend, though you don't need to spend this much for a good facial moisturizer. The formula is best for dry skin and it contains some beneficial plant extracts as well as antioxidant vitamins and a tiny amount of repairing ingredients. Its only drawbacks include the rose flower extract and a small amount of fragrance ingredients that have the potential to cause irritation. The rose flower is the bigger cause for concern; fragrance-free is the preferred way to go for all skin types, including when you're struggling with signs of aging (see the Appendix for details).

☺ GOOD $$$ **Multivitamin Power Firm** *($53 for 0.5 fl. oz.)* contains mostly silicones, thickeners, vitamin E, vitamin A, antioxidants, anti-irritant, plant oils, plant extracts, and vitamin C. It's a good antioxidant serum for all skin types, but has no special benefit (and is not emollient enough) for the lips. Lips will feel silkier and smoother with this serum on them, but they will not be firmer (but you may get a slight filling benefit if you're concerned about vertical lines on the lips). As for the eye area, the flavor this product contains isn't what you want to be using so close to the eyes.

☺ GOOD $$$ **Pure Light SPF 30** *($60 for 1.7 fl. oz.)*. It's wonderful that this daytime moisturizer with sunscreen contains titanium dioxide and zinc oxide in a silky, lightweight base formula with some very good antioxidants and a cell-communicating ingredient. What rains a bit on this parade is the lack of substantiated research about the peptide that Dermalogica claims will treat discoloration and the inclusion of fragrant, but irritating, ylang-ylang oil (listed by its Latin name *Canaga odorata*). There isn't much of this fragrant oil present, but its inclusion means that what would've been a brilliant sunscreen is instead just a very good sunscreen, but not for sensitive skin.

☺ GOOD $$$ **Pure Night** *($75 for 1.7 fl. oz.)*. Although there is a lack of serious research that the peptide in this product will lighten skin discolorations, this is, for the most part, an outstanding moisturizer for dry to very dry skin. It contains a copious amount of antioxidants (including some that rarely show up in other products), cell-communicating niacinamide, and skin-conditioning emollients. The only drawback (and the reason this is not rated Best) is the inclusion of ylang-ylang oil, listed by its Latin name *Canaga odorata*. Although the small amount present is not likely to cause irritation, it serves no purpose for skin and contains potentially irritating fragrant components.

☹ AVERAGE $$$ **Age Reversal Eye Complex** *($75 for 0.5 fl. oz.)*. Before we discuss the formula, you need to know that you don't need a separate product for the skin around your eyes (see the Appendix to find out why). If you're still curious about this eye cream, which makes all the usual claims of reducing dark circles, puffiness, and wrinkles, it does contain several anti-aging ingredients that will benefit skin anywhere on your face. The texture is light and silky, and it works well under makeup. Despite containing superstar ingredients, such as retinol, green tea, and vitamin C, this eye cream loses points for including a fairly high amount of radish root, which is a skin irritant. That means there is the potential for irritation (which hurts skin's healing process and causes collagen breakdown), even though there are also some great ingredients.

☺ AVERAGE $$$ **Barrier Repair** *($38 for 1 fl. oz.)* is a silicone-based moisturizer that contains several great antioxidants and a high amount of anti-irritant oat kernel oil. Other anti-irritants are present, too, and these along with the silicones and evening primrose oil help reinforce and repair skin's barrier. The problem comes from the inclusion of ginger root extract because this plant can be irritating and won't help sensitive skin improve. As for the claim that this formula protects skin from reactive ozone... well, it doesn't. First, what does the company mean by "reactive ozone"? Ozone is highly reactive all by itself, and depending on the source, is all around us. The antioxidants this contains can help to a point, but they cannot block the action of ozone on our skin, so this isn't a security blanket for skin exposed to ground-level forms of this gas.

☺ AVERAGE $$$ **C-12 Concentrate** *($90 for 1 fl. oz.)*. This water- and silicone-based serum's only unique ingredient is oligopeptide-34, an ingredient that allegedly is responsible for improving skin clarity and treating discolorations. It comes from raw material supplier Caragen, and the only information pertaining to its efficacy also comes from Caragen, which makes it not much to go on. You can consider the claim unsubstantiated and completely biased. All in all, this is just an ordinary (and we mean really ordinary) serum for normal to dry skin, with nothing to offer for skin discolorations or any other skin concern. For the health and appearance of your skin, you should opt for a product whose lightening ingredients have a better track record than those that Dermalogica chose. For the same amount of money you can get a prescription for a hydroquinone product with copious research proving its efficacy for treating skin discolorations, including melasma. Or, in the cosmetics realm, for this kind of money, selecting a product loaded with antioxidants (especially vitamin C given its role in mitigating sun-induced skin discolorations), cell-communicating ingredients like niacinamide, and skin-identical ingredients, which this one sorely lacks, would be far better!

☺ AVERAGE $$$ **Dynamic Skin Recovery SPF 30** *($62 for 1.7 fl. oz.)* deserves credit for combining an in-part avobenzone sunscreen with several state-of-the-art ingredients known to help skin look and function better. This would have rated higher if it did not contain problematic feverfew extract along with several irritating fragrant oils. The oils are present in meager amounts, but why include them at all?

☺ AVERAGE $$$ **Total Eye Care SPF 15** *($42 for 0.5 fl. oz.)* lists only titanium dioxide as the active ingredient, making this a gentle sunscreen to use around the eyes. Iron oxides, talc, and mica provide a brightening effect to shadowed areas, while lightweight emollients moisturize. The formula lacks significant amounts of antioxidants and interesting skin-identical ingredients, but is an option for normal to dry skin.

☹ POOR **Active Moist** *($54 for 3.4 fl. oz.)* contains several irritating plant extracts including lavender, ivy, and arnica. All these are problematic ingredients for skin. This is otherwise a very bland, lightweight moisturizer lacking any state-of-the-art ingredients to justify its price. Note that this contains the sunscreen ingredient ethylhexyl methoxycinnamate which, when combined with the irritating plant extracts, increases the likelihood of stinging and burning when applied near the eyes.

The Reviews D

☹ POOR **Clean Start Brighten Up SPF 15** *($24 for 2 fl. oz.)* lacks the UVA-protecting ingredients of titanium dioxide, zinc oxide, avobenzone (also known as butyl methoxydibenzoylmethane), ecamsule, or Tinosorb and is not recommended. Also, nothing in this formula is capable of refining or purifying pores. If anything, the triglyceride base can contribute to clogged pores.

☹ POOR **Clean Start Welcome Matte SPF 15** *($24 for 2 fl. oz.)* lacks the UVA-protecting ingredients of titanium dioxide, zinc oxide, avobenzone (also known as butyl methoxydibenzoylmethane), ecamsule, or Tinosorb and is not recommended. Even if this did contain reliable UVA-protecting ingredients, it also several irritating plant oils, and irritation increases oil production in the pore (see the Appendix for details). This product is 100% incapable of banishing breakouts and cleaning pores. The small amount of salicylic acid and the pH won't allow any exfoliation to occur, and the other aspects of the formula give it a somewhat matte finish, but that doesn't hold up as the day goes by.

☹ POOR **Clearing Mattifier** *($42 for 1.3 fl. oz.)* does contain 2% salicylic acid, yet the pH of 4.7 doesn't allow it to function as an exfoliant. The silicones in this product leave a soft matte finish, but the amount of cinnamon bark extract is cause for concern, making this unhelpful BHA product a poor option—not to mention an expensive one, considering that several products can provide a matte finish just like this one does and they also exfoliate to improve clogged pores, blackheads, and breakouts. You'll find examples on our list of Best BHA Exfoliants at the end of this book.

☹ POOR **Extra Firming Booster** *($48 for 1 fl. oz.)* contains irritating bitter orange flower and only makes skin feel firmer because of the PVP (a hairstyling film-forming agent) it contains. The ylang-ylang oil (listed as *Cananga odorata*) can cause contact dermatitis and itchy skin, which isn't what you want from any product. This also contains other irritating plant extracts and ultimately isn't a product we can recommend, at least not for anyone who wants skin that look and acts younger.

☹ POOR **Extra Rich Faceblock SPF 30** *($48 for 1.7 fl. oz.)* would have been an excellent, in-part zinc oxide moisturizing sunscreen for normal to dry skin, but it contains irritating essential oils of sandalwood, eucalyptus, and geranium. Without these troublesome ingredients, this would be highly recommended due to its antioxidant and cell-communicating ingredient content.

☹ POOR **Gentle Soothing Booster** *($48 for 1 fl. oz.)* could have earned highly recommended status due to its roster of genuinely soothing plant extracts. However, the St. John's wort *(Hypericum perforatum)* extract can cause severe phototoxic reactions on sun-exposed skin, and that's hardly gentle (Source: naturaldatabase.com). Ideally, this formula should also contain skin-repairing ingredients such as fatty acids, cholesterol, ceramides, and glycerin to help repair and replenish skin's surface.

☹ POOR **Intensive Eye Repair** *($48 for 0.5 fl. oz.)* should not be used around the eyes because it contains fragrant rose extract as well as arnica. Neither is a good ingredient for skin anywhere on the face, but especially not in a product applied so close to the eyes. What a shame, because even though you don't need an eye cream (see the Appendix to find out why), this version for normal to dry skin contains numerous beneficial ingredients, including lots of antioxidants and repairing ingredients.

☹ POOR **Multivitamin Power Concentrate** *($54 for 45 capsules)* has antioxidant finesse and a nonaqueous formula, but it's sabotaged by irritating citrus oils of lime, orange, and grapefruit.

This is a dangerous product to apply to skin if it will be exposed to sunlight. See the Appendix to learn how daily use of highly fragrant products like this hurt your skin.

☹ POOR **Oil Control Lotion** *($38 for 2 fl. oz.)* contains 1% salicylic acid at an effective pH of 3.6, but this is not recommended because it also contains irritating balm mint, camphor, and menthol. What a shame! And none of the plant extracts in this lotion can have any effect on skin's oil production. If anything, the irritation from the menthol and camphor can stimulate excess oil production at the base of pores, quickly making oily skin worse. What a shame, because this contains several intriguing ingredients capable of helping blemish-prone skin.

☹ POOR **Oil-Free Matte Block SPF 20** *($45 for 1.7 fl. oz.)* includes titanium dioxide for UVA protection and comes in a lotion base that contains some good antioxidants. Unfortunately, it also contains enough grapefruit peel oil to be irritating and possibly cause a sensitizing reaction on sun-exposed skin.

☹ POOR **Power Rich** *($180 for 1.5 fl. oz.)* is an obscenely expensive product that is little more than a moisturizer. As far as moisturizer formularies go, this is pretty standard, which is really embarrassing given the sky-high price. Dermalogica and countless other cosmetics companies sell equivalent or better moisturizers for a fraction of what this costs, and there is no legitimate reason the price needs to be so high (or that products priced as this one is are automatically better or more powerful for your skin). Power Rich has a notably silky, slightly spackle-like texture and contains several ingredients of benefit for those with dry skin (the company mentions this being great for mature skin, but age is not a skin type), yet it contains some potent irritants, too. Regardless of your age or concerns, no one's skin should be subjected to ginger, grapefruit, and jasmine oils. All these fragrant plant oils contain volatile constituents capable of causing skin irritation—and none of them are proven to benefit skin that has lost its firmness or elasticity (Source: naturaldatabase.com). If anything, daily use of this product may lead to collagen breakdown, which isn't what you want if your goal is to look younger, longer.

☹ POOR **Redness Relief SPF 20** *($43 for 1.3 fl. oz.)* is a daytime moisturizer with sunscreen that provides broad-spectrum sun protection with its in-part zinc oxide sunscreen. That's great but it's a problem that a sheer, moisturizing tint designed to reduce redness contains sensitizing ginger root. Ginger offers some benefits for skin, but it's one of those plant extract whose pros and cons don't add up to a smart choice for sensitive skin (Source: *Journal of Environmental Pathology, Toxicology, and Oncology*, Volume 18, 1999, pages 131–139). Also, the green tint this has isn't something you'd want to apply all over your face, as it tends to give the complexion a seasick appearance that must be covered with makeup to look normal.

☹ POOR **Sheer Moisture SPF 15** *($43 for 1.3 fl. oz.)* includes zinc oxide for reliable UVA protection, but also contains lavender oil. Lavender smells great but its fragrant components cause a number of problems for skin, which we discuss in the Appendix.

☹ POOR **Skin Hydrating Booster** *($54 for 1 fl. oz.)* contains balm mint (melissa) and lavender oil, making this far too irritating for all skin types. How disappointing, because the formula contains some notable skin-repairing ingredients and has a lightweight texture those with oily skin would appreciate. See the Appendix for details on the problems lavender oil can cause.

☹ POOR **Skin Smoothing Cream** *($58 for 3.4 fl. oz.)* contains a potentially irritating amount of arnica as well as sensitizing ylang-ylang oil. Even if you wanted to tolerate these

👁 Did you know you don't need an eye cream? It's true! See the Appendix to find out why.

ingredients, the moisturizer is an overall boring formula with a paltry amount of antioxidants. See the Appendix to learn how daily use of highly fragrant products damages skin.

☹ POOR **Super Rich Repair** *($78 for 1.7 fl. oz.)* isn't as rich as the name states, mostly because the dry-finish solvent isohexadecane is the second ingredient. This moisturizer has an impressive assortment of emollients, water-binding agents, skin-identical substances, cell-communicating ingredients, and antioxidants. That's wonderful for dry skin at any age, so why the bad rating? Dermalogica added a slew of fragrant plant oils that are proven to irritate your skin. The daily irritation this moisturizer causes may lead to collagen breakdown and hurt your skin's healing process, and that's no way to look younger! True, the amount of fragrant oils is small compared to the beneficial ingredients, but (especially for this amount of money) your skin deserves all the good stuff and none of the bad!

☹ POOR **Super Sensitive Faceblock SPF 30** *($45 for 1.7 fl. oz.)* contains lavender oil, which is completely unsuitable for "super sensitive" skin. It's good that the active ingredients are only titanium dioxide and zinc oxide, and the formula has some well-researched antioxidants and soothing agents, but the lavender oil trumps them all (see the Appendix for details).

☹ POOR **Ultracalming Serum Concentrate** *($52 for 1.7 fl. oz.)* contains some skin-silkening and repairing ingredients that anyone with a compromised skin barrier needs, sensitive or not. The formula also includes some plant-based antioxidants and soothing agents. But, despite this good news, Dermalogica missed the opportunity to make this a truly effective product for sensitive skin because they included a problematic plant extract along with fragrance ingredients and, believe it or not, the irritant sage oil. Although sage oil has some beneficial properties, they are countered by several problematic components of the plant, including camphor, which is one of the must-avoid ingredients for all skin types because of the irritation it causes, and we know that irritation causes collagen to break down, impairs healing, and increases redness. Far from being ultra-calming, this serum is a mistake for anyone with sensitive, reddened skin.

☹ POOR **Ultra Sensitive Faceblock SPF 25** *($33 for 1.7 fl. oz.)* contains balm mint (*Melissa officinalis*), which may make skin ultra-sensitive and irritated. This sheer tinted daytime moisturizer with sunscreen lists titanium dioxide as its sole active ingredient. That's great and capable of providing gentle, broad-spectrum protection, but the formula also assaults skin with several other ouch-inducing essential oils, including thyme, rosewood, and orange. It's a classic example of a product marketed to sensitive skin that actually contains ingredients known to make this skin type worse.

DERMALOGICA SUN CARE

☹ POOR **After Sun Repair** *($32 for 3.4 fl. oz.)* contains far too many irritating plant extracts and fragrant plant oils to be even slightly capable of repairing sun-exposed skin. If anything, the irritant potential of the fragrant oils will further damage skin and negatively affect the healing process. What was Dermalogica thinking? And lastly, if you're taking ideal care of your skin you should be doing whatever you can to minimize excess sun exposure—so products like this won't be needed.

☹ POOR **Solar Defense Booster SPF 30** *($43 for 1.7 fl. oz.)* contains avobenzone, so this one has good UVA protection! However, it also contains balm mint and lemon extracts plus lavender oil, all skin irritants. See the Appendix for details on how lavender oil harms skin.

☹ POOR **Solar Defense Wipes SPF 15** *($22 for 15 wipes)* not only lack the correct UVA-protecting ingredients (see the Appendix for details), but also contain balm mint and several irritating essential oils, including spearmint.

DERMALOGICA SPECIALTY SKIN-CARE PRODUCTS

✓☺ BEST $$$ **Extreme C** *($85 for 0.3 fl. oz.)*. This liquid powder product would be an interesting way to experiment with stabilized vitamin C. The form of vitamin C is magnesium ascorbyl phosphate. Based on its concentration, there is reason to believe you will see some improvement in skin discolorations, although the research is clear that the results will not be as impressive as what you'd get from a hydroquinone-based product. It's good that there are other antioxidants, a cell-communicating ingredient, and some skin-identical ingredients included, too, because without them this would have been a one-note product not worth its price. Although this is still on the extremely pricey side (you're only getting 0.3 ounce, making this about $250 per ounce), it's a good formula in stable packaging and is suitable for all skin types.

☺ AVEARGE $$$ **Clean Start Hit the Spot** *($22 for 0.3 fl. oz.)*. This water-based anti-acne gel is similar to Dermalogica's Clean Start Bedtime for Breakouts below, but it bests that product because it omits irritating camphor and includes a much greater amount of anti-irritants. That's helpful for inflamed skin, but this still isn't much of a spot treatment for breakouts because it doesn't contain the ingredients necessary to kill acne-causing bacteria or to exfoliate dead skin cells. Oleanolic acid, a component of plants, is present and has a mild antibacterial potential, but the ingredients it was compared with (none are in this product) did much better (Source: *Phytomedicine*, August 2007, pages 508–516).

☹ POOR **Clean Start Bedtime for Breakouts** *($22 for 2 fl. oz.)* is supposed to be your bedtime answer for preventing breakouts before they surface and lead to a series of bad skin days. It contains 2% salicylic acid as the active ingredient, but the pH of this product is too high for exfoliation to occur. Even if the pH were within range, the base formula contains camphor, which is exceedingly irritating and will increase oil production in the pore. Some of the plant extracts have antibacterial action, but, with the exception of tea tree oil, none of them have convincing research proving their effectiveness against acne-causing bacteria (Sources: *Phytomedicine*, August 2007, pages 508–516; *Pharmazie*, March 2005, pages 208–211; and *African Journal of Medicine and Medical Sciences*, September 1995, pages 269–273). As for the tea tree oil being useful, the amount this product contains is too low for it to have a positive impact on breakouts.

☹ POOR **Concealing Spot Treatment** *($25 for 0.33 fl. oz.)* contains 5% sulfur, a potent disinfectant that can be unusually drying and irritating for skin (though it is a potent disinfectant for acne-causing bacteria). This also contains a large amount of witch hazel and other irritants, including camphor and cinnamon bark. Because the formula is so drying and irritating, applying this to a breakout is likely to make it look much worse than if you had used nothing, and its finish isn't the most attractive, which may leave you to wonder why you bothered.

☹ POOR **Multivitamin Power Recovery Masque** *($45 for 2.5 fl. oz.)* includes some very good plant oils and antioxidants, but those are countered by irritating plant extracts as well as the potent menthol derivative menthoxypropanediol, making this impossible to recommend for any skin type. See the Appendix to learn how irritation hurts skin.

☹ POOR **Overnight Clearing Gel** *($45 for 1.7 fl. oz.)* has a pH of 4, which is borderline for allowing its 2% salicylic acid to exfoliate skin. Although some exfoliation will occur, this product contains several irritating plant extracts and oils, including sage, rosemary, and citronella. Camphor is also in the mix. That's really disappointing because without the copious amounts of irritants, this would have been an above-average BHA option for all skin types.

☹ POOR **Sebum Clearing Masque** *($42 for 2.5 fl. oz.)* is a clay mask that contains several irritating ingredients including menthol and camphor, which makes it a problem for all skin types. Menthol and camphor have no effect on oil production or absorption, and the pH of 4.5 prevents the salicylic acid from clearing clogged pores, not to mention the amount of salicylic acid is on the low side for efficacy. Even without the irritants and with a lower pH to ensure the salicylic acid worked, this mask's blend of thick clays, wax, and a high amount of oil make it difficult to rinse. Did anyone at Dermalogica try this before releasing it to consumers (and skin-care professionals) who look to this line for skin-care solutions?

☹ POOR **Skin Hydrating Masque** *($38 for 2.5 fl. oz.)* is based around irritating bitter orange flower extract and also contains irritating ivy, pellitory, and arnica extract, all of which cancel out the effect of the anti-irritant plant extracts in this well-intentioned but problematic mask. Antioxidant vitamins are present, but in amounts too low to offer much benefit, especially not when combined with the problematic plant extracts.

☹ POOR **Skin Refining Masque** *($38 for 2.5 fl. oz.)* contains the same irritating plant extracts as the Skin Hydrating Masque above, but makes matters worse by adding menthol and sage to the mix. It is not recommended for even occasional use.

☹ POOR **Special Clearing Booster** *($44 for 1 fl. oz.)* is a needlessly expensive topical disinfectant with 5% benzoyl peroxide as the active ingredient. This water-based solution is not recommended because it contains several irritating plant extracts including lavender, St. John's wort, sage, lemon, and ivy. All these have the potential to worsen redness and stimulate excess oil production at the base of the pores, leading to oily skin and breakouts getting worse, not better.

☹ POOR **UltraCalming Relief Masque** *($42 for 2.5 fl. oz.)* is bound to make sensitive skin worse, or at least leave it confused. The formula contains some calming ingredients, including oatmeal and matricaria flower, but they're joined by fragrant plant irritants such as ginger and radish roots. When sensitive, reddened skin is your concern, avoiding needless irritants must be priority number one. Regrettably, that means using this mask is a step in the wrong direction. Also, for sensitive skin, keep in mind that daily skin care is far more important than the benefits you may get from using a mask once or twice per week.

DERMALOGICA LIP CARE

☺ GOOD $$$ **Clean Start Smart Mouth Lip Shine** *($16 for 0.3 fl. oz.)*. Other than the fact that it contains a small amount of fragrance ingredients, this is a well-formulated lip moisturizer. Its smooth texture is lighter than traditional oil–based balms, though it still works to prevent chapping and keep lips soft.

☺ GOOD $$$ **Renewal Lip Complex** *($26 for 0.06 fl. oz.)* is a somewhat unconventional lip balm because it has a lighter texture than standard wax- or oil–based balms. Both of those substances (wax and oil) show up in Renewal Lip Complex (which is good because they help keep lips moist and have tenacity) along with vitamin E, emollients, plant oil, and some peptides. It is the peptides that Dermalogica claims are responsible for preventing signs of aging caused by AGEs (advanced glycation end-products), but there is no proof they can do this. It is not yet known whether applying small amounts of ingredients that inhibit AGEs in a petri dish or on cultured cells can do the same thing in a cosmetic product. Realistically, this balm will keep lips smooth and help prevent chapping, but that's all you can legitimately rely on.

☹ POOR **Climate Control Lip Treatment** *($7.50 for 0.15 fl. oz.)* cannot shield lips from environmental pollutants or protect it from reactive ozone (ozone is bad to breathe, too, so how does this lip balm protect us from that?). It's an oil- and wax-based formula that would have been recommended for dry to very dry lips if it did not contain several fragrant plant extracts whose irritation potential can make dry, chapped lips look and feel worse. Of particular concern is comfrey (*Symphytum officinale*) because this plant extract can cause liver problems when ingested (Source: naturaldatabase.com). The likelihood you'll ingest some of it from this lip balm is there, and the amount present in the formula is definitely cause for concern.

DHC

Strengths: Several inexpensive products; many fragrance-free products; complete product ingredient lists on their website; several worthwhile cleansers and makeup removers; an effective AHA product; antioxidant olive oil and olive leaf extract are present in many products.

Weaknesses: Mostly unexciting toners; an effective BHA product that regrettably contains an irritant; no skin-lightening options with a roster of proven ingredients; huge assortment of products, many with repetitive or gimmicky formulas; products with nanoparticles of silver (completely useless for skin), which can cause permanent skin discoloration (who wants to absorb silver into their skin given that it can be toxic when consumed?).

For more information and the latest DHC reviews, visit CosmeticsCop.com.

DHC CLEANSERS

✓☺ BEST **Cleansing Milk** (*$24 for 6.7 fl. oz.*) is an excellent, detergent-free cleansing lotion for dry to very dry or sensitive/rosacea-prone skin. It removes makeup easily, but you'll have to use a washcloth to avoid leaving a film on your skin.

✓☺ BEST **Make Off Sheet** (*$8 for 50 sheets*) consists of cotton wipes soaked in a cleansing base that's similar to detergent-enhanced liquid makeup removers. These are fragrance-free and are an option for all skin types. The only issue is that these tend to be ineffective for removing long-wearing or waterproof makeup. These types of makeup are best removed with a silicone- or oil–based formula, be it a cleanser or product labeled makeup remover.

☺ GOOD **Cleansing Foam** (*$9 for 2.1 fl. oz.*) is a standard, foaming water-soluble cleanser that is a good option for normal to oily skin, as the amount of potassium hydroxide makes it potentially drying for those with normal to dry skin. We disagree with their claim that this formula is "gentle enough for multiple daily cleansings," because it isn't, not to mention that washing your face more than twice daily is not only unrealistic for most people, but also incredibly drying and stripping for skin. Frequent cleansing doesn't improve skin, although with these ingredients it can disrupt the skin's protective barrier if used several times in a day.

☺ GOOD **Washing Powder** (*$10 for 1.7 fl. oz.*) is a detergent-based powder that forms a water-soluble, foaming cleanser when mixed with water. The amount of papain is much too small to provide enzymatic exfoliation, not to mention that papain is an unreliable ingredient for exfoliating skin because it has stability issues. If the novelty of this is appealing, it's a good fragrance-free option for normal to oily skin.

☺ GOOD **$$$ Face Wash** (*$29.50 for 6.7 fl. oz.*) would earn a higher rating if it did not contain fragrant rosemary oil (which isn't "rejuvenating" as claimed). The amount is small enough that it isn't likely cause for concern, but you should be extra careful using this water-soluble cleanser around the eyes. The detergent-based formula removes makeup easily and is best for normal to oily skin.

☺ AVERAGE **Pure Soap** (*$10.50 for 2.8 fl. oz.*) is very similar to DHC's Olive Soap reviewed below, except this version has less olive oil and a lighter texture, making it suitable for oily skin. It is fragrance-free, but still not preferred to an effective and gentle water-soluble cleanser.

☺ AVERAGE **Salicylic Acne Wash** (*$16.50 for 4 fl. oz.*) cannot banish acne blemishes because its active ingredient (2% salicylic acid) is rinsed down the drain before it has a chance to work. This is otherwise a very ordinary cleanser/scrub hybrid for normal to oily skin. Keep in mind that acne cannot be scrubbed away, nor can blackheads. In fact, using a scrub over acne lesions can worsen the inflammation and slow the healing process.

☺ AVERAGE $$$ **Deep Cleansing Oil** *($26 for 6.7 fl. oz.)* is said to be the company's most popular product the world over, but the formula doesn't support the claim (and just think of all the ordinary products that enjoy enduring popularity). The olive oil–based formula is blended with a surfactant/emulsifying agent (sorbeth-30 tetraoleate) that provides greater cleansing ability than oils alone (which aren't really that cleansing, but can remove makeup) and also helps make this oil easier to rinse than you might expect, though it can still leave a film. The rosemary oil is a potential irritant, especially when used around the eyes, but this is still a workable option.

☺ AVERAGE $$$ **Olive Soap** *($22 for 3.1 fl. oz.)* is a soap-free bar cleanser that contains detergent cleansing agents buffered by olive oil and glycerin. Although this is better than traditional soap, it can be drying for dry or sensitive skin, and isn't preferred to a good water-soluble cleanser.

☹ POOR **Mild Soap** *($15.50 for 3.1 fl. oz.)* is mild in name only. This is a very standard bar soap formula that can be too drying for all skin types, not to mention that it leaves a residue on skin that can build up and make for a dull-looking complexion.

☹ POOR **Mild Touch Cleansing Oil** *($14 for 5 fl. oz.)* contains skin-damaging lavender oil. Lavender oil causes skin-cell death and increases oxidative damage (Sources: *Contact Dermatitis*, September 2008, pages 143–150; and *Cell Proliferation*, June 2004, pages 221–229). Because this cleansing oil leaves a residue on skin, some of the lavender oil remains, and that's not good news.

☹ POOR **Q10 Facial Film Soap** *($11 for 40 sheets)* consists of dry sheets steeped in a dehydrated cleansing solution that is activated by mixing with water. They can be too drying and irritating for all skin types because the main ingredient is sodium lauryl sulfate (which is listed on the label as sodium laurate, another name for sodium lauryl sulfate, something that perhaps the company was trying to hide).

DHC EYE-MAKEUP REMOVER

✓☺ BEST **Eye & Lip Makeup Remover** *($12.50 for 4 fl. oz.)* is a very good, fragrance-free makeup remover that contains a tiny amount of a plant extract (amor cork) known for its anti-inflammatory action. The dual-phase formula (which means you must shake this before each use) contains silicone to help remove stubborn and long-wearing makeup, including waterproof mascara. It is a great option for all skin types.

DHC TONERS

✓☺ BEST $$$ **CoQ10 Lotion** *($35 for 5.4 fl. oz.)*. Although you don't need to spend nearly this much for a great toner, this is a fairly impressive formula from DHC. It contains the antioxidant coenzyme Q10 (listed as ubiquinone) along with some good water-binding agents, repairing ingredients, and soothing ingredients. It is best for normal to dry or sensitive skin. Those with slightly dry skin may find this is the only "moisturizer" they need during warmer weather when skin is less likely to look or feel dry.

☺ GOOD $$$ **Q10 Lotion** *($36 for 5 fl. oz.)* is a water-based toner that contains some good anti-irritants and water-binding agents along with a tiny amount of antioxidants, including ubiquinone (coenzyme Q10). Much is known about the antioxidant activity of Q10 when ingested, but there is only a small amount of in vitro research demonstrating its effect on skin cells. From what's known, it appears that ubiquinone not only has antioxidant activity that allows it to protect skin from sun damage, but also can inhibit MMP-1, a matrix metalloproteinase that causes collagen breakdown (Sources: *Journal of Cosmetic Dermatology*, March 2006, pages 30–38; and *Biofactors*, 2005, pages 179–185, and 1999, pages 371–378). Note that the Biofactors studies were conducted by researchers working for Beiersdorf, and one of their brands (Nivea) sells products that contain ubiquinone. More important, the concentration of ubiquinone used in the studies was likely much greater than the tiny amount present in skin-care products, including this one. As long as you don't expect this toner to keep your skin looking wrinkle-free, it's a suitable option for normal to dry skin.

☺ AVERAGE **Acerola Lotion** *($17 for 3.3 fl. oz.)* contains some good water-binding agents and a tiny amount of placental protein, an animal-derived ingredient that some of you may wish to avoid. Acerola is a poor source of vitamin C because of how it is processed (which likely destroys the vitamin C content that it had when in pure form), but this is still a decent toner for normal to dry skin. It contains fragrant plant extracts.

☺ AVERAGE **Balancing Lotion** *($24 for 6 fl. oz.)* contains less than 1% glycolic acid, which is a shame, because this toner's pH of 3.9 would have allowed exfoliation to occur if the AHA were present at a higher concentration. As is, this toner underwhelms, and also contains two problematic plant extracts (horsetail and lemon), making it a "Why bother?" for any skin type.

☺ AVERAGE $$$ **Acerola 100** *($22.50 for 1 fl. oz.)* does contain a minute amount of acerola, which is a source of vitamin C; however, acerola included in a cosmetic is unlikely to be a good source of vitamin C because much of the vitamin is destroyed during the drying and processing (Source: naturaldatabase.com). Plus, for the money, there is not enough of the showcased ingredient present to maintain healthy skin; the skin is more complicated than that, just like vitamin C isn't the only vitamin you need in your diet. This is just a bare bones fragrance-free toner for normal to dry skin.

☺ AVERAGE $$$ **Alpha-Arbutin White Lotion** *($44 for 3.3 fl. oz.)* contains mostly water, slip agents, water-binding agent, plant extract, alpha-arbutin, more water-binding agents, pH adjusters, and fragrant flower extracts. Alpha-arbutin has some research showing it can lighten skin discolorations, but the research was on a 5% concentration, while this product has less than a 2% concentration. Hydroquinone is still the ingredient with the most research showing efficacy for skin-lightening, but as an alternative, a 5% alpha-arbutin product is an option. It's just that this product doesn't qualify.

☺ AVERAGE $$$ **Mild Lotion** *($35 for 6 fl. oz.)* is merely water, glycerin, slip agent, cucumber juice, placental protein (an ingredient many cosmetics companies no longer use due to pressure from animal rights advocates), and preservatives. The price is insulting for what is nothing more than an exceedingly ordinary toner.

☺ AVERAGE $$$ **Mild Lotion II** *($29 for 4 fl. oz.)*. This alcohol-free toner is supposed to be an advanced version of the company's original Mild Lotion. Neither the original nor the Mild Lotion II deserve to be labeled "advanced," at least not when their ingredient lists are measured against what published research shows that all skin types need. For example, instead of treating skin to a range of skin-repairing and cell-communicating ingredients, Mild Lotion II contains a frustrating mix of fragrant plant extracts with no research showing they are beneficial for skin. It does contain some plant-based anti-irritants, but not enough to help the claim. This toner ends up being a mixed bag for all skin types; it contains nothing to minimize pore size or help normalize pore function, and it's mostly lacking in the types of ingredients aging skin needs to look and act younger. At best, this is an OK toner for normal to dry skin.

☺ AVERAGE $$$ **Olive Leaf Lotion** *($39 for 4 fl. oz.)* is a boring, overpriced toner for all skin types. While it's good that they omitted fragrance, there isn't much to extol here, unless you believe olive leaf extract is the best antioxidant around (which, of course, it isn't).

☺ AVERAGE $$$ **Q10 Water Mist** *($29 for 5 fl. oz.)* is an unimpressive, overpriced toning mist that contains mostly water, slip agent, anti-irritant, and preservative. The amount of ubiquinone (coenzyme Q10) is too insignificant for your skin to notice. It is fragrance-free.

☹ POOR **Platinum Silver Nanocolloid Lotion** *($27 for 4 fl. oz.)*. With a name like this product has, you'll either wonder what in the world it's supposed to do or assume that the mystery behind the name must mean an antiwrinkle miracle is in store. "Nanocolloid," what does that mean? Regrettably, the answer is depressing rather than enlightening. This toner-like product contains mostly water, slip agent, and alcohol. Alcohol causes free-radical damage, irritation, and dryness. This also contains a small amount of other problematic ingredients, including the plants angelica and arnica, both irritants, and pure silver, which can cause a permanent bluish discoloration on skin (Source: naturaldatabase.com).

☹ POOR **Salicylic Acne Toner** *($16.50 for 5.4 fl. oz.)* contains 2% salicylic acid as an active ingredient, but the pH is above 4, so it will not function very well, if at all, as an exfoliant. This is otherwise a below-average toner whose rosemary oil content can irritate skin. The irritation this toner is capable of causing can trigger more oil production at the base of your pores, making oily skin, redness, and acne worse instead of better.

☹ POOR **Skin Softener** *($33.50 for 3.3 fl. oz.)* contains a high amount of coltsfoot extract, a plant whose chemical constituents are considered carcinogenic and toxic when administered orally, and it has no documented benefit for skin (Source: naturaldatabase.com).

☹ POOR **Soothing Lotion, For Drier Skin** *($19 for 6 fl. oz.)* contains alcloxa, an ingredient that has constricting properties, which is certainly not helpful for dry skin, and it can be irritating. The glycolic acid is present at too low a concentration to exfoliate skin, but the pH of 4.4 would inhibit that from occurring anyway.

DHC EXFOLIANTS & SCRUBS

✓☺ BEST **Renewing AHA Cream** *($39 for 1.5 fl. oz.)* contains a blend of 10% AHAs (mostly lactic acid) and the pH of 3.8 allows exfoliation! The lightweight, fragrance-free lotion base is great for normal to dry skin, and this contains antioxidant olive oil along with a couple of impressive water-binding agents.

☺ GOOD **Salicylic Face Milk** *($21 for 2 fl. oz.)* contains 2% salicylic acid and has a pH of 3.8, so exfoliation will occur. Although this is an effective BHA product for blemishes, signs of aging, and blackheads, it also contains a couple of potentially troublesome ingredients (rosemary and perilla extracts). Neither is present in significant amounts, however, so this is still worth considering as a BHA product for normal to slightly dry or slightly oily skin. Those looking for well-formulated BHA products that contain soothing anti-irritants to calm redness may want to consider the options from Paula's Choice. Each is fragrance-free and designed to perfect your skin without causing irritation. As with all well-formulated BHA products, the options from Paula's Choice also stimulate collagen production for younger-looking skin.

☺ AVERAGE $$$ **Facial Scrub** *($16.50 for 3.5 fl. oz.)* is a substandard scrub for normal to dry skin because the abrasive agent is apricot seed powder. This is not preferred to polyethylene or jojoba beads, which are spherical, because the apricot seed powder particles may have sharp edges that leave your skin with microscopic, skin-damaging scratches. The potassium-based ingredients add unnecessary dryness, making this less preferred to most other facial scrubs.

DHC Moisturizers (Daytime & Nighttime), Eye Creams, & Serums

☺ GOOD **Antiox C** *($34.50 for 1.4 fl. oz.)* is worth considering if you have normal to dry skin and are looking for a stably packaged moisturizer with stabilized vitamin C. The vitamin C and olive oil are the only antioxidants of note in this moisturizer. The inclusion of anti-irritant licorice is thoughtful, and the formula is fragrance-free.

☺ GOOD **CoQ10 Face Milk** *($38 for 3.3 fl. oz.)*. This lightweight moisturizer contains some very good ingredients for normal to slightly dry skin. The lotion texture slips over skin and leaves a smooth finish while treating your skin to proven plant-based antioxidants. What's disappointing is that half of the most beneficial ingredients (including the coenzyme Q10, listed by its technical name ubiquinone) are listed after the preservative, so they don't count for much. Still, the fact that this is fragrance-free makes it great for all skin types, and the price is reasonable given that the amount of product provided is greater than most facial moisturizers.

☺ GOOD **Q10 Eye Cream** *($24 for 0.88 fl. oz.)* has a well-rounded formula and packaging that will keep the many antioxidants it contains stable. The drawback is that most of the antioxidants (and the alpha-arbutin, which doesn't lighten dark circles) are present in meager amounts. That's disappointing, but this is still a good fragrance-free moisturizer for dry skin anywhere on the face (you don't need an eye cream; see the Appendix to find out why).

☺ GOOD **Q10 Neck Cream** *($24 for 0.88 fl. oz.)* contains the same ingredients as the DHC Q10 Eye Cream above, and holds no special benefit for skin on the neck. How odd that nearly identical formulas are positioned for two different areas, but undoubtedly there are some women who will buy into that foolishness. The best neck cream a person can use is a well-formulated sunscreen that provides sufficient UVA protection. No neck-area products we've ever seen can forestall aging, slackening skin if sun protection isn't used daily.

☺ GOOD $$$ **Vitamin C Essence** *($38 for 0.84 fl. oz.)* is a very good lightweight, fragrance-free serum with stabilized vitamin C (magnesium ascorbyl phosphate) as the second ingredient. Although really a one-note product for all skin types, it is a formidable option for those interested in seeing what a vitamin C-exclusive product can do for their skin. Do keep in mind, however, that skin needs far more than one beneficial ingredient, however great it may be.

☹ AVERAGE **Acerola Cream** *($23 for 1.4 fl. oz.)*. DHC boasts about the antioxidant content of this moisturizer for normal to dry skin, but then neglected to use air-tight packaging to keep them stable. The jar packaging allows the antioxidants to deteriorate after opening, but that isn't a big issue because there aren't many antioxidants in this product anyway. This is an OK moisturizer, but forget about any benefits from the acerola (a type of cherry that's rich in vitamin C), which could have been helpful if a larger amount were included and if it were in better packaging. By the way, the placental protein in this moisturizer, which is most likely derived from cows, offers no special benefit for skin.

☹ AVERAGE **Acerola Extract** *($22.50 for 1 fl. oz.)* is merely water, butylene glycol, and acerola fruit extract. The fluid texture contains a small amount of acerola, which is a good source of vitamin C when taken orally, but not in a skin-care product. Much of acerola's potency is destroyed during the process of drying and getting it into the product (Source: naturaldatabase.com). Aside from stability issue, there isn't enough of the showcased ingredient present to maintain healthy skin. Plus, your skin needs a lot more than vitamin C, no matter what the form or how stable, because skin is far more complicated than that; just like vitamin C isn't the only vitamin you need in your diet. This is just a bare bones fragrance-free moisturizer for normal to slightly dry skin that leaves it hungry for more.

☺ AVERAGE **Acerola Gel** (*$17 for 1.4 fl. oz.*) contains a bit of acerola and little else. This is a mediocre gel moisturizer for normal skin. Acerola is not a wonder ingredient for skin; plus, the manner in which it is processed and packaged depletes any potential efficacy.

☺ AVERAGE **Alpha-Arbutin White Milk** (*$44 for 2.7 fl. oz.*) contains alpha-arbutin as well as mulberry extract, both of which have in vitro research demonstrating their potential effectiveness for lightening skin discolorations. Although this product comes in packaging that will keep these light- and air-sensitive ingredients stable once opened, what's questionable is whether DHC used these ingredients in amounts great enough to improve discolorations. Research on alpha-arbutin points to a 5% concentration being necessary for results, and we're skeptical this product contains that amount. Still, unless you're bothered by the inclusion of placental protein (an animal-derived ingredient), this is worth considering by those with normal to dry skin that has mild discolorations.

☺ AVERAGE **Ceramide Cream** (*$35 for 1.4 fl. oz.*) doesn't contain any ceramides; if it did they would have to be listed because ceramides are individual ingredients, not delivery systems like liposomes. Despite the misleading name, the formula contains some excellent skin-identical ingredients. Unfortunately, this moisturizer for normal to dry skin will see its antioxidants break down shortly after the jar is opened, and that's not good news (see the Appendix for details).

☺ AVERAGE **Ceramide Milk** (*$29.50 for 2.7 fl. oz.*) is a standard lightweight yet emollient moisturizer for normal to dry skin. The formula does not list any ceramides, which makes the name misleading. Although this contains antioxidants (mostly from olive oil), the translucent bottle packaging demands careful storage to keep it protected from exposure to light. Ceramide Milk is fragrance-free.

☺ AVERAGE **Concentrated Eye Cream** (*$31.50 for 0.7 fl. oz.*) is a basic, lightweight eye cream whose rosemary leaf extract content (although a good source of antioxidants) may be too irritating for use near the eyes. None of the plants in this cream can diminish drooping skin or lighten dark circles. In fact, the antioxidant potency of these plants is lessened due to jar packaging (see the Appendix for details), making this a merely average option for normal to slightly dry skin.

☺ AVERAGE **CoQ10 Gel** (*$32 for 1.4 fl. oz.*). Despite the "gel" name, this product is a lightweight, fragrance-free lotion with enough plant oil to make those with oily, breakout-prone skin nervous. It's a fairly basic moisturizer that's best for normal to slightly dry skin that's also sensitive; you also can use this if you have normal to oily skin, but you want to avoid the oily areas. Half of the most beneficial ingredient (coenzyme Q10, listed by its technical name ubiquinone) is listed after the preservative, which means there isn't really enough of it in this product to warrant the product's name or emphasis. That's disappointing, but not a deal-breaker if you're a fan of DHC and need a lightweight moisturizer that provides smoothing hydration for dry areas.

☺ AVERAGE **Emollient Balm** (*$35 for 3.3 fl. oz.*) is a basic emollient moisturizer for normal to dry skin not prone to breakouts. It contains some good, if gimmicky, water-binding agents and the primary antioxidant is olive oil. The translucent glass bottle means this should be stored away from light to keep the antioxidants stable during use. The amount of retinol is too small to matter, while the addition of coltsfoot extract is potentially problematic.

☺ AVERAGE **Extra Nighttime Moisture, For Everyone's Skin** (*$32.50 for 1.5 fl. oz.*) is not for everyone—those with acne-prone skin will not appreciate the oil content of this moisturizer. It is otherwise a basic, minimal frills moisturizer for normal to slightly dry skin. The jar packaging will compromise the antioxidant potential of the olive oil; the other antioxidants are present in amounts too small for skin to benefit.

☺ AVERAGE **Eye Bright** *($21.50 for 0.52 fl. oz.)* is mostly water and cucumber juice with slip agents and the plant *Isodonis japonicus*, whose terpene content can be irritating to skin, especially around the eyes. You'd be better off using plain, fresh cucumber slices to soothe the eye area, though that home remedy isn't all it's cracked up to be either! See the Appendix to find out why products like this are absolutely not needed.

☺ AVERAGE **Eye Off-Shade** *($19 for 0.21 fl. oz.)* tries to convince you it is the solution for dark, puffy eyes, but it contains not a single ingredient that can alleviate either condition. The plant extracts referred to as brightening agents are present in the tiniest amounts imaginable, while the crux of the formula relies on placental protein. Growth factors from animal and human placentas appear to play a role in wound-healing, but that is completely unrelated to the cause of dark circles or puffy eyes.

☺ AVERAGE **Olive Leaf Milk** *($39 for 2.7 fl. oz.)* claims to be the daytime moisturizer for environmentally damaged (including sun-damaged) skin. What a joke! This contains nothing that's not also in most of DHC's other moisturizers, and without a sunscreen it is an impractical choice for daytime use (unless your foundation is SPF 15 or greater and you apply it evenly and liberally). This is an OK moisturizer for normal to dry skin that relies on olive oil and its extract as the main antioxidants. It does contain a tiny amount of the cell-communicating ingredient lecithin, but the amount of sodium hyaluronate is insignificant. Olive Leaf Milk contains fragrance in the form of floral extracts.

☺ AVERAGE **Olive Virgin Oil** *($39 for 1 fl. oz.)* is pure virgin olive oil. Even if virgin olive oil were a great skin-care ingredient (and it does have benefits for dry skin), why would you bother buying this from a cosmetics company for such an absurd amount of money, as opposed to buying the exact same thing from a grocery store for a fraction of the price? Olive oil is a good antioxidant moisturizing oil for dry skin, but that's about it. DHC does their best to convince consumers that this offering is somehow special and superior to the olive oil you'd use for cooking, but it absolutely is not.

☺ AVERAGE **Tocophero E Cream** *($31 for 1.2 fl. oz.)* contains an impressive amount of vitamin E along with some other known antioxidants. However, jar packaging won't keep them stable during use, relegating this to ho-hum status as a moisturizer for normal to dry skin not prone to blemishes. The amount of rosemary extract poses a slight risk of irritation, and note that the placental protein (which is most likely derived from cows) has no special benefit for skin.

☺ AVERAGE **Water Base Moisture** *($16.50 for 2 fl. oz.)* is a simple, ultra-light moisturizer for normal to oily skin. It supplies some skin-identical substances and other water-binding agents such as placental protein and serine, along with tiny amounts of anti-irritants. Although inexpensive, your skin deserves more than this can provide.

☺ AVERAGE **White Sunscreen SPF 25** *($24 for 1 fl. oz.)* has more pros than cons. The pros include titanium dioxide and zinc oxide as active ingredients, making this a potential option for sensitive skin. It also has a lightweight, silky texture and absorbent matte finish suitable for oily skin, and it works well under makeup. The cons include a slight white cast from the amount of mineral sunscreen ingredients and the inclusion of silver, which has potentially unpleasant, permanent side effects for skin. The amount of silver is barely worth mentioning, but it really should not be included in skin-care products.

The Reviews D

☺ AVERAGE $$$ **Alpha-Arbutin White Cream** *($47 for 1.2 fl. oz.)* claims to be a one-of-a-kind skin-lightening product because it contains alpha-arbutin. However, this potential skin-lightening agent isn't unique to this product or to DHC. Alpha-arbutin can block the pathways involved in causing melanin to form, but this product doesn't contain the 5% concentration that has been shown in some research to be effective. Plus the jar packaging DHC uses will not keep this ingredient stable! See the Appendix to learn why jar packaging is a bad idea for products like this.

☺ AVERAGE $$$ **CoQ10 Eye Cream** *($39 for 0.88 fl. oz.)*. This emollient eye cream for dry skin sounds exciting but ends up being a rather ordinary option. It is also further proof that the ingredients in eye creams rarely differ from those used in facial moisturizers, proving once again why eye creams are unnecessary additions to your skin-care routine (see the Appendix for details). Supposedly, this contains 10 times more of the antioxidant coenzyme Q10 (listed as ubiquinone) than other eye creams DHC sells. If that's true, why is DHC continuing to sell those other products? Shouldn't they admit this is the one to buy if you want the benefits of coenzyme Q10? As it turns out, this antioxidant is but one of many to consider. It isn't the best.

☺ AVERAGE $$$ **EGF Cream** *($89 for 1.2 fl. oz.)* claims to combat signs of aging with a peptide linked to epidermal growth factors. We think it's a good thing the peptide in question is barely present. Why? Because the research examining the topical effects of epidermal growth factors has been short term and concerned primarily with their effect on wound-healing. Wrinkles and discolorations (common signs of aging) are not wounds, and although the claim that you can "heal" a wrinkle like a wound by treating it with growth factors is good theory, the research hasn't been done to prove such efficacy (or safety). In theory, epidermal growth factors (hormones that induce skin-cell production), when applied topically, may trigger repair mechanisms in skin that have become faulty due to age and sun damage (DNA damage caused by sun exposure). However, theory isn't fact. The problem is, we don't know for sure which growth factors work best, how much is needed, and whether or not long-term use is safe (Sources: *Skin Research and Technology*, August 2008, pages 370–375; and *The Surgeon*, June 2008, pages 172–177). In addition, it's well known that epidermal growth factors administered orally as an adjunct or alternative to chemotherapy cause a variety of skin problems, from rashes to acne (Source: *Clinical Journal of Oncology Nursing*, April 2008, pages 283–290). In short, until more is known about formulary protocols for epidermal growth factors in skin-care products, we don't advise using them as part of your anti-aging skin-care routine, no matter how small an amount is in the product. Although the small amount means that it is probably not going to have any effect at all, pro or con, why take the risk? As mentioned, this DHC moisturizer claims to contain a peptide classified as an epidermal growth factor, but that designation isn't clear in any research; rather, it appears to be strictly a marketing claim. That leaves you with an emollient moisturizer whose plant oil and antioxidant efficacy will suffer due to the jar packaging (after all those claims, using jar packaging is just an unwise decision, as we explain in the Appendix). This ends up being a grandiose-sounding product that's essentially just a basic moisturizer for dry skin.

☺ AVERAGE $$$ **Extra Concentrate** *($42 for 1 fl. oz.)* plays on the popular myth that topically applied collagen can add to the collagen content of wrinkled, sun-damaged skin. It doesn't work that way, but most of the ingredients in this "concentrate" have hydrating ability.

The plant extracts include a mix of anti-irritants and irritants, so in effect they cancel each other out.

☺ AVERAGE $$$ **Eye Treatment Essence Peptides** *($39.50 for 1 fl. oz.)* wants you to believe the tiny amount of peptides it contains will stimulate collagen production to rejuvenate skin's support structure. There is no proof peptides can do this, though they appear to have worth as cell-communicating ingredients, assuming that enzymes in the skin don't destroy them before they reach their target cells. Even so, the peptide content of this product is really disappointing, and it is otherwise a do-nothing gel for normal to oily skin.

☺ AVERAGE $$$ **Q10 Cream** *($47 for 1 fl. oz.)* contains more antioxidants than what DHC typically puts in their moisturizers, which makes it all the more shameful that jar packaging was chosen. You're paying a hefty price for this moisturizer for normal to dry skin, but most of what you're paying for will be wasted as the antioxidants degrade in the jar packaging (see the Appendix for details).

☺ AVERAGE $$$ **Retino A Essence** *($38 for 0.51 fl. oz.)* contains a very small amount of vitamin A as retinyl palmitate. It is otherwise a lightweight, silky moisturizer for normal to slightly dry skin not prone to blemishes. If you're looking for a vitamin A product, there are better options from Neutrogena and Paula's Choice, among other brands. And please remember that skin care is never as simple as one ingredient. Vitamin A (specifically when used as retinol) is beneficial, but so are numerous other ingredients skin needs to look its healthy, youthful best (that's the approach Paula's Choice and select other cosmetics companies take, because it's what your skin needs).

☺ AVERAGE $$$ **Wrinkle Essence** *($45 for 0.67 fl. oz.)* is no more the "essence of youthful skin" than cosmetic surgery is the best solution for personal relationship issues. This blend of water with slip agents and water-binding agents is about as unexciting as it gets. Almost all the ingredients appear in myriad DHC products, making this an expensive extra that can be ignored, mostly because it doesn't work as claimed.

☹ POOR **Neck Treatment Essence Peptides** *($39.50 for 1 fl. oz.)* is a ridiculously ineffective product to consider if you're concerned about slackening skin on the neck. First, there is no research proving any peptide can shore up and tighten loose skin (and the amount of peptides in this product is embarrassingly low); second, there is far more preservative than interesting ingredients in this product; and third, nothing in this formula can improve the appearance of sun-damaged skin on the neck or chest All this adds up to is a waste of time and money.

☹ POOR **Olive Leaf Cream** *($39 for 1.4 fl. oz.)* is an emollient moisturizer that indeed does contain olive oil, which can be a beneficial, nonirritating plant oil for dry skin. However, the moisturizing goes astray because of the pointless inclusion of menthol, which is irritating, and jar packaging, which won't keep the olive-based antioxidants stable during use. What could've been a very good moisturizer for dry skin gets tripped up by a potent irritant and problematic packaging.

☹ POOR **Platinum Silver Nanocolloid Cream** *($25 for 1.5 fl. oz.)* makes claims that have no substantiated research behind them, and also contains several plant ingredients that are a distinct problem for skin, including angelica, arnica, and perilla. In addition, it contains silver, which can cause bluish skin discolorations, and platinum powder, which has no benefit for healthy, intact skin. The silver is even more of a problem if DHC is serious about it being nano-sized, as this will enhance its penetration into the skin, which is not a good thing.

☹ POOR **Platinum Silver Nanocolloid Milky Essence** *($25 for 2.7 fl. oz.)* is the lotion version of the Platinum Silver Nanocolloid Cream above, and the same comments apply.

DHC SUN CARE

☺ GOOD **Body Sunscreen Milk SPF 30+** *($19 for 2.7 fl. oz.)*. Offering a sunscreen designed for the body in such a small size is truly problematic and possibly dangerous, but at least this is a gentle, fragrance-free formula whose sole active ingredient is titanium dioxide. Because you have to apply a sunscreen liberally, 2.7 ounces isn't going to last very long for anybody and that can start getting expensive. It has a milky lotion texture that sets to a soft matte finish and also includes some beneficial extras, though none of them are present in impressive amounts. This definitely has potential, but given the fairly ordinary formula there are far better and less expensive options to consider.

DHC LIP CARE

☺ GOOD **Lip Cream** *($7.50 for 0.05 fl. oz.)* is an emollient, lanolin-based lip balm packaged in a lipstick-style container, making for a portable, convenient way to keep dry, chapped lips to a minimum. This is fragrance-free, and contains antioxidant olive oil, too, putting it above many other balms.

☺ GOOD **Vitamin C White Stick** *($22 for 0.05 fl. oz.)* is a lip balm for aging lips; its main ingredient is ascorbyl tetraisopalmitate, a form of vitamin C with limited research pertaining to its antioxidant ability (Sources: *International Journal of Pharmaceutics*, October 2007, pages 181–189; and *Photochemistry and Photobiology*, May-June 2006, pages 683–688). Because this is not an acidic form of vitamin C, it shouldn't cause irritation. However, it isn't the all-in-one anti-aging savior DHC makes it out to be; it's just a potentially effective antioxidant for skin. This is otherwise a standard, wax-infused lip balm that puts a slight white cast on lips due to the zinc oxide it contains.

DHC SPECIALTY SKIN-CARE PRODUCTS

☺ GOOD **$$$ Alpha-Arbutin White Powder** *($20.50 for 0.17 fl. oz.)* is meant as a spot treatment for small areas of discoloration. The amount of alpha-arbutin is potentially effective, but there isn't a lot of research proving this is the best skin-lightening agent to choose. Still, if you're curious and will diligently wear a sunscreen as well, this is an option for all skin types and may be used with any other skin-care product.

☺ GOOD **$$$ Mineral Mask** *($37 for 3.5 fl. oz.)* is a standard clay mask containing enough water-binding agents to help offset the clay content that can make skin feel too dry or tight. It is a good option for normal to oily skin.

☺ GOOD **$$$ Wrinkle Filler** *($27.50 for 0.52 fl. oz.)* doesn't fill wrinkles in the same way some silicone-based primers can, and would be better described as an oil–based moisturizer for dry to very dry skin that is also sensitive. Antioxidant benefit is provided from the olive and rice oils along with vitamin E. This also contains a licorice-based soothing agent, and is fragrance-free. On balance, though, the formula isn't as well-rounded as what aging skin needs, so this is no longer one of our top picks for anti-aging products.

☹ AVERAGE **Alpha-Arbutin White Mask** *($12 for 5 sheets)* is a gimmicky sheet-style mask you place over your face and remove after several minutes. The amount of alpha-arbutin is inconsequential for lightening skin discolorations, not to mention that this ingredient is best left on skin in order for it to work, so it's silly to include it in a short-term application product meant for occasional use.

☹ AVERAGE **Eyelash Tonic** *($13 for 0.21 fl. oz.)* does not contain a single ingredient that can discourage lash breakage or create a "more robust lash line." Instead, this contains problematic plant extracts, including comfrey and watercress. Interestingly, the main plant ingredient, *Swertia japonica*, is one of several herbs listed as plant sources for a substance that helps inhibit the conversion of testosterone to its more potent form, dihydrotestosterone, which causes men to lose their hair. That fact is unrelated to keeping eyelashes from falling out (men who go bald typically don't lose their eyelashes along with scalp hair), and the fact remains that there is no proof this plant extract has any effect, pro or con, on eyelashes.

☺ AVERAGE **Q10 Mask** *($14 for 4 sheets)* are gimmicky sheets meant to work as a mask; you place it over your face and then remove it after several minutes. The water-based formula is OK for normal to oily skin, but if you were hoping to get a mega-dose of coenzyme Q10 (ubiquinone), keep shopping—it is barely present in this formula, and is of little use to skin when used short term. Plus, it is not the only ingredient skin needs (any more than it is the only nutrient needed in your diet).

☺ AVERAGE **Tourmaline Pack** *($37 for 3.5 fl. oz.)* is a standard clay mask that contains a lot of tourmaline, which DHS maintains energizes skin and delves deep into pores to rid them of embedded impurities. It sounds like a marvelous mask, which makes you wonder why DHC needs so many other masks, none of which contain tourmaline. The truth is the whole notion is bogus, and the only revving-up your skin will see is from the irritation possible due to the inclusion of capsicum (pepper) extract.

☹ AVERAGE **$$$ Clarifying Pore Cover Base** *($19 for 0.42 fl. oz.)*. This mattifier is designed to keep excess shine at bay for those with oily skin. The blend of silicone polymers and silicones does a fairly good job at this, but the formula would be even better if truly absorbent ingredients like magnesium carbonate were present in greater amounts. Still, this has a silky, weightless texture that smoothes easily over skin, and its somewhat spackle-like texture helps temporarily diminish the appearance of large pores. Two cautions: This contains a sunscreen ingredient (ethylhexyl methoxycinnamate) that can be a problem for use near the eyes or on sensitive skin. It also contains fragrant rose extract, though the amount is likely low enough to not be much of a problem. Ultimately, this ends up being expensive for so-so results; you may want to consider superior oil-absorbing options such as Paula's Choice Shine Stopper Instant Matte Finish.

☹ POOR **Acne Spot Therapy** *($14.50 for 0.52 fl. oz.)* contains 3% sulfur as the active ingredient, which makes this too drying and irritating for all skin types. A couple of the plant extracts are also irritating and lack efficacy for acne-prone skin, but sulfur is the main concern. Benzoyl peroxide is a better (and better tolerated) topical disinfectant for killing the bacteria that contribute to acne.

☹ POOR **Revitalizing Moisture Strips: Eyes** *($8 for 6 strips)* consist of crescent-shaped paper strips that you moisten and affix to the under-eye area, hoping they'll impart "brightness and vibrancy to weary-looking eyes." About the only thing these strips impart is irritation, which results from a high amount of salt-based film-forming agents and starch. And while the irritation is occurring, your skin is also being constricted by alcloxa; there is very little going on that is actually helpful, let alone revitalizing. This is one to ignore!

☹ POOR **Revitalizing Moisture Strips: Mouth** *($9.50 for 6 strips)* shares the same application method and formulary inadequacies as DHC's Revitalizing Moisture Strips: Eyes. That means little benefit to skin around the mouth, but lots of irritation from the salt-based film-forming agent and the constricting alcloxa.

☹ POOR **Revitalizing Moisture Strips: Neck** *($11 for 6 strips)* shares the same application method and formulary inadequacies as DHC's Revitalizing Moisture Strips: Eyes, and the same concerns apply. In addition, the tartaric acid the Neck version has can also be irritating.

DHC FOUNDATIONS & PRIMERS

☺ GOOD **Velvet Skin Coat** *($21)* is said to be a DHC customer favorite, and it's not hard to see why: Its silky, silicone-based formula leaves all skin types feeling incredibly soft and smooth. It can minimally fill in pores and superficial lines and helps facilitate makeup application. The problem is in how basic the formula is—the blend of silicones and a tiny amount of olive oil isn't nearly as impressive as similar primer/line filler–type products from lines such as Good Skin (reviewed on CosmeticsCop.com), Estee Lauder, Smashbox, and even the Regenerist serums from Olay. All of these can make your skin feel equally silky, yet they offer several more beneficial ingredients. This DHC product is an option if you need a lightweight moisturizer or want to try a basic foundation primer; it's just not as noteworthy as competing products.

☺ GOOD **$$$ Q10 Base Makeup Moisture Care Liquid Makeup** *($28)*. This initially creamy liquid foundation smoothes on skin easily and provides medium yet natural-looking coverage. Once blended into skin, it feels significantly drier than the luminous finish appears. The finish and the formula make this a good option for normal to combination skin, but it likely will leave any dry areas feeling drier. Those looking for more moisture or for anti-aging benefit (indicated in the product's Q10 Moisture Care name) likely will want to supplement this product with a well-formulated moisturizer packed with skin-beneficial ingredients, because this foundation contains only a small amount of them, and the moisturizing benefit is lacking.

DHC CONCEALER

☺ GOOD **Q10 Concealer** *($12)*. This cream concealer feels deceptively lightweight on skin despite the medium to full coverage it provides without feeling heavy or greasy. Application and blending are easy because the texture is on the moist side, but it has a soft matte finish once it sets. This isn't recommended for use over blemishes or acne-prone skin because it contains several ingredients that potentially can clog pores and make matters worse. However, this would be a very good option for use under the eye or for other skin discolorations. Both shades are in the light to medium skin-tone range, which is workable, but leaves those with dark skin tones without options.

DHC POWDERS

✓☺ BEST **$$$ Q10 Face Powder** *($17)*. This talc-based powder has a beautifully airy texture and gives skin a polished look without being the least bit dry or powdery. Recommended for all but very oily skin, this powder's shades are nearly interchangeable because all go on translucent. Despite the name, the amount of coenzyme Q10 (listed by its technical name, ubiquinone) is too small to be of any benefit for your skin.

☹ AVERAGE **$$$ Q10 Moisture Care Powder** *($16)*. This standard pressed powder feels slightly chalky on skin and imparts only the sheerest hint of color. There are some moisturizing ingredients in the formula that do give the powder a somewhat creamy texture, but the hydration is negligible because the main ingredient (talc) absorbs moisture, which means the hydrating ingredients don't do much. This powder is best for those with slightly dry or combination skin looking for a dusting of powder to set their makeup, but you can't rely on this for coverage or oil control.

DHC EYESHADOW

✓☺ BEST **Eye Shadow Moon** *($6)* is DHC's single eyeshadow option, and it applies smoothly and covers well, with noticeable color impact from one stroke of the brush. Every shade has some amount of shine, and for most the shine is quite pronounced, so this isn't recommended for a less-than-taut eye area because shiny eyeshadows enhance the appearance of wrinkles. The Misty Khaki shade looks greener than it applies, which is a good thing (no one should wear vivid green eyeshadow unless they're the Wicked Witch of the West). Avoid the tricky-to-work-with Misty Bordeaux.

DHC EYE & BROW LINERS

✓☺ BEST **Eyeliner Perfect Pro Pencil** *($7)*. Before we comment on the pencil itself, please note that the price for the pencil does not include an attachment to hold the pencil—it is just for the pencil head. We know that sounds strange, but that's the way it's sold, and you definitely need the attachment piece for the pencil to work. Why DHC doesn't offer this as an assembled pencil is odd, but you can purchase their Eyeliner Perfect Pro Holder for an additional price, so the cost is basically equivalent to that of other eyeliner pencils sold at the drugstore. If you don't mind the contrivance, you'll find this a superior automatic eye pencil for drawing thin, precise lines that last.

☺ AVERAGE **Eyebrow Perfect Pro Pencil** *($5.50)*. This automatic, retractable eyebrow pencil requires you to purchase DHC's Eyebrow Perfect Pro Holder + Brush for an additional price (the brush is nothing more than a small mascara head) if you want to use this as an intact, complete pencil. The combined price isn't bad, and although this pencil has a powder finish that stays in place, it's tough to apply and tends to hurt because you must use so much pressure to define your brows. Far better powder brow pencils are available from the drugstore.

☺ AVERAGE **Eyebrow Perfect Pro Powder** *($7.50)*. This brow powder is applied with a pointed sponge-tip applicator that touches a reservoir of powder every time you take it out of its case. You can use this alone or elongate it to normal pencil size by purchasing DHC's Eyebrow Perfect Pro Holder. This is an OK way to softly define brows with powder, but a pencil with a powder finish is more versatile, especially if you need to better define your brows without adding much thickness or color.

☺ AVERAGE **Eyeliner Perfect Pro Powder** *($7)* must be used with DHC's Eyeliner Perfect Pro Holder, available for purchase separately. It would have been far better and more logical if DHC just provided a product you could use without assembling anything. What you end up with is an inadequate pointed sponge-tip applicator, and it's a poor way to apply powder eyeshadow. A regular eyeshadow and eyeliner brush is distinctly preferred, but this setup is passable for a soft, diffused effect.

DHC LIP COLOR

✓☺ BEST **Lip Color Perfect Pro Creme** *($11)*. This lipstick is sold by itself in a lipstick tube or you can purchase a sleek refillable case at an additional cost. True to its name, this is a creamy lipstick. It feels lush and moisturizing on lips while imparting full color and a soft sheen finish. It isn't nearly as slick as DHC's Lip Color Perfect Pro Long Last, and as a result it lasts longer! One drawback: DHC offers only three shades, which is definitely limiting.

✓☺ BEST **Moisture Care Lipstick** *($14.50)*. If you're looking for a moisturizing lipstick in a soft shade, this is worth checking out. It applies luxuriously smooth and imparts a comfort-able amount of moisture without leaving lips feeling too slick. The small amount of shimmer it contains gives lips an attractive sheen without leaving large flecks of sparkle behind. The formula boasts an assortment of beneficial moisturizers and no added fragrance or flavoring. Of the eight shades, it would be hard to go wrong with any one of them!

☺ GOOD **$$$ Lip Color Perfect Pro Long Last** *($12)* is sold by itself in a lipstick tube or you can purchase a sleek refillable case at an additional cost. The slick, creamy formula feels lighter than traditional cream lipsticks, and imparts rich color with a satin finish. The slickness doesn't dissipate, and as a result this won't be anyone's go-to cosmetic when you want a long-lasting lipstick. This is recommended if you don't mind routine touch ups and you find one of the few shades DHC offers appealing.

☺ AVERAGE **$$$ Moisture Care Liquid Lip Color** *($17)*. This sheer lip gloss imparts plenty of moisture, but deposits far less color than you might expect because it looks quite opaque in the clear tube packaging and on DHC's website. The elongated sponge-top applicator takes some getting used to, as it's very easy to apply too much and create gooey lips.

DHC MASCARAS

✓☺ BEST **$$$ Mascara Perfect Pro Double Protection** *($17.50)*. There isn't anything about this mascara that makes it more "pro" than any other great mascara, but wow does it produce copious length and thickness without clumps! The polymer–based formula forms tiny tubes around each lash. Initial application is wet, but if you're careful this won't smear as it sets and then it's locked in place until you use water and gentle pressure to loosen the tubes (no cleanser needed). It's quite impressive that this stays on when you splash your face, but then comes off with plain water and slight agitation. Note: This dries quickly so if any comb-through is needed, be swift.

DIOR

Strengths: It's all in the makeup: some extraordinary foundations, some of which include sunscreen; the liquid concealer; very good loose powder, and powder eyeshadows; some great mascaras; brow gel; elegant creamy lipsticks and several good lip glosses.

Weaknesses: Expensive; lackluster moisturizers and serums that contain more fragrance and preservatives than elegant ingredients; irritating toners and self-tanners; ordinary masks; lack of products to address the needs of those with blemishes or skin discolorations; some foundations with SPF ratings that are too low; mostly average makeup brushes.

For more information and reviews of the latest Dior products, visit CosmeticsCop.com.

DIOR CLEANSERS

☺ GOOD **$$$ Gentle Foaming Cleanser for Dry and Sensitive Skin** *($32 for 4.2 fl. oz.)* is a good, though overpriced, cleanser that's best for normal to dry or combination skin. It is not suitable for sensitive skin because it contains fragrance, but at least the fragrance isn't as potent as the scent of many other Dior cleansers, but that's not saying much. The water-soluble formula removes excess oil and makeup without leaving skin dry, and it has a soft, slightly creamy texture that rinses completely. Of course, there is no reason in the world to spend this much for a good cleanser, but, if for some reason you cannot imagine buying any brand but Dior, this is an option.

☹ AVERAGE **$$$ Instant Cleansing Water** *($36 for 6.7 fl. oz.)* is a very basic water-soluble cleanser whose formula is closer to a makeup remover than a regular facial cleanser. It is preposterously overpriced for what you get, or rather, for what you're NOT getting!

☹ AVERAGE **$$$ Gentle Cleansing Milk, Dry or Sensitive Skin** *($32 for 6.7 fl. oz.)* is a mineral oil–based cleansing lotion and is as ordinary and out-of-date as you can get. While it does have some cold cream–like merit for very dry skin, it isn't suitable for sensitive skin because it contains synthetic and plant-based fragrance that can be irritating for all skin types, but especially sensitive skin. Like many mineral oil–based cleansing lotions, this works well to remove makeup when wiped off, but it doesn't rinse well.

☹ POOR **DiorSnow White Reveal Gentle Purifying Foam** *($40 for 3.7 fl. oz.)*. This foaming cleanser (which cannot whiten skin) has a rich, creamy texture, but because its cleansing base includes soap-like ingredients it is too drying for most skin types, and definitely not purifying (though you certainly will be clean). Adding to this potential problem is the amount of fragrance included, which is unusually high for a cleanser (fragrance isn't skin care). This also contains the irritating menthol derivative menthoxypropanediol, which has no skin-care benefits whatsoever and, in fact, can have a negative impact on skin due to the irritation it causes. Who thought this cleanser was a good idea? See the Appendix for details on the numerous problems this cleanser presents.

☹ POOR **Purifying Cleansing Milk, Normal or Combination Skin** *($32 for 6.7 fl. oz.)* is a lightweight cleansing lotion which is overpriced, and it's worrisome that the formula includes irritating iris root extract, which isn't good for any skin type. It works well to remove makeup, but so do lots of other cleansers that cost less and omit the needless irritants.

DIOR EYE-MAKEUP REMOVER

☺ AVERAGE **$$$ Instant Eye Makeup Remover** *($28 for 4.2 fl. oz.)* is an exceptionally basic eye-makeup remover! Although it works, there is no logical reason to spend so much money on a product like this. Please see our list of Best Makeup Removers for effective, less expensive options.

DIOR TONERS

☺ AVERAGE **$$$ DiorSnow White Reveal Lotion 1 Fresh** *($50 for 6.7 fl. oz.)* is a very expensive toner containing some intriguing ingredients for dry skin, including glycerin, antioxidant vitamin C, and nonfragrant plant oil. The vitamin C may have some lightening ability, which is nice, but the additions of numerous fragrance ingredients that can cause irritation make it not worth the benefit. Those interested in using vitamin C as a skin lightener (and there is a viable reason to do so) should consider the serums from Paula's Choice RESIST, SkinCeuticals, and MD Skincare instead of this toner and its mixed bag of results.

☺ AVERAGE **$$$ DiorSnow Lotion White Reveal Lotion 2 Riche** *($32 for 4.2 fl. oz.)* misses the mark thanks to its frustrating mix of beneficial and problematic ingredients. Because the DiorSnow line is all about lightening skin, it's good that this toner contains a helpful amount of vitamin C (ascorbyl glucoside) because this ingredient is known to improve brown spots and uneven skin tone. The vitamin C is the most exciting element of this hydrating toner for normal to dry skin. All the other exciting ingredients are listed after the preservative and fragrance, so they don't count for much. Speaking of fragrance, the chief negative element of this toner is the amount of fragrance ingredients it contains. See the Appendix to learn about the problems associated with daily use of fragrant products.

☺ AVERAGE **$$$ Gentle Toning Lotion, Dry or Sensitive Skin** *($32 for 6.7 fl. oz.)* contains a fragrant plant extract that has no real benefit and may cause irritation. On balance, this is a poor choice for those with sensitive skin, and merely an OK option for normal to dry skin.

DIOR EXFOLIANTS & SCRUBS

☺ GOOD **$$$ Instant Gentle Exfoliant** *($38 for 2.6 fl. oz.)* is worth considering if you like facial scrubs and have money to waste. The formula is suitable for all skin types except sensitive (due to the fragrance it contains) and the abrasive polyethylene (plastic) granules are indeed gentle. However, it is an understatement to say that there are other scrubs that function just as well as, if not better than, this for a fraction of the price.

☺ AVERAGE $$$ **Capture Totale Peeling Lumiere Multi-Perfection Resurfacing Peel Radiance +** *($95 for 1.7 fl. oz.)* is billed as a peel, but this highly fragranced product is really a scrub containing a small amount (less than 1%) of the BHA exfoliant salicylic acid. The pH of this scrub is too high for the salicylic acid to exfoliate skin, and it's rinsed from your skin before the salicylic acid has much chance to work. Most likely the abrasive agent is silica beads, and they are quite gentle. This works as a scrub for normal to dry skin, but it's overpriced for what you get. Besides, a leave-on exfoliant with salicylic acid or the AHA glycolic acid, would produce superior results, including enhanced collagen production, which scrubs don't provide.

DIOR MOISTURIZERS (DAYTIME & NIGHTTIME), EYE CREAMS, & SERUMS

☺ GOOD $$$ **DiorSnow Protection UV White Reveal Shield SPF 50** *($50 for 1.3 fl. oz.)* is a daytime moisturizer with sunscreen that contains a whopping 19% zinc oxide along with the synthetic sunscreen active octinoxate. You'll notice it leaves a distinct, lingering white cast on skin. We suppose that's fine if you're looking to whiten your skin all over (a desire in some Asian and Indian cultures), but most Westerners will find the effect off-putting. Dior provides no other pigments to adjust the tint this white sunscreen has, which limits its appeal. That said, this provides brilliant broad-spectrum protection and has a supremely silky texture that glides over skin. It contains antioxidant vitamin C as ascorbyl glucoside, although this form of vitamin C doesn't have the wealth of research regarding its ability to lighten skin to support its use over pure vitamin C and other C derivatives. Still, all forms of vitamin C have antioxidant benefit for skin, but the antioxidant hoopla stops there; all the other antioxidants in this product are present in such teeny-tiny amounts that your skin isn't likely to benefit. This product contains fragrance ingredients known to irritate skin and potentially cause problems when skin is exposed to sunlight, although the high amount of sun protection is likely to mitigate the latter problem. In the end, this is a fairly good option for normal to slightly dry skin not prone to blemishes, but it's definitely something to test before buying.

☺ AVERAGE $$$ **Capture Totale Haute Nutrition Rich Creme** *($135 for 1.7 fl. oz.)* is an emollient moisturizer with a silky texture and contains some beneficial emollients for dry skin, but it's way overpriced for what you get. The plant oils and tiny amounts of antioxidants won't remain potent for long due to the jar packaging, which is disappointing at any price point (see the Appendix for further details). The youth-promoting plants Dior boasts about in this product have no research proving they can make skin look younger, by one day or even by one minute. Besides, they're present in token amounts, which is typical for Dior's skin-care products. This contains several fragrance ingredients known to cause irritation.

☹ AVERAGE $$$ **Capture Totale Multi-Perfection Concentrated Serum** *($140 for 1 fl. oz.)* is an average water- and silicone-based serum containing enough film-forming agent to make skin look smoother temporarily. For the money, it is not preferred to the truly state-of-the-art serums from Olay, Paula's Choice, Estee Lauder, or Clinique.

☺ AVERAGE $$$ **Capture Totale Multi-Perfection Creme** *($135 for 1.7 fl. oz.)* is an incredibly overpriced, yet incredibly average, emollient moisturizer for normal to dry skin, which contains far more fragrance than legitimate beneficial ingredients (and the jar packaging won't help keep the tiny amount of antioxidants stable once this is opened; see the Appendix for details).

☺ AVERAGE $$$ **Capture Totale Night Ritual Intensive Night Restorative Cream** *($145 for 1.7 fl. oz.)* takes a cue from competitor Chanel's ultra-pricey Sublimage Essential Regenerating Cream, claiming that its rare, revitalizing plant, longoza, is "grown only in Madagascar" and, therefore, must have phenomenal benefits for aging skin. Why is it that such ingredients never seem to show up in Peoria or Houston? Why only in exotic locales? Are exotic plants automatically better for skin? The mystique makes it sound like you're buying something unique or special. The marketing myths about plants, or rare species of seaweed, from remote countries or islands where they're gathered by tribal harvesting practices, and on and on, seem never-ending. Speaking of marketing nonsense, Longoza is actually a city in Madagascar, and the plant of that name appears to be a form of wild ginger. Yet it's not present anywhere in this product. That's OK, though, because there's no evidence that any species of ginger can "turn back the clock" for your skin. This ends up being a silky-textured but basic moisturizer that's a mediocre option for normal to slightly dry skin.

☺ AVERAGE $$$ **Capture Totale UV Protect SPF 35** *($53 for 1 fl. oz.)* is a daytime moisturizer with an in-part avobenzone sunscreen that has a silky, lightweight texture and smooth finish those with normal to slightly dry or slightly oily skin will appreciate. This is an expensive way to get sun protection, and because you have to apply all sunscreens liberally to get the SPF benefit on the label, you have to ask yourself how liberally you'll apply this, knowing that if you apply it correctly you'll be replacing it fairly often, and that could add up to spending more than $600 per year on a facial sunscreen. We wish we could tell you that the price is justified because this product is brimming with state-of-the-art ingredients, but it isn't. The mica adds a subtle glow to skin, but that's a cosmetic effect, and all the antioxidants are listed after the preservative and fragrance, making them merely a dusting.

☺ AVERAGE $$$ **DiorSnow D-NA Control White Reveal Essence** *($120 for 1.7 fl. oz.)* is a water-based serum with a beguiling description; you're not getting a well-proven ingredient for your money. Dior includes ascorbyl glucoside (a form of vitamin C) as the key whitening agent in this product. If you removed the vitamin C from this formula, the result would be a very basic, overpriced option. For the money, you're better off investing in a vitamin C serum with proven forms of this vitamin or a skin-lightening product with hydroquinone.

☺ AVERAGE $$$ **DiorSnow White Reveal Illuminating Eye Treatment** *($69 for 0.5 fl. oz.)* is housed in an elegant squeeze tube. This lightweight moisturizer is suitable for slightly dry skin anywhere on the face. It contains a good amount of vitamin C (in the form of ascorbyl glucoside), but offers little else of interest to anyone hoping to address sun-damaged skin. Nothing in this eye cream will reduce dark circles or puffiness, but this does contain ingredients that leave a soft white cast on skin, which is where the "brightening" element comes into play. It's strictly a cosmetic effect, but it can minimize the appearance of dark circles to a modest degree. For some reason, Dior opted to include fragrance in this product. Fragrance isn't skin care, but it's definitely best to avoid it in any product meant for application near the eyes. See the Appendix to find out why, in truth, you don't need an eye cream.

☺ AVERAGE $$$ **Hydra Life Pro-Youth Protective Fluid SPF 15** *($56 for 1.7 fl. oz.)* contains sunscreen and that is the only youthful attribute of this daytime moisturizer, which isn't bad, but is way overpriced for what you get. Avobenzone is included for reliable UVA protection and it is formulated in a lightweight lotion base suitable for normal to slightly dry skin.

☹ POOR **21 Night Renewal Treatment** *($230 for 1 fl. oz.)* promises to give you younger-looking skin after 21 nights. This mega-pricey 3-product set provides a one-week supply of three vials of serum (each a different formula) that, taken together, add up to 1 ounce of product. Now that's what we call sticker shock! As it turns out, despite the fancy packaging, this treatment is far from exciting and absolutely not worth the money. If you're curious (but please drop all curiosity after reading this review), here's how the set breaks down, week by week. **Week 1** is essentially a fluid that contains the AHA glycolic acid, but the amount of this exfoliating ingredient (likely 2–3%) isn't enough to make much difference on sun-damaged skin, even though the serum's pH is within range for exfoliation to occur. This also contains salicylic acid, but likely too low an amount to offer much benefit. What really makes this a no-go is the inclusion of alcohol. As the second ingredient, it makes Week 1 of this 3-week treatment about as far from anti-aging as you can get, because alcohol causes collagen breakdown and hurts the skin's ability to heal (see the Appendix to find out why irritation from alcohol is such a problem). **Week 2**'s serum is similar to that of the Week 1 product, minus the salicylic acid and with only a dusting of glycolic acid. It's mostly water, alcohol, slip agents, and a citrus extract that, like all citrus, poses a risk of irritation. Once again, the alcohol makes this pro-aging rather than anti-aging, and the formula contains too few beneficial ingredients to make it worth your time or money. Finishing the trio is the **Week 3** serum, which is just a lightweight moisturizer that contains a small amount of alcohol (definitely less cause for concern than the amount of alcohol present in the Week 1 and Week 2 serums). This product is not the brilliant capper of a 21-night treatment; on its own, it's barely passable as a moisturizer, and definitely puts your skin at risk of irritation from the amount of citrus extract and fragrance it contains. You can save a lot of money by avoiding this misnamed treatment and consider a well-formulated AHA or BHA exfoliant instead (or, for what this costs, a professional AHA or BHA peel from a dermatologist). Check out the Best Products chapter for our top exfoliant picks.

☹ POOR **Capture Totale Eyes Essential Eye Zone Boosting Super Serum** (*$70 for 0.5 fl. oz.*). Claiming to be the first cellular regenerator sounds like just the boost your eyes need, but that term is meaningless because "cellular" isn't something you can regenerate. Clever marketing is never skin care, and that is exactly the case for this product. What you're getting here is mostly water, slip agents, thickener, and film-forming agents that have a hairspray-like effect on skin. So, although you may perceive skin as being tighter or firmer, it's strictly a cosmetic effect. Plus, this is potentially irritating when used around the eyes. This contains some intriguing anti-aging ingredients, but as is often the case with Dior products, the state-of-the-art ingredients are a minor part of the formula. Fragrance takes center stage and, in fact, is a problem for use near the eyes. See the Appendix for details on the problems fragrance presents for all skin types. Ultimately, this eye serum cannot make good on its claims and really isn't worth considering at all because you're getting so few beneficial ingredients. One more point: You don't need a special product for the eye area (see the Appendix to learn why).

☹ POOR **Capture Totale Multi-Perfection Eye Treatment** (*$85 for 0.5 fl. oz.*) has a light-weight yet hydrating texture that's suitable for slightly dry skin, but, ultimately, it contains too many potential troublemakers to make it worth considering. Even if the formula didn't have the problems it does, the truth is you don't need an eye cream (see the Appendix to learn why), especially not one that costs as much as this and provides so few benefits.

☹ POOR **Capture Totale One Essential Skin Boosting Super Serum** (*$95 for 1 fl. oz.*) is, according to Dior, their most advanced and scientifically proven serum. So, you ask, does that mean that their other products are not as advanced or scientifically proven? Of course not, they're not going to stop selling all their other anti-aging serums and moisturizers that make similar fantastic-sounding claims, which should give you pause. And what about a few months down the road, when yet another "essential" serum is launched? We're all for improving products to keep in step with current scientific research, but the research Dior seems to be relying on isn't going to result in younger-looking skin; in fact, possibly just the opposite. This serum is primarily water, slip agents, and alcohol. Alcohol causes free-radical damage and collagen breakdown—it's hard to imagine what scientific research Dior is actually relying on. There are some impressive ingredients in here, but there is also a lot of fragrance. All in all, the alcohol is a deal breaker because it is a serious problem for skin (see the Appendix for details). There are lots of well-formulated serums without the negatives this "one" presents.

☹ POOR **DiorSnow D-NA Reverse Night** *($124 for 1 fl. oz.)* is sold as an intensive whitening concentrate, but the only thing concentrated about this skin lightener is the skin-damaging alcohol it contains (see the Appendix for details). A couple of potentially helpful skin-lightening ingredients are included, but their benefit is lost due to the problems that this much alcohol causes for your skin. If persistent discolorations are a concern, you would be much better off using a prescription hydroquinone product or an over-the-counter skin lightener from Paula's Choice or Alpha Hydrox, which are available for a fraction of what this product costs!

☹ POOR **Hydra Life Pro-Youth Comfort Creme** *($56 for 1.7 fl. oz.)* is a truly basic, mundane moisturizer for normal to dry skin. Its age-fighting ability is nonexistent because it contains only a paltry amount of anything that helps combat wrinkles. Even if it were well-formulated, the jar packaging won't keep the antioxidants stable.

☹ POOR **Hydra Life Pro-Youth Protective Creme SPF 15** *($56 for 1.7 fl. oz.)* contains sunscreen and that is the only youthful attribute of this daytime moisturizer. Avobenzone was included for reliable UVA protection and it is formulated in a lightweight but substantial cream base. The jar packaging, however, not only is unsanitary, but also compromises the potency of the tiny amount of antioxidants Dior did include. Your normal to dry skin deserves better—there are plenty of less expensive moisturizers with sunscreen that provide a lot more than this.

☹ POOR **Hydra Life Pro-Youth Sorbet Creme** *($56 for 1.7 fl. oz.)* has a texture for normal to dry skin that is indeed reminiscent of sorbet, but does that really matter when the formula is nearly void of youth-promoting ingredients and is packaged in a jar? See the Appendix to learn of the problems jar packaging presents. Save your money: This isn't the moisturizer to buy.

☹ POOR **Hydra Life Pro-Youth Sorbet Eye Creme** *($49 for 0.5 fl. oz.)* has a lightweight cream texture and contains enough film-forming agent to make skin anywhere on the face look temporarily smoother. The formula is completely average and it's packaged in a jar, which allows the minimal amount of antioxidants to degrade shortly after opening.

☹ POOR **Hydra Life Skin Energizer Pro-Youth Hydrating Serum** *($73 for 1.6 fl. oz.)* contains way too much skin-damaging alcohol. When it comes to looking youthful, this type and amount of alcohol is not what you want. It causes free-radical damage and leads to collagen breakdown. The result? More wrinkles. Knowing this, it's really difficult to take Dior's "Pro-Youth" designation seriously. Even without all the alcohol, the utter lack of proven anti-aging ingredients in this serum is shocking.

☹ POOR **Hydra Life Skin Perfect Pore Refining Perfecting Moisturizer** *($65 for 1.7 fl. oz.)* lists alcohol as the second ingredient, so this barely hydrating formula is only "perfect" for causing dryness and irritation that hurts your skin's healing process and causes collagen breakdown, because that's what alcohol does to skin in the amount included in this formula. This does contain some intriguing ingredients, but because there's more alcohol and shine (mica, which has no skin-care benefit; it just adds shine) than beneficial ingredients, your skin will be left wanting (and needing) a lot more.

DIOR SUN CARE

☹ POOR **Dior Bronze Self-Tanner Natural Glow, Body** *($33 for 4.4 fl. oz.)* lists alcohol as the second ingredient, and contains the same ingredient (dihydroxyacetone) found in most self-tanning products. Knowing this, why subject your skin to irritation from this much alcohol?

☹ POOR **Dior Bronze Self-Tanner Natural Glow, Face** *($31 for 1.8 fl. oz.)* contains far too many potentially irritating fragrance ingredients to make it worth choosing over countless other self-tanning products, not to mention the needlessly high price for a very basic formula.

☹ POOR **Dior Bronze Self-Tanner Shimmering Glow, Body** *($33 for 4.5 fl. oz.)* is similar to the Dior Bronze Self-Tanner Natural Glow, Face above, and the same review applies.

DIOR LIP CARE

☺ AVERAGE $$$ **Dior Addict Lip Glow SPF 10** *($30)* is a moisturizing balm that also packs a punch of color while leaving lips feeling soft and smooth. This pink balm quickly turns a brighter hue once applied to lips, and also leaves a stain after the product's balm-like feel wears off. Unfortunately, it also comes only in one color, which may not look great on everyone. Dior claims that their "Addict Lip Glow reacts directly with the unique chemistry of each woman's lips before releasing its color ingredient...," which harkens back to the day of mood lip glosses. Remember those? For 89 cents, back in the day, a color turned a shade when it came in contact with your lip color and body heat. Now you get the same hype with little substance for a heftier price tag. For women with pale lips, the shade can develop into a deep, bright-pink hue, whereas those with darker pigmentation may experience an overall deepening and brightening of their natural lip color. Body chemistry or not, you still have to like the color it becomes. The SPF 10 is below what's recommended by every dermatology board in the world, and does not contain the UVA-protecting ingredients of titanium dioxide, zinc oxide, avobenzone, Tinosorb, Mexoryl SX, or ecamsule to deliver broad-spectrum protection.

☹ POOR **Creme de Rose Smoothing Plumping Lip Balm SPF 10** *($26.50)* feels velvety smooth on the lips, while also adding a touch of pink color and sunscreen. Unfortunately, these positives are far outweighed by the negatives. In a turn for the worse, the formula contains a rose scent that is not only potentially irritating, but also unpleasant for anyone who doesn't want to smell hints of potpourri all day long. It also doesn't "re-plump" lips as claimed. The SPF rating is too low for you to rely on it during the day (medical boards around the world recommend at least an SPF 15), although it does include avobenzone (listed as butyl methoxydibenzoylmethane) for reliable UVA protection.

☹ POOR **Dior Addict Lip Maximizer** *($30)* fails miserably as a lip plumper. The mint flavoring creates a slight, cooling, tingling effect that makes you think it's working, but in reality this is just a gloss with potentially irritating ingredients. Save your money (and your lips)!

DIOR SPECIALTY SKIN-CARE PRODUCTS

☺ GOOD $$$ **DiorSnow Pure UV Ultra-Whitening Spot Corrector SPF 50 PA+++** *($46 for 0.63 fl. oz.)* contains almost 20% titanium dioxide, along with other sunscreen actives, which assures you of significant broad-spectrum sun protection. Sold as a spot treatment, this whitens skin cosmetically (the titanium dioxide and iron oxides provide concealer-like coverage) and is best paired with a skin-tone-correct foundation. This is an OK, though very expensive, option for normal to oily skin not prone to blemishes.

☺ AVERAGE $$$ **DiorSnow White Reveal Fresh Creme** *($90 for 1.7 fl. oz.)* is just like many other Dior products claiming to lighten skin, this product contains the form of vitamin

C known as ascorbyl glucoside. There is emerging research pertaining to this ingredient's ability to lighten skin, at least compared with other forms of vitamin C or ingredients such as hydroquinone or niacinamide. But, assuming that ascorbyl glucoside was a great option for lightening discolorations, the fact that Reveal Fresh Creme is packaged in a jar means the stability and potency of the vitamin C will be squandered shortly after opening because vitamins and plant extracts, among other beneficial ingredients, break down in the presence of air. This overpriced skin lightener has little hope of working, and is not preferred to countless others.

☺ AVERAGE **$$$ Hydra Life Beauty Awakening Rehydrating Mask** *($38 for 2.5 fl. oz.)* is a standard, but good, moisturizing mask for normal to dry skin. It doesn't treat skin to anything particularly special or "awakening," but will make skin feel smooth and comfortable. Of all the Hydra Life products, this one is the most intriguing, but that's still not saying much.

DIOR FOUNDATIONS & PRIMERS

☺ GOOD **$$$ DiorSkin AirFlash Spray Foundation** *($62)* is an aerosol foundation that can be tricky to use, but with a little patience the results are rewarding. The coverage you get depends on your application. Spraying it in your hand at close range and then applying to the face will net medium to full coverage that looks surprisingly natural, and is far less messy than holding it 12 inches or more from your face (as the Dior makeup artist we spoke to recommended). Either way it provides a sheer veil of color and coverage. Once sprayed on, AirFlash dries, well, in a flash—so blending must be quick. Luckily, this blends evenly and sets to a long-wearing, silky matte finish that will require more than a water-soluble cleanser to remove. The shades are excellent, with options for fair to medium skin. Although this is pricey, it is a unique twist on liquid foundations and does indeed feel weightless, which is ideal for oily to very oily skin. By the way, since this foundation can get on your clothing or hairline as you spray it (especially given that you should keep your eyes closed when doing so), it is best applied before dressing, with your hairline protected by a towel or headband, because if you aren't careful it can get all over. The mist this produces is ultra-fine, but some spotting can occur when spraying from the distance that Dior recommends, and do make sure the opening doesn't clog or a mess will ensue.

☺ GOOD **$$$ Diorskin Crystal Nude Natural Matte Skin Perfecter** *($40)* works well as a primer when applied under foundation. The directions say it can also be used over foundation, but that can wreck your makeup. The silky texture blends imperceptibly into skin, smoothing over pores to make them slightly less noticeable.

☺ GOOD **$$$ DiorSkin Eclat Satin** *($47)* is Dior's foundation for those with dry skin, and it delivers—with a creamy, moisturizer-like texture that has a natural affinity for skin. It provides medium to almost full coverage, yet does so without looking thick or cakey and leaves an attractive dewy finish. There are some attractive shades available, but watch out for any with unflattering peach or rose undertones. The fact that this foundation is highly fragranced keeps it from earning a better rating.

☺ GOOD **$$$ Diorskin Forever Compact Flawless Perfection Fusion Wear Makeup SPF 25** *($49)* is a fragrance-free pressed-powder foundation including sunscreen that blends a synthetic active (octinoxate) with a very low amount of titanium dioxide. Because octinoxate doesn't provide sufficient UVA (think anti-aging) protection on its own, you're left with

---

� Highly fragranced products smell good, but won't help your skin! See the Appendix for details.

a foundation whose sunscreen isn't up to par for daytime protection in comparison to many. Despite the disappointingly low amount of titanium dioxide, the truth is that with expensive products, like this one, you're not likely to apply enough of it to obtain the level of sun protection stated on the label. That's why we recommend viewing products like this as an adjunct to another product rated SPF 15 or greater that provides broad-spectrum protection. Sunscreen issues aside, this powder foundation has a beautifully soft texture that glides over skin and meshes with it so well the effect is amazingly natural, yet you get light coverage to blur minor redness and other imperfections. The satin-matte finish enlivens skin without making it look the least bit dry or cakey. Overall, the formula is best for normal to dry skin. Dior's shade range is impressive, with a good mix of neutral to warm-toned colors suitable for fair to tan skin tones.

☺ GOOD $$$ **Hydra Life Pro-Youth Skin Tint SPF 20** *($40)* is a tinted moisturizer with sunscreen that has a velvety liquid texture which feels light on the skin and blends well while providing medium coverage. It eventually sets to a semi-matte finish and has the potential to last sufficiently well throughout the day, and its sunscreen includes titanium dioxide for sufficient UVA protection. The color selection is limited, but if you can find one that works for you, this tinted moisturizer has its strong points (although price isn't one of them).

☺ AVERAGE $$$ **Capture Totale Radiance Restoring Serum Foundation SPF 15** *($80)* is an overpriced, highly fragranced liquid foundation for normal to dry skin claiming to combine the skin-improving benefits of makeup with the anti-aging ingredients present in other Dior Capture Totale skin-care products, which actually isn't saying much. Although this hits the right marks for broad-spectrum sun protection along with an elegant texture, it doesn't contain ingredients that make it anti-aging or an all-in-one solution for wrinkles over and above the sunscreen it contains—not even close! This has a fluid, slightly creamy texture that is easy to blend. It sets to a smooth, satin-like finish that adds a subtle glow and provides medium to full coverage. As for the shades, more than half of the shades are too peach, pink, orange, or rose; the best shades are those for fair to light skin tones. Considering the claims, the formula contains only a dusting of anti-aging ingredients. None of the exotic-sounding plant extracts in this foundation can "correct all visible signs of aging." There is no single ingredient or blend of ingredients that can "correct" every sign of aging, and there's no research proving otherwise. Besides, if this foundation were all it took to correct all signs of aging, what are all the other Dior Capture Totale products for; this should be all you need, right?

☺ AVERAGE $$$ **DiorSkin Forever Flawless Perfection Fusion Wear Makeup SPF 25** *($47)* is a liquid foundation with an amazingly silky, fluid texture that blends readily, setting (quickly) to a lasting matte finish those with normal to oily skin will love. The finish is incredibly skin-like, yet provides light to medium coverage to even skin tone and softly blur imperfections. What's more, the sunscreen is in-part titanium dioxide, so broad-spectrum protection is assured. With all this praise, why didn't this fantastic foundation get a higher rating? Alcohol. This skin irritant is the third ingredient, so it's present in an amount that has the potential to cause irritation that hurts skin's ability to heal and produce healthy collagen. Adding to this issue is that this foundation is also very fragrant, and fragrance isn't skin care. The range of shades presents some excellent options for fair to tan skin tones, but beware that not every shade is aces. What a shame a couple of formulary drawbacks keep this otherwise stellar foundation from earning our top rating!

☺ AVERAGE $$$ **DiorSkin Nude Natural Glow Hydrating Makeup SPF 10** *($47)* has an SPF rating that's below the standard recommended by all major health organizations and that's unfortunate. SPF 10 isn't terrible, but SPF 15 or greater is preferred. The fluid texture of this foundation has an elegant slip that makes blending a breeze, and the satin matte finish looks incredibly skin-like. It provides sheer to light coverage, but layers well for trouble spots, although you'll still need a concealer to mask red spots or dark circles. Dior's shade range has improved, but despite their efforts, some duds remain. This foundation is best for normal to slightly oily skin. Note: The amount of alcohol, while seemingly high, is not cause for concern. The same holds true for the fragrance ingredients (such as limonene) in this foundation. Of course, the formula would be better without these ingredients!

☺ AVERAGE $$$ **DiorSkin Nude Natural Glow Creme-Gel Makeup SPF 20** *($49)* fails to provide sufficient UVA protection because it doesn't include the UVA-protecting ingredients of titanium dioxide, zinc oxide, avobenzone, Mexoryl SX, Tinosorb, or ecamsule. This oversight leaves your skin vulnerable to the sun's aging rays. Just about every other aspect is impressive, although without question you don't have to spend nearly this much for a great foundation. This has a smooth, gel-cream texture that isn't slick and applies evenly, offering sheer to medium coverage and a lightweight semi-matte finish. Dior offers options for light to dark skin tones, but watch out for shades with an unflattering peach undertone. This fragranced foundation is best for normal to slightly dry or slightly oily skin.

☺ AVERAGE $$$ **DiorSkin Nude Natural Glow Sculpting Powder Makeup SPF 10** *($50)* is a pressed-powder foundation offering three strips of powder in one compact. The shades in each compact are tone-on-tone, and at least one strip in each shade contains shimmer. More visually appealing than practical, this smooth powder is best used by swirling a brush (either the one Dior includes, which is workable, or your regular powder brush) over the entire powder. Doing so results in a finish that feels matte but looks shimmery, which isn't the best look for those with oily skin. If oily skin isn't a concern, this powder foundation provides light to medium coverage. The SPF rating is too low to be counted on for sufficient sun protection (SPF 15 is considered the minimum by most medical boards around the world), but it does include titanium dioxide for reliable UVA protection, so if paired with a moisturizing sunscreen underneath or a pressed powder with sunscreen, that would make it passable. Turning to the shades, almost all are too peachy to look convincing when applied all over the face but are best used to highlight skin or, if preferred, as a peach-tinged bronzing powder with strong shimmer. Overall, this is a pricey product with fairly mediocre performance.

☺ AVERAGE $$$ **DiorSkin Sculpt Line-Smoothing Lifting Makeup SPF 20** *($55)* doesn't contain anything to make lines look smoother, at least not any more so than any other foundation, but that cosmetic effect is a poor substitute for wrinkle prevention, which is where an effective sunscreen comes in. Unfortunately, this anti-aging makeup misses the mark by not including UVA-protecting ingredients. That's truly a shame, because it has a creamy-smooth texture and a beautiful application perfect for those with normal to dry skin who prefer a slightly moist finish and medium to full coverage. In terms of sculpting or lifting, don't count on such benefits, especially with insufficient sun protection. This does contain a tiny amount of peptides, but they're listed after the preservative, meaning their benefit to skin will be minimal at best. There are enough positives to make this worth considering, but not over similar foundations that get the critical issue of sun protection right.

☺ AVERAGE $$$ **Skinflash Radiance Boosting Makeup Primer** *($42)* is a tinted water-based primer with a thin texture leaving a radiant, albeit dry, finish on skin. Packaged like an oversized click-style pen, the primer can be stroked on directly with the adequately sized synthetic brush or with your fingertips (the former does produce a surprisingly smooth and even application). The problem with this primer is that even though it does adequately "prime" the

The Reviews D

face (by evening out the skin tone and providing a smoother surface that helps foundation look better), it doesn't provide added skin-care benefits. In fact, the formula doesn't contain much in the way of skin-redeeming ingredients, and the amount of alcohol is potentially a concern (see the Appendix for details). Also, the fragrance ingredients this contains are known to cause irritation, making this a product to avoid applying around the eyes.

☺ AVERAGE **$$$ DiorSnow UV Shield BB Crème SPF 50 PA+++** *($50)* contains an in-part titanium dioxide sunscreen and has a somewhat thick but silky formula that's best for normal to slightly dry skin. BB creams are supposed to contain a range of ingredients that go beyond what most tinted moisturizers offer, yet almost without exception, they're little more than tinted moisturizers with sunscreen. This formula contains vitamin C (ascorbyl glucoside) and a teeny-tiny amount of antioxidants, but that's about it in terms of unique ingredients. As usual with Dior products, this is fragranced and contains fragrance ingredients known to cause irritation. Only one shade is offered, and it's a soft, slightly sheer peach that's best for light to light-medium skin tones. This provides sheer to light coverage and a satin matte finish that helps blur imperfections, just like most tinted moisturizers. The "PA" followed by plus signs (PA+++, for example) is a designation used in Japan for rating the UVA protection of a sunscreen. The SPF number is about the sun's UVB rays; there are very few countries that have a UVA rating reference. Three plus symbols after the "PA" indicate the highest level of UVA protection, which can be as low as PA+, which means some UVA protection. The PA standard is not accepted or used in other countries, but because this Dior product originated in Japan, it includes the PA statment on the labeling. The concept is interesting, but ultimately the SPF rating and the active ingredients matter far more because the method of assessing UVA protection is not widely accepted, primarily because it is very difficult to get agreement from scientists on what tests to use and what they mean.

☹ POOR **DiorSkin Nude Natural Glow Fresh Powder Makeup SPF 10** *($46)* is a loose-powder foundation with a gossamer-light texture and silky, sheer application. Things go awry with the finish, however, which casts an ethereal, whitish glow. This is apparent with all the shades, despite their perceptible depth of color when viewed in the package. If that isn't odd enough, for some reason Dior chose to add the potent menthol derivative menthoxypropanediol to the formula. Between that, the strange way each shade "reads" on skin, and the low SPF rating, this isn't recommended.

DIOR CONCEALERS

✓☺ BEST **$$$ DiorSkin Sculpt Lifting Smoothing Concealer** *($35)* is expensive, but there's no denying that this is a formidable concealer worthy of your attention. The silky, silicone-enhanced formula begins slightly thick, but blends very well. It has minimal slip, so it does a great job of staying precisely where you place it, drying to a satin matte finish that provides significant coverage. Dark circles and redness are easily erased, but this concealer never looks too thick and it creases only minimally. It comes in three superb shades, though only for fair to medium skin tones. Forget about the sculpting and lifting claims because they are mere fantasy, but the rest is as real as it gets.

☺ AVERAGE **$$$ DiorSkin Nude Skin Perfecting Hydrating Concealer** *($30)* comes in a range of flattering shades that offer medium to full coverage while feeling silky-smooth on skin. This liquid concealer blends evenly without tugging or pulling at skin, and offers a dewy finish. But therein lies the problem: The finish easily slips into fine lines and is too emollient for those with oily, blemish-prone skin. Unfortunately, fine lines, oily skin, and blemishes are an issue most of us struggle with, but if you are one of the lucky few who don't have to worry about those issues, then this is a good option for a moisturizing concealer. Adding a sheer layer of powder helps set the concealer for improved wear, though you may still get some creasing into lines.

DIOR POWDER

☹ AVERAGE **$$$ DiorSkin Forever Wear-Extending Invisible Retouch Powder SPF 8** *($42)* is a talc-based pressed powder with a smooth, sheer texture that also feels a bit waxy and can end up looking heavy on your skin. Each of the three soft shades (best for fair to medium skin tones) leaves a natural matte finish, but this is definitely a powder to try in the store before purchasing. As for the sunscreen, not only is SPF 8 below the minimum SPF 15 rating recommended by medical boards worldwide, but also it does not include the ingredients needed to shield your skin from the sun's entire range of damaging UVA rays, which is essential for anti-aging benefits. See the Appendix for further details.

DIOR BLUSHES & BRONZERS

✓☺ BEST **$$$ Bronze Harmonie de Blush** *($44)* is an attractive pressed bronzing powder featuring multiple colors in one compact. The idea is to swirl the brush over the entire cake, which transfers an even application of sheer bronze tones to your skin. The texture is wonderfully smooth and the sheer colors leave a soft shine finish. This is worth exploring if you normally combine powder blush and bronzer.

✓☺ BEST **$$$ DiorBlush** *($42)* is superlative, and most of the available colors are excellent, with several soft choices that apply evenly. Each shade is infused with shine, but it's not too intrusive. This blush has that extra something that pushes it above and beyond the best.

✓☺ BEST **$$$ Dior Bronze Matte Sunshine SPF 20** *($46)* is expensive. However, if the price doesn't deter you, it performs quite well. The sunscreen is in-part titanium dioxide, so this can serve as a helpful adjunct to an SPF-rated product applied to your entire face, something you wouldn't want to do with a bronzing powder. But remember, you must apply it liberally to achieve the SPF rating on the label. This has a sublimely silky texture that goes on beautifully smooth, leaving a dimensional matte (yes, this is a matte bronzing powder) finish.

☺ GOOD **$$$ Dior Bronze Original Tan** *($46)* is a pressed bronzing powder that delivers an impressive amount of color in just one stroke of the brush. It blends evenly to a shimmer finish with a pinch of sparkle—just enough to give you a healthy glow without looking overly done. Watch out for shades with an overtly peach or reddish-brown undertone.

DIOR EYESHADOWS

✓☺ BEST **$$$ 1-Couleur Eyeshadow** *($29)* has an enviably silky, almost creamy texture. The application is excellent, as is the color saturation, making these single shadows a pleasure to work with. The drawback for those with wrinkles is the amount of shine. If wrinkles aren't a concern and you want shine, there are some attractive shades to consider.

✓☺ BEST **$$$ 5-Couleur Eyeshadow Palette** *($59)*. The texture of these is like powdered sugar and the fragrance-free, talc-based formula doesn't crease. Each shade applies very smoothly, doesn't flake, and provides more coverage (and definitely has a stronger color payoff) than most powder eyeshadows. You can truly be an "artiste" with these shadows and a good set of eyeshadow brushes—and most sets have a color dark enough to work as powder eyeliner, not to mention these shadows work wet or dry. The ongoing problem is Dior's often contrasting or overly trendy color combinations. Sadly, these tend to outnumber the workable sets, though there are some worth considering. These shadows are predominantly shiny, but if that's your thing, the shine in many sets is on the soft side and clings beautifully. It's still too shiny for wrinkled or drooping eyelids, but younger women with the means to afford these eyeshadow sets will be impressed. Note: The tiny applicators that come with each set should be discarded in favor of full-size professional brushes.

☺ GOOD $$$ **3 Couleurs Smoky Ready-to-Wear Smoky Eyes Palette** *($48)* isn't quite as nice as Dior's five-color eyeshadow palettes. Each sleek compact holds three powder eyeshadows and two sponge-tip applicators, which you can toss in favor of using full-size professional brushes. Most of the trios are well coordinated, with each containing a light, medium, and dark shade that doubles as eyeliner. The smooth, non-powdery texture glides on and blends evenly, yet the light and medium shades are surprisingly sheer, which means you must layer them for more intense shading or coverage. These shadows have shine, and the darkest shade in each trio has glitter instead of low-glow shimmer (be aware that the glitter will flake a bit during wear).

☹ AVERAGE $$$ **5-Couleurs Designer All-in-One Artistry Palette** *($59)* is housed in a sleek mirrored compact with five eyeshadows. Four are silicone-based and laced with varying degrees of shine, while the darkest shade is essentially a cream eyeliner with an almost-matte finish and enough depth to work as eyeliner. The shadows have a unique silky, airy texture that's like an ultra-light powder, and they apply beautifully without flaking. Even better, the color, which goes on soft but builds easily, really lasts and resists creasing. The cream eyeliner works great and doesn't veer toward being greasy or looking smeared. One drawback, especially considering this palette's price, is that the shadows and liner can dry out quickly (for example, all the open testers at our Sephora store were dried out and unusable). Also, layering the various shades can result in a muddy look rather than smooth gradations of color possible from powder eyeshadows. If you decide to try this, be sure to keep it tightly closed between uses (you may even want to close it between applying each shade).

DIOR EYE & BROW LINERS

✓☺ BEST $$$ **Liquid Eyeliner** *($34)* is brilliantly designed to offer precision and ease of use. The calligraphy-style fine-tip applicator evenly dispenses product through the soft, flexible brush hairs. Because the hairs taper to a fine point, the result is meticulous detailing, but you also can apply more pressure to fan the brush and make a thicker line. The product dries quickly and stays put all day, without flaking or smearing.

☺ GOOD $$$ **DiorLiner Precision Eyeliner** *($34)* is a long-lasting liquid liner that comes with a good brush that makes even application easy. The bottom of the pen houses the liquid and you have to click the base to feed the brush. If Dior sold refills, this would be an option; since they don't, this is absurdly overpriced for what you get, though still deserving of a Good rating.

☺ GOOD $$$ **DiorShow Liner Waterproof** *($29)* is an automatic, retractable eye pencil that never needs sharpening and has a wonderfully smooth application. It sets within seconds to a long-wearing finish that's slightly prone to smearing—but this also allows you to use a brush to soften or "smoke out" the line before it sets and refuses to budge. Once set, this is really difficult to remove! You'll need a silicone- or oil–based eye-makeup remover as well as a fair amount of pressure to make sure you're getting every trace of this eyeliner off.

☺ GOOD $$$ **Sourcils Poudre Powder Eyebrow Pencil** *($29)* has a soft powder texture that fills in and defines brows without looking heavy (no Joan Crawford arches here!) and comes in three beautiful shades. Although an automatic, twist-up brow pencil or a powder eyeshadow with a thin brush is easier to use to create realistic eyebrow definition, this remains one of the better standard brow pencils. The mascara brush at the opposite end of the pencil is a nice touch for softening the result.

☺ AVERAGE **$$$ DiorShow Brow Styler Ultra-Fine Precision Brow Pencil** *($29)* certainly lives up to its name in terms of allowing for precise detailing. This fine-point, retractable pencil has a semi-stiff texture that doesn't smudge or smear. The conveniently attached spoolie brush allows you to further refine your look by combing and taming brows. On the downside, some may find this pencil requires too much time and effort to apply because the point is so fine and because there is only one shade, Universal Shade, which is a dark brown. Dark brown is hardly universal; what about women who have red, blonde, or black hair? In this case, one shade does not fit all.

DIOR LIP COLOR & LIPLINERS

✓☺ BEST **$$$ RougeLiner Automatic Lip Liner** *($29)* never needs sharpening, is retractable, and has a beautifully smooth application. Another strong point is how long-lasting the color is: Some of the shades have such a strong stain they take considerable effort to remove! It is definitely an excellent lip pencil to consider if you don't mind spending this much.

☺ GOOD **$$$ Dior Addict Ultra-Gloss** *($28)* has an emollient, lanolin-based formula that is great for dry lips and provides a smooth, glossy finish that isn't sticky. The sheer- to light-coverage colors are a tantalizing mix, with options for the color-shy and for those with a flair for the dramatic.

☺ GOOD **$$$ Rouge Dior Lipcolor** *($32)* makes all sorts of claims in terms of long wear and amplified color technology, but for all the hype this is nothing more than a standard, but good, creamy lipstick. It offers enticing shades with medium opacity and a soft glossy finish. The pigments in this lipstick are more concentrated than usual, which means the colors last longer. However, you'll likely be ready for a touch-up before then because the glossy finish is short-lived.

☺ AVERAGE **$$$ Dior Addict Lip Polish** *($30)* is said to be a lip primer and polish in one, but in reality it's nothing more than a standard lip gloss. The sponge-tip applicator is designed to spin across your lips as it is applied, which is fine, but there is no advantage over using a traditional applicator. This lip gloss is offered in flattering shades, all of which have an ample glossy (and non-sticky) finish.

☺ AVERAGE **$$$ Dior Addict Lipstick** *($30)* is a greasy, slick lipstick that can quickly look messy and easily migrate into lines around the mouth. Coverage from each of the many shades is light to moderate, which means you're getting only a slight stain, so these colors don't go the distance (and for this much money, they should). The finish is wet-look gloss and the fragrance is, thankfully, subtle.

DIOR MASCARAS

✓☺ BEST **$$$ DiorShow Iconic Mascara** *($28.50)* has a unique rubber-bristled brush that does a fantastic job of extending and curling every last lash, all without clumps. This doesn't build the wow-factor thickness of the original Diorshow Mascara, but has a cleaner, more precise application that refuses to falter (and gets incrementally better) with successive coats.

✓☺ BEST **$$$ DiorShow Waterproof Mascara** *($25)* is Dior's best waterproof mascara to date. Although the brush is enormous and can be difficult to work with, you will find it produces copious length and respectable thickness without clumps or smears. The formula is tenaciously waterproof, but easier than most to remove, making this highly recommended if your mascara budget extends to Dior's price point.

☺ GOOD **$$$ DiorShow Black Out Spectacular Volume Intense Black-Kohl Mascara** *($25)* has a large brush that can be difficult to control and apply evenly, but with patience this builds dramatically thick, full lashes. This is also one of the blackest mascaras around; the color really makes an impact. You'll appreciate how soft this keeps lashes, plus it wears beautifully yet removes easily with a water-soluble cleanser. A less cumbersome brush would have earned this a higher rating.

☺ GOOD **$$$ DiorShow Black Out Waterproof Mascara** *($25)* does a beautiful job of coating lashes a dramatically dark shade of black, minus clumps, flakes, or smearing. This mascara excelled on our waterproof test, and while it may not deliver the level of thickness and length of today's best mascaras, it's still a good option for those looking for a stay-put mascara that meticulously defines lashes.

☺ GOOD **$$$ DiorShow Mascara** *($25)* has one of the largest brushes we've ever seen on a mascara wand, which makes it a bit tricky to work with, and nearly impossible to reach the small lashes near the eye's inner and outer corners, but with patience and practice every lash can be covered. The payoff is extraordinarily long, thick lashes with minimal to no clumping, and beautiful separation. Beyond the cumbersome brush, the only caveat with this mascara is its potent fragrance. There is no reason for mascara to contain fragrance, but then again, this is Dior.

☺ GOOD **$$$ DiorShow Maximizer Lash-Plumping Serum** *($28)* is primarily a lash primer, despite the name, meaning it is applied before mascara, but it doesn't deposit any color. It is meant to add bulk and oomph to lashes so the mascara that's applied over it works even better. The good news is it really works and it goes on smooth, quick, and clump-free. However, you don't really need a lash primer if you are using a really great mascara, which you should be. But for those who insist a lash primer is a must, this offering from Dior is worth your attention (whether or not it's worth your money is up to you). To warrant the hefty price tag Dior claims that this product acts as "a nourishing serum treatment that promotes long-term lash growth." It doesn't promote anything in the way of lash growth—this is just colorless mascara—and the formula doesn't include any ingredients known to stimulate lash growth. It's mostly water with wax and wax-like thickening agents. The tiny amounts of vitamin E, soy protein, sodium hyaluronate, and the crustacean extract artemia have absolutely no ability to influence lash growth or strength.

☹ AVERAGE **$$$ DiorShow Extase Mascara** *($28.50)* doesn't deposit mascara evenly (more like every third lash), and the unusually thick formula goes on too wet and heavy. This is an OK option if you've got the patience and the desire to tame this unruly mascara with a separate eyelash comb or brush. This does offer impressive staying power (perhaps due to the inclusion of shellac), as it didn't budge, flake, or smear even through a full-blown, allergy-induced eye-rubbing fit. Sadly, staying power really doesn't matter if the product doesn't look great in the first place!

☹ AVERAGE **$$$ DiorShow Unlimited Ultra-Lengthening Curving Mascara** *($24.50)* thickens better than it lengthens, and nothing about its performance deserves "ultra" status. Application tends to be a bit uneven and slightly wet, so you'll get some smearing unless you're meticulous (or wipe down the wand beforehand).

☹ POOR **DiorShow Iconic Extreme Waterproof Mascara** *($28.50)* produces prodigious length quickly and cleanly; there's no denying that. Thickness is minimal, but it builds decently if you have the patience to apply several coats. Lashes are left with a soft curl that lasts. Despite these impressive traits and the fact that this won't flake, it isn't waterproof. Simply splashing your eyes with a bit of water causes the formula to break down and run. Didn't anyone at Dior test this product before they decided to label it waterproof?

DIOR FACE & BODY ILLUMINATORS

✓☺ BEST $$$ **DiorSkin Ultra Shimmering All Over Face Powder** *($44)* is a pressed shimmer powder that's an ideal find for those who want a soft, glowing sheen rather than "look at me!" sparkles. The super-smooth texture makes it a joy to apply, and it blends evenly to a finish that's tailor-made for highlighting skin. The multiple tones in this powder are best swirled together with your brush so they come off as one uniform shade on skin.

☺ GOOD $$$ **Skinflash Radiance Booster Pen** *($37)* promises "professional lightworks in a flash." What this really ends up being is merely a click-pen applicator set up so that you need to twist the base of the component to feed product onto the attached synthetic brush. This produces a flesh-toned liquid that at first appears to be a concealer. Yet once it's applied to skin it practically vanishes into it, providing minimal coverage as it sets to a natural matte (in feel) finish. Basically, this is a sheer highlighter with a touch of shimmer to help light reflect more evenly off skin. To some extent, this can soften minor flaws and subtle discolorations. It is best for creating soft highlights under the eye, on the brow bone, and down the bridge of the nose, and the fact that this blends so well into skin makes it a pleasure to work with, especially if you're attempting a complex highlighting/contouring makeup application. Each shade is initially pink or peach, but "neutralizes" once blended.

DIOR BRUSHES

☺ GOOD $$$ **Dior Brushes** *($20–$52)* are respectable but by no means perfect or worthy of must-have status. Given Dior's vast selection of makeup, it's surprising their brush choices are so limited.

DOVE (SKIN CARE ONLY)

Strengths: Inexpensive; available in every major drugstore and mass-market store.

Weaknesses: The bar cleansers may be soap-free and contain moisturizing ingredients, but they can still leave a residue and are not preferred to gentle, water-soluble cleansers.

For more information and reviews of the latest Dove products (including their body-care products), visit CosmeticsCop.com.

DOVE CLEANSERS

☹ POOR **Beauty Bar, Pink** *($11.99 for 8 bars)* is standard-issue, no-frills bar soap. Yes, it does contain a detergent cleansing agent and moisturizing stearic acid, but the overall effect on skin is still drying, and it doesn't rinse easily.

☹ POOR **Beauty Bar, White** *($11.99 for 8 bars)* is a standard issue bar cleanser that contains elements of traditional soap with detergent cleansing agents. Despite some moisturizing ingredients, the overall effect on skin is drying and the soap leaves a residue that is difficult to rinse, so expect it to impede the performance of other, leave-on skin-care products. Bar soaps are always a bad idea for skin because in addition to leaving residue behind, the ingredients that keep these types of soaps in bar form can clog pores and trigger irritation. You can find gentle, yet effective liquid cleanser recommendations on our Best Cleansers list at the end of this book.

☹ POOR **Gentle Exfoliating Beauty Bar** *($11.99 for 8 bars)* is a standard bar cleanser that does not contain any exfoliant ingredients (the former version did). It is similar to Dove's other Beauty Bars, and as such is not recommended.

☹ POOR **Go Fresh Burst Beauty Bar** *($11.99 for 8 bars)* is similar to Dove's Beauty Bar, White, only with a lot more fragrance, which isn't skin care. Otherwise, the same review applies. The same comments also apply to Dove's **Go Fresh Cool Moisture Beauty Bar**, **Go Fresh Energize Beauty Bar**, and **Summer Care Beauty Bar**.

☹ POOR **Nourishing Care Shea Butter Beauty Bar** *($11.99 for 8 bars)* is similar to Dove's Beauty Bar, White, only with the inclusion of shea butter. Otherwise, the same review applies.

☹ POOR **Sensitive Skin Beauty Bar, Unscented** *($11.99 for 8 bars)* is similar to Dove's other Beauty Bars and is not recommended. Although this bar cleanser is fragrance-free, it still contains soap constituents that can be drying for skin and definitely do not rinse well. The residue this cleanser leaves on skin can impede the performance of leave-on products such as exfoliants and moisturizers.

DR. DENESE NEW YORK

Strengths: Several well-formulated serums and moisturizers that are reasonably priced; a very good matte-finish, tinted sunscreen with zinc oxide; uses well-researched, proven ingredients that truly benefit skin, and uses them in higher concentrations than most skin-care lines.

Weaknesses: Problematic toner; inclusion of unnecessary irritants such as lavender oil and menthol; limited options for sun protection; a few gimmicky, multistep kits and specialty products that are easily replaced by other products in her line.

For more information and reviews of the latest Dr. Denese products, visit CosmeticsCop.com.

DR. DENESE NEW YORK CLEANSERS

☺ AVERAGE **$$$ Hydrating Cleanser** *($22 for 6 fl. oz.)* is a cleansing lotion that requires a washcloth for complete removal. It doesn't contain any coenzyme Q10 as claimed, but no matter: It and the vitamins this does contain are mostly rinsed down the drain. This is an OK cleanser for dry skin not prone to breakouts. This removes makeup fairly well, but ends up being pricey for what you get.

☺ AVERAGE **$$$ Hydroshield Cleansing Cream** *($22 for 8 fl. oz.)*. This silky, oil-like cleanser contains a blend of silicones to remove makeup. It contains a gentle cleansing agent and plant oil to assist the silicones, but the latter are doing the brunt of the work as you slide this over your skin. Because of the silicone-heavy formula, this isn't a true cleansing cream, but rather is closer to a cleansing oil with a standard liquid texture; indeed, the main ingredient is a form of silicone that has a very fluid, runny consistency. What's intriguing is the number of anti-aging ingredients in this cleanser. Even retinol is on board, although retinol can present problems if used too close to the eye. Because this cleanser is difficult to remove without leaving a residue, it's likely some of the anti-aging ingredients will remain on your skin. Of course, that also means that traces of the two fragrant plant extracts this contains also will be left on your skin, so it's good the amounts are low enough that the risk of irritation is very low. Ultimately, this cleanser is unique, but not as easy to use as a creamy, water-soluble cleanser. It definitely removes all types of makeup and the silicones leave dry skin feeling smooth—if only removing this were easier.

DR. DENESE NEW YORK TONER

☹ POOR **Pore Refining Toner** *($19 for 8 fl. oz.)* is a water- and aloe-based toner that would have been much better for skin if it didn't include irritating witch hazel, lavender oil, and several citrus extracts. This toner does contain AHAs, but the pH of 6 prevents them from functioning as exfoliants. This product is not recommended; see the Appendix for further details on lavender oil.

DR. DENESE NEW YORK EXFOLIANTS & SCRUBS

☺ GOOD $$$ **SkinPerfect Rx Glycolic Transforming Peel** (*$45 for 1 fl. oz.*). When we called Dr. Denese's customer service team to ask about the percentage of AHAs in this product, we were told it was proprietary information. That kind of response is not uncommon, but it doesn't help consumers who are looking for a good AHA exfoliant. There's no need to keep this information secret because it's only part of the formula, and the percent determines its efficacy. We suspect the concentration of lactic and glycolic acids is about 10%, and we know the pH of 3.6 is within range for exfoliation to occur. This water-based gel contains some very good antioxidants and soothing agents, but the presence of citrus extracts (which do not function like AHAs, nor do maple or sugarcane) keeps this from earning a Best Product rating. This is a good, but overpriced, option for all skin types except sensitive, but the price is out of the ballpark given the well-formulated options available from Alpha Hydrox and Paula's Choice.

☺ AVERAGE $$$ **Damage Reversal Pads** (*$45 for 60 pads*) contain a solution of 2% hydroquinone in a waxy base that will be a problem for anyone whose skin is prone to break-outs or blackheads. The fact that these pads are packaged in a jar means the hydroquinone will quickly become inactive, as will the plant extracts and antioxidants. There really isn't any compelling reason to consider this over skin-lightening products with hydroquinone that come in better packaging. The list of Best Skin-Lightening products at the end of this book presents several options.

☺ AVERAGE $$$ **Resurface & Glow Treatment Face Wash** (*$22.50 for 8 fl. oz.*). Despite the lengthy claims that make this cleanser/scrub hybrid sound like the fast track to perfect skin, it's merely a scrub, and a rather ordinary one at that—nothing else. The alumina it contains is not the same as what is used in microdermabrasion, but even if it were, you wouldn't want to attack your skin with that kind of barrier-damaging granules on a daily basis. The inclusion of glycolic acid is pointless because you rinse this scrub from your skin, so it won't be in contact long enough to have any benefit; the same is true for the antioxidant vitamins that are present. This is an OK scrub for normal to dry skin, but the emollients don't make it a cinch to rinse.

☹ POOR **Advanced Firming Facial Pads** (*$48 for 100 pads*) contain 10% glycolic acid and have a pH of 3.8 to ensure efficacy (this was confirmed by the company and our own testing). Interestingly, although menthol is no longer listed on the ingredient statement, these pads have a noticeable mint smell and definitely cause your skin to tingle while providing an intense cooling sensation. The tingle can occur with use of an effective AHA product (which this qualifies as), but the cooling effect is not indicative of how AHAs should feel. We called the company to ask about this discrepancy, and were told that the pads do, in fact, still contain menthol. Therefore, they are still not recommended. The addition of a couple of peptides doesn't change the fact that these pads add extra irritation to the skin and still have poor aesthetics.

☹ POOR **Firming Facial Light Resurfacing Peel** (*$33.25 for 2 fl. oz.*). This peel's pH is within the range for the AHAs it contains (lactic and glycolic acids) to exfoliate, but there's not much of them in here, which is surprising for this brand. Other than the amount of film-forming agent (think hairspray that you can peel off) that's in here, which can temporarily make skin look smoother, there is no compelling reason to consider this orange-tinted facial peel.

☹ POOR **Firming & Resurfacing Eye Pads** (*$28 for 60 pads*). These pads contain a potentially effective amount of the AHA glycolic acid, but the pH is too high for it to function as an exfoliant. More troubling is the amount of triethanolamine in these pads. As the second ingredient, this pH-adjusting ingredient is too irritating to use so close to the eyes

(Source: cosmeticsinfo.org). Last, the jar packaging won't keep key ingredients stable during use; see the Appendix for further details.

☹ POOR **Neck Saver Neck Firming Pads** *($31 for 60 pads)*. Although these pads contain an effective amount (likely 10%) of the AHA glycolic acid (along with a smaller amount of the BHA salicylic acid), they're steeped in a formula that contains irritating ingredients such as witch hazel distillate, menthol, and lavender oil. Each of these presents problems for your skin; see the Appendix for details. There are antioxidants in this formula, but because these pads are packaged in a jar, these helpful ingredients will quickly deteriorate (refer to the Appendix foe details). One more comment: You don't need a special exfoliant for your neck. Any well-formulated AHA or BHA exfoliant you're using on your face can be used on your neck, too.

DR. DENESE NEW YORK MOISTURIZERS (DAYTIME & NIGHTTIME), EYE CREAMS, & SERUMS

✓☺ BEST **FirmaTone Rx RetinolMax Chin and Neck Firming Serum** *($48.50 for 1 fl. oz.)*. Although this serum's formula deserves our top rating, it must be said that you do not need a special product for your neck and chin! In fact, this serum does not differ in any meaningful way from those Dr. Denese offers for all-over facial use. And there is no reason you can't apply this "chin and neck firming serum" all over your face, including around the eyes. The fragrance-free formula has a silky, silicone-enriched texture that contains an exciting blend of retinol, peptides, vitamin-based antioxidants, and some good skin-repairing ingredients.

✓☺ BEST **$$$ FirmaTone Rx Eye Puff and Circle Minimizer** *($36 for 0.2 fl. oz.)*. This lightweight serum for the eye area (though there's no reason this couldn't be used all over the face) is essentially a souped-up, better version of Clinique's All About Eyes Serum De-Puffing Eye Massage. It even has the same cylindrical packaging with a metal roller-ball applicator that dispenses the product around the eye area. Denese's version is chock-full of antioxidants, skin-identical hyaluronic acid, and anti-inflammatory caffeine. When applied topically, caffeine serves as an anti-inflammatory and has a constrictive effect on skin, which may lead to reduced puffiness, assuming it arises from edema (swelling) and not aging (Sources: *Planta Medica*, October 2008, pages 1548–1559; and naturaldatabase.com). The main differences between this and the Clinique All About Eyes Serum is that Denese's version contains a much greater amount of the mineral pigment mica. The mica adds shine to the skin, which can have a cosmetic brightening effect, but shine isn't skin care. In addition, Denese omits the fragrant citrus extract that Clinique uses in an amount that's potentially irritating. Yes, you're paying more for Denese's product and you don't get as much product as Clinique provides (0.2 ounce versus 0.5 ounce), but Denese has the better formula. Despite the claim of improving dark circles, this doesn't contain ingredients that can do that. However, the barrier repair and antioxidant ingredients will certainly improve the condition of skin anywhere on the face, so in the case of dark circles, you may notice some improvement simply because the skin is in better shape. This product cannot address puffiness related to aging, where the fat pad beneath the eye has shifted and skin develops a pooch. This type of puffiness can only be corrected with cosmetic surgery. Interestingly, one of the plant extracts in this product can cause vasodilation, which means it increases circulation. That can be good, but not when dark circles are the concern, at least not if the dark circles are from excess blood vessels underneath skin. Another plant extract in this product has a relaxing action on blood vessels, so most likely the two cancel each other out (Source: naturaldatabase.com). Other exotic-sounding plant extracts in this product have no research relating them to skin care, though some such as *Bletilla striata* (a species of orchid) are a source of fragrance. One more note: This product does not contain retinol as claimed. However, that doesn't change its status as a very good gel-type serum for all skin types.

✓☺ BEST $$$ **FirmaTone Rx RetinolMax Firming Serum** *($79.92 for 1 fl. oz.)*. Is a higher concentration of retinol better? That's the assertion this fragrance-free, silicone-based serum makes, along with boldly stating that "nothing on the market is more effective for firming the appearance of skin." That's an interesting claim, especially when you consider that Dr. Denese sells numerous other serums and other products with retinol, and all of them claim to be the bee's knees, too. Does the good doctor not believe her own claims, or is she just hoping you'll pay attention to one of these products and overlook the similar claims made for all the rest? We won't go on record and state this retinol serum is the most potent around, because it isn't. Most likely, the amount of retinol is between 0.5–1%, which is plenty of potency for most people (though you can find products with even higher amounts of retinol, even though that's not necessarily better for your skin). For the record, high potency retinol products are generally considered to be those with a retinol content of 0.4-1.6%, so Denese is hardly the only brand offering such potency. Interestingly, low amounts of retinol (as low as 0.1%) have been shown to increase epidermal thickness and reduce signs of aging (Sources: *Skin Pharmacology and Physiology*, July 2009, pages 200–209; and *Archives of Dermatology*, May 2007, pages 606–612). Denese is absolutely right in claiming that the retinol in this serum may sting and cause peeling when you first begin using it. For some this may be a temporary problem; others will find these effects intensify with further use, and don't let up as long as you continue using the product. The reaction is completely dependent on an individual's response to retinol—this product is hardly the only one capable of causing such side effects. That said, this is yet another antiwrinkle serum with retinol to consider. It is recommended for normal to dry skin and is beautifully packaged to keep the retinol stable during use.

✓☺ BEST $$$ **HydroShield Eye Serum** *($58.50 for 1 fl. oz.)* contains silicone, antioxidants, ceramides, retinol, several fatty acids, and preservatives. This fragrance-free serum is an outstanding formulation that is recommended for all skin types. It may be used around the eyes or anywhere on the face. Its lightweight texture and matte finish make it well suited for those with oily skin looking for the benefits of antioxidants and retinol without heaviness. Despite our enthusiasm, in truth, you don't need a special serum for use around your eyes (see the Appendix to find out why).

✓☺ BEST $$$ **HydroShield Ultra Moisturizing Face Serum** *($65 for 1 fl. oz.)* contains a brilliant assortment of ingredients, including skin-silkening silicone, ceramides, cell-communicating ingredients, and vitamins, and all without added fragrance or irritants. Interestingly, the company offers this serum in three different packages. The 1-ounce version is in a frosted glass bottle with a dropper applicator. If you opt for this version, the bottle must be stored in a cool, dark place to protect the antioxidants from degrading with ongoing light exposure. The 0.5-ounce version is sold in an opaque pump bottle and is exclusive to QVC, where the Denese brand is primarily sold. In addition, for $181, this serum comes in a 4-ounce opaque bottle with a pump. Prices notwithstanding, for convenience, ease of use, and preserving the activity of the anti-aging ingredients, the 0.5- and 4-ounce sizes have the better packaging.

✓☺ BEST $$$ **SPF 30 Defense Day Cream** *($49 for 2 fl. oz.)* features an in-part zinc oxide sunscreen and is slightly tinted to offset the white cast this ingredient can leave on skin. The product is described as being able to "intensely hydrate" the skin, but the inactive ingredients don't support this claim because they are primarily dry-finish silicones, aloe, and talc. The jar packaging won't keep the antioxidants in the formula stable during use, so avoid that option (available in a 2-ounce size). Instead, go for the larger 4-ounce size packaged in an opaque tube or, if your budget is limited, they also offer a 1.5-ounce tube for $34. This fragrance-free sunscreen is best for normal to slightly oily skin not prone to blemishes. It feels wonderful and is tenacious, so be sure you remove it with a washcloth and/or silicone-based makeup remover.

☺ GOOD $$$ **FirmaTone RetinolMax Neurotrophic Night Cream** (*$199 for 1.7 fl. oz.*). This emollient moisturizer for dry skin is exceedingly expensive, and although you don't need to spend anywhere near this much for a good moisturizer, at least this formula contains several intriguing ingredients. Antioxidant vitamins (including a good amount of retinol) are paired with cell-communicating peptides and skin-repairing ingredients to help your skin look and act younger while stimulating collagen production. All of that is great, but again, these benefits are available from many other moisturizers that cost significantly less. You may be wondering what "neurotrophic" in this product's name means. The term refers to how nerves in the body influence tissue (think skin) nutrition. It sounds medicinal and scientific until you realize that, in one way or another, most beneficial ingredients in skin-care products have some sort of effect on nerves in your skin. It stands to reason because nerves influence many processes skin uses to defend itself from problems. For example, if you touch a hot stove with your bare hand, nerves in your skin receive a message from your brain to remove your hand from the heat source. Even the act of massaging a moisturizer over skin involves nerves, because they're what provide the sensation you associate with applying skin-care products. In the end, the term doesn't really convey anything special about this product. This moisturizer also contains the ingredient telomerase. That's a first, as this ingredient isn't listed in any of the cosmetic ingredient databases we consult when we review products. Telomerase is an enzyme made of proteins and bits of RNA that influence chromosomes in the body. It plays a powerful role in the body because it regulates the lifespan of cells. In babies, telomerase is quite active as it influences development; however, in adults, telomerase mostly lies dormant because, left unchecked, it can lead to uncontrolled cell division, which is the blueprint for cancer. Telomerase is tied to anti-aging studies because we know that as telomerase diminishes or becomes inactive, cells stop replicating and eventually lose the ability to divide and multiply. This leads to a cascading series of events that ultimately end in death (without viable cells, our bodily systems cannot function to keep us alive). The simplified explanation above doesn't explain whether or not telomerase in skin-care products is helpful for skin in any way (or whether or not that would be a good or bad thing), but given that this enzyme could potentially influence cellular division and lifespan, it isn't something you want to find in your moisturizer if it does work. Do you really want to apply an untested ingredient that may negatively influence cell division and longevity? Interestingly, the active component in green tea (known as EGCG) has been shown to interrupt the influence of telomerase on tumor cells, thus reducing the growth of cancer and having amazing benefits, both when applied topically and taken orally (Sources: *Biochemical Pharmacology*, December 2011, pages 1807–1821; and treatment-skincare.com/ Telomerase/Structure.html). The good news is that no research has shown topical application of telomerase has a negative impact on skin. However, there isn't any research proving it's helpful, either. Knowing this, the question of whether or not to use a product with telomerase comes down to erring on the side of caution.

☺ GOOD **$$$ Wrinkle Rx 76% Peptide Solution Concentrate** *($147.36 for 1 fl. oz.)*. Let's assume for a moment that a 76% concentration of peptides is what's needed to help with deep wrinkles and other signs of aging; well, you wouldn't be getting anywhere near that concentration from this water-based serum. This does contain more peptides than you normally see in serums and moisturizers, but absolutely not 76%, not even 2%. Besides, there's no research proving that any amount or any combination of peptides can make deep wrinkles, or any wrinkles, a thing of the past. Despite the ludicrous price and the overly hyped claims, this serum is on balance well-formulated. It contains an impressive mix of the types of ingredients you should be using to help remedy signs of aging and allow your skin to repair itself. You just don't need to pay this much for the results, and the peptides are better for marketing claims than for your skin. What's better for your skin is that Dr. Denese packaged this so the ingredients remain stable and do retain their potency. This serum would earn a Best Product rating if it did not contain fragrant bitter orange peel oil. The amount is small, but it still carries a potential risk for irritation without a benefit, which is never the goal, especially not at this price.

☺ GOOD **$$$ Wrinkle Rest Expression Line Peptide Concentrate** *($75 for 1.7 fl. oz.)* is a silicone- and glycerin-based serum that primarily claims to moisturize skin by infusing the top layers with lipids (fats). However, it doesn't contain any lipids, and the peptides aren't as concentrated as they are in other Denese products. This contains an ingredient listed as pinacolyl-trans retinoate, which the company making it says is a retinol derivative. The only information about this ingredient (trade name RETexture Granactive RD-101) comes from the manufacturer, which is about as reliable as McDonald's saying hamburgers are nutritional powerhouses. It likely has antioxidant ability similar to other forms of vitamin A, but there's no proof it is as efficacious as tretinoin (Retin-A) without the irritation. This serum won't put wrinkles to rest, but is a good option for normal to slightly dry skin.

☺ GOOD **$$$ Wrinkle Rx Deep Wrinkle Environmental Shield Serum** *($49.50 for 1.7 fl. oz.)* contains enough titanium dioxide to give skin a brightening effect (described as a "youthful, healthy glow") when applied, while the mineral pigments bismuth oxychloride and mica provide shine. Shine isn't skin care, regardless of your age, although this minimally hydrating serum does contain some good anti-aging ingredients, including retinol and several well-researched antioxidants. It contains fragrance in the form of ethylene brassylate and fragrant floral extracts. This is a good serum with retinol for normal to oily skin, although someone with oily skin may not appreciate the shine this leaves.

☺ GOOD **$$$ Wrinkle Rx Extreme Pro-Peptide Gel** *($64.56 for 1.7 fl. oz.)*. Dr. Denese is very excited about this gel-textured serum, claiming it is "the one" for tackling expression lines, be they around the eyes, between the brows, or on the forehead. The expression lines are supposedly eliminated thanks to the peptides and vitamin C this serum contains, but this isn't Botox in a bottle. There is no substantiated research proving that any of the peptides in this product can relax expression lines, and the same goes for the apple stem cell technology Denese brags about (but that's a good thing, because if this stem cell worked as claimed, it could cause more problems than benefits). Despite the claims being more fantasy than reality, this is actually an exceedingly well-formulated serum that can, to some extent, help mitigate signs of aging and stimulate collagen production. The amount of vitamin C is impressive, as is the retinol. The serum is loaded with peptides, which have theoretical cell-communicating ability, and antioxidants are plentiful. Its only drawback (and what keeps it from earning a Best Product rating) is the inclusion of biter orange oil. There isn't much of it in the product, but its presence is still discouraging. Still, this is recommended if you have normal to oily skin and aren't expecting deep wrinkles to vanish. It will likely prove to be too active for those with sensitive skin.

☺ GOOD $$$ **Wrinkle Rx Extreme Retinol Eye Gel** *($45 for 0.5 fl. oz.)* is a very good silicone-based serum that treats skin anywhere on the face to a blend of vitamin C (in the form of ascorbic acid, which may be too irritating for use around the eyes), retinol, peptides, and a form of retinol known as hydroxypinalactone retinoate. The "Stem-bio technology" ingredient referred to in the claims is Domestica Fruit Cell Culture. It's touted by the manufacturer, and by the cosmetics companies that have thrown it into their formulas, as being able to restore skin. The Domestica Fruit Cell Culture is claimed to be from a rare Swiss apple tree (of course it has to be rare; the marketing story wouldn't be nearly as interesting if the apple tree were in Detroit or Chicago) and is based on plant callus cells. Plant callus cells are formed when a plant is wounded. The cells surrounding the wound turn back into stem cells, meaning they change and become cells that can produce wound-healing plant tissue. After the wound has healed, these callus cells remain stem cells (they are totipotent) and can continue to make whatever type of cells the plant needs. The Swiss apple tree in question also has substances that give the tree longevity. That's really good news for the plant, but whether or not it is good news for your skin is simply a guessing game, supported only by the in vitro research performed by the ingredient manufacturer, who claims that it shows some protective benefit. If this ingredient really did have some protective potential for skin cells, then it would be just like the protective benefit you get from hundreds of other ingredients, from sunscreens to antioxidants and cell-communicating ingredients such as retinol or niacinamide. This is neither a miracle nor the new must-have ingredient for skin. There simply isn't any published, peer-reviewed research showing benefit or even demonstrating that there are no risks. Besides, if this ingredient is such an anti-aging miracle, why doesn't Dr. Denese include it in all her moisturizers and serums? The unknowns about daily use of plant stem cells on skin keep this fragrance-free serum from earning a Best rating.

☹ AVERAGE **Baggage Lost Puff Reducing Eye Gel** *($23 for 1 fl. oz.)* is a lightweight moisturizer that doesn't contain anything that can noticeably reduce puffiness or dark circles under the eye. Classic "deflating" ingredients such as cucumber show up, but no topical ingredient or blend can address the cause of age-related puffy eyes. The second ingredient, sweet almond seed extract, has soothing properties—nice, but not a cure-all for under-eye woes. See the Appendix to find out why, in truth, you don't need a special product for the eye area.

☹ AVERAGE **Wrinkle Rx Moisture Surge Day Cream** *($34.90 for 1.7 fl. oz.)* isn't suitable for daytime use on its own because it does not provide sun protection. Forget the concept of using a separate "day cream" along with a sunscreen. Unless your skin is exceptionally dry, you don't need both, because many daytime moisturizers with sunscreen provide enough hydration to eliminate the need for a separate "daytime" moisturizer. Although this moisturizer for dry skin contains some great ingredients to ease dryness and provide anti-aging benefits, many of the most exciting ingredients (including the retinol) won't remain stable because this product is packaged in a jar (see the Appendix for details), and the research is clear on what jar packaging does to delicate, light- and air-sensitive ingredients. Because the key ingredients will begin losing their effectiveness shortly after this product is opened, it isn't a moisturizer worth purchasing.

☹ AVERAGE $$$ **Firming Facial Age Corrector Cream** *($43.50 for 1.7 fl. oz.)*. This lushly textured moisturizer for normal to dry skin contains several beneficial ingredients for skin. Unfortunately, those ingredients (which include retinol) won't remain potent for long due to the jar packaging. See the Appendix to learn why jar packaging is a problem for products like this. Also, the amount of glycolic acid in this moisturizer is too low for it to exfoliate skin, plus the product's pH isn't within the correct range for that to occur.

☺ AVERAGE $$$ **HydroShield Eye Fix Duo** *($30 for 1 fl. oz.).* The Denese line sells several products for the eye area, but if any of them worked as claimed, you'd only need one, right? This unnecessary option includes two products: one for the upper-eye area and one for the skin beneath the eye. **Upper Eye Lid Care** is a creamy moisturizer that contains some very good antioxidants and cell-communicating ingredients, but the jar packaging will reduce their potency after opening. The **Under Eye Care** is a silicone-based serum that has a mild, spackle-like effect on superficial lines. It contains some good antioxidants and mineral pigments that provide a cosmetic brightening effect. Unfortunately, this product is also packaged in a jar, so the antioxidants won't do much for your skin. This isn't a great solution or fast fix for "the total eye area," or any area of the face for that matter. See the Appendix to learn why, in truth, you don't need an eye cream.

☺ AVERAGE $$$ **HydroShield Hydrating Dream Cream** *($43.50 for 3.4 fl. oz.)* may seem like a dream cream because of the silky-smooth texture that makes skin feel amazing, but it's a crying shame that most of the state-of-the-art ingredients in this moisturizer for dry skin will see their efficacy suffer due to the jar packaging. Dr. Denese supposedly is a research-oriented physician and it's her research that led to the creation of these products. That doesn't explain why she routinely overlooks the importance of packaging as it relates to formulas containing light- and air-sensitive ingredients (exposure to air deteriorates all plant extracts, vitamins, antioxidants, peptides, and on and on). It's also disappointing that this product contains fragrance and coloring agents, because a physician should know both are common sources of skin allergies (with fragrance being the bigger offender) and have no value as skin-care ingredients.

☺ AVERAGE $$$ **RestorEyes Eye Cream** *($45 for 0.5 fl. oz.)* is an even better formulation than the HydroShield Eye Serum above, so why the average rating? Jar packaging. Thanks to that poor choice, the many antioxidants in this product (plus its retinol) will be useless shortly after the product is opened. In truth, though, you don't need an eye cream—whether it comes in a jar or not (see the Appendix to find out why).

☺ AVERAGE $$$ **Triple Strength Eye Wrinkle Smoother** *($49.50 for 0.5 fl. oz.)* contains a very high amount of an acrylate-based film-forming agent. It can make skin around the eyes appear smoother and feel "tighter," but there is concern that this amount of acrylate can be irritating for your skin, especially when used around the eyes (Source: ctfa.org). By the way, absolutely nothing in this product is "triple strength" or unique for skin around the eyes. In fact, see the Appendix to find out why you don't need a special product for the eye area.

☺ AVERAGE $$$ **Triple Strength Wrinkle Smoother** *($54 for 2 fl. oz.)* won't help reduce lines resulting from facial expressions, but it does contain a powerhouse of helpful ingredients and the formula is suitable for normal to dry skin. The level of acrylate film-forming agent in this moisturizer does lend a slight tightening and "firming" effect to skin, but this tactile benefit is temporary and incapable of keeping expression lines at bay. The problem is that despite several intriguing ingredients, the amount of acrylates can be irritating, especially if applied near the eyes.

☺ AVERAGE $$$ **Vitamin C Line Filling Radiance Cream** *($38 for 1 fl. oz.).* Curse the jar packaging that is this product's downfall! In better packaging (such as an airless jar or an opaque tube with a pump dispenser), this would be an affordable way to treat normal to dry skin to an antioxidant-rich moisturizer with a beautifully silky texture. The silkiness doesn't depend on the packaging, so you'll still get a beautifully smooth texture and finish, but nearly

The Reviews D

all the beneficial ingredients in this product (including retinol) will deteriorate with the repeated exposure to light and air. By the way, vitamin C plays only a minor role in this formula; Vitamin E is present in a much greater amount, so the name isn't logical.

☹ POOR **Cellular Firming Serum** *($64 for 1 fl. oz.)* is one of several serums in the Dr. Denese line, and it is one you should avoid. Although this contains some intriguing ingredients to help lighten discolorations, the second ingredient is a form of alcohol that will cause dryness, irritation, and free-radical damage. The formula also contains menthol, which only serves to cause further irritation. Dr. Denese should know better! Lastly, the AHAs and BHA in this serum cannot exfoliate your skin because this serum's pH is too high.

☹ POOR **CellRenew Rx Cell Recharging Gold Serum** *($99 for 1 fl. oz.)*. This very expensive serum from Dr. Denese likely owes its price to the inclusion of gold. Although gold sounds luxurious, as it turns out gold in any amount is not a precious ingredient for your skin. In fact, it is a relatively common allergen that can induce dermatitis on the face and eyelids (Sources: *Inflammation and Allergy Drug Targets*, September 2008, pages 145–162; *Dermatologic Therapy*, volume 17, 2004, pages 321–327; and *Cutis*, May 2000, pages 323–326). Gold compounds are associated with many side effects. For example, gold compounds used to treat arthritis have been shown to cause birth defects and to pass into breast milk; can interact with other drugs; and can cause sun sensitivity, dizziness, nausea, vomiting, fainting, and increased sweating. There is zero research proving topical application of gold has any antiwrinkle or rejuvenating effect on skin, but clearly it causes problems. (Please see the Appendix for details on why irritants like gold are a problem for all skin types.) Because of this, we cannot recommend this serum, despite the fact that it contains an impressive range of beneficial ingredients.

☹ POOR **High Potency Dark Circle Rx Eye Formula** *($29.80 for 0.5 fl. oz.)*. This fragrance-free eye-area product contains some interesting ingredients, including moisturizing plant oils and a small amount of arbutin, a skin-lightening ingredient whose effect on dark circles is unknown. If your dark circles are caused by excess melanin (skin pigment) production, which can be either genetic or a consequence of sun damage, then skin-lightening ingredients such as arbutin may help. But if the underlying cause of your dark circles is a combination of thin skin, heredity, and how blood pools beneath your eye, then skin-care ingredients are of little use. The truth is dark circles are very frustrating to treat. Where this product goes astray is the inclusion of a high amount of film-forming agents (think hairspray), which can cause undue irritation despite giving the sensation, as they dry, of eye-area skin feeling tighter. Ultimately, the irritation potential from the amount of film-forming agents, coupled with the fact that this product offers little hope for dark circles, makes it tough to recommend. Please see the Appendix for details on the problems irritation causes for all skin types.

☹ POOR **Wrinkle Rx Instant Wrinkle Press** *($20 for 0.5 fl. oz.)*. The name for this serum makes it seem as though you can apply it and, voila, your wrinkles and deep creases will be ironed out, like pressing a pair of slacks. Regrettably, the second ingredient in this product is sodium silicate. It is a highly alkaline and potentially irritating antiseptic and mineral used in cosmetics (Source: *American Journal of Contact Dermatitis*, September 2002, pages 133–139). Given the lack of redeeming ingredients in this product (retinol is included, but Dr. Denese uses retinol in almost all her serums, so there's no need to settle for this one), it isn't worth considering.

DR. DENESE NEW YORK SELF-TANNER

✓☺ BEST $$$ **Glow Younger Clear Self-Tanner for Face and Body** *($21 for 6 fl. oz.)*. This fragrance-free self-tanner is a wonderful option for all skin types. It feels light and silky, absorbs quickly, and supplies skin with small amounts of several cell-communicating ingredi-ents, which is more than what most self-tanners provide. Ignore the wrinkle-reducing claims, but consider this an above-average self-tanner.

DR. DENESE NEW YORK SPECIALTY SKIN-CARE PRODUCTS

☺ AVERAGE **$$$ Pro C Illuminating Cell Defense Pads** *($49.50 for 100 pads).* Although these pads contain an impressive amount of vitamin C along with lots of other beneficial anti-aging ingredients, none of that will matter due to the jar packaging which exposes these sensitive ingredients to light and air (see the Appendix for details). Regardless of the antioxidant content, no skin-care products can guarantee complete protection from free-radical attack. Antioxidants can help a great deal, but lots of bodily systems (such as respiration) rely on a certain amount of free-radical damage in order to work. (You do want to keep breathing, right?)

☹ POOR **Wrinkle RX Deep Wrinkle Treatment with Retinol** *($25 for 1 fl. oz.)* is sold as a weekly mask to add firmness to skin. Although it contains some good anti-aging ingredients, such as retinol, the amounts are in short supply compared with the amount of problematic ingredients. Chief among them is sodium silicate, the second ingredient, a highly alkaline and potentially irritating antiseptic mineral that is not going to help you look younger (Source: *American Journal of Contact Dermatitis*, September 2002, pages 133–139). A product like this hurts the credibility of Denese's line, which mostly has helpful products for those concerned with aging skin.

DR. DENESE NEW YORK FOUNDATION

☺ GOOD **$$$ Age Corrector Firming & Retexturizing Foundation** *($31.50).* If the name isn't a giveaway, this liquid foundation is designed with anti-aging in mind. It is said to instantly firm skin while giving instant perfection. Admittedly, the formula is laced with several ingredients that typically show up in antiwrinkle products, but none of them have a miracle firming or tightening effect on skin. This foundation also contains stem cells from apples, but there is no proof that apple stem cells are the answer for wrinkles. The real reason to consider this foundation is for its silky texture and air-brushed matte finish. You'll get sheer to light coverage and a formula that does a good job of not slipping into lines, although it can crease a bit under the eyes if not blended well. Only three shades are available, and they're not the most neutral. Medium has a peach cast that's hard to soften, but it may work for some skin tones. Light is too dark for fair skin but OK for light skin. If one of the shades works for you, this foundation is best for normal to slightly dry or slightly oily skin.

DR. DENESE NEW YORK CONCEALERS

☺ GOOD **Body Perfect Concealer** *($28.50 for 2 fl. oz.).* This generously sized concealer in a tube is a nonaqueous, silicone-based formula that has a silky texture and smooth, even application. It's meant to conceal spider veins and discolorations on legs, hands, and chest, but you can apply it to the face as well. Overall, it's better at covering smaller discolorations than applying over a road map of spider veins. It doesn't conceal purplish varicose veins at all. This blends readily and provides very good coverage, but it isn't opaque like Dermablend, and it lasts. The silicone base provides a relatively budge-proof and water-resistant finish. We wish more than two shades were offered because what's available will work only for those with light to medium skin tones.

☺ GOOD **$$$ Damage Reversal Treatment Stick** *($28 for 0.16 fl. oz)* is the only concealer we know of that contains hydroquinone as an active ingredient, let alone with 2% hydroquinone. As such, it's worth considering as a skin-lightening and concealing product in one. The dual-sided component includes two shades of lipstick-style cream concealer. Both shades are neutral and work well on light skin tones used separately or blended together. The texture is thick and this doesn't have much slip, but it covers well and stays in place. It is fragrance-free.

DR. DENESE NEW YORK POWDER

☺ AVERAGE $$$ **HydroShield Hydrating Treatment Powder** *($23)*. This talc-based pressed powder isn't hydrating in the least! Talc is the first ingredient, but the second is an acrylic, the third is boron nitride, and then there are other absorbing ingredients. Calling this hydrating is akin to calling a tricycle a car. You'll find this has a smooth, dry texture that provides a sheer matte finish, although the finish doesn't feel hydrating at all. The colors veer toward being too warm, so each has an overtone of peachy gold that's tricky to soften. If you decide to try this, it's best for normal to oily skin. There is a tiny amount of cell-communicating ingredients and an antioxidant, but the container won't keep them stable.

DR. DENESE NEW YORK LIP COLOR

☺ AVERAGE $$$ **HydroShield Lip Intensive Balm** *($16)*. Although the price for this sheer lipstick (or, if you prefer, tinted lip balm) is high, at least you're getting two lipsticks. The question is whether you'll like the emollient, greasy texture. The two-pack provides the same color, a warm nude with a sheer peach tinge. You'll get a glossy finish that feels comfortable but is fleeting, and this absolutely creeps into lines around the mouth.

DR. DENESE NEW YORK FACE ILLUMINATOR

☺ GOOD **Sheer Glow Face Brightener with Pro-Peptide Factor** *($24.50 for 1.5 fl. oz.)*. The glow you get from this product isn't what most people would consider sheer. This lightweight lotion provides a moderate amount of peachy gold shimmer anywhere it's applied. It looks best when mixed with a moisturizer or liquid foundation because then the shine is downplayed and you get what the product name states, a sheer glow. For some reason, the sunscreen ingredient ethylhexyl methoxycinnamate is a major ingredient in this product. Although that's not a bad thing, you should use caution if applying this near your eyes, and certainly do not apply it to your eyelid area due to the risk of irritation if the sunscreen ingredient gets into your eyes.

DR. DENESE NEW YORK SPECIALTY MAKEUP PRODUCTS

☺ AVERAGE $$$ **Lash Faker Eyelash & Brow Enhancer** *($30 for 0.2 fl. oz.)* is merely a cosmetic without any capacity to change one hair on your face. The ingredients in this product will moisturize and condition eyelashes and brow hair, but that's about all you can expect and that won't change how they look in the least. Do not confuse this product with those that contain prostaglandin analogues, the class of ingredients included in some lash-enhancing products that actually do affect lash growth and their resulting length and color. If your expectation is simply to apply a blend of conditioning agents to make lashes and brows softer, this will work. If you want longer, thicker lashes without using mascara, then you'll need to use one of the lash-enhancing products that contain drug ingredients whose side effects include lash growth and darkening. An example of such a product is Latisse, available by prescription.

DR. HAUSCHKA

Strengths: None for skin care; the powder blush and regular lipstick are good, though not worth a special trip to the health food store.

Weaknesses: Every skin-care product contains at least one volatile fragrant component that can be irritating to skin as well as causing increased sensitivity when skin is exposed to sunlight; sunscreens; the moisturizers are mostly redundant and easily replaced by plain, nonfragrant oils; no products to successfully address even the most basic skin-care concerns.

For more information and reviews of the latest Dr. Hauschka products, visit CosmeticsCop.com.

DR. HAUSCHKA CLEANSER

☹ POOR **Cleansing Milk, for All Skin Conditions** *($36.95 for 4.9 fl. oz.)* lists alcohol as the second ingredient, which is hardly gentle. Also problematic is the inclusion of essential-oil fragrance. See the Appendix to learn why alcohol and fragrance are bad news for all skin types.

DR. HAUSCHKA TONERS

☹ POOR **Clarifying Toner, for Oily or Blemished Skin** *($34.95 for 3.4 fl. oz.)* contains too much alcohol to soothe irritated skin, although several of the plant extracts have documented research showing that they have soothing benefits when applied topically.

☹ POOR **Facial Toner, for Normal, Dry or Sensitive Skin** *($34.95 for 3.4 fl. oz.)* contains less alcohol than Dr. Hauschka's Clarifying Toner, for Oily or Blemished Skin above, but lacks any interesting ingredients, and the essential-oil fragrance prompts irritation, which is not what sensitive (or any) skin needs. See the Appendix to learn why irritation from fragrance is a serious problem for all skin types.

DR. HAUSCHKA SCRUB

☺ AVERAGE **$$$ Cleansing Cream, For All Skin Conditions** *($26.95 for 1.7 fl. oz.)* is a substandard facial scrub that contains almond meal as the abrasive agent. Although definitely natural, almond meal (or other ground nuts or shells) is not preferred to synthetic polyethylene beads for exfoliation. This is because the synthetic beads are rounded and smooth to minimize skin damage, while nuts and shells may have sharp, uneven edges that cause microscopic tears. This is an OK scrub for normal to slightly dry skin, but quite expensive when you consider a washcloth used with your cleanser can do a better job.

DR. HAUSCHKA MOISTURIZERS (DAYTIME & NIGHTTIME), EYE CREAMS, & SERUMS

☺ AVERAGE **$$$ Daily Revitalizing Eye Cream, for All Skin Conditions** *($51.95 for 0.42 fl. oz.)* is a good but needlessly expensive eye-area moisturizer, and the amount of alcohol may be problematic for this area. If the skin around your eyes is dry, using plain avocado oil would be a safer, less expensive option. Besides, in truth you don't need an eye cream (see the Appendix to find out why).

☹ POOR **Eye Contour Day Balm, for All Skin Conditions** *($51.95 for 0.34 fl. oz.)* is a castor oil–based balm that contains St. John's wort, which is contraindicated for topical use because it may cause a phototoxic reaction (Sources: *Photochemistry and Photobiology*, August 2006, ePublication; and *Photodermatology, Photoimmunology, and Photomedicine*, June 2000, pages 125–128). The essential-oil fragrance is also a problem because such volatile substances are best left off skin, especially around the eyes. See the Appendix for further details and to find out why you don't need an eye cream.

The Reviews D

☹ POOR **Eye Solace, for All Skin Conditions** *($32.95 for 1.7 fl. oz.)* lists eyebright extract as the second ingredient and also contains fennel extract, which can be a skin irritant (Source: *Allergy and Immunology*, April 2002, pages 135–140). Eyebright has a history of anecdotal use, but is considered possibly unsafe for topical or ophthalmic use, not to mention the lack of evidence that it is a curative for puffy eyes (Source: naturaldatabase.com).

☹ POOR **Moisturizing Day Cream, for Normal, Dry or Mature Skin** *($39.95 for 1 fl. oz.)* lacks sunscreen, so it's not suitable for daytime application, and it contains some problematic plant extracts, including St. John's wort, witch hazel, and irritating fragrant components from essential oils. See the Appendix to learn why high amounts of fragrance are a problem for all skin types.

☹ POOR **Normalizing Day Oil, for Oily, Blemished and Mature Skin** *($42.95 for 1 fl. oz.)* contains mostly goldenrod extract, plant oils, plant extracts, and fragrance. You can find plant oils like this in your kitchen cabinet (almond, wheat germ, and jojoba) and they are just fine for dry skin. What is strange is that this product is recommended for blemished skin to "balance oil production, heal blemishes, and reduce redness and sensitivity." We can't imagine anything less helpful for oily skin or blemishes than more oil, and not a single ingredient in this product is capable of reducing oil production or healing blemishes.

☹ POOR **Quince Day Cream, for Normal, Dry or Sensitive Skin** *($35.95 for 1 fl. oz.)* contains some good emollients but quince has no special benefit for skin, though the seeds contain enough cyanide to be potentially toxic (Source: *Herb Contraindications and Drug Interactions*, Eclectic Medical Publications, Second Edition, 1998). Further, the essential-oil fragrance irritates skin due to its volatile components (including eugenol, which should make anyone with sensitive skin nervous).

☹ POOR **Regenerating Day Cream** *($79.95 for 1.35 fl. oz.)* is an emollient, oily moisturizer that would've been an option for dry to very dry skin if it did not contain fragrant plants that have no established, proven benefit for skin. This also contains an unidentified essential-oil fragrance (so who knows what you're putting on your skin) as well as several fragrance ingredients that are known irritants. All these ingredients are listed before the key ingredients that Dr. Hauschka claims will support "natural cellular regeneration." Skin cannot regenerate when it is subjected to topical irritants that don't offer an overwhelming extra benefit. This is not a product that's worth the time or expense. If you have dry skin and want to go natural, consider using pure olive and/or almond oil (go ahead and buy organic) instead of this moisturizer, your skin and budget will be far better off if you do.

☹ POOR **Regenerating Serum** *($85 for 1 fl. oz.)* is one of the most unimpressive serums around. The second ingredient is alcohol, so expect irritation, inflammation, and free-radical damage (because that's what alcohol causes on contact with skin; see the Appendix for details). Quince seed has no special benefit for skin, and most of the other plant extracts are there for fragrance, not anti-aging efficacy (fragrance is not skin care). Actually, quince seed has constricting properties and as such can be an irritant (Source: naturaldatabase.com). This serum is absolutely not recommended.

☹ POOR **Rhythmic Conditioner, Sensitive, for Sensitive Skin** *($89.95 for 0.9 fl. oz.)* lists fragrance (essential oil) as the second ingredient, so not only do you not know what you're really putting on your skin, it's likely to be very irritating. One of the plant extracts (southernwood) has so little documentation of its alleged benefits that it is rarely used. See the Appendix to find out why daily use of highly fragranced products is bad for all skin types.

☹ POOR **Rhythmic Night Conditioner, for All Skin Conditions** (*$89.95 for 0.9 fl. oz.*) contains mostly water, rose oil, witch hazel, royal jelly, and silver. Silver can be a skin irritant with long-term use, as can rose oil and witch hazel. As for the royal jelly, claims for it have never been substantiated.

☹ POOR **Rose Day Cream, for Dry, Sensitive or Mature Skin** (*$42.95 for 1 fl. oz.*) contains St. John's wort, which may cause a phototoxic reaction when applied topically. Even without this risk, the essential-oil fragrance and its volatile components spell trouble for skin, especially if this is used as a daytime moisturizer (which it shouldn't be since it leaves your skin vulnerable to sun damage).

☹ POOR **Rose Day Cream Light** (*$42.95 for 1 fl. oz.*) is primarily water, sesame oil, and alcohol. The rose petal extract adds fragrance only, not anything nurturing or protecting for dry skin. Moreover, the fragrant components (in the form of essential oils) are irritating for skin and problematic in the presence of sunlight. See the Appendix for further details on the problems excess fragrance causes for all skin types.

☹ POOR **Toned Day Cream, for Normal, Dry or Sensitive Skin** (*$39.95 for 1 fl. oz.*) is similar to the Rose Day Cream, for Dry, Sensitive or Mature Skin above, and the same review applies.

DR. HAUSCHKA LIP CARE

☹ POOR **Lip Balm, for All Skin Conditions** (*$16.95 for 0.15 fl. oz.*) ranks below standard even though it has some good emollient ingredients for dry lips. There's no reason to consider this due to the sensitizing potential of St. John's wort and several volatile fragrant components that serve no purpose for lips. Equally bad is the **Lip Care Stick, for All Skin Conditions** ($13.95 for 0.16 fl. oz.).

DR. HAUSCHKA SPECIALTY SKIN-CARE PRODUCTS

☹ POOR **Cleansing Clay Mask, for All Skin Conditions** (*$49.95 for 3.1 fl. oz.*) is nothing more than clay with a plant extract, witch hazel, and cornstarch. The clay works as an absorbent and is beneficial for oily areas, but the plant extract (nasturtium) contains the volatile component benzyl mustard oil, which can cause contact dermatitis (Source: *The Complete German Commission E Monographs: Therapeutic Guide to Herbal Medicines*, American Botanical Council, 1998).

☹ POOR **Facial Steam Bath, for All Skin Conditions** (*$34.95 for 3.4 fl. oz.*) is an aqueous solution that contains daisy extract as the second ingredient. Also known as tansy, this extract can cause severe contact dermatitis, and that's not at all helpful for any skin type or condition (Source: naturaldatabase.com).

☹ POOR **Firming Mask, for All Skin Conditions** (*$52.95 for 1 fl. oz.*) won't firm skin at all and contains several fragrance ingredients that irritate skin and hurt its healing process. This contains nonfragrant plant oils, too, but when mixed with fragrant plants, their benefits are muted.

☹ POOR **Intensive Treatment 01** (*$89.95 for 1.3 fl. oz.*) is a terribly formulated product. It contains several known irritants, including witch hazel distillate (a way to sneak alcohol onto your skin), a potentially drying amount of mineral salts, and a lot of essential-oil fragrance (the essential oils the fragrance contains are kept secret, which goes against cosmetics regulations from every country in the world). None of this can help teens or adults regain a balanced complexion during "transitional periods" in their lives. Whether you believe the unfounded hype for this brand or not, the company can't provide one source of proof that the natural ingredients in this specialty product can work as claimed. It is also shocking that the formula isn't worth pennies per ounce. The teeny amount of silver in here can actually cause damage to skin; but the amount in here is only good for story telling, not helping skin. Hauschka products have a cult following of those who want to believe they are only using the purest and most natural ingredients possible that are best for their skin; that isn't the case with this line in any way, shape, or form.

☹ POOR **Intensive Treatment 02** *($89.95 for 1.3 fl. oz.)* this formula is little more than eau de cologne and alcohol; ignore the absurd claims and marketing. The sparse plant extracts aren't capable of what is asserted on the label. Those considering this "treatment" are supposed to believe that the few plants and minerals in this product are "rhythmitised dilutions." This made-up word is meant to allude to a magical concept of putting ingredients into some kind of rhythm to enhance their efficacy. There is no chemical, recipe, or cosmetic process known as rhythmitising, but we're sure Hauschka's marketing team had a good time coming up with the concept. The plants and minerals in this product won't reduce inflammation and promote clear skin and not at the age they've established for this product (25 years or older). They could have only arrived at that age by lottery. What's even hokier, however, is the process they claim to use so that the plants and minerals will behave on skin as claimed. This is just another poor formulation from Dr. Hauschka that has no anti-inflammatory effect whatsoever.

☹ POOR **Intensive Treatment 03** *($89.95 for 1.3 fl. oz.)*. Those considering this "treatment" are supposed to believe that the plants in this specialty product have been rhythmically combined and, therefore, are able to cleanse the skin, minimize acne, and relieve redness. None of it is true, especially not with the problematic ingredients in this specialty product. How fragrant rose flower water, irritating witch hazel, and an unidentified essential-oil fragrance are going to help anyone's skin is a good question as there is no research anywhere in the world proving otherwise—but suffice it to say this is not the way to obtain clear, soothed skin. This product is little more than eau de cologne and perfume. There are plenty of redness-reducing plants Dr. Hauschka could've chosen—it is possible to make a naturally soothing product—but the company seems intent on offering their customers products that smell far better than they could ever work to improve skin.

☹ POOR **Intensive Treatment 04** *($89.95 for 1.3 fl. oz)* is waste-of-time product and there just aren't any nice words we can use to describe it. How a cosmetics company can convince aestheticians and the public that an overly fragrant blend of sandalwood and essential oils (none of which are identified, so who knows what you're putting on your skin) is revitalizing therapy for aging skin is snake oil salesmanship at its slickest. This is not supportive, nurturing, or able to "work with skin's natural rhythms." Sandalwood distillate (sandalwood and alcohol) can cause contact dermatitis and has no proven benefit for skin of any age (Source: naturaldatabase. com). In fact, none of the ingredients in this treatment are the least bit helpful for anyone's skin. Using this "treatment" is akin to dousing your skin with perfume, nothing more.

☹ POOR **Intensive Treatment 05** *($89.95 for 1.3 fl. oz.)*. Nothing in this product is going to bring things into balance or make a noticeable improvement in the changes skin goes through during menopause. As for the black cohosh, there is no research showing it has any benefit when applied topically, though there is research showing that oral consumption can help relieve some menopausal symptoms (Source: herbmed.org).

☹ POOR **Moisturizing Mask, for Dry, Sensitive and Mature Skin** *($52.95 for 1 fl. oz.)* lists quince seed extract as the second ingredient, which means this is too irritating for all skin types. It contains some very good nonvolatile plant oils, but why not spare your skin the irritation (and skip the expense) and use plain sunflower or olive oil as a mask?

☹ POOR **Rejuvenating Mask, for All Skin Conditions** *($52.95 for 1 fl. oz.)* won't rejuvenate skin, but will irritate it due to the amount of alcohol and quince seed it contains, along with an essential-oil fragrance. See the Appendix to find out why irritation is a problem for all skin types.

☹ POOR **Soothing Mask** *($52.95 for 1 fl. oz.)* contains the ingredient witch hazel water (which is mostly alcohol) high up on the list, which doesn't start things out well. Emollients are sandwiched between other unhelpful ingredients such as alcohol and several fragrance ingredients that also are known to cause irritation. This mask will "transform red, irritated skin," but not in the way you may be hoping because it will only make matters worse!

DR. HAUSCHKA FOUNDATION

☹ POOR **Translucent Make-Up** *($36.95)* lists alcohol as the second ingredient and that is in no way nourishing for skin. Because of the alcohol and the fact the colors tend to turn pink or rose, this foundation is not recommended. See the Appendix to learn why alcohol is a problem for all skin types.

DR. HAUSCHKA CONCEALER

☹ POOR **Concealer** *($24.95)* is a liquid concealer dispensed through an angled sponge-tip applicator for spot camouflage, but apart from the packaging, problems abound. The formula is knock-your-socks-off fragrant, and the second listed ingredient is alcohol. That alone makes this a poor choice for all skin types, and absolutely not recommended for use around the eyes. The alcohol creates a thin texture that nets spotty coverage and a flat matte finish that isn't nearly as attractive as today's best concealers.

DR. HAUSCHKA POWDER

☺ AVERAGE **$$$ Translucent Face Powder, Loose** *($36.95)* is a talc-free sheer powder that has a soft, but overly dry, texture that can feel grainy. Tapioca starch is used in place of talc, and the texture difference is apparent. Only one shade is available, and it is fine for fair to light skin.

☹ POOR **Translucent Face Powder, Compact** *($36.95)* contains rose petals and silk powder, which nevertheless look thick, dry, and chalky on skin, especially in the single available shade. The texture is not finely milled, and the result is a pressed powder that makes skin look made-up and flat rather than polished and dimensional.

DR. HAUSCHKA BLUSHES & BRONZERS

☺ GOOD **$$$ Rouge Powder** *($29.95)* claims to contain nourishing ingredients to balance the skin, but is just a soft, sheer, matte-finish blush that comes in three warm-toned colors. This powder blush has a much better texture than Dr. Hauschka's Translucent Face Powder, Compact, but is still overpriced for what you get.

☺ AVERAGE **$$$ Bronzing Powder** *($36.95)* is a smooth-textured pressed bronzing powder whose main problem is that its sole shade doesn't resemble a bronze or tan tone in the least. Instead, it's predominantly peach with an undertone of pink. Not bad for blush, but inappropriate for use as an all-over bronzing powder, which is how this is being sold. This is also very fragrant and the ingredient list indicates several volatile fragrant irritants. If a natural bronzing powder is your goal, check out the superior options from Physician's Formula Organic Wear.

☀ Sunscreens must provide reliable UVA (anti-aging) protection. See the Appendix for details.

☹ POOR **Rouge Powder Duo** *($29.95)* is a fragrant pressed-powder blush with a smooth, but dry, texture. Application is sheer, but it builds well, and the finish is soft matte. As for the fragrance, it's natural, but that's not a green light; the fragrance includes chemicals known to be irritating to skin, including eugenol and linalool. Considering that drawback and the eyebrow-raising price, this isn't the powder blush to set your sights (or cheeks) on.

☹ POOR **Translucent Bronze Concentrate, for All Skin Conditions** *($39.95 for 1 fl. oz.)* contains alcohol along with the irritating fragrance ingredients linalool, limonene, eugenol, and citronellol. It is also overpriced and no match for other cosmetic bronzing gels or good self-tanning lotions.

DR. HAUSCHKA EYESHADOWS

☹ POOR **Eyeshadow Palette** *($44.95)* is a talc-based set of four powder eyeshadows that comes in a selection of neutral shades that are workable for most fair to medium skin tones. As for the formula, it's a shame Dr. Hauschka added fragrance ingredients known to be irritating. For this reason, despite some impressive attributes, Eyeshadow Palette is not recommended.

☹ POOR **Eyeshadow Solo** ($19.95) is a pressed-powder eyeshadow that contains several irritating fragrance ingredients, including eugenol. Eyeshadow does not need fragrance; there are numerous powder eyeshadows that not only cost less and perform better, but also omit the irritating fragrance.

DR. HAUSCHKA EYE & BROW LINERS

☺ AVERAGE $$$ **Eyeliner** *($17.95)* is a standard, needs-sharpening pencil, but one that goes on soft while not being too creamy. That means you have to layer to build eye-defining intensity, but the pencil has more longevity than many others. If you don't mind routine sharpening, it's worth a look, but watch out for the blue and green shades.

☺ AVERAGE $$$ **Eyeliner Duo** *($29.95)* is a standard dual-sided pencil that needs routine sharpening. One end offers a dark shade for defining the eyes; the other end is a white for highlighting. Both have a creamy texture that tends to smudge easily, and the white shade looks too harsh (using white to line the eyes is a theatrical technique that rarely looks good in daylight or for daily makeup).

☹ POOR **Liquid Eyeliner** *($21.95)* is ridiculously priced, and a huge setback. The long, thin brush is relatively easy to use, but the color tends to bleed and takes longer than it should to set. The result is an uneven line that tends to look sooty rather than sophisticated. This also smells strongly of rose, which isn't what you want to apply so close to the eye.

DR. HAUSCHKA LIP COLOR & LIPLINERS

☺ GOOD $$$ **Lipstick** *($23.95)* is rose-scented and has a smooth, creamy, texture and an attractive group of colors that range from nude pinks to rich burgundies. Although these go on nearly opaque, the colors have minimal stain.

☺ GOOD $$$ **Lipstick Novum** *($23.95)* is available in a small range of brown-toned shades. It's a creamy lipstick with a smooth, emollient texture and nearly opaque coverage with a soft gloss finish. It leaves a good stain after application, so it has enough staying power to make it through a few hours of wear. This is not, however, for those prone to lipstick bleeding into lines around the mouth.

☺ AVERAGE $$$ **Lipliner** *($17.95)* is routine fare. This needs-sharpening pencil has a soft, but not too creamy, texture and a soft, dry finish to help keep lipstick in place. There are six shades that coordinate decently with the company's lipstick colors.

☺ AVERAGE **$$$ Novum Lip Gloss** *($19.95)* is a very sheer lip gloss with a thin texture that feels surprisingly moist and leaves a soft gloss finish. Shorter-lived on lips than most glosses, this comes in only two shades, which is limiting. Still, it contains plenty of natural oils (including many found in other lip glosses) and it isn't as fragranced as many other makeup products this line offers.

DR. HAUSCHKA MASCARAS

☺ AVERAGE **Mascara** *($25.95)* imparts minimal length and absolutely no thickness. You may be wondering why you bothered…we know we were! In addition, the alcohol in this mascara will eventually make lashes feel dry and brittle.

☺ AVERAGE **$$$ Volume Mascara** *($29.95)* does a reasonably good job of (slowly) building moderate thickness. This excels at lengthening without clumping or smearing, leaving lashes defined and perfectly separated from root to tip. Despite these positives, the unconventional formula contains several synthetic fragrant components along with rose essential oil. These ingredients aren't ideal for use so close to the eyes, even though the amounts of each are relatively low. Given that there are far superior mascaras available from the drugstore for one-third the price, there isn't much reason to choose this.

DR. HAUSCHKA BRUSHES

☹ AVERAGE **$$$ Face Powder Brush** *($57.95)*. The shape and density of this brush is quite good, as is the overall craftsmanship. But for the money, the natural hair isn't as soft as it should be. Lines such as M.A.C., Bobbi Brown, and Trish McEvoy offer powder brushes in this price range that are wiser investments because they have the luxury feel and extra performance that this powder brush lacks, despite its strong points. The **Rouge Powder Brush** ($41.95) feels noticeably scratchy on skin, and its semi-flat shape tends to apply powder blush in a stripe rather than as a soft wash of color. Density is good, but overall this brush has too many drawbacks (including the price) to make it worth strong consideration.

E.L.F. COSMETICS

Strengths: Inexpensive; praiseworthy powder blush and eyeshadows; brow gel/clear mascara; oil-blotting papers are a steal; great brushes in the Studio line.

Weaknesses: Mostly average formulas in smaller packaging than what's typical; terrible concealers; limited options for foundation; average to not-worth-it-at-any-price brushes (in e.l.f.'s main line).

For more information and reviews of the latest e.l.f. products, visit CosmeticsCop.com.

E.L.F. COSMETICS CLEANSER

☺ GOOD **Makeup Remover Cleansing Cloths** *($3)* contain a silicone and emollient blend that works quite well to remove makeup, including waterproof formulas. The fragrance-free formula is a nice change of pace, too, not to mention the price! These cloths would earn Best Product rating if they didn't contain the Kathon CG blend of preservatives. Because these preservatives are irritating if left on skin, you'll need to rinse after using these cloths.

E.L.F. COSMETICS EYE-MAKEUP REMOVER

☺ GOOD **Eye Makeup Remover Pads** *($1 for 18 pads)* offer a very gentle, fragrance-free formula infused onto small round pads. They produce a slight lather and should be rinsed from the skin (or used before cleansing), but they work well to remove non-waterproof makeup.

E.L.F. COSMETICS SPECIALTY PRODUCTS

✓☺ BEST **Shine Eraser** *($1 for 50 sheets)* is the best value around for oil-blotting papers. These powder-free sheets work quickly to mop up excess shine before touching up with powder.

☺ GOOD **Radiance Enhancer** *($3)* is an affordable way to experiment with this style of highlighting. Available in three shades, the thin liquid dispenses from a brush applicator that you can sweep onto any part of your face that you would like to reflect light. Once blended, the slightly moist fluid sets to a matte finish, but you'll still see the luminous shimmer beneath. Of the three shades, Golden is the trickiest to use because of its strong orange and yellow undertones.

☺ GOOD **Wrinkle Refiner** *($3 for 0.16 fl. oz.)* is a click-pen wrinkle filler that is dispensed via a smooth, angled tip. The formula is nothing to write home about, but it's a decent blend of silicones whose spackle-like texture helps to temporarily fill in and smooth superficial (not deep) lines and wrinkles. The formula contains a small amount of antioxidants, including vitamins A and E, and none of the plant extracts are known irritants, which is good news. This would work well around the eyes, as it does not contain fragrance. Considering the low price, this is worthy of a test run.

E.L.F. COSMETICS FOUNDATIONS & PRIMERS

☺ GOOD **Tinted Moisturizer SPF 15** *($1)* provides broad-spectrum sun protection thanks to its in-part titanium dioxide sunscreen. It has a strong fragrance, and a sheer, slightly moist texture that gives minimal coverage. Its satin matte finish is best for those with normal to dry skin. Among the six sheer shades, only Spice (Tone 3) should be considered carefully. All told, despite getting less than half an ounce of product, this inexpensive tinted moisturizer is worth considering.

☺ GOOD **Mineral Foundation SPF 15** *($5)* is one of the least expensive, loose-powder mineral foundations available; it's mostly impressive for the money. In the plus column are its titanium dioxide and zinc oxide active ingredients. The formula is also fragrance-free so it's great for sensitive or rosacea-affected skin. It also feels and looks lighter than many competing mineral makeups yet provides medium coverage. In the minus column are its shiny finish imbued with sparkles, its component (because it plays up the messy element of loose powder foundation), and the fact that three of the five shades (Warm, Dark, and Deep) are terrible. The Fair shade is slightly pink but workable, while the Light shade fares best. This mineral makeup has its strong points, but its drawbacks significantly limit its appeal.

☹ AVERAGE **Mineral Face Primer** *($6)* is a good primer product, but other than having silicones for a silky texture, it's no frills. That's about on par with what one should expect for $6, but on balance there are lots of value primers (and serums, which double as primers so you don't need two products) that offer your skin a lot more. This fragrance-free primer is best for normal to oily skin.

☹ AVERAGE **Personal Blend Foundation SPF 15** *($8)* addresses the trickiness of precise shade-matching because e.l.f. developed this makeup with four chambers of loose powder foundation in different shades and undertones that can be mixed and blended to match your skin tone. While it does have a mineral-based sunscreen, the packaging and the product's texture are problematic. The sifter opening at the top of each chamber is too small to get product out easily. Add to that a slightly clumpy texture, and it's even more challenging to get enough powder out or to blend it easily with another shade. It also takes effort to get the color blended the same way each time. The clumping also makes even application difficult, but once blended (if you have the patience), the finish left behind is slightly luminous and feels somewhat creamy, while the coverage is light. The formula and finish work for all skin types.

☹ POOR **All Over Cover Stick** *($1)* is a very tiny stick foundation with an unattractively thick, greasy texture that blends decently but still looks heavy on skin (sort of like theatrical greasepaint). The waxlike thickening agents put acne-prone skin on the fast track for more blemishes, and two of the three shades are very peach.

☹ POOR **Tinted Moisturizer SPF 20** *($3)* might sound like a great find, but in this case it's too good to be true. This is inexpensive and has a very good in-part titanium dioxide-based SPF, but it falls down in other important areas. Its initially creamy texture quickly becomes dry, which makes even application and blending difficult. Its soft matte finish leaves a hint of glow, but ultimately it isn't hydrating enough for dry skin. The shade range is limited, but even if you find a great match, the colors tend to oxidize and turn slightly to noticeably orange shortly after application.

E.L.F. COSMETICS CONCEALERS

☺ AVERAGE **Mineral Concealer SPF 15** *($5)* has a loose-powder texture that is messy to apply as concealer (dusting it all over as a powder foundation is easier) and it suffers from shades that don't resemble real skin tones and look either too peach, ghostly, or ashen. Warm and Light fare best, but that certainly limits this product's appeal. If you decide to try this, it has a smooth, soft texture that provides moderate coverage and leaves a shiny finish. This is dry enough to emphasize lines around the eyes.

☹ POOR **Concealer Pencil & Brush** *($3)* is a dual-sided pencil with one end being a cream concealer and the other being a firm brush for blending. The pencil is medicated with 2% salicylic acid but the nonaqueous formula prevents a pH from being established, so this has no effect on acne. Even if it did, the waxes and oils in this formula are absolutely not what anyone struggling with acne should be applying to their breakouts. Not only does the concealer end look too thick and heavy on skin, but all the colors veer toward peach.

☹ POOR **Corrective Concealer** *($3)* isn't a product any professional makeup artist would have in his or her kit. You get two shades of peach concealer, one pastel pink color, and a mint green shade. Although these have a light cream texture, coverage is sparse and they remain creamy enough to crease and fade in short order. Don't bother!

☹ POOR **Tone Correcting Concealer** *($1)* has a silky, moist texture that never sets, so this liquid concealer is prone to fading and creasing. Combined with its spotty coverage and three fairly peach colors, this is a concealer to avoid.

☹ POOR **Under Eye Concealer & Highlighter** *($3)* is a dual-sided liquid concealer with a matte finish and a complementary liquid highlighter that has a fluid texture with a bit too much slip. Although the color pairings are workable and the concealer provides OK coverage, both formulas contain sensitizing preservatives not recommended for use in leave-on products. They definitely pose a risk of irritating delicate skin around the eyes.

E.L.F. COSMETICS POWDERS

☺ GOOD **Clarifying Pressed Powder** *($1)* claims to help treat and prevent breakouts, but it contains absolutely nothing that is capable of doing that. This is a very good, talc-based pressed powder with enough mineral oil and petrolatum to create a satin-smooth texture best for normal to dry skin. It applies sheer, all four colors are great, and it leaves a satin matte finish that doesn't look the least bit powdery. The Tone 3 and Tone 4 shades function as bronzing powders for light to medium skin tones.

The Reviews E

☺ GOOD **Translucent Matifying Powder** *($3)* is a talc-based pressed powder that's available in only one shade. It is supposed to go on translucent, but instead leaves a soft pink cast that works best on fair to light skin tones. The powder has a silky texture and fine, natural-looking finish on skin. It isn't the best for keeping skin matte, but is suitable for all skin types, provided you have a light skin tone, too.

E.L.F. COSMETICS BLUSHES & BRONZERS

✓☺ BEST **Studio Blush** *($3)* is a smash hit and includes a selection of beautiful shades with a subtle, radiant glow. The soft, suede-smooth, pressed-powder texture blends on flawlessly and adheres well to skin. The colors go on lightly, but are easily layered for more intensity without looking chalky or cakey. We'd put this up against any expensive department store blush!

✓☺ BEST **Studio Cream Blush** *($6)* has a spongy, mousse-like texture that blends beautifully on skin and sets to a soft powder finish. Unlike some cream blushes, this one doesn't settle into pores. Instead, the range of attractive, highly pigmented shades offers a nice pop of color, and a little goes a long way.

☺ GOOD **Bronzer** *($3)* is a mica- and talc-based, pressed bronzing powder that includes four squares of color (without dividers) in one compact. Swirled together with a brush, the colors come off as one uniform bronze shade. All three of the Bronzers are recommended, though this isn't rated Best due to its drier-than-usual texture. It finishes matte, which is unusual for bronzing powders.

☺ GOOD **Contouring Blush & Bronzing Powder** *($3)* is a pressed-powder blush and pressed bronzing powder in one compact. Both products leave a shiny finish and share the same talc-based formula. The colors look best when blended together, using the golden brown bronzer first and the peachy-pink blush next. The bronzing powder is suitable for contouring light to medium skin tones, but generally speaking, it isn't a great idea to contour with a shiny powder (you want contour to be subtle). The shiny finish affords a shimmer that lasts and sparkling particles that have a slight tendency to flake.

☺ GOOD **Mineral Blush** *($5)* is an inherently messy loose-powder blush, packaged in a standard jar with a non-closable sifter. However, this is still a very good option to consider. The colors are soft and beautiful, and include muted and bright shades, each with a soft glow finish. Application is smooth and even, while the overall texture is dry due to the minerals it contains.

☺ GOOD **Natural Radiance Blusher** *($1)* is a pressed-powder blush with a smooth, slightly thick texture. It applies evenly and imparts sheer color with a soft glow for a soft shine finish. The pigmentation of the shades is best for fair to medium skin tones.

☹ AVERAGE **All Over Color Stick** *($1)* is a tiny, twist-up color stick meant for use anywhere on the face. The sheer, shimmer infused colors are best for highlighting features, such as the brow bone or top of the cheekbone, and the fragrance-free formula is best for normal to dry skin. This product is not emollient enough to use on your lips (nor are the colors well suited for lips) and applying it to your eyelid area guarantees creasing due to the moist finish.

☹ AVERAGE **Healthy Glow Bronzing Powder** *($1)* is a talc-based, pressed bronzing powder that has an initially smooth texture; however, it can apply unevenly because it tends to grab onto your skin. Its dry finish (enhanced by clay) also makes it difficult to blend.

☹ POOR **Essential Blush** *($2)* has a dry, chalky texture that doesn't cling well to skin, which hinders its wearability. There are several attractive shades, but they impart color so sheer you really have to layer it to see much of a difference. Even then, you'll only notice a slight, subtle glow from this powder blush.

E.L.F. COSMETICS EYESHADOWS & PRIMERS

☺ GOOD **Brightening Eye Color** *($1)* presents a selection of eyeshadow quads packaged with sponge-tip applicators, which should be tossed out. These quads are an amazing value for the money, especially if you prefer sheer colors and don't mind shine (every quad has some amount of shine, but none are outright glittery). They have a reasonably smooth texture and apply evenly, and every set has at least one shade that can serve as powder eyeliner. The best sets include Matte Mauve (it's almost matte), Butternut, Drama, and Nouveau (the olive-green shade in this one goes on khaki and blends well with the other colors). You can find eyeshadows that last longer and have a texture that's more elegant, but you'll pay a lot more for the privilege.

☺ GOOD **Custom Eyes** *($1)* are powder eyeshadows sold singly giving you the option to customize a quad set of your own. The compact holds four colors, and it can also hold the Custom Lips and Custom Face shades, too. These eyeshadows have a different formula than the Brightening Eye Color above. They're powder-free and based on oil and waxes, which result in a smooth, creamy-feeling texture that applies like a powder, but unfortunately are also prone to creasing and fading, especially if your eyelids are oily. These are still worth testing because they blend well and go on sheer. The best shades (all with some amount of shine) are Pink Ice, Wisteria, Mocha, Ivory, Dusk, and Moondust.

☺ GOOD **Mineral Eyeshadow** *($3)* is a mica-based loose-powder eyeshadow with a mark-edly dry texture that applies surprisingly smooth. The shade range is extensive and presents some beautiful options whether you want to go with soft or bold colors. All of them have shine, and many have shiny particles that tend to flake. Others omit the shiny particles and leave a metallic sheen instead. The company claims this formula is hydrating, but it absolutely isn't. No powder can be hydrating because the ingredients composing a powder are absorbent by nature. This eyeshadow also will not "minimize the appearance of fine lines." Just the opposite is true: The shiny finish these have will emphasize lines. However, those without lines around the eyes and who have a preference for loose-powder eyeshadow may want to give this affordable option a go.

☹ AVERAGE **Essential Eyelid Primer** *($1)* has a lightweight, liquid texture that sets to a matte finish. We did a split face test and noticed that shadow held up slightly better throughout the day (in terms of being more resistant to creasing and smudging) on the eye that had the primer, though the results weren't all that dramatic. A good, matte-finish concealer plus pressed powder can provide the same (if not better) results, but if you still want to give this a go, at this price you don't have much to lose.

☹ AVERAGE **Eyeshadow** *($1–$5)* are typically packaged in palettes ranging from four to four dozen shades! Their eyeshadows have three basic finishes: frost, sparkle, and satin. Regrettably, they all have a dry texture that requires a lot of patience to apply if you don't want it to flake or look uneven. On balance, the satin shades perform best because they have the most color payoff and minimal flaking. The sparkly shades contain large flecks of shine that inevitably will end up all over your face. The shades run the absolute gamut, from soft nudes to bold brights, but for every good shade, there are two to avoid. Given the bargain price and the bevy of bright colors, this is a fun option for young girls, but it's probably not for women who want a classic or elegant finish.

☹ AVERAGE **Mineral Eyeshadow Primer** *($3)* goes on as a slick liquid that takes way too long to set. The result is sheer coverage and a translucent peach cast that feels tacky to the touch once it finally dries. The finish isn't the easiest to apply shadows over, and this isn't preferred to a good matte finish liquid concealer.

The Reviews E

☺ AVERAGE **Studio Matte Eyeshadow** *($3)*. This loose-powder eyeshadow is messy to apply because it drips everywhere (including onto the skin below the eyes), and the finely milled pigments grab skin unevenly. Despite claims that this is a "pigment-rich" eyeshadow, the colors go on sheer and require extra layering to build intensity. The shade selection is a mixed bag of classic and trendy colors, all of which have a nice matte finish, but they tend to dissipate as the day wears on. This loose eyeshadow really isn't worth the trouble; pressed eyeshadows are much easier to use.

☹ POOR **Essential Duo Eye Shadow Cream** *($1)* is touted as a "long-wear and crease-resistant" formula, but that simply isn't true. The super creamy texture glides across skin and blends beautifully, but on the flipside, it tends to travel into creases and lines almost instantly. Also, some of the shades go on too sheer and then dissipate as the day wears on. Most of the colors offered come in shade combinations that do not complement each other, which makes this duo eyeshadow even harder to work with; in addition, each has a shiny finish that will draw more attention to wrinkles.

☹ POOR **Eye Primer & Liner Sealer** *($3)* is a dual-sided product that includes an oil–based eye primer on one end and a water-based liquid on the other. The flesh-toned Eye Primer winds up like a lipstick and has a thick, creamy texture that covers poorly. Its oil base doesn't improve eyeshadow application or wearability, and it looks obvious on skin. The Liner Sealer takes too long to dry and ends up removing a portion of whatever you've used to line your eyes … and this is supposed to be helpful?

☹ POOR **Eyeshadow Duo** *($1)* is an inexpensive powder eyeshadow option that is, unfortunately, flaky and dry with negligible color payoff. All the color combinations contain excessive shimmer and shine, which makes the powder's tendency to flake all the more unacceptable.

☹ POOR **Eye Transformer** *($3)* is nothing more than a quad set of pastel-tinged shiny eyeshadows. Each has a dry texture that flakes during application and none of the shades are that attractive whether worn alone, mixed together, or applied to "transform" other shades of eyeshadow. No matter how you slice it, this isn't a transformation for the better!

☹ POOR **Studio Cream Eyeshadow** *($3)* is unimpressive on many levels. The shade range is limited and void of flattering, neutral colors. The shimmery finish of this creamy eyeshadow contains glitter, which is distracting, and the shininess will accentuate wrinkles. Shades go on with varying intensities depending on which one you select, but the majority are sheer and tend to dissipate as the day wears on. It isn't crease-proof, either.

☹ POOR **Studio Pigment Eyeshadow** *($3)* is a complete mess to work with. The colors go on very sheer, which is ironic given that "pigment" is part of the name. It's nearly impossible to prevent the loose-powder formula from chipping onto the skin below the eyes during application. The shade selection has a couple neutral options, but is based mainly around jewel tones with a metallic finish.

E.L.F. COSMETICS EYE & BROW LINERS

✓☺ BEST **Essential Waterproof Eyeliner Pen** *($1)*. True to claim, this liquid eyeliner is water-resistant and has impressive staying power. The flexible, felt-tip pen offers just enough control without being so fine that you have to apply several layers. It dispenses deeply saturated color in a smooth, even flow without dragging or skipping. It's important to give the wet formula ample time to set, otherwise it will smear if you touch it, but once dry, this eyeliner isn't going anywhere and will not flake off throughout the day.

✓☺ BEST **Studio Cream Eyeliner** *($3)*. This gel-cream eyeliner applies with super smooth ease and can be blended upon initial application for a smokey effect. The formula is smudge-proof and water-resistant once set, and it holds up well throughout the day. The shade range includes options in both classic and trendy colors, some of which have a metallic finish. Note: The included brush doesn't work well for applying this eyeliner.

☺ GOOD **Eyebrow Kit** *($3)* features a pressed brow powder and creamy brow tint in one compact. The brow powder is silky and works well to fill in and define brows with soft color. The creamy brow tint, which is incorrectly labeled as a gel, is oil–based and imparts soft color that goes on sheer. The sheerness is good because the brow tint's hue is considerably darker than the brow powder. Used together this is a smart way to enhance brows and help keep stray hairs in place. The limited shades are best for light to medium brown eyebrows.

☺ GOOD **Eyebrow Treat & Tame** *($3)* is a dual-sided product offering a tinted brow gel (labeled as "Tame") on one end and a clear, brush-on "Regrowth Treatment" on the other. The sheer brow gel works great and comes in three very good colors for dark blonde to medium brown brows. The brush-on clear gel doesn't contain anything capable of stimulating hair growth, so ignore that claim. It functions best as a brush-on setting gel for unruly brows, and it has a non-sticky finish.

☹ AVERAGE **Eye Widener** *($1)* is a creamy, standard, pencil with a sharpener built into the cap. You're instructed to stroke the pencil along the upper lash line and on the inside rim of the lower lash line to create the illusion of larger eyes. This is a theatrical makeup technique that tends to look obvious in person (and in daylight), not to mention the risk of putting a cosmetic product so close to the eye itself. This is an OK option as a soft white shimmer pencil for the upper lash line.

☹ AVERAGE **Liquid Eye Liner** *($1)* has one of the widest liquid eyeliner shade selections (9 in all!) at an affordable price. These inkwell-style liquid eyeliners are worth an audition if you have patience and a steady hand. Note that these are not for novice liquid eyeliner users; overdoing it causes the color to bleed and the formula has a longer-than-usual dry time, which makes for a tricky and potentially messy application. Setting aside application risk, these are vibrant and long-lasting, and they feature a sturdy applicator brush that rivals those in high-end packaging.

☹ POOR **Eyebrow Lifter & Filler** *($3)* is a dual-sided, slightly chunky pencil that includes a brow pencil one end and a creamy highlighter on the other. The pinky peach color and thick texture of the highlighter are wholly unattractive and the product tends to sit on top of skin, looking artificial. The brow pencil isn't terrible, but it has a soft, creamy texture that isn't pre-ferred to brow pencils that have a smooth, dry texture and powder finish.

☹ POOR **Mineral Eye Liner** *($3)* in an automatic, retractable eye pencil with a trace amount of minerals; however, minerals are absolutely not key to an eyeliner's performance. This pencil has an oil–based formula that's noticeably greasy. It glides on, but tends to smear and fade quickly.

E.L.F. COSMETICS LIP COLOR & LIPLINERS

✓☺ BEST **Mineral Lip Gloss** *($3)* is a standard lip gloss with a thin but moisturizing texture, smooth application, and soft gloss finish that doesn't feel the least bit sticky. The mineral oil–based formula includes a well-edited selection of versatile shades, including a colorless option (Crystal Clear). It is also fragrance- and flavor-free. Well done and wonder-fully affordable!

✓☺ BEST **Mineral Lipstick** *($5)* is a creamy lipstick that has an edge if you're looking for a formula that's all natural and doesn't contain fragrance. It has a smooth, slightly stiff texture that feels creamy and not the least bit slippery, so it tends to wear well and fade evenly. Color deposit is great and the shade range presents several enticing options.

✓☺ BEST **Studio Lip Lock Pencil** *($3)* is an automatic, retractable lipliner designed to help prevent lipstick from feathering, and it indeed does just that. The waxy texture applies smoothly without feeling greasy and helps stop lipstick from bleeding into lines around the mouth. The fact that it's colorless means you can wear it with any lipstick shade. The claims that this also can keep lip gloss in check are false, as gloss has too much movement and no pencil can keep it from slipping into lines around the mouth. Otherwise, this is a great product for anyone struggling with lipstick bleeding into lines around the mouth.

✓☺ BEST **Studio Lip Stain** *($3)* does a phenomenal job of imparting opaque color that lasts for hours and goes on evenly and smoothly. One end of the dual-sided applicator contains a fluid lip stain that sets to a matte finish; the other end has a clear gloss, allowing you to add a moisturizing, shiny finish. This lip stain is smudge-proof, easy to use, wears for hours, and comes in a variety of attractive shades. With all that and its great price, what's not to love?

☺ GOOD **Custom Lips** *($1)* are single pans of lip color that you add to a compact. You can add up to four shades, or you can mix and match with e.l.f.'s Custom Eyes and Custom Face shades. These have a thick texture with a slight slip and minimally emollient finish. Every color, even the deep reds and plums, applies very sheer. The only issue with a product like this is that it requires finger application unless you're willing to tote a lip brush.

☺ GOOD **Essential Lipstick** *($1)* has a satiny smooth texture that glides across lips and feels moisturizing. The deeply pigmented shades offer several attractive options, each of which has a slightly shiny finish. If you tend to have issues with lipstick feathering into fine lines around your mouth, this isn't the lipstick for you. Otherwise, this is a good, budget-friendly option.

☺ GOOD **Hypershine Lip Gloss** *($1)* applies smoothly and leaves a non-sticky, moderately glossy finish. The click-pen with brush applicator works well and, though this gloss offers only a small selection of shades, they go on nearly transparent, making these a safe bet to apply over any color of lipstick.

☺ GOOD **Lip Liner & Blending Brush** *($3)* is just what the name states, housed in a dual-ended pencil cartridge. The **Lip Liner** is a wind-up, retractable pencil with a creamy texture and easy application. The **Blending Brush** is flexible, nicely tapered, and works well should you wish to soften the result from the Lip Liner. Only one shade is offered, but it's one many women will find quite wearable.

☹ GOOD **Super Glossy Lip Shine SPF 15** *($1)* used to offer sufficient broad-spectrum sun protection, but the formula changed, and it now lacks adequate UVA protection. What disappointing news! If this bargain lip gloss still interests you, you'll find it's an oil–based lip gloss in sheer colors.

☺ AVERAGE **Essential Shimmer Lip Gloss** *($2)* is a basic, somewhat sticky lip gloss that is applied with a sponge-tip applicator. Interestingly, it was a bit of a chore to get enough of the product out of the tube and onto the applicator to evenly coat the lips (it took several dips of the wand). Once applied, the result is a subtle shimmer with just the right amount of sparkle and shine. This gloss has a fruity flavor.

☺ AVERAGE **Feather Proof Moisturizing Lip Liner** *($1)* has a formula that is way too greasy to prevent feathering, and needs routine sharpening. This is an OK lip pencil that comes in a mostly pink-tinged range of shades, but spending a bit more at the drugstore will open the door to several superior lip pencils.

☺ AVERAGE **Luscious Liquid Lipstick** *($1)* is a standard, slightly thick lip gloss housed in a click-pen applicator that includes a built-in synthetic brush. The mineral oil–based formula feels smooth and has a strong vanilla/mint fragrance, though it doesn't make lips tingle, which is good (tingling = irritation). The mostly sheer colors are fine.

☺ AVERAGE **Matte Lip Color** *($3)* is a twist-up, retractable, fragrance-free lipstick in "pencil" form. It doesn't need sharpening and the slightly wide but pointed tip makes application fairly easy. True to its name, this provides a matte finish. Shortly after application, it begins to feel dry and becomes more uncomfortable the longer it's worn (though it stays on quite well and doesn't have a strong tendency to bleed into lines around the mouth). Topping this with lip gloss is an option, but the trade-off is less longevity. The color selection is small but workable, comprised of nude and soft pink tones, though each shades applies opaque. If you're a fan of matte lipsticks this is worth considering (the price is hard to beat), but it isn't among the most elegant or comfortable options available.

☺ AVERAGE **Mineral Lip Liner** *($3)* is an oil–based, automatic, retractable pencil that applies smoothly, but is too creamy to last. It does an okay job of defining lips, but cannot stop lipstick or gloss from bleeding into lines around the mouth.

☺ AVERAGE **Pout Perfector** *($3)* is an ultra shiny glossy paste meant for the lips. It is sold as a product to make lips look fuller by placing the shine to the center of your bottom lip using the wand applicator. From a makeup point-of-view it is a standard technique, but this product fails to deliver really impressive results. The gloss' texture is thick (like frosting), so it's difficult to blend over lip color and virtually impossible to use on bare lips alone. A dollop of a pearlescent or shimmery shade of your favorite gloss or a white shiny eyeshadow would work even better to create this visual effect.

☹ POOR **Essential Lip Stain** *($2)* has a felt-tip marker–style applicator that comes to a fine point to allow precise control. The major issue is getting the actual liquid formula to come out of the applicator so you can apply it to your lips! It takes several applications to get the color to fully cover your lips, and even then it can look streaky if you're not careful.

☹ POOR **Lip Primer & Plumper** *($3)* is a dual-sided product; one side is an oil–based cream concealer for lips and the other side is a clear lip balm. The concealer portion (labeled **Primer**) is supposed to function as a lip base for your lipstick to keep color from smudging. It doesn't do that. Instead, it places a thick, opaque layer over lips that interferes with lipstick application and doesn't stay it in place. The lip balm doesn't list any plumping ingredients, but smells strongly of cinnamon, which will plump lips via strong irritation. This is one to leave on the shelf!

☹ POOR **Plumping Lip Glaze** *($1)* is a waxy-feeling, dual-sided lip gloss that contains a lot of menthol, which plumps lips by virtue of irritation but ends up being too irritating for frequent use (and touch-ups with this very sheer gloss would definitely be frequent). See the Appendix to learn why irritation is bad for your lips (and skin).

☹ POOR **Studio Lip Balm SPF 15** *($3)*. There are two major flaws in this lip balm with sunscreen. One: The tingling sensation and flavoring are an indication that this is an irritating formula, which is a problem for lips. Two: The formula's sunscreen lacks adequate UVA protection to keep lips protected from the sun's most aging rays. As is, we cannot recommend this product, despite its pleasantly smooth, lightweight texture and attractive colors.

E.L.F. COSMETICS MASCARAS

✓☺ BEST **Studio Lash Extending Mascara** *($3)* does an excellent job of defining lashes while adding length. The lightweight, flake-free, smudge-proof formula gives a natural but enhanced look and does a decent job of holding curl. The brush is designed with short bristles on one side and longer bristles on the other, so you can apply it according to your preference and easily coat those hard-to-reach lashes. If you are looking for thickness, this isn't the mascara to buy, but otherwise it is a brilliant option.

✓☺ BEST **Wet Gloss Lash & Brow Clear Mascara** *($1)* houses a clear gel formula in a dual-sided, dual-brush component. One end is for eyebrows (the brush is suitable for brow application) and the other for lashes (with an equally suitable brush). The gel applies smoothly, is non-sticky, and does a great job of grooming brows or providing slight lash enhancement while leaving a subtle glossy finish. All this for $1? Sold!

☺ GOOD **Regular & Waterproof Mascara Duo** *($1)* is an extremely affordable dual-sided mascara. One side is regular mascara, the other is waterproof. The regular mascara is surpassingly good, allowing quick and dramatic lengthening of lashes with minimal clumps and delivering a long-lasting finish. In contrast, the waterproof version (which has the same brush as the regular mascara) goes on thin, doesn't build much length, doesn't thicken, and is only mildly waterproof. Although not equally impressive, for the price, even half of this mascara is a beauty steal.

☺ GOOD **Studio Exact Lash Mascara** *($3).* The "exact" portion of this mascara's name stems from its ability to provide precise application, and that's exactly what you get. The short, stout, angled brush allows you to coat hard-to-reach lashes. Due to its small size, some may find this brush easier to use on the bottom lashes than traditional mascara brushes. While this offers softly defined, fringed lashes that hold curl, don't count on much added length or volume. We experienced a tiny amount of flaking, but no smudging. The tube this comes in is smaller than average, perhaps because e.l.f. knows many people will use this only on their bottom lashes or as an accent for the hard-to-reach lashes. Given the extremely low price point, this is still a bargain!

☺ GOOD **Studio Volume Plumping Mascara** *($3)* delivers volume and bold lashes. You'll also get some clumping along the way, but nothing that can't be smoothed out with an eyelash comb. Not everyone will appreciate the oversize brush, but if that's not an issue for you, this is a great thickening mascara. As an added bonus, the flake-free, smudge-free formula doesn't leave lashes feeling hard and crunchy.

☺ GOOD **Volumizing Mascara** *($2)* is a beauty bargain! As long as you can forgo the "volume" portion of the name, this mascara is excellent. It builds little thickness, but lengthens and defines lashes without clumping or smearing. In just a few swipes of the somewhat bushy brush you can have long, separated lashes with a slight curl—and they stay that way all day. We also like that this formula leaves lashes soft rather than brittle. That's a lot of great benefits for a rock-bottom price!

☹ AVERAGE **Essential Lengthening & Defining Mascara** *($1)* applies in such a light-weight manner that it takes several layers to build length, but surprisingly you still get clump-free, defined lashes, with minimal thickness. The smudge-proof formula holds up well throughout the day, although there is a bit of flaking. In a turn for the worse, it contains two preservatives (methylisothiazolinone and methylchloroisothiazolinone), which are not recommended for use

---

⊘ Think "hypoallergenic" means safe for sensitive skin? See the Appendix to find out the truth.

in leave-on products due to their irritation potential. All things considered, we don't recommend this mascara over other inexpensive options, although we acknowledge the price is tempting!

☺ AVERAGE **Lengthening & Volumizing Mascara** *($3)* is incapable of providing fuller, thicker lashes. It goes on evenly but very thin, so at best you'll get modest length without clumps or smearing. It wears well and is easy to remove, but contains two preservatives (methylisothiazolinone and methylchloroisothiazolinone) not recommended for use in leave-on products due to their irritation potential.

☺ AVERAGE **Mineral Infused Mascara** *($3)* has a lot going for it, despite the deceiving mineral name (the only minerals to speak of are the same mineral-based cosmetic pigments used in countless mascaras). The rubber-bristled brush deposits mascara evenly and cleanly, with barely a clump in sight. Lashes are quickly defined and beautifully lengthened for a flutter-worthy effect. Thickness is slight and not easily built, so this is best thought of as a lengthening formula. Unfortunately, it begins breaking down due to the amount of emollient caprylic/capric triglyceride, so this isn't the mascara to turn to if you're looking for long wear and no midday cleanups along the upper lashline.

☺ AVERAGE **Waterproof Lengthening & Volumizing Mascara** *($3)* builds modest length and hints at some thickness, but never progresses beyond average regardless of how many coats are applied. The formula is waterproof and removes easily with a water-soluble cleanser. It also wears well without flaking, and is an OK option if you're not one for much lash impact.

E.L.F. COSMETICS FACE & BODY ILLUMINATORS

✓☺ BEST **Mineral Glow** *($8)* is an excellent illuminating loose mineral powder. It has a soft, smooth texture that applies and adheres well without flaking. Like all loose powders, this can come off on clothing, so use caution if you're applying this from the neck down. Both shades are attractive and cast a subtle glow wherever they're applied.

☺ GOOD **Shimmering Facial Whip** *($1)* comes in a tiny tube and dispenses as a lotion that tends to drag a bit during application. It sets to a slightly moist finish that imparts gleaming shimmer that's too strong for daytime unless blended very well. Most of the sheer shades are best for the cheeks or for highlighting lips; Toasted and Citrus are good options for eyeshadow, but be sure to set this with a powder eyeshadow to avoid creasing.

☺ AVERAGE **Tone Correcting Powder** *($3)* is a mica-based, shiny pressed powder that includes four sheer, pastel shades in one compact. The shine is moderate, but the dry texture means results don't last long, not to mention the pastel finish is trickier to work with.

E.L.F. COSMETICS BRUSHES

✓☺ BEST **11 Piece Studio Brush Collection** *($30)* includes almost every brush e.l.f. Studio offers. All the brushes in this set are also sold separately for $3 each, so with the kit's 11 brushes you're essentially getting the carrying case plus one brush for free. The zippered case is made of a soft synthetic fabric and has room for every brush in this set. As for the brushes themselves, they are each made of synthetic Taklon hair and are surprisingly good considering their low cost. Each one is exquisitely soft and well made, with sleek handles that feel great. It's really hard to believe such quality brushes are so darn cheap! The best brushes in the set (and again, all the brushes are sold individually) are the **Complexion Brush**, **Small Smudge Brush**, **Concealer Brush** (though we prefer one with a more pointed tip), **Small Precision Brush** (great for lining the eyes when a smoky eye design is being done), and the **Small Angled Brush** (which works great for brows or eyelining). Fans of applying foundation with a brush should check out the **Angled Foundation Brush**. The **Contour Brush** isn't the best and the **Powder Brush** is cut straight across, which isn't the easiest way to dust on loose or pressed powder (this type of cut makes it easy to over-powder).

☺ GOOD **Blush Brush** *($3)* is a synthetic hair blush brush that is more than respectable for the money. It has a good shape and is extremely soft plus it picks up and holds color well. Ideally it should be denser and the hairs should be a bit longer to cover the full cheek area (someone with large cheeks or a full face will find this brush way too small). However, if the size and cut works for you, the price cannot be beat.

☺ GOOD **e.l.f. Brushes** *($1–8)* are sold individually. As you may have expected, the quality isn't top of the line. What's missing from many of them is soft, dense hair that allows precision application of color and expert blending. Still, some of these are surprisingly good for the money (they beat any pre-assembled brush set from major drugstore lines). The ones to consider are the **Eyelash and Brow Wand**, **Brow Comb and Brush**, **Defining Eye Brush** (best for shadow, not for applying powder eyeliner), and the synthetic **Eyeliner Brush**.

☺ GOOD **Eyelash Curler** *($3)*. Whether you need a mini eyelash curler to handle the corner lashes or a regular sized one to take on a full row of eyelashes, these metal curlers with a rubber strip work as well as any to make lashes look uplifted and fringed. These curlers aren't of the same craftsmanship as those from, say, Shu Uemura, but they cost a lot less.

☺ GOOD **Kabuki Brushes-Mineral** *($5–$8)*. e.l.f. Mineral offers a **Face Kabuki Brush** and a **Body Kabuki Brush**. Both are composed of synthetic Taklon fiber and feel wonderfully soft. They're not as dense as many other Kabuki brushes we've seen, but they're shaped well and do a good job of applying loose or pressed powder in even, sheer layers. We're skeptical of the antibacterial claims made for these brushes, so these should be washed every few months or so depending on frequency of use. At the very least, you need to remove the facial oils that can build up on brushes over time. The **Kabuki Brushes-Studio** *($6–$8)* are very similar and the same comments apply.

☹ AVERAGE **Professional 5-Piece Brush Collection** *($10)* includes basic brushes for powder, blush, and eyeshadow, but none of them are good enough to make this your primary brush set, even though the price is right.

☹ AVERAGE **Professional 9-Piece Master Set** *($15)* includes the **Total Face Brush**, **Blushing/Bronzing/Blending Brush**, **Foundation Brush**, **Defining Eye Brush**, **Blending Eye Brush**, **Smudge Eye Sponge**, **Eyelash/Brow Wand**, **Brow Comb/Brush**, and **Lip Defining Brush**, all packaged in a deluxe roll-up case. A couple of the tools are great, but the rest are average to poor, making this a sketchy set to consider.

E.L.F. COSMETICS SPECIALTY MAKEUP PRODUCTS

☺ GOOD **Natural Lash Kit/Dramatic Lash Kit** *($1)*. These kits are a good, inexpensive way to experiment with false eyelashes. Both kits present a full set and include a tiny tube of adhesive, which is convenient. The kits are aptly named based on the results they provide, although getting false eyelashes to look natural isn't an easy feat.

☹ AVERAGE **Mini Makeup Collection** *($15)* is right up your alley, if you love e.l.f.'s Studio makeup kit. You get nine shades of eyeshadow, one cream eyeshadow, a blush, bronzer, brow powder, mini eye pencil, mini applicators, and lots of lip gloss in one small, square plastic box. The cream eyeshadow is mostly useless because it deposits almost no color, but the powder eyeshadows, each quite shiny, are smooth with the medium to dark shades having a good color deposit. There are two green shades that are best avoided. The eye pencil and mini applicators are a joke, but the brow powder, powder blush, and bronzing powder are fine (though the blush and bronzer are shiny). Although not everything in this kit is brilliant, it remains a good value overall, assuming you have full-sized brushes already!

☹ POOR **SPF 45 Sunscreen UVA/UVB Protection** *($6)*. Despite the name, this product isn't a sunscreen lotion or cream; it's a loose powder that provides a high level of sun protection from an unusually prodigious amount of the mineral sunscreen actives titanium dioxide and zinc oxide. Although the mineral actives provide admirable broad-spectrum sun protection, they also lend this powder a heavy, chalky texture and dry finish that makes skin look dull rather than dimensional. The finish magnifies wrinkles (even so-called "fine lines") and any bit of dry skin you may have, even though it blends fairly well. Those with oily skin or oily areas will find this powder grabs and can be tricky to sheer out (even more so if you apply it with the enclosed puff rather than a powder brush). Only one shade is available, and it's a peachy-pink tint that helps offset the white cast the high amount of mineral actives have. Unfortunately, the tint isn't a great compromise, as it looks obvious on fair to light skin and just plain odd on medium to tan skin tones. Note that the color e.l.f. displays on their website looks much more neutral than what you get. The sun protection and price are great, but esthetically, this loose powder is impossible to recommend.

EAU THERMALE AVENE (SKIN CARE ONLY)

Strengths: Good cleansers; moisturizers with retinaldehyde, an effective derivative of vitamin A; every sunscreen provides reliable UVA protection; a good lip balm.

Weaknesses: Mostly overpriced for what you get; no products to manage skin discolorations; repetitive moisturizer formulas, none of which are impressive; products for sensitive skin that contain fragrance or other potentially irritating ingredients; the redness-reducing products simply trade one problem for another.

For more information and reviews of the latest Eau Thermale Avene products, visit CosmeticsCop.com.

EAU THERMALE AVENE CLEANSERS

☺ GOOD **Clean-AC Cleansing Cream** *($18 for 6.76 fl. oz.)* was created for those whose skin is irritated or dehydrated from acne treatments. Although acne treatments should never cause excess irritation or dehydration, sadly, many do, because their formulas contain drying, irritating ingredients. But, you can treat acne without causing undue stress to your skin, and when you do that you won't need a special cleanser to deal with the side effects from problematic anti-acne products; any gentle, water-soluble cleanser will do. That being said, this is a good cleanser for normal to dry skin, whether blemishes are an issue or not. It contains gentle cleansing agents in a slightly creamy, lotion-like base that comforts without leaving skin tight or dry.

☺ GOOD **Cleanance Soap-less Gel Cleanser** *($18 for 6.76 fl. oz.)* is a very good water-soluble cleanser suitable for all skin types, except sensitive. It does a reasonably good job of removing makeup, though you may need to use a washcloth with it to remove long-wearing formulas. This isn't recommended for sensitive skin because it contains fragrance. Although all skin types do better with fragrance-free products, those with sensitive skin should take extra care to avoid fragranced products.

☺ GOOD **$$$ Diacneal Soap-Free Gel Cleanser** *($24 for 6.76 fl. oz.)* is a gentle yet effective formula that's fine for normal to oily skin. There is no reason this version needs to cost as much as it does, though it is fragrance-free.

☺ GOOD **$$$ Gentle Milk Cleanser** *($18 for 6.76 fl. oz.)* is a simply formulated, yet gentle detergent-free cleansing lotion for dry to very dry skin. It removes makeup easily yet doesn't rinse well without the aid of a washcloth. It's disappointing that this contains fragrance because it is designed for sensitive skin.

☺ GOOD **$$$ Micellar Lotion Cleanser & Makeup Remover** *($19 for 6.76 fl. oz.)* contains fragrance (not the best for those with sensitive skin); however, this is a very good, mild eye-makeup remover and/or cleanser for normal to dry skin. Its formula is similar to that of many baby shampoos, and so is not adept at removing silicone-based or long-wearing makeup. If that's not your concern, however, this is recommended.

☹ AVERAGE **Cold Cream Ultra-Rich Soap-Free Cleansing Bar** *($9 for 3.52 fl. oz.)* isn't as bad for skin as traditional bar soap, but it doesn't rinse easily and the film it leaves on skin may cause dryness, and it certainly impedes the action of any moisturizers or serums you apply to your skin after cleansing.

☹ AVERAGE **$$$ Cold Cream** *($17 for 1.2 fl. oz.)* is an old-fashioned cold cream containing mostly mineral oil, water, and beeswax. You could easily replace this greasy formula with pure mineral oil and do far better, and save a lot of money. This is a dated way to remove makeup, and its cleansing ability is minimal. It definitely requires the use of a washcloth to avoid leaving a greasy film. This is only for dry skin not prone to blemishes.

☹ AVERAGE **$$$ Gentle Gel Cleanser** *($18 for 6.76 fl. oz.)* is soap-free, but that doesn't necessarily make it a gentle option. Considering this product is aimed at those with sensitive skin, it should be fragrance-free, and it's not. This is a basic but effective water-soluble gel cleanser that is best for normal to slightly dry skin.

☹ AVERAGE **$$$ Tolerance Extreme Cleansing Lotion, No-Rinse, Tissue-Off Formula** *($32 for 1.69 fl. oz.)* is a cold cream–style cleanser for dry skin sold as a special product meant to be used for three weeks. Why the magic number of three weeks is a good question, but the answer is nothing more than marketing caprice. This is little more than a glycerin and mineral oil, very basic, detergent-free cleanser suitable for delicate or sensitive skin, and it removes makeup well, though you'll need to use a washcloth to avoid leaving a greasy residue. For the money, you're getting a shockingly small amount of product. (Really, water, glycerin, and mineral oil means this couldn't be more than a 50-cent formula.)

☹ POOR **Cold Cream Emollient Cleansing Gel** *($24 for 13.52 fl. oz.)* has an interesting mix of ingredients that you see in water-soluble and cold cream–type cleansers. The result removes makeup and rinses quite well, though you may need a washcloth for complete removal. Ignore the thermal spring water claims because spring water doesn't make one difference your skin will notice. This was previously recommended as a great option for normal to very dry skin, but since the formula now includes irritating fragrant oils from orange and rosemary, it is no longer worth buying. These fragrant oils are a problem for use around the eyes and also make this a no-go for sensitive skin.

☹ POOR **Extremely Gentle Cleanser for Intolerant Skin** *($19 for 6.76 fl. oz.)* lists the second ingredient as a disinfectant and antifungal agent most often used as a preservative. O-phenyl phenol is known to be irritating for skin and eyes and has no business in a product for "hypersensitive skin" (Source: *Contact Dermatitis*, April 2006, page 332). Avoid this cleanser!

EAU THERMALE AVENE EYE-MAKEUP REMOVER

☹ AVERAGE **$$$ Gentle Eye Make-Up Remover** *($18 for 5.07 fl. oz.)* isn't all that gentle given that the second ingredient is triethanolamine and the fourth ingredient is an acrylate. In addition, the amount of cleansing agent is really low compared with other makeup removers, which means you have to work harder to take your eye makeup off. Given the price, this isn't worth considering over the outstanding makeup removers from Almay or Neutrogena, both of which are great for sensitive skin.

EAU THERMALE AVENE TONERS

☹ POOR **Gentle Toner** *($18 for 6.76 fl. oz.)* is mostly water and fragrance, and has no redeeming value for skin, sensitive or not, because it is little more than eau de cologne. Applying this is like putting perfume on your face, and that is never a good idea.

☹ POOR **Cleanance Anti-Shine Purifying Lotion** *($18 for 7 fl. oz.)* claims to be "astringent," and it is, thanks to the alcohol it contains. Although the amount of alcohol isn't as great as in many other toners for oily skin, it's still potentially problematic. See the Appendix to learn how irritation from alcohol can make oily skin and enlarged pores worse. Contrary to claim, this toner does not contain ingredients that leave skin shine-free. If anything, its combination of glycol with plant oils will leave skin shiny. The amount of salicylic acid is too low for it to function as an exfoliant, but even if present in a greater amount, it wouldn't exfoliate because the pH of this toner is too high. This fragranced toner ends up being not much better than standard alcohol-based toners for oily skin. A far superior option to improve skin and reduce enlarged pores is Paula's Choice Skin Balancing Pore-Reducing Toner.

☹ POOR **Thermal Spring Water** *($11 for 5.29 fl. oz.)* is marketing at its best. There is no reason to consider this toner unless you believe that Avene's thermal spring water is the answer for your skin. Despite the purity claims, in the world of skin care, water is water and regardless of where it came from, it's necessarily purified to prevent microbial contamination. No type of water can leave a soothing barrier on skin. The water that doesn't penetrate the skin will evaporate, leaving compromised skin right back where it was when you started. The comparative studies done on Avene's thermal spring water merely indicate that patients prefer it to other spray-on waters and to a random group of skin-care products for soothing their skin after a cosmetic corrective procedure, and all the studies were done by Avene. What we don't know is whether or not some other product, such as a silicone-based gel with anti-irritants, would've performed much better (Sources: *Journal of Cosmetic Dermatology*, March 2007, pages 31–35; and *Journal of Drugs in Dermatology*, September 2007, pages 924–928). As for the nitrogen, it is used as a propellant in this product and has no established benefit for skin. However, nitrogen can generate free-radical damage and cause cell death (Sources: *Cellular and Molecular Biology*, April 15, 2007, pages 1–2; *Mechanisms of Ageing and Development*, April 2002, pages 1007–1019; and *Toxicology and Applied Pharmacology*, July 2002, pages 84–90).

EAU THERMALE AVENE EXFOLIANTS & SCRUBS

☺ AVERAGE $$$ **Gentle Purifying Scrub** *($18 for 1.76 fl. oz.)* is a very standard scrub that contains ground-up plastic as the scrub agent and a small amount of detergent cleansing agent. It is suitable for normal to oily skin; those with sensitive skin should avoid scrubs, especially ones like this that contain fragrance.

☺ AVERAGE $$$ **Cleanance K Cream-Gel** *($22 for 1.44 fl. oz.)* is chiefly an AHA exfoliant meant for acne-prone skin. Although AHA ingredients can be helpful for breakouts, BHA (active ingredient salicylic acid) is preferred because it can penetrate oil to better dislodge blockages inside the pores. BHA is also mildly antibacterial and has anti-inflammatory properties, while AHAs do not have these traits. Although this product does contain BHA, it's present in too small an amount to be of much benefit. The AHA ingredients are present in an amount capable of exfoliating, and the pH of 3.6 ensures these ingredients will exfoliate, which is the goal. Although the AHAs are helpful, most struggling with breakouts will get better results from a BHA exfoliant. As for this product being a better choice for sensitive, easily irritated skin, it isn't. Not only is the amount of AHAs a potential problem for extra sensitive skin, but also the inclusion of fragrance isn't a good idea because fragrance itself can be irritating. See the Appendix for further details on why fragrance isn't good for skin. This ends up being an OK but pricey option as an AHA exfoliant for normal to slightly dry skin, and a questionable option for breakout-prone skin.

EAU THERMALE AVENE MOISTURIZERS (DAYTIME & NIGHTTIME), EYE CREAMS, & SERUMS

☺ GOOD **Cream for Intolerant Skin** *($26 for 1.35 fl. oz.)* is for those with sensitive skin that's also dry. Those with this kind of skin may wish to consider this mineral oil–based, gentle moisturizer. The formula isn't very exciting, but it is extremely unlikely to make sensitive skin react negatively. It is fragrance-free, which, combined with its benign formula, makes it of value for sensitive skin.

☺ GOOD **$$$ TriXera Emollient Cream** *($29 for 6.84 fl. oz.)* is a good, though relatively standard, moisturizer for dry to very dry skin. What is most interesting, despite the fact that it's being sold as a face and body moisturizer (which explains the larger size), is that it's better formulated than most of Avene's smaller-sized and far more expensive face products. Actually, when you think about it, that's a bit shocking; perhaps they thought no one would notice. This is fragrance-free and an option if dryness and sensitive, reactive skin are your chief concerns. The evening primrose oil is a respectable addition because its fatty acid profile is rich in cell-communicating linoleic acid. Evening primrose oil is also a good source of antioxidant vitamin E.

☺ AVERAGE **Clean-AC** *($16 for 1.35 fl. oz.)* is a very basic, below-standard moisturizer described as a special treatment for acne-prone skin experiencing bothersome dryness. The amount of fatty acids (thick, wax-like ingredients) and oils will remedy dryness, but at the potential risk of making blemishes worse. It's such a bland formula that we can't imagine anyone would have a sensitizing reaction to it, but that's not about helping acne-prone skin. There are dozens of other moisturizers that ease dryness, but that are less likely to exacerbate blemishes (and that also offer blemish-prone skin some anti-irritants to reduce redness and/or niacinamide, which has research showing it can reduce breakouts).

☺ AVERAGE **Clean-AC Hydrating Cream** *($20 for 1.35 fl. oz.)*. Although this unnecessarily fragranced formula contains some notable emollients and an anti-irritant, there are better moisturizers that offer a range of antioxidants, more anti-irritants, proven skin-repairing ingredients, and cell-communicating ingredients to help normalize healthy cell production. This is an OK option for normal to dry skin, although the emollients and the amount of plant oil make it potentially problematic for breakout-prone skin.

☺ AVERAGE **Cleanance Anti-Shine Regulating Lotion** *($18 for 1.35 fl. oz.)* has a soft matte finish, and the slip agents it contains provide lightweight hydration. This won't keep shine under control for long (a matte-finish foundation and powder would last longer), but it's an OK moisturizer for oily skin with dry patches. The tiny amount of salicylic acid provides no benefit toward exfoliation and it can't help reduce blemishes.

☺ AVERAGE **Emulsion Ultra High Protection for Sensitive Skin SPF 50+** *($29.95 for 1.7 fl. oz.)* does not list active ingredients, but given that its primary distribution is in Europe, that omission is acceptable because sunscreens are not regulated as over-the-counter drugs in European Union countries and they aren't required to list the active ingredients separately. This product contains Tinosorb (listed by its chemical name methylene bis-benzotriazolyl tetra-methylbutylphenol) for sufficient UVA protection along with a tiny amount of zinc oxide. The base formula is an OK option for normal to dry skin, but it lacks significant antioxidants and other ingredients that skin needs as part of a state-of-the-art routine. The amount of vitamin E in this product is minimal.

☺ AVERAGE **High Protection Mineral Cream SPF 50** *($21 for 1.69 fl. oz.)* includes titanium dioxide and zinc oxide as active ingredients, so it's great for reliable sun protection. The formula is also slightly tinted to offset the white cast a high amount of mineral actives often has. These active ingredients are preferred for those with sensitive skin; however, Avene also included fragrant orange oil (although only a small amount), thus reducing the appeal for those with sensitive skin. In addition, there's a very low amount of antioxidants. This is still an OK but not exceptional choice for those with normal to slightly dry or slightly oily skin not prone to blemishes.

☺ AVERAGE **Hydrance Optimale Hydrating Cream SPF 25, for Normal to Dry Skin** *($36 for 1.35 fl. oz.)* is a daytime moisturizer with an in-part titanium dioxide sunscreen. It's an option for normal to dry skin, but it's hardly an exciting one, especially considering the price. Broad-spectrum sun protection is assured, but the lightly emollient base formula elicits more of a "so what?" than an "oh, wow!" reaction. The amount of antioxidants is paltry, but at least this comes in packaging that will help keep them stable during use.

☺ AVERAGE **Hydrance Optimale Light Hydrating Cream, for Normal to Combination Skin** *($28 for 1.35 fl. oz.)* is an average moisturizer suitable for normal to dry skin, but too emollient to use over oily areas if combination skin is your skin type.

☺ AVERAGE **Hydrance Optimale Riche, Rich Hydrating Cream for Dry to Very Dry Sensitive Skin** *($28 for 1.35 fl. oz.)* is a slightly more emollient version of Avene's Hydrance Optimale Light Hydrating Cream, for Normal to Combination Skin above, and the same review applies.

☺ AVERAGE **Redness Relief Soothing Cream, for Sensitive Skin, SPF 25** *($33 for 1.35 fl. oz.)* would be far better if it contained only mineral actives (i.e., titanium dioxide and zinc oxide) because they are the least likely to cause a reaction. Although this sunscreen contains titanium dioxide, it is paired with other synthetic active ingredients that make it a questionable choice for those with truly sensitive skin. This product also contains fragrance, another no-no when sensitive skin is your target audience. Lastly, the green tint of this product will slightly tone down redness, but at the expense of leaving your skin looking as though you're seasick. A better solution for reducing redness would be to use a yellow-toned foundation with a tita-nium dioxide–based sunscreen over a well-formulated moisturizer that contains anti-irritants, antioxidants, and skin-identical (repairing) ingredients.

☺ AVERAGE **Rich Compensating Cream** *($32 for 1.37 fl. oz.)* is a moisturizer for normal to dry skin with an enviably silky texture; however, the formula isn't impressive. Basic emol-lients and thickeners help ease dryness, but it is woefully short on beneficial antioxidants, skin-identical ingredients, or cell-communicating ingredients. Moreover, the tiny amount of antioxidants it does contain will deteriorate once this jar packaging is opened.

☺ AVERAGE **Soothing Eye Contour Cream** *($24 for 0.34 fl. oz.)* is a basic, mineral oil–based, fragrance-free moisturizer, an OK option for dry skin anywhere on the face. This contains bisabolol (an anti-irritant derived from chamomile), but it cannot alleviate puffy eyes.

Puffy eyes are caused by allergies, fat pads pouching through lax muscles, or fluid retention, and skin-care products are often of little help for relieving these causes of puffiness (and of no help when the puffiness is due to age-related factors such as fat pads shifting beneath the skin). See the Appendix to find out why, in truth, you don't need an eye crema.

☹ AVERAGE **Ystheal Cream, for Dry to Very Dry Skin** ($38 for 1.01 fl. oz.) is a very basic, mineral oil–based, emollient moisturizer that's suitable for its intended skin type, but that's it. The amount of retinal (also known as retinaldehyde, an effective derivative of vitamin A) and vitamin E is embarrassingly low. Any less expensive moisturizer with retinol from RoC, Neutrogena, Paula's Choice, or Alpha Hydrox is preferred to this.

☺ AVERAGE **Ystheal+ Emulsion Lotion, for Normal to Combination Skin** ($38 for 1.01 fl. oz.) is a lighter-weight version of Avene's Ystheal Cream, for Dry to Very Dry Skin. In addition to the lighter texture, it lacks the retinal (a derivative of vitamin A) that's present in the Cream version. As for the vitamin E, the amount is so low that its impact on skin will be negligible. That leaves you with an ordinary emollient moisturizer for normal to dry skin that doesn't earn its anti-aging stripes.

☺ AVERAGE **Ystheal+ Eye Contour Care** ($34 for 0.5 fl. oz.) is an OK, mineral oil–based moisturizer for dry skin anywhere on the face. It is fragrance-free, so has an edge for the eye area when compared with Avene's moisturizers with fragrance. As for the retinal (a derivative of vitamin A), it's barely present and ends up not counting as an "antiwrinkle" ingredient. See the Appendix to learn why, in truth, you don't need an eye cream!

☺ AVERAGE $$$ **Diroseal Anti-Redness Skincare Lotion** ($46 for 1.03 fl. oz.) is an overpriced moisturizer differing little from the majority of moisturizers sold by Avene. The only significant difference here is this lotion has a green tint that is intended to minimize redness. Although it can mask redness to an extent, the trade-off is green-tinged skin that you have to cover up with another product. You'd be better off using a regular moisturizer loaded with anti-irritants that neutralize redness without just trying to cover it up. Examples of well-formulated moisturizers with anti-irritants are Clinique's Super Rescue Antioxidant Night products or those from Paula's Choice RESIST and Skin Recovery lines.

☺ AVERAGE $$$ **Eluage Cream** ($42 for 1.01 fl. oz.). The only anti-aging ingredients of note in this moisturizer for normal to dry skin are sodium hyaluronate and retinal, the latter also known as retinaldehyde, an effective derivative of vitamin A. Unfortunately, both ingredients are present only in teeny-tiny amounts (there is more fragrance and preservatives than either of these ingredients), so this isn't what we'd consider anti-aging or a product with "advanced technology." On the plus side, this is packaged so that the retinal remains stable during use. Eluage Cream misses the mark by not including a range of anti-aging ingredients that help repair skin, encourage healthier cell production, and soothe irritation. It's little more than an average moisturizer, and your skin deserves (and, in fact, needs) better.

☺ AVERAGE $$$ **Eluage Eye Contour Care** ($38.50 for 0.5 fl. oz.) is nearly identical to Avene's Eluage Cream, which is sold as a facial moisturizer. The eye cream is fragrance-free, and that's great, but that's the most significant difference (and it must be said that, whether around the eyes or elsewhere, skin does better with fragrance-free products). Given its strong similarity to the Eulage Cream facial moisturizer, we're reminded once again that eye creams aren't necessary (see the Appendix for details). Otherwise, the same review applies.

☺ AVERAGE $$$ **Retrinal Cream 0.05** ($61 for 1 fl. oz.) is nearly identical to Avene's other Retrinal Creams except for a slightly different concentration of "retinal" as indicated on the label. Also known as retinaldehyde, retinal is similar to retinol (we have no idea why the name of the product is retrinal as there is no skin-care ingredient on their label called retrinal). Retinaldehyde is a worthwhile ingredient for skin, as it can reportedly be better used by skin than retinol because it takes fewer steps in the conversion process for it to become the active form of vitamin A after it is absorbed. Retinaldehyde is also supposedly better tolerated than retinol though there is limited information on that. However, all forms of vitamin A can cause undesirable side effects such as flaking and dryness (Source: *Dermatologic Therapy*, September-October 2006, pages 289–296). How much retinol or retinal is needed for skin isn't firmly established. Higher percentages can cause unwanted side effects, but too little and it is questionable whether or not it is effective. Other than the retinaldehyde, this is a very standard, unimpressive moisturizer for normal to dry skin. It is worth considering if you are looking for a vitamin A product for your skin; just keep in mind the skin needs more than one ingredient to be healthy and function like younger skin. It is just like your diet: No matter how healthy green tea is, if that was all you drank you would be malnourished.

☺ AVERAGE $$$ **Retrinal Cream 0.1** *($69 for 1 fl. oz.)* is nearly identical to Avene's other Retrinal Creams except for a different concentration of "retinal" as indicated on their ingredient label. It is worth considering if you are looking for a vitamin A product for your skin, just keep in mind the skin needs more than one ingredient to be healthy and function like younger skin.

☺ AVERAGE $$$ **Retrinal H.A.F. Firming Gel** *($46 for 0.5 fl. oz.)* is an alleged skin-firming product with a lotion rather than gel texture. Its ordinary, water and wax formula does not add up to firming benefits in any way, shape, or form. One of the last ingredients listed is retinal. Not to be confused with retinol, retinal is a derivative of vitamin A, also known as retinaldehyde. Amounts of 0.05% and above have been shown to build collagen fibers after skin samples were exposed to UV light, but that was in controlled laboratory settings on human skin samples—and the amount of retinaldehyde in this product is most likely less than 0.05%, so we wouldn't count on similar results with daily use of this product (Source: *Dermatology*, Supplement, 1999, pages 43–48). This remains an OK moisturizer for normal to dry skin, nothing more.

☺ AVERAGE $$$ **Retrinal H.A.F. Gel** *($46 for 0.5 fl. oz.)* has a lotion texture rather than a gel texture, and its wrinkle-reducing benefits are dubious at best, especially given that the retinal is one of the last ingredients listed. This remains an OK moisturizer for normal to dry skin, nothing more. If you're curious to see what retinaldehyde can do for your skin, consider Avene's Retrinal Cream 0.1 instead.

☺ AVERAGE $$$ **Serenage Nutri-Redensifying Day Cream** *($47 for 1.4 fl. oz.)* is an average, overpriced moisturizer that's merely an OK option for dry skin. It is said to contain "pre-tocopheryl," but that ingredient actually isn't on the ingredient label. There is some research showing pre-tocopheryl (meaning a precursor of vitamin E) can be a good antioxidant when combined with other ingredients, but again, this formula doesn't have any so it's a moot point. Perhaps Avene is referring to the avocado oil and shea butter this contains because they are natural sources of vitamin E, but that's just a guess. In the long run, vitamin E in the form of tocopherol or a blend of tocotrienols is by far the most stable and bioavailable form of vitamin E for skin. Regardless of the puzzling claim, this moisturizer doesn't have what it takes to qualify as an anti-aging treatment. A greater range of skin-repairing ingredients, antioxidants, and the addition of cell-communicating ingredients would make that description and price more realistic.

The Reviews E

☺ AVERAGE **$$$ Serenage Nutri-Redensifying Vital Serum** *($51 for 1.01 fl. oz.)* is a rather ordinary serum said to contain "hyaluronic acid fragments" that help "redensify" skin and fight sagging. Hyaluronic acid in skin-care products cannot do that (see the Appendix to learn why anti-sagging products don't work as claimed), but even more bizarre is that this product doesn't contain any form of hyaluronic acid, fragments or otherwise. Many lines add hyaluronic acid (or its salt form, sodium hyaluronate) to their products because it is an excellent skin-repairing ingredient, but what it cannot do (regardless of the amount or the claims) is work topically to plump wrinkles and strategically lift skin as it does when it is injected (think dermal fillers). When done correctly by a good cosmetic dermatologist, dermal fillers absolutely can add density to skin and, to a certain degree help give skin a slight lift without surgery. This serum (whose texture is closer to a lotion-like moisturizer) contains some good ingredients for dry skin, but it lacks an array of antioxidants or skin-repairing ingredients that would at least justify a bit of the cost—as is, there is nothing special or really worth the price.

☺ AVERAGE **$$$ Thermal Spring Water Gel** *($22 for 1.5 fl. oz.)* is incapable of moisturizing skin because it is nothing more than water, gel-based thickener, and baking soda—that's it. Unless you absolutely believe Avene's thermal spring water is the only ingredient your skin needs to satisfy all manner of skin-care needs (and that would be a truly mistaken belief), you're better off massaging plain tap water on your skin and following with a well-formulated serum or moisturizer. Although spring water is supposed to be pH-neutral, we're concerned that the baking soda will raise this product's pH to an alkaline level, which would make it potentially drying, not hydrating, for skin.

☺ AVERAGE **$$$ Thermal Spring Water Soothing Serum** *($34 for 1.01 fl. oz.)* is an ordinary, lightweight, gel moisturizer for normal to oily skin. Like most Avene products, it is woefully short on antioxidants, skin-identical ingredients, and cell-communicating ingredients. There are more preservatives and acrylates in here than beneficial ingredients. This ends up being more of a "why bother" than anything else. One more comment: the amount of alcohol is likely too low to be cause for concern, though it's disappointing this moisturizer contains more alcohol than state-of-the-art ingredients.

☺ AVERAGE **$$$ Tolerance Extreme Soothing Cream** *($36 for 1.7 fl. oz.)* contains a mundane mix of mineral oil, plant oil, and thickeners, an option for dry, sensitive skin; but on the other hand, your skin deserves so much more. The formula is fragrance- and preservative-free, which is helpful, but to be truly beneficial it should contain state-of-the-art ingredients that restore skin's barrier, including antioxidants, anti-irritants, and skin-identical ingredients. If a less-is-more approach is your idea of skin care, this fits the bill. This product is an option, albeit an unexciting one, if your skin is dry and extremely sensitive to most moisturizers.

EAU THERMALE AVENE SUN CARE

☺ GOOD **Sunscreen Spray SPF 20** *($21 for 6.76 fl. oz.)* is a lightweight, spray-on sunscreen lotion providing sufficient UVA protection thanks to its in-part titanium dioxide sunscreen. It is recommended for normal to dry skin, but would've been rated higher if it contained appreciable amounts of antioxidants.

☺ GOOD **$$$ Moisturizing Self-Tanning Lotion** *($22 for 3.38 fl. oz.)* is a very standard, but good, self-tanning lotion for normal to dry skin. Its silky texture contains the same tanning ingredient (dihydroxyacetone) found in almost all self-tanners. This is pricey considering it works about as well as most other sunless tanning products, which cost less and come in bigger sizes. Still, it does the job.

EAU THERMALE AVENE LIP CARE

☺ GOOD **Cold Cream Lip Balm** *($12 for 0.14 fl. oz.)* is an emollient lip balm whose oil–based formula is excellent for dry, chapped lips. It would be better if it was fragrance-free, but at least Avene omitted the common lip balm irritants (e.g., menthol) that show up in many other products like this.

☺ GOOD **$$$ Cold Cream Lip Cream** *($14 for 0.4 fl. oz.)* is a tube-packaged lip balm that is a very good option to help improve dry, chapped skin on your lips. Its rich lanolin and Vaseline-base does indeed have a cold cream–like texture and it's relatively easy to smooth over the lips. The mix of oils and waxes helps protect against moisture loss while the mineral pigment mica leaves a subtle shimmer finish. This lip balm contains fragrance, although the amount is low so it shouldn't be cause for concern.

EAU THERMALE AVENE SPECIALTY SKIN-CARE PRODUCTS

☺ GOOD **$$$ Akerat S Psoriasis Skin Cream** *($28 for 3.38 fl. oz.)* is designed to treat the symptoms of psoriasis, of which the most pervasive is dry, scaly skin. The active ingredient is 2% salicylic acid, but the pH of the product is above 4, so this won't be as effective as it could have been for reducing the scaling so common to psoriasis. What makes this product helpful is its urea content. Urea is a moisturizing agent that is known to reduce the hyperproliferation of psoriatic skin cells. When coupled with emollients and oils, urea can offer relief to dry, itchy skin while also helping to reduce inflammation (Sources: *Clinics in Dermatology*, July-August 2008, pages 380–386; and *Acta-Dermato Venereologica*, September 1996, pages 353–356). Because of urea's known track record for psoriasis, this product is recommended; however, there are less expensive urea-based and salicylic acid–based moisturizers available at the drugstore (ask your pharmacist if you cannot locate them in the skin-care aisle).

☹ AVERAGE **Soothing Moisture Mask** *($24 for 1.69 fl. oz.)* is a mundane, boring mask. Other than oils (mostly mineral oil) and emollients that make dry skin look and feel better, there isn't much of interest or benefit about this creamy mask. It doesn't contain even one state-of-the-art ingredient!

☹ AVERAGE **$$$ Cleanance Purifying Mask** *($20 for 1.5 fl. oz.)* is a decent yet overpriced clay-based mask for those with normal to oily skin. Although it contains the AHA glycolic acid and the BHA salicylic acid, the clay (kaolin) keeps this mask from having the acidic pH level necessary for exfoliation to occur. A potential issue with this mask is that the thickening agents it contains keep the clay from being as absorbent as it could be. These thickeners prevent the mask from being too drying, but those with very oily skin aren't going to find much benefit. It is best for those with slightly oily or combination skin.

☹ AVERAGE **$$$ TriAcneal** *($60 for 1.01 fl. oz.)* is a very expensive anti-acne product that contains glycolic acid. The company states it's present at 6%, which, coupled with this product's pH, means exfoliation will occur. Although AHA in the form of glycolic acid can absolutely be helpful for breakouts, research shows that when acne is the concern, salicylic acid (BHA) is preferred to glycolic acid because it is oil-soluble and also has antibacterial and anti-inflammatory properties, three important needs for someone with blemish-prone skin. TriAcneal also contains a form of retinaldehyde, known as retinal, but the amount is merely a dusting; there is more red dye in here than retinal. The company states they're using 0.1% retinal, but the ingredient list doesn't necessarily jibe with that. Assuming it's close, there is research showing 6% glycolic acid and 0.1% retinal can be helpful for breakouts. This ends up being an acceptable yet overpriced product whose acne-improving ability, including improving the appearance of acne marks, is limited but may be worth a look if your skin doesn't respond well to a BHA exfoliant. Note: The amount of alcohol this contains is likely too low to be cause for concern. What's certain, though, is that alcohol won't help improve acne or signs of aging.

ELIZABETH ARDEN

Strengths: Moderately priced; some excellent serums (including the ceramide capsules) and moisturizers; good cleansers for normal to dry skin; good concealer, eyeshadow, and lipsticks.

Weaknesses: No products for those battling blemishes; no effective skin-lightening products; no AHA or BHA products; several products whose sunscreen lacks sufficient UVA protection; most of the foundations with sunscreen fail to provide sufficient UVA protection; lackluster eye and brow pencils; some problematic lip color products; jar packaging.

For more information and reviews of the latest Elizabeth Arden products, visit CosmeticsCop.com.

ELIZABETH ARDEN CLEANSERS

☺ GOOD $$$ **Hydra-Gentle Cream Cleanser, for Dry/Sensitive Skin** *($19.50 for 5 fl. oz.)* would be better for its targeted sensitive-skin customer if it did not contain fragrance; however, this is a very good, silky cleansing lotion that removes makeup and does not contain detergent cleansing agents.

☺ GOOD $$$ **Intervene 3-in-1 Daily Cleanser Exfoliator Primer** *($21.50 for 5 fl. oz.)* is a copiously foaming cleanser that does a much better job of cleansing skin than exfoliating it. The scrub particles are polyethylene beads, but their presence in this product isn't as prominent as in many other (less expensive) cleanser/scrub options available at the drugstore. Consider this a good cleanser for normal to oily skin; it's capable of removing makeup, but the scrub particles aren't for use over the eye area.

☹ AVERAGE $$$ **Ceramide Purifying Cream Cleanser** *($27.50 for 4.2 fl. oz.)* is a basic, water- and mineral oil–based cleansing lotion that contains barely any ceramides. The tiny amount of sandalwood oil isn't great for skin or for use in the eye area, but is not likely a cause for concern. This will require a washcloth for complete removal and is suitable for normal to dry skin.

ELIZABETH ARDEN TONERS

☹ POOR **Ceramide Purifying Toner** *($27.50 for 6.7 fl. oz.)* lists alcohol as the second ingredient and also contains some potentially irritating plant extracts, all of which undermine the effectiveness of the ceramides and other skin-identical ingredients in this misguided toner.

ELIZABETH ARDEN EXFOLIANTS & SCRUBS

☹ AVERAGE $$$ **Ceramide Plump Perfect Gentle Line Smoothing Exfoliator** *($27.50 for 3.4 fl. oz.)* is a very rich, creamy scrub that is best for those with dry to very dry skin. Rounded polyethylene beads buff the skin, and they're cushioned by plant oil plus several emollients. The emollience of the formula makes this scrub tricky to rinse, but it can be done. This came close to earning a Best rating, but Arden added several fragrant plant and fragrance ingredients known to cause irritation. Between that fact and the price, it is perfectly fine to leave it alone. Those with dry skin will be better off using a creamy cleanser with a washcloth. You'll get the same results, but almost zero risk of irritation.

ELIZABETH ARDEN MOISTURIZERS (DAYTIME & NIGHTTIME), EYE CREAMS, & SERUMS

✓☺ BEST $$$ **Ceramide Gold Ultra Restorative Capsules** *($68 for 0.95 fl. oz.)* are an interesting way to provide normal to very dry skin with a short but very effective roster of ingredients that can restore a healthy skin-barrier function, all while supplying elements that skin needs to look and act younger. Cell-communicating ingredients and skin-restoring ceramides join two forms of antioxidant vitamin A as well as some vitamin E. As claimed, these capsules are fragrance- and preservative-free. They are definitely a consideration for those dealing with eczema or rosacea (assuming your rosacea-prone skin is not also oily).

✓☺ BEST $$$ **Extreme Conditioning Cream SPF 15** *($38.50 for 1.7 fl. oz.)* provides UVA protection with its in-part avobenzone sunscreen and comes in an emollient, silky, antioxidant-enriched base. Both packaging options (some retailers carry this product in an opaque pump bottle and others carry it in a squeeze tube) will keep the light- and air-sensitive ingredients stable, so this is an all-around exceptional daytime moisturizer for normal to dry skin.

☺ GOOD $$$ **Ceramide Gold Ultra Lift and Strengthening Eye Capsules** *($52 for 60 capsules)* is a silicone-based serum packaged in capsules housed in a jar container, and the capsules contain many impressive ingredients, including ceramides, several antioxidants, and cell-communicating ingredients. All of these can help improve skin-cell production, but none are capable of lifting skin that has begun to sag. One problem in an otherwise exemplary formula is the amount of witch hazel extract. This is not a great ingredient for skin, especially around the eyes, and unfortunately, there is more of it in these capsules than there is of the aforementioned beneficial ingredients. Still, the extract form of witch hazel isn't as bad as the distillate or pure form—but it's enough to keep this product from earning a higher rating. There's no reason Arden's regular Ceramide capsules cannot be used around the eyes, too.

☺ GOOD $$$ **Ceramide Plump Perfect Targeted Line Concentrate** *($65 for 0.5 fl. oz.)* has a lot of wonderful things going for it, including a supremely silky texture and nearly weightless finish suitable for all skin types. The pump-dispensed serum is packed with antioxidants and ingredients that mimic the structure and function of healthy skin, as well as lesser amounts of a couple of cell-communicating ingredients. The only drawback keeping it from earning a higher rating is the volatile fragrant components, which can be irritating. Their presence is minimal, but they ding this product compared to similarly well-formulated serums from Estee Lauder, Paula's Choice, Olay, and Clinique.

☺ GOOD $$$ **Intervene Timefighting Radiance Serum** *($49.50 for 1 fl. oz.* is a good option for normal to slightly dry skin. It's no more concentrated than several other well-formulated serums, so ignore that attempt to make Intervene seem as though it's the only answer for your aging skin. However, it's a worthwhile serum that can help smooth the appearance of lines and encourage a healthy barrier function, although reversing the hands of time is not in its bag of tricks. The downsides to this serum are a couple of potentially irritating plant extracts (clover and narcissus) along with some fragrance ingredients that can be troublesome for all skin types, especially sensitive skin or skin affected by rosacea. Their inclusion isn't a deal-breaker for this serum, but they do keep it from earning a Best Product rating.

☺ GOOD $$$ **Overnight Success Skin Renewal Serum** *($49 for 1 fl. oz.)* promises to resurface and regenerate skin's appearance, giving your skin enhanced clarity and a less blotchy appearance. Yet the best thing this serum has going for it is that its silicone base will leave skin

The Reviews E

🍸 Did you know alcohol in skin-care products is a big problem? See the Appendix to learn more.

feeling exceptionally silky. In terms of enhanced clarity, there is nothing in the product that can make skin clearer. However, because silicones can even out your skin's texture you may perceive more clarity. This is because of how silicone functions on skin: smooth-textured skin is better able to reflect light, which does improve its appearance, but that's a cosmetic effect, not an anti-aging breakthrough. Arden wisely filled this serum with several very good skin identical ingredients and antioxidants, ingredients you should expect to see in any serum (or moisturizer), especially in this price range. Even better, packaging for this product will ensure that the antioxidants remain stable during use. The inclusion of the Australian flower extract *Centipedia cunninghamii* (also known by its less appealing garden name, old man weed) is curious, because it is commonly used as a medicinal remedy for colds and chest pain (Source: naturaldatabase.com). Reliable, substantiated information about this extract's effect on skin doesn't seem to exist. The extract does not appear to be harmful or irritating, but there are no proven studies pertaining to its usefulness as an antiwrinkle ingredient. Our one complaint is the intense fragrance. We don't often comment on a specific skin-care product's scent, but this serum's perfumey scent lingers on the skin long after it has been absorbed. Both Clinique and Paula's Choice have similar products that are fragrance-free and less expensive, but this product is definitely an option for all but sensitive skin types seeking either a lightweight moisturizer or antioxidant product.

☺ GOOD $$$ **Prevage Day Ultra Protection Anti-Aging Moisturizer SPF 30 PA ++** *($129 for 1.7 fl. oz.)* is a good, though exceedingly overpriced, daytime moisturizer with sunscreen for normal to dry skin. UVA protection is assured thanks to the inclusion of stabilized avobenzone, and the base formula is creamy and provides enough emollients to keep those with dry skin happy. This also works well under foundation. As for the claims, there is no published, substantiated research proving that idebenone (listed as hydroxydecyl ubiquinoyl dipalmitoyl glycerate) is "the most powerful and effective antioxidant." Even the concept is ludicrous, because there are hundreds of antioxidants, and comparisons among different antioxidants are few and far between. The few comparative studies that have been done refute the claim, demonstrating instead that other antioxidants such as L-ergothioneine (also present in this product but not promoted like idebenone) and resveratrol (not in this product) are in fact more potent than idebenone (Source: *Journal of Cosmetic Dermatology*, March 2008, pages 2–7; and September 2007, pages 183–188). Another published study compared the photoprotective (i.e., sun-protective) effect of idebenone with that of other antioxidants, including vitamins C and E. Although the study was paid for by Skinceuticals (which sells an antioxidant-laden product that competes with Prevage), it was well designed and ably proved that idebenone doesn't offer much photoprotection in comparison with other antioxidants (Source: *Journal of Investigative Dermatology*, March 2006, pages 1185–1187). The bottom line is: Idebenone is one of many good antioxidants to look for in skin-care products, but it isn't the best or most potent. No single antioxidant is the best, which is why many researchers believe that a cocktail approach is best when applying antioxidants topically. This product contains fragrance ingredients that pose a slight risk of irritation and it also contains cosmetic pigments that lend a soft shine to skin.

☺ GOOD $$$ **Prevage Eye Advanced Anti-Aging Serum** *($100 for 0.5 fl. oz.)* is an eye-area serum that has a lot going for it. But, before you get too excited, know that the price is outrageous. What's more, this serum contains nothing (and we mean nothing) that is special or unique for the eye area. If you're using one of the well-formulated "facial" products from Prevage (or any recommended facial moisturizer or serum), there's no reason you cannot apply it around the eyes, too (see the Appendix for further details). You may be tempted to try this serum because it claims to address every eye-area woe, from wrinkles to dark circles to puffiness. Although it contains an impressive assortment of skin-repairing, smoothing, and antioxidant ingredients, none of them are proven to improve dark circles or puffy eyes. The anti-aging ingredients can help improve the appearance of wrinkles and other signs of sun damage, but they're not unique to this product. What about the "revolutionary" antioxidant idebenone (listed as hydroxydecyl ubiquinoyl)? Despite the claim that its performance is "unsurpassed," it's not true. Idebenone was shown in limited research to out-perform a handful of some well-known antioxidants, but subsequent research has shown that idebenone isn't the best (Source: *Journal of Cosmetic Dermatology*, March 2008, pages 2–7, and September 2007, pages 183–188). The truth is there are hundreds of brilliant antioxidants for skin, and your skin needs more than one great antioxidant anyway, just like your diet requires a variety of healthy ingredients. If you decide to try this product, its silky texture is best for normal to slightly oily or combination skin, but it won't provide much moisture for dry areas. Note that this contains the mineral pigment mica to add shine around the eyes. To some extent, that can help reflect light so dark circles are less apparent. But shine isn't skin care, it's makeup, so if dark circles are your concern, you'll get more mileage from a great concealer than from a skin-care product that imparts shine.

☺ GOOD $$$ **Prevage Face Advanced Anti-Aging Serum** *($159 for 1.7 fl. oz.)* continues the carefully orchestrated launch of Prevage, which was first marketed to physicians and is now available in what is termed an "over-the-counter" version, marketed under the Elizabeth Arden name. Arden partnered with Allergan, the company that makes Prevage, to create a product that contains the "powerful" antioxidant idebenone (listed on the ingredient list as hydroxydecyl ubiquinone). What is the difference, you ask, between the dermatologic version and the one sold at the Arden counter? The original Prevage formula is billed as "physician-strength" and contains 1% idebenone, while Arden's cosmetics-counter version contains 0.5% idebenone. The physician-strength angle is bogus because idebenone is not a drug of any kind, nor is it regulated or akin to any type of prescription treatment. There is no reason it can't be sold in any retail channel. Such positioning and exclusivity is clever marketing on Allergan's part (the company also distributes Botox and Latisse, and markets the M.D. Forte skin-care line). The study that showed idebenone has the antioxidant muscle to surpass others involved only 30 subjects, and compared idebenone to vitamins C and E, alpha lipoic acid, coenzyme Q10, and kinetin. The study did not, however, compare the effects of idebenone to many of the hundreds of other potent antioxidants that commonly appear in other skin-care products, nor did it compare the effects of idebenone with the effects of a combination of antioxidants. Perhaps a cocktail of antioxidants would far surpass idebenone—we don't know. The world of antioxidants is far more complex than the mere handful that Allergan compared to idebenone. To date, there are still no published, peer-reviewed studies that support idebenone's alleged superiority. This does not mean idebenone is not a valid antioxidant for skin. Given what we know about how ubiquinone performs in the body, it is definitely not a throwaway ingredient. What is fairly certain, however, is that it is neither the best nor the most potent antioxidant around. Comparing Allergan's original Prevage formula to Arden's is like comparing night and day. Arden's water-in-silicone version is silky-smooth, and with a formula that's nearly identical to that of Allergan's "medically positioned" (however inaccurate that is) Prevage MD. Both Prevage products are water-in-silicone serums that contain several skin-friendly ingredients, including glycerin, phospholipids, green tea, sodium hyaluronate, and algae. Which Prevage product to choose isn't a tough decision, given that efficacy levels for idebenone have not been established. The fact that Arden's product contains 50% less than the original Prevage is inconsequential, and there is no research proving that 1% idebenone is preferred to Arden's 0.5%. Is Arden's readily available version worth the money? Despite its elegant formula, the answer is "no." Considering that idebenone is not the definitive antioxidant and that many companies are producing antioxidant serums and lotions that contain a cocktail of antioxidants, Arden's price point is undeservedly high. The product is a worthwhile option, and the formula is suitable for all skin types—unless you're sensitive to fragrance. But money-wise, lots of companies have antioxidant-loaded products that cost less (in some cases, much less) and, due to their blend of antioxidants, potentially offer skin a greater complement of benefits. One last note: The mica in both Prevage products lends a slight shimmer to skin, which the companies describe as enhancing skin's radiance; it's just shine, nothing more.

☺ AVERAGE **Eight Hour Cream Skin Protectant** *($19.50 for 1.7 fl. oz.)* lands on many fashion magazines' "best of beauty" lists for its long-standing history and versatility. However, it's just a blend of emollients with fragrance, salicylic acid (incapable of exfoliating in this product because the pH is too high), plant oil, vitamin E, and preservatives. (So much for the validity of the "best" lists in fashion magazines!) Plain Vaseline, which makes up the bulk of this formula, would work just as well. One more thing: The "protectant" in the product name is especially misleading, since the best way to really protect skin is by using a product with an effective UVA/UVB sunscreen.

☺ AVERAGE $$$ **Ceramide Plump Perfect Ultra All Night Repair and Moisture Cream for Face and Throat** *($62 for 1.7 fl. oz.)* has a long ingredient list for a moisturizer for normal to dry skin, but almost all the beneficial ingredients are wasted due to the jar packaging. See the Appendix to learn why jar packaging is a problem. In better packaging, this moisturizer would be an easy, though pricey, one to recommend. One more comment: Despite containing some state-of-the-art ingredients, nothing in this moisturizer can lift, re-sculpt, or re-contour sagging skin.

☺ AVERAGE $$$ **Ceramide Plump Perfect Ultra Lift and Firm Moisture Cream SPF 30** *($68 for 1.7 fl. oz.)*. The chief anti-aging element of this daytime moisturizer for normal to dry skin is its sunscreen, which includes avobenzone for sufficient UVA protection. Beyond sun protection, this has an impressive roster of antioxidant vitamins, antioxidant-rich plant extracts, and skin-identical ingredients such as ceramides, lecithin, and phospholipids. Regrettably, this also contains clover flower, a plant extract that can cause irritation, as well as numerous fragrance ingredients known for their irritating properties. For these reasons, we cannot assign a higher rating to what's otherwise a very well-formulated daytime moisturizer with sunscreen.

☺ AVERAGE $$$ **Ceramide Premiere Intense Moisture and Renewal Overnight Regeneration Cream** *($95 for 1.7 fl. oz.)*. In so many ways this is a truly well-formulated moisturizer for dry skin. The emollients are excellent and it is stocked with skin-repairing ingredients. What it lacks is an impressive array (and greater amounts of) antioxidants necessary to reduce free-radical damage, which means you won't see as much collagen renewal as the product claims. What doesn't add up in comparison to the price tag is the jar packaging. Though it is beautiful, an attractive container doesn't translate to skin-care benefit. Jar packaging is a disaster because it won't keep the good ingredients stable (see the Appendix to understand the problems jar packaging creates). One other point: The only radiance this product provides is from the mica it contains. Mica is a shiny mineral used in thousands of products claiming to brighten skin. Other than the cosmetic benefit you may see after applying this product, shine particles don't have anything to do with skin care.

☺ AVERAGE $$$ **Ceramide Premier Intense Moisture Renewal Regeneration Eye Cream** *($68 for 0.5 fl. oz.)*. Giving up jar packaging is something many cosmetics companies refuse to do. They prefer selling formulas in attractive containers that have no ability to keep the ingredients they contain stable. It is well known among researchers and scientists that jar packaging is not only unsanitary, but also almost all beneficial ingredients break down in the presence of air. What a waste! Aside from the jar packaging that this fragrance-free eye cream comes in, you don't need a separate product labeled as an eye cream for your eye area. We know that sounds shocking, but check out the Appendix to see why you can save money giving up this erroneous belief. The formula is an emollient moisturizer for dry skin containing an impressive blend of skin-repairing ingredients, though it lacks an array of antioxidants that would really aid in building new collagen. It claims to replenish skin with sea minerals, but the small amount of *Fucus serratus* it contains (sea algae) isn't all that helpful for skin and there isn't any research showing what it provides, either. One other point: The only radiance this product provides is from the mica it contains. Mica is a shiny mineral used in thousands of products claiming to brighten skin. Other than the cosmetic benefit you may see after applying this product, shine particles don't have anything to do with skin care.

☺ AVERAGE $$$ **Intervene Anti-Fatigue Eye Cream** *($38.50 for 0.5 fl. oz.)* is another eye cream packaged in a jar, not what the world needs, but they just keep coming! You can check out the Appendix to find out why you don't need an eye cream and why jar packaging is something you should never buy. But what about the actual formula, can it help with dark circles and "fatigue"? From a makeup perspective, the silky, almost spackle-like texture of this eye cream can help improve the appearance of dark circles by creating a smoother surface. Smooth surfaces reflect light better, so shadowed areas appear less dark. This eye cream also contains the mineral pigment mica for shine, but shine isn't skin care; it's makeup. Adding shine isn't going to do much to make dark circles less apparent, and it may make wrinkles more noticeable. Arden included several fragrant plant extracts, all of which pose a risk of irritation, especially in the eye area. Irritating ingredients can hurt healthy collagen production, which isn't anti-aging in the least.

☺ AVERAGE $$$ **Intervene Stress Recovery Night Cream** *($49.50 for 1.7 fl. oz.)* is a relatively unimpressive moisturizer. It has the requisite silky texture and some mica that adds a soft shine to your skin, but it's disappointing that several state-of-the-art ingredients will have their potency muted due to jar packaging (see the Appendix to learn why jar packaging is a problem). An intriguing ingredient in this product is Teprenone, which is described as an active ingredient whose multiple functions include limiting skin-cell senescence (cell death). As it turns out, this ingredient is a drug that Arden appears to be using off-label (meaning it is really a pharmaceutical), which my research indicates is against FDA regulations. Teprenone is the brand name for a drug known as geranylgeranylacetone, which is used to treat gastric ulcers and is being researched as an option for slowing age-related hearing loss (Sources: *Brain Research*, May 2008, pages 9–17; and *Digestion*, October 2007, pages 215–224). What do hearing loss and ulcers have to do with aging skin? One of the key ways geranylgeranylacetone works is by influencing heat shock proteins. These proteins help other proteins interact as they should at the cellular level, which affects many systems in the body. Heat shock proteins are most active during times of stress, such as exposure to cigarette smoke and exposure to sunlight. When heat shock proteins are reduced (which is ultimately what you want because that means reducing inflammation), cells appear to live longer. I suppose Arden theorized that geranylgeranyl acetone (as Teprenone) may also have a helpful effect when applied topically.

After all, the skin is a source of heat shock proteins, and it is certainly exposed to enough stressful situations where an ingredient that helps these proteins function more efficiently would be a benefit. However, there's no research proving that topically applied geranylgeranylacetone has any effect on heat shock proteins within skin. Moreover, as previously mentioned, Arden is using a drug ingredient in a cosmetic product, which means the consumer is the guinea pig. For that reason, Intervene Stress Recovery Night Cream is not a product we can recommend, though the formula doesn't deserve a Poor rating.

☺ AVERAGE $$$ **Prevage Day Intensive Anti-Aging Moisture Cream SPF 30** (*$129 for 1.7 fl. oz.*) is an exceedingly overpriced daytime moisturizer with sunscreen for normal to dry skin. It gets the important issue of UVA protection right thanks to the inclusion of stabilized avobenzone, and the base formula is creamy and provides enough emollients to keep those with dry skin happy. In addition to the problem expensive moisturizers with sunscreen presents—that is, given the cost, you're not likely to apply it liberally enough to get the rated protection—the antioxidants this contains, including the publicized idebenone, won't remain stable because this is packaged in a jar, which is ludicrous. Please see the Appendix for details on the problems jar packaging presents. As for the claims, there is no published, substantiated research proving that idebenone (listed as hydroxydecyl ubiquinoyl dipalmitoyl glycerate) is the best antioxidant. Even the concept is silly, because there are hundreds of brilliant antioxidants for skin, and comparisons among different antioxidants are few and far between.

☺ AVERAGE $$$ **Prevage Night Anti-Aging Restorative Cream** (*$132 for 1.7 fl. oz.*) attempts to carry on the theme that idebenone (listed on the package as hydroxydecyl ubiquinoyl dipalmitoyl glycerate) is the best antioxidant to exert an anti-aging, reparative effect on skin. See the review for Prevage Day Ultra Protection Anti-Aging Moisturizer SPF 30 PA ++ for more details. What cannot be ignored, however, is the jar packaging, a bad decision that means the key antioxidants, including idebenone, won't remain stable during use (see the Appendix for further details), which makes this a poor choice all around.

☹ POOR **Ceramide Time Complex Moisture Cream SPF 15** (*$52 for 1.7 fl. oz.*) lacks the UVA-protecting ingredients of titanium dioxide, zinc oxide, avobenzone, Tinosorb, or Mexoryl SX, and is not recommended. Without getting this step right, no daytime moisturizer can legitimately be called "anti-aging."

☹ POOR **Intervene Radiance Boosting Moisture Cream SPF 15** (*$49 for 1.7 fl. oz.*). The only radiance this product provides is from the mica it contains. Mica is a shiny mineral used in thousands of products claiming to brighten skin. Other than the cosmetic benefit you may see after applying this product and the beautiful jar packaging (it really is stunning), there isn't much reason to consider using this moisturizer. Keep in mind that pretty packaging and a shiny ingredient isn't skin care. You do get UVA sun protection from the avobenzone it contains, but it lacks octocrylene, which is one of the ingredients that helps keep avobenzone stable (and based on the formula, we're not sure what Arden is using to keep the avobenzone stable). Also the SPF 15 is the minimum required for adequate sun protection; it has become standard among dermatologists to recommend higher SPF numbers to be sure you're getting enough sun protection (because most of us aren't applying enough sunscreen each day). As far as moisturizing benefits are concerned, this is nicely formulated for barrier repair ingredients and the urea provides exfoliation. However, it would have been far better with an array of antioxidants. A major disappointment is the jar packaging, which won't keep the good ingredients in here stable. Another drawback is the amount of fragrance this contains. Wafting aroma isn't skin care and, in fact, can cause irritation, which is a problem for skin. (See the Appendix to find out why fragrance and jar packaging are problems). Overall, this moisturizer has more drawbacks than benefits.

☹ POOR **Prevage Eye Ultra Protection Anti-Aging Moisturizer SPF 15 PA++** *($100 for 0.5 fl. oz.)*. The notion that there is one antioxidant that is better than all others is absolutely not true. Current research makes it 100% clear that skin can benefit from a wide range of antioxidants, along with other beneficial ingredients, so buying a product with one showcased ingredient, however hyped, is really shortchanging your skin. Aside from the idebenone hype, this eye cream with sunscreen is a big disappointment. Not only is it exceedingly overpriced (remember, you must apply sunscreen liberally to get the SPF protection on the label), but also the sunscreen portion fails to provide sufficient UVA protection because it doesn't contain the UVA-protecting ingredients of avobenzone, Tinosorb, zinc oxide, titanium dioxide, or ecamsule (Mexoryl SX). That means your eye area will remain vulnerable to wrinkles and other signs of aging. Last, you don't need an eye cream! There is no research proving that the skin around the eye area needs something different from skin elsewhere on the face, jaw, or chest (see Appendix for details). What you get when you buy an eye cream like this is a small container of product (often half the size of a container of face product) that is twice as expensive. One more point: To add insult to injury, this eye cream is packaged in a jar, so any of the good ingredients will not remain stable because they deteriorate in the presence of air, and jar packaging lets air in every time you open it. What an expensive mistake!

ELIZABETH ARDEN LIP & SMILE CARE

☹ POOR **Eight Hour Cream Lip Protectant Stick SPF 15** *($19.50 for 0.13 fl. oz.)* won't protect lips from the sun's UVA rays because it lacks any of the UVA-protecting ingredients of titanium dioxide, zinc oxide, avobenzone, Tinosorb, or Mexoryl SX. In addition, the sheer colors can't provide the physical-type block that opaque lipsticks offer, so this product is not recommended.

ELIZABETH ARDEN SPECIALTY SKIN-CARE PRODUCTS

☺ GOOD $$$ **Prevage Clarity Targeted Skin Tone Corrector** *($125 for 1 fl. oz.)* is a specialty skin-care product that promises to provide even skin tone, but, unfortunately, it doesn't deliver in the way the claims assert. This doesn't instantly fade discolorations, and even over the long run, the results likely will disappoint, especially if you don't use this religiously with a sunscreen during the day. With a lightweight, silky, serum-like texture, it does contain some very good antioxidants and a form of vitamin C (ascorbyl glucoside) that has a small amount of research showing it can be helpful for improving skin discolorations, but we don't know how much is needed in skin-care products to obtain results. Still, it's a helpful antioxidant and the formula contains some good moisture-binding ingredients, too. This also contains a blend of shiny pigments and other coloring agents to visibly "brighten" skin, but that's a makeup effect, not skin care. Whether or not you want to pay this much for benefits that are more in line with makeup than with skin care is up to you, but we don't recommend it. This product definitely contains some good skin-care ingredients, but if an uneven skin tone and/or brown discolorations are your concern, this isn't the most exciting solution.

ELIZABETH ARDEN FOUNDATIONS

✓☺ BEST $$$ **Pure Finish Mineral Tinted Moisturizer SPF 15** *($30)*. Forget the mineral portion of this product's name—that's just Arden jumping on the mineral makeup bandwagon. Besides, there is nothing particularly "mineral" about this makeup. Nonetheless, this tinted moisturizer is worthy of your attention for better reasons, starting with its in-part titanium dioxide sunscreen. The texture is light yet creamy and the finish decidedly moist, almost to the point of being glow-y, but this doesn't contain obvious shimmer. You'll get sheer to light coverage on par with what most tinted moisturizers provide. Formula-wise, it's a nice touch that this contains some skin identical ingredients and antioxidants, while also being fragrance-free. It is best for normal to dry skin, and all the shades are worth considering.

☺ GOOD **$$$ Ceramide Ultra Lift and Firm Makeup SPF 15** ($42) cannot lift your skin in the least. Sagging skin cannot be corrected by skin-care or makeup products. We wish that weren't the case, but it's true. The numerous factors that lead to sagging (sun damage, muscle laxity, bone loss, fat pads shifting, and gravity) cannot be addressed by skin-care products; you need cosmetic corrective procedures for genuine improvement. Lifting claim aside, this foundation offers a soft, lightweight cream texture that's a breeze to blend. Its subtle satin finish enlivens skin without adding shine, and it has only a slight tendency to slip into lines around the eye. Coverage is in the light to medium range, and this builds without looking heavy over areas that may need a bit more camouflage. The mostly neutral shade range is extensive and offers options for fair to tan skin tones; the best shades are those for fair to light skin. Avoid the ashy rose Mocha II, the rosy Cameo, and the slightly pink Cream, which will only emphasize a ruddy complexion. The only drawback is the jar packaging. Normally that's not a problem for a foundation because most foundations do not contain light- or air-sensitive ingredients. However, this one includes several antioxidants and a handful of other ingredients that don't hold up well when constantly exposed to air (oxygen) and light. The Good rating pertains to this foundation's overall performance; in different, opaque packaging, this would earn our highest recommendation.

☺ GOOD **$$$ Flawless Finish Mousse Makeup** ($33) is the original mousse foundation. It's packaged in a metal can that uses a propellant to distribute an airy, bubbly, flesh-toned foam, which blends on better than you might expect, though you might end up wasting some product until you get used to the dispensing method. Coverage is sheer, and the texture has enough slip to allow for adequate blending. This dries to a soft matte finish and is an option for normal to slightly oily or dry skin. If you're prone to breakouts, you will appreciate the absence of potentially pore-clogging thickening agents in this formula. Nine shades are on hand, including some great colors for fair skin tones, but avoid Melba, Bisque, and Natural. Ginger is slightly pink, and should be considered carefully.

☹ AVERAGE **$$$ Flawless Finish Bare Perfection Makeup SPF 8** ($33). Although this has an SPF rating that's too low and is without adequate UVA protection, it is actually an impressive foundation suitable for normal to dry skin. With a smooth, moist texture and satin finish capable of delivering sheer to light coverage, it's worth a look, but it's not recommended over foundations that go the distance to protect skin with SPF 15. There are nine shades to consider, including a couple of good options for darker skin tones. The shades that should be avoided due to overtones of peach, orange, or pink are Cameo, Honey, Mocha II, and Fawn. Buff is slightly peach, but may work for some light skin tones.

☹ AVERAGE **$$$ Flawless Finish Dual Perfection Makeup SPF 8** ($33) is a talc-based pressed-powder foundation with a silky feel and a very smooth finish. The SPF rating is embarrassingly low—by itself this is a no-no for daytime—but the in-part titanium dioxide would add some extra protection if you paired it with an effective SPF 15 sunscreen. The formula works best for someone with normal to slightly dry or slightly oily skin, and most of the 12 colors are excellent. The only ones that should be avoided due to their peach casts are Buff and Cameo.

☺ AVERAGE **$$$ Intervene Makeup SPF 15** *($36)* is another look-younger-now foundation whose anti-aging claims are immediately discredited because the sunscreen does not provide sufficient UVA protection, one of the most significant aspects of keeping skin young. Arden, come on! Everything else about this foundation (well, almost everything—some of the shades arc duds) is outstanding, from its silky-smooth texture that provides light moisture to its satin finish suitable for normal to dry skin. Coverage goes from light to medium, and this offers plenty of time to blend before it sets. If you decide to try this (and doing so requires you to pair it with a broad-spectrum sunscreen rated SPF 15 or greater), the shade to avoid is Soft Cognac. Soft Shell and Soft Cameo are borderline pink and should be considered carefully.

ELIZABETH ARDEN CONCEALERS

✓☺ BEST **$$$ Ceramide Ultra Lift and Firm Concealer** *($19.50)* is a creamy concealer that sets to a soft matte finish and blends effortlessly on skin. It camouflages skin imperfections such as dark circles, redness, and blemishes with medium to full coverage and stays put throughout the day. All the colors are excellent and best for fair to medium skin tones. See the Appendix to find out why the lifting claims this concealer mentions won't come true.

☺ GOOD **$$$ Flawless Finish Maximum Coverage Concealer** *($18)* is excellent in most respects! Although the maximum coverage claim is open to debate, without question this cream concealer housed in a sleek compact is an extremely smooth option whose slightly thick texture is a pleasure to blend. It doesn't magnify pores or dry patches (but those with dry skin will want to prep with moisturizer or serum) and it provides medium to nearly full coverage with a beautiful, skin-like finish. Its only drawbacks are that it creases slightly into lines around the eye and tends to fade after a few hours of wear. Arden offers three shades, all of them wonderfully neutral. The darkest shade (Deep) isn't for truly dark skin tones, but the lighter shades are workable for fair to medium skin tones. This concealer is great for disguising dark circles as well as for muting redness or minor discolorations, although its creamier formula makes it iffy for use over acne-prone areas.

ELIZABETH ARDEN BLUSHES & BRONZER

✓☺ BEST **$$$ Ceramide Cream Blush** *($24)* is a cream blush with a subtle satin finish, but it is pricey, but a little goes a long way. Color payoff is remarkable, but this is easy to blend without having it slip into areas where blush shouldn't be. Best for normal to dry skin that's not prone to blemishes, it comes in four beautiful shades that add translucent vibrancy to your cheeks.

☺ AVERAGE **$$$ Color Intrigue Cheekcolor** *($22)* is a collection of pressed-powder blushes, each with a slightly dry, grainy texture and sheer, blendable application. Every shade has some amount of shine, but the truly underwhelming texture doesn't make this worth considering over blushes rated with a Good rating or greater.

☹ POOR **Color Intrigue Bronzing Powder Duo** *($32)* is a talc-based, pressed-powder bronzer that features two shiny colors in one compact. Each shade has a dry, slightly grainy texture but sheer application. The overall performance doesn't come close to matching the price, and this makes it not worth considering over countless other bronzing powders.

ELIZABETH ARDEN POWDERS

☺ GOOD **$$$ Ceramide Skin Smoothing Loose Powder** *($30)* is a talc-based loose powder containing several ceramides, but in a powder we're skeptical that the benefits of those ingredients are helpful given that the packaging isn't airtight. For aesthetics it has an obviously shiny finish. If you're OK with or want a very shiny loose powder, this does have a gossamer texture, weightless finish, and comes in four workable shades that go on translucent.

☺ GOOD **$$$ Flawless Finish Ultra Smooth Pressed Powder** *($24.50)* competes nicely with other talc-based pressed powders that leave a silky, sheer, real-skin finish rather than looking dry or chalky. It comes in four shades, though each is so sheer the color is almost a non-issue. One more thing: This deposits so minimally on skin that someone with very oily areas will be disappointed and need to find a more absorbent powder.

ELIZABETH ARDEN EYESHADOWS & EYE PRIMERS

✓☺ BEST **Color Intrigue Eyeshadow** *($15)* is ideal. Each shade has a wonderful, satin matte, non-powdery finish and a texture that blends and layers beautifully. Every shade has at least a touch of shine, but the good news is the shiniest shades leave more of a sheen than glitter or sparkles, and these shadows don't flake.

✓☺ BEST **$$$ Color Intrigue Eyeshadow Duo** *($24.50)* is a powder eyeshadow with a very smooth texture and beautifully even application that blends well and provides ample color saturation. Each duo has shine, but in most cases it's more of a soft sheen than all-out sparkles. Regrettably, most of the color pairs aren't the easiest to work with. The best duos are Pink Clover and Autumn Leaves.

☺ GOOD **Color Intrigue Eyeshadow Quad** *($29.50)* shares the same formulary and application traits as the single Eyeshadow above, but here you get four shades in one compact. We wish the color combinations were more thoughtful; the quads we saw weren't the easiest shades to work with, and all were very shiny. The shades tend to change seasonally, so keep your eyes open for an attractive grouping where you can realistically use more than two colors!

☹ AVERAGE **Advanced Eye-Fix Primer** *($21.50 for 0.25 fl. oz.)* is supposed to be a sheer cream for the eyelid to prevent makeup creasing; it's basically water, silicone, talc, and wax. Forget this boring, superfluous product and just use a good matte finish concealer, which would work as well, if not better, than this product.

ELIZABETH ARDEN EYE & BROW LINERS

☹ AVERAGE **$$$ Color Intrigue Eyeliner** *($16)* wins points for being an automatic, retractable pencil with an easy-glide application, but because it stays creamy you'll find that it fades and smears easily. All the shades have a slight to strong metallic finish, which can be a fun departure, though perhaps too distracting for day-to-day wear. If you decide to try this, it works best to create a smoky eye, rather than a long-lasting line.

☹ AVERAGE **$$$ Smoky Eyes Powder Pencil** *($16.50)* is definitely powdery, and best used to draw a thick line that you then smudge for a smoky appearance; otherwise this will smudge on its own. It needs routine sharpening but applies without pulling or tugging—always a plus.

☹ POOR **Dual Perfection Brow Shaper and Eyeliner** *($18)* has a dry, grainy texture and is meant to be used wet, yet once dry the powder tends to flake. There are much easier, longer-lasting ways to shape and define the eyebrow and line the eye.

ELIZABETH ARDEN LIP COLOR & LIPLINERS

✓☺ BEST **$$$ Color Intrigue Effects Lipstick** *($19.50)* comes in almost two dozen shades. The color selection favors bolder, shimmer-infused colors, and includes some decadent reds and rich browns. As for the lipstick itself, it is creamy-smooth without feeling a bit slick or greasy. This is one of the few creamier lipsticks that won't immediately creep into lines around the mouth, and it sets to a semi-matte finish that allows for reasonably long wear (it helps that these lipsticks have lots of pigment, too!).

☺ GOOD $$$ **Ceramide Ultra Lipstick** *($22.50)* is a creamy lipstick that goes on velvety smooth and comes in an extensive shade range that includes gorgeous berry, red, pink, and nude beige hues. Elizabeth Arden included an impressive mix of skin-identical ingredients, antioxidants, and cell-communicating ingredients, but in this type of container many of those ingredients won't remain stable; as a result they'll provide limited to no benefit. This lipstick doesn't make lips look any fuller or plumper than any other good creamy lipstick.

☺ GOOD **High Shine Lip Gloss** *($15)* doesn't distinguish itself as a "must-have" lip gloss, but it's a workable option with a medium-thick texture and slightly sticky finish. The sheer shades are infused with sparkles, and luckily they don't make lips feel grainy as the moisturizing effect wears off.

☹ AVERAGE $$$ **Smooth Line Lip Pencil** *($16)* is a standard, needs-sharpening pencil that slides over lips without tugging or skipping. It is more creamy than greasy, and would have been rated higher if routine sharpening weren't required. Arden included a lip brush on the opposite end of the pencil, and it's surprisingly good.

☹ POOR **Crystal Clear Lip Gloss** *($14)* is a very thick, sticky gloss that is flavored with spearmint, which tastes nice but can be irritating for the lips.

ELIZABETH ARDEN MASCARAS

✓☺ BEST $$$ **Ceramide Lash Extending Treatment Mascara** *($20)*. Arden is playing up this mascara by mentioning their ceramide complex, which is said to lengthen, define, and revitalize lashes. Although this contains some ingredients not seen in many other mascaras, the ceramides compose only a small part of the formula. They likely have some conditioning benefit for lashes, but this isn't lash revitalization in a tube and ceramides can't grow or change lashes in any way. The ingredients that lengthen and define lashes are standard and, of course, the brush plays an even more important role in how mascara applies than almost any other part of the product. In this case, claims notwithstanding, you will be impressed with the clean, swift application that lengthens and separates lashes evenly. Unless you were trying for mondo thickness, we can't imagine someone being disappointed with this mascara's performance, and it leaves lashes feeling soft.

☺ GOOD $$$ **Double Density Maximum Volume Mascara** *($19)* is a mascara whose name conflicts with the actual results you'll notice. This isn't a poor mascara—far from it. But if your definition of "dramatically" thickened lashes is textbook, you'll see that this mascara is primarily about clump-free lengthening. You will get some thickness, with effort, but not an effect most people would call dramatic. This mascara is worth trying if your expectations are not as lofty as Arden's claims.

ELIZABETH ARDEN BRUSHES

✓☺ BEST **Face Powder Brush** *($28)* is a synthetic hair brush that's exceptionally soft and dense. It's ideal for applying all types of powder, including powder foundations. The slightly angled cut allows the brush to easily fit the contours of the face. As a bonus, Arden includes a tiny version of this brush that's so small as to be impractical, but we suppose it's OK in a pinch.

ELIZABETH ARDEN SPECIALTY MAKEUP PRODUCTS

☺ AVERAGE $$$ **Advanced Lip-Fix Cream** *($21.50 for 0.5 fl. oz.)* is supposed to prevent lipstick from feathering. Packaged in a tube, it goes on like a moisturizer and must dry before

The Reviews E

you put on your lipstick, which is not convenient for touch-ups during the day. Anti-feathering products that come in lipstick or lipliner forms mean there's no waiting between applications, and you don't need to remove what you have on to reapply more, and those options make Arden's version less enticing.

ESTEE LAUDER

Strengths: Some of the most state-of-the-art moisturizers and serums around; excellent sunscreens; some good cleansers, toners, and makeup removers; several categories of makeup excel, including some extraordinary foundations (that include shades for darker skin tones), concealers, powders, blush, and eyeshadows; a mostly good selection of eye, brow, and lip pencils; their long-wearing lip color and some of the lipsticks (including Double Wear) are supremely good.

Weaknesses: Several items are highly fragranced; incomplete and/or problematic products for anyone battling blemishes; no effective AHA or BHA products; many of the Re-Nutriv products are priced too high given similar, less expensive options from Lauder; some of the sunscreens and foundations with sunscreen lack sufficient UVA protection; the mascaras; the brushes aren't on par with those from other Lauder-owned lines, such as Bobbi Brown or M.A.C.; some superfluous specialty products and problem pencils; jar packaging.

For more information and reviews of the latest Estee Lauder products, visit CosmeticsCop.com.

ESTEE LAUDER CLEANSERS

✓☺ BEST **$$$ Verite LightLotion Cleanser** *($23.50 for 6.7 fl. oz.)* is an emollient, cold cream–style cleanser that is an option for someone with dry, sensitive, or reddened skin not prone to breakouts. Its merit for sensitive skin earns its Best Product rating.

☺ GOOD **$$$ Perfectly Clean Light Lotion Cleanser** *($23 for 6.7 fl. oz.)* is a water-based emollient cleansing lotion that does not contain detergent cleansing agents, so it is a good option for dry to very dry skin. This product can do a reasonably good job of removing makeup, but you may need to pair it with a washcloth or wipe it off altogether to ensure complete removal.

☺ GOOD **$$$ Re-Nutriv Intensive Hydrating Creme Cleanser** *($45 for 4.2 fl. oz.)* is an emollient, creamy cleanser for dry to very dry skin. It's pricey for what you get, but will hydrate and remove makeup efficiently (though not without the aid of a washcloth).

☺ GOOD **$$$ Soft Clean Moisture Rich Foaming Cleanser** *($20 for 4.2 fl. oz.)* is a creamy, cushiony cleanser whose potassium-derived cleansing base can produce a copious foam, although that has little to do with a product's cleansing abilities. This can be a good, water-soluble cleanser for normal to slightly dry or slightly oily skin. It contains more fragrance than Lauder's other cleansers.

☺ GOOD **$$$ Soft Clean Tender Creme Cleanser** *($20 for 4.2 fl. oz.)* is a standard cleansing cream for normal to dry skin. It does not contain detergent cleansing agents, but it can remove most types of makeup without the aid of a washcloth. Used around the eyes (to remove eye makeup or mascara), it can leave a greasy film that is not preferred, especially when compared with a silicone-based makeup remover or water-soluble cleanser.

☹ AVERAGE **$$$ Nutritious Purifying 2-in-1 Foam Cleanser** *($20 for 4.2 fl. oz.)* is a foaming cleanser that contains some plant oil and extracts that are nutritious when consumed

---

Ɫ Lavender oil smells great, but fragrance isn't skin care! Find out why in the Appendix.

as part of a healthy diet, but have no effect when massaged over skin and quickly rinsed off. Some of the potassium-based cleansing agents in this product are constituents of soap and as such they can be drying unless your skin is oily to very oily. This cleanser is an effective makeup remover.

☺ AVERAGE $$$ **Perfectly Clean Splash Away Foaming Cleanser** *($20 for 4.2 fl. oz.)* lists alkaline and drying potassium myristate as the main cleansing agent, so this will be a problem cleanser for all skin types except very oily. It does remove makeup completely, but is nearly akin to washing with standard bar soap.

☹ POOR **Sparkling Clean Oil-Control Foaming Gel Cleanser** *($23 for 6.7 fl. oz.)* is a somewhat drying water-soluble cleanser that would have been an option for oily skin, but the inclusion of irritating menthyl lactate makes it a less than sparkling option.

☹ POOR **Sparkling Clean Purifying Mud Foam Cleanser** *($20 for 4.2 fl. oz.)* is a water-soluble foaming cleanser that contains soap-based potassium myristate as its main cleansing agent. It can be drying for all but very oily skin, especially with the "mud" (clay) thrown in. The deal-breaker is the addition of irritating menthyl lactate, which won't purify skin in the least.

ESTEE LAUDER EYE-MAKEUP REMOVERS

☺ GOOD **Take It Away Total Makeup Remover** *($23 for 6.7 fl. oz.)* is a water and wax concoction with a lotion texture that does an efficient job of removing most makeup without irritating skin.

☺ GOOD $$$ **Gentle Eye Makeup Remover** *($15.50 for 3.4 fl. oz.)* is a very standard, but effective, fragrance-free, detergent-based eye-makeup remover. Several less expensive versions at the drugstore easily replace this, but it's an option if you want to spend more.

☺ GOOD $$$ **Take It Away LongWear Makeup Remover Towelettes** *($18 for 45 towelettes)* feature a formula that is remarkably similar to that of the Gentle Eye Makeup Remover above, only steeped into disposable towelettes. This product is not adept at removing long-wearing or waterproof makeup and ideally should be rinsed from skin because, left on, the detergent cleansing agent can be drying.

ESTEE LAUDER TONERS

☺ GOOD $$$ **Re-Nutriv Intensive Softening Lotion** *($45 for 8.4 fl. oz.)* has a lot to benefit all skin types, including antioxidants and cell-communicating ingredients. If you're going to spend a lot of money on a toner, this option has visible rewards! A couple of cautions: Lauder included gold in this product, likely to reinforce their marketing of Re-Nutriv as luxury skin care. If you have metal allergies (such as to nickel), this may be a problem; research has shown those with nickel allergies often have a similar though less-intense response to skin contact with other metals, including gold (Source: *Clinical and Experimental Immunology*, December 2006, pages 417–426). The second concern is the clear plastic bottle packaging. Once you have this at home, you must store it away from light sources to protect the efficacy of the antioxidants and plant extracts. Do not leave this sitting on your vanity counter.

☺ GOOD $$$ **Soft Clean Silky Hydrating Lotion** *($21.50 for 6.7 fl. oz.)* is one of the most original and skin-beneficial toners in the Estee Lauder line, and would be a great option for normal to dry skin. It is alcohol-free and contains mostly water, silicone, thickener, slip agent, plant extracts (including fragrant floral extracts), skin-identical ingredients, emollient, anti-irritant, Vaseline, film-forming agent, fragrance, and preservatives. The tiny amount of caffeine is unlikely to be a problem, but this toner is a bit too fragrant for someone with very sensitive skin.

☹ POOR **Perfectly Clean Fresh Balancing Lotion** *($21.50 for 6.7 fl. oz.)* won't balance your skin in the least. It's mostly water and slip agent with plant extracts. Some of the plants are fragrant and serve no benefit for skin while others have anti-inflammatory activity. That's nice, but the anti-inflammatory plants will be fighting against the irritation caused by the menthol in this toner. In short, it's not recommended.

☹ POOR **Sparkling Clean Mattifying Oil-Control Lotion** *($21.50 for 6.7 fl. oz.)* lists alcohol as the second ingredient, which is drying and irritating for skin, plus it stimulates oil production at the base of your pores. This also contains the alkaline ingredient barium sulfate, which is a potential skin irritant. Keep in mind that you can't "dry up" oil because it isn't wet. Drying ingredients also negatively affect skin cells, and that doesn't help skin in the least. Products such as Paula's Choice Shine Stopper Instant Matte Finish work much better to control shine.

ESTEE LAUDER SCRUB

☺ AVERAGE $$$ **Idealist Dual-Action Refinishing Treatment** *($49.50 for 2.5 fl. oz.)* is really just a scrub with a fancy name, said to combine the benefits of microdermabrasion with a 30% glycolic acid (AHA) peel. Interestingly, the formula doesn't contain any AHAs; instead, it contains acetyl glucosamine and salicylic acid, which is a BHA. Acetyl glucosamine doesn't have convincing research proving its exfoliating ability (only the Lauder companies seem to think it works in this manner), and the salicylic acid cannot exfoliate because the product pH is well above 4. The pH is above 4 because the main ingredient is magnesium sulfate, which when mixed with water forms a solution with a pH of approximately 6 (Source: drugs.com). The warming sensation on your skin is the result of a chemical reaction that occurs when magnesium sulfate is mixed with water. The warmth may feel nice and may make you think it's doing something for your skin, but it doesn't do a thing; it's just a high school chemistry class demonstration. Lauder claims this product opens pores, but pores cannot be opened and closed like window blinds, although this myth perpetuates like so many others. If anything, the heat this product generates can cause capillaries to surface and that can be a problem. In no way is this product similar to any 30% AHA peel; in fact, it isn't even close to being a good scrub. The silicone in this product makes it difficult to rinse, but it does leave a smooth finish.

ESTEE LAUDER MOISTURIZERS (DAYTIME & NIGHTTIME), EYE CREAMS, & SERUMS

✓☺ BEST $$$ **Advanced Night Repair Concentrate Recovery Boosting Treatment** *($85 for 1 fl. oz.)* serves as a partner product to Lauder's enduring Advanced Night Repair serum. This concentrated version (supposedly with five times the amount of patented recovery complex than the original Advanced Night Repair) is meant to be used for three weeks, after which you revert to your usual routine of applying original Advanced Night Repair. Considering that the price for the Concentrate is double that of the original Advanced Night Repair, you may wonder if this allegedly more potent version is worth the upgrade. It turns out that the formulas are similar in some ways, but the differences are notable enough to definitely make Advanced Night Repair Concentrate the superior product, and not only for three weeks. Its silicone content gives the Concentrate a silkier texture than the original, but the big difference is in the larger amount of antioxidants Lauder packed into the Concentrate version. This is enough of a difference to consider the original antiquated. Whether or not the extras are worth the money is up to you (Paula's Choice RESIST Super Antioxidant Concentrate Serum is a brilliant alternative to this for a fraction of the price). Clinique offers serums that are just as well-formulated. A major ingredient in the Advanced Night Repair Concentrate and in the original

Advanced Night Repair is bifida ferment lysate. The bifida portion refers to bifidobacteria, a strain of bacteria found in the human body and believed to provide immune protection and prevent gastrointestinal problems (in other words, it's a friendly strain of bacteria). How does it relate to skin care? Claims made for this ingredient are that it can do for the face what it does for the body, enhance the immune system and decrease bad bacteria. There is no published information establishing that to be true. Oral consumption of this bacteria (it is often present in yogurt and can be purchased in supplement form) has a couple of studies that show it can be of benefit in helping with infant eczema, but that's about it when it comes to skin (Source: naturaldatabase.com).

✓☺ BEST **Nutritious Vita-Mineral Moisture Lotion** *($38 for 1.7 fl. oz.)* isn't any more "nutritious" for your skin than any other well-formulated moisturizer, but it contains the usual Lauder assortment of beneficial ingredients. Skin is treated to a lightweight, slightly creamy texture that is best for those whose complexion is normal to dry (this is too emollient for oily areas). Several antioxidants are included plus cell-communicating ingredients and some intriguing water-binding agents. The minerals in this product are scant and do not offer protection against irritants (my goodness, what claim isn't attached to minerals these days?), but the combination of ingredients in this moisturizer will strengthen skin's barrier and help it to become healthier.

✓☺ BEST $$$ **Nutritious Vita-Mineral Radiance Serum** *($40 for 1 fl. oz.)* is very similar to other serums from Lauder owned brands. The mix of bells and whistles differs between the serums, with Lauder's Nutritious containing more food-based ingredients such as soy, pomegranate, and corn. However, both serums are shining examples of how to formulate a state-of-the-art product that treats all skin types to many of the ingredients they need to maintain and ensure healthy functioning. Antioxidants and cell-communicating ingredients are present in appreciable amounts, which is what you want to see in a serum at any price point. This serum cannot increase natural cell turnover, so don't mistake it for an exfoliant. This does contain fragrance, while several other serums from Lauder brands do not.

✓☺ BEST $$$ **Perfectionist [CP + R] Wrinkle Lifting/Firming Serum** *($65 for 1 fl. oz.)*. This reformulation of Lauder's former Perfectionist [CP+] adds an "R" to the product name but otherwise not much has changed. The CP + R stands for correct, prevent, and repair; those who used the previous formula won't notice a big difference from this updated version, but it remains a formidable, ultra-silky serum to consider in the battle against signs of aging. Unlike the previous version, the [CP + R] formula is a bit thinner and perhaps a touch silkier and less fragrant. The updated version still contains silicones (lots of them, which is why this feels so amazingly silky). It's easy to spread and sets quickly to a smooth, slightly powdery finish. Otherwise, the same comments we made for the previous version of Perfectionist [CP +] apply here, too: This rated highly not on the basis of its wrinkle-dashing or lifting claims but because it contains numerous skin-repairing ingredients and plenty of antioxidants that help improve the way skin looks and feels. In that sense, which is what matters most for your skin, Perfectionist [CP+ R] Wrinkle Lifting/Firming Serum is a powerhouse option for all skin types (but those with dry skin should be aware this is NOT a hydrating serum). Just like the previous version of Perfectionist serum, Lauder claims it's their most effective wrinkle-fighting formula ever (if that's the case, why are they also selling numerous other ultra-pricey antiwrinkle/ lifting products in their Re-Nutriv line or La Mer line?) because it begins stimulating collagen production in just two hours. There's no proof of that (Lauder never makes their research available for public scrutiny), but we do know that when skin is protected from sun damage and treated to the ingredients it needs to restore and defend itself, it will make plenty of healthy collagen on its own (skin loves making collagen and would do so in a controlled, manner if we would just stop preventing that from taking place). It's not as though you can begin using this serum and within weeks your skin will have generated so much collagen that even the deeper, etched wrinkles will be a thing of the past. Besides, if this serum were as adept at generating collagen as claimed that would eventually be to your skin's detriment; too much collagen can result in bumpy skin that doesn't move naturally. Don't forget, excess collagen production is the basis of many scars, including surgical incision scars and deep wounds. Perfectionist [CP + R] is supposed to blur and smooth lines with its "flexible elastomer" which is a fancy way of saying this serum contains a polymer that works to temporarily fill in superficial lines by forming a flexible, invisible mesh (sort of like a girdle) on your skin's surface. Such technology and ingredients aren't unique to Lauder; you'll find it in similar serums that make firming or lifting claims; however, the effect is always temporary and how long it lasts depends on how expressive you are. Despite some anti-aging claims that still qualify as over-the-top, there's no question that this is a sophisticated formula that does an excellent job of combining and supplying skin with a wide complement of beneficial ingredients. Some of those ingredients can notably improve your skin's appearance, and, yes, reduce the signs of aging, including, to some extent, wrinkles. If you're looking for peptides, this serum contains them, but they're certainly not front and center. Perhaps this is Lauder's way of acknowledging that peptides aren't the antiwrinkle wonder many companies make them out to be. They do have theoretical cell-communicating ability, but whether or not they can last in skin long enough to penetrate to where they could do the most good is unlikely. This serum does contain mineral pigments that cast a subtle ethereal glow, but that is a cosmetic effect not a skin care benefit. As with most Lauder products, it is fragranced. Note: A 1.7-ounce size is also available; it retails for $95.

✓☺ BEST **$$$ Re-Nutriv Intensive Lifting Serum** *($185 for 1 fl. oz.)* boasts some lofty anti-aging claims, but does this live up to that lofty assertion? Without question, there are some extraordinary ingredients in this fragranced serum that can make a difference in the health, resilience, and appearance of skin (though your budget will suffer!). The packaging is such that the many antioxidants and the cell-communicating ingredients this contains will remain stable during use, but you don't need to spend this much to get the advantageous ingredients that make this silky-textured product a winner. Lauder's Advanced Night Repair Concentrate Recovery Boosting Treatment offers similar benefits (albeit with different textures), and Clinique has equally impressive options in their Repairwear line, all for a lot less money than Lauder's Re-Nutriv line. Should you decide to over-spend and purchase this serum, the base formula is preferred for normal to dry skin.

✓☺ BEST **$$$ Time Zone Line & Wrinkle Reducing Lotion SPF 15** *($58 for 1.7 fl. oz.)*. The curiosity about the Time Zone products comes from the attention-getting claim that they take 10 years off the look of your skin in 4 weeks. That would certainly grab our attention, but if you stop and think, it really isn't a claim we haven't heard before, from Lauder and numerous other lines. If your skin is rough and dry and you put a moisturizer on it, you're going to look younger, but it doesn't take this product to achieve that. Examining the ingredient list for this Time Zone product reveals it truly isn't different from most other daytime moisturizers with sunscreen, sold by Lauder and other companies. So do all of those take 10 years off, too? Our advice: Ignore the decade-erasing claim because it won't show up in the mirror no matter how long you use this product. It provides sufficient sun protection (which is the only legitimate wrinkle-reducing claim that can be made for this product) and it has a creamy texture suitable for normal to dry skin. However, unlike Lauder's other Time Zone moisturizers, which are packaged in jars, this is packaged in an opaque pump bottle. That means that in addition to an in-part avobenzone sunscreen, you're getting lots of antioxidants, cell-communicating ingredients, and some decent water-binding agents and they will remain stable once you start using it. The base formula isn't as light as many with combination skin would prefer, but it's acceptable and certainly worth a trial run. Despite our enthusiasm for the formula and the packaging, as mentioned, there isn't much difference between the Time Zone daytime moisturizers and those with sunscreen from Lauder's other sub-brands. If you're using DayWear or Resilience Lift with good results, there's no need to try Time Zone—it isn't the one group of Lauder products finally telling you the truth about youth in a bottle. And keep in mind that any well-formulated daytime moisturizer with sunscreen can do what this product claims to do (and we don't mean subtracting 10 or more years from your face): It can protect your skin from sun damage while allowing it to repair past damage (to an extent), and can encourage a healthy barrier function so your skin is better able to defend itself against future signs of aging. Now that's the kind of time zone we'd prefer to live in, and Lauder doesn't have a corner on this arena!

✓☺ BEST $$$ **Verite Special EyeCare** *($45 for 0.5 fl. oz.)* is a very emollient, water-based moisturizer that contains a good mix of skin-identical ingredients, antioxidants, and cell-communicating ingredients. Like all Verite products, this is fragrance-free. Despite the impressive rating, in truth you don't need a special product for the eye area (see the Appendix to find out why).

☺ GOOD $$$ **Advanced Night Repair Synchronized Recovery Complex** *($80 for 1.7 fl. oz.)* bears striking formulary similarities to the original Advanced Night Repair product (which has been discontinued). Both have the same base formula consisting of water, a type of friendly bacteria (bifida ferment lysate), slip agents, and thickener. The Synchronized Recovery Complex adds three new ingredients, which are discussed below. Needless to say, this serum isn't a must-have for anyone's skin and certainly doesn't break new ground for state-of-the-art products or for Lauder, either. We suspect Lauder simply realized (though what took them so long is anyone's guess) that their original Night Repair product was getting long in the tooth, especially when compared with their other offerings, and needed an update. One of the new ingredients is *Arabidopsis thaliana*, a small flowering plant that has in vitro research showing its protein fragments may enhance the skin's ability to protect itself from UVB damage. Preliminary research also suggests it may function as a cell-communicating ingredient; however, research on intact human skin is lacking and this plant is far from the only ingredient to offer these potential benefits (Sources: *Biochemistry*, April 2008, pages 4583–4596; and *FEBS Letters*, July 2007, pages 3356–3362). Tripeptide-32 is another new ingredient in this serum, and it also has research showing it, like many other peptides, has theoretical cell-communicating ability. It's theoretical because getting a peptide to reach its target site within the skin is difficult due to the presence of enzymes in skin that work to break down the peptide before it has a chance to work as claimed. However, tripeptide-32 appears to have a protective effect against proteins that damage cells, though there is no research proving it works when applied in small amounts to intact human skin (Sources: *Neuroscience Letters*, Volume 419, 2007, pages 247–252; and *Folia Pharmacologica Japonica*, Volume 129, 2007, page 18P). Still, it's a step in the right direction and clearly shows Lauder put some thought into the formula. The last new ingredient of note is lactobacillus ferment, another strain of friendly bacteria. Although this ingredient has multiple health benefits when consumed orally, there is no research proving its merit for topical application on skin (Source: naturaldatabase.com). All told, although this serum is an improvement over Lauder's original Advanced Night Repair product (and deserving of a good rating), it doesn't join the ranks of today's best serums and doesn't have what it takes to make good on its dramatic, reparative claims. This fragrance-free serum is suitable for all skin types, and leaves a slightly tacky finish on skin.

☺ GOOD **$$$ DayWear Advanced Multi-Protection Anti-Oxidant Lotion SPF 15** *($45 for 1.7 fl. oz.)* has a fluid, non-greasy texture and a lightweight feel on the skin. The sunscreen actives include avobenzone for reliable UVA (think anti-aging) protection, which is great. This is not a matte-finish sunscreen, and there's no way to guarantee it won't cause breakouts (this is true of all sunscreens), but it is worth auditioning if you have oily skin and have not been able to find a daytime moisturizer with sunscreen that works for you. The packaging will definitely keep the many antioxidants stable much longer than the jar-packaged DayWear Cremes, and this also contains some intriguing cell-communicating ingredients. Ordinarily, a product like this would earn our top rating; however, it contains fragrance ingredients known to cause irritation. The amounts are most likely too low to be cause for concern, but their presence is enough to keep this from the Best Products list.

☺ GOOD **$$$ Hydrationist Maximum Moisture Lotion** *($40 for 1.7 fl. oz.)* is part of Lauder's endless parade of moisturizers, though the claims aren't all that astounding or much different from what they've stated for dozens upon dozens of their other moisturizers. You'd think we'd get tired of the same old song, but it seems that with moisturizers, the tune continues, with few people noticing that the lyrics remain the same. Lauder states that moisture "is one of skin's key defenses against signs of aging that appear too soon," but when skin begins to show signs of aging (e.g., wrinkles, fine lines, or discolorations), what it needs is not more moisture, but more of the substances that help skin to maintain its moisture balance. Years of sun exposure (even if you use sunscreen) destroy the key components in skin that it needs to maintain its moisture balance, firmness, tone, skin color, and a host of other aspects of skin whose loss we associate with aging. In short, sun-damaged, irritated skin isn't able to retain its moisture reserves in an effort to look better. Of course, that's where a well-formulated moisturizer comes into play; it gives skin the substances that sun and environmental stressors have depleted. And, of course, when wrinkles are the concern, sun protection is critical, too. Everything about the Hydrationist moisturizers is designed to make skin look younger, just as many moisturizers claim to do. And without question, using any moisturizer over dry, wrinkled skin is going to make it look better. Whether you choose to improve your skin with Hydrationist or not is up to you, but it's important to note that this is the only Hydrationist moisturizer worth considering. The reason: Because every other Hydrationist moisturizer is packaged in a jar and that doesn't keep the worthwhile ingredients stable. This version is in far better packaging and as such the numerous antioxidants it contains will remain stable and effective during use. That's great news, but ideally Lauder should've used this type of packaging for every Hydrationist moisturizer. The Maximum Moisture Lotion formula is best for normal to slightly dry or slightly oily skin. It has a beautifully silky texture and works great under makeup (assuming your foundation contains sunscreen). This is not rated a Best Product because a few of the plant extracts have the potential to be irritating. The beneficial ingredients outweigh this risk, but it still deserves mention.

☺ GOOD **$$$ Idealist Cooling Eye Illuminator** *($58 for 0.5 fl. oz.)* is essentially a silky, thin-textured cream packaged in a small tube that's outfitted with an angled ceramic-tip applicator. The ceramic tip stays cool, so as you dispense the product and use the tip to massage it around your eye area, it feels refreshing. To some extent, the coolness of the tip can help reduce puffy eyes—at least the kind of puffiness that results from allergies or fluid retention, but only temporarily, until the irritation and swelling from those problems return. If your puffiness is age-related (meaning it's a result of fat pads beneath the skin slipping out of place, resulting in a pouched look), products like this have no effect. Of course, Lauder maintains this product is great for dark circles and wrinkles, too, but it only helps with dark circles because the creamy lotion has a pale golden, opalescent pink shimmer to reflect light from the shadowed areas. The effect is a cosmetic trick, not skin care, and it's no match for what a great concealer can accomplish. Besides, the finish quickly emphasizes wrinkles or crepey skin around the eyes, so you'll want to camouflage it with a creamy concealer anyway. If this provided broad-spectrum sun protection, the dark circle-diminishing claim would carry more weight (unprotected sun exposure absolutely makes dark circles worse). Although this doesn't contain fragrance per se, it does contain fragrant plant extracts (including tangerine), which pose a risk of irritation whether used around the eyes or elsewhere on the face, and irritation can cause collagen to break down. The formula also contains some very good antioxidants and skin-repairing ingredients, but they don't make up for the irritating ingredients, any more than eating broccoli makes up for eating chocolate cake. Aside from the uniqueness of the ceramic-tip applicator, this Idealist product (which is offered in two shades, though both go on very sheer and impart the same type of shine) isn't all that special. The anti-aging ingredients it contains are found in numerous other products, including facial moisturizers and serums. The truth is you don't need an eye cream (see the Appendix for details), although if occasional puffiness is your concern, you may find a product like this worth the expense.

☺ GOOD $$$ **Idealist Even Skintone Illuminator** *($85 for 1.7 fl. oz.)* is said to improve what many women struggle with as they age: an uneven skin tone. If the promise of improved skin tone isn't convincing enough, this silky skin-lightening serum is also supposed to correct red marks from acne and sun-induced skin discolorations without the proven yet controversial ingredient hydroquinone. Although this serum feels great going on and leaves a super-smooth finish, texture-wise it isn't too far removed from Lauder's Idealist Pore Minimizing Skin Refinisher. Both products have similar ingredients, and they even have the same lingering citrus-tinged fragrance, which isn't the best for skin because fragrance, natural or synthetic, can cause irritation (see the Appendix for details). As it turns out, Idealist Even Skintone Illuminator is almost identical to Lauder-owned Clinique's Even Better Clinical Dark Spot Corrector. Lauder's version costs more (because Lauder maintains more of a prestige positioning, whereas Clinique is marketed to the masses) and contains fragrance (not a skin-care benefit), but other than that, the only difference is that Lauder's version adds an illuminating, subtle golden shimmer to your skin. Shine isn't skin care, it's makeup, but undoubtedly many women will like the soft golden glow this leaves behind. Because this product is nearly identical to Clinique's Even Better Clinical Dark Spot Corrector, the same basic comments apply (please refer to that review for details). One ingredient in this product deserves further explanation: dimethoxytolyl propylresorcinol. This ingredient is a chemical compound from the *Dianella ensifolia* plant. It is known to inhibit tyrosinase, which is the enzyme in skin that spurs melanin production. There are many ingredients research has shown to inhibit the action of tyrosinase, as this is believed to be a fairly efficient way to control hyperpigmentation. Examples of such ingredients are various types of mushrooms, grape seed, 1-propylmercaptan, and arbutin. To date, there is no conclusive research proving that dimethoxytolyl propylresorcinol is the best one, or that its efficacy is comparable to that of hydroquinone. According to research published in *Drugs of the Future* (volume 33, 2008, pages 945-954), dimethoxytolyl propylresorcinol inhibited pigmentation on reconstituted human skin and animal models. How this ingredient works on reconstituted skin isn't identical to how it will work on intact, alive human skin, but at least it gives researchers some idea of how it works and how it may be used in skin-care products. Still, this bit of information isn't a lot to go on. It's an understatement to mention that it pales in comparison to the reams of published research on hydroquinone! What about the salicylic acid? Although this BHA ingredient can improve skin-cell turnover to help fade discolorations faster, the amount Lauder includes in this product is likely less than 1%, and the pH of 4.4 io above the ideal of 3.5 to 4, which would make it a more effective exfoliant. When all is said and done, there's only a tiny bit of research supporting the skin-lightening claims made for this product. You may experience some good results from this product, but those with melasma or more widespread hyperpigmentation issues should consider (or stick with) prescription hydroquinone products, in addition to being neurotic about daily sun protection, which is essential if your goal is to reduce discolorations. One final comment: Although some of the ingredients in this product can help fade red marks from acne, these aren't exceptional for that purpose. A well-formulated BHA product, along with a fragrance-free, antioxidant-rich moisturizer, plus daily sun protection is a better way to go if lingering red marks are your concern.

☺ GOOD $$$ **Idealist Pore Minimizing Skin Refinisher** *($48.50 for 1 fl. oz.)* is Lauder's all-in-one solution to problems such as large pores, flaky skin, redness, and, of course, fine lines. Lauder claims that this product makes pores appear one-third smaller, instantly, and that this version contains three times more acetyl glucosamine than the original Idealist formula. It does indeed contain more acetyl glucosamine, but is that an advantage? Derived from sugar, acetyl glucosamine doesn't have known exfoliating properties (Lauder claims it helps unglue the bonds that hold dead skin cells to the surface, something a well-formulated AHA or BHA product accomplishes). Acetyl glucosamine's primary constituents are mucopolysaccharides and hyaluronic acid. Found in all parts of the skin, it has value as a repairing ingredient and is effective (in high concentrations) for wound-healing. There is also research (*Cellular-Molecular-Life-Science*, 53(2), February 1997, pages 131–140) showing that chitins (also known as chitosan, which is composed of acetyl glucosamine) can help in the complex process of wound-healing. However, that is a few generations removed from acetyl glucosamine being included in a skin-care product. Procter & Gamble has published research on the skin-lightening effect of acetyl glucosamine when used at concentrations of 2% or more in combination with niacinamide (such as in their Olay Definity products), but although Lauder is likely using that amount, they left out niacinamide (Source: *Journal of Cosmetic Dermatology*, March 2007, pages 20–26). There are some notable ingredients in here, but in terms of making skin look better and pores appear smaller, it does so mostly by cosmetic trickery. For example, the strong silicone base instantly makes skin look smoother, so it reflects light better, and it can temporarily fill in large pores and superficial lines. Cosmetic pigments (iron oxides, mica, and titanium dioxide) provide a brightening effect, imparting a "glow" to your skin. Beyond the light show, plant-based anti-inflammatory ingredients help minimize minor redness, and antioxidants such as green tea help keep skin protected from free-radical damage. What's not good news is the inclusion of lavender and orange along with the fragrant ingredients limonene and linalool. They're present in an amount that may be potentially irritating, which keeps this from earning a Best Product rating. If you decide to give this a go, it is best for normal to oily skin.

☺ AVERAGE **Nutritious Vita-Mineral Moisture Gel Creme** *($38 for 1.7 fl. oz.)* is a silky-textured, water-based moisturizer suitable for normal to slightly dry or slightly oily skin. The jar packaging ends up negating the potency of the pomegranate and other antioxidants that make more than a cameo appearance in this product. In better packaging, this moisturizer would be highly recommended.

☺ AVERAGE $$$ **Advanced Night Repair Eye Synchronized Complex** *($49.50 for 0.5 fl. oz.)* is the partner product to Advanced Night Repair Synchronized Recovery Complex. As is typical for Lauder's moisturizers, this eye-area moisturizer (which doesn't contain a single ingredient that would make it unique for the skin around the eyes) is loaded with beneficial ingredients for your skin. It has a beautifully silky texture and is fragrance-free. The problem is that Lauder packaged it in a jar, which is a shame (see the Appendix for details). One more point: You have to wonder why, if this eye cream takes care of every eye-area concern, as Lauder claims, they continue to sell so many other eye creams (and gels and serums and on and on) claiming to do the same thing? If just one of them worked to vanquish dark circles, puffiness, dryness, and wrinkles, they wouldn't need dozens more, right? Refer to the Appendix to learn why you don't need an eye cream (or gel).

☺ AVERAGE $$$ **Day Wear Advanced Multi-Protection Anti-Oxidant Creme Oil-Free SPF 25** *($45 for 1.7 fl. oz.)* has what it takes to keep skin protected from sun damage, but the formula's numerous antioxidants, which could be incredibly beneficial for skin, will degrade upon opening because this product is packaged in a jar (so much for "the most advanced anti-oxidant power ever"). The formula is best for normal to dry skin; although oil-free, it contains oil-like and emollient ingredients that will feel heavy and slick over oily areas.

☺ AVERAGE $$$ **DayWear Advanced Multi-Protection Anti-Oxidant Creme SPF 15 Dry Skin** *($43 for 1.7 fl. oz.)* has what it takes to keep skin protected from sun damage, but the formula's numerous antioxidants, which could be incredibly beneficial for skin, will degrade upon opening the jar packaging. The formula is best for normal to dry skin.

☺ AVERAGE $$$ **Hydra Complete Multi-Level Moisture Eye Gel Creme** *($38.50 for 0.5 fl. oz.)* is just like most of Lauder's moisturizers, whether they're sold for use in the eye area or not. It has a beautifully silky texture and contains an impressive amount of antioxidants along with some notable skin-identical and cell-communicating ingredients. Unfortunately, those ingredients (which skin needs) won't remain potent once this product is in use, and that's because of the jar packaging (see the Appendix for details). You're left with a moisturizer for slightly dry skin anywhere on the face, but that's it. The algae extract in this eye cream won't reduce puffiness over time. If it could, why not just use the pure substance on skin instead of the tiny amount in this product?

☺ AVERAGE $$$ **Hydrationist Maximum Moisture Creme, Dry Skin** *($40 for 1.7 fl. oz.)*. It's disappointing that Lauder once again opted for jar packaging. This moisturizer is loaded with antioxidants (some of which have irritant potential) and numerous plant extracts, but they won't remain stable once this product is opened. The thickeners and emollients this contains are great for dry skin and the formula contains some cell-communicating and skin-identical ingredients, too (just like most Lauder moisturizers), but a large portion of the formula is wasted due to the jar packaging, not to mention the hygiene issue of repeatedly dipping fingers into a jar.

☺ AVERAGE $$$ **Hydrationist Maximum Moisture Creme, Normal/Combination Skin** *($38 for 1.7 fl. oz.)* is a lighter-weight, silkier version of Estee Lauder's Hydrationist Maximum Moisture Creme, Dry Skin above, and the same review applies. The only Hydrationist moisturizer worth considering is the Maximum Moisture Lotion because it isn't packaged in a jar.

☺ AVERAGE $$$ **Hydrationist Maximum Moisture Creme SPF 15, Normal/Combination Skin** *($40 for 1.7 fl. oz.)* is supposed to provide maximum moisture, but what about Lauder's many other almost identical products? They're still selling their DayWear, Resilience, and Time Zone products, all of which have formulary traits similar to those of Hydrationist.

These other moisturizers also make the same claims in terms of moisturizing skin, so how is a consumer to choose? That's where marketing claims come into play, not quality, and that's where Hydrationist fits in because there isn't much to extol. Essentially, all Lauder is stating is that using this product daily will result in younger-looking skin that's better able to hold on to moisture because its barrier function is improved. That sounds (and is) great for skin, but the fact is such a statement is applicable to any well-formulated moisturizer with sunscreen—and Lauder doesn't have an ace up their sleeve that no one else does, despite their mostly excellent moisturizers. Although we can't fault this moisturizer's in-part avobenzone sunscreen or antioxidant-enriched silky formula, it falls down hard due to one critical issue: Packaging. Putting this brilliant formula in a jar means that the numerous light- and air-sensitive ingredients won't remain stable once this is opened. In better packaging, this would be a great option for normal to dry skin (someone with combination skin will find this too emollient for oily areas).

☺ AVERAGE $$$ **Nutritious Vita-Mineral Infusing Eye Gel** *($36 for 0.5 fl. oz.)* is a lightweight gel moisturizer that contains several beneficial plant extracts. The concern is that a couple of the plants (such as rosemary and tangerine) pose a risk of irritation for skin, and this risk increases when they're in a product meant for use in the eye area. Ironically, even though this eye gel has "mineral" in its name, the only mineral in the formula is manganese, and it's barely present. Manganese isn't a must for skin, but if you're going to position this product as containing minerals, they deserve more prominence. There are several antioxidants in this formula, including from plant sources. However, the jar packaging Lauder chose won't keep them stable during use, which is disappointing. See the Appendix to find out why you don't need an eye cream (or gel) and certainly not one packaged in a jar.

☺ AVERAGE $$$ **Re-Nutriv Creme** *($350 for 16.7 fl. oz.)* is a very emollient, mineral oil–based moisturizer for dry skin. It does contain some good skin-identical ingredients and antioxidants, but jar packaging won't keep the antioxidants stable. See the Appendix to learn why jar packaging is a problem.

☺ AVERAGE $$$ **Re-Nutriv Intensive Lifting Creme** *($170 for 1.7 fl. oz.)* is a good moisturizer with lots of good skin-identical ingredients, antioxidants, and anti-irritants; however, there is nothing in it that will lift skin anywhere, and the price is nothing less than obscene given the ingredient list and jar packaging. See the Appendix to learn why jar packaging is a problem.

☺ AVERAGE $$$ **Re-Nutriv Intensive Lifting Eye Creme** *($90 for 0.5 fl. oz.)* is a very emollient eye cream for dry to very dry skin, but it won't lift skin or reduce dark circles. It comes up comparably short in antioxidants, but even if they were there in abundance, jar packaging wouldn't keep them stable once the product is opened. See the Appendix to learn more about the problems jar packaging presents and why, in truth, you don't need an eye cream.

☺ AVERAGE $$$ **Re-Nutriv Intensive Lifting Lotion** *($170 for 1.7 fl. oz.)* cannot work remotely as claimed—this isn't any closer to a face-lift-in-a-bottle than any other moisturizer or serum from Lauder's vast stable of options (hundreds at last count). If anything, although this contains some impressive ingredients to improve skin's health and appearance, it also contains some standout problem ingredients as well. Chief among them is gold, which we're sure helps with the luxury, prestige positioning that Lauder strives for with Re-Nutriv, but the reality is that gold is a relatively common allergen that can induce dermatitis about the face and eyelids (Sources: *Inflammation and Allergy Drug Targets*, September 2008, pages 145–162; *Dermatologic Therapy*, volume 17, 2004, pages 321–327; *Cutis*, May 2000, pages 323–326; and naturaldatabase.com). There isn't much gold in here, but its benefit for skin is void, so why include it at all, other than for image and marketing fluff? Lauder offers dozens of other moisturizers (most priced lower than this) that omit the problematic ingredients and that overall are better formulated.

☺ AVERAGE $$$ Re-Nutriv Lightweight Creme *($350 for 16.7 fl. oz)* is an emollient but overall lackluster formula compared to most other Lauder moisturizers, including those selling for half this price. The "Lightweight" portion of the name is misleading due to this moisturizer's oil content.

☺ AVERAGE $$$ Re-Nutriv Replenishing Comfort Creme *($135 for 1.7 fl. oz.)*. Like many cosmetics companies, Lauder won't give up jar packaging. The cosmetics industry stubbornly sells formulas in attractive containers that have no ability to keep the ingredients they contain stable. It is well known among researchers and scientists that jar packaging is not only unsanitary, but many beneficial ingredients breakdown in the presence of air. What a waste! (See the Appendix to find out all the problems associated with jar packaging). On the other hand, as is true for many of Lauder's moisturizers, this is a well-formulated blend of antioxidants, skin-repairing and cell-communicating ingredients, and emollients. The assortment of these ingredients is truly impressive. Regrettably, this could have been a beautiful option for dry skin if the ingredients were in the kind of packaging that holds them stable and effective once you open it.

☺ AVERAGE $$$ Re-Nutriv Replenishing Comfort Eye Creme *($80 for 0.5 fl. oz.)* is nearly identical to Lauder's Re-Nutriv Replenishing Comfort Creme above, and the same review applies. Please see the Appendix to learn why you don't need an eye cream.

☺ AVERAGE $$$ Re Nutriv Ultimate Lift Age Correcting Creme *($260 for 1.7 fl. oz.)* is a very good moisturizer for dry to very dry skin, but the price and packaging are a problem. Also on the edge of ludicrous are the claims, but more on that in a moment. Formula-wise, this earns praise for including proven emollients along with several antioxidants, some cell-communicating ingredients, and a nice mix of skin-identical ingredients. Note that the state-of-the-art ingredients in this moisturizer also are found in many others moisturizers (including others from Lauder) that don't come with Re-Nutriv's high blood pressure–inducing price tag. As exciting as the formula is, the jar packaging is a problem, and a big disappointment given the price. See the Appendix to learn why jar packaging is a problem. Turning to the claims, they're indeed spellbinding, but you have to wonder: If this is Lauder's "ultimate" answer to aging skin (they promote it as being the most amazing formula ever), then what are all their other antiwrinkle/lifting/firming products for? Is Re-Nutriv the real deal, and the other, less expensive products and the products from other Lauder lines such as La Mer or Clinique just a waste of money? You may be impressed that this moisturizer contains gold. Yes, gold is luxurious and expensive, and a hallmark of the Re-Nutriv line—but it doesn't have any benefits for your skin. In fact, applied topically, gold can cause contact dermatitis (Sources: *Inflammation and Allergy Drug Targets*, September 2008, pages 145–162; *Dermatologic Therapy*, volume 17, 2004, pages 321–327; and *Cutis*, May 2000, pages 323–326). That means this serum stands a fairly good chance of being problematic, potentially hurting your skin's healing process, and hindering healthy collagen production. You're also getting a lot of shine with this moisturizer, but a shiny finish isn't skin care, it's just shine, the same you get from a luminescent foundation or powder, and it's not enough of a light show to make anyone think you're looking younger. What about this being able to lift your skin? Sorry, not possible. We wish that weren't the case, but it's true. The multiple factors that lead to sagging (e.g., sun damage, bone loss, fat pads shifting, muscle movement, gravity) simply cannot be addressed by any skin-care product, regardless of price tag or claim. Lauder's claim of your skin looking "more lifted" implies you'll get the results you're looking for, but the way the claim is worded, it doesn't actually state that any lifting is taking

The Reviews E

place. Making skin look "more lifted" doesn't mean your skin will actually *be* lifted. Even if it were lifted, where would the excess skin go? Not surprisingly, no one at the Lauder counter had a plausible answer to this question! Ask them next time you're there, and see how they respond.

☺ AVERAGE **$$$ Re-Nutriv Ultimate Lift Age Correcting Eye Creme** (*$115 for 0.5 fl. oz.*) is the eye cream partner to Lauder's Re-Nutriv Ultimate Lift Age Correcting Creme above. Not surprisingly, the formulas have no significant differences, and the minor differences have nothing to do with the skin around your eyes. This is further proof of why eye creams are a waste of money and completely unnecessary (see the Appendix for details).

☺ AVERAGE **$$$ Re-Nutriv Ultimate Lift Age Correcting Mask** (*$100 for 2.5 fl. oz.*) will not lift or correct even one month off your age. What is ultimate is how emollient and rich this plant oil and Vaseline-based mask will feel on dry to very dry skin. It also has an interesting mix of skin-repairing ingredients and antioxidants. While not as loaded with beneficial ingredients as many other Lauder products, this isn't quite a slacker, either. But before you pull out your charge card, what is problematic is the amount of sandalwood extract it contains. There is more of this fragrant extract than almost any of the ingredients that really benefit aging skin. Though exceptionally aromatic, sandalwood is a fragrance ingredient that is not the best for skin. See the Appendix to learn why fragrance is a problem for all skin types. One more point: This also contains pearl powder. What you'll find online about pearl powder in cosmetics is a long list of claims from companies using it, but there is no research supporting any of those promises. Anecdotes of mystical Chinese preparations or secrets of Cleopatra are as realistic as thinking the world is flat. In the real world, pearls are nothing more than calcium carbonate and, like gold, they have no benefit for skin. This would be worthwhile as a mask or leave-on moisturizer for dry skin if it weren't for the fragrance. Though even ignoring that shortcoming, this much money for a mask with no chance of lifting your skin is something that should give you pause.

☺ AVERAGE **$$$ Re-Nutriv Ultimate Lift Age Correcting Serum** (*$210 for 1 fl. oz.*) claims to have "5 times the levels of potent lifting, tightening, and repair ingredients." It makes you wonder what their other products are for if this one is so powerful. Regrettably, the formula for this serum tells another story. Like most of Lauder's serums, this contains several antioxidants along with lesser amounts of cell-communicating and skin-repairing ingredients. Yet, for all the good that antioxidants do for our skin, none of them can lift sagging skin or make it "tighter and more toned," at least not beyond the fleeting sensation of skin feeling tighter, which isn't the same as actually making skin tighter. See the Appendix for details on why products like this cannot help sagging skin. The gemstones in this product may sound exotic, but there is no research showing that such ingredients can do anything for wrinkles, or for any other skin problem for that matter. Although this serum contains lots of antioxidants and has a silky texture, the amount of gold is a potential problem. Yes, gold is luxurious and expensive, and a hallmark of the Re-Nutriv line—but gold doesn't have any benefits for your skin. In fact, applied topically, gold can cause contact dermatitis (Sources: *Inflammation and Allergy Drug Targets*, September 2008, pages 145–162; *Dermatologic Therapy*, volume 17, 2004, pages 321–327; and *Cutis*, May 2000, pages 323–326). That means this serum stands a fairly good chance of being problematic, potentially hurting your skin's healing process, and hindering healthy collagen production. You're also getting a lot of shine with this serum, but a shiny finish isn't skin care, it's just shine, and it's not enough of a light show to make anyone think you're looking younger. In the end, this serum isn't worth the expense—Lauder and many other companies offer better options, all of which are on our Best Serums list at the end of this book.

☺ AVERAGE **$$$ Resilience Lift Firming/Sculpting Eye Creme** *($55 for 0.5 fl. oz.)* has an intriguing formula that supplies several good emollients and numerous anti-aging ingredients (the same ones they include in their facial moisturizers, which means you're not getting anything special by purchasing a product labeled "eye cream"; see the Appendix for further info). What's sad (and happens all too often with Lauder's eye creams) is that many of the ingredients will break down due to the jar packaging. That means you're not getting the anti-aging benefits that the skin anywhere on your face needs, making this eye cream much less appealing. Please see the Appendix to learn of the problems jar packaging presents. As for the claims, this eye cream doesn't contain anything capable of lifting skin, at night or any other time. Many of the ingredients can stimulate healthy collagen production, but the jury is out as to how well they stimulate elastin production. This is because we have a finite number of elastin fibers; once they're damaged (think of a rubber band being stretched to the breaking point), the body doesn't generate new elastin, so the best we can hope for is elastin repair. As anyone who's tried to patch together a snapped rubber band knows, it never goes back to its original strength. The "luminizing optics" Lauder refers to as being able to blur the look of lines is just a fancy way to describe shine. Shine isn't skin care—it's makeup, and most will find that applying shine to wrinkles tends to emphasize them rather than downplay them.

☹ AVERAGE **$$$ Time Zone Anti-Line/Wrinkle Eye Creme** *($45 for 0.5 fl. oz.)* is the eye-area counterpart to Lauder's overhyped Time Zone facial moisturizers. Other than being more emollient, there is nothing about it that makes it specially formulated for the eye area. The claims mention that this eye cream is "so powerful" that every woman showed a reduction in the look of lines and wrinkles. That sounds mighty impressive until you realize that simply improving the look of lines and wrinkles, which any moisturizer will do, is a cosmetic effect. Not to mention how many times we've heard this before about countless other products the Lauder Corporation sells. See the Appendix to learn why the jar packaging this come in is a problem.

☹ AVERAGE **$$$ Time Zone Line & Wrinkle Reducing Moisturizer SPF 15 Dry Creme** *($58 for 1.7 fl. oz.)* provides good broad-spectrum sun protection and contains some great ingredients for anti-aging, but it's all for naught because this is packaged in a jar. See the Appendix to find out the multiple problems jar packaging presents.

☹ AVERAGE **$$$ Time Zone Line & Wrinkle Reducing Moisturizer SPF 15 Normal/Combination Creme** *($58 for 1.7 fl. oz.)* is similar to the Time Zone Line & Wrinkle Reducing Moisturizer SPF 15 Dry Creme above, except it has a lighter texture. Otherwise, the same comments apply and this is not the Lauder moisturizer to buy.

☹ AVERAGE **$$$ Time Zone Night Anti-Line/Wrinkle Creme** *($62.50 for 1.7 fl. oz.)* adds nothing to what Lauder already offers, which is really disappointing given a fairly decent price point for any of the Lauder companies (remember Lauder owns Aveda, Origins, Clinique, Bobby Brown, and La Mer). Although Lauder generally does moisturizers better than most of its competitors, in this case the jar packaging means the beneficial anti-aging ingredients will have their potency diminished with each use (to say nothing of the bacterial contamination that occurs each time you dip your finger into the jar). If any of Lauder's stable of antiwrinkle creams produced the results they promise, the company wouldn't have to keep creating new antiwrinkle products, but that's not the reality. Because hope springs eternal, most women keep

The Reviews E

🔻 Wondering why that product claiming to lift sagging skin didn't work? See the Appendix!

coming back to the cosmetics counters for the next antiwrinkle miracle. We realize this sounds dismal (and to the extent that women waste their money on such products, it is), but the truth is that a well-formulated moisturizer (e.g., lotion, cream, serum, gel) can be a brilliant way to help skin look and act younger. No, your wrinkles won't be gone and you won't look a decade younger in one week, but with the right routine (sunscreen, exfoliant, and other products targeted for your skin-care concerns, such as acne, rosacea, oily skin, dry skin), you will see an improvement. But products packaged in jars like this aren't the way to get that improvement.

☹ POOR **Clear Difference Advanced Oil-Control Hydrator** *($32.50 for 1.7 fl. oz.)* lists alcohol as the second ingredient, and that makes this otherwise fine moisturizer a problem for all skin types. See the Appendix to find out all the problems alcohol causes for your skin. This product does not contain ingredients that can keep skin "hydrated inside, perfectly matte outside." Rather, the predominance of alcohol keeps the moisturizing ingredients from doing their job. How unfortunate, because the price is downright affordable (for a Lauder moisturizer, anyway) and this contains some excellent skin-identical ingredients (though few antioxidants).

☹ POOR **Re-Nutriv Ultimate Lift Age Correcting Creme for Throat and Decolletage** *($120 for 1.7 fl oz.)*. The only thing ultimate about this moisturizer is the price tag. Where to begin? Let's start with the claim that this formula is somehow specially formulated for your chest and neck area. There is no research showing your neck and chest require anything different than the face, not even one ingredient. If anything, because this moisturizer doesn't contain sunscreen it would be a problem for use during the day, leaving that area of your body exposed to the sun's damaging rays. Moving on, while this does contain a truly impressive array of antioxidants and skin-repairing ingredients along with silky, rich emollients, it doesn't out-perform other Lauder moisturizers costing far less. The entire Re-Nutriv line is all about pricing and prestige positioning, not about superior formulations for "mature" skin. Another issue is that Lauder won't give up jar packaging and this product is no exception. The cosmetics industry in general stubbornly sells formulas in attractive containers that have no ability to keep the ingredients they contain stable. It is well known among researchers and scientists that jar packaging is not only unsanitary, but also almost all beneficial ingredients break down in the presence of air. What a waste! Claiming to lift skin and reduce crepiness and discolorations sounds great, but this is really just a potentially great moisturizer for evening (remember it lacks sunscreen so daytime use is out). The teeny amount of gold this contains is a relatively common allergen that can induce dermatitis on the face and eyelids (Source: *Cutis*, May 2000, pages 323–326). There is no research showing it has any benefit when applied topically to skin. In the real world of facts, gold's only benefit is collecting it, selling it, or wearing it, not applying it to your skin. One more point: This also contains pearl powder. What you'll find online about pearl powder in cosmetics is a long list of claims from companies using it, but there is no research supporting any of those promises. Anecdotes of mystical Chinese preparations or secrets of Cleopatra are as realistic as thinking the world is flat. In the real world, pearls are nothing more than calcium carbonate and, like gold, they have no benefit for skin.

☹ POOR **Resilience Lift Firming/Sculpting Face and Neck Creme SPF 15** *($75 for 1.7 fl. oz.)* is a facial moisturizer with sunscreen that uses "neck" in the name. In truth, you should be able to apply any well-formulated facial moisturizer with sunscreen to your neck, too (and chest, if this area of skin will be exposed to daylight). Regrettably, this isn't a well-formulated product, at least not from the sunscreen angle. To provide the best broad-spectrum protection, any SPF-rated product should contain one or more of the following active ingredients: titanium dioxide, zinc oxide, avobenzone, Mexoryl SX (ecamsule), or Tinosorb. Without at least one of these, your skin isn't getting sufficient UVA protection, so it remains vulnerable to the sun's most aging rays. This is not recommended.

ESTEE LAUDER SUN CARE

☺ GOOD **Bronze Goddess Golden Perfection Self Tanning Lotion for Face** (*$22.50 for 1.7 fl. oz.*) is a very standard, but good, self-tanning lotion. It turns skin tan with dihydroxyacetone, the same ingredient in most self-tanners. This comes in a lotion base that's best for normal to dry skin. It contains several fragrant plants, which likely mute the effectiveness of the beneficial ingredients, such as the soothing agents and skin-identical ingredients. This self-tanner is tinted with cosmetic pigments so you get instant, shimmering color as your sunless tan develops.

☺ AVERAGE **Bronze Goddess Sun Indulgence Lotion for Face SPF 30** (*$22 for 1.7 fl. oz.*) is a tinted sunscreen with shimmer that contains avobenzone for sufficient UVA protection. Because the Bronze Goddess products are all about the seduction of tropical, exotic scents, this product is highly fragranced. It contains the usual assortment of beneficial ingredients we've come to expect from Lauder, but their effect on skin will be limited because the skin has to defend itself from the irritation caused by the amount of fragrance and the many fragrant plants in this product. This isn't one of Lauder's better sunscreens, but it's an acceptable option for normal to slightly dry skin.

☹ AVERAGE **$$$ Bronze Goddess Self Tanning Milk for Body** (*$26.50 for 5 fl. oz.*) contains a skin-unhealthy amount of fragrance along with numerous fragrant plants. That makes it a tough sell compared with several other self-tanners that turn skin color using the exact same ingredient, dihydroxyacetone. It's nice that this contains cosmetic pigments for instant color (and shine) as your tan develops, but lots of self-tanners offer this benefit without the significant amount of fragrance. See the Appendix to learn why excess fragrance is a problem for all skin types.

☺ AVERAGE **$$$ Bronze Goddess Tinted Self-Tan Golden Perfection Tinted Self-Tanning Gelee for Body** (*$28.50 for 5 fl. oz.*) is a very fragrant self-tanning lotion that has a silky, gel-like texture. It turns skin tan with dihydroxyacetone, the same ingredient found in hundreds of self-tanners. This option from Lauder also contains cosmetic pigments that add instant bronze color and shimmer to skin. The amount of fragrance and fragrant plants isn't smart skin care, but this does leave an attractive bronze sheen on skin. One caution: The sugars in this formula (fructose, sucrose) may play a role in activating advanced glycation end-products (AGE), which progressively damage skin's elasticity.

ESTEE LAUDER SPECIALTY SKIN-CARE PRODUCTS

✓☺ BEST **$$$ Resilience Lift Extreme Ultra Firming Mask** (*$40 for 2.5 fl. oz.*) is a powerhouse formula for dry to very dry skin and is best left on as a moisturizer rather than used occasionally as a mask to be rinsed off. This mask is supposed to revitalize skin with advanced lifting and firming technology, but it can't do that. It doesn't even contain ingredients to create a temporary tightening effect, and that are often used in products to convince you that your skin really is being firmed and lifted. However, as long as you're not banking on this product being a face-lift in a tube, it is without question a formidable moisturizer that treats dry skin to a bevy of ingredients that will improve its feel and appearance.

☺ GOOD **$$$ Perfectionist [CP+] Targeted Deep Wrinkle Filler** (*$39.50 for 0.5 fl. oz.*) is said to be a "powerful daily treatment for your deepest wrinkles." It's designed to be used on lines around the eye, creases in the forehead, furrows between the brow—anywhere you have lines that don't go away when your face is expressionless. This type of product isn't anything new; for example, Lauder-owned Good Skin (sold at Kohl's department stores) sells TriAktiline Instant Deep Wrinkle Filler. All these are silicone-based serum-like products that serve as a soft spackle for wrinkles and large pores. You pat the product into and over creases, and it provides a superficial, temporary filling effect. How long results last depends on the formula and, more critically, on how expressive you are. And, of course, none of these products have even a fractional ability to work like Botox or dermal fillers, but that's another story. This "filler"-type serum has a silky, thick texture that dispenses from a pointed rubber-tipped applicator. We suppose that's for precise application into lines, but you still need to pat and smooth it over your skin. It sets quickly to a soft, powder-like matte finish laced with subtle sparkles, which some may not appreciate. Despite the shine, the filling effect is impressive. It really did a good job of smoothing superficial lines, including those around the eyes and mouth. There's a significant caveat to this product, however. It doesn't work well when used with a liquid foundation that contains silicones (which is roughly 85% of liquid foundations sold today). Applying a silicone-enhanced foundation over Perfectionist looks terrible. It makes foundation look patchy and, over the course of several hours, looks progressively worse. With this pairing, skin actually looks older! What to do? Well, you can experiment with other filler-type products or be sure to pair Perfectionist with a silicone-free foundation. Still, you shouldn't have to give up your favorite foundation (or concealer) to experience the benefits (however temporary) that Perfectionist offers. The overall formula contains several outstanding ingredients for all skin types, including copious amounts of antioxidants and lesser amounts of skin-identical and cell-communicating ingredients. This would be rated a Best Product if the fragrance wasn't so potent. We suspect many will have trouble using this product around the eyes (which is where most will apply it) because the fragrance can be sensitizing.

☺ GOOD $$$ **Re-Nutriv Intensive Lifting Mask** *($70 for 1.7 fl. oz.)* is a very good moisturizing mask for normal to dry skin, but for the money, the formula cannot compete with Lauder's superior, less expensive Resilience Lift Extreme Ultra Firming Mask above.

☹ AVERAGE $$$ **Resilience Lift Instant Action Lift Treatment** *($65 for 1 fl. oz.)* is essentially a wrinkle filler sold as a way to give sagging skin a tightened, lifted look whenever you want. Housed inside a tube-like component with a built-in applicator is a thick, serum-like product whose silicone-based, film-forming agents serve as a soft spackle for wrinkles. How any of this is supposed to lift skin is a good question—in reality, it isn't possible. Please see the Appendix to learn why products like this cannot lift skin, either instantly or over the long term. This product will make skin feel silky and can temporarily fill in and smooth minor lines and wrinkles, but how long the effect lasts depends on how expressive you are and what other products you may be applying at the same time. The film-forming agents it contains can make skin feel tighter, but that's not the same as actually tightening sagging skin (which is what certain cosmetic corrective procedures, such as Fraxel or Ulthera, can do). Resilience Lift Instant Action Lift Treatment contains several beneficial ingredients to help skin look and act younger, and the packaging helps keep these ingredients stable during use, which is what you want. Unfortunately, it also contains a gum resin from the plant *Commiphora mukul*. This plant has some intriguing research about its properties when consumed orally, and it appears to have antioxidant and anti-inflammatory benefits when applied to skin; however, it is also known to cause numerous skin reactions, ranging from redness to what's described as "bulbous lesions," depending on how much is applied at one time (Source: naturaldatabase.com). In short, this isn't a great ingredient to see in skin-care products, as its potential for irritation cannot be ignored (and Lauder isn't using just a tiny amount of it). It's possible that the swelling this plant may cause will make wrinkles less apparent, but it's a backward approach: The irritation caused by topical application has the potential to damage healthy collagen production and hurt skin's ability to heal. There are other "filler"-type products that can produce the same wrinkle-softening results as this product, but without the potential for irritation. An example is Good Skin's TriAktiline Instant Deep Wrinkle Filler, which is sold at Kohl's.

ESTEE LAUDER FOUNDATIONS & PRIMERS

✓☺ BEST $$$ **Invisible Fluid Makeup** *($35)*. This fragrance-free liquid foundation's big claim is "see no makeup, feel no makeup," but you'll feel something (however light) and to some extent this does look like makeup, albeit a very sheer one. The fluid texture is on the runny side, and demands vigorous shaking before each use or you will notice separation and have trouble getting this to blend on evenly. Once shaken well, you dispense it from a fine-point tip and blend... and keep blending because this has quite a bit of slip and takes longer than usual to set. The finish is matte with a subtle sheen and a translucent to sheer coverage that won't exaggerate large pores or wrinkles. This foundation's best attribute is how natural it looks, yet the trade-off is minimal coverage. This isn't the makeup to choose if you have an uneven skin tone, brown spots, or redness you'd like to soften. It helps to some extent, but really you're getting less coverage than most tinted moisturizers provide. For some, that may be just perfect. The formula is best for normal to oily or combination skin. It does not provide enough moisture for dry areas, though you can prep with an emollient moisturizer (with sunscreen, because this foundation doesn't offer sun protection) first. As for the shades, there are great options for light to dark skin tones, with none to avoid. However, many of the shades go on a bit pink or peach, so you'll need to choose carefully. The pink and peach tones aren't worth avoiding because the overall effect from this makeup is so sheer. There are no colors for very light skin, but the darker shades are outstanding.

✓☺ BEST $$$ **Matte Perfecting Primer** *($32 for 1 oz.)* has a silky texture just like most foundation primers. But this goes the extra mile by offering skin a good range of beneficial ingredients, making it more advantageous if you prefer to prep your skin with a product labeled "primer" instead of one labeled "serum." In truth, any well-formulated serum does double-duty as a primer, but perhaps the serum you prefer has a texture that doesn't pair well with your foundation. In that case, a primer like this is worth a look, especially if you have normal to oily or combination skin. This does a very good job of smoothing the skin's texture while slightly filling in large pores and leaving a soft, slightly absorbent matte finish that works (for a couple of hours at least) to keep excess shine at bay. In terms of filling in large pores, the effect is minor but noticeable, and of course, it's temporary, lasting a few hours or less depending on how oily your skin is and the type of foundation you apply after this primer. One last attribute of this primer is that it's fragrance-free. It contains many of the same great anti-aging ingredients Lauder includes in their serums, but most of their serums contain fragrance, which isn't helpful for anyone's skin.

✓☺ BEST $$$ **Resilience Lift Extreme Radiant Lifting Makeup SPF 15** *($37.50)* is a liquid foundation with an in-part titanium dioxide sunscreen and an antioxidant-rich formula that contains several other beneficial ingredients, although given that the frosted glass packaging won't protect them from light degradation, you must carefully store this away from light; that is, don't leave it out on your vanity if your bathroom has a window. Despite some formulary

The Reviews E

improvements, this foundation isn't going to lift skin anywhere, although it will help protect skin against further signs of aging because of the sun protection it provides. It also has a gorgeous, silky texture that's slightly creamy and a pleasure to blend. Women with normal to dry skin are bound to find this foundation's satin finish elegant; it really beautifies skin without looking heavy or like a layer of makeup, although no one is going to think you've gone au naturel with this on. Coverage is moderate to full, and most of the shades are exemplary. Although the lifting claims are a bust, everything else about this foundation is superior, making it worth strong consideration.

✓☺ BEST **$$$ Resilience Lift Extreme Ultra Firming Creme Compact Makeup SPF 15** *($37.50)* is one of the best, if not the best, cream foundation we've seen in years. Lauder has crafted a compact foundation with an in-part titanium dioxide sunscreen that has an extraordinarily smooth texture. As such, it is a dream to blend, and sets to a natural matte yet slightly moist finish capable of providing medium to nearly full coverage without looking waxy or mask-like. The formula is best for normal to dry skin not prone to blemishes, and almost all the shades are recommended. Bravo!

☺ GOOD **$$$ DayWear BB Anti-Oxidant Beauty Benefit Creme SPF 35** *($38 for 1 fl. oz.)* is Lauder's contribution to the trend of BB creams and also is one of the better options to try. However, it must be said that BB creams typically hold no advantage over other foundations or tinted moisturizers that contain extra ingredients such as antioxidants. Antioxidants are plentiful in this formula, and you also get reliable broad-spectrum sun protection (though the amount of titanium dioxide is on the low side for sufficient UVA protection, which is why this missed our top rating). Ultimately, think of BB creams as tinted moisturizers with a smattering of other skin-friendly ingredients. They do not reduce or prevent blemishes. The texture dispenses quite thick, but once you blend it softens and smoothes easily over skin, providing sheer to light coverage and a soft matte finish that looks natural. Best for normal to oily skin and suitable for breakout-prone skin, this fragranced BB cream comes in two warm-toned shades. Light is too dark for fair skin but suitable for light to light-medium skin tones; Medium is acceptable for its intended skin tone. A few of the plant extracts in the formula pose a slight risk of irritation, but for the most part they're outweighed by the number of beneficial ingredients this DayWear product contains.

☺ GOOD **$$$ Re-Nutriv Intensive Lifting Makeup SPF 15** *($70)* is elegantly packaged in a frosted-glass jar complete with golden cap and trim, and includes a titanium dioxide sunscreen. This has a silky, silicone-based formula that blends down to a satin matte finish that is not at all emollient—nor something those with dry skin would enjoy. It's best for those with normal to slightly dry or slightly oily skin seeking medium coverage and a whatever-it-may-cost makeup. The shades are impressively neutral. Like its companion product, this foundation is not capable of lifting the skin, but it will lift lots of money from your bank account.

☺ GOOD **$$$ Re-Nutriv Ultimate Lifting Creme Makeup SPF 15** *($80)* is one of Lauder's most expensive foundations, and your first question may be, "Is it worth the money?" Although this creamy foundation has a lot going for it, the answer is "no." It has a titanium dioxide–based sunscreen, which is great for protecting skin, but so do countless other foundations that cost significantly less. Lauder goes on and on about the skin-care technology behind this foundation, but it won't lift skin in the least. The base formula isn't nearly as exciting as many of their well-formulated moisturizers, plus the jar packaging won't keep the antioxidants in here stable. Texture-wise, this is extra rich, almost to the point of being greasy. It slides over skin and is easy to blend, but doesn't ever set, so you're left with a creamy finish that must be set with powder. You'll get medium coverage without much effort, and it's hard to get less than that, even if you apply a sheer layer (but don't do that because you'll cheat your skin of the sun protection it needs). Most of the shades are very good. Based on the emollience of this foundation, we recommend it only for someone with dry to very dry skin, assuming you're willing to pay the exorbitant price.

☺ GOOD **$$$ Re-Nutriv Ultimate Radiance Makeup SPF 15** *($80)* is one of the most expensive foundations sold in department stores, and the extra expense gets you a lavish silver box (which you'll recycle or discard) and a pretty, though standard, frosted-glass bottle that complements other makeup products in the Re-Nutriv line. But, given that none of that paraphernalia goes on your face, it is a waste and not what you should pay attention to. The foundation itself includes an in-part titanium dioxide sunscreen, just like lots of other foundations. That's the only anti-aging element you can count on, but it doesn't have to cost this much. This has a slightly creamy texture reminiscent of a lightweight moisturizer. It blends easily and sets to a radiant finish suitable for normal to dry skin. Lauder salespeople like to point out that this foundation is different because it contains precious gemstones, but adding ruby, gold, or sapphire powder to makeup doesn't bestow a special benefit on skin of any age, not to mention that the amount is so trivial as to be nothing more than a dusting. The small range of shades is mostly neutral, though a few have a slightly pink cast. Although this foundation deserves a Good rating, Lauder sells other foundations that are just as good (or better) for almost one-third the price.

☺ AVERAGE **$$$ Double Wear Light Stay-in-Place Makeup SPF 10** *($35)* misses being assigned a Good rating because its SPF rating is below the benchmark for daytime protection. The sole active is titanium dioxide, and it's present in an amount that suggests a higher SPF rating was attainable—so why Lauder assigned a paltry SPF 10 is odd. This fluid foundation isn't as sheer as the description states. Yes, it feels much lighter than Lauder's original Double Wear foundation, but it loses none of its predecessor's formidable staying power. Application is smooth, but blending must be swift because it sets quickly to a long-wearing matte finish (applying it to small areas at a time works best). This really does stay on like few other foundations do, whether you're perspiring or simply have oily skin. Coverage is light to medium—trying to apply this sheer still nets noticeable coverage, so don't mistake this for a tinted moisturizer, because it isn't. All the shades are very good. For daytime wear, this is best for those with normal to very oily skin who want a budge-proof foundation, but are willing to apply a sunscreen rated SPF 15 or greater first. One more comment: the strong matte finish of this foundation tends to magnify large pores.

☺ AVERAGE **$$$ Double Wear Maximum Cover Camouflage Makeup for Face & Body SPF 15** *($33.50)* has a more fluid texture, with enough slip to make controlling the application tricky. It doesn't provide as much coverage as the name indicates, but it does cover well, provides a titanium dioxide sunscreen, and blends to a solid matte finish. The range of shades is limited but commendable, with only one shade being a bit too peach.

☺ AVERAGE **$$$ Double Wear Stay-in-Place Makeup SPF 10** *($34)* is great—at least when it comes to a terrific matte finish that doesn't move. If you have normal to oily skin, you'll be impressed with the application and the way it holds up over a long day, and the texture isn't as thick and hard to move as it once was. The SPF is too low for it to be your sole source of daytime protection, but it is pure titanium dioxide. If you have oily skin and want to give this a try, pair it with a matte-finish sunscreens with UVA protection such as those from Paula's Choice or Peter Thomas Roth. There are several shades offered. Shell and Ecru are excellent for fair skin, and darker skin tones are well served, too. The shades to steer clear of due to pink, orange, or peach tones are Suede and Rich Cocoa.

☹ AVERAGE **$$$ Futurist Age-Resisting Makeup SPF 15** *($37.50)* leaves out the most important anti-aging weapon anyone can have: a sunscreen with sufficient UVA-protecting ingredients! How disappointing that a foundation with such a superlative texture and luminous finish has this as its major flaw. Almost as upsetting is that the base formula was modified to include several state-of-the-art ingredients (if ever there was a foundation that functions like skin care, this is it), yet Lauder didn't improve the deficient sunscreen element. Sigh! If you have normal to dry skin and are prepared to wear a sunscreen underneath, you will get a great medium-coverage foundation. Unusual for Lauder is that more than half of the available shades are too rose, orange, or copper for most skin tones, so choose carefully and inspect the results in natural light before deciding to buy.

☹ AVERAGE **$$$ Illuminating Perfecting Primer** *($32 for 1 oz.)* isn't as good as Lauder's Matte Perfecting Primer reviewed above, mostly because it lacks the range of beneficial ingredients the Matte version has in abundance. The sheer, soft cream texture smoothes on easily and leaves a radiant (non-sparkling) glow. Its slightly moist finish isn't nearly as silky as that of most primers, though we appreciate that it's fragrance-free, because fragrance isn't skin care. This is an OK option for normal to dry or combination skin, but is not preferred to prepping your skin with a well-formulated serum.

☹ POOR **Double Matte Oil Control Makeup SPF 15** *($35)* does not offer the UVA-protecting ingredients of titanium dioxide, zinc oxide, avobenzone, Tinosorb, or Mexoryl SX, and also has other undesirable traits (including the irritant balm mint and a preponderance of peachy shades), which make it a poor choice for all skin types.

☹ POOR **Lucidity Light-Diffusing Makeup SPF 8** *($35)* does not include the UVA-protecting ingredients of titanium dioxide, zinc oxide, avobenzone, Tinosorb, or Mexoryl SX and its SPF is much too low for adequate daytime protection. In addition, this has become a dated liquid foundation with few redeeming qualities.

ESTEE LAUDER CONCEALERS

☺ GOOD **$$$ Ideal Light Brush-On Illuminator** *($26.50)* is sold as a concealer and radiance-reviving product in one. The click-pen applicator feeds product onto a synthetic brush tip. This makes spot application easy, but it is possible to dispense too much product, and there's no way to put it back. This concealer works better as a highlighter due to its sheer texture. Coverage is not sufficient enough to hide darkness under the eyes, camouflage redness, or blur sun-induced discolorations. It layers well for areas that do need more coverage, but why bother when a standard concealer does that with considerably less product? As a highlighter, this product adds a soft-focus effect to skin, sets to a satin matte finish, and actually works better when paired with a regular concealer (applied afterward). You can dab it on to highlight under the eyes, the brow bone, or bridge of the nose. Several shades are offered for your preference.

☺ GOOD **$$$ Smoothing Creme Concealer** *($22)* comes in a squeeze tube, so be cautious of dispensing too much. It has a soft, creamy texture and a natural finish that allows for medium coverage with minimal chance of creasing. This can easily look too thick and heavy if not blended well; with practice, you'll find it a workable option. Among the shades, there are options for fair to deep skin tones.

☺ AVERAGE **$$$ Double Wear Stay-in-Place Flawless Wear Concealer SPF 10** *($22)* is a matte finish concealer that provides nearly full coverage and includes a plethora of neutral-toned shades ranging from fair to deep. The texture has minimal slip and delivers a matte finish that stays put throughout the day, ideal for normal to oily or breakout-prone skin. Seamless application is obtainable, but you must blend quickly before the formula has a chance to set. Once it dries, this is tricky to soften as it has very little movement. Despite containing titanium dioxide sunscreen for broad-spectrum sun protection with anti-aging benefits, it's disappointing that the SPF stopped at 10. The recommended minimum by medical boards all over the world is SPF 15, so SPF 10 just doesn't cut it. Had the SPF been higher we would have given this a better rating. Still, this is worth considering for extra sun protection around the eyes, and it's great for those with dark circles.

☹ POOR **Re-Nutriv Intensive Concealing Duo** *($38)* is one of the thickest, greasiest concealers around, and although it provides sufficient coverage, it looks heavy and creases endlessly. Don't bother!

ESTEE LAUDER POWDERS

☺ GOOD **$$$ Double Wear Mineral Rich Loose Powder Makeup SPF 12** *($35)* is a finely milled loose powder that offers broad-spectrum sun protection (thanks to titanium dioxide), while also providing light to medium buildable coverage. The incredibly silky-dry finish has the slightest hint of shimmer, but it's so subtle you'll hardly notice. The shade selection ranges from light to medium-dark in a variety of flattering tones. We don't recommend using the powder puff that comes with this powder to apply it. Instead, apply it with a brush; it blends beautifully on skin. This gets a nod from us, but with one caution: We don't recommend this or any other loose (or pressed) powder as your sole source of sun protection. All sunscreens must be applied liberally, and applying a pressed or loose powder liberally can make it look thick and cakey. Also, the SPF 12 is below the minimum standard recommended by most medical boards worldwide (SPF 15 is the minimum). However, if you use this in combination with your daytime moisturizer or foundation that does have a sunscreen (SPF 15 or greater), this is a very good option to consider; hence, it earns a positive rating.

☺ GOOD **$$$ Lucidity Translucent Loose Powder** *($31)* is talc-free and has an intriguing texture that's difficult to describe because Lauder opted not to use talc alternatives such as mica and cornstarch. The texture is very light and feels weightless and smooth on skin. It leaves a soft, radiant shine, which is supposed to downplay wrinkles, but doesn't really have that effect. Still, this is recommended for normal to dry skin and it comes in beautiful shades, including options for dark (but not very dark) skin.

☺ GOOD **$$$ Re-Nutriv Intensive Comfort Pressed Powder** *($50)* offers more coverage and a longer-lasting matte (in feel) finish than the Re-Nutriv Intensive Smoothing Powder reviewed below. The shine is also toned down compared to the loose version, but still visible. All told, this is a very good, though pricey, powder for normal to very dry skin. It doesn't look the least bit powdery, and comes in four excellent shades.

☺ GOOD **$$$ Re-Nutriv Intensive Smoothing Powder** *($50)* has a supremely silky, almost creamy feeling, talc-based texture. It meshes perfectly with skin and leaves a polished finish complete with a noticeable amount of shine. We suppose that part is what Lauder hopes will distract you from noticing that your wrinkles aren't really smoothed, but at least it's not blatant sparkles. If you're going to spend too much money on a loose powder, this is definitely one of the better ones to consider. The shades are soft and neutral, imparting just a hint of color.

☹ AVERAGE **$$$ Double Matte Oil-Control Pressed Powder** *($27)* has a talc- and silica-based formula. The texture is similar to that of the Lucidity Translucent Pressed Powder reviewed below, but with an even drier, slightly chalky finish. Although that can be a problem for some skin tones, a powder this dry is a boon for those with very oily skin. All the shades are good, and include options for dark (but not very dark) skin.

☺ AVERAGE **$$$ Double Wear Stay-in-Place Powder Makeup SPF 10** *($35)* lists titanium dioxide as its sole active ingredient, but the SPF rating is below the benchmark, making this talc-based powder best as an adjunct to another product (foundation or moisturizer) rated SPF 15 or greater. It has a very smooth but thick texture that blends well and provides slight to medium buildable coverage. The strong matte finish has a bit of chalkiness to it that primarily affects the darker shades, which tend to go on or turn ash. Among the shades are some great neutral options for fair to medium skin. The absorbency and matte finish make it best for oily to very oily skin.

☺ AVERAGE **$$$ Lucidity Translucent Pressed Powder** *($27)* has a talc-based formula that goes on smoothly but quite dry. It leaves skin looking powdered and doesn't do a thing to soften the appearance of lines, but that's not a realistic quality to look for in powder anyway. The six sheer shades tend to be a bit peach or pink, but that's not really noticeable on skin.

ESTEE LAUDER BLUSHES & BRONZERS

✓☺ BEST **$$$ Pure Color Blush** *($28)* lives up to its name in terms of richly pigmented shades that add a true flush of color. The soft and silky pressed-powder texture blends on beautifully smooth and leaves a radiant glow. The color range is extensive, with options for every skin tone, and you have your choice of satin or shimmer finishes.

✓☺ BEST **$$$ Signature Satin Creme Blush** *($26)* has an exquisite texture that applies smoothly, setting to a silky soft powder finish that feels slightly moist. Ideal for normal to dry skin, the colors go on translucent and build well if you want more intensity. The only drawback is the limited range of shades, but hopefully they will remedy that. By the way, what's available now contains only traces of shine, so this is suitable for daytime makeup.

☺ GOOD **$$$ Bronze Goddess Soft Duo Bronzer** *($32)* is a pressed-powder bronzer that provides two shades (without dividers) in one compact. You get a soft, fleshy peach shade along with a medium bronze shade. The included brush is soft, but the odd cut and flat shape doesn't produce results as foolproof as using a full size blush or powder brush. The powder has a smooth, dry texture and soft, even application that works well to produce a convincing tan without excess shine. Also recommended are Lauder's **Bronze Goddess Soft Matte Bronzer** ($32) and **Bronze Goddess Soft Shimmer Bronzer** ($32). Both work best on light to medium skin tones, or to complement the color you get from self-tanner.

ESTEE LAUDER EYESHADOWS & PRIMERS

✓☺ BEST **Double Wear Stay in Place Eyeshadow Base** *($16)* looks like a pale peach cream concealer in its glass pot, but applies silky-smooth and almost colorless. The powdery solvents and clay that comprise the bulk of this formula lend a matte base to eyelids, and this works well to enhance eyeshadow application and longevity. Although this works as claimed (it even kept a cream eyeshadow crease-free all day), you can get the same results by applying a matte-finish concealer before brushing on your eyeshadows.

✓☺ BEST **$$$ Pure Color EyeShadow** *($20)* is remarkable. It has an enviable silkiness and ultra-smooth texture that meshes with skin rather than looking like powder sitting on top of it. The shades labeled matte are almost matte (there's just a hint of shine), those labeled Satin have soft shine (OK for wrinkled areas when applied sparingly), those labeled Shimmer have strong shine, and those labeled Metallic are glittery and the trickiest to work with (plus the glitter tends to flake). The best shades are Chocolate Bliss, Wild Truffle, Lavish Mink, Provocative Plum, Sandbar Beige, Mischievous Mulberry, Summer Linen, and Wild Sable. Each shade is packaged in a flat compact that includes a built-in mirror and throwaway sponge-tip applicator (the applicator should be tossed in favor of full-sized eyeshadow brushes).

✓☺ BEST $$$ **Pure Color EyeShadow Duo** *($30)* has a buttery-smooth, beautifully silky texture that's a pleasure to apply. These blend superbly and deposit enough color that you'll want to apply in sheer layers unless a more dramatic effect is desired. Most of the duos are well coordinated and each shade has a moderate to intense shimmer finish. The shine doesn't flake, but as with all shiny eyeshadows, they can emphasize wrinkles or sagging skin around the eyes. Duos to consider include Platinums, Cobblestones, Khakis, and Shells.

☺ GOOD $$$ **Double Wear Stay-in-Place ShadowCreme** *($18.50)* is housed in a cumbersome glass pot and is a very good cream-to-powder eyeshadow. Application is impressive: it has just the right amount of slip to allow for smooth, controlled blending. Its crease-free finish is matte in feel, but appearance-wise it's shiny as all get-out. Those with wrinkles around the eye won't appreciate how this cream shadow magnifies them, but if that doesn't apply to you (or you only blend this on the brow bone), then this is recommended.

☺ GOOD $$$ **Pure Color Five Color EyeShadow Palette** *($45)* seems pricey, but the cost isn't as hard to take since you're getting five shades of powder eyeshadow in one sleek compact—and a handful of the sets are coordinated for a beautiful eye design. The enclosed sponge-tip applicators can be tossed because they're too small and you'll get much better results from eyeshadow brushes. Unlike Lauder's Pure Color single and duo eyeshadows, these have a softer color deposit that must be layered for good intensity (though the darker shades go on quite dark even when applied sheer). The texture is smooth and the formula blends well, which is what you want when you're applying several shade of eyeshadow. Each Palette has at least one matte-finish shade and almost all of them have a color that's dark enough to use for eyelining. The most versatile palettes are Film Noir, Desert Heat, and Bronze Dunes.

☺ GOOD $$$ **Pure Color Gelee Powder EyeShadow** *($24)* has a smooth cream-to-powder feel that adheres nicely to skin and won't flake. All the shades have a finely milled shimmering glow that's on the metallic side, and some of the colors go on richly whereas others go on sheer, so you'll need to experiment to see which you prefer. With an untraditional color palette, including vivid shades of teal, silver, and copper among others, it's a great idea to play with these at the counter before you consider purchasing them—especially at this price.

ESTEE LAUDER EYE & BROW LINERS

✓☺ BEST $$$ **Double Wear Stay-in-Place Gel Eyeliner** *($21.50)* is fantastic. The creamy texture glides on without clumping and you have plenty of time to blend before it sets in place for its all-day (really) finish. The colors go on boldly and include classic and trendy options. Watch out for the occasional bright blue and green shades, at least if you want a classic eye design rather than a shocking pop of color. As with all long-wearing gel eyeliners, this requires a good makeup remover when you're ready to take it off.

✓☺ BEST $$$ **Double Wear Zero-Smudge Liquid Eyeliner** *($21.50)* is an excellent liquid liner with a precision felt tip that applies color evenly and easily. This takes several seconds to set, but once it does, it won't move until you're ready to take it off. An interesting twist to this liner is that the shades have a slight glossy finish. Most of the shades are classics, but they do have a touch of sparkle that's not distracting.

☺ GOOD **$$$ Automatic Brow Pencil Duo** *($23.50)* comes in elegant, refillable packaging with an angled brow brush. The pencil has a dry but smooth texture that applies evenly without being too thick or greasy, nor does it deposit too much color at once. The shade selection includes options for blondes and redheads, but the brow brush is too stiff and scratchy for consistent, comfortable use.

☺ GOOD **$$$ Automatic Eye Pencil Duo** *($23.50)* is a standard, twist-up, retractable pencil in an elegant container that features a pointed sponge tip for softening and blending. Although pricey, the refills are a bargain and then you have the sexy container. The formula sports a drier finish, making these less prone to smearing or fading. Classic, attractive shades are offered, and you are bound to find one that flatters your skin tone and eye color.

☹ AVERAGE **$$$ Pure Color Intense Kajal EyeLiner** *($20)* delivers a smooth, even line of color that is easy to blend for a smokey effect, but its creamy texture means it's best to set it with a powder eyeshadow if you want it to stay in place. The shades are richly pigmented, but ultimately this eyeliner pencil isn't worth its price.

ESTEE LAUDER LIP COLOR & LIPLINERS

✓☺ BEST **$$$ Double Wear Stay-in-Place Lip Duo** *($25)* has a formula, application process, and performance identical to that of (Lauder-owned) M.A.C.'s Pro Longwear Lipcolour. As such, this and M.A.C.'s version take first place as the best long-wearing lip colors on the market, although for this category of lip products, the term "best" is relative. We've tested every major contender in this group, from the original Max Factor Lipfinity (no longer available) to copycat versions from Cover Girl, L'Oreal, Lancome, Maybelline New York, Revlon, and Smashbox. Most of them have similar positive attributes and all of them wear longer than traditional lipsticks (even those with a matte finish). Lauder and M.A.C.'s versions excel because they have the smoothest textures and the most even wear. When the color starts to fade (and exactly when that occurs depends greatly on the type of food—greasy or messy—you eat), it does so without chipping or flaking. In addition, the glossy top coat feels light and is completely non-sticky, while others run the gamut from thick and syrupy to super-slick. There are drawbacks to be sure, such as needing to routinely reapply the top coat to ensure comfortable wear, but that's a much simpler task than touching up lipstick, where in most cases you need a mirror (especially if you wear reds or other strong colors). Speaking of color, Lauder's shade selection is smaller than M.A.C.'s, but there's not a bad one in the bunch!

✓☺ BEST **$$$ Double Wear Stay-in-Place Lipstick** *($25)* is a truly matte lipstick! It goes on surprisingly creamy and then dries down to a long-wearing, non-slip finish. No worry about slippage into lines around the mouth, that's for sure. For those who are used to creamy or glossy lipsticks, you will not be happy with this one, but if you would like to stop using lipsticks that quickly run into lines, then this should be high on your list. Because this has a dry finish, you may be tempted to apply a gloss over it, but that negates the benefit of a matte lipstick and the same potential problems will ensue. Lauder's shade range is beautiful and every color provides full coverage.

✓☺ BEST **$$$ Signature Hydra Lustre Lipstick** *($22.50)* is a very good cream lipstick that doesn't feel too slick or slippery and as a result has reasonably good staying power. This remains comfortably creamy with a moist finish that's not noticeably glossy. The shade range is

---

✍ Buying skin-care products packaged in jars? See the Appendix to learn why that's a bad idea.

enticing, and offers your choice of cream, shimmer, or very sparkly finishes. Yes, this is pricey; but if you're going to spend this much for lipstick, you should be buying those that go the distance, and this one fills the bill!

☺ GOOD $$$ **Pure Color Gloss Stick** *($22.50)* provides a good balance between a lipstick and a lip gloss. The creamy gloss texture leaves lips feeling velvety smooth and shiny, while adding color in varying intensities and shades. Colors range from bright corals and pinks to more subdued nude hues and deep shades of plum. Because of its glossy nature, Pure Color Gloss Stick doesn't have much staying power, but if you are looking for a product that supplies color, hydration, and shine without being overly glossy, this is a great hybrid option.

☺ GOOD $$$ **Pure Color Long Lasting Lipstick** *($25)* is a very good, albeit pricey lipstick. It's too creamy to make good on its long-lasting claim (rather than the 4 hours it claims, you can count on about 2), but the colors are richly luxurious and this has a beautifully smooth application that feels creamy without being greasy. Remarkably, it isn't too slick either, which means there's much less chance of it feathering into lines around the mouth, although that will occur if paired with lip gloss. The shade selection is enticing, with shimmer, cream, and frost finishes in rich vibrant colors.

☹ AVERAGE $$$ **Automatic Lip Pencil Duo** *($23.50)* is a standard, twist-up, retractable lipliner, but the tip of the pencil comes out of a wider-than-normal opening, which makes it too thick to be capable of drawing a thin outline around the mouth. That's not a deal-breaker, but what you may not like is that this pencil stays creamy, diminishing its longevity. The built-in lip brush is a nice touch, but not enough to warrant a higher rating.

☹ AVERAGE $$$ **Double Wear Stay-in-Place Lip Pencil** *($19)* needs sharpening and can we all agree that we shouldn't have to take time to sharpen our pencils every morning to get our makeup on? Were it not for the need for routine sharpening, this pencil would be a great option, albeit a pricey one given how many great pencils there are at the drugstore. The texture is comfortably firm with a suede-smooth application that makes perfect liplining nearly effortless.

☹ AVERAGE $$$ **Pure Color Gloss** *($22.50)* is a standard gloss that happens to be highly fragranced, which isn't great for your lips because fragrance causes irritation. You'll smell this gloss when it's on because the strong scent will be right below your nose. This has a thick but spreadable texture and wet-look gloss finish with some residual stickiness.

ESTEE LAUDER MASCARAS

✔☺ BEST $$$ **Double Wear Zero-Smudge Lengthening Mascara** *($21)* has a different, larger brush whose shape and bristle layout allows for equal measures of length and thickness (Clinique's Lash Power, which is similar, isn't much for building thicker lashes). This is easily one of Lauder's most impressive mascaras, and it wears tenaciously. The bonus, at least compared to other long-wearing/waterproof mascaras, is how easy this is to remove. Warm water and agitation alone will do it, but for best results you should follow with your regular cleanser or makeup remover.

✔☺ BEST $$$ **Sumptuous Bold Volume Lifting Mascara** *($21)* has an uneven application, which tends to deposit too much mascara to the outer lashes, but this gives way to smooth results and supremely long lashes that are perfectly defined. Want more? Successive coats not only smooth through minor clumps, but also build appreciable thickness. The formula wears without smearing and flaking, and removes easily with a water-soluble cleanser.

✔☺ BEST $$$ **Sumptuous Waterproof Bold Volume Lifting Mascara** *($21)*. With most waterproof mascaras you get appreciable length, but then you have to trade off on thickness. That's because the ingredients that add thickness to lashes don't always hold up well, and in a waterproof formula, holding up is the goal. In this case, you can have the best of both worlds without clumps or flaking during wear. You'll see impressive results with just a few strokes, and you can keep building for fullness and definition without creating spidery-looking or spiky lashes. True to claim, this is waterproof. It requires a separate eye-makeup remover to take it off; Paula's Choice Gentle Touch Makeup Remover works beautifully, or you can explore other options recommended throughout this chapter.

☺ GOOD $$$ **Sumptuous Extreme Lash Multiplying Volume Mascara** *($23.50)* has a large brush, which, if you can get past (or get used to) it, does a great job of making lashes longer, thicker, and flutter-worthy. Application is almost perfectly even, and the slight clumping is easily combed through for beautifully separated lashes. If you apply several coats, this comes close to creating a false lash effect, but it's not as dramatic as the claims imply. This mascara wears without a hitch (but be careful of getting excess mascara on your lash line during application) and it comes off easily with a water-soluble cleanser.

☺ AVERAGE $$$ **Lash Primer Plus** *($20)* is sold as a pre-mascara conditioning base for lashes, but that is an unwarranted step given the industrywide availability of superior one-step mascaras. The formula closely matches that of most mascaras, save for the addition of a tiny amount of nut oils.

☺ AVERAGE $$$ **MagnaScopic Maximum Volume Mascara** *($21)* supposedly makes lashes 300% thicker. Lauder even refers to it as "the fast track to thick lashes." If that's the case, then it must be a poorly traveled track, because thickness was hard to come by even after successive applications, and there were clumps along the way. Where this really excels (beyond its clever name) is for lengthening and long wear. If you're willing to put up with a slightly uneven application and have the patience to separate clumped lashes, this is a good (but not great) option.

☺ AVERAGE $$$ **Sumptuous Two Tone Eye Opening Mascara** *($28)*. The premise behind the "two tone" portion of this dual-ended mascara's name is that it offers two colors and two brushes in one component. In each case, Lauder recommends using the classic black mascara on the top lashes. For the bottom lashes, you are supposed to use the colored mascara (brown, dark blue, or deep plum), which comes with a brush that is shorter in length and has short bristles. The result is supposed to be an "eye-brightening" effect, and while we didn't notice any of that going on, the idea to use a softer color than black on the lower lashes isn't a bad one. (In fact, that's exactly what we recommend for eyeliner on the upper and lower lash line.) On top lash, black mascara adds volume and length, whereas the bottom lash mascara offers softly defined, smudge-proof lashes. The problem is this mascara is flaky no matter which way you use it. Had that not been the case, it would've received a higher rating.

ESTEE LAUDER FACE & BODY ILLUMINATORS

✓☺ BEST $$$ **Signature 5-Tone Shimmer Powder for Eyes, Cheeks, Face** *($38)* is an easy-to-apply pressed powder with shine! It has a buttery smooth texture and nearly foolproof application that adds soft, sheer colors and a radiant finish that enlivens skin without overdoing the sparkles. It is excellent used over blush, on its own as a cheek color/highlighter, or dusted over smaller areas. Lauder offers ivory-pink or soft bronze options, and both palettes are beautiful, particularly for fair to medium skin tones.

ESTEE LAUDER BRUSHES

☺ GOOD $$$ **Estee Lauder Brushes** *($20-$42)* have improved over the years in terms of shape, density, and softness, but they're still not as elegant, functional, or attractive as those from Lauder-owned M.A.C., Bobbi Brown, or Aveda. At Lauder's price points, we expected, but didn't observe, higher quality. Still, they have improved and are a viable option if you're keen on exploring brushes with the Lauder logo.

EUCERIN (SKIN CARE ONLY)

Strengths: Inexpensive and widely distributed; fragrance-free cleansers.

Weaknesses: Anti-redness products that added questionable ingredients instead of increasing the anti-inflammatory agents; nothing for acne-prone skin; jar packaging.

For more information and reviews of the latest Eucerin products (including their body-care products), visit CosmeticsCop.com.

EUCERIN CLEANSER

✓☺ BEST **Redness Relief Soothing Cleanser** *($8.79 for 6.8 fl. oz.)* is a gentle, fragrance-free, water-soluble cleansing gel whose simple formula is ideal for those with sensitive, easily irritated skin. It contains licorice root extract, a good anti-irritant, but considering the amount of it here and the limited time it's in contact with your skin, it will not lead to "immediate redness relief." However, this cleanser isn't apt to make persistent facial redness worse. It is best for normal to slightly dry or slightly oily skin.

EUCERIN MOISTURIZERS (DAYTIME & NIGHTTIME), EYE CREAMS, & SERUMS

☺ AVERAGE **Everyday Protection Face Lotion SPF 30** *($8.99 for 4 fl. oz.)* has two things going for it: an in-part mineral sunscreen (titanium dioxide and zinc oxide with other actives) and a fragrance-free formula. The synthetic sunscreen actives, while important, don't qualify this product as nonirritating, so this isn't a surefire bet for those with sensitive skin or rosacea. It is also disappointing that antioxidants are completely absent. Still, this provides reliable broad-spectrum sun protection in a creamy base and ends up being an affordable, though unexciting, option.

☺ AVERAGE **Q10 Anti-Wrinkle Sensitive Skin Creme** *($11.79 for 1.7 fl. oz.)* contains some well-documented antioxidants in a light yet creamy base formula. Unfortunately, jar packaging won't keep the antioxidants stable, leaving you with an average choice for normal to dry skin. See the Appendix to learn why jar packaging isn't the way to go for moisturizers.

☺ AVERAGE **Redness Relief Daily Perfecting Lotion SPF 15** *($14.99 for 1.7 fl. oz.)* deserves praise for including titanium dioxide for sufficient UVA protection, but there are problems with this formula, especially for those with reddened, easily irritated skin. The active ingredients are two synthetic sunscreens, which, while generally well tolerated, are not the best for someone with sensitive skin. Eucerin would have been wise to use just titanium dioxide and/or zinc oxide as the active(s). Another issue is the inclusion of denatured alcohol. There's not a lot of it in the product, but for someone with red, sensitive skin, it's cause for concern. The alcohol is more prevalent than the played-up licorice extract, which is present in such a small amount its soothing benefit is negligible. Finally, this lotion is tinted mint green in an effort to cancel facial redness. Such color-correction rarely looks convincing, but in this case, it's so sheer as to be barely noticeable on skin, so it doesn't matter one way or the other. This moisturizing sunscreen is an OK option for normal to dry skin that is not affected by redness or sensitivity, but it's certainly not what current research indicates is a state-of-the-art formula.

☺ AVERAGE **Redness Relief Soothing Night Creme** *($14.99 for 1.7 fl. oz.)* doesn't have much to it, though it is fragrance-free, which is great for sensitive skin. Given what we know about what skin needs to look and feel healthy, whether it is sensitive or not, this jar-packaged moisturizer lacks interest. Consisting primarily of water, glycerin, panthenol, and triglycerides, it's an extremely simple, slightly emollient formula for normal to slightly dry skin. What's missing are antioxidants, cell-communicating ingredients, and a more sophisticated mix of ingredients that mimic the structure and function of healthy skin. It does contain licorice extract for its anti-irritant properties, but given the small amount, we're skeptical that someone with persistent redness or rosacea will notice their symptoms abating. Still, if you're curious, this bland formula shouldn't make reddened, sensitive skin worse. Check out the Appendix to find out why moisturizers in jar packaging aren't the best idea.

☹ POOR **Q10 Anti-Wrinkle Sensitive Skin Lotion SPF 15** *($10.99 for 4 fl. oz.)* does not contain the UVA-protecting ingredients of titanium dioxide, zinc oxide, avobenzone, Tinosorb, or Mexoryl SX, and is not recommended. No antioxidant around can make up for an omission like this, at least if your goal is to keep skin from wrinkling and sagging.

EUCERIN LIP CARE

✓☺ BEST **Aquaphor Lip Repair** *($4.29 for 0.35 fl. oz.)* is a very good (though hard to find) emollient lip balm that comes in a squeeze tube. The fragrance-free formula is gentle and does an excellent job of taking care of dry, chapped lips. Eucerin included a small, but potentially effective, amount of antioxidants, an anti-irritant, and a cell-communicating ingredient, all of which can contribute toward making your lips healthier. Formula- and cost-wise, this is a great, portable lip balm!

EUCERIN SPECIALTY SKIN-CARE PRODUCTS

✓☺ BEST **Aquaphor Healing Ointment** *($5.99 for 1.75 fl. oz.)* is a gentle formula that does a formidable job of protecting skin that is dry, cracked, or irritated, although this isn't much more than a classic ointment. Aquaphor Healing Ointment may be used anywhere on the face, including the lips. It is excellent for severely dry hands and feet. The price and size mentioned in this review refers to the tube. Aquaphor also comes in a larger jar, but this tends to be messier. This deserves our highest rating due to its value for compromised skin and as an aid for sensitive skin. It is a dermatologist favorite for good reason! **Aquaphor Baby Healing Ointment** ($8.28 for 3 fl. oz.) is nearly identical to the original Aquaphor Healing Ointment, and the same comments apply.

GARNIER NUTRITIONISTE (SKIN CARE ONLY)

Strengths: The eye roller is an intriguing product.

Weaknesses: Lack of sufficient UVA protection from the sunscreens; average to below average moisturizers; mostly irritating cleansers; no products for blemish-prone skin; no products to address uneven skin tone or skin discolorations; ineffective BHA products; jar packaging.

For more information and the latest Garnier Nutritioniste product reviews, visit CosmeticsCop.com.

GARNIER NUTRITIONISTE CLEANSERS

☹ POOR **Moisture Rescue Fresh Cleansing Foam** *($5.99 for 6.8 fl. oz.)* contains some potentially drying cleansing agents as well as a high amount of potassium hydroxide (that's lye), an alkaline ingredient that can destroy skin's protective barrier and leave your skin feeling dry and tight, a sensation that doesn't mean your skin is clean. Add to that the strong kick of fragrance and the claim that this cleanser is hydrating and it becomes a bad joke. If you're shopping for water-soluble cleansers at the drugstore, look to those from CeraVe, Olay, or most of those from Neutrogena instead.

☹ POOR **Refreshing Remover Cleansing Towelettes, Oil-Free** *($6.79 for 25 towelettes)* have minimal cleansing ability (they don't remove mascara, as claimed) and end up being irritating to skin thanks to the amount of peppermint steeped in each cloth.

☹ POOR **Skin Renew The Brusher Gel-Cleanser, Oil-free** *($7.99 for 5 fl. oz.).* Garnier has created what can be described as a poor woman's Clarisonic. Unlike Clarisonic's expensive battery-powered facial brush, Garnier's option includes a built-in brush that is powered only by your hand as you massage it over your face. The bristles are relatively soft and composed of synthetic fiber, which essentially is just a glorified washcloth. As it turns out, although the brush isn't a problem, the gel cleanser is. It is highly fragrant and contains irritants such as witch hazel and peppermint as well as the potent menthol derivative menthoxypropanediol. Garnier maintains this is gentle enough for daily use, but that must mean they haven't seen the research about what risks these ingredients pose for skin. The novelty of a built-in brush isn't enough to make this worth a try—not if you want to keep your skin healthy.

☹ POOR **Skin Renew The Brusher Microbead Cleanser, Combination Skin** *($7.99 for 5 fl. oz.)* not only contains scrub particles to do a more thorough job, but the cleanser itself is dispensed onto a built-in brush, ready to massage over your face. The scrub granules plus the brush can be exfoliation overkill (especially if you're too zealous while using), but what really makes this a poor option is the cleansing formula. It is loaded (and we mean loaded) with fragrance ingredients known to be irritating. Also on hand for more irritation is peppermint and a potent form of menthol known as menthoxypropanediol. All this irritation can lead to dry, flaky, tight skin.

☹ POOR **The Ultimate Cleanser 3-Way Clean, Oil-free** *($7.99 for 5 fl. oz.).* The "3-way" part of this product's name refers to the fact that it can be used as a cleanser, a scrub, or a mask. The formula is closest to that of an absorbent clay mask for oily skin, and that's how it works best—but there are warnings all the way around no matter how you use it. As a cleanser, this is tricky to use, and it doesn't contain much in the way of cleansing ingredients. It isn't adept at removing makeup, either. As a scrub, it contains standard polyethylene (plastic) scrub beads, but the clay base makes it harder to use than a regular facial scrub that also contains cleansing agents because it is hard to move around on your skin and it's difficult to rinse. Although this may seem like a convenient product, no matter how you use it, your skin will suffer irritation from peppermint and menthol. This kind of irritation causes collagen to break down and can stimulate oil production at the base of the pore. Last, but not least, whether used as a mask, cleanser, or scrub, this is difficult to rinse.

GARNIER NUTRITIONISTE SCRUB

☹ POOR **Expert Exfoliator Daily Exfoliating Gel, Oil-free** *($6.49 for 5 fl. oz.).* Although this cleanser/scrub hybrid has its strong points, they're weakened by the inclusion of several problematic ingredients, including the drying cleansing agent TEA-lauryl sulfate and an irritating amount of peppermint, not to mention the menthol, which cannot deep clean or refine pores as claimed. See the Appendix to learn why irritants like these are a problem for all skin types.

GARNIER NUTRITIONISTE MOISTURIZERS (DAYTIME & NIGHTTIME), EYE CREAMS, & SERUMS

☺ GOOD **Skin Renew Anti-Puff Eye Roller** *($13.49 for 0.5 fl. oz.).* The best part of this product is the metal roller-ball applicator, which glides along the curvature of the under-eye area with ease, depositing a thin layer of water based liquid. The two ingredients associated with reducing puffiness and dark circles are escin (a component of horse chestnut), due to its circulation-stimulating abilities, and caffeine, due to its constricting abilities. Regrettably, neither ingredient's association with reducing puffy eyes has any solid research to support the claim, although both are notable antioxidants (Source: naturaldatabase.com). This does have a temporary smoothing and tightening effect on skin, but not to the extent that puffy eyes will be visibly deflated. The mica casts a slight shimmer on skin, which reflects light away from dark circles, but a concealer would work much better. At best, this is a novel way to apply a light film of moisture-binding agents and antioxidants to skin. The fragrance-free formula is suitable for all skin types.

☺ AVERAGE **Skin Renew Radiance Moisture Cream** *($13.99 for 1.7 fl. oz.)* is among Garnier's most interesting formulas, but that's not exactly high praise because most of their moisturizers are average to below average at best. Although the texture feels great, it fails to supply your skin with the range of important ingredients it needs to look and act younger. Garnier did include a small amount of some good antioxidants (including a form of vitamin C), but they won't remain stable once this jar-packaged moisturizer is opened. See the Appendix to learn why jar packaging is a problem. Also disappointing is the range of fragrance ingredients present. These include benzyl salicylate, geraniol, and limonene, all of which put your skin at risk of irritation that causes collagen to break down and hurts the skin's ability to fight wrinkles. This also contains mica for a shiny glow, but shine isn't skin care, it is merely a makeup effect.

☺ AVERAGE **Ultra-Lift 2-in-1 Wrinkle Reducer Serum + Moisturizer** *($16.99 for 1.7 fl. oz.).* Housed in one container is a swirled moisturizer and serum said to firm skin and reduce wrinkles. But far from being a 2-in-1 miracle, this product, whose texture is more moisturizer than serum, is mostly disappointing. It contains a standard roster of slip agents and thickeners to create a cushiony feel, but the state-of-the-art ingredients are in short supply. This is said to contain "pro retinol from nature," but the form of vitamin A used is retinyl linoleate, which may be natural or synthetic. This form of vitamin A is retinol combined with linoleic acid, and both are good cell-communicating ingredients. However, there is considerably more research on pure retinol benefiting skin than retinyll linoleate, and even so, Garnier isn't using much retinyl linoleate in this product. Along with the retinyl linoleate is a tiny amount of antioxidant vitamin E, likely not enough to offer any anti-aging impact. This serum plus moisturizer makes some big promises, but the formula simply isn't capable of fulfilling them. For certain, it cannot lift sagging skin; no skin-care product or ingredient can do that because the multiple factors that lead to sagging cannot be completely addressed by skin-care products. In terms of instant firming, this contains enough film-forming agents to make skin feel a bit firmer, perhaps even a little tighter, but skin feeling firmer or tighter isn't the same as it actually becoming firmer or tighter—it's just a tactile sensation that may make you think the product is doing something. If you decide to try this, it's best for normal to dry skin.

☺ AVERAGE **Ultra-Lift Anti-Wrinkle Firming Eye Cream** *($14.99 for 0.5 fl. oz.)* doesn't contain any ingredients capable of lifting or noticeably firming skin, but it has a silky cream texture many will find appealing. What's not so appealing is the low amount of retinyl linoleate (a form of retinol) and the fact that the waxes in this eye cream make it somewhat of an antiquated formula. In short, this eye cream cannot lift wrinkles around the eye. Even if it could, where would the excess skin go? Cosmetic surgery is the only solution for sagging skin around the eyes. Lastly, we know it's surprising but the truth is you don't need an eye cream (see the Appendix to find out why).

☺ AVERAGE **Ultra Lift Pro Gravity Defying Cream Intensive** (*$16.99 for 1.5 fl. oz.*) differs little from several others Garnier Nutritioniste offers. It contains mostly water, silicone, glycerin, plant oil, thickeners, film-forming agent, and preservative. None of these ingredients can lift or re-sculpt skin. If it really worked as claimed, cosmetic surgeons would be closing shop left and right—yet that's not happening. This contains a handful of intriguing ingredients, but most of them will be diminished because Garnier chose jar packaging. At best, this is a mediocre option for normal to dry skin, assuming you don't expect even a fraction of the claims to become reality. See the Appendix to learn of the problems jar packaging presents.

☹ POOR **Moisture Rescue Lightweight UV Lotion SPF 15** (*$8.39 for 4.5 fl. oz.*) does not provide sufficient UVA protection because it doesn't contain titanium dioxide, zinc oxide, ecamsule, Tinosorb, or Mexoryl SX. The only lightweight aspect of this lotion is that it's light on beneficial ingredients. Its formula is so stunningly basic it makes white bread look exciting in comparison. It's mostly water, silicone, glycerin, film-forming agent (think hairspray), fragrant plant extracts, and enough fragrance ingredients to cause irritation, which won't help skin's barrier remain healthy and able to retain moisture. If anything, your skin needs rescuing from this product! See the Appendix to learn why daily use of fragranced products like this hurt your skin.

☹ POOR **Moisture Rescue Refreshing Gel-Cream** (*$7.99 for 1.7 fl. oz.*). How moisturizing can a product that lists alcohol as its third ingredient be? Well, given that alcohol dries out the skin, it's obviously not very moisturizing, although this fact seemingly wasn't apparent to Garnier. Between the alcohol, which causes free-radical damage and collagen breakdown, and a shockingly basic, highly fragranced formula, this is a terrible moisturizer for all skin types.

☹ POOR **Skin Renew Anti-Dark-Circle Eye Roller** (*$13.49 for 0.5 fl. oz.*). This lightweight serum is packaged in a tube with one end having a metal roller-ball applicator. You're supposed to massage it over dark circles for quick relief, but don't count on instant or long-term improvement, or any dark circle-related benefit from this type of packaging. It would be great if we could instantly roll away dark circles, but it's just not possible. Massaging skin to stimulate circulation isn't the answer in this case, because increasing blood flow to the under-eye area can actually make dark circles look even darker. Also, some types of dark circles are due to pigmentation issues that are either hereditary or from sun damage. These types of dark circles don't respond to massage or any of the ingredients in this product. Although the roller-ball applicator is a "neat-o" factor, what's dispensed is far more problematic than exciting. The formula contains a high amount of alcohol and the sunscreen ingredient ethylhexyl methoxycinnamate. The alcohol causes collagen breakdown and hurts skin's healing process—two things guaranteed to make dark circles worse—and the sunscreen ingredient isn't the best for use so close to the eye itself (it can cause stinging). You would be far better off treating your eye area with a fragrance-free serum loaded with collagen-stimulating antioxidants and keeping it protected daily with a sunscreen rated SPF 15 or greater. Those steps will help your dark circles considerably more than this product ever could!

☹ POOR **Skin Renew Anti-Sun Damage Daily Moisture Lotion SPF 28** (*$13.49 for 2.5 fl. oz.*) provides avobenzone for sufficient UVA protection, which is great. What's not so great is the inclusion of alcohol as the third ingredient. The previous version of this daytime moisturizer with sunscreen did not contain alcohol, and the formulary change isn't a boon for anyone's skin. Adding to the irritation and potential for collagen breakdown from the alcohol is the inclusion of several fragrance ingredients known to cause irritation. Given the number of SPF-rated moisturizers that omit needless irritants, why bother with this one?

☹ POOR **Skin Renew Miracle Skin Perfector B.B. Cream SPF 15** *($11.99)* is among the least impressive of the numerous BB creams the cosmetics industry offers. Its sunscreen fails to provide sufficient UVA protection, so right from the start a key benefit (broad-spectrum sun protection) falls short and leaves your skin vulnerable to wrinkles. This has a lightweight, thin cream texture that feels more like a lotion when applied, and it is easy to blend. It sets to a satin finish that feels slightly moist, making this preferred for normal to dry skin. Two shades are offered, both of which are on the peachy side. Since this isn't as sheer as a tinted moisturizer, the peachy tint can look more obvious (the formula provides light coverage). Although Garnier has printed some impressive-looking before-and-after photos on the box for this BB cream, the reality is that this effect is best achieved with a good foundation, not a product whose shades tend to look off and whose formula slips easily into lines and large pores. One more drawback, and this is a big one: this BB cream is intensely fragranced and contains numerous fragrance ingredients known to cause irritation. Between that, the lack of sufficient UVA protection, and the paltry amount of beneficial extras (BB creams are supposed to contain beneficial ingredients like antioxidants and skin-lightening agents), this is not recommended.

☹ POOR **Ultra-Lift Anti-Wrinkle Eye Roller** *($14.99 for 0.5 fl. oz.)*. This lightweight serum is packaged in a tube with one end having a metal roller-ball applicator. You're supposed to massage it around the eye area to reduce wrinkles (specifically, crow's-feet at the edges of the eyes), but the formula is incredibly problematic and not the least bit anti-aging. Despite the coolness factor from the roller-ball applicator, what it dispenses exposes your skin to a strong dose of irritation. The amount of alcohol plus citrus extracts, ginger root, and a sensitizing preservative causes collagen breakdown and hurts skin's healing process. That is not uplifting in the least.

☹ POOR **Ultra-Lift Anti-Wrinkle Firming Moisturizer, SPF 15** *($14.99 for 1.6 fl. oz.)* continues L'Oreal's (parent company of Garnier) frustrating predilection for launching sunscreens that lack sufficient UVA-protecting ingredients. They know better, and have for years, so products like this are in no way deserving of a purchase or even a second glance. Even if this daytime moisturizer with sunscreen supplied the type of UVA protection you need if your goal is to prevent wrinkles, the overall formula is stunningly basic and contains a couple of fragrance ingredients that pose a risk of irritation.

☹ POOR **Ultra-Lift Anti-Wrinkle Firming Night Cream** *($14.99 for 1.7 fl. oz.)* contains several ingredients that are necessary to make dry to very dry skin look and feel better, including glycerin and shea butter. Although those and the thickening agents in this moisturizer serve dry skin well, the product's jar packaging compromises the effectiveness of the antioxidants, and that's ultra-disappointing. Also a letdown is the inclusion of fragrance ingredients known to cause irritation. See the Appendix to learn why jar packaging and fragrance are a problem, and to learn what you can do to help sagging skin.

☹ POOR **Ultra-Lift Daily Targeted Wrinkle Treatment** *($14.99 for 1 fl. oz.)* is said to target deep wrinkles at their source, but that's not possible because deep wrinkles (the kind you see after years of sun damage and facial expressions) have their source in the dermis, beyond where moisturizers can really have an impact. As it turns out, this is another below average moisturizer from L'Oreal-owned Garnier. Although it contains some good emollients and antioxidants (along with retinyl linoleate, which is a form of retinol), it also contains several fragrance ingredients known to cause irritation. See the Appendix to learn why daily use of highly fragrant products like this is a mistake for all skin types.

☹ POOR **Ultra Lift Intensive Deep Wrinkle Night Cream** *($16.99 for 1.5 fl. oz.)*. Claiming to plump deep wrinkles while you sleep is the enticing promise this relatively inexpensive product wants you to believe is possible. So, will you wake up in the morning looking like you've had a face-lift or had dermal fillers injected into your lines? No. Not only won't this product perform that outstanding feat, the formula is an utter disappointment and an overall problem for skin. Despite a silky texture, the amount of alcohol is a serious cause for concern (alcohol causes free-radical damage and collagen breakdown) and the formula is practically void of antioxidants and key antiwrinkle ingredients (i.e., those that can stimulate healthy collagen production and skin's natural repair process so wrinkles truly look better). Even if those ingredients were present, the jar packaging wouldn't keep them stable so it doesn't matter anyway.

GARNIER NUTRITIONISTE SPECIALTY SKIN-CARE PRODUCT

☹ POOR **Skin Renew Dark Spot Corrector Clinical** *($16.99 for 1.7 fl. oz.)* contains pure vitamin C (ascorbic acid) to help lighten brown spots from sun damage. The amount of vitamin C is impressive, and there is research proving it is a viable option for lightening discolorations (Sources: *Archives of Pharmacal Research*, May 2011, pages 811–820; and *American Journal of Clinical Dermatology*, April 2011, pages 87–99). However, there is a concern over the amount of potassium hydroxide (lye), which can cause dryness and irritation, as can the numerous fragrance ingredients in this gel. Irritation in turn can make stubborn discolorations (including red or brown marks from acne) worse because it hurts skin's ability to heal and repair itself. Although this product has the potential to improve discolorations, it may also make them last longer—and do you really want to risk that?

GIORGIO ARMANI (MAKEUP ONLY)

Strengths: Outstanding foundations, superb powder textures, a brilliant shimmer fluid, great primers; perfect bronzers; a neutral palette of complexion enhancers make this line's makeup a must-see.

Weaknesses: Expensive; the skin care (reviewed on CosmeticsCop.com) is more gimmicky than useful, though some of the textures are beautiful; foundations with sunscreen that do not provide sufficient UVA protection; mascaras that aren't as impressive as they should be.

For more information and reviews of the latest Giorgio Armani products, visit CosmeticsCop.com.

GIORGIO ARMANI FOUNDATIONS & PRIMERS

✔☺ BEST **$$$ Designer Shaping Cream Foundation SPF 20** *($65)* earns a place on the ever-growing list of Uber-pricey foundations, but at least there is a lot to love about this particular option. Its higher-than-usual sunscreen is in-part titanium dioxide, and this is one of the creamiest yet lightweight foundations for dry to very dry skin you're likely to find. Its emollient texture feels decadently silky and blends very well, though it takes time to set to a soft satin finish. Dry skin is left with a radiant glow, while coverage stays in the medium range. The silk fibers and oil in this foundation do not contour skin, so don't mistake this for a face-lift in a jar (though that's likely how the lofty price was determined). It is a rich yet not heavy-feeling cream foundation with a superb blend of ingredients to replenish dry skin while leaving a soft glow.

✓☺ BEST **$$$ Lasting Silk UV Compact SPF 34** *($59)* is an impressive powder foundation with sunscreen! The texture is elegantly silky and it blends to a beautiful smooth finish while offering medium coverage. The shade range is typical Armani, which means excellent! They offer seven flattering colors, with options for fair to tan skin. All that and broad-spectrum sun protection in an easy-to-use pressed powder for all skin types! What more could you ask for? OK, the price is needlessly high, but if you are willing to splurge, this is a great powder foundation with sun protection. Those on a budget, fear not: Maybelline New York's Age Rewind Protector Finishing Powder SPF 25 is equally fantastic (and don't forget, L'Oreal owns Giorgio Armani and Maybelline).

✓☺ BEST **$$$ Light Master Primer** *($57)* is an outstanding thin-textured fluid product that gives skin a subtle lit-from-within glow. Its texture is light and silky, and it leaves a minimally moist finish. Applied under foundation, it helps enliven the complexion and adds heightened dimension to skin. It may also be used over foundation to highlight key areas. The light-show claims Armani makes for this primer are over-the-top, but if you're shopping Armani for primers and don't mind the expense for a cosmetic facial pick-me-up, this is worth a trial run.

☺ GOOD **$$$ Designer Lift Smoothing Firming Foundation SPF 20** *($65)* is a very good liquid foundation with an in-part titanium dioxide sunscreen. Broad-spectrum sun protection is assured, but in terms of lifting or firming skin, the formula cannot do that. For the most part, this contains a similar roster of ingredients you'll find in most modern liquid foundations. Armani includes some vitamin E (tocopherol) and a tiny amount of the cell-communicating ingredient adenosine, but these won't do much to firm skin and they absolutely cannot correct sagging. The company claims "12 hours of lifting action," but really the only lifting that occurs is when you pick up the glass bottle to dispense the foundation! Designer Lift has a silky, elegant, fluid texture that provides medium, buildable coverage and sets to a soft, semi-matte finish. Like all Armani's liquid foundations, this blends beautifully. The smooth, almost weightless finish improves skin's appearance without sinking into lines around the eyes or magnifying large pores, but it is not quite as natural-looking as Armani's Luminous Silk Foundation. The shade range is mostly impressive, though the majority of colors skew toward being yellow-toned rather than true neutrals. That's not necessarily bad, but it can make finding an exact match trickier. The best shades are those for fair (but not porcelain) to light/medium skin tones, and consider the slightly peach shade 8 carefully. The darkest shade, 11.5, is a workable option, but is also slightly red with a copper undertone, which limits its appeal. Shade 7 is a great example of a classic beige with just a hint of pink. Note: The shades go on at least one notch darker than they appear in the bottle, and, as the Armani makeup artist explained to us, the colors tend to oxidize (darken) during wear. We noticed this as well, and in fact were told that the company was likely going to tweak the formula to correct this color issue. This missed our highest rating due to the inclusion of fragrance ingredients known to cause irritation. Although they're not present in a high amount, their inclusion isn't a plus, and can make this foundation iffy to use around the eyes. This foundation is best for normal to oily or combination skin.

☺ GOOD **$$$ Fluid Master Primer** *($56)* is a clear, silicone-based primer that spreads easily over skin and leaves a beautifully silky finish. You're not getting anything extra for your money, other than the Armani name. This primer doesn't "hold" makeup better than most others, and its formula is comparable to silicone-based primers from many other brands, from Lancome to Smashbox.

☺ GOOD **$$$ Luminous Silk Foundation** *($59)* is the foundation every Armani makeup artist we spoke to raves about. It's not hard to see why, because this liquid foundation has a fluid, ultra-smooth texture that floats over the skin and dries to a natural, slightly matte finish with a faint hint of shine. It's a really beautiful foundation that enhances rather than masks skin. For light coverage and an unbelievably skin-like result that comes in over a dozen mostly gorgeous colors for fair to dark skin, this foundation is tough to beat. Luminous Silk Foundation is best for normal to slightly dry or slightly oily skin. This was formerly given our highest rating but has been downgraded a bit because the formula (which we previously hadn't closely examined) contains fragrance ingredients known to cause irritation. Their inclusion also makes this foundation iffy for use near the eyes. The fragrance ingredients aren't present in high amounts, but this foundation would certainly be better without them. One more potential cause for concern is the amount of alcohol this product contains, but in all likelihood its low enough to be a minor issue.

☺ AVERAGE $$$ **Master Corrector** *($36)* is a series of color-correcting liquids packaged in slim, shapely components and outfitted with a precision brush applicator. The thin, light texture is easy to blend, but the two colors are too obvious on skin, so you end up substituting one color "flaw" for another. Pink and Orange are workable but only if carefully applied and deftly blended. We suspect most women won't want to bother with this product.

☹ POOR **Lasting Silk UV Foundation SPF 20** *($59)*. Although UVA protection is assured thanks to the in-part titanium dioxide sunscreen, alcohol is the third ingredient. Sometimes, depending on the formula, that isn't an issue, but in this case, you can smell the alcohol and feel its tingle on your skin—and that's never a good sign because alcohol causes free-radical damage and irritates skin, which is not silky, but rather rough and unpleasant on skin. This liquid foundation has a sheer, fluid texture that blends well and sets to a satin matte finish, but so do many other foundations that don't cause the problems this one does. For significantly less money and no irritation, consider L'Oreal True Match Super Blendable Makeup SPF 17 (L'Oreal owns Giorgio Armani).

GIORGIO ARMANI CONCEALER

☺ AVERAGE $$$ **High Precision Retouch** *($36)* is a liquid concealer applied with the type of long, thin brush usually reserved for liquid eyeliners. You can indeed be precise with the brush, but it's not the best for covering large areas, such as darkness under the eye. Its fluid texture provides medium coverage and blends decently, but because it never really sets, it won't last long before fading and creasing. The three shades are good if you're willing to put up with this concealer's drawbacks (and price).

GIORGIO ARMANI POWDERS

✓☺ BEST $$$ **Luminous Silk Powder** *($47)* is an outstanding talc-based pressed powder whose pigments and talc are finely milled so you get a silky, sheer application that meshes with skin and provides a matte finish that's not powdery or dry. Note that this powder is laced with a tiny amount of sparkles, but their subtlety makes this suitable even for daytime wear. Each of the seven shades is recommended, and there are options for fair to dark (but not very dark) skin. If you're going to spend top dollar on a pressed powder, you should be looking at products like this (but you also should be aware that L'Oreal and Maybelline offer competitive pressed powders at the drugstore for one-fourth the price).

✓☺ BEST $$$ **Micro-fil Loose Powder** *($49)* has an airy, ultra-fine texture and a seamless finish that is incapable of looking too dry or powdery on skin. The three colors are excellent, though each one leaves a very soft sparkle—something those with oily skin will not be thrilled with, but that those with dry skin will find attractive.

GIORGIO ARMANI BLUSHES & BRONZER

☺ GOOD **$$$ Blending Blush Duo** *($60)* is a cream-to-powder blush and highlighter in one compact. Both formulas are supposed to morph into a fluid when they come in contact with your skin, but that doesn't happen. The blush and highlighter blend easily and supply soft color with a delicate powder finish. You'll notice subtle sparkles, so keep that in mind if you don't want shiny cheeks. Shade 3 is an attractive peach/bronze duo for summer.

☺ GOOD **$$$ Sheer Bronzer** *($49)* is a collection of three pressed bronzing powders, each with a silky but dry texture that is tightly pressed, so the application is sheer. These brush on evenly and leave a soft, shimmering finish. It's not as natural as a true tan (which doesn't glisten), but the believable colors compensate for that. Shade #1 is tricky because it tends to look a bit too brown, but it works as a soft contour color.

☺ AVERAGE **$$$ Blushing Fabric Second Skin Blush** *($38)* is a cross between a cream and a gel blush with a smooth, silky feel. This blush blends beautifully on skin for an even, streak-free application. At first glance, the color can look shockingly bright, but as you blend it into your skin, it imparts a translucent, vivid color. The soft matte finish stays put throughout the day, so there is no need for touch-ups.

☺ AVERAGE **$$$ Sheer Blush** *($44)* is a good powder blush with a silky, dry texture and smooth application that imparts minimal color. For this amount of money, you should expect (and get) a bigger color payoff. As is, the palette of nude and soft pastel tones provides a bit too much shine for daytime wear.

GIORGIO ARMANI EYESHADOWS

✓☺ BEST **$$$ Maestro Eye Shadow Quads** *($59)* are powder eyeshadows whose texture is very smooth and blends on slightly creamy, leaving a soft satin finish. Each shade goes on softer than it looks in the compact, but they layer well for enhanced shading. Every quad is recommended except number 1, which has mostly obvious blue tones, not for everyday use. One more note: The colors have dividers between them and the strips are wide enough to accommodate regular-size eyeshadow brushes, which is a nice touch.

☺ GOOD **$$$ Eyes to Kill Intense Silk Eyeshadow** *($32)* has an unusual speckled and swirled appearance that combines two shades for one unique effect. Its texture is a cross between a dry powder and a cream eyeshadow. Truly unique, this applies smoothly yet intensely, regardless if used wet or dry (wet application is definitely more intense). The finish is high color and shine, and flaking is minimal. Because the shimmer finish is so strong, these shadows magnify wrinkles or loose skin around the eyes. The shade ranges are attractive, with several options to shape and shade the eye. Watch out for Blast of Blue, Sweet Fire, Lust Red, and Purpura. All these trendy colors are tricky to work with and end up making the eye area look more clownish than classy.

☺ GOOD **$$$ Maestro Eye Shadow** *($30)* has an extremely silky texture that blends beautifully. The collection of shades tends to emphasize sparkling shine, despite claims that there are matte and satin shades, too (the only matte shade we saw was number 11). Oddly, almost all of them apply more sheer than they look, including the darker browns and grays. This ends up being a good, though needlessly expensive, powder eyeshadow.

GIORGIO ARMANI EYE & BROW LINERS

☺ GOOD **$$$ Maestro Liquid Eye Liner** *($31)* is packaged like a fountain pen, and its brush allows for a precise, controlled application. The dry time is average; ideally, liquid eyeliner should dry faster than this does to reduce the chance of smearing. However, once set, this has a matte finish and stays in place really well.

☺ AVERAGE $$$ **Eye Brow Defining Pencil** *($29)* needs sharpening, but for those who don't mind the inconvenience, this has a smooth, dry application and soft powder finish that really stays in place. The two shades present no options for dark brown or red/auburn brows, a strange oversight from a line of this nature.

☺ AVERAGE $$$ **Smooth Silk Eye Pencil** *($28)* is a standard pencil (in that it needs regular sharpening), but otherwise it has a wonderfully silky application that sets to a reasonably solid finish. For the money, this is above average, though it's not preferred to automatic pencils. Unless you're interested in using eye pencil for shock value, avoid numbers 3 and 6.

GIORGIO ARMANI LIP COLOR & LIPLINERS

✓☺ BEST $$$ **Lip Shimmer** *($27)* is a splurge, but one you may not mind making if a fantastic lip gloss tops your list of makeup must-haves. This elegant, lightweight, and completely non-sticky lip gloss is applied with a brush and comes in a beautiful selection of colors, each with varying degrees of shimmer.

✓☺ BEST $$$ **Rouge D'Armani Lipstick** *($30)* is a beautiful lipstick with several stunningly gorgeous shades, including nudes, pinks, plums, mauves, reds, and more, in varying intensities of sheer to opaque color. The satin-cream texture glides on lips with velvety smoothness and leaves a slightly shiny finish, some of which also contain a subtle hint of shimmer. Armani claims this "long-wear formula results in up to 8 hours of intense color." The color certainly doesn't last that long before needing a touch-up, but it does stay on better than your average creamy lipstick.

☺ GOOD $$$ **Lip Wax** *($27)* is described as a modern version of lip color that is essentially a thick, waxy lipstick melted into a pot. Applied with a brush (which must be purchased separately) or a clean fingertip, this has a balm-like texture and leaves lips with a soft wash of color. Depending on how much you apply, the finish varies from soft matte to low-glow sheen. This is nice but it isn't as convenient as popping open a lipstick and slicking it on lips.

☺ AVERAGE $$$ **Gloss D'Armani The Cinema Lacquer** *($28)* is not worth paying extra for. It initially goes on velvety smooth, but can feel thick and heavy once it sets. Each shade contains finely milled glitter that adds to the shiny, luminescent finish, and there is an extensive range of attractive, sheer colors. Armani claims this gloss holds up "for eight hours without fading or migrating," but it wears off just like a regular gloss.

☺ AVERAGE $$$ **Smooth Silk Lip Pencil** *($26)* is a needs-sharpening lip pencil that feels creamy without being slick and applies smoothly. Pigmentation is stronger than usual, so each of the attractive shades has a good stain and impressive staying powder. This would earn a Good rating if it didn't require routine sharpening. You can find lip pencils at the drugstore that perform as well as this for a fraction of the price.

GIORGIO ARMANI MASCARAS

✓☺ BEST $$$ **Eyes to Kill Exceptional Volume Mascara** *($30)* is great if your goal is impressive length combined with moderate thickness that doesn't veer into overly dramatic lashes. The large brush has expertly spaced bristles that allow surprisingly nimble application,

👁 Did you know you don't need an eye cream? It's true! See the Appendix to find out why.

even to hard-to-reach lashes. In just a few strokes, lashes are richly defined, separated without annoying clumps, and beautifully fringed. If you're going to spend more than is necessary for a great mascara, this is one to consider. It wears without flaking or smearing and comes off with a water-soluble cleanser.

✓☺ BEST $$$ Eyes to Kill Lash Stretching Mascara ($30) is expensive and for what this mascara costs, it should really impress—and it does! You can interpret the "lash stretching" portion of the name to mean dramatic length, as this mascara allows you to quickly lengthen and define each lash. The formula applies without a clump and doesn't flake during wear, which is great. This is also easy to remove with a water-soluble cleanser. You won't see a lot of thickness, but this won't disappoint if your goal is longer, separated lashes with a soft fringe.

☺ GOOD $$$ Eyes to Kill Mascara ($30) promises weightless volume, but once you brush on several coats, lashes take on a distinctly heavy feel that differs from the feel you get with most mascaras. Interestingly, this mascara's component and cap are surprisingly heavy, too. If these trade-offs don't bother you, Eyes to Kill Mascara produces strikingly dramatic results. With just a few strokes, lashes are amazingly long, thick, and slightly curled. Even if you're careful during application, some clumping is inevitable; however, it is easy to smooth through and this mascara wears well throughout the day. Results are comparable to wearing false eyelashes, but this is easy to remove with a water-soluble cleanser.

☺ AVERAGE $$$ Maestro Instant Volume Mascara ($28) is another comb mascara. Although it does create instant volume, the best-looking result required more work than a mascara should. The variegated mini-combs deposit a lot of mascara on lashes, but their layout doesn't allow for even application. Therefore, brushing through lashes with a clean mascara wand is necessary to make things look clean yet full. If you're curious to try this type of mascara, L'Oreal's Volume Shocking Mascara is half the price and has a much better application.

GIORGIO ARMANI FACE & BODY ILLUMINATOR

✓☺ BEST $$$ Fluid Sheer ($59) is similar in texture and application to Armani's Luminous Silk Foundation, but is meant to "sculpt" and "illuminate" the complexion. For a touch of radiant shine or to softly highlight or shadow your features in the evening, these are fine and they blend well with foundation or moisturizer. The shade range presents potential options for blush, contour, or bronzing—and, of course, highlighting. Best of all, the shine effect doesn't flake and stays in place on all but the oiliest skin.

GIORGIO ARMANI BRUSHES

☺ GOOD $$$ Giorgio Armani Brushes ($25–$56). Armani's brushes have been improved, but they weren't that deficient in the first place. Overall, it's a functional, well-assembled brush collection without any glaring omissions, though the price point doesn't make them preferred to less expensive brushes. The **Face Brush** and **Blush Brush** are full, soft, and luxurious (which they should be at this price), while the **Large Eye Contour Brush** and **Blender Brush**, which Armani recommends for applying foundation, are also standouts for their versatility. **Lip Brush** ($25) is too standard for the money, and because it's a nonretractable brush without a cap, portability is a problem.

GUERLAIN

Strengths: Lavish packaging (if that appeals to you); some great foundations with sunscreen; the Terracotta bronzing powders; some good lipsticks and blush; impressive eyeshadow singles.

Weaknesses: Very expensive; over-reliance on jar packaging; pervasive fragrance; lack of products to deal with acne or skin discolorations (Guerlain does sell a "whitening" line outside the United States and Canada); irritating toners; several products laced with irritating plant extracts; limited shade ranges.

For more information and reviews of the latest Guerlain products, visit CosmeticsCop.com.

GUERLAIN CLEANSERS

☺ AVERAGE $$$ **Secret de Purete Cleansing Creme** *($62 for 6.5 fl. oz.)* is a very basic, cold cream–style cleanser that's an OK option for dry to very dry skin. It requires a washcloth for complete removal—and this does need to be completely removed, because some of the fragrance ingredients can be irritating if left on skin.

☺ AVERAGE $$$ **Secret de Purete Cleansing Foaming Cream** *($47 for 5 fl. oz.)* has a great name but an average formula that is so basic the price is a joke. This can be a good, water-soluble cleanser for normal to oily skin, but so are most water-soluble cleansers at the drugstore.

☺ AVERAGE $$$ **Secret de Purete Cleansing Milk** *($47 for 6.8 fl. oz.)* is a very basic, water- and mineral oil–based lotion cleanser that requires a washcloth for complete removal. This contains fragrance ingredients (including eugenol) that can be irritating if left on skin.

GUERLAIN EYE-MAKEUP REMOVER

☺ AVERAGE $$$ **Secret De Purete Eye and Lip Make-up Remover Bi-Phasic** *($50 for 4.2 fl. oz.)* is an exceptionally standard, silicone-based makeup remover that is easily replaced by less expensive versions from Clinique, Neutrogena, and Paula's Choice. The lily extracts this contains can be potential irritants for the eye area, but the amounts are so small it may not be a problem.

GUERLAIN TONERS

☺ AVERAGE $$$ **Orchidee Imperiale Toner** *($128 for 4.5 fl. oz.)*. We had to check and recheck to make sure we were seeing clearly because the price of this toner is so far out of line given its basic formula. Guerlain refers to this as a precious toner, but the only thing precious about it is the claims. This basic glycol- and glycerin-based liquid does have mushroom and orchid extract, but the research about either of these helping skin just doesn't exist, though there is the possibility orchid can actually be a skin irritant. What you are certainly getting is far more perfume and preservative than beneficial ingredients. If only it were loaded with antioxidants, skin-repairing ingredients, or cell-communicating ingredients, then the price might be a bit easier to swallow. As is, it makes us choke a bit. By the way, the notion that the formula helps prepare your skin for the "bioassimilation" of the orchid extract is like suggesting ice cubes in a martini shaker help prepare your body to "bioassimilate" the gin. A potentially irritating ingredient like orchid extract is not a good thing. While this isn't a terrible formula, given the price it should have been at least somewhat age-defying with an array of antioxidants as the claims suggest.

☹ POOR **Purifying Iris Toner** *($45 for 6.8 fl. oz.)* lists alcohol as the second ingredient and also contains irritating iris extract and fragrance ingredients. Guerlain recommends this for oily skin, but the thickeners and plant oil won't keep skin matte for long, and irritation doesn't work for any skin type. See the Appendix to find out why irritation is a problem for oily skin.

☹ POOR **Success Model Smoothing Toner** *($50 for 6.7 fl. oz.)* talks of how it should be considered "a real firming treatment for skin," but with alcohol as the second ingredient and more preservatives than helpful ingredients, this is yet another Guerlain toner to avoid.

⊗ POOR **Super Aqua-Lotion Toner, Optimum Hydration Resistance** (*$48 for 6.7 fl. oz.*) begins as a basic toner with some moisturizing ingredients, but then includes the irritating menthol derivative menthoxypropanediol, which definitely is not "optimum" for skin. See the Appendix to learn why irritation is a problem for skin.

GUERLAIN SCRUB

⊗ POOR **Secret De Purete Gentle Polishing Exfoliator** (*$57 for 4.2 fl. oz.*). The only secret about this formula is how utterly ordinary and boring it is. Actually, given the price, the formula is downright insulting. This mineral oil- and wax-based cleanser uses synthetic beads to exfoliate skin. If it were only wax and exfoliating beads, it would at least get an "average" rating, but in this case the amount of fragrance is so wafting you can barely breathe. Even if you liked the aroma, fragrance isn't skin care. In fact fragrance is a problem for all skin types (see the Appendix to find out why). You would be far better off using just plain mineral oil (it's the first ingredient in this product) with a washcloth rather than this concoction. This product contains two extracts of lilies, one from the Nile and the other from India. As exotic as this might sound, they have no properties that are helpful for skin. Even if they did, the amount this contains is infinitesimal.

GUERLAIN MOISTURIZERS (DAYTIME & NIGHTTIME), EYE CREAMS, & SERUMS

☺ AVERAGE **$$$ Abeille Royale Youth Serum Firming Lift** (*$141 for 1 fl. oz.*) is a water-based serum that is betting on bees as the fountain of youth. More specifically, Guerlain wants you to believe that royal jelly, a milky substance secreted by worker bees, can heal your skin while lifting and firming it along the way. Sigh. We thought royal jelly had fallen by the wayside; it didn't work for wrinkles and signs of aging in the 1980s and it doesn't work now. The fact that it's French royal jelly may up its chic profile, but still doesn't make this effective. Regardless of where the royal jelly is sourced, its chemical breakdown is mostly water, followed by proteins, sugars, and a tiny amount of fats. The rest includes trace amounts of vitamins, amino acids, and salts. None of this is the key to lifted, firmer skin, though components in royal jelly can function as water-binding agents (Source: naturaldatabase.com). Not surprisingly, topical application of this bee-produced ingredient can cause contact dermatitis and irritation. Honey is the third ingredient, and it's another by-product from bees. More so than royal jelly, honey has benefit for your skin, but its primary benefit has to do with wound-healing, and wrinkles aren't wounds. Bottom line: You're not getting anything spectacular for your money. In fact, beyond the honey, there's far more fragrance and preservative in this serum than anti-aging ingredients.

☺ AVERAGE **$$$ Happylogy Eye Glowing Eye Care** (*$77 for 0.5 fl. oz*) contains nothing that will make dark circles and puffiness "fade away," but the mineral pigments in this eye-area serum will cast a soft glow that reflects light from shadowed areas. You can achieve the same thing from a concealer with a soft shimmer, such as those from Estee Lauder or L'Oreal.

☺ AVERAGE **$$$ Issima Secret Divin Skin Perfecting Serum, Anti-Ageing** (*$100 for 1 fl. oz.*) is a standard, water-based serum with silicone. The third ingredient is hydrolyzed *Adansonia digitata* extract, from a plant whose leaf extract has been studied in animals (via oral administration), but that has no research or proof pertaining to its benefit for skin (Source: *Pakistan Journal of Biological Sciences*, 2004, pages 870–878). Most of the intriguing ingredients in this serum appear well after the preservatives and fragrance.

☺ AVERAGE **$$$ Orchidee Imperiale Cream** (*$400 for 1.7 fl. oz.*) has at its center a story about the orchid, which is emblematic of Guerlain's skin care (odd, because so few of its products contain orchid). It is said that this flower's secrets of longevity have been revealed and formulated into this ultra-pricey, jar-packaged moisturizer. Considering the price, you'd think orchid extract would be front and center in all their products, but it isn't. In fact, even in this namesake formula, preservatives and fragrance play a much greater role, making the orchid more of an afterthought than the catalyst Guerlain claims it to be. Topping it off, there is no research anywhere showing that orchid extract has any positive effect on skin, let alone being capable of redefining facial contours and minimizing wrinkles. This isn't worth indulging in, but it's an OK moisturizer for dry skin.

☺ AVERAGE $$$ **Orchidee Imperiale Exceptional Complete Care Eye and Lip Cream** *($185 for 0.5 fl. oz.)* contains next to no orchid extract, but that's fine because it has no positive impact on aging skin anyway. This is a lightweight moisturizer for slightly dry skin whose most intriguing ingredients are given short shrift compared with the amount of preservatives and fragrance—which means this isn't money well spent!

☺ AVERAGE $$$ **Orchidee Imperiale Exceptional Complete Care Fluid** *($280 for 1 fl. oz.)* is the lotion version of the Orchidee Imperiale Cream above, and the same basic comments apply, except this product's texture is better for normal to slightly oily skin.

☺ AVERAGE $$$ **SOS Creme** *($70 for 1 fl. oz.)* is a good emollient moisturizer for dry to very dry skin. The jar packaging isn't an issue because this formula is devoid of antioxidants or other light- and air-sensitive ingredients. Considering its SOS name and skin recovery claims, that omission is a disappointment.

☺ AVERAGE $$$ **SOS Serum, for Sensitive and Intolerant Skins** *($89 for 1 fl. oz.)* is somewhat similar to Estee Lauder's Advanced Night Repair serums, both of which are a better choice for the money than this product. The antioxidants and cell-communicating ingredients are given low priority relative to the preservative. And where are the soothing agents to justify the product name and claims?

☺ AVERAGE $$$ **Super Aqua-Eye** *($93 for 0.5 fl. oz.)* is an OK moisturizer for dry skin, but is not the best for use around the eye because of the fragrant plant extracts. The most beneficial ingredients in this product are found in countless others sold at much more affordable prices. Besides, you don't need an eye cream (see the Appendix to find out why).

☺ AVERAGE $$$ **Super Aqua-Eye Eye Serum** *($98 for 0.5 fl. oz.).* Just to be clear from the get-go, you don't need a separate product labeled as an eye cream for your eye area, which we know sounds shocking but check out the Appendix to see why you can save money giving up this erroneous belief. There is nothing "unprecedented" about this formula unless you take that to mean extraordinary claims with an extraordinarily basic formula. This emollient moisturizer for dry skin contains a mostly antiquated mixture of water, glycol, and waxes with a decent smattering of skin-repairing ingredients. What it lacks is a significant amount of antioxidants that would really be helpful for the eye area or any part of the face. Although it contain peptides, the amounts are miniscule and are far exceeded by the amount of preservative. One of the more ridiculous claims this product asserts is that it contains fragments of hyaluronic acid. Guerlain states "Known for its volumizing, plumping and smoothing power, hyaluronic acid is a molecule capable of retaining the equivalent of 1,000 times its volume in water." First, the amount of hyaluronic acid in this product is so minute that a 1,000 times increase wouldn't be enough water for an ant. Moreover, dry skin isn't about water content, but about repairing skin so it can maintain its natural balance of water. In truth, a 1000 times increase would be damaging for skin. Just because you soak in a tub of water doesn't mean your skin is moisturized; if anything, it will make skin drier. Perhaps the best part of this formula is that it is one of the only ones from Guerlain that doesn't contain fragrance. Not sure how that happened, but it is the first step in the right direction from Guerlain we've seen in years.

☺ AVERAGE $$$ **Super Aqua Day Triple Protection Shield SPF 30** *($85 for 1.3 fl. oz.)* does a decent job of achieving the SPF rating with an OK amount of the UVA-protecting ingredient titanium dioxide, but that's where the good news stops. From any angle, there is no triple protection in this formula. When it comes to sunscreen, the price itself should be a deterrent because of the need to apply sunscreen liberally. How liberally is anyone going to apply a sunscreen costing this much? Other than the price, the rest of the mattifying formula is at best mediocre with fragrance and preservative outpacing any of the potentially good ingredients (of which there is only a handful anyway).

☹ POOR **Abeille Royale Day Cream-Normal to Combination Skin** *($102 for 1.7 fl. oz.).* Abeille means "bees" in French and this product is all about the miraculous benefits honey, beeswax, and royal jelly can have for your skin. If you want to buy into the claim that those ingredients are essential for skin care, then you might as well waste your money on this concoction because this overly expensive moisturizer definitely contains a mix of bee by-products. While those ingredients are on the label, this also contains almost as much fragrance and preservative as anything bees create. See the Appendix to find out why this much fragrance is a serious problem for skin. In terms of your skin-care routine, there is no research showing any substances from bees are good or even needed for skin. All you are getting is as an overly fragranced, absurdly expensive formula that is easily replaced by dozens of other far less pricy options. The paltry amount of antioxidants, skin-repairing ingredients, and cell-communicating ingredients it contains is shameful.

☹ POOR **Abeille Royale Day Cream-Normal to Dry Skin** *($102 for 1.7 fl. oz.)* is similar to the Abeille Royale Day Cream-Normal to Combination Skin above, and the same review applies.

☹ POOR **Abeille Royale Lotion** *($61 for 5 fl. oz.)* is similar to the Abeille Royale Day Cream-Normal to Dry Skin above, only with a lotion texture. Otherwise, the same comments apply.

☹ POOR **Abeille Royal Night Cream** *($171 for 1.7 fl. oz.)* is similar to the Abeille Royale Day Cream-Normal to Dry Skin above, only with a thick, creamy texture. Otherwise, the same comments apply—and this is absurdly overpriced for what you're not getting!

☹ POOR **Abeille Royale Up-Lifting Eye Care** *($120 for 0.5 fl. oz.).* If you are concerned about wrinkles and dry skin around your eyes, we recommend you look elsewhere. This formulation is strangely less emollient than the Abeille facial moisturizers from Guerlain. High up on the ingredient list is aluminum starch octenylsuccinate, an absorbent ingredient rarely seen in products for dry skin. For the few beneficial ingredients this does contain, the jar packaging won't keep these air-sensitive ingredients stable. See the Appendix to find out all the problems associated with jar packaging. Aside from the jar packaging, you don't need a separate product labeled as an eye cream for your eye area, which we know sounds shocking, but check out the Appendix to see why you can save money giving up this erroneous belief.

☹ POOR **Midnight Secret Late Night Recovery Treatment** *($110 for 1 fl. oz.)* is a lightweight moisturizer that doesn't hold any sort of secret for fatigued skin. This isn't a party-all-night-yet-look-refreshed-in-the-morning elixir. It's actually a problem for skin due to the irritating plant extracts it contains, including arnica and St. John's wort.

☺ AVERAGE $$$ **Orchidee Imperiale Longevity Concentrate** *($490 for 1 fl. oz.).* If only beautiful packaging, exaggerated claims, and over-the-top pricing could determine quality, then this offering from Guerlain would be a no-brainer for us to favorably review. As is, we would have to be brain-dead to recommend you do anything except pass this by and hope we saved you from wasting your money. For $490 this product should be brimming with state-of-the-art, potent antioxidants and cell-communicating ingredients, but it isn't. On a positive note, this does have a beautiful, silky texture and would work well for normal to dry skin, but that can be said for hundreds of skin-care products. However, what it lacks is far more significant than what it contains. Other than the orchid extract, which has no research showing it has any benefit for skin, this contains more perfume and preservative than anything your skin truly needs to be healthy and younger. For decades, cosmetics companies have been trying to pass off one ingredient as a miracle, but it is advertising nonsense. Miracle ingredients come and go and, in reality, skin and its needs are far more complicated than any single ingredient.

☹ POOR **Orchidee Imperiale Neck and Decollete Cream** *($365 for 2.5 fl. oz.)*. If only women could decipher an ingredient label before they spent their money, they would quickly see that the only thing imperial about this product is the name and the empty claims on the label. The imperial orchid molecular extract it is supposed to contain is a contrived name because everything is made of molecules. Moreover, there isn't any research showing orchids of any kind have benefit for skin. As a matter of fact, orchid extract can be a skin irritant, which is certainly a problem for skin anywhere on your body. What you are really getting in here is water, waxes, and lots of perfume and preservatives. The small amount of truly beneficial ingredients it contains won't remain stable due to the jar packaging (see the Appendix to find out why jar packaging is a problem). It is also important to mention that there is no research anywhere in the world showing the neck or chest area needs one ingredient different from the face. In fact, because most neck and chest products don't contain sunscreen, you would actually be risking more crepey, discolored skin if you used it during the day without sunscreen over it.

☹ POOR **Orchidee Imperiale White Age Defying Brightening Serum** *($465 for 1 fl. oz.)*. We wonder sometimes if companies selling such ridiculously overpriced products with such truly poor formulations as this one snicker every time one is sold. All we can do is try not to eat lunch when we have to tell you about how sick it makes us that products like this are being sold and that women will actually buy them. What you end up getting with this serum is mostly water, waxes, and alcohol. This much alcohol can potentially be damaging because it can cause free-radical damage (see the Appendix to find out why alcohol is such a serious problem for skin). Guerlain refers to the sensation it imparts as refreshing but alcohol is not refreshing; it's irritating and drying. The orchid extract sounds pretty but there is no research showing it has benefit for skin, whether it is for skin-lightening or otherwise, though it can be a skin irritant. There is a tiny amount of lactic acid in here but not enough for it to be effective as an exfoliant. This contains an even tinier amount of a licorice extract, a plant that can have skin-lightening properties, but for this kind of money and the paltry amount, it's barely worth mentioning. The few other beneficial ingredients in here are nice and the packaging will keep them stable, but overall you're getting far more preservative and perfume than anything helpful for skin.

☹ POOR **Super Aqua-Serum** *($162 for 1 fl. oz.)*. Guerlain labels this a modern-day classic. We'd label it an abject disappointment. There are far better serums available for a lot less money.

GUERLAIN SPECIALTY SKIN-CARE PRODUCTS

☺ AVERAGE **$$$ Super Aqua-Mask Intensive Mask, Optimum Hydration Revitalizer** *($105 for 6 masks)* isn't intensive or all that hydrating due to its silicone content, and it tends to leave a silky, powder-dry finish. The amount of emollients is small, while exciting ingredients are, as usual with Guerlain, in short supply. This is an OK mask for normal to slightly dry skin. The amount of cedar bark extract poses minimal to no risk of irritation. Guerlain's **Super**

Aqua-Mask Mask, Optimum Hydration Revitalizer ($62 for 2.5 fl. oz.) is also not worth the price, but is an OK option for normal to dry skin.

☹ POOR **Orchidee Imperiale Mask** (*$365 for 2.5 fl. oz.*). Even if we could say something positive about this exceptionally ordinary mask, the jar packaging wouldn't keep any of the potentially helpful ingredients stable. Though this is a rather emollient formula for dry skin, it lacks appreciable amounts of antioxidants or skin-repairing ingredients. The orchid extract sounds pretty, but when it comes to your skin there is no research showing it can do anything except emit fragrance and fragrance isn't skin care. Guerlain suggesting orchid can impart longevity to skin is little more than a fantasy. Overall, this isn't a terrible formula, but for the money you should expect (and get) a beautiful formulation! One more point: The only thing revitalizing about this product is the mica it contains. Mica is a shiny mineral used in thousands of products claiming to brighten skin. Other than the cosmetic benefit you may see after applying this product, shine particles don't have anything to do with skin care.

GUERLAIN FOUNDATIONS & PRIMERS

☺ GOOD $$$ **Lingerie de Peau Invisible Skin Fusion Foundation SPF 20** (*$58*) is an excellent liquid foundation that looks beautifully natural and very skin-like. Its silky texture glides over skin and blends perfectly to a natural matte finish with just a hint of glow. Coverage is in the light to medium range, and this won't crease into lines or magnify large pores. Those looking for sun protection from their foundation will be pleased that this provides critical UVA screening from titanium dioxide. Most of the shades are beautiful, and include options for fair to medium skin tones (Guerlain doesn't cater to women of color). The only shades to avoid are the orange-tinged Dore Naturel 23 and the slightly rose Rose Naturel 13. With all the accolades, you may be wondering why this didn't receive our top rating. Two reasons: The amount of alcohol in the formula is potential cause for concern and this contains several fragrance ingredients known to cause irritation. Neither of these drawbacks are deal-breakers (though the price should give you pause), but they're enough of a concern to prevent an unequivocal recommendation. If you decide to try this foundation, it is best for normal to oily skin.

☺ AVERAGE $$$ **Meteorites Perles Light-Diffusing Perfecting Primer** (*$66*) has opulent packaging that catches the eye and carries a price tag that must mean it's the cream of the crop. Don't be fooled by the glam and particularly not by this primer. While most primers are silicone-based, this one relies on water and standard slip agents, neither of which justifies the price. It has a liquidy texture that imparts very sheer color and imbues skin with crystalline sparkles that will be noticeable in daylight. The finish is smooth and weightless, but no one will believe your skin is "lit from within" given such obvious sparkles. In this instance, and in so many other instances with Guerlain, pretty packaging does not translate into an impressive product superior to others in any given cosmetic category.

☹ POOR **Parure Extreme Luminous Extreme Wear Foundation SPF 25** (*$58*) is an overpriced liquid foundation that makes two mistakes we cannot look past: Despite the SPF 25 rating, no active ingredients are listed. That means you cannot rely on this for sun protection. The second mistake is the amount of alcohol the formula contains. It's the third ingredient, and the odor is apparent. The high amount of film-forming agents this contains ensure long wear, but you can achieve this benefit from foundations that don't cause irritation, which hurts your skin and causes it to look older than it is. Even with a better formula and reliable sun protection, this still contains numerous fragrance ingredients capable of causing irritation. It is not recommended.

GUERLAIN POWDER

☺ GOOD **$$$ Meteorites Travel Touch Voyage Powder** *($52)* is a very sheer loose powder that comes in a jar with a built-in sponge applicator, which is awkward to use but does keep this powder from getting too messy. It leaves skin looking smooth and refined without being too matte. The single pale pink shade enlivens skin with a subtle shimmer.

GUERLAIN BRONZERS

☺ GOOD **$$$ Terracotta Bronzing Powder Moisturizing and Long-Lasting** *($47)* presents eight mostly believable, tan-toned colors (Shade No. 2 is a bit coppery; shades 3 and 4 are best). Three of the four have noticeable shine that negates the natural look—real tanning doesn't yield iridescence—while Shade No. 4 is more of a low-glow shimmer. If you decide to splurge and deal with the shine, you will find Terracotta has a smooth texture and applies evenly, though a little goes a long way. The formula is talc-based and contains fragrance.

☺ AVERAGE **$$$ Terracotta Light Sheer Bronzing Powder** *($50)* is one of the most expensive pressed bronzing powders around, and the talc-based formula isn't worth the expense. Although the shine is subdued, the texture is dry enough to hinder application. Three sheer shades are available, with Brunette 02 being too orange to look convincing. For less than five dollars, Wet 'n Wild's Bronzer has this beat hands down.

GUERLAIN LIP COLOR

☺ GOOD **$$$ Kiss Kiss Precious Colours Lipstick** *($30)* is Guerlain's most elegant, creamy lipstick, with a smooth texture and full-coverage colors. It is slick enough to bleed into lines around the mouth. The price is indulgent, but once you see the container this lipstick is housed in, you'll know why.

GUERLAIN MASCARA

✓☺ BEST **$$$ Le2 de Guerlain Two Brush Mascara** *($36)* comes in a sculptural, modern art-inspired, gold-colored tube that houses two different mascara brushes (both of which have the same mascara formula). You get a regular-size and a mini-size mascara brush, the latter being Step 2, which you use to reach the lashes at the inner corner of the eye (or to further emphasize the lash's outer fringe). The regular-size brush has rubber bristles and works brilliantly to make lashes defined, long, and voluminous. We didn't think the smaller brush was needed at all, but used it anyway and was able to reach the tiny lashes toward the tear duct that many mascara wands cannot. However, defining these tiny lashes can look odd on some people, and their proximity to the tear duct can encourage this water-soluble mascara to break down and smear. This is one expensive mascara that just happens to deliver in a way that makes a splurge very tempting, but we would still consider Cover Girl's Lash Blast (orange tube) over this one any day!

GUERLAIN FACE & BODY ILLUMINATORS

☺ AVERAGE **$$$ Meteorites Perles Illuminating Powder Pure Radiance** *($58)* is described as "celestial, luminous and inventive." Flowery language aside, these multicolored powder beads have a slight to moderately intense shine. This does not provide coverage, even the skin tone, or do much to keep oily areas in check, yet it is a perennial best-seller for Guerlain (and has been since its launch in 1987). Given that several less expensive powders produce similar and in some cases superior results, we can only surmise that the continued popularity of these powder beads is due to the luxurious, well-heeled image Guerlain has created.

☹ POOR **L'Or Radiance Concentrate with Pure Gold** *($71)* is not only absurdly over-priced, but this gold shimmer gel goes on too wet, feels slick, and doesn't set. It imparts minimal shine but leaves skin feeling sticky. With all these drawbacks, do you really care that Guerlain used particles of 24-carat gold? … Neither do we! By the way, pure gold, as luxurious as it sounds for skin care, is a known contact allergen!

☹ POOR **Precious Light Rejuvenating Illuminator** *($49)* is Guerlain's version of Yves Saint Laurent's Touche Eclat Radiant Touch. The results from this brush-on highlighter will make you wonder why you spent so much money for a product that tends to sit on your skin unattractively, magnifying uneven skin texture and wrinkles. The finish is too powdery and matte for a natural-looking highlighter, and all three shades add an eerie whitish cast to skin.

GUERLAIN BRUSHES

☺ AVERAGE $$$ **Meteorites Brush** *($36)* is sold to use with their pastel powder beads. It is well constructed and features an elegant handle and a take-along case, but the hair itself is too stiff and slightly scratchy when compared to the best powder brushes.

JANE IREDALE (MAKEUP ONLY)

Strengths: Lip balm with SPF 15; the makeup is mostly excellent, particularly the powder-based products, which include Iredale's contribution to mineral makeup; mostly great makeup brushes.

Weaknesses: Many of the claims made for these products are not supported by solid research; the Circle/Delete concealer, poor eye pencils; LipColours SPF 18 contain irritating peppermint; some superfluous specialty products.

For more information and reviews of the latest Jane Iredale products, visit CosmeticsCop.com.

JANE IREDALE FOUNDATIONS & PRIMERS

✓☺ BEST $$$ **Amazing Base Loose Minerals SPF 20** *($42)* contains titanium dioxide and zinc oxide as the active sunscreen ingredients and these definitely contribute to the powder's opacity, cling, dry finish, and long-wearing capabilities. This loose-powder foundation is talc-free and has a very smooth texture that tends to get drier in feel and appearance the longer it's worn. You can use it dry or can mix it with a moisturizer to approximate a liquid foundation or to allow for easier application over drier skin. (Keep in mind, however, that mixing it will diminish the powder's sunscreen properties.) Either method can be messy, which is true for any loose-powder application, and that's a definite drawback. Amazing Base provides medium to full coverage. The smooth, dry texture and comparatively lighter finish (though it still looks like powder makeup) with a faint bit of shine is preferable to many other mineral makeups. It is much less shiny than the bareMinerals foundation from bare escentuals. Most of Iredale's shades are superbly neutral, but some go on a bit lighter or darker than they appear, so testing them on your skin is imperative. The only shade to be careful of, due to its slight peach-rose tone, is Honey Bronze. The Global shades for darker skin tones are worth considering, but careful testing is a must because the high mineral content can cause these shades to look ashen on some skin tones. Despite some minor drawbacks discussed above, this is still worthy of our highest rating because it is great for sensitive or rosacea-affected skin.

✓☺ BEST $$$ **PurePressed Base Mineral Foundation SPF 20** *($40–$52)* is a pressed-powder version of the Amazing Base above, except this one is more matte and not as thick, so oilier skin will be less likely to experience a heavy, caked look once the skin's oil and the powders mix. The sunscreen is pure titanium dioxide and zinc oxide. The same basic comments made for Amazing Base apply here as well; however, this offers a much tidier application and a broader range of shades, including some exemplary options for darker skin tones. Of the shades, the only ones to consider avoiding are Honey Bronze, Butternut, and Teakwood. The vast majority of skin-true shades here are gorgeous, just as they are for Amazing Base.

☺ GOOD $$$ **Liquid Minerals** *($48 for 1.01 fl. oz.)* combines "light-diffusing, soft focus" minerals with "ingredients that replenish the cellular layers of the epidermis." That sounds tempting until you realize that lots of ingredients in liquid foundations (such as glycerin and cholesterol) offer this benefit. This non-powder entry from Iredale is a bit tricky to dispense from its pump applicator, but it has a silky, water-light texture and provides a smooth, sheer-coverage matte finish. The minerals (pigment) are encapsulated and dispense somewhat chunky, which makes blending a bit more difficult. However, once you get the hang of it, this foundation applies well with a sponge or synthetic brush. Among the shades, a few (Golden Glow, Autumn, and Honey Bronze) are a bit too peach for some medium skin tones, but are still worth considering. Warm Sienna is slightly gold, while the rest of the shades are beautifully neutral and appropriate for fair to dark skin. This is a much lighter alternative to either of the powder-based mineral foundations and, although it contains some great water-binding agents, the matte finish makes it best for normal to slightly oily or oily skin.

☺ AVERAGE $$$ **Absence Oil Control Primer SPF 15** *($37)* seems to be the product those with overactive oily skin have been searching for—yet the formula doesn't give much credibility to the oil-control and regulating claims. Although it's nice that the sunscreen (available only in the Absence 2 shade) is pure titanium dioxide and zinc oxide, some of the major ingredients (including candelilla wax and fatty acids from macadamia nut oil) in this cream-to-powder primer won't help oily skin. The colorless base of the original Absence (this does not offer sun protection) slips over skin and sets to a matte finish, but those with truly oily skin will find it doesn't last as long as they'd like. Absence 2 has a sheer peach tint (not tan, as described) that is borderline problematic for medium skin tones. Both versions are an OK option to prep your skin with a matte-finish product; just don't expect it to regulate your skin's oil production.

☹ POOR **Dream Tint Moisture Tint SPF 15** *($36)* isn't a dream tint unless almost no coverage is on your checklist. Even if very sheer coverage is what you're looking for, this fluffy cream-textured product is no longer worth checking out. In mid-2010, the company reformulated the product due to what they maintained was "an unpleasant natural smell." Their solution was to add skin-damaging lavender oil (see the Appendix to learn why this plant oil is bad), which knocked this tinted moisturizer from its former status as Best Product. Considering the number of fragrant extracts Iredale could've used to improve the former version's scent, it's a shame that a formerly very good product is now impossible to recommend, despite its pure titanium dioxide sunscreen.

JANE IREDALE CONCEALERS

☺ GOOD $$$ **Disappear** *($26)* is positioned as "the ultimate in camouflage creams" and is designed to conceal tattoos. It doesn't provide that much coverage, but does a great job concealing minor redness and other bothersome discolorations. The semi-liquid consistency has just enough slip to blend well, and once dry its matte finish stays put. The formula contains several antioxidants, but the "blemish control botanicals" are a far cry from tried-and-true anti-blemish actives such as benzoyl peroxide or salicylic acid. Iredale maintains that the green tea extract in this concealer combats acne, but research does not support this assertion when green tea extract is applied topically instead of consumed in the diet. All five shades are outstanding and best for fair to medium/tan skin.

☺ AVERAGE $$$ **Active Light Under-Eye Concealer** *($27)* is a thick liquid concealer dispensed from a click-pen applicator and applied with the built-in synthetic brush. The smooth texture blends readily and provides nearly full coverage with a slightly flat, opaque finish. Creasing is minimal and the formula contains several skin-friendly ingredients—though it includes too many waxes for use over breakouts. The major problem is with the colors, half of which look nothing like skin and, when used over dark circles, essentially trade one discoloration problem for another. Avoid shades 4, 5, and 6, all of which are too pink or peach. Shades 1, 2, and 3 are yellow-toned options, but only for very fair to light skin tones.

☹ POOR **Circle/Delete** *($30)* comes in a pot with two colors; a lighter tone and a medium tone. The texture is quite thick and creamy and you will get opaque coverage. This will definitely crease, and applying one of the mineral powders over it tends to look heavy and obvious. Last, the three duos have colors that are a far cry from real skin tones, and blending them together is tricky.

☹ POOR **Zap&Hide Blemish Concealer** *($26)*. We admire the concept behind this dual-sided product packaged to resemble a smaller-than-usual lipstick. The **Zap** portion is a colorless balm designed to disinfect breakouts, while the **Hide** portion is a cream concealer meant to camouflage unsightly redness from the blemish. Things begin to unravel from there. The Zap portion is based around shea butter, an emollient ingredient that isn't what someone struggling with acne needs because it is extremely emollient and greasy. It also contains a potentially effective amount of tea tree oil, but Iredale also included fragrant oils of geranium, ylang-ylang, and lavender, which cause irritation; they don't kill acne-causing bacteria. Meanwhile, the Hide portion shares the same formulary drawbacks. It would be nothing more than a happy accident if you saw any sign of blemish relief using this well-intentioned, but poorly formulated, product.

JANE IREDALE POWDERS

☺ GOOD $$$ **Brush-Me Matte** *($46)* involves a loose powder housed in a component that's affixed with a powder brush for convenient, on-the-go application. The brush is quite good, and the closure mechanism keeps the bristles from splaying and the mess to a minimum. The powder has a fine, dry texture that mattifies skin while imparting subtle sparkle (not exactly what oily skin needs). It goes on translucent, and as such is suitable for all skin colors. Note that the second listed ingredient in this powder is rice starch, a food ingredient that can feed the bacteria that contribute to acne.

☺ AVERAGE $$$ **PureMatte Finish Powder** *($30)* feels matte and has a light, dry texture oily skin will love, but it contains more shine than either of Iredale's foundation powders. There is one shade and it's suitably neutral, although limited to light skin.

JANE IREDALE BLUSHES & BRONZERS

✓☺ BEST $$$ **PurePressed Blush** *($27)* has a silky texture that goes on exceedingly smooth. The color range is impressive, offering equally good options for light and dark skin tones, but note that each shade has a touch of shine.

☺ GOOD $$$ **Quad Bronzer** *($48)* is a very expensive pressed bronzing powder that features four segments of color: pale pink, rose, bronze, and copper. The result when all are swirled together with a brush is a soft rosy bronze tone that looks best on light to medium skin tones. The powder has a smooth, dry texture and is best brushed on sheer, because more than a sheer application results in the powder grabbing and looking uneven on skin.

☺ GOOD $$$ **So-Bronze** *($42)* is a talc-free, pressed bronzing powder that comes in two shades. The number 1 option is best for fair to light skin and features minimal shine, while number 2 is darker and has a separate, crescent-shaped shiny powder segment that really lays on the sparkles. Both options have a smooth but dry texture and apply evenly (just use them sparingly).

☺ AVERAGE $$$ **In Touch Cream Blush** *($27)* has a smooth, almost slick texture and comes in a portable, twist-up stick. Each blush shade is sheer and leaves skin with a moist-glow finish. The drawbacks are that this won't last the whole day, you get a surprisingly small amount of product for the money, and the artificial chocolate scent and flavor will be off-putting for many.

☺ AVERAGE $$$ **Brush-Me Bronze** *($44)* is an overpriced loose-powder bronzer. The mica-based, talc-free formula has a soft, dry texture and more opacity than most bronzing powders due to its titanium dioxide and zinc oxide content (note that this product does not come with an SPF rating). The result is color that doesn't enliven skin the way the best powder bronzers do. Instead, skin looks a bit flat, but the mica lends a sheen that makes the finish less drab than it would otherwise be. Two shades are available, and both are acceptable bronze tones for light to medium skin. Overall, this is a messier and definitely pricey way to use bronzing powder!

JANE IREDALE EYESHADOWS & PRIMERS

✓☺ BEST $$$ **PurePressed Eye Shadows** *($19)* applies evenly without flaking or skipping, and tends to go on color-true. Each shade has at least a slight amount of shine, but it is downplayed to a soft glow in many. The shiniest shades tend to deposit the least amount of color, and are best for highlighting the brow bone.

☺ GOOD $$$ **Lid Primer** *($18.50)* comes with your choice of two cream-to-powder shades, a soft pearlized ivory or a shimmering pink. Both apply easily, have a slight tendency to crease, and offer significant coverage. Despite the shine, these are good choices if you have any discoloration on your eyelid and don't like the look you get using concealer and powder prior to eyeshadow.

☺ AVERAGE $$$ **Triple Eye Shadows** *($28)* suffer from mostly poor or exceedingly shiny color combinations, despite having a great, smooth texture. The only workable sets are Triple Cognac and Cloud Nine, but two of the three shades in Pink Bliss are good.

☺ AVERAGE **Highlighter Pencil** *($15.50)* is a standard chunky pencil with a pale pink shade on one end and an opalescent white shade on the other. The shine is intense without being glittery, and the only issue is that the creamy texture doesn't last too long around the eye, so some fading and creasing are unavoidable.

☺ AVERAGE **Eye Gloss** *($15.50)*. Housed in small plastic tubes are various colors of Iredale's lightweight, sheer liquid eyeshadow. Every shade piles on the shine and has enough slip to allow blending to be smooth yet controllable. Once set this has a tendency to settle into lines and eye creases, so this isn't the best option for long-wearing eye makeup.

JANE IREDALE EYE & BROW LINERS

☺ GOOD $$$ **Liquid Eye Liner** *($21)* goes on slightly wetter than most, but the brush is great, being flexible enough to glide easily along the lash line, yet it lets you maintain control.

The Reviews J

Dry time is slower than average, but once set the formula stays in place and wears well. We encourage you to explore the liquid eyeliner options from L'Oreal or Almay first, but this is an option if you want to spend more money.

☺ GOOD **$$$ PureBrow Fix & Mascara** *($21)* is a standard, clear brow gel that works as well as those sold at the drugstore. The only advantage is that this comes with two brushes, though most will find one preferable.

☺ AVERAGE **$$$ Cream to Powder Eyeliner** *($27)* includes one matte and two shimmer-finish, cream-to-powder shades in a single compact. Each applies smoothly and sets to a relatively solid powder finish, though it isn't impervious to smudging and smearing. All in all, this doesn't compare to the long-wearing, gel-type eyeliners from Bobbi Brown, M.A.C., or Stila.

☹ POOR **Eye Pencils** *($11)* are creamy, run-of-the-mill pencils that apply a bit too thick and smudge easily. Don't bother.

JANE IREDALE LIP COLOR & LIPLINERS

☺ GOOD **$$$ Lip Fixation** *($30)* includes a lip paint and softly tinted gloss in one dual-sided component. The lip paint is applied to clean, dry lips and sets within a minute. Because this type of lip color supplies little slip and no moisture, following with the glossy top coat is mandatory for comfortable wear. Iredale refers to her lip paint as **Lip Stain**, and the thin-textured, pigment-rich formula does indeed seem to stain lips. Once set, this stuff isn't budging! Unlike less expensive options from Cover Girl or Maybelline, the **Lip Gloss** top coat has a thick, syrupy texture and noticably sticky finish. Lips are left glistening, and thankfully the stickiness softens with time. Because the Lip Gloss is tenacious, you don't have to reapply it as often. That fact is the sole plus for those considering this product over less expensive options. Otherwise, like most of its drugstore counterparts, Lip Fixation provides long wear that doesn't flake or chip. You may notice a bit of color peeling at the sides of the mouth, but this is easily remedied with a very sheer application to this area. The shade selection is spartan, but the combinations are attractive.

☺ AVERAGE **Lip Definer** *($11)* has a creamy texture and attractive colors, but is otherwise standard and requires routine sharpening.

☹ POOR **PureMoist LipColours SPF 18** *($20)* are one of the few lipsticks with sunscreen that offer UVA protection (Iredale uses zinc oxide), but this plus is sidelined by the irritating peppermint extract that is also included. Granted, these lipsticks don't have the most elegant texture, but the boon of sun protection would have made them worth trying if not for the irritating peppermint.

☹ POOR **PureGloss for Lips** *($20)* is a sheer, minimally sticky gloss available in some enticing colors, but the inclusion of ginger root oil produces a tingly-warm sensation that means lips are being irritated, not cared for.

JANE IREDALE MASCARAS

☺ GOOD **$$$ Longest Lash Thickening and Lengthening Mascara** *($33)*. We have no idea why this Iredale mascara costs twice as much as her other lash-enhancing options because the results certainly aren't worth the price. That's not to say this isn't a good mascara, because it most certainly is—lashes are appreciably lengthened, separated without clumps, and left with a soft fringe. Any thickness is hard to come by, so ignore all claims that this brings lashes to their fullest potential. We can think of several mascaras at the drugstore whose all-around performance beats this handily, so there is no reason to spend this kind of money.

☺ AVERAGE **$$$ PureLash Lengthening Mascara** *($18)* builds moderate length with a very clean, clump-free application. Thickness is scarce, and this isn't what we would call dramatic mascara, but it does the job and stays on all day.

☺ AVERAGE **$$$ PureLash Mascara** *($16)* offers decent (but unimpressive) length with a soft curl. This doesn't thicken lashes in the least, but it wears well and removes easily.

☺ AVERAGE **$$$ PureLash Conditioner** *($16.50)* is essentially a basic mascara formula without pigment. Used as a primer, it bulks up lashes prior to mascara application, although it's no better than applying two or three coats of mascara. This does contain conditioning agents, but lashes don't need conditioning the same way hair does (and conditioning lashes will not help them grow).

JANE IREDALE FACE & BODY ILLUMINATORS

☺ GOOD **$$$ Moonglow** *($48)* comes with four pressed shimmer powder wedges in one compact. There are no dividers between the colors, but each is big enough to use alone with most eyeshadow brushes. Using a blush or powder brush is tricky and will result in one color (a soft golden bronze with a hint of copper—shades having nothing to do with the moon), but the effect is flattering for evening or glamour makeup.

☺ AVERAGE **24-Karat Gold Dust** *($12.50)* is just mica, iron oxides, and real gold flakes. Combined, they make this simply a shiny loose powder whose glistening effect works nicely for evening glamour, though application is messy.

JANE IREDALE BRUSHES

✓☺ BEST **Deluxe Eye Shader** *($24)* is great and definitely worth considering for eyeshadow application. Also recommended and rated ☺ GOOD **$$$** are the **Foundation Brush** ($41), **Handi Brush** ($45), and **Chisel Powder** ($30). Less expensive but recommended are the **Eye Shader** ($16), **Eye Contour** ($15), **Angle Liner/Brow** ($11.50), and **Camouflage Brush** ($17). The **White Fan Brush** ($15) has little practical purpose and is easily replaced by other brushes.

JANE IREDALE SPECIALTY MAKEUP PRODUCT

☺ AVERAGE **$$$ Corrective Colors** *($22)*. Housed in one palette are four shades of creamy-bordering-on-greasy color correctors. You get a Yellow, Peach, Beige, and Lilac shade along with a brief explanation of what color each shade is supposed to cancel or neutralize. The Yellow and Beige shades are acceptable and yellow tones do help cancel red tones (much better than mint green does). The Peach and Lilac shades share the same issue, which is that both look unnatural on skin and replace one coloration problem with another. Regardless of shades, the texture is thick and tends to look heavy and obvious on skin, even with careful blending.

JASON NATURAL (SKIN CARE ONLY)

Strengths: Inexpensive; several very good, value-sized water-soluble cleansers; outstanding eye-makeup remover; a few moisturizers and serums that qualify as beauty bargains; one good AHA product.

Weaknesses: Jar packaging for many antioxidant-rich products; boring to irritating toners; no product to effectively address the needs of acne-prone skin; potentially problematic topical scrubs; most of the lip products contain peppermint oil; several otherwise top-notch products ruined by inclusion of one or more irritating plant extracts.

For more information and reviews of the latest Jason Natural products, visit CosmeticsCop.com.

The Reviews J

JASON NATURAL CLEANSERS

✓☺ BEST **Red Elements Hydrating Lotion Cleanser, for Normal to Dry Skin** *($12.49 for 7.25 fl. oz.)* is an excellent gentle cleansing lotion that is suitable for normal to dry skin. As with most cleansing lotions, you must use a washcloth to ensure it's completely rinsed off. It's fragrance-free and does not contain any irritating plant extracts.

☺ GOOD **Aloe Vera Satin Soap, for Hands and Face** *($8.39 for 16 fl. oz.)* is a standard, generous-sized, water-soluble cleanser (it isn't soap at all) that's not as moisturizing as claimed, but still a very good option for normal to oily skin. The amount of sage extract isn't cause for concern in terms of irritation.

☺ GOOD **Apricot Satin Soap, for Hands and Face** *($8.37 for 16 fl. oz.)* is similar to the Aloe Vera Satin Soap, except its oil content makes it preferred for normal to slightly dry skin.

☺ GOOD **Chamomile Satin Soap, for Hands and Face** *($8.39 for 16 fl. oz.)* is similar to the Aloe Vera Satin Soap, minus the sage extract and plus some anti-irritants. Otherwise, the same review applies.

☺ GOOD **Ester-C Super-C Cleanser Gentle Facial Wash** *($8.89 for 6 fl. oz.)* is a good, water-soluble cleanser for normal to oily skin that would be even better if it did not contain orange extract and a mysterious, unidentified blend of fragrant oils. Still, it rinses without residue and removes makeup easily.

☺ GOOD **Glycerine & Rosewater Satin Soap, for Hands and Face** *($8.37 for 16 fl. oz.)* is similar to the Aloe Satin Soap above, except for the inclusion of fragrant rose water. Otherwise, the same review applies.

☺ GOOD **Lavender Satin Soap, for Hands and Face** *($8.39 for 16 fl. oz.)* is similar to the Apricot Satin Soap above, except this contains lavender extract, though not in an amount likely to cause problems for skin. Otherwise, the same review applies.

☺ GOOD **Mango Satin Soap, for Hands and Face** *($8.39 for 16 fl. oz.)* is nearly identical to the Apricot Satin Soap above, except with mango instead of apricot. Otherwise, the same review applies.

☺ GOOD **Red Elements Exfoliating Scrub** *($13.49 for 4 fl. oz.)* doesn't contain any abrasive agents, so this doesn't work as a facial scrub. It's best described as a creamy cleanser, and the amount of plant oil it contains makes it difficult to rinse. Still, it's an OK, fragrance-free cleansing option for someone with dry to very dry skin.

☺ GOOD **Red Elements Gentle Gel Cleanser, for Normal to Oily Skin** *($12.49 for 7.25 fl. oz.)* is worth an audition if you prefer a gentle, fragrance-free gel cleanser and have sensitive skin. This product's lack of detergent cleansing agents makes it a poor choice for removing excess oil or makeup, but it's fine for those with normal to dry skin who use minimal to no makeup.

☹ POOR **Herbal Extracts Satin Soap, for Hands and Face** *($8.39 for 16 fl. oz.)* contains problematic amounts of plant extracts such as comfrey, clove, and sage, and isn't worth considering over the Satin Soaps from Jason Natural.

☹ POOR **Tea Tree Satin Soap, for Hands and Face** *($8.37 for 16 fl. oz.)* contains a lot of tea tree oil, which lends it a medicinal smell. It would have been a much better option for oily skin were it not for the orange oil and eucalyptus. See the Appendix to learn why irritation makes oily skin worse.

JASON NATURAL EYE-MAKEUP REMOVER

✓☺ BEST **Quick Clean Makeup Remover Pads** *($8.95 for 75 pads)* do an excellent, clean-sweep job of removing most types of eye makeup (waterproof makeup won't budge with this product). The gentle formula contains some notable soothing agents and is fragrance-free.

JASON NATURAL TONERS

☺ GOOD **Red Elements Calming Toner** *($13.01 for 4.5 fl. oz.)* provides skin with the antioxidant red tea as well as several water-binding agents. It contains tiny amounts of alcohol and witch hazel, but not really enough to cause irritation. Without them, however, this product would have earned a Best Product rating.

☹ POOR **Ester-C Super-C Toner** *($7.97 for 6 fl. oz.)* contains the irritants witch hazel and orange oil, which makes this a non-super choice for any skin type.

JASON NATURAL MOISTURIZERS (DAYTIME & NIGHTTIME), EYE CREAMS, & SERUMS

☺ GOOD **Aloe Vera Pure Beauty Oil** *($6.39 for 1 fl. oz.)* cannot protect against sun damage as claimed because it lacks sunscreen ingredients. However, it will relieve dry skin on contact due to its oil content.

☺ GOOD **Jojoba Pure Beauty Oil** *($6.39 for 1 fl. oz.)* is just jojoba oil, an excellent, non-volatile plant oil for dry to very dry skin thanks to its chemical makeup, which is very similar to the skin's own oil (sebum). But that similarity explains why jojoba oil can be a problem for blemish-prone skin, and why Jason's claim that this oil "works great for minimizing the appearance of blemishes and large pores" is completely false and misguided.

☺ GOOD **Vitamin K Creme Plus Intense Skin Nourishing Creme** *($18.97 for 2 fl. oz.)* is a very good moisturizer for normal to dry skin, but the claims it makes about vitamin K improving circulation and eliminating surfaced capillaries are unsubstantiated. It does contain methylsulfonylmethane (MSM); please refer to the Cosmetic Ingredient Dictionary online at CosmeticsCop.com for more information.

☺ GOOD **$$$ Ester-C Hyper-C Serum Anti-Aging Therapy** *($34.38 for 1 fl. oz.)* is a lotion-style serum that's a good option for those with normal to dry skin looking to experiment with a vitamin C product. It's a shame the other antioxidants (all of which have impressive research supporting their topical application) are included in lesser amounts than Jason's fragrance blend.

☺ AVERAGE **5,000 I.U. Vitamin E Revitalizing Moisturizing Creme** *($6.39 for 4 fl. oz.)* is fairly similar to the 25,000 I.U. Vitamin E moisturizer reviewed below, and the same review applies.

☺ AVERAGE **14,000 I.U. Vitamin E Pure Beauty Oil** *($6.39 for 1 fl. oz.)* is just vitamin E and some plant oils. That makes it a good, though greasy, moisturizer for dry skin. While 14,000 I.U. sounds like a lot, it ends up being less than 0.33 ounce. How much of any antioxidant skin needs is unknown, but this makes it sound like you're getting a whole lot when you're not. Research has shown that vitamin E is not helpful for healing scars, and as a lone ingredient isn't the one answer for skin.

☺ AVERAGE **32,000 I.U. Vitamin E Pure Beauty Oil** *($8.97 for 1 fl. oz.)* is similar to the 14,000 I.U. Vitamin E Pure Beauty Oil above, but this contains more vitamin E.

☺ AVERAGE **25,000 I.U. Vitamin E Age Renewal Moisturizing Creme** *($11.49 for 4 fl. oz.)* sounds like a powerhouse of this well-known antioxidant, but the 25,000 I.U. of vitamin E amounts to only 0.67 ounce. Plus, in any amount, the jar packaging won't keep the vitamin E and other antioxidants in this emollient moisturizer stable. See the Appendix to learn more about the problems jar packaging presents.

☺ AVERAGE **Aloe Vera 84% Ultra-Comforting Moisturizing Creme** *($8.65 for 4 fl. oz.)* is an OK moisturizer but compared to many other moisturizers, it's not exactly state-of-the-art. This has potential for normal to dry skin but the jar packaging won't keep the antioxidant ingredients stable (see the Appendix for details).

The Reviews J

☺ AVERAGE **Cocoa Butter Intensive Moisturizing Creme** *($6.39 for 4 fl. oz.)* has very little cocoa butter and is misnamed. This is an OK emollient moisturizer for dry skin that, once again, won't prevent stretch marks during pregnancy.

☺ AVERAGE **Tea Time Anti-Aging Moisturizing Creme** *($14.43 for 4 fl. oz.)* has a lot going for it in terms of antioxidants, so it's a shame jar packaging was chosen because that won't keep them stable during use (see the Appendix for further details). This is otherwise an average emollient moisturizer for normal to dry skin.

☺ AVERAGE **Vitamin E Oil 45,000 I.U. Pure Beauty Oil** *($11.49 for 2 fl. oz.)* would be the best Jason vitamin E oil to consider if you're curious about what this vitamin can do for skin. In addition to vitamin E, the product contains some very good, nonvolatile plant and nut oils, including several whose linolenic and linoleic acid content is very helpful for dry to very dry skin. Although the label on this clear glass bottle shields the product somewhat from light, it's best to store it in a dark place to preserve the effectiveness of the ingredients.

☺ AVERAGE $$$ **Ester-C Creme Anti-Aging Moisturizer** *($14.99 for 2 fl. oz.)* has a standard cream texture and is composed of basic thickening agents, but the real stars of this moisturizer are vitamin-based antioxidants. Unfortunately, jar packaging won't keep them stable once it's opened, making this a less impressive option for normal to dry skin.

☺ AVERAGE $$$ **Red Elements Hydrating Night Creme** *($19.94 for 1.5 fl. oz.)* is nearly identical to the Red Elements Lifting Eye Creme below, although this product isn't quite as thick because it contains more glycerin. Otherwise, the same review applies, including the jar-packaging comments.

☺ AVERAGE $$$ **Red Elements Lifting Eye Creme** *($19.94 for 0.5 fl. oz.)* contains some great antioxidants, but the choice of jar packaging leaves them susceptible to breaking down shortly after this emollient eye cream is opened. We've seen more elegant formulas, but this product is suitable for dry skin anywhere on the face, assuming you want to settle for less.

☹ POOR **Ester-C Ultra-C Eye Lift** *($19.99 for 0.47 fl. oz.)* contains some very good antioxidants in stable packaging, but the company took the citrus theme too far. The tangerine oil's prominence in this product makes it too irritating, especially for use around the eyes. See the Appendix to learn why irritation is a problem for all skin types and why, in truth, you don't need an eye cream.

☹ POOR **Ester-C Vita-C Max Instant Facial** *($34.38 for 4 fl. oz.)* contains menthol, which makes this triglyceride-based moisturizer for dry to very dry skin not worth the experience (and it's about as close to an instant facial as McDonalds is to gourmet dining).

☹ POOR **Red Elements Daily Moisturizing Creme SPF 15, for Normal to Dry Skin** *($17.49 for 2 fl. oz.)* does not contain the UVA-protecting ingredients of titanium dioxide, zinc oxide, avobenzone, Tinosorb, or Mexoryl SX and is not recommended. Even with sufficient UVA protection, this product's jar packaging compromises the effectiveness of the antioxidants it contains (see the Appendix for further details).

☹ POOR **Red Elements Daily Moisturizing Lotion SPF 15, for Normal to Oily Skin** *($17.49 for 2 fl. oz.)* does not contain the UVA-protecting ingredients of titanium dioxide, zinc oxide, avobenzone, Tinosorb, or Mexoryl SX, and is not recommended. What a shame, because this is otherwise a well-packaged, antioxidant-rich lightweight lotion.

☹ POOR **Tea Tree Oil Pure Oil** *($10.47 for 1 fl. oz.)* claims to be nothing but 100% pure tea tree oil, which, if that's accurate, is a problem for skin. There is preliminary evidence that high concentrations of tea tree oil can cause ototoxicity (ear problems), and there are case reports of 100% tea tree oil causing contact dermatitis and inflammation (Source: naturaldatabase.com).

Tea tree oil in 2%–5% concentrations is generally well tolerated and has merit for acne-prone skin; a 100% concentration is a recipe for disaster.

☹ POOR **Vitamin E Oil 5,000 I.U. Pure Beauty Oil** ($6.39 for 4 fl. oz.) is similar to the 14,000 I.U. Vitamin E Pure Beauty Oil above, except this contains less vitamin E and an unidentified "essential oil blend" that is likely problematic for skin.

☹ POOR **Wild Yam Balancing Moisturizing Creme** ($15.29 for 4 fl. oz.) contains irritating lavender extract as the second ingredient, along with wild yam. Wild yam, when applied to skin, does not have a "harmonizing" effect. A study published in *Climacteric: The Journal of the International Menopause Society*, reached the following conclusion: "Wild yam applied topically appears to be no better than placebo for relieving vasomotor symptoms such as hot flashes and night sweats in menopausal women using wild yam cream for 3 months. It doesn't appear to cause changes in serum follicle stimulating hormone (FSH), estradiol, or progesterone." Further, wild yam has no other established benefit for skin.

JASON NATURAL SUN CARE

✓☺ BEST **Sunblock Mineral SPF 30** ($14.95 for 4 fl. oz.). Although some of the claims for this sunscreen are dubious, without question it is an excellent option for those with dry, sensitive skin. The sole actives—zinc oxide and titanium dioxide—are gentle and provide reliable (and necessary) broad-spectrum protection. Jason Natural claims this doesn't leave a white cast on skin, but it does, especially on those who have medium to dark skin tones. This is an unavoidable side effect, given how much titanium dioxide is in the formula. This fragrance-free sunscreen contains several antioxidants and soothing agents. Note that you can apply this to the face as well as the body. Two claims to debunk: First, this is not a chemical-free sunscreen. Every cosmetic ingredient, even the natural ones, are technically chemicals. It doesn't help the consumer when cosmetics companies misuse the word "chemical" to scare you into thinking their product is better or preferred. Second, the term "hypoallergenic" is meaningless; see the Appendix to find out why.

☺ GOOD **Sunblock Facial SPF 20** ($12.39 for 4 fl. oz.) is an emollient sunscreen for normal to dry skin not prone to blemishes. It includes an in-part titanium dioxide sunscreen, but lacks the complement of antioxidants found in today's best sunscreens.

☺ GOOD **Sunblock Kids Natural SPF 45** ($11.20 for 4 fl. oz.). There is nothing, and we mean nothing, about this sunscreen formula that makes it preferred for kids or sensitive skin, and it's not even vaguely natural. The active sunscreen ingredients it contains can cause tearing and stinging if the sunscreen gets into your child's eyes, and it isn't hypoallergenic (see the Appendix to learn why "hypoallergenic" is meaningless). What you are getting with this sunscreen is reliable broad-spectrum protection, including sufficient UVA protection from titanium dioxide. The fragranced base formula is fine for normal to dry skin, and, of course, it can be used by kids as well as adults. Although this sunscreen contains some soothing natural ingredients (plant extracts), labeling it a "natural sunblock" is misleading. This sunscreen contains several synthetic ingredients, including most of the actives that are providing the sun protection. That's not bad for skin; it just isn't natural as the company claims.

☺ GOOD **Sunblock Sport SPF 45** ($9.87 for 4 fl. oz.) is a good sunscreen that provides broad-spectrum protection and is best for those with normal to dry skin. Critical UVA protection (think anti-aging) is supplied by titanium dioxide, which is joined by higher levels of several synthetic sunscreen ingredients. The formula is an option for active individuals, but just like any water-resistant sunscreen, you must reapply after swimming or perspiring heavily.

Also, because this sunscreen contains synthetic sunscreen ingredients, it will irritate your eyes once you start sweating. For the eye area it is far better to use a sunscreen that contains only the mineral active sunscreen ingredients—titanium dioxide or zinc oxide, or both—on your face. Synthetic sunscreen ingredients, while effective, can irritate the eyes.

JASON NATURAL SPECIALTY SKIN-CARE PRODUCTS

☺ GOOD **Ester-C C-Lite Skin Tone Balancer** *($17.49 for 1 fl. oz.)* is designed to reduce age-inflicted skin discolorations, but neither of the ingredients it contains can do much of that, since one has only minimal research supporting its skin-lightening benefit (kojic dipalmitate), while the other (vitamin C) is present in an ineffective amount. This is a good serum for normal to slightly dry skin, and contains enough antioxidants to make it a consideration.

☺ AVERAGE $$$ **Ester-C Hydrating Mask** *($16.79 for 2.75 fl. oz.)* claims it will completely rehydrate skin in 15 minutes, but contains too much clay to do that (and it takes more than hydration to nourish skin). This is an OK, slightly moisturizing mask for slightly dry skin not prone to blemishes.

☺ AVERAGE $$$ **Red Elements Red Clay Masque** *($15.76 for 4 fl. oz.)* doesn't contain anything that increases collagen production as claimed, and is actually a confusing formulation. Water and clay (for oily skin) are mixed with several plant oils (for dry skin), so we're not sure which skin type the company had in mind. In any case, your skin is likely to be confused by this product (the clay and oils sort of cancel each other out). It's nice that antioxidants were included, but given the short amount of time this mask is on the skin, and the fact that it's likely to be used infrequently, they are of little benefit.

KATE SOMERVILLE (SKIN CARE ONLY)

Strengths: Provides complete ingredient lists on their website; good topical disinfectant for acne; some fantastic serums and moisturizers chock-full of beneficial ingredients.

Weaknesses: Expensive; irritating cleansers and scrubs; several products contain irritating ingredients with no proven benefit for skin.

For more information and reviews of the latest Kate Somerville products, visit CosmeticsCop.com.

KATE SOMERVILLE CLEANSERS

☺ AVERAGE $$$ **Detox Daily Cleanser** *($32 for 4 fl. oz.)* gets things off to an irritating start because this water-soluble cleanser for normal to oily skin contains tangerine peel oil. The glycolic, lactic, and salicylic acids may seem impressive, but in a cleanser they are rinsed down the drain before they can benefit your skin. Ditto for the tea tree oil in this cleanser, though there's too little of it to work as a disinfectant for blemishes anyway. Given the high price and the potential for irritation, especially if used around the eyes, this cleanser is a tough sell.

☹ POOR **Gentle Daily Wash** *($32 for 4 fl. oz.)* is far from gentle! Not only does this water-soluble wash contain a drying detergent cleansing agent, it assaults skin with irritating sage, bergamot, and lavender oils. And Somerville has the audacity to claim this concoction calms skin; 'gentle' must be a euphemism of some kind! This highly fragranced cleanser is not recommended.

☹ POOR **Purify Clarifying Cleanser** *($32 for 4 fl. oz.)* is not recommended because it contains a drying cleansing agent and several potent irritants, including a form of menthol and citrus and mint oils. None of these ingredients helps skin and they are troublesome when used around the eyes. An aesthetician should know better than to offer such a problematic cleanser—and not be selling such a poor formula at such an outrageous price!

KATE SOMERVILLE EYE-MAKEUP REMOVER

☺ GOOD $$$ **True Lash Lash Enhancing Eye Makeup Remover** *($35 for 1.7 fl. oz.)* is said to have the added benefit of creating "more voluminous lashes," a claim that's open to interpretation, but many will conclude it means using this will give you thicker lashes, which absolutely isn't the case. This contains ingredients that work to remove makeup, even waterproof mascara, but none of the plant oils, extracts, or the peptide this contains have any research proving they do something to enhance lash growth or volume. This is a good, fragrance-free option for removing makeup, but without question it is overpriced for what you're getting.

KATE SOMERVILLE TONER

☺ AVERAGE $$$ **Clarifying Treatment Toner** *($24 for 5 fl. oz.)* contains witch hazel, which can be almost as irritating as alcohol due to its drying, astringent qualities. This toner contains a tiny amount of lactic acid (AHA), but not enough to function as an exfoliant. Instead, the lactic acid joins the other water-binding agents to hydrate the skin, somewhat offsetting the dryness witch hazel can cause. Somerville claims the phytic acid this contains can reduce post-acne scars, but there's no research proving it has this benefit. Instead, the only research on phytic acid's skin-lightening ability examined rice bran extract (a natural source of phytic acid and other antioxidants) and found it had some skin-lightening benefit, but no mention was made of the type of discoloration that can occur after a blemish has healed (Source: *Pharmaceutical Biology*, February 2012, pages 208–224). Phytic acid is typically derived from corn, but is also found in grains, soy, and legumes. It is a good antioxidant and is often used in cosmetics as a chelating agent (an ingredient that bonds to metal molecules, preventing them from interacting negatively with other ingredients). This toner is a mixed bag that ends up having more pros than cons, but the con (witch hazel) is a considerable one, especially given it's the third ingredient. That makes this toner a less compelling option for oily, problem skin.

KATE SOMERVILLE EXFOLIANTS & SCRUBS

☺ GOOD $$$ **ExfoliKate Acne Clearing Exfoliating Acne Treatment** *($65 for 2 fl. oz.)* combines elements of an AHA and BHA exfoliant with a standard scrub and a clay mask. More scrub than anything else, you're directed to use it once or twice weekly, massaging skin for 30 seconds and then leaving the product on for another minute before rinsing. We wish we could state this is an ingenious way to get breakouts under control, but instead it exposes skin to numerous irritating ingredients that can make acne and its accompanying redness worse, not better. The formula is medicated with 0.5% salicylic acid, but the pH of this product is not within range for it to function as an exfoliant. The same holds true for the AHA ingredients, and none of these are of much help in a product whose contact with skin is so brief (in contrast, breakouts often respond well to a leave-on BHA exfoliant with 1–2% salicylic acid). Irritating ingredients steal the show here, yet none of the fragrant plant oils have research proving they help acne, either by clearing breakouts or preventing new ones. This product is an expensive mistake and absolutely not recommended for anyone, regardless of skin type or concern. See the Appendix to learn why irritation is a problem for all skin types, especially oily skin.

☹ POOR **Clinic-To-Go Resurfacing Peel Pads** *($48 for 16 pads)*. These AHA exfoliating pads are meant for twice-weekly use to rejuvenate skin's appearance. Apparently, this treatment is similar to seeing Somerville herself for a facial, but if the ingredients these pads are steeped in is what she uses for in-clinic resurfacing, cancel your appointment! Although the pads contain an effective amount (likely 10–12%) of the AHA lactic acid and the pH allows it to function as an exfoliant, with each use you're exposing skin to irritants. Witch hazel, myrtle, sage, and disinfectant sulfur are not the path to skin improvement. All these can cause irritation that leads to dry, flaky skin and damaged collagen production. The numerous fragrance ingredients in the formula only worsen the effects of the aforementioned irritants. Once-weekly use of a well-formulated AHA exfoliant with a higher amount of AHAs can improve numerous signs of aging, and you can do this with products that don't expose your skin to irritants. One example is Paula's Choice RESIST Weekly Resurfacing Treatment; you'll find others on our list of Best AHA Exfoliants at the end of this book and on CosmeticsCop.com.

☹ POOR **ExfoliKate Gentle Exfoliating Treatment** (*$65 for 2 fl. oz.*) would be a decent scrub for dry skin if it did not contain numerous fragrant oils, but the price is beyond obnoxious—it's downright offensive! Somerville recommends it for sensitive skin, but the fragrant oils make it inappropriate for all skin types. The AHA lactic acid is included, too, and in a respectable amount, but this ingredient doesn't do much in a product that you rinse from your skin. As for the enzymes papain and bromelain, they are notoriously unstable and most likely lose their efficacy during the manufacturing process, unless they are specially modified, which doesn't appear to be the case with this product (Sources: *Protein Engineering, Design, and Selection*, June 2010, pages 457–467; *Biochemistry*, December 2009, pages 1337–1443; and *Pharmazie*, April 2003, pages 252–256). Moreover, both of these enzymes can cause contact dermatitis, especially for those allergic to latex (Source: naturaldatabase.com). Lastly, the amount of oils in this scrub makes it difficult to rinse. Talk about an expensive mistake!

☹ POOR **ExfoliKate Intensive Exfoliating Treatment** (*$85 for 1.7 fl. oz.*) is billed as the next best thing to seeing Kate Somerville for an appointment. Well, we don't think so, not even remotely so. Packaged in an airless jar, this ordinary topical scrub contains plastic beads as the scrub particles, plus lactic acid. You're supposed to apply it to your skin and leave it on for 20–30 seconds, then rinse. That's not much time for the lactic acid to work, but the pH of this scrub is too high for exfoliation to occur regardless of how long you leave it on your skin. Actually, leaving this on your skin for even one second is a mistake: it's fraught with irritants, including geranium, rosewood, cinnamon, orange, and patchouli oils. No wonder the company states that redness may appear several minutes after removing this from skin; it's not "increased circulation" in a healthy sense—it's increased circulation as a direct response to intense irritation, and that's bad for skin (see the Appendix to find out why).

☹ POOR **Micro Glycolic Polisher** (*$90 for 1.7 fl. oz.*). We suppose if you're going to be charging this much money for a exfoliant whose abrasive agent is soy flour, you need to make sure consumers know it's a "clinic favorite" that can "peel away the years," and the rest will take care of itself. You need to know there is nothing professional-grade about this product, and nothing unique, special, or all natural. There is no ingredient in this product that other companies don't have access to. Once you wipe away all the hype and nonsense, this ends up being a potentially irritating mix of witch hazel water (which is mostly alcohol) and AHAs that likely won't have a chance to work before they are rinsed away. In addition, the bergamot oil is also irritating, and would completely negate any anti-inflammatory activity that the touted blue lotus extract may have. This is a great big overpriced mistake for all skin types, even among those who don't bat an eye at the price.

KATE SOMERVILLE MOISTURIZERS (DAYTIME & NIGHTTIME), EYE CREAMS, & SERUMS

✓☺ BEST **$$$ Line Release Under Eye Repair** (*$125 for 0.5 fl. oz.*) won't send your wrinkles into retreat, but this is nevertheless a remarkable formula for slightly dry or slightly oily skin anywhere on the face. Fragrance was excluded, and this contains a blend of skin-silkening silicones and hefty amounts of cell-communicating ingredients, ceramides, and, to a lesser but still noteworthy extent, antioxidants. The silicone base works well under makeup. However, expecting your eyes to appear lifted and contoured is not realistic; that achievement remains in the realm of cosmetic surgery or cosmetic corrective procedures, the very services that Kate's spa provides to her clients, despite the products she sells Despite our rating and comments for this product, the fact is you don't need a special product for the eye area (see the Appendix to find out why).

✓☺ BEST $$$ **Quench Hydrating Face Serum** *($65 for 1 fl. oz.)* is one of the better products Somerville sells. It has a beautifully smooth, silicone-based texture that makes skin feel like silk, and it provides potent cell-communicating ingredients and antioxidants, including retinol, all in stable packaging. The formula is fragrance- and preservative-free (preservatives are not required because the product is nonaqueous) and assuredly one of the better serums out there. Now this would be money well spent, though you can find less expensive, equally well-formulated serums with retinol, including Paula's Choice RESIST Intensitve Wrinkle-Repair Retinol Serum which, on balance, offers more benefits than Somerville's option.

✓☺ BEST $$$ **SPF 55 Serum Sunscreen** *($45 for 2 fl. oz.)*. This in-part avobenzone sunscreen is not a serum. Rather, it's a lightweight, thin-textured lotion that spreads easily on skin and leaves a soft matte finish. The formula is fragrance-free and contains some notable antioxidants though it would better if they were present in greater amounts. Still, this is an excellent option for those with normal to oily skin seeking a sunscreen with a higher SPF rating for longer days in the sun (though keep in mind that reapplication is essential to maintain protection).

☺ GOOD $$$ **Deep Tissue Repair With Peptide K8** *($150 for 1 fl. oz.)* is sold with so many superlatives on its label you'd swear this was the answer to every anti-aging concern (but if that were the case, why would they sell all these other antiwrinkle products; companies never explain that inconsistency). The claims literally state that you can watch your wrinkles "lift away," but you'll be standing in front of the mirror into the next millennium if you're waiting for that to happen. Housed in airless jar packaging, this is just a very expensive moisturizer for dry to very dry skin. The peptide is almost nonexistent, and even if there were a pound of the stuff in here, it cannot encourage cellular repair, reverse damage, or significantly change a wrinkle. The thickeners and the emollient, nonfragrant plant oils will ease and help prevent dryness while restoring smoothness to skin, and it contains some ingredients that reinforce skin's barrier effectively, but that's as deep as it gets. The grapefruit peel oil keeps this from being rated a Best Product, but the amount is likely too low to cause irritation (be careful if you wear this during daylight hours without a sunscreen; grapefruit oil can cause a phototoxic reaction).

☺ GOOD $$$ **Goat Milk Cream** *($55 for 1.7 fl. oz.)* is a very good emollient moisturizer for dry to very dry skin not prone to breakouts. Goat's milk may have anecdotal information about its use by ancient Egyptians, but those same Egyptians also used lead as eyeliner and didn't know a thing about sun damage or skin cancer (so much for the credibility of ancient beauty secrets). This contains some antioxidant-rich plant ingredients, and the airless jar packaging will keep them stable during use. Goat Milk Cream does contain a tiny amount of fragrant plant extracts.

☺ GOOD $$$ **Neck Tissue Repair Cream with Peptide K8** *($150 for 1.7 fl. oz.)*. The cosmetics industry wants consumers to think that the neck requires a special product. Most women don't realize that the same products and routines they use to keep their facial skin in top shape should also work for their neck, if the skin is the same type. Skin is skin, everywhere on the body, and depending on its type (dry or oily), it needs the same state-of-the-art ingredients, from head to toe. Taking care of the skin on your neck does not mean you need to buy special neck creams (your facial products will work just fine), and this product is a perfect example. Not surprisingly, this neck moisturizer doesn't contain a single ingredient that doesn't also show up in facial moisturizers, and its texture isn't any different, either. This contains lots of emollient thickeners along with some good water-binding agents, skin-repairing and cell-communicating ingredients, and antioxidant plant oils. All told, this is a well-formulated product that can help skin anywhere on the body look and act younger, but it is not unique to the needs of aging skin on the neck. This missed our top rating due to the inclusion of grapefruit seed oil along with fragrance ingredients known to cause irritation. The amounts are small, but without question, this product would be better off without them. Note: Although this is packaged in a jar, it is a specially designed airless jar that does not expose the delicate ingredients to light and air.

☺ GOOD $$$ **Quench Oil-Free Hydrating Face Serum** *($65 for 1 fl. oz.)* contains a high amount of the plant extract *Plumeria acutifolia*. Although research on this plant's benefit for skin is scant, we know that it contains chemical constituents with anti-inflammatory action, which is helpful (Source: *Planta Medica*, November 2008, pages 1749–1750). The formula, which is oil-free as claimed, also contains some good hydrating ingredients, though the blend of the ingredient propanediol coupled with a film-forming agent lends a slightly tacky finish. As for the peptides, they are cell-communicating ingredients that do not have substantiated research proving their worth for reducing expression lines or wrinkles—this isn't liquid Botox. On balance, this is a good, though pricey, fragrance-free serum for normal to oily or combination skin. The claims are somewhat over-the-top (for example, the tightening actin this has is from the film-forming agent, not your skin actually becoming tighter or being lifted), but it contains enough repairing and replenishing ingredients to merit consideration.

☺ AVERAGE $$$ **HydraKate Line Release Face Serum** *($150 for 1 fl. oz.)* is mostly a blend of silicones with a repairing ingredient, film-forming agent, and preservative. It's absurdly overpriced for what you get, and contains more sodium hydroxide (a pH adjuster) than beneficial ingredients. Kate Somerville offers better, less expensive serums that stand a much better chance of helping skin than this product. The tightening effect this offers comes from pullulan, a yeast-derived starch ingredient whose tightening effect is temporary and strictly cosmetic. In many ways this formula is just embarrassing, and the price is deplorable considering what you get.

☺ AVERAGE $$$ **Oil Free Moisturizer** *($65 for 1.7 fl. oz.)* is a surprisingly disappointing fragrance-free moisturizer, especially considering the cost. It has a lightweight texture suitable for normal to slightly dry skin, but outside of some sugar- and algae-based water-binding agents, it doesn't offer much significance for skin. The airtight jar packaging helps keep the sea-based ingredients stable during use, but the formula really should include some potent antioxidants and a cell-communicating ingredient or two. The tightening and toning claims are possible thanks to the amount of film-forming agent (think hairspray) in this moisturizer but that isn't the best for skin. However, that effect is more tactile than a benefit, and those with oily areas shouldn't expect this to work well as an absorbent moisturizer.

☹ POOR **CytoCell Dark Circle Corrective Eye Cream** *($75 for 0.5 fl. oz.)* has a smooth, lightweight texture, and is a completely ordinary combination of fatty acids and water. It has no discernible ability to reduce the appearance of dark circles other than the strictly cosmetic effect from mineral pigments, such as titanium dioxide, and "optical brighteners," like mica. These mineral ingredients add a reflective, shiny opaque finish on the skin around the eyes, making dark circles somewhat less obvious, but they don't treat or lighten dark circles, they simply make them less apparent. You'll get better results using a full-coverage concealer. As for treating puffiness, this doesn't work. Skin-care products are not the solution, no matter their cost or what they claim. Puffiness around the eyes results primarily from fluid retention, allergies, fat pads shifting, or irritation—there are no skin-care creams that can address these issues. However, not using products that contain irritating ingredients, like this one does, would be a good place to start (along with not sleeping in your makeup). Plus, you do not need a separate eye cream (see the Appendix to find out why). This fragrance-free eye cream also contains two preservatives—methylisothiazolinone and methylchloroisothiazolinone (known as Kathon CG)—known to be sensitizing and not recommended for use in leave-on products. Given that the eye area can be more sensitive anyway, it doesn't make sense to use products that contain sensitizing preservatives in an eye cream.

☹ POOR **CytoCell Dermal Energizing Treatment** (*$150 for 1.7 fl. oz.*) is supposed to contain a special peptide that stimulates stem-cell activity in skin. Thankfully, that isn't remotely possible, because in real life that wouldn't be a good thing for your skin. As with so many things in the cosmetics industry, budding scientific research is contrived and spun to make a skin-care product sound worthy of your attention. Cosmetics companies seem to have "breakthrough" discoveries long before modern medicine and science can report a breakthrough and attest to its safety. Of course, that's because cosmetics are not regulated and the companies can get away with making almost any cleverly couched claim they dream up, no real proof required. That's not even close to the way stem cells are being studied and tested in the scientific and medical realms. But, as you know, it hasn't stopped many cosmetics companies from heralding stem-cell stimulation as the next fountain of youth. (Who needs proof to believe their skin will be ageless, right?) As it happens, this moisturizer has the tiniest amount of peptide imaginable, and there's not a shred of evidence demonstrating that this peptide, or any peptide, or any other ingredient, has any effect on the activity of stem cells in your skin. What we do know is that this moisturizer contains potent irritants that keep your skin from looking younger due to the collagen breakdown they can cause, among other problems. The lavender oil causes skin-cell death and enhances oxidative damage (see the Appendix), and the bergamot oil contains volatile components that can cause skin discolorations in the presence of sunlight (Sources: *Contact Dermatitis*, September 2008, pages 144–150; *Cell Proliferation*, June 2004, pages 221–229; and naturaldatabase.com). This product is packaged in a jar, which is a problem for delicate ingredients. See the Appendix to learn why jar packaging for skin care is a bad idea.

☹ POOR **Nourish Daily Moisturizer** (*$65 for 1.7 fl. oz.*) has a lot going for it, including lightweight emollients, a selection of peptides, and some good antioxidants. However, the inclusion of fragrant lavender extract plus orange oil makes this could-have-been-nourishing moisturizer an irritating experience for normal to dry skin (and it's disappointing the fragrant ingredients are present in a larger amount than the antioxidant vitamins and peptides, all of which qualify as anti-aging, but not so much in this formula). By the way, this is not "the perfect daily moisturizer for those interested in preventing and reversing the signs of aging" because it does not provide sun protection. What a disingenuous, blatantly inaccurate statement! As an aesthetician, Somerville should know better. Without sun protection, no skin-care product can reverse signs of aging and of course aging itself cannot be reversed.

⚥ Highly fragranced products smell good, but won't help your skin! See the Appendix for details.

☹ POOR **Total Vitamin Antioxidant Face Serum** (*$65 for 1 fl. oz.*) contains significant amounts of vitamin C, anti-irritant chamomile, and green tea, but the addition of fragrant geranium and lavender oils makes this water-based serum too irritating for all skin types. Calling this "total vitamin" is misleading, as it includes only two vitamins, and there are lots of vitamins that can be beneficial for skin when applied topically. Without the fragrant oils (and fragrance ingredients such as geraniol and linalool), this would be one of Somerville's better products, especially for sensitive skin. See the Appendix for further details on lavender oil.

KATE SOMERVILLE SPECIALTY SKIN-CARE PRODUCTS

✓☺ BEST **$$$ Anti Bac Clearing Lotion** (*$39 for 1.7 fl. oz.*) deserves consideration as an effective topical disinfectant for acne, at least if you don't mind spending this much. This contains 5% benzoyl peroxide along with some plant antioxidants. One of them (*Argania spinosa*) has limited information about topical use, but oral consumption has shown it to have anti-inflammatory potential in animals (Source: *Annals of French Pharmaceutics*, 1998, pages 220–228). Anecdotally, extracts from this tree are said to be effective against pimples, but it's a good thing benzoyl peroxide is on hand to provide results you can rely on. This fragrance-free product is an option for all skin types dealing with acne. Labeling this "prescription-quality" is meant to make it sound special, but all benzoyl peroxide products could make this claim because benzoyl peroxide is an over-the-counter drug that is also available by prescription. Note that the small amount of alcohol this contains is not cause for concern, though it's disappointing to see it listed before the skin-repairing ingredients of ceramides and cholesterol.

✓☺ BEST **$$$ Complexion Correction Spot Reducing Concentrate** (*$48 for 0.5 fl. oz.*) is an excellent, though expensive, skin-lightening product whose formula is best for normal to dry skin. The slightly creamy, lotion-like texture is medicated with 2% hydroquinone, the gold standard active for lightening brown spots and other discolorations from sun damage. Kudos to Somerville for omitting fragrance and fragrant plants and for including additional anti-aging ingredients such as retinol and vitamin-based antioxidants. For what this costs those extra yet essential ingredients should be present in greater amounts, but that doesn't change the fact that this is an overall well-done formula for those struggling with discolorations.

☺ GOOD **$$$ Complexion Correction Daily Discoloration Perfector** (*$80 for 2 fl. oz.*) contains alternatives to hydroquinone (the gold-standard for skin lightening), such as alpha-arbutin, a form of resorcinol, and retinol. Although these ingredients have some research pertaining to their ability to lighten discolorations, that research isn't as impressive as it is for hydroquinone. Still, if you're looking for alternatives, this product has merit. A couple of issues to consider with this product are that it includes citrus extracts as well as a form of resorcinol, both of which pose a risk of irritation. In all likelihood, the amount of resorcinol in this product doesn't pose a risk (Source: *Contact Dermatitis*, April 2007, pages 196–200), but it probably doesn't impact skin color, either. That leaves the citrus extracts as the wild cards in terms of irritation, and we can't say for certain that they won't be a problem.

☺ GOOD **$$$ Complexion Correction Overnight Discoloration Perfector** (*$70 for 1 fl. oz.*). Other than containing a small amount of fragrant plant extracts that pose a slight risk of irritation, this is a good, though pricey, skin-lightening product for normal to dry skin. Rather than being medicated with hydroquinone, for this version Somerville opted for alpha-arbutin and a form of vitamin C (tetrahexyldecyl ascorbate), though the amount of the latter is likely too low to have much impact on brown spots. Still, the alpha-arbutin is potentially helpful due to its relation to hydroquinone, and keeps this skin-lightening product on our list of good options, though you don't need to spend this much to get a well-formulated skin-lightening product. For example, Paula's Choice has three options that stand just as good a chance of working, but for a lot less money.

☺ GOOD $$$ **Quench Hydrating Mask** *($45 for 2 fl. oz.)* is an intriguing mask that has potential for dry skin. It isn't brimming with great ingredients, but between the sodium PCA and urea, it is unique enough to consider. It would have been more interesting if the really impressive ingredients were higher up on the ingredient list, but there is enough in here to help your skin.

☺ AVERAGE $$$ **24 Hour Pimple Punisher** *($28 for 0.5 fl. oz.)*. Housed in a dual-sided component, this anti-acne product consists of one product meant for use in the morning and one for application at night. For daytime, we have the **AM Blemish Clearing Gel**, a lightweight formula containing some great anti-inflammatory ingredients and fatty acids that may help skin reduce breakouts, though the research on this isn't definitive. For nighttime, you're sup-posed to dab on the **PM Acne Treatment Clay**, which is medicated with anti-acne superstar salicylic acid. Unfortunately, the amount of clay can make this treatment drying and keeps the salicylic acid from functioning as an exfoliant (salicylic acid needs an acidic pH to work against acne, while clay pushes a product's pH toward the alkaline range). Although the salicylic acid won't work as intended, this contains most of the same soothing ingredients found in the AM Blemish Clearing Gel. The clay will help absorb excess oil and "dry out" a blemish, but keep in mind that drying out a blemish isn't the best approach because it can impede healing—and prolonged (such as overnight) contact with clay can exacerbate this dryness. This leaves us with a dual-sided product in which one end is worth using and the other isn't, at least not every night. There are better ways to "punish" pimples without causing unwanted side effects, which is where this product falls down, but it's effective enough to warrant consideration, assuming the price doesn't bother you.

☹ POOR **Clearing Mask** *($45 for 2 fl. oz.)* is an overpriced clay mask that offers little hope of making blemished skin clearer, and may only end up confusing it due to its blend of clay, emollient thickener, and oil. The lavender oil is a source of skin irritation and has no effect on acne, other than potentially making it worse by stimulating oil production at the base of the pores. See the Appendix for more details on lavender oil.

☹ POOR **DermalQuench Liquid Lift Advanced Wrinkle Treatment** *($95 for 2.5 fl. oz.)* is overpriced and contains several problematic ingredients for all skin types. It supposedly gives your skin the "signature glow" Kate Somerville bestows upon the celebrity clients who see her for facials, but the glow comes from ingredients that cause free-radical damage and those that can be acutely irritating. This propellant-based product is housed in a metal canister to which you affix a long, slightly curved wand before dispensing over key areas of your face. You're di-rected to apply this morning and evening, holding the applicator can one-half inch away from your face, then "striping" the product across the cheekbone, from mouth to ear, and along the jawline. It dispenses as a slightly runny foam, and you must shake the can repeatedly through-out the process to make sure the foam texture maintains itself. Once applied, you're told to massage the product into your face and neck area. The ingredients are then said to go to work improving wrinkles, sagging, and uneven skin tone (all signs of aging many of us struggle with).

You may be wondering if all this effort is worth it, and the answer is no. As mentioned above, Liquid Lift Advanced Wrinkle Treatment contains several problematic ingredients. One of them is the plant extract *Tropaeolum majus*. Also known as nasturtium, this plant is a good source of vitamin C but one of its principal ingredients is benzyl mustard oil, a fragrant oil that can cause acute irritation and contact dermatitis (Source: naturaldatabase.com). It also contains fragrant lavender oil, which you can read about in the Appendix. These irritants may create a "glow" to skin, but that effect isn't worth the damage that's taking place beneath skin's surface. Over time, it can lead to skin that looks older, not younger or refreshed.

This product also contains oxygenating ingredients that may provide a radiance boost (sort of like the slight flush you get after exercising), but these oxygenating ingredients only increase free-radical damage on skin, which is a key component of aging (Source: *Journal of the American Academy of Dermatology*, March 2012, ePublication). Although this product also contains vitamin-based antioxidants, they will likely degrade and be of little help to your skin in the presence of the potent oxygenating ingredients. Needless to say, Liquid Lift cannot lift skin and it isn't advanced, at least not if your goal is looking younger.

☹ POOR **EradiKate Acne Treatment** *($22 for 1 fl. oz.)* lists 10% sulfur as its active ingredient. Without question, sulfur is a potent topical disinfectant and there is research showing it can be an effective treatment for breakouts and even rosacea. However, in this amount and in a base of irritating isopropyl alcohol and camphor, it becomes a potent, skin-damaging irritant. You may get initial benefit, but with the trade-off of dry, flaky skin that can look red and inflamed, along with impaired healing due to the damage caused as a result of this cocktail of potent irritants.

KIEHL'S (SKIN CARE ONLY)

Strengths: Kiehl's staff is generous when it comes to providing samples and product information; some good cleansers; a worthwhile selection of sunscreens with avobenzone for UVA protection; a reliable lip balm; many fragrance-free items.

Weaknesses: Expensive for what you get; the Blue Herbal products are terrible for acne; no products to successfully address skin discolorations; the toners; the self-tanner; jar packaging.

For more information and reviews of the latest Kiehl's products, visit CosmeticsCop.com.

KIEHL'S CLEANSERS

✓☺ BEST **$$$ Ultra Facial Cleanser, For All Skin Types** *($18 for 5 fl. oz.)* is an excellent, fragrance-free water-soluble cleanser for all skin types. Effective yet gentle, this product foams slightly and can remove all but the most tenacious makeup. Now this is how to formulate a cleanser (but please note that you don't have to spend this much to get an equally good cleanser).

☺ GOOD **Gentle Foaming Facial Cleanser, for Dry to Normal Skin Types** *($18 for 8.4 fl. oz.)* is accurately named. This standard, water-soluble cleanser doesn't have much to it, but it's fragrance-free and does the job for its intended skin types.

☺ GOOD **Washable Cleansing Milk, for Dry, Normal to Dry or Sensitive Skin Types** *($17.50 for 8.4 fl. oz.)* is a lotion cleanser that is an option for normal to dry skin, though it isn't all that washable without the help of a washcloth. The trace amounts of milk and vitamins in this product are barely detectable.

☺ AVERAGE **$$$ Photo-Age Deep Activating Exfoliating Cleanser** *($22 for 3.4 fl. oz.)* is a very mundane, almost substandard foaming cleanser that claims to immediately break apart surface discolorations, which means they want you to believe that you can just scrub away your uneven skin tone. It isn't possible—wouldn't it be nice if it really were that easy? This cleanser contains typical polyethylene beads to provide a scrub effect, but this kind of scrub doesn't do much to remove the layers of skin that can impact skin color. Successful lightening requires diligent and consistent application of products with hydroquinone or other ingredients such as arbutin or various forms of vitamin C. Even then, you also must be diligent about sun protection and, whenever possible, avoid direct exposure to sunlight. Using any skin-lightening product with an AHA (glycolic or lactic acid) or BHA (salicylic acid) exfoliant can speed results and can provide other anti-aging benefits. As for this cleansing scrub, it is less desirable than many others because it contains a high amount of potassium hydroxide (lye), which is extremely irritating and drying, and several fragrance ingredients known to cause irritation. Last, the price is obnoxiously out of line for what (and how much) you get.

☹ POOR **Acai Damage-Minimizing Cleanser** *($24.50 for 5 fl. oz.)* is a terrible formulation in many ways. Let's start with the price, which is considerably more than anyone needs to spend on any facial cleanser, but even more absurd when it is as ordinary and badly formulated as this one. Turning to the formula, it is fraught with irritants. From its orange fruit water base to the potentially irritating amount of alcohol and fragrant oils of rosemary and lavender. This cleanser won't minimize signs of damage, but may cause it. Acai may be a great antioxidant, but its benefit is lost in a cleanser that is rinsed down the drain.

☹ POOR **Blue Herbal Gel Cleanser** *($21 for 8.4 fl. oz.)* contains 1.5% salicylic acid, but in a cleanser this ingredient is wasted because it's not left on the skin long enough to have an effect. The real problem with this cleanser is the inclusion of ginger, cinnamon, menthol, and camphor. If you are using this product, please reconsider!

☹ POOR **Ultra Facial Oil-Free Cleanser** *($18 for 5 fl. oz.)* definitely gets your face clean and removes makeup, but with the potential trade-off of leaving skin feeling tight and dry. The formula contains some drying, soap-like ingredients, including a fairly high amount of potassium hydroxide (that's lye). Those with very oily skin may find this cleanser a good option, but keep in mind that the irritation caused by the cleansing agents can stimulate more oil production at the base of your pores—so the matte finish this cleanser leaves will be short-lived and your skin can suffer in the long run.

KIEHL'S EYE-MAKEUP REMOVER

☺ GOOD **$$$ Supremely Gentle Eye Make-Up Remover** *($16.50 for 4.2 fl. oz.)* has gentle written all over it, but they should have added "greasy," too, because the amount of oil in this remover leaves a discernible film on skin. This is best for dry skin, and best used before a standard, water-soluble cleanser. It will remove makeup with minimal effort.

KIEHL'S TONERS

☺ AVERAGE **$$$ Photo-Age Activated Toner** *($26 for 6 fl. oz.)* is a decent, though only minimally beneficial, option for normal to dry skin. The amount of vitamin C it contains is potentially helpful for lightening discolorations, but you'll need more than this to achieve truly noticeable results. Many of the effective ingredients in this toner aren't present in significant amounts, and there are enough preservatives and fragrance high up in the ingredient list to prevent us from giving it a good rating.

☺ AVERAGE **$$$ Ultra Facial Oil-Free Toner** *($16 for 8.4 fl. oz.)* is a fragrance-free toner for all skin types that couldn't be more basic, and ends up being a waste of money, even though it doesn't contain problematic ingredients like alcohol or fragrant oils as many toners do. What's missing (and what your skin needs from a toner) is a range of skin-repairing ingredients along with antioxidants and ingredients that encourage healthier skin cells. This toner is mostly water, glycerin, and preservative. Kiehl's included a couple of novel plant extracts, but neither of them has research proving any benefit for skin, so they amount to a "why bother?" rather than a must-have. Also the amounts are so small they end up being merely window dressing. The tiny amount of sodium hyaluronate (a good repairing ingredient found naturally in healthy skin) is likely too low to provide any benefit for your skin.

☺ AVERAGE **$$$ Ultra Facial Toner, For All Skin Types** *($16 for 8.4 fl. oz.)* has its name all wrong, because if this is the ultra (as in "ultimate") toner for all skin types, then the formulators at Kiehl's haven't updated their notes since, oh, the early 1970s. This toner for normal to dry skin consists primarily of water, slip agents, emollient, and preservatives. The tiny amount of vitamin C and plant oils doesn't compensate for the ho-hum ingredients that precede them.

☹ POOR **Acai Damage-Protecting Toning Mist** *($26 for 6 fl. oz.)* lists citrus water and alcohol as the main ingredients, making this spray-on toner anything but protective. Citrus water is useless for skin and alcohol causes free-radical damage, cell death, and irritation (see the Appendix for further details). The only redeeming ingredient in this product is the antioxidant fruit acai; however, it is left to flounder amidst lots of problematic ingredients.

☹ POOR **Calendula Herbal-Extract Toner, Alcohol-Free, for a Normal to Oily Skin Type** *($35 for 8.4 fl. oz.)* is such a basic, nearly do-nothing toner that the price is ludicrous. If you're interested in calendula for skin care, buy a bottle of the oil from a health food store or steep the plant in hot water, let it cool, and bottle your own. Either option is an improvement over this product.

☹ POOR **Cucumber Herbal Alcohol-Free Toner, for Dry or Sensitive Skin** *($16 for 8.4 fl. oz.)* contains balm mint, juniper, pine needle, and arnica, making it too irritating for all skin types, especially sensitive skin. See the Appendix to find out why irritation is a problem for everyone's skin.

☹ POOR **Herbal Toner with Mixed Berries and Botanical Extracts, for Normal to Oily Skin Types** *($25 for 8.4 fl. oz.)* contains berries supposedly placed in each bottle by hand, but aside from looking kind of neat, they have no impact on skin. What will affect skin (negatively) is the peppermint in this poorly formulated toner.

☹ POOR **Rosewater Facial Freshener-Toner, for Normal to Oily Skin** *($16 for 8.4 fl. oz.)* lists alcohol as the second ingredient and contains too little of anything of redeeming value for skin. The alcohol will make oily skin worse by triggering more oil production at the base of your pores.

KIEHL'S EXFOLIANTS & SCRUBS

☺ GOOD **$$$ Epidermal Re-Texturizing Micro-Dermabrasion** *($41 for 2.5 fl. oz.)* is your basic microdermabrasion-in-a-jar topical scrub, with alumina as the abrasive agent. The emollients and silicone in this product help protect skin from the alumina, which can be rough on your skin if not used very gently. Although pricey, this is a good, fragrance-free scrub for normal to dry skin.

☺ GOOD **$$$ Over-Night Biological Peel** *($46 for 1.7 fl. oz.)* is supposed to be as potent as a 10% glycolic acid product, but it contains no AHAs, or BHA for that matter. Instead, this water- and silicone-based fluid contains urea, which is indeed an exfoliant, albeit a far less sexy version than AHAs or BHA because it's derived from urine (though most cosmetics companies use a synthetic version). Urea definitely has exfoliating and water-binding properties when used on skin, and unlike AHAs and BHA, its efficacy is not pH-dependent. Much as AHAs do, it can cause a stinging sensation on application. Urea can be beneficial for those with dry skin because, although the manner in which it works isn't fully understood, it has proven very effective at reducing moisture loss from the epidermis (Source: *Dry Skin and Moisturizers Chemistry* *and Function*, Loden & Maibach, 2000, pages 235–236). Kiehl's ingredient list also points to HEPES as an enzyme activator. However, this ingredient (hydroxyethylpiperazine ethane sulfonic acid) functions as a buffering agent, which should help reduce any potential irritation from the urea. Although this peel is pricey and not necessarily superior to an AHA (or BHA) product, it is nevertheless a novel approach to exfoliating skin if you're curious to try something different, or if your skin has not responded favorably to AHA products.

☹ AVERAGE **$$$ Milk, Honey and Almond Scrub** *($20.50 for 6 fl. oz.)* is a rather inelegant, from-the-kitchen scrub that contains almond-seed meal and grain flours to exfoliate skin. The honey base makes this somewhat sticky while the plant oils impede rinsing, which adds up to a passable but barely worthwhile scrub for normal to dry skin.

☹ AVERAGE **$$$ Pineapple Papaya Facial Scrub, Made with Real Fruit** *($28 for 3.4 fl. oz.)* relies partly on pineapple enzymes to exfoliate skin. The enzymes are unreliable exfoliants. The corncob powder is a low-tech exfoliant, but is what saves this scrub for normal to oily skin from being a total waste of time and money.

KIEHL'S MOISTURIZERS (DAYTIME & NIGHTTIME), EYE CREAMS, & SERUMS

☺ GOOD **$$$ High-Potency Skin-Firming Concentrate** *($56 for 1.7 fl. oz.)* is a lightweight, fragrance-free, serum-type moisturizer with a fairly modern assortment of helpful ingredients for skin. Of course, none of them are capable of addressing "multiple skin firmness concerns," but they can help skin restore a healthy barrier and prevent moisture loss.

☺ GOOD **$$$ Line-Reducing Eye-Brightening Concentrate** *($41 for 0.5 fl. oz.)* contains mostly slip agent, silicone, vitamin C (as ascorbic acid, which can be irritating if used around the eyes), glycerin, thickeners, and more silicones. Kiehl's claims the vitamin C content is 10.5%, and it may well be, but there is no research proving this is the magic number needed to reduce wrinkles or under-eye circles. Still, it's a good antioxidant for skin and comes in opaque packaging to keep it stable during use. This isn't a slam-dunk for use around the eyes, but should be OK for use on other areas of the face by all skin types. Fragrance in the form of orange flower extract is one more reason to keep this away from the eye area—and check out the Appendix to find out why you don't need a special product for the eye area.

☺ GOOD **$$$ Powerful Strength Line Reducing Concentrate** *($58 for 1.7 fl. oz.)* is mostly slip agent, silicone, vitamin C, more silicones, film-forming agent, and the cell-communicating ingredient adenosine. Although this is a one-note product, it's an option if you want a stably packaged vitamin C serum.

☺ GOOD **$$$ Ultra Moisturizing Eye Stick SPF 30** *($20 for 0.18 fl. oz.)* is a rich, fragrance-free, balm-like sunscreen stick that contains an in-part avobenzone sunscreen. The amount of synthetic active ingredients may be too high to use around the eyes, but this can be a very good sunscreen for other exposed areas, such as the ears, scalp, or the top of your feet.

☹ AVERAGE **Abyssine Lotion + SPF 15** *($48 for 2.5 fl. oz.)* provides an in-part titanium dioxide sunscreen in an incredibly ho-hum base formula for normal to slightly dry or slightly oily skin. This contains some good antioxidants and a couple of cell-communicating ingredients, but in amounts too small for skin to notice.

☹ AVERAGE **Creme D'Elegance Repairateur, Superb Tissue Repairateur Creme** *($50 for 4 fl. oz.)* is nothing more than an average emollient moisturizer for dry skin. The name is fancy, but the formula is outdated, and the most intriguing ingredients amount to less than a dusting.

☹ AVERAGE **Panthenol Protein Moisturizing Face Cream, for Normal to Dry and Dry Skin Types** *($26 for 4 fl. oz.)* is an OK but dated emollient moisturizer for its intended skin type. Most of the interesting ingredients are listed well after the preservative, so they don't count for much.

☺ AVERAGE **Sodium PCA "Oil Free" Moisturizer** *($18 for 2 fl. oz.)* is oil-free but also very boring, offering little for normal to oily skin other than silicone and thickeners. The tiny amount of antioxidants will deteriorate quickly due to jar packaging; see the Appendix for further details on the problems jar packaging presents.

☺ AVERAGE **$$$ Abyssine Cream +** *($48 for 1.69 fl. oz.)* contains a meager amount of exciting ingredients for skin, and what little there is will quickly break down once this jar-packaged cream is opened. At best, this is an extremely average, overpriced moisturizer for normal to dry skin.

☺ AVERAGE **$$$ Abyssine Eye Cream +** *($37 for 0.5 fl. oz.)* contains mostly water, glycerin, silicone, several thickeners, and a preservative. The called-out "survival molecule" ingredients are barely present, but even if they were somehow special and unique, they are barely present in this formula and won't remain stable once this jar-packaged eye cream is open. This is a barely passable fragrance-free option for normal to dry skin anywhere on the face, but check out the Appendix to find out why you don't need an eye cream.

☺ AVERAGE **$$$ Cryste Marine Firming Cream** *($49.50 for 1.7 fl. oz.)* makes a big deal out of the Mediterranean-sourced flower (*Crithmum maritimum*, or rock samphire) extract it contains. Supposedly, this flower can increase the renewal rate of skin cells, but there is no information to support this claim. Even if it had such an effect, the amount in this product is minuscule (there's more preservative than flower extract). That leaves you with a pricey moisturizer that has some respectable qualities, yet remains an ordinary choice when compared to similarly priced products from other lines, such as Clinique, Estee Lauder, and Paula's Choice. Nothing in this product is capable of firming skin.

☺ AVERAGE **$$$ Cryste Marine Firming Eye Treatment** *($38 for 0.5 fl. oz.)* is incapable of firming skin and the jar packaging will render the tiny amounts of antioxidants ineffective shortly after you open the product. At best, this will make dry skin anywhere on the face feel softer and smoother. For the money, you should expect more, not to mention this is further proof of why you don't need to use an eye cream (see the Appendix to find out why).

☺ AVERAGE **$$$ Cryste Marine "Ultra Rich" Lifting and Firming Cream** *($51 for 1.7 fl. oz.)* makes a claim that conflicts with basic physics. According to Kiehl's, this rather boring but emollient moisturizer for normal to dry skin contains "Hyaluronic Filling Spheres." The sponge-like absorbency of these spheres is said to trap the skin's own water, causing the molecules to expand, which "immediately" lifts skin. Assuming the spheres work as claimed (although the amount of sodium hyaluronate in this product is next to nothing), the effect would not be to lift skin but rather to stretch it or make it puffy. When you look at it that way, the appeal pretty much vanishes.

☺ AVERAGE **$$$ Photo-Age Corrective Moisturizer** *($45 for 2.5 fl. oz.)* is a moisturizer for normal to slightly dry skin that is supposed to produce a more even skin tone. The only ingredient present in this formula that can possibly help improve skin color is a form of vitamin C that doesn't have a lot of great research behind it. That doesn't mean it's not an option, but it does mean there are better options out there. Other than the vitamin C, this is a very basic moisturizer that can make minor dry areas feel better, but it lacks the state-of-the-art ingredients that all skin types need to look their best.

☺ AVERAGE **$$$ Rosa Arctica Youth Regenerating Cream with Rare "Resurrection Flower"** *($60 for 1.7 fl. oz.)* has a lackluster, overpriced formula, like most of Kiehl's moisturizers. Its star ingredient, "Rosa arctica," is barely present and the tiny amount of antioxidants it does contain will break down due to the jar packaging (see the Appendix to learn more about why jar packaging is a problem). At best, this will make dry skin feel somewhat better, but your skin deserves much more, such as healing and skin-repairing ingredients, environmental protection, and on and on!

☺ AVERAGE **Ultra Facial Cream** *($24.50 for 1.7 fl. oz.)* provides another story about two special ingredients extracted from remote locations, also claimed to be valuable for skin because they can survive in harsh climates (lots of plants can survive harsh climates, but rubbing them on your skin is not going to help you with sun damage or with frigid conditions). It also doesn't help that these miracle plants are present in such tiny amounts, and the jar packaging won't keep any of the token amount of antioxidants stable during use. This is definitely more ordinary than ultra for normal to dry skin.

☺ AVERAGE **Ultra Facial Moisturizer** *($18 for 2.5 fl. oz.)* remains a very popular product for Kiehl's, sort of like the original Dramatically Different Moisturizing Lotion remains a hot seller for Clinique. Both products cover the basic needs of someone with normal to dry skin, but lack anything truly beneficial or state-of-the-art for skin. The tiny amounts of plant oils and vitamins in this moisturizer will have little to no impact, though it is fragrance-free.

☹ POOR **Abyssine Cream + SPF 23** *($45 for 1.7 fl. oz.)* provides an in-part avobenzone sunscreen, but otherwise has a formula that's similar to the boring Abyssine Cream + from Kiehl's. Although this provides great broad-spectrum sun protection, the inclusion of several fragrant oils makes it too irritating for all skin types, plus the jar packaging won't keep the tiny amount of antioxidants stable during use. See the Appendix to learn more about why fragrance and jar packaging are bad news for your skin.

☹ POOR **Acai Damage-Correcting Moisturizer** *($45 for 2.5 fl. oz.)* is mostly water, alcohol, plant oils, and thickeners. The amount of alcohol is cause for concern because it's quite likely to cause irritation and free-radical damage, which is what alcohol does. The main plant oils are of the nonfragrant variety, but their effectiveness on dry skin is muted due to the prevalence of alcohol. Adding to this problem is the inclusion of irritating rosemary and lavender oils. This contains the antioxidant fruit acai, but given the problematic ingredients it's keeping company with, you are better off correcting the mistake of purchasing this product sooner rather than later.

☹ POOR **Acai Damage-Repairing Serum** *($49 for 1.7 fl. oz.)* is an overpriced serum that contains mostly water, fragrant water, and alcohol. How any of that is supposed to repair visible skin damage is a mystery and, in reality, completely impossible. Orange fruit water is orange juice, and that is a skin irritant, and the third ingredient is alcohol, which causes free-radical damage, cell death, and irritation. This also contains fragrant lavender and rosemary oils, which serve to damage, not repair, skin. The amount of antioxidant acai is impressive, but it's fighting an uphill battle against the irritants and skin-damaging ingredients that dominate this faulty serum. See the Appendix to learn how irritation hurts everyone's skin.

☹ POOR **Blue Herbal Moisturizer** *($23 for 3.4 fl. oz.)* is an ultra-light, matte finish moisturizer for oily skin which contains 0.5% salicylic acid as its active ingredient. Although the pH makes the salicylic acid content minimally effective as an exfoliant, what keeps this from earning a recommendation is the inclusion of menthol and plant irritants such as cinnamon and ginger. Irritation is a problem for all skin types, causing collagen to breakdown and increases oil production in the pore. This is not preferred to Clinique's Mild Clarifying Lotion or any of the BHA products from Paula's Choice.

☹ POOR **Eye Alert** (*$21.50 for 0.5 fl. oz.*) is a water-based eye gel which contains little that's helpful for your skin, but it does supply a large amount of alcohol! As usual with Kiehl's skin-care products, the "star" ingredients called out on the label are present in the tiniest amounts imaginable, which means they won't help your skin in any significant way. Moreover, there isn't any reliable research proving vitamins, caffeine, or cucumber help your eye area look more alert, and even if they were able to do that, they aren't unique to this product. See the Appendix to learn more about the problems alcohol presents and why, in truth, you don't need an eye gel.

☹ POOR **Midnight Recovery Concentrate** (*$43 for 1 fl. oz.*) contains a few helpful ingredients for dry skin, but it is loaded with irritating fragrant oils. Restoring skin's healthy appearance overnight isn't going to happen with this product. Coriander, lavender, and rosemary are the biggest offenders; they all present problems for your skin, including irritation and collagen breakdown. Please … save your skin and your cosmetics budget and ease your dryness with a well-formulated fragrance-free moisturizer coupled with a nonfragrant plant oil such as olive or evening primrose.

☹ POOR **Midnight Recovery Eye** (*$36 for 0.5 fl. oz.*) is a problematic mix of beneficial ingredients and problematic irritating ingredients. Irritation is always bad for skin; even when you can't see it on the surface, it is causing damage underneath, especially around the eyes (see the Appendix for details and to find out why you don't need an eye cream). This moisturizing formula begins well, using nonfragrant emollient plant oils that would work for dry skin, but alcohol is rather high on the list and several fragrant extracts are in here, too. Fragrance is a culprit for causing irritation that can make eye-area concerns worse, not better.

☹ POOR **Ultra Facial Moisturizer SPF 15** (*$21 for 2.5 fl. oz.*) lacks the UVA-protecting ingredients of titanium dioxide, zinc oxide, avobenzone, Tinosorb, or Mexoryl SX, and is not recommended. Even if this had sufficient UVA protection, it is an exceptionally boring moisturizer for the money.

☹ POOR **Ultra Facial Oil-Free Gel Cream** (*$26 for 1.7 fl. oz.*) has a lightweight, silky texture, but this moisturizer contains enough alcohol to make it a problem for all skin types. See the Appendix to learn why irritation is so bad for your skin. Even without the alcohol, this is a lackluster formula that falls short of providing your skin with what it needs to look and act younger.

☹ POOR **Ultra Facial Oil-Free Lotion** (*$26 for 4.2 fl. oz.*) is a lightweight moisturizer that contains enough alcohol (it's the third ingredient) to make it a problem for all skin types. Alcohol causes dryness and free-radical damage, and impairs healthy collagen production. Along with the alcohol comes irritation from menthol, which makes this moisturizer even more of a problem. Please see the Appendix for additional facts on why irritation is so bad for your skin. The plant extracts this contains do not have documented benefit for skin, making this more of a "why bother?" than a must have.

☹ POOR **Ultra Facial Tinted Moisturizer SPF 15** (*$24.50 for 2.5 fl. oz.*) comes in three sheer shades and has a much more interesting (though still lackluster) formula than the Ultra Facial Moisturizer SPF 15 above. However, the absence of sufficient UVA protection makes this a poor choice for daytime anti-aging benefits.

KIEHL'S SUN CARE

☺ GOOD **Vital Sun Protection Lotion SPF 30** (*$19.50 for 5 fl. oz.*) is a very good, in-part avobenzone sunscreen for UVA protection; it is appropriate for someone with normal to slightly oily skin. It contains a film-forming agent that provides water resistance, which Kiehl's advertises on the product label. Our only point of contention with this sunscreen is the claim that "minimal chemical ingredients" are used, which we're betting they've chosen to say to try to imply that their sunscreen is superior to others, and it just isn't true. It contains 18% active ingredients—all of them synthetic sunscreen agents—and synthetic preservatives and film-forming agents. Kiehl's claim of using a "minimal" amount doesn't add up to anything like a genuine definition and is a completely disingenuous statement. This product is fragrance-free and does contain vitamin E for some antioxidant benefit.

☺ GOOD **Vital Sun Protection Lotion SPF 40** *($19.50 for 5 fl. oz.)* is similar to the Vital Sun Protection Lotion SPF 30 above, except that it contains a higher concentration of active ingredients and a larger amount of film-forming agent for water resistance. Otherwise, the same comments apply regarding formula and skin type.

☺ GOOD **$$$ Creme de Corps Light-Weight Body Lotion with SPF 30 Sunscreen** *($27 for 8.4 fl. oz.)* is a good sunscreen for the body if you're looking for a lightweight texture, smooth finish, and UVA protection courtesy of stabilized avobenzone. There are few beneficial extras to speak of, and the price is out of line for what you get, but this does provide sun protection without the heavy, sometimes thick feel you get from some sunscreens for the body.

☺ AVERAGE **$$$ Super Fluid UV Defense SPF 50+** *($34.50 for 1.7 fl. oz.)* is a very basic, ultimately disappointing sunscreen with a price that is likely to discourage the liberal application that is essential. Stabilized avobenzone is on hand for reliable UVA protection, but alcohol plays a fairly strong supporting role in this sunscreen, which would be to your skin's detriment. Alcohol is always irritating and drying and causes free-radical damage, not the best for skin. Plus, the price tag and the small quantity make it unlikely you will apply this liberally from the neck down, which is how sunscreen must be applied. Super Fluid does have a silky texture and nearly weightless finish, but it's too short on redeeming qualities to make it a worthwhile purchase. As for the "prevent 90% of skin aging" claim, that can be said of any well-formulated sunscreen that provides broad-spectrum protection—and Super Fluid UV Defense SPF 50 doesn't qualify as the best sunscreen around.

☹ POOR **Sun-Free Self-Tanning Formula** *($22.50 for 5 fl. oz.)* doesn't distinguish itself performance-wise from other self-tanners containing dihydroxyacetone. However, it can be irritating to skin because it contains many volatile fragrant oils and extracts.

KIEHL'S LIP CARE

☺ AVERAGE **Lip Balm #1 SPF 4** *($7 for 0.5 fl. oz.)* is a very standard, Vaseline-based lip balm that contains a good blend of emollients to prevent dry, chapped lips. It is fragrance-free. The SPF rating is just embarrassing, as most dermatologists are advising at least SPF 15 and many are encouraging SPF 30 as the minimum, even for lips.

☹ POOR **Lip Balm SPF 15** *($9.50 for 0.5 fl. oz.)* is an emollient lip balm available in clear or tinted shades, but none of them provide sufficient UVA protection, which leaves lips vulnerable to sun damage. See the Appendix to learn more about which UVA-protecting ingredients are best.

KIEHL'S SPECIALTY SKIN-CARE PRODUCTS

☺ AVERAGE **Acne Blemish Control Daily Skin-Clearing Treatment** *($30 for 1 fl. oz.)* contains 1.5% salicylic acid (BHA) as its active ingredient, but unfortunately its pH is too high for exfoliation to occur. You may get minimal results using it, but it doesn't compete favorably with better and far less expensive BHA products from Paula's Choice. If it were formulated within the proper pH range, this lightweight lotion would've been an excellent product to help combat acne and blackheads.

☺ AVERAGE **$$$ Photo-Age High Potency Spot Treatment** *($50 for 1 fl. oz.)* is a specialty product that makes claims that are beyond this formula's capacity. It contains mostly water, followed by slip agents, silicone, thickeners, and the antioxidant ellagic acid. Ellagic acid is a potent antioxidant compound present in pomegranate and in most berries. Research has shown that, like many other antioxidants, it can reduce the signs of sun damage, including keeping collagen intact when skin is exposed to UVB light. There is also limited research showing that ellagic acid can interrupt the process that causes excess melanin formation in skin (Sources: *Experimental Dermatology*, August 2010, pages 182–190; *and International Journal of Cosmetic Science*, August 2000, pages 291–303). The problem with this formula is that ellagic acid is the only worthwhile ingredient present in any appreciable amount. Your skin needs an array of beneficial ingredients to truly fight sun damage and wrinkling—there isn't any single miracle ingredient. If ellagic acid were the best ingredient, why doesn't Kiehl include it in all their Photo-Age products, or other antiwrinkle products for that matter? Your skin won't be happy with the fragrance and peppermint leaf extract this product contains because of the irritation they can cause. See the Appendix to learn why irritation is a problem for all skin types.

☺ AVERAGE **Rare Earth Deep Pore Cleansing Masque** *($23 for 5 fl. oz.)* is a very basic clay mask that's an OK (but needlessly pricey) option for oily skin. It contains some good absorbent ingredients and is fragrance-free, which is a nice change of pace.

☺ AVERAGE **Soothing Gel Masque** *($19.50 for 2 fl. oz.)* is a lightweight gel mask suitable for normal to oily skin experiencing dry patches. The green tea has soothing benefits, but the jar packaging won't keep it stable for long. See the Appendix to learn why jar packaging is a problem.

☹ POOR **Blue Herbal Spot Treatment** *($16 for 0.5 fl. oz.)* lists alcohol as the second ingredient, and farther down the list are a slew of other irritants, including menthol, camphor, witch hazel, cinnamon, and ginger. What was Kiehl's thinking? See the Appendix to learn why the irritants in this spot treatment are a nightmare for oily, breakout-prone skin.

☹ POOR **Clearly Corrective Dark Spot Solution** *($49.50 for 1 fl. oz.)* is a water-based serum said to lighten dark spots with vitamin C. Although there's vitamin C in this serum (a novel form, explained below), the formula contains a potentially problematic amount of alcohol and also comes in clear packaging that won't keep the vitamin C stable during use (see below for details). Alcohol causes dryness and free-radical damage, and hinders skin's ability to look and act younger. Vitamin C, either as pure ascorbic acid or as the derivative that Kiehl's uses (3-O ethyl ascorbic acid, which breaks down to pure vitamin C on skin) is a wonderful antioxidant and there's a good amount of research showing how it helps reduce dark spots and other brown discolorations on skin, most of which come from sun damage. But because all forms of ascorbic acid are susceptible to deteriorating in the presence of light and air, opaque packaging is a must. A clear bottle just doesn't cut it. The China-based company that supplies this form of vitamin C to cosmetics lines has their own research showing this ingredient is stable after 90 days of light and air exposure, but without seeing the study, it's difficult to know the control factor, not to mention that the company selling this ingredient to cosmetics firms likely won't go on record claiming it's unstable. This somewhat tacky-textured serum also contains fragrant

⚘ Exposing oily skin to irritating ingredients makes it worse! See the Appendix to learn more.

lavender oil, a plant oil that even in small amounts can cause irritation that hurts skin's ability to repair itself and generate healthy collagen. The citrus extracts this contains aren't good news for your skin, either. As for the peony root extract that Kiehl's promotes for this skin-lightening product, it has no established benefit for skin. Even if it did, the amount this serum contains is minuscule. Clinique, philosophy, and Paula's Choice are among the brands that offer superior skin-lightening products that stand a great chance of lightening dark spots.

☹ POOR **Double Strength Deep Wrinkle Filler** *($39 for 0.68 fl. oz.)* is a thin-textured wrinkle filler that is a problem for all skin types and not recommended. The alcohol it contains causes dryness, irritation, and free-radical damage, which hurts your skin's ability to heal and limits its ability to produce healthy collagen. This isn't the way to strengthen aging skin or improve the appearance of wrinkles. The two types of hyaluronic acid Kiehl's mentions in their claims as being important to the formula are barely present, so don't expect them to help your skin; neither is capable of acting like the hyaluronic acid used in dermal fillers.

KISS MY FACE (SKIN CARE ONLY)

Strengths: Inexpensive; generous sizes; some very good sunscreens, occasional use of anti-oxidants without troublesome plant extracts; some fragrance-free products.

Weaknesses: Nearly all products contain one or more problematic plant extracts or volatile plant oils; no products to successfully treat acne or lighten skin discolorations; several bar soaps; no reliable AHA or BHA products; irritating toners.

For more information and reviews of the latest Kiss My Face products, visit CosmeticsCop.com.

KISS MY FACE CLEANSERS

☺ AVERAGE **Clean for a Day Creamy Face Cleanser** *($15 for 4 fl. oz.)* contains tangerine oil and other fragrant plants that, organic or not, are a problem for your skin. The cleansing agent may be naturally derived, but the fragrant plant extracts are not the best for skin. This could have been a great option for normal to dry skin if Kiss My Face had chosen plants that aren't known to be problematic for skin.

☺ AVERAGE **Olive & Aloe Soap** *($2.99 for 4 oz. bar)* is an olive oil–based soap in which the oil has been saponified (that is, it's been turned into soap). It is an OK option for normal to slightly dry skin but does not rinse easily, and the residue can lead to dull skin. It is also more drying than most water-soluble cleansers that come in a lotion form.

☺ AVERAGE **Pure Olive Oil Soap** *($2.99 for 4 oz. bar)* is similar to the Olive & Aloe Soap above, and the same review applies. The same review, price, and size also applies to the **Olive & Chamomile Soap**, **Olive & Green Tea Soap**, and **Olive & Honey Bar Soap**.

☹ POOR **Olive & Lavender Soap** *($2.99 for 4 ounce bar)* contains lavender, and is not recommended for any skin type. See the Appendix to learn why lavender is among the worst ingredients for skin.

☹ POOR **Start Up Exfoliating Face Wash** *($15 for 4 fl. oz.)* contains problematic amounts of several fragrant oils that are a distinct problem for your skin. It really doesn't matter if they're organic or not because the source of irritating, skin-damaging ingredients doesn't make them any more or less of a problem for skin.

KISS MY FACE TONER

☹ POOR **Balancing Antioxidant Toner for All Skin Types** *($15 for 5.3 fl. oz.)*. This spray-on toner is loaded with irritating ingredients, including witch hazel, which contains about 14%

alcohol and causes irritation, free-radical damage, and dryness. This is a clear case of natural not being inherently better for your skin. Thinking otherwise and not paying attention to which natural ingredients are helpful and which are a problem is likely to put your skin on the fast track to irritation. Paula's Choice Earth Sourced Purely Natural Refreshing Toner is a superior option that treats your skin to proven, gentle natural ingredients.

KISS MY FACE MOISTURIZERS (DAYTIME & NIGHTTIME), EYE CREAMS, & SERUMS

✓☺ BEST **Face Factor Face + Neck SPF 30** *($12.95 for 2 fl. oz.)* is a truly outstanding product in the Kiss My Face line! This in-part zinc oxide sunscreen for normal to dry skin contains a very good array of antioxidants, soothing agents, emollients, and cell-communicating ingredients. Well done, and it's fragrance-free, too! This formula should be suitable for those struggling with dry skin and occasional breakouts; however, as with any skin-care product, it takes experimentation to discover what works best for you.

☺ AVERAGE **Eyewitness Eye Repair Creme for All Skin Types** *($19 for 0.5 fl. oz.)* contains some helpful plant oils and anti-irritants, but loses credibility because it contains problematic irritating plant extracts and lavender oil, although not very much. Overall, this formula's mix of good and not so good ingredients is what earns it an average rating. See the Appendix to find out why, in truth, you don't need an eye cream.

☺ AVERAGE **Honey Calendula Natural Ultra Moisturizer** *($4.99 for 4 fl. oz.)* would be better without the potentially irritating plant extracts, but is an OK option for dry skin not prone to blemishes. It contains antioxidant grape seed oil and a tiny amount of water-binding agents.

☺ AVERAGE **Intensive Repair Night Creme** *($23 for 1 fl. oz.)* is a good emollient moisturizer with a few problematic fragrant plant oils that can cause irritation, but probably not enough to be of concern. Nothing about the formula is intensive or special for skin at night.

☺ AVERAGE **Olive & Aloe Moisturizer, for Sensitive Skin** *($4.99 for 4 fl. oz.)* contains many ingredients that are helpful for dry skin, including olive oil, almond oil, vitamin E, lecithin, and even wax. However, the number of fragrant plant extracts makes it unsuitable for sensitive skin, and additional fragrance is thrown in, too. See the Appendix to learn why daily use of fragrant skin-care products is problematic.

☺ AVERAGE **Under Age Ultra Hydrating Moisturizer** *($21 for 1 fl. oz.)*. It's unfortunate that Kiss My Face has a propensity for commingling helpful and potentially harmful natural ingredients in their products. Without the problematic plant extracts, particularly lavender, which is high up on the ingredient list, this would've been a good emollient moisturizer for dry skin. As is, it's not worth strong consideration over many others in this price range.

☹ POOR **Brightening Day Creme with SPF 4** *($23 for 1 fl. oz.)*. Not only is SPF 4 a dangerously low rating, but also the price and claims for this product are offensive given the formulation and the fact that the active ingredients aren't listed on the label as they are supposed to be according to FDA regulations. It does contain titanium dioxide and zinc oxide, but the lack of active status and the meager SPF rating adds up to a big zero. This is not a daytime moisturizer worth trying, for many reasons, including the irritants of peppermint, clary sage, and melissa, which are damaging to skin.

☹ POOR **C the Change Ester C Serum for All Skin Types** *($21 for 1 fl. oz.)* contains a stabilized form of vitamin C and is packaged to ensure stability, but it contains far too many potentially problematic irritating ingredients, including lemon and grapefruit oils. Those ingredients are indeed natural, but being natural has nothing to do with whether or not it is good for your skin. See the Appendix to learn why irritation from fragrance hurts everyone's skin.

☹ POOR **Cell Mate Facial Creme and Sunscreen SPF 10 Normal to Oily Skin** *($21 for 1 fl. oz.)* does not provide sufficient UVA screening and the SPF 10 is too low to provide sufficient daytime protection according to every medical board in the world. Even if it had an SPF 15 rating, this product is questionable because it contains a lot of lavender oil, and that's not good news. Lavender oil may smell appealing, but scent isn't skin care. See the Appendix to learn why lavender is among the worst ingredients for skin.

☹ POOR **Face Factor Face & Neck SPF 50** *($13.95 for 2 fl. oz.)*. One unique aspect of this daytime moisturizer with sunscreen is its inclusion of avobenzone and zinc oxide, two active ingredients the FDA does not permit to be combined in one product. This combination is approved for use in most other parts of the world, and we suspect the FDA will permit it (along with titanium dioxide plus avobenzone) at some point, but for now, it appears Kiss My Face goes against FDA regulations. We called the company numerous times to ask for an explanation of its choice of actives in this product, but we didn't get an answer. Other than the regulatory issue mentioned above, which is really only a problem for regulators, not for your skin, the formula is rather ordinary, except that it also contains lavender oil. This fragrant plant oil is a problem for all skin types, even in small amounts, as is the case with this product. All in all, this is not something you want to kiss your face with. See the Appendix to learn why lavender oil makes this product one to avoid.

☹ POOR **Lavender & Shea Butter Ultra Moisturizer** *($4.99 for 4 fl. oz.)* contains lavender oil, which makes it a distinct problem for all skin types. As we've stated before, topical application of lavender oil can cause skin-cell death (Source: *Cell Proliferation*, June 2004, pages 221–229), among other problems, all discussed in the Appendix.

☹ POOR **Olive & Aloe Ultra Moisturizer Fragrance-Free, for Extra Sensitive Skin** *($4.99 for 4 fl. oz.)* is not fragrance-free because it contains several fragrant plant extracts, including orange blossom and lavender (which are not great for any skin type, especially extra sensitive). See the Appendix to learn why daily use of fragranced products is a problem for skin.

☹ POOR **Peaceful Patchouli Moisturizer** *($4.99 for 4 fl. oz.)* contains a significant amount of patchouli oil, whose volatile components (including eugenol) can be irritating to skin. Far from being a peaceful experience for anyone's skin, this moisturizer also contains several other plant extracts and oils known to be irritating, and the heavy thickeners it contains can quickly clog pores. Patchouli oil may smell appealing, but fragrance isn't skin care, especially for someone with sensitive, reddened skin.

☹ POOR **Peaches & Creme Ultra Moisturizer 4% Alpha Hydroxy** *($4.99 for 4 fl. oz.)* contains fruit extracts that do not function in the same manner as AHAs, though the citrus ingredients can cause needless irritation. This product also contains numerous fragrant plant extracts that cause irritation, an almost surefire way to cause skin problems rather than improve them.

☹ POOR **Vitamin A & E Moisturizer** *($4.99 for 4 fl. oz.)* contains standard emollients for dry skin, but has an unusually greasy texture that is not suited for dry skin prone to breakouts. Actually, given the problematic plant extracts this contains, it's a poor choice for any skin type. The vitamins A and E referred to in the claims makes it seem as though this moisturizer contains a large amount of those antioxidant vitamins. In truth, it contains roughly the same amount as countless other moisturizers.

KISS MY FACE SUN CARE

✓☺ BEST **Kids Natural Mineral Sunblock Lotion SPF 30** *($14.99 for 4 fl. oz.)*. Unlike some other sunscreens Kiss My Face markets to kids, this version doesn't contain fragrant irritants. Instead, you get gentle, broad-spectrum protection from the mineral sunscreen actives titanium dioxide and zinc oxide. This lightweight yet emollient lotion base, which is best for normal to dry skin, contains several antioxidant-rich plant ingredients. This is also fragrance-free, which is a benefit for all skin types, especially sensitive and children's skin. We have a winner, and its price isn't too bad, either! Note: Although this sunscreen contains many natural ingredients, it isn't all natural. That's fine, though, because in most instances the best products include a blend of natural and synthetic ingredients proven to be safe and effective.

✓☺ BEST **Oat Protein Complex Sun Screen SPF 18** *($11.95 for 4 fl. oz.)* is an excellent fragrance-free, water-resistant sunscreen for those struggling with dry, sensitive skin or rosacea. The active ingredients of titanium dioxide and zinc oxide are effective and gentle, while the base formula has a creamy lotion texture that contains anti-irritants and antioxidant-rich plant oils. Note that the amount of mineral actives leaves a slight white cast that requires thorough blending.

✓☺ BEST **Sun Spray Lotion SPF 30** *($15.95 for 8 fl. oz.)* contains an in-part zinc oxide sunscreen for reliable broad-spectrum protection. The fragrance-free formula also contains some proven antioxidants in the form of plant oil and extracts. It applies smoothly, is water-resistant, and is an all-around great choice for active adults or kids. The formula is best for normal to dry skin.

☺ GOOD **Hot Spots with SPF 30** *($8.95 for 0.5 fl. oz.)*. This wax-based sunscreen stick contains avobenzone for sufficient UVA protection. It's a good, emollient option for use on sun-sensitive areas, as indicated in the claims.

☺ GOOD **Oat Protein Sun Screen SPF 30** *($12.95 for 4 fl. oz.)* is a basic, in-part zinc oxide water-resistant sunscreen that is a very good option for normal to dry skin not prone to blemishes. The formula contains some helpful antioxidants and a tiny amount of soothing agents in a creamy lotion base suitable for use from head to toe.

☺ AVERAGE **Sun Spray Oil SPF 30** *($12.95 for 4 fl. oz.)*. This fragrance-free spray-on sunscreen is such a mixed bag, it doesn't rise above average. It's great for your skin that Kiss My Face didn't add fragrance (natural or synthetic, fragrance can be a source of irritation), but not so great that for a sunscreen rated SPF 30, the amount of avobenzone is only 1%. Avobenzone is on hand for its role in providing critical UVA (think anti-aging) protection, but ideally you want to see at least 2% in a product rated above SPF 15. The emollient, silky formula feels great and leaves skin with a smooth sheen, but lacks antioxidants your skin needs for optimal environmental defense. True to claim, the formula is water-resistant, but its wrinkle-reducing prowess is tied only to the sunscreen—something that can be said about most SPF-rated products. If you decide to try this, it is best suited for normal to dry skin that's not prone to breakouts.

☹ POOR **Everyday SPF 15 Moisturizer** *($12.95 for 11 fl. oz.)* does not contain the UVA-protecting ingredients of titanium dioxide, zinc oxide, avobenzone, Tinosorb, or Mexoryl SX, and is not recommended. This also contains several fragrant plant extracts that can cause irritation. See the Appendix to learn more about irritation's effects on skin.

☹ POOR **Kids 100% Natural Blue Sun Stick SPF 30** *($10.99 for 0.5 fl. oz.)* contains citrus oils that make this too potentially irritating for a kid's, or an adult's, skin, so it's not recommended. See the Appendix for details on why irritation is a problem for everyone's skin. One more comment: This sunscreen stick has a neat feature in that it applies blue, and then lightens over time, indicating when it's time to reapply. The "fun" blue color may appeal to kids, and parents may like the visual reminder that it's time to reapply, but this chemistry trick doesn't change the fact that this sunscreen contains fragrant irritants. With the exception of the different colors, the same review applies to the **Kids 100% Natural Pink Sun Stick SPF 30** ($10.99 for 0.5 fl. oz.) and **Kids 100% Natural White Sun Stick SPF 30** ($10.99 for 0.5 fl. oz.).

☹ POOR **Sport Spray SPF 50** *($16.99 for 8 fl. oz.)* provides broad-spectrum protection that includes avobenzone for UVA protection, but the amount of this UVA-protecting ingredient is atypically low. That isn't a deal-breaker, but the amount of alcohol in the base formula most certainly is a problem for skin. What a shame, because this antioxidant-rich sunscreen would otherwise be worth considering.

KISS MY FACE LIP CARE

☹ POOR **Coconut Pineapple Lip Balm SPF 15** *($3.49 for 0.15 fl. oz.)* may taste like a pina colada, but choosing a lip balm based on flavor isn't a good idea because it encourages lip-licking, which worsens chapping. Flavor issue aside, the real problem is that the sunscreen actives in this lip balm do not provide sufficient UVA protection, leaving your lips vulnerable to the sun's most aging rays (see the Appendix for further details). The bottom line: This inexpensive lip balm isn't worth considering. The same deficient sunscreen issue and poor rating also applies to the **Cranberry Orange Organic Lip Balm SPF 15**, **Ginger Mango Organic Lip Balm SPF 15**, **Sliced Peach Organic Lip Balm SPF 15**, **Strawberry Organic Lip Balm SPF 15**, and **Vanilla Honey Organic Lip Balm SPF 15** (each costs $3.49 for 0.15 fl. oz.).

☹ POOR **Sport Lip Balm SPF 30** *($3.49 for 0.15 fl. oz.)*. Although this wax-based lip balm protects lips from UVA damage with its in-part avobenzone sunscreen, it contains lime and spearmint oils along with menthol, which makes it exceedingly irritating to lips. Lime Oil can cause a phototoxic reaction that can discolor skin (and lips) and a sunscreen may not be enough to stop this (because no sunscreen blocks 100% of UV light). Your lips deserve adequate UVA protection in a moisturizing formula that doesn't contain potentially harmful ingredients.

☹ POOR **Treat Mint Organic Lip Balm SPF 15** *($3.49 for 0.15 fl. oz.)* is similar to the Sport Lip Balm SPF 30 above, and the same review applies.

KISS MY FACE SPECIALTY SKIN-CARE PRODUCTS

☹ POOR **Break Out Botanical Acne Gel** *($19 for 1 fl. oz.)*. The second ingredient in this product is irritating peppermint oil, and that's followed by witch hazel extract, which contains about 14% alcohol for more irritation. What follows that is essentially a rogue's gallery of irritants, none of which alleviate acne or promote clear skin; in fact, because irritation can increase oil production and hurt the skin's healing process, it can make matters worse. Just reviewing this ingredient list is enough to make a person break out!

☹ POOR **Pore Shrink Deep Cleansing Mask** *($15 for 2 fl. oz.)* is a clay mask that dips below standard because of its many irritating plant extracts and oils. It is capable of causing irritation, which hurts the skin's healing process and stimulates oil production in the pore, which will in turn lead to pores becoming enlarged (probably not what you had in mind).

KORRES NATURAL

Strengths: An excellent powder blush; some good cleansers and makeup removers.

Weaknesses: Blatantly dishonest claims; several products contain irritating ingredients, including volatile fragrant components; no products for successfully managing acne or skin discolorations; jar packaging; average moisturizers, including some with disappointing SPF ratings; lackluster masks; the foundation primer contains potent irritants; standard eye pencil; some of the plant extracts are from endangered species of plants.

For more information and reviews of the latest Korres Natural products, visit CosmeticsCop.com.

KORRES NATURAL CLEANSERS

☺ GOOD **$$$ Milk Proteins 3 in 1 Cleansing Toning and Eye Make-Up Removing Emulsion** *($21 for 6.76 fl. oz.)* is an effective, albeit greasy, way to remove makeup and cleanse dry to very dry skin. Its toning properties are questionable and, contrary to claims, you will want to use this with water (and a washcloth) to avoid leaving a greasy residue on your skin. Surprisingly, this is fragrance-free and suitable for sensitive skin. The amount of milk protein (listed as whey protein) is so small your skin won't notice it. In the long run, there is little reason to use this instead of pure sunflower oil or canola oil, which is in essence all you are buying.

☺ GOOD **$$$ Milk Proteins Cleansing & Demake Up Wipes** *($12 for 25 wipes)* is a lightweight cleansing solution infused into soft, disposable wipes. They don't remove long-wearing or matte-finish makeup very well, but they're fine for removing lightweight makeup or for refreshing normal to dry skin. For less money, consider using fragrance-free baby wipes. The milk protein in these Korres wipes is listed last on the ingredient list, and clearly is an afterthought, not the emphasis the name implies.

☺ GOOD **$$$ Milk Proteins Foaming Cream Cleanser** *($21 for 5.07 fl. oz.)*. Like many so-called natural products, this cleanser is a mix of natural and synthetic ingredients. That's great, because this combination often produces the best results in terms of product performance, aesthetics, and stability. What's disappointing is how expensive this cleanser is for what amounts to a fairly standard foaming formula. It's an option for normal to combination or oily skin if you don't mind the fragrance and are willing to look past the claims that the milk proteins are doing anything special (they're not, at least not in the tiny amounts Korres uses). Those with dry skin will likely find this cleanser isn't as creamy as it should be to combat dryness. This cleanser works well to remove makeup and rinses without a residue.

☺ GOOD **$$$ Pomegranate Cleansing & Make Up Removing Wipes** *($12 for 25 wipes)*. These soft cloths don't remove long-wearing or matte-finish makeup very well, but they're fine for removing lightweight makeup or for refreshing normal to dry skin. For less money (each Korres wipe costs you $0.48), consider using fragrance-free baby wipes.

☺ GOOD **$$$ White Tea Facial Fluid Gel Cleanser** *($21 for 6.76 fl. oz.)* is a standard, but good, water-soluble cleanser for all skin types except sensitive. It would be rated a Best Product if it did not contain fragrance but the amount is low, which helps to minimize the risk of irritation (especially around the eyes). This removes makeup easily.

KORRES NATURAL TONER

☹ POOR **Pomegranate Toner, Oily to Combination Skin** *($20 for 6.75 fl. oz.)* lists alcohol as its second ingredient. Please see the Appendix to find out why alcohol is a problem for all skin types, especially oily skin. As for the pomegranate, despite its prominence in the product's name, it is barely present in the formula. Fragrance got higher billing, but fragrance isn't skin care.

KORRES NATURAL SCRUB

☺ AVERAGE **$$$ Pomegranate Deep Cleansing Scrub** *($21 for 1.35 fl. oz.)* uses ground olive seeds as the abrasive agent. Although natural, the problem with this ingredient is that the particle edges cannot be refined so they move smoothly over skin. As a result, these types of scrub ingredients can be abrasive and end up doing more harm than good, especially if used too often or too aggressively. The relatively creamy ingredients keep the olive seed scrub particles suspended, which helps keep them from being too much of a problem, but ideally, a washcloth is gentler. And for superior results, a well-formulated AHA or BHA product beats any scrub, any time. If you decide to try this, it is best for normal to dry skin not prone to breakouts.

KORRES NATURAL MOISTURIZERS (DAYTIME & NIGHTTIME), EYE CREAMS, & SERUMS

☺ AVERAGE $$$ **Evening Primrose Eye Cream** (*$30 for 0.68 fl. oz.*) is an OK eye cream whose formula is mostly thickeners and zinc oxide. The amount of zinc oxide is high enough so that this goes on slightly white, which some will find helps improve the appearance of dark circles (though the effect is strictly cosmetic). For the most part, the only ingredient of interest is evening primrose oil though this contains a few other beneficial ingredients, too. The issue is none of the ingredients in this fragranced eye cream are special for the eye area. If anything, this product is simply more proof of why eye creams are not needed (see the Appendix to find out why).

☺ AVERAGE $$$ **Evening Primrose Eye Cream SPF 6** (*$38 for 1.01 fl. oz.*) is underwhelming with its disappointing SPF rating, even though it's pure zinc oxide (SPF 15 is the standard from medical boards worldwide). The base formula is suitable for normal to dry skin, but it is exceedingly ordinary, not particularly natural, and because it contains fragrance makes it a poor choice for use near the eyes. See the Appendix to learn why you don't need a special product for the eye area.

☺ AVERAGE $$$ **Pomegranate Balancing Cream-Gel Moisturizer** (*$32 for 1.4 fl. oz.*). This moisturizer's mix of natural and synthetic ingredients creates a lightweight cream-gel texture, but contains too many oil–based ingredients to make it a winning choice for use on oily areas of combination skin. Best for normal to slightly dry skin, the texture is appealing, but the overall formula is lacking the kind of ingredients all skin types need to look and act younger and healthier. More disappointing is that jar packaging will hurt the effectiveness of the plant-based oils and antioxidants. The formula also contains several fragrance ingredients that are known to cause irritation. See the Appendix to learn why daily use of fragrant products and jar packaging are problems. Bottom line: This is an average formula that feels good but cannot balance oily areas or have any positive impact on sebum (oil) production.

☺ AVERAGE $$$ **Quercetin & Oak Antiageing & Antiwrinkle Day Cream SPF 4 for Normal to Dry Skin** (*$48 for 1.69 fl. oz.*). SPF 4? Are they kidding? Not only is that rating embarrassing dated, it flies in the face of the minimum SPF of 15 recommended by most medical boards around the world. The active ingredients in this product do not supply sufficient UVA protection, which means your skin is left vulnerable in more ways than one to the sun's most aging rays. Interestingly, this contains avobenzone (listed as butyl methoxydibenzoylmethane), but because it isn't part of the active ingredients, it cannot be relied on for sun protection. What about quercetin and oak being proven natural alternatives to retinol? Not true, at least not by the standards published scientific research is held to—and that's what you want in terms of reliable (rather than marketing-based) information. Besides, technically, it could be argued that retinol is a natural ingredient, too (though the retinol used in most cosmetic products is synthetic to improve stability and offer enhanced efficacy). Retinol occurs in many animal foods, such as beef, eggs, and certain fish. And in this particular product, the amount of quercetin (a good antioxidant) and oak is almost nil. The emollient base formula for normal to dry skin contains several good natural ingredients, but this isn't a daytime moisturizer we can encourage anyone to use due to its low SPF rating.

☺ AVERAGE $$$ **Quercetin & Oak Antiageing & Antiwrinkle Eye Cream** *($42 for 0.51 fl. oz.)* contains some excellent ingredients to moisturize dry skin anywhere on the face. Unfortunately, none (and we mean not a single one) of the ingredients in this product will help improve dark circles or puffiness. And nothing in this eye cream is special for use around the eyes. If anything, this product's fragrance and inclusion of fragrant plant extracts such as myrtle and rosemary make it a problem to use near the eyes themselves! For what this costs, it's disappointing that most of the intriguing antioxidant plant extracts are listed after the fragrance and preservatives. This includes the alleged "star" ingredients quercetin and oak. Far from a truly advanced formula capable of making a dramatic difference, at best this will plump wrinkles (as any moisturizer can) and smooth fine, dry lines. See the Appendix to learn why, in truth, you don't need to bother with eye cream.

☺ AVERAGE $$$ **Quercetin & Oak Antiageing & Antiwrinkle Face Serum** *($62 for 0.91 fl. oz.)*. We would love to see the "clinical proof" Korres mentions in the claims for this pricey, water-based serum. They maintain that antioxidants quercetin and oak simulate the anti-aging effects of retinol, but that isn't borne out by any published, documented research. In contrast, there are hundreds of studies attesting to retinol's benefits for skin. Besides, just because something is an alternative doesn't mean it's as good or even that it works in the same way. For example, chicken is an alternative to salmon, but both have their own flavor, texture, and nutritional profiles. This contains some intriguing ingredients and many of them are natural, but synthetic film-forming agents are in here too, so please don't mistake this for an all-natural anti-aging miracle. It offers subtle line-smoothing and a dose of hydration, but lacks an impressive range of proven anti-aging ingredients to help your skin look and act younger. The film-forming agents may make skin feel tighter, but they are not actually tightening loose or sagging skin. This does contain two forms of stabilized vitamin C in decent amounts, so it's worth considering if vitamin C is what you're after—but you can find better products with this ingredient plus a range of other proven age-fighters. SkinCeuticals, Dr. Dennis Gross Skincare, and Paula's Choice RESIST are but a few lines to consider for better anti-aging options.

☺ AVERAGE $$$ **Quercetin & Oak Antiageing & Antiwrinkle Night Cream** *($52 for 1.35 fl. oz.)*. This emollient moisturizer for dry skin has a silky, lush texture that feels great. It contains several beneficial plant extracts, too, though the amount of the antioxidant flavonoid quercetin is disappointingly low. Even if quercetin were more prominent, however, this product's jar packaging will render it and the other plant ingredients unstable shortly after you open it because all those ingredients deteriorate on exposure to air. In better packaging, this would be a very good moisturizer to consider. There is no substantiated research proving the antioxidants quercetin and oak rival retinol.

☺ AVERAGE $$$ **Wild Rose 24-Hour Moisturising & Brightening Cream, Normal to Dry Skin** *($35 for 1.35 fl. oz.)* is a standard moisturizer for normal to dry skin. It contains some helpful plant extracts, but they will not remain stable after opening because of jar packaging. See the Appendix for further details. The claims made for the plant *Imperata cylindrica* are not supported by published research, meaning there's no evidence it can regulate "the moisture equilibrium of skin." At best, this will make dry skin feel smoother and softer, but so can lots of other moisturizers that cost less, have better formulas, and are packaged to keep important ingredients stable during use.

☺ AVERAGE $$$ **Wild Rose 24-hour Moisturiser SPF 6** *($32.50 for 1.4 fl. oz.)*. SPF 6 is an embarrassingly low and harmful SPF rating! Despite titanium dioxide as the sole active ingredient, this isn't a daytime moisturizer we can recommend for sufficient sun protection, and it wouldn't be recommended by any medical board in the world because SPF 15 is considered minimum and higher is better. This does contain some beneficial plant oils and extracts, but much of their potential is diminished due to the jar packaging, which won't keep those ingredients stable. This also contains several fragrance ingredients known to cause irritation, so keep that in mind if you find yourself drawn to this moisturizer's scent. See the Appendix to learn why jar packaging and fragrance aren't wise ways to pick skin-care products.

☺ AVERAGE $$$ **Wild Rose Face and Eye Serum** *($41 for 1.01 fl. oz.)* isn't "ultra-concentrated" as claimed, unless they're referring to it being concentrated with water, which is the main ingredient and among the most common cosmetic ingredients used. Witch hazel water, which is a known irritant (though the water form of this plant is the least concerning in terms of irritation), is the second ingredient. Otherwise, for a brand that fronts natural ingredients, this serum contains an abundance of synthetic ingredients. That's not bad; it just makes the company's marketing angle misleading. They want you to think the natural ingredients are perfecting your skin, but synthetic ingredients are doing most of the work. This ends up being an OK serum for normal to oily skin, though the inclusion of some fragrant plant extracts plus the aforementioned witch hazel makes this an iffy product to use around the eyes (besides, you don't need a separate product for the eye area; see the Appendix for details). The formula contains some helpful antioxidants, including a form of vitamin C and rose hips oil, which is a natural source of vitamin C. That's nice but ultimately not enough to earn this serum a higher rating.

☺ AVERAGE $$$ **Wild Rose + Vitamin C Advanced Brightening Sleeping Facial** *($48 for 1.35 fl. oz.)*. This moisturizer for dry skin is sold as a treatment for dark spots yet its formula contains few ingredients known to make an improvement. Chief among them is vitamin C (listed as ascorbyl tetraisopalmitate), but the amount is so low you're not likely to see much, if any, difference. Far from "a breakthrough in beauty sleep," most of the exciting ingredients in this moisturizer won't remain stable after you open it because of jar packaging. Even stable forms of vitamin C, which this product contains, will eventually break down with daily exposure to light and air. It is also disappointing that the formula contains more alcohol than beneficial ingredients for skin. Although the amount of alcohol is likely too low to cause irritation, its presence combined with fragrance makes this a less desirable choice—and again, this isn't worth considering at all if your concern is lightening dark spots. It simply won't work, either in 14 days as claimed or even after 14 months.

☹ POOR **Pomegranate Mattifying Treatment, Oily to Combination Skin** *($38 for 1.35 fl. oz.)*. Rather than use elegant, dry-finish silicones or similar ingredients to create a silky, absorbent mattifier, Korres uses rice starch, alcohol, and witch hazel. Two of those three are irritating for skin, and problematic for oily skin because irritation triggers more oil production at the base of the pores, making oily skin worse. The same is true for oily areas when you have combination skin, so this mattifier is a poor choice no matter how much oil you're struggling with. The formula also contains the irritating menthol derivative, menthyl lactate, whose cooling sensation may feel refreshing but it's your skin signaling it's being irritated—even if you cannot see the damage taking place. The problematic ingredients in this mattifier are especially disappointing because this does contain some helpful ingredients, including antioxidants, soothing agents, and ingredients that have a mild antibacterial action.

☹ POOR **Quercetin & Oak Antiageing & Antiwrinkle Mattifying Fluid Texture Lotion** *($50 for 1.69 fl. oz.)*. This intensely fragranced mattifying fluid contains some lightweight ingredients, but nothing to absorb excess oil and entrap it so skin stays shine-free. In fact, considering the product name and claims, it's surprising that the formula contains a high amount of oil and fatty acids that, you guessed it, make oily skin look, feel, and act oilier! One could argue that this has merit as a lightweight moisturizer, but again, the fragrance is knock-your-socks-off strong and fragrance isn't skin-caring in the least! Plus, some of the plant extracts in this mattifying fluid can cause irritation that leads to more oil production—not what you want if your goal is to reduce shine and keep skin matte.

☹ POOR **Wild Rose Serum** *($41 for 1.01 fl. oz.)*. Irritating, drying witch hazel distillate, which contains alcohol, is the second ingredient in this poorly formulated serum, and alcohol causes free-radical damage, irritation, and impairs the skin's ability to heal. Beneficial plant ingredients and other antioxidants are in short supply, while fragrance ingredients present the risk of further irritation. See the Appendix to learn why irritation is a problem for all skin types.

KORRES NATURAL LIP CARE

☺ GOOD **Lip Butters** *($12 for 0.21 fl. oz.)*. Korres offers several flavors of the same basic emollient lip balm formula. Whether you choose **Guava**, **Quince**, **Plum**, **Pomegranate**, **Jasmine**, **Mango**, or **Wild Rose**, the only difference is the fragrance and a token amount of the namesake plant extract. These lip balms have a thick but smooth consistency and a glossy finish that works well to keep lips moist and protected. Note that these lip balms are packaged in jars, most likely due to the thickness of the formula, which would not work successfully in a ChapStick-style component.

KORRES NATURAL SPECIALTY SKIN-CARE PRODUCTS

☺ GOOD $$$ **Pomegranate Purifying Natural Clay Mask** *($27 for 1.35 fl. oz.)* is a very good, though needlessly expensive, clay mask for oily or breakout-prone skin. The blend of clay (kaolin) with glycerin allows the clay to absorb excess oil without causing excess dryness, and also aids with rinsing. The tiny amount of jojoba oil is not cause for concern and in fact may benefit skin due to the anti-inflammatory properties this nonfragrant plant oil has. Of minimal cause for concern is the benzyl alcohol, as this alcohol can be a problem when used in higher amounts and the amount in this mask is potentially borderline, but in all likelihood not an issue. If you were expecting this mask's name meant it was brimming with the antioxidant benefit of pomegranate, it isn't. Clearly the pomegranate name was appealing, but its presence in the formula was an afterthought.

☹ POOR **Yoghurt Instant Soothing Gel** *($38 for 1.01 fl. oz.)*. Applying yogurt to skin may be a Greek tradition but there isn't much research supporting yogurt's benefit for skin when applied topically rather than ingested. Yogurt contains components that can help soothe skin, but this gel contains the potent irritant menthyl lactate, which isn't the least bit soothing, especially on sunburned skin. If you're curious to see how yogurt may help sensitized, irritated, or sunburned skin, apply plain Greek yogurt from your grocery store, not this product! One more comment: The emollient shea butter this contains is thick enough to trap heat beneath skin, yet this heat needs to dissipate when you're sunburned or skin cannot heal properly and the burn may worsen.

KORRES NATURAL FOUNDATIONS & PRIMERS

✓☺ BEST $$$ **Wild Rose Mineral Foundation SPF 30** *($28)*. Although mineral makeup is nothing special (truly, the ingredients used for mineral makeup are present in most powders), this is one of the better mineral foundations with sunscreen to consider. It feels unbelievably light especially since it contains over 30% mineral sunscreens as the active ingredients. The texture is beautifully silky, almost gossamer, and meshes well with skin, providing light coverage and a glow-y, radiant finish. You can layer this for a bit more coverage, but that intensifies the sheen this leaves, which won't please those with oily skin or oily areas. Because of the finish, this loose-powder foundation is best for normal to dry skin. A small range of shades is offered for fair to medium skin tones and each is excellent. As with any loose-powder foundation with sunscreen, we don't recommend relying on it as your sole source of sun protection. That's because you're not likely to apply this liberally enough to get the amount of protection stated on the label. However, it works well layered over your daytime moisturizer or liquid foundation with sunscreen. One caution: The component is a standard pot with a sifter and screw-on cap. Once the plastic shield over the sifter is open, this can get messy, so it's not the type of foundation you'd want to travel with or tote around in your daytime bag.

☺ GOOD $$$ **Wild Rose Foundation SPF 20** *($30)* has a thin, fluid texture that smoothes easily over skin, setting to a finish that feels moist but looks matte. The liquid formula is best for normal to slightly dry or slightly oily skin. The shade range is mostly great, but there are no options for dark skin tones. Avoid WRF6 due to its strong peach cast. This foundation provides sheer to light coverage and has a lingering scent. The sunscreen is in-part titanium dioxide; so, as long as you apply this liberally and evenly, it can serve as your daytime facial sun protection.

☺ AVERAGE $$$ **Pomegranate Mattifying Primer** *($33 for 1.01 fl. oz.)*. This highly fragrant primer has a silky, cream-gel texture that glides over skin, setting to a soft matte finish that feels a bit tight but is tolerable under makeup. To some extent, this helps smooth the appearance of enlarged pores and helps keep excess shine at bay, but for how long depends on what other products you use and how oily your skin is. Most will find the results last for a few hours, assuming you follow with a matte finish foundation and powder. It's a shame witch hazel water is one of the main ingredients, as this can be irritating due to its astringent qualities (though the irritation is less than from more concentrated forms of witch hazel). Between this and the likely irritation from the fragrance, this product presents the risk of stimulating nerve endings in skin to produce more oil, which isn't the goal. Companies such as Smashbox, OC Eight, and Paula's Choice offer fragrance-free mattifiers that function as primers, too—assuming your goal is reducing oily shine and minimizing pores. The fragrance from Pomegranate Mattifying Primer really lingers, and fragrance, whether natural or synthetic, isn't skin care. Last, in terms of this primer being "loaded with antioxidants," it isn't. Antioxidants are present, but not in amount that would qualify as "loaded."

☹ POOR **Face Primer** *($28)*. Korres makes a big deal about the fact that this primer is silicone-free, as if silicone were some evil ingredient for skin, which is especially disingenuous for a line whose products are filled with synthetic ingredients. Silicone is not a problem for skin; if anything, research shows it has remarkable healing properties (and it absolutely does not suffocate skin). Whether or not this product is or isn't natural doesn't tell you anything about its benefit for skin. Claims aside, this could have been a worthwhile pre-makeup moisturizer for those with normal to slightly dry skin. Unfortunately, it contains a high amount of melissa, a plant whose various parts are irritating for skin. Melissa has antioxidant benefit, but so do many other plants that don't come with the inherent risk of irritation. This also contains grapefruit peel oil, which also is irritating.

☹ POOR **Quercetin & Oak Face Primer Antiageing Primer** *($33 for 1.01 fl. oz.)* is a very basic emollient moisturizer that is being sold as a primer. Nothing about this is anti-aging save for the product name which, sadly, won't help your skin. The big deal-breaker with this primer is the inclusion of grapefruit oil, a citrus oil whose volatile components cause irritation, especially on sun-exposed skin. This product is a must to avoid—countless primers are worth considering before this, assuming you even want to bother with a primer (in most cases, a well-formulated serum is a perfect primer, too).

☹ POOR **Vitamin E Face Primer** *($28 for 1.01 fl. oz.)*, despite the name, contains a nearly insignificant amount of vitamin E). It otherwise has the same concerns as the Quercetin & Oak Face Primer Antiageing Primer, and the same review applies.

KORRES NATURAL CONCEALERS

☺ AVERAGE **$$$ Quercetin & Oak Antiageing/Antiwrinkle Concealer** *($22)* has a thick, creamy consistency and a semi-moist finish suitable for those with normal to dry skin. You can achieve full coverage, but beware: This concealer's creaminess means it's prone to settling into fine lines unless you take care to set it with powder. The shade range includes four colors, for light to tan skin tones; the Medium Tan shade is not recommended due to its unflattering orange undertone. Although Korres makes some unusual claims about the ingredients in this concealer, they're mostly fiction.

☺ AVERAGE **$$$ Wild Rose Concealer** *($20)*. Housed in a click-pen applicator with a built-in synthetic brush is this slightly thick yet smooth concealer. It blends well with just enough slip and sets to a satin matte finish that's moderately crease-prone unless set with powder. Compared with similarly packaged concealers, each of its acceptable shades provides average coverage.

KORRES NATURAL POWDERS

☺ GOOD **$$$ Wild Rose Mineral Illuminating Powder** *($18)* is a sheer, loose powder designed to add shine to the skin. Its pale pink color works for fair to light skin tones and the smooth finish is laced with sparkles you'll see in daylight (so you may want to consider this for evening makeup unless you want a noticeable sparkling face during the day). The powder is lightweight and applies smoothly, yet ultimately loose powders with shine are trickier (and messier) to work with than adding shine to your face with a liquid or cream product.

☺ GOOD **$$$ Wild Rose Mineral Setting Powder** *($18)* is a very good, weightless loose powder. Its talc-free formula melds with skin to provide sheer coverage and a refined appearance without looking chalky. The single shade is soft and pale, yet goes on translucent so it's workable for all but very dark skin tones. The one drawback (which ultimately comes down to personal preference) is that the powder contains a lot of shine. You'll see visible sparkles on your skin, so oily areas end up looking oilier. If you don't mind (or if you want) shine with a polished finish, this powder is recommended. The only mineral it contains is silica, which isn't unique or special for skin, so you can basically ignore the mineral marketing angle. This powder is suitable for all skin types, and is fragrance-free.

☺ AVERAGE **$$$ Wild Rose Compact Powder** *($28* has a soft, smooth texture that adheres nicely to skin and provides sheer coverage. The shade range is somewhat limited, with only four colors, and even the darkest shade is only a light tan, but each is neutral and flattering. Korres claims this powder's namesake ingredient, wild rose (which is listed as *Rosa canina* fruit oil) "works to repair fine lines and wrinkles and brighten uneven skin tone." You can forget that because the wild rose isn't present in a high enough concentration to do much of anything, not to mention that one ingredient is never the anti-aging answer; plus, in this kind of packaging, it won't remain stable anyway. A bigger issue is the inclusion of fragrance, which can be irritating and problematic for skin. Please see the Appendix to learn why fragrance can be a problem for all skin types.

KORRES NATURAL BLUSHES

✓☺ BEST **$$$ Zea Mays Blush** *($24)*. The powder blush from Korres is one of the highlights of the makeup line. Although each shade has some degree of shine, the creamy smooth texture and near-seamless application are commendable. Other strong points include the color payoff (a little goes a long way) and the way each shade enlivens cheeks without looking dry or powdery. This is a blush to check out if you don't mind (or want) shiny cheeks.

☺ AVERAGE **$$$ Blush** *($24)* doesn't stand out in any significant way so its price isn't justified. The mica-based powder formula has a sheer yet slightly dry texture that goes on smooth but quite sheer. You will need to layer to see much color, but on the other hand the sheer application prevents you from overdoing it. Still, this isn't a blush that shows up well on medium to dark skin tones. As for the shades, each is laced with a hint of shine, and the few colors offered are the same ones you've seen many times over from countless other makeup lines. See what we mean about this being nothing special?

KORRES NATURAL EYESHADOW PRIMERS

☺ GOOD **$$$ Quercetin & Oak Antiageing Eye Primer** *($21)* has a soft, initially slick texture that sets in a flash to a smooth powder finish. Its sheer matte finish has a subtle peach tint that helps to brighten the eye area, though you can get a better overall effect from a liquid highlighter or liquid concealer with a hint of shine. The fragrance-free formula contains a dusting of anti-aging ingredients, but nothing to really justify the expense. As with most eyeshadow primers, this helps enhance eyeshadow application and wear. We wouldn't put it above what a good matte finish concealer or foundation can do, but if you don't use these types of products yet do need something to help your eye makeup last longer, then this is a good, though pricey, option.

KORRES NATURAL LIP COLOR

✓☺ BEST **Lip Butter Glaze** *($14)* is a cross between a lip gloss and a lip balm. Housed in a squeeze tube with a slanted plastic applicator tip, the fluid texture feels oily but isn't super-slick. It moisturizes like a balm while leaving a wet-looking, high-gloss shine without a trace of stickiness. The colors are beautiful whether you want sheer pink, coral, or deep red (each goes on softer than they look when dispensed from the tube). This contains fragrance in the form of jasmine extract.

✓☺ BEST **$$$ Cherry Full Color Gloss** *($17)* is packaged with a wand applicator, and appears to be just like countless other glosses. However, it isn't. You'll notice its balm-like texture that keeps lips protected from moisture loss is its main point of difference. It feels substantial without being sticky and leaves a wet shine finish that doesn't immediately slide right off the lips. We disagree that the colors are "full" (as in full coverage) because they aren't; however, Plum 27 is a must-see if you're looking for a stunning plum-red to wear alone or over lipstick.

☺ GOOD **$$$ Raspberry Antioxidant Liquid Lip** *($22)* provides the coverage of a standard cream lipstick with the shiny finish of a lip gloss. Packaged like many lip glosses, color is applied via an angled sponge-tip applicator. The fragrance-free formula's thin texture moisturizes without feeling greasy and is minimally sticky, so it's comfortable. The shades include nude pinks and berry tones, and among those are a couple of gorgeous reds (one with a blue

☀ Sunscreens must provide reliable UVA (anti-aging) protection. See the Appendix for details.

base, the other with an orange base). As for antioxidants, this contains a tiny amount of them, including raspberry oil, but likely not enough to make a big difference.

☺ AVERAGE $$$ **Mango Butter Lipstick SPF 10** *($18)*. We wish this lipstick had a higher SPF rating because its in-part avobenzone sunscreen is terrific. This sheer lipstick has a smooth, moisturizing texture and glossy finish. The colors are well edited, at least if you prefer rose and pink tones. It's worth considering if you want a sheer lipstick with sunscreen. The SPF rating is why this lipstick received an Average rating instead of a Good one.

KORRES NATURAL MASCARA

☺ GOOD $$$ **Provitamin B5 & Rice Bran Mascara** *($18)*. We weren't expecting to like this mascara as much as we did. Formula-wise, it's nothing special and many of the ingredients aren't the least bit natural, which is true for most of Korres products. Still, the brush allows for nimble lash separation and soft definition with appreciable length and no clumps. Thickness isn't much to speak of, but this is worth a try if you want long, defined lashes that look great all day. Note: This product is also known as **Deep Colour Mascara**. One more comment: There isn't enough Pro-vitamin B5 (panthenol) in this to condition one eyelash.

L'OCCITANE

Strengths: Provides complete ingredient lists for some of its products on company website; some very good cleansers, including for sensitive skin; some facial sunscreens provide sufficient UVA protection.

Weaknesses: Expensive; many products are heavily fragranced or contain irritating fragrance ingredients; jar packaging is prevalent, which won't keep ingredients stable; the products are not all natural.

For more information and reviews of the latest L'Occitane products, visit CosmeticsCop.com.

L'OCCITANE CLEANSERS

✓☺ BEST $$$ **Ultra Comforting Cleansing Milk** *($22 for 6.7 fl. oz.)* does not contain any fragrance or fragrant plants, which makes it a very good option for sensitive skin. This fluid yet milky cleanser feels soothing, removes makeup, and rinses better than expected, though some may find they need to use a washcloth for complete removal. It is fragrance-free and also does not contain preservatives, at least if the ingredient list on the package is accurate. That lack of preservatives is slight cause for concern because a water-based product like this should have a reliable preservative system, although this is packaged so that the product remains hygienic during use. By the way, if this product that's formulated without fragrance is good for sensitive skin, does that mean that all the other L'Occitane products laden with fragrance are bad for sensitive skin, by L'Occitane's own standards? Just a question to ask yourself if you are considering purchasing from this line.

☺ GOOD $$$ **Almond Apple Cleansing Oil** *($22 for 6.7 fl. oz.)* is an emollient fluid cleanser that changes into a milky emulsion when mixed with water. It's a suitable, though overly fragrant, cleanser and makeup remover for dry to very dry skin.

☺ GOOD $$$ **Immortelle Brightening Cleansing Foam** *($26 for 5.1 fl. oz.)* is a standard, fairly unnatural, water-soluble cleanser that cannot lighten your complexion, which is its big selling point. L'Occitane wants you to think that because the Immortelle flower does not wither or lose its color even after it's been picked, that applying its oil to your skin will somehow provide the same benefit and help it resist signs of aging. Whatever prevents the Immortelle flower from withering and fading cannot be transferred to your skin or body, and there is no research proving otherwise. Actually, L'Occitane's claim is not all that unusual; over the years other product lines also have attributed interesting properties to various plant extracts, trying to convince you that they can be passed on to your skin—those were gimmicks, too. The flower and fruits chosen do not have any research showing them to be powerhouse lightening solutions for skin discolorations. Although even if they did, the effect would be severely compromised because this is a rinse-off product and the ingredients are rinsed down the drain. As a cleanser, this foams (for those who like a foaming wash) and is a good, though fragrant, option for normal to slightly dry or slightly oily skin. It is capable of removing makeup, which is always a plus.

☺ AVERAGE $$$ **Foaming Rice Cleanser** *($20 for 6.7 fl. oz.)* is an ordinary, unnatural water-soluble cleanser with an unusual formula because its main cleansing agent is very mild, but there's more acrylate film-forming agent (think hairspray) than there is in almost any other cleanser. Considering L'Occitane makes such a to-do about being all natural this is just a really odd misstep. True to its name, this does foam, but that has no bearing on how clean your skin will be when you're done. The inclusion of vinegar and lime peel extract negates the initial gentleness of this cleanser, making it a tough recommendation for any skin type, though we suppose it's an OK option for normal skin as long as you don't use it around your eyes.

☺ AVERAGE $$$ **Immortelle Milk Makeup Remover** *($27 for 6.7 fl. oz.)* is a very basic blend of thickeners and glycerin, so it's essentially a modified version of cold cream. It works well to remove makeup with or without water (though you'll definitely want to rinse it to avoid leaving a greasy film and to ensure all your makeup is gone). It is an acceptable, though needlessly pricey, option for dry skin. The flower extract in this product is from the daisy family and has a scent reminiscent of curry. There is nothing about this that makes it preferred over many cleansers available at the drugstore.

☹ POOR **Angelica Cleansing Gel** *($20 for 6.7 fl. oz.)* is a standard, detergent-based formula that would be suitable for normal to oily skin if it did not contain peppermint oil and angelica extract. Both of these ingredients are irritants and the irritation they cause can stimulate excess oil production at the base of pores. This is less of an issue in a rinse-off product like this, but given the number of wonderfully gentle cleansers for oily skin, why use one that's potentially troublesome?

L'OCCITANE TONERS

☺ AVERAGE $$$ **Immortelle Essential Water for the Face** *($27 for 6.7 fl. oz.)* has a great name to describe a really ordinary, boring toner for normal to dry skin! Some of the plant extracts it contains are beneficial, but the problem is the number of fragrance ingredients that dull the positives and that also pose a risk of irritation. In the end, this toner doesn't deserve consideration. Estee Lauder offers far better toner formulas for those looking to spend in this price range, or for less money you can consider the state-of-the-art toners from Paula's Choice.

☹ POOR **Angelica Face Toner** *($20 for 6.7 fl. oz.)* is little more than water, glycerin, and fragrance. It's closer to perfume than skin care, and not recommended. Even without the high amount of fragrance, the plant extracts in this toner, including peppermint, are known irritants. This product is a classic example of why many people find toners don't improve their skin—there are great toners out there, but this isn't one of them!

☹ POOR **Immortelle Brightening Water** *($27 for 6.8 fl. oz.)* is not recommended because it contains a high amount of daisy flower extract, known to cause severe contact dermatitis (Source: naturaldatabase.com) and has no known benefit for skin. This toner also contains numerous fragrance ingredients known to cause irritation. See the review for L'Occitane's Immortelle Brightening Cleansing Foam for an explanation of the immortelle flower claim.

☹ POOR **Olive Tree Toning Face Mist** *($22 for 5.1 fl. oz.)* is a spray-on toner that lists spearmint oil as the second ingredient and contains enough alcohol to make it a problem for all skin types. Even if the alcohol posed minimal risk, the amount of spearmint oil is a deal-breaker, because irritation is always damaging for skin. See the Appendix for further details.

☹ POOR **Purifying Rice Toner** *($20 for 6.7 fl. oz.)* is a dual-phase toner containing mattifying silica, but ultimately is a confusing and irritating experience for oily skin. The amount of rice vinegar and lemon peel oil is reason enough to completely avoid this toner because there is no research showing those ingredients to be beneficial for any skin type, especially if your goal is to reduce the inflammation acne causes. See the Appendix to learn why irritation is a big problem for oily skin.

L'OCCITANE SCRUB

☺ AVERAGE $$$ **Ultra Rich Face Scrub with Shea Butter** *($34 for 3.4 fl. oz.)* is unhygienic due to its jar packaging. With regular use, you'll be dipping wet fingers into the container, stressing the preservative system and, well, making a mess. The thick texture of this product is likely what mandated jar packaging, but this product's texture is also ill-suited to a scrub—at least when it comes time to rinse! This is among the least impressive scrubs because instead of gentle exfoliating granules, it contains walnut shell powder. The rough, irregular edges of these shells can scratch and tear at skin, making dryness, flaking and oily areas worse. This scrub is a so-so option for dry skin (the shea butter helps cushion the rough nature of the walnut shells), but optimally you will get much better results from using an AHA (such as glycolic acid) or BHA (such as salicylic acid) exfoliant than any scrub.

L'OCCITANE MOISTURIZERS (DAYTIME & NIGHTTIME), EYE CREAMS, & SERUMS

☺ AVERAGE **Shea Butter Ultra Rich Face Cream** *($10 for 0.5 fl. oz.)* is a decent moisturizer to consider, if you're sold on the benefits of shea butter for dry skin, but it certainly isn't all natural and isn't an improvement over pure shea butter, which you can buy for a fraction of the cost at the drugstore. However, we wouldn't encourage anyone to seek out any one key emollient at the expense of other critical ingredients to help skin look and feel its best, such as antioxidants, cell-communicating ingredients, and skin-repairing ingredients. Unfortunately, choosing this product is saying yes to one-note skin care, not to mention that you're exposing your skin to several potentially irritating fragrance ingredients. By the way, assuming this cream really does contain 25% shea butter, the jar packaging will routinely expose this fatty acid-based emollient to oxygen, which will cause it to become rancid over time. See the Appendix for more facts about jar packaging.

☺ AVERAGE $$$ **Almond Apple Velvet Concentrate** *($42 for 1.7 fl. oz.)* has some impressive ingredients and it will take care of dry skin in terms of helping it feel smoother and softer. The reason for the neutral rating is the jar packaging, which diminishes the effectiveness of the antioxidants it contains (see the Appendix for details).

☺ AVERAGE $$$ **Immortelle Precious Cream** *($58 for 1.7 fl. oz.)* is a standard, emollient moisturizer for normal to dry skin and a product that contains far more fragrance and preservative than the natural ingredients that L'Occitane wants you to focus on. L'Occitane wants you to think that because the Immortelle flower does not wither or lose its color even after it's been picked, that applying its oil to your skin will somehow provide the same benefit and help it resist signs of aging. Whatever prevents the Immortelle flower from withering and fading cannot be transferred to your skin or body, and there is no research proving otherwise. There are several good ingredients in here (particularly antioxidants), but there also is an overly generous supply of ingredients that aren't helpful or precious in the least. And when it comes to natural, polyester is looking more like an eco-friendly material than this product. Add to this L'Occitane's choice of jar packaging and you end up with a product that is anything but precious—rather it is an ersatz zirconium. See the Appendix to learn why jar packaging is a problem.

☺ AVERAGE **$$$ Immortelle Precious Fluid** *($48 for 1 fl. oz.)* has a formula where almost all the good stuff is listed after the fragrance and preservative. At least it feels silky and has a soft, powder-like finish that's slightly hydrating. As such, it is best for normal to slightly dry or slightly oily skin but your skin deserves better. Aside from the overly hyped nonsense about the Immortelle flower (discussed in the review for Immortelle Precious Cream above), the formula is a mix of synthetic and natural ingredients, just like countless others. You're not getting a lot of beneficial ingredients proven to improve signs of aging.

☺ AVERAGE **$$$ Shea Butter Fabulous Serum** *($42 for 1 fl. oz.)* has a texture that's much closer to a moisturizer than a serum, making this a good moisturizer for those with normal to dry skin. Shea butter is a wonderful emollient with antioxidant properties, and L'Occitane includes some good skin-identical ingredients and a mixed bag of beneficial and questionable plant extracts. Although that's good news, this serum/moisturizer hybrid (again, it's really more of a moisturizer than a serum) loses points because it includes lots of fragrance ingredients known to cause irritation. If you're hooked on L'Occitane, this may still be worth considering, but overall your skin will do better with a well-formulated, fragrance-free serum and moisturizer.

☺ AVERAGE **$$$ Shea Butter Ultra Rich Eye Balm** *($34 for 0.5 fl. oz.)* contains coconut oil and shea butter as the main ingredients, so the "ultra rich" name is apropos. Although both ingredients are helpful for dry skin anywhere on the face, the amount of fragrant orange flower water is cause for concern. Orange flower water is nothing more than a way to add fragrance to a product, and an eye cream is one skin-care product where fragrance should be omitted, or at least minimized. Believe it or not, the jar packaging isn't a big issue for this product. That's because the formula sorely lacks antioxidants, which is the group of ingredients (along with skin-identical ingredients and cell-communicating ingredients) that your skin really needs, and why this doesn't deserve better than an average rating. You can get the same if not better results just using pure shea butter, which you can buy at most drugstores for a fraction of this price—and check out the Appendix to find out why you don't need an eye cream.

☹ POOR **Angelica Eye Roll-On** *($28 for 0.33 fl. oz.)* is a lightweight fluid for the eye area that's housed in a small bottle outfitted with a roller ball applicator. It is a basic hydrating formula that is not unique in any way for eye-area concerns. If anything the inclusion of angelica extract and oil plus the fragrance ingredient limonene makes this a mistake to use around the eyes. Angelica oil contains chemical constituents that can be phototoxic, including bergapten, imperatorin, and xanthotoxin. Although some components of angelica oil have antioxidant ability, it is a risky ingredient to use on skin if it is exposed to sunlight (Sources:naturaldatabase. com; and *Journal of Agricultural and Food Chemistry*, March 2007, pages 1737–1742). Consider this further proof of why you don't need a special product for around the eyes (see the Appendix for details).

☹ POOR **Angelica Hydration Cream** *($42 for 1.7 fl. oz.)* has a lush, creamy texture that feels great over dry skin. Unfortunately, its namesake plant (angelica) is its major downfall.

This contains angelica extract and oil, discussed in the review for Angelica Eye Roll-On above. If that wasn't bad enough, the formula also contains irritant peppermint oil and, in many ways, is short on the type of ingredients all skin types need to look and feel their youngest and healthiest. The jar packaging for this moisturizer is also a problem, which we discuss in the Appendix. There is no research showing the angelica plant stimulates aquaporins, which are proteins in skin that play a role in regulating water content between skin cells.

☹ POOR **Angelica Protective Lotion SPF 15** *($38 for 1 fl. oz.)* contains synthetic active ingredients, including avobenzone for reliable UVA protection. What's odd about that is it's counterintuitive to L'Occitane's natural positioning—why not use titanium dioxide or zinc oxide instead (though there's nothing wrong with the actives they chose)? Although this lightweight lotion is capable of providing broad-spectrum sun protection, its formula is weak on antioxidants and other repairing ingredients. Instead of those beneficial ingredients, you're getting irritants such as angelica and peppermint oils, neither of which is the least bit helpful for anyone's skin. There are numerous other daytime moisturizers with sunscreen that are preferred to this disappointing formula.

☹ POOR **Angelica UV Shield SPF 40** *($38 for 1 fl. oz.)* contains titanium dioxide as its sole active ingredient, which is great because on its own, titanium dioxide provides reliable broad-spectrum sun protection. What's not so great is this silky daytime moisturizer's inclusion of problematic plants such as angelica and peppermint oils. Angelica oil is a particularly bad choice for daytime use because the oil contains chemical constituents that can be phototoxic, discussed in the review for Angelica Eye Roll-On above. Granted, this product contains sunscreen to protect skin from UV damage, but why chance the irritation when there are so many daytime moisturizers whose formulas don't present the problems this does—and in fact contain a much better array of anti-aging ingredients?

☹ POOR **Divine Cream** *($95 for 1.7 fl. oz.)* is expensive! The only thing divine about this product is the price, and that's assuming that divinity is correlated somehow with a high price tag. Labeling this product as "complete regenerating skin care" is so far off the mark you can't even see the target. More to the point, if this is a "complete regenerating" product, what are all the other Immortelle products for? Is this their best option for being "immortelle"? Also, because it doesn't contain sunscreen, it assuredly is not a complete option for daytime! Although this moisturizer has its share of impressive beneficial ingredients, the amount of synthetic and natural fragrance ingredients is cause for concern because they are irritants, as are some of the plant extracts and the myrtle oil. According to the Natural Medicines Comprehensive Database, myrtle oil used topically can cause "bronchial spasm, asthma-like attacks, or respiratory failure in infants and children." Granted, this isn't a product for kids, but why bother including such a problematic, unimpressive ingredient that doesn't have any research showing it has any benefit for skin? The jar packaging issue isn't even worth going into detail about because this is just a really bad, overpriced product.

☹ POOR **Divine Extract** *($108 for 1 fl. oz.)* contains myrtle oil and, according to Natural Medicines Comprehensive Database (naturaldatabase.com), when used topically on children it can cause asthma-like attacks and there is absolutely no research showing it has any benefit for skin. What were they thinking? Sadly, there was potential here because this contains some good antioxidants, nonfragrant emollient plant oils, and skin-repairing ingredients, but the myrtle extract along with other problematic ingredients such as fragrance and irritating plant extracts add up to one big headache of a product. See the Appendix to learn why fragrance and irritation are a problem for all skin types.

⊗ POOR **Divine Eyes** *($72 for 0.5 fl. oz.).* Even though this eye cream is far better for-mulated (and practically void of the problematic fragrant extracts L'Occitane uses in their products), it still contains myrtle oil and other problematic ingredients discussed in the review for Divine Extract above. It's not recommended, and you don't need an eye cream (see the Appendix to find out why).

⊗ POOR **Immortelle Brightening Moisture Cream** *($58 for 1.7 fl. oz.)* contains a fair number of problematic ingredients. The *Helichrysum italicum* flower oil is a natural source of the fragrance ingredients nerol, linalool, and limonene, each of which is irritating for all skin types. Moreover, this plant and the daisy flower extract are distinct problems for anyone with ragweed allergies (Source: naturaldatabase.com). As far as the good ingredients are concerned, the jar packaging won't keep them stable. See the Appendix to learn about the problems jar packaging presents.

⊗ POOR **Immortelle Brightening UV Shield SPF 40** *($56 for 1 fl. oz.)* is a confusing mix of ingredients both beneficial and detrimental to skin. For example, high up on the in-gredient list is wild daisy flower extract and, while that might be attractive in an open field, on your skin it can cause a negative reaction if you are allergic to ragweed, chrysanthemums, marigolds, daisies, and many other herbs. In short, this is not an ingredient you want on your face. Although there are some great plant oils in here and the sunscreen is mineral-based with an impressive amount of titanium dioxide, there is also way too much fragrance that skin doesn't need. The natural and synthetic fragrant components this contains can cause irritation and that is always bad for skin. In terms of sun protection, it is important to be aware that you always have to apply sunscreen liberally to get the benefit of the SPF rating on the label. Pricey sunscreens might deter you from doing so and that would detrimental for your skin. Adding to this product's problems is that despite the presence of plant oil that would be great for dry skin (assuming the other problematic ingredients weren't in here), it also contains a high amount of cornstarch, an ingredient which is absorbent and better for oily skin.

⊗ POOR **Immortelle Precious Eye Balm** *($38 for 0.5 fl. oz.)* is a water- and rosehip-based moisturizer with a light texture and contains enough film-forming agent (a type of ingredient typical in hairsprays) to help make wrinkles look temporarily smoother. The film-forming agent (polymethyl methacrylate) is about as natural as polyester and it can be an irritant in high amounts. The plant extracts are mostly ordinary and innocuous, but the inclusion of ivy extract isn't good news. Combine this with a lack of significantly helpful ingredients and jar packaging and this eye balm is best left on the shelf, especially considering that it offers no special benefit for dark circles or puffy eyes. See the Appendix to learn more about jar packag-ing and why, in truth, you don't need to bother using an eye cream.

⊗ POOR **Immortelle Precious Night Cream** *($70 for 1.7 fl. oz.)* contains nothing inherently "precious," nor does it offer any special action during the night. It contains several emollient ingredients and nonfragrant plant oils that are wonderful for dry to very dry skin, but the plant oils' antioxidant benefits won't remain stable once this moisturizer is opened because it's packaged in a jar. See the Appendix for details on the other problems jar packaging presents. What about the claim that this night cream fills wrinkles? Don't count on it, at least no more than what you'd see from many other emollient moisturizers. Simply put, moisturizing dry skin always makes wrinkles less apparent, though you won't see much, if any, filling effect. (That's a result you'll get only from dermal injections, not skin-care products.) Although jar packaging is a problem for this moisturizer, a bigger concern is the fragrant oils it contains. Although L'Occitane includes nonfragrant oils that are fine on their own, they also included fragrant oils, each of which is known to cause irritation, especially for sensitive skin (Source: naturaldatabase. com). The fragrant components may make this moisturizer smell good, but a pleasant scent isn't always pleasing to your skin. See the Appendix for details on the problems fragrant oils present.

☹ POOR **Immortelle Precious Protection SPF 20** *($58 for 1.7 fl. oz.)* is a daytime moisturizer with a pure titanium dioxide sunscreen that contains several problematic natural ingredients! What a shame. It contains some good natural ingredients, too, but so do lots of other moisturizers that don't expose your skin to fragrant oils and plant extracts known to cause allergic reactions (Source: naturaldatabase.com). Fragrance ingredients are included, too, so you end up getting a product that can irritate your skin, hurt your skin's healing process, damage collagen, and incite free-radical damage. The SPF 20 is well done, with titanium dioxide as the active, but the beneficial ingredients that could possibly make this an interesting sunscreen to consider if none of the negative ingredients were present, will deteriorate on opening due to the jar packaging (see the Appendix for details). None of that is precious or protective!

☹ POOR **Immortelle Very Precious Regenerating Concentrate** *($58 for 1 fl. oz.)* is a concentrated, triglyceride-based moisturizer for dry to very dry skin containing some wonderful emollient, antioxidant, and soothing plant ingredients. Unfortunately, it also contains some really irritating plant extracts, such as citrus oils and sandy everlasting, listed by its Latin name *Helichrysum italicum*. The latter is a distinct problem for all skin types due to its irritant potential and is not recommended for anyone allergic to ragweed (Source: naturaldatabase.com). Your dry skin will be much better off if you treat it to plain evening primrose or borage seed oil, and you can mix either one with your regular moisturizer for times when you need a more emollient product. See the Appendix to learn why fragrance, natural or synthetic, is bad for skin.

☹ POOR **Rice Ultra-Matte Face Fluid** *($26 for 1 fl. oz.)* is a lightweight, silky moisturizer with a suitably matte finish for oily skin; however, the amount of rice vinegar (which has no benefit for skin) and the lemon peel oil make it too irritating for even occasional use. Mattifying products from Smashbox, Clinique, and Paula's Choice omit the irritants and supply skin with a shine-free finish and with the ingredients it needs to function in a healthy manner.

L'OCCITANE LIP & SMILE CARE

☹ POOR **Shea Butter Lip Balm Stick** *($10 for 0.17 fl. oz.)* is a lip balm that contains some excellent ingredients to improve dry lips and prevent moisture loss that leads to chapping and flaking. Regrettably, it is highly fragranced and contains numerous fragrance ingredients known to cause irritation. That means potentially drier, more chapped lips even though you're diligently applying this balm to relieve those symptoms. Please refer to our list of Best Lip Products at the end of this book for superior options with and without sunscreen.

L'OCCITANE SPECIALTY MAKEUP PRODUCTS

☺ AVERAGE **$$$ Immortelle Cream Mask** *($62 for 4.4 fl. oz.)* is for dry to very dry skin not prone to breakouts. Although it contains some substantial emollients to help dry skin look and feel better, there's also a lot of fragrance, and most of the really intriguing ingredients (such as antioxidant vitamins and nonfragrant plant oils) are barely present. Even if these extras were included in greater amounts, the choice of jar packaging won't keep them stable once this mask is in use (see the Appendix for further details).

☹ POOR **Immortelle Brightening Essence** *($56 for 1 fl. oz.)* contains only one worthwhile ingredient for those looking to brighten their complexion and that is ascorbyl glucoside. This form of vitamin C can be helpful, but no more than many other ingredients—an assortment of effective ingredients would be far better. The vitamin C is in a water base formulated with standard slip agents to improve application, but that's the only good news and it isn't all that good. Immortelle Brightening Essence contains far too much fragrance and too many problematic plants to make it worth considering. The *Helichrysum italicum* flower oil is a natural source of the fragrance ingredients nerol, linalool, and limonene, each of which is irritating for all skin types. Moreover, this plant and the daisy flower extract are distinct problems for anyone with ragweed allergies, and are known to cause contact dermatitis (Source: naturaldatabase.com). This may smell divine, but please repeat after us: Fragrance isn't skin care!

☹ POOR **Immortelle Brightening Moisture Mask** *($62 for 4.4 fl. oz.)* is a confusing mix of beneficial and detrimental ingredients. For example, high up on the ingredient list is wild daisy flower extract. That might be attractive in an open field, but on your skin it can cause a negative reaction if you are allergic to ragweed, chrysanthemums, marigolds, daisies, and many other herbs. In short, this is not an ingredient you want on your face. Although there are some good plant oils in here, there is also a great deal of fragrance, both synthetic and natural, which can cause irritation. If that wasn't bad enough, the few good ingredients in here won't stay stable due to the jar packaging (see the Appendix for details).

L'OREAL PARIS

Strengths: Inexpensive, some good water-soluble cleansers; nice assortment of self tanning options; one of the best, most comprehensive makeup collections at the drugstore, with superb options in almost every category; L'Oreal's mascaras (along with those from sister company Maybelline New York) are a tough act to follow.

Weaknesses: Jar packaging; many of the daytime moisturizers with sunscreen lack sufficient UVA protection; no products to successfully combat blemishes (at least not without causing more irritation); no effective skin-lightening options that don't contain problematic ingredients; boring to problematic toners; several foundations with sunscreen still lack sufficient UVA protection.

For more information and reviews of the latest L'Oreal Paris products, visit CosmeticsCop.com.

L'OREAL PARIS CLEANSERS

☺ GOOD **go 360° Clean Deep Facial Cleanser for Sensitive Skin** *($6.99 for 6 fl. oz.).* The only point of interest to this standard, but well-formulated cleanser is the "Scrublet" device that L'Oreal includes. It's an oval-shaped soft rubber disc outfitted with several nubs designed to provide a more thorough cleansing experience. You can consider this an alternative to using a washcloth, although the washcloth lets you cover more surface area faster. L'Oreal omitted the irritating and skin-damaging menthol and fragrance they included in their other go 360° cleansers, so this is indeed better for sensitive skin.

☺ GOOD **Age Perfect Rich Restorative Cream Cleanser for Mature Skin** *($6.69 for 5 fl. oz.).* Nothing about this cleanser represents a special formula for mature skin. In fact, it isn't a special formula for anyone's skin at any age; it is just a standard lotion-style, water- and oil–based formula that contains a small amount of detergent cleansing agent that would work well for someone with normal to dry skin. (But keep in mind that not everyone with mature skin, whatever that means, has dry skin!) Combined, they do a thorough job of cleansing normal to dry skin and removing makeup. The calcium in here is a gimmicky ingredient that cannot strengthen skin the way drinking calcium-rich beverages (milk) can strengthen bones. Skin is not affected by topically applied calcium. All in all, a very good cleanser with a great price tag but with really misleading, fabricated claims.

☺ AVERAGE **Revitalift Radiant Smoothing Wet Cleansing Towelettes** *($6.69 for 25 towelettes)* are cloths soaked in a cleaning lotion whose alcohol concentration (as in denatured alcohol, not the benign cetyl or stearyl alcohol fatty acids) is a slight cause for concern. But coupling that with the many fragrance ingredients included makes these towelettes a source of potential irritation if skin is not rinsed afterward. Since part of the convenience of using cleansing cloths is not having to rinse, why bother with these when there are plenty of better options at the drugstore? Even fragrance-free baby wipes would be a better option than this.

☺ AVERAGE **Revitalift Radiant Smoothing Cream Cleanser** *($6.69 for 5 fl. oz.)* is a good, though very basic, water-soluble cleanser for normal to slightly dry skin. It cannot nourish skin or boost radiance, both strange claims to make for a cleanser because the nourishing part (even if it could do that) would be rinsed down the drain, and the radiance part is just clean skin, something most cleansers can do. The salicylic acid in this cleanser is too low to function as an exfoliant, not to mention you rinse it from skin before it has a chance to work. The fragrance in here is pretty intense, and there is a lot of titanium dioxide, which makes the product look white but also makes it harder to rinse. All in all, it's just an okay cleanser with a great price

☹ POOR **go 360° Clean Anti-Breakout Facial Cleanser** *($6.99 for 6 fl. oz.)* is a water-soluble cleanser for oily, breakout-prone skin that contains irritating peppermint and menthol, making it a problem. The "scrublet" that accompanies this product is cute but will only exacerbate the irritating ingredient's effects on your skin, not to mention scrub devices like this should not be used over acne lesions. See the Appendix to learn why irritation is a big problem for oily, acne-prone skin.

☹ POOR **go 360° Clean Deep Cream Cleanser** *($6.99 for 6 fl. oz.)*. The only point of interest to this standard, overly fragranced cleanser is the "Scrublet" device that L'Oreal includes. It's an oval-shaped soft rubber disc outfitted with several nubs designed to provide a more thorough cleansing experience. You can consider this an alternative to using a washcloth, although the washcloth lets you cover more surface area faster. As for the cleanser itself, it is not recommended because it contains menthol and also is highly fragranced, which is an additional problem for skin (see the Appendix for details on how irritation hurts skin).

☹ POOR **go 360° Clean Deep Facial Cleanser** *($6.99 for 6 fl. oz.)*. is nearly identical to the go 360° Clean Deep Cream Cleanser above, and the same review applies.

☹ POOR **Youth Code Foaming Gel Cleanser** *($7.99 for 6.7 fl. oz.)*. This fragranced, water-soluble gel cleanser is an average option for normal to oily or combination skin. The salicylic acid in this cleanser cannot exfoliate skin due to its brief contact (you'll rinse this before it has a chance to work). Of most concern is the amount of fragrance ingredient p-anisic acid and the inclusion of skin-irritant menthol. These additions make this cleanser a tough sell, especially considering that other drugstore brands offer gentler cleansers one shelf over.

L'OREAL PARIS EYE-MAKEUP REMOVER

✓☺ BEST **Clean Artiste Waterproof & Long Wearing Eye Makeup Remover** *($6.99 for 4 fl. oz.)* is a very good dual-phase eye-makeup remover that also happens to be exceptionally gentle and fragrance-free. It works quickly and efficiently to remove all types of makeup, including waterproof mascara. The price is great, too!

L'OREAL PARIS TONER

☹ POOR **HydraFresh Toner** *($6.29 for 8.5 fl. oz.)* lists alcohol as the third ingredient, which isn't terrible, but it's not helpful either. What follows is barely interesting for skin and makes this a toner you should ignore.

L'OREAL PARIS SCRUB

☺ GOOD **go 360°** Clean Deep Exfoliating Scrub *($6.99 for 6 fl. oz.)* includes L'Oreal's "Scrublet," a tiny, oval-shaped rubber disc outfitted on one side with tiny nubs. The goal is to achieve a more thorough scrub experience, but given that this product also contains scrub particles (polyethylene beads and a tiny amount of apricot seed powder), using it with the Scrublet can be irritating to the skin, which is detrimental—irritation does not equal deep cleansing. This is a good scrub on its own, and it's good the apricot seeds are only a tiny portion of the formula. In contrast to rounded polyethylene beads, seed and nut powders can scratch and tear skin, which is damaging and not necessary for exfoliating skin.

L'OREAL PARIS MOISTURIZERS (DAYTIME & NIGHTTIME), EYE CREAMS, & SERUMS

☺ GOOD **Revitalift Complete Anti-Wrinkle and Firming Moisturizer SPF 30 Day Lotion** *($13.99 for 1.7 fl. oz.)* includes an ample amount of avobenzone for reliable UVA protection. This moisturizer for normal to slightly dry skin has a silky, fluid texture that works beautifully under makeup. We also were impressed with the range of antioxidants, water-binding agents, and the addition of the cell-communicating ingredient adenosine, but our enthusiasm was dampened by the inclusion of several fragrance ingredients. The fragrance ingredients are known to cause irritation, and coupled with the amount of synthetic sunscreen actives, have the potential to make this daytime moisturizer more irritating than it would be without fragrance. Still, this deserves a Good rating because the pros outweigh the cons, and the price isn't out of line, either. This doesn't contain pure retinol, but instead contains retinyl palmitate, a blend of retinol with a fatty acid. The small amount isn't likely to have much antiwrinkle effect, but it still should provide antioxidant benefit to skin.

☺ GOOD **Youth Code Eye Cream** *($24.99 for 0.5 fl. oz.)*. If the claims for L'Oreal's Youth Code products and their GenActiv technology sound familiar, that's because Lancome (which L'Oreal owns) claimed almost the same thing in 2010 when they launched their Genifique products. No one on the Paula's Choice Research Team was surprised when Youth Code was announced, as it's common for L'Oreal and Lancome to offer similar products whose only significant differences are price and retail location. Please see the review below for L'Oreal's Youth Code Day Lotion SPF 30 for a discussion of the gene-stimulating claims. This well-packaged, fragrance-free eye cream (it comes in a squeeze tube with a built-in, smooth-tip applicator) is a pretty good formula. It does not contain anything special for the eye area, and you don't need an eye cream (more on that in a minute), but overall this is a better formula than most of L'Oreal's other eye-area moisturizers. This eye cream is packaged in a jar as part of L'Oreal's Youth Code Starter System. Given the jar packaging and weaknesses of the other Youth Code products packaged in this system, it is not recommended. Our review only applies to the eye cream as sold separately.

☺ AVERAGE **Age Perfect Anti-Sagging & Ultra-Hydrating Eye Cream** *($16.99 for 0.5 fl. oz.)* is an emollient moisturizer for normal to dry skin that loses points for its jar packaging and the mere dusting of antioxidants. This contains mineral pigments that leave a soft shine finish on skin, but that won't diminish wrinkles (though it does "brighten"). See the Appendix to learn why jar packaging is a problem and why, in truth, you don't need an eye cream.

☺ AVERAGE **Age Perfect Anti-Sagging + Anti-Age Spot Hydrating Moisturizer Night Cream** *($15.99 for 2.5 fl. oz.)* is actually sold with the tag line of being a new menopause innovation, which it absolutely isn't. Such a boring skin-care product cannot address the physiologic changes a woman's skin endures during menopause, as these affects are related to hormonal loss, something this moisturizer cannot correct. This ends up being another standard, jar-packaged moisturizer from L'Oreal. It's an OK option for normal to dry skin but offers little in the way of anti-aging ingredients and contains nothing that can correct sagging or lighten a single age spot. By the way, sagging skin is not (we repeat, NOT) an issue any skin-care products can fix, regardless of the claim or ingredients. Acknowledging this will save you a lot of time, money, and frustration. At best, this moisturizer will make skin smoother and softer, though it does so by risking irritation due to the fragrance ingredients and fragrant jasmine extract it contains. One last note: The jar packaging isn't a formulary issue here due to the lack of antioxidants, but it's still a hygiene issue when you consider that you need to stick your fingers into the product every day.

☺ AVERAGE **Age Perfect Hydra-Nutrition Day/Night Cream for Mature, Very Dry Skin** *($16.99 for 1.7 fl. oz.)*. The claims and statistics for this "age imperfect" moisturizer look impressive, but without knowing the standards of how they arrived at their conclusions, it's mostly marketing mumbo jumbo. For example, after 2 weeks, 98% of testers felt this product restored comfort to their skin. That sounds great, but the fact is that any moisturizer can do that: Apply it to dry skin on your arm for the same period of time and don't apply moisturizer to the other arm; the one that has been moisturized will feel more comfortable, right? The other claims follow the same logic, and there's no convincing research anywhere that calcium is as essential for your skin when applied topically. (Skin isn't bone, so the association of helping bones is irrelevant for skin.) As it turns out, this jar-packaged moisturizer harkens back to the 1950s thanks to its water, oil, and wax formula. How dated can you get? There's nary an intriguing anti-aging ingredient to be found, but L'Oreal added lots of fragrance ingredients known to cause irritation and artificial coloring agents for a pretty appearance in the jar. For this product, jar packaging doesn't matter much, because it is void of state-of-the-art ingredients. One more point: The only difference between a day cream and a night cream is sun protection, so this product is completely inappropriate for daytime use; in this case, it is also not worthwhile at night.

☺ AVERAGE **Collagen Moisture Filler Day/Night Cream** *($11.49 for 1.7 fl. oz.)* is moisturizer for dry skin that has a formula closely matching several from Lancome, except L'Oreal (Lancome's parent company) products have a price point that's much easier to accept. Still, it really blows to pieces the prestige image Lancome strives for when you realize you can buy essentially the same moisturizer from L'Oreal for $16 instead of $100 (and up) at the Lancome counter! This moisturizer has a silky, emollient texture, but the forms of collagen it contains cannot fuse with the collagen in your skin and plump wrinkles from the inside out. You'll see a reduction in the appearance of lines, just as you do with most emollient moisturizers, but that's it. This product lacks a selection of state-of-the-art ingredients that skin needs to restore and repair itself as well as to fend off free-radical damage.

☺ AVERAGE **Revitalift Anti-Wrinkle Concentrate** *($15.79 for 1 fl. oz.)*. You have every right to expect a brilliant, advanced formula owing to L'Oreal's claim that this product is their most potent antiwrinkle serum ever. But because L'Oreal historically (more often than not) likes making lofty claims without backing them up with superior formulas, all you really end up with is wordplay and a product that is better left on the shelf. This is nothing more than an average water-based serum that possesses a silky texture suitable for normal to slightly dry or slightly oily skin, but that's about it. Antioxidants are in woefully short supply (their use

---

⊘ Think "hypoallergenic" means safe for sensitive skin? See the Appendix to find out the truth.

of retinyl palmitate is not the same as retinol, despite their labeling it as "Pro-Retinol A"), skin-identical and cell-communicating ingredients are lacking, and the pH of this serum won't permit the salicylic acid to function effectively as an exfoliant. You're getting more shiny mineral pigments than the anti-aging ingredients L'Oreal touts on the packaging. This does contain several fragrance ingredients that pose a risk of irritation. Any of the serums from Olay or Paula's Choice are distinctly preferred to this far-from-advanced (and incapable of lifting even one skin cell) serum.

☺ AVERAGE **Revitalift Clinical Repair 10 Day Treatment SPF 20** *($24.99 for 1.7 fl. oz.).* L'Oreal claims this moisturizer with an in-part avobenzone sunscreen fights the 10 visible signs of aging. They mention just about every sign-of-aging concern a person may have, from wrinkles to loss of firmness and sagging, yet the truth is that no single product (or ingredient) can address all those issues. Think of it like your diet and how there isn't one powerhouse meal you can eat that addresses all aspects of your health. Perhaps L'Oreal is banking on the fact that their "Clinical Strength Retinol" is the does-it-all ingredient, but retinol cannot amend everything that happens to our skin with age (although it would be great if that were true). Besides, there are no standards for "Clinical Strength" when it comes to retinol, so most likely L'Oreal is describing it that way hoping consumers will think this product is somehow more potent. This product provides the broad-spectrum sun protection that's necessary to keep skin from suffering the aging effects of sun exposure. The base formula is a lightweight cream that contains standard thickening agents along with antioxidant soybean oil and retinol. It's not a very exciting formula, but some may find it convenient to have retinol in a product with sunscreen. What can be problematic is the combination of the synthetic sunscreen actives with retinol and several fragrance ingredients L'Oreal added to the formula. This is not a daytime moisturizer with sunscreen for those with sensitive skin, and it's capable of causing irritation if applied around the eyes (where sun protection is most definitely needed). All told, you're getting sun protection with light hydration for normal to slightly dry skin and a decent dose of retinol, but this combination isn't enough to make good on L'Oreal's claims of fighting 10 signs of aging. Plus, the potential for irritation from the fragrance ingredients can be a step backward in the fight for younger-looking, more radiant skin.

☺ AVERAGE **Revitalift Complete SPF 30 Day Lotion with Photo-Aging Complex** *($13.99 for 1.7 fl. oz.).* If this is supposed to be L'Oreal's "most complete" Revitalift product (the implication being that this does it all), then why do they continue to sell all their other Revitalift products? Of course, as it turns out, this isn't the complete answer to your skin-care needs. The main anti-aging benefit you get from this product is sun protection from avobenzone, which provides critical shielding from the sun's UVA rays. L'Oreal also includes antioxidants and cell-communicating ingredients associated with helping you look younger, but the small amounts are disappointing. As for the "Pro-Retinol A" (retinyl palmitate) and elastin, neither is present in an amount that makes this the best anti-aging moisturizer around. Besides, elastin in skin-care products cannot fuse with the elastin in your skin and somehow make it firmer and less prone to sagging; it just isn't possible (although we all wish that weren't the case). At best, what this product provides is broad-spectrum sun protection in a lightweight lotion base that's best for normal to oily skin. This is not rated higher because its numerous fragrance ingredients are cause for concern. All are known to irritate skin, and irritation is always a problem, especially if your goal is younger-looking skin.

☺ AVERAGE **Revitalift Complete Eye Cream** *($15.99 for 0.5 fl. oz.)* is a water- and silicone-based moisturizer for normal to dry skin anywhere on the face. It is fragrance-free, as claimed. The tiny amount of vitamin A is the only antioxidant, though jar packaging won't keep it stable (see the Appendix for details and to learn why you don't need an eye cream). Of course, nothing in this product will lift skin or reduce puffy eyes.

☺ AVERAGE **Revitalift Complete Night Cream** *($15.99 for 1.7 fl. oz.)* is shockingly similar to most of the other night creams L'Oreal (and sister company Lancome) sell. Housed in a jar is a formula that's mostly water, silicone, glycerin, thickeners, plant oil, and emollients followed by fragrance ingredients, wax, and more fragrance ingredients. The truly intriguing ingredients are present in very tiny amounts, and the jar packaging degrades their effectiveness, not to mention the hygiene issue jar packaging presents. This very fragranced moisturizer offers little in terms of anti-aging benefit, and its irritant potential is not something to take lightly.

☺ AVERAGE **Revitalift Deep-Set Wrinkle Repair 24 HR Eye Repair Duo** *($19.99 for 0.4 fl. oz.)* is a dual-sided product that includes an eye cream with sunscreen for A.M. application and an eye cream without sunscreen for use at night. The **A.M. Formula** includes an in-part avobenzone sunscreen, though avobenzone and the other sunscreen actives in this formula aren't the best for use in the immediate eye area (titanium dioxide and/or zinc oxide are preferred). Still, it provides broad-spectrum sun protection. We wish the base formula were at least a little exciting, but it isn't. The amount of alcohol and the lack of truly state-of-the-art ingredients make it a very disappointing eye cream or face cream. It does contain cosmetic pigments that impart a subtle brightening effect. The **P.M. Formula** is a basic emollient moisturizer suitable for dry skin anywhere on the face. There are some intriguing ingredients in this eye cream, but none of them are present in amounts worth getting excited about. In the end, this is just another lackluster antiwrinkle product from L'Oreal. It cannot repair deep wrinkles and neither product contains a significant amount of vitamin A. L'Oreal refers to it as Pro-Retinol A, but the actual name is retinyl palmitate, an antioxidant that shows up in hundreds of moisturizers and is hardly the only helpful ingredient for skin. See the Appendix to learn why, in truth, you don't need an eye cream.

☺ AVERAGE **Revitalift Deep-Set Wrinkle Repair Night Creme** *($19.99 for 1.7 fl. oz.)*. L'Oreal describes this moisturizer, packaged to have a medical look, as a luxurious cream, and in terms of texture, that's correct. If only silky emollients and thickening agents could thwart expression lines and deep, etched wrinkles! Because they can't, they are good only for temporarily smoothing dry skin; they can't enhance the skin's barrier or protect the skin from free-radical damage. So in this case you're left with an ordinary but decent moisturizer for dry to very dry skin, nothing more. What's particularly disappointing is the preponderance of fragrance ingredients; they're even listed before L'Oreal's touted Pro-Retinol A (retinyl palmitate), which is truly disappointing. Having met L'Oreal's spokesperson Andie McDowell, we can attest to how stunning she is, but it isn't because of L'Oreal, and especially not because of this product.

☺ AVERAGE **Revitalift Double Eye Lift** *($15.99 for 0.5 fl. oz.)* packages two products in one dual-chambered pump container. You're supposed to apply both products in sequence, because one is designed to reduce wrinkles while the other firms and lifts—an odd instruction given how many individually packaged L'Oreal moisturizers claim to do the same thing at once. Step 1 is the **Under Eye Anti-Wrinkle Cream**. This emollient, cushy moisturizer with a silky finish will improve the appearance of dry skin (and fine lines caused by it) under the eye. However, the only compelling antioxidant is retinyl palmitate (not retinol, as claimed), so this isn't as exciting as it could have been, though it is fragrance-free. Step 2 is the **Upper Eye Lifting Gel**, a mix of water, silicone, glycerin, thickener, film-forming agent, vitamin E, and the cell-communicating ingredient adenosine. This won't lift skin but it is a decent lightweight moisturizer. Combined, this duo is more impressive than what L'Oreal usually produces, but that isn't saying much. Of course, this won't "stop the signs of aging … for 40ish skin," or skin of any age.

☺ AVERAGE **Revitalift Face & Neck Day Cream** *($15.99 for 1.7 fl. oz.)* has some emollient properties and a silky texture suitable for normal to dry skin, but it's inappropriate for daytime use unless you pair it with a foundation rated SPF 15 or greater. The soy and vitamin A antioxidants won't last long once this jar-packaged product is opened, and the volatile fragrant components may cause irritation. It is very disappointing to see that fragrance ingredients such as amyl cinnamal and benzyl cinnamate are more prominent in this product than good-for-skin ingredients such as retinyl palmitate and soy protein, plus those won't remain stable for long once this jar-packaged moisturizer is opened.

☺ AVERAGE **Youth Code Day Lotion SPF 30** *($24.99 for 1.7 fl. oz.)*. If the claims for L'Oreal's Youth Code products and their GenActiv technology sound familiar, that's because Lancome (which L'Oreal owns) claimed almost the same thing in 2010 when they launched their Genifique products. Before we discuss the "breakthrough claims" and the technology behind this product, you need to know that this product is merely a lightweight daytime moisturizer with an in-part avobenzone sunscreen (the avobenzone is stabilized by octocrylene, which is great). L'Oreal got the critical UVA protection issue right this time, something they often leave out of their formulas here in the United States. Other than that, this product, which is best for normal to slightly dry or slightly oily skin, doesn't break any new ground. In fact, the overall formula is average when compared with the other options you'll find on our Best Moisturizers with Sunscreen list at the end of this book. The crux of Youth Code is the claim that it stimulates genes in your skin that supposedly are responsible for its regenerating power. It is absolutely true that there are genes in our skin responsible for generating proteins. These proteins create antioxidant pathways that protect skin from intrinsic (internal) and external signs of aging. As we age (actually, as we accumulate more sun damage from years of exposure), these genes become less able to "express" themselves in a healthy manner. That leads to oxidation within the skin and a decreased ability for the gene-generated proteins and enzymes to handle oxidative stress. The result of these deficiencies is damaged collagen, inflammation, and unwanted changes to skin texture, such as roughness, increased sensitivity, and, yes, wrinkles (Sources: *Planta Medica*, October 2008, pages 1548–1559; *Pigment Cell & Melanoma Research*, February 2008, pages 79–88; and *Free Radical Biology & Medicine*, August 2008, pages 385–395). L'Oreal's solution is a yeast ingredient known as bifida ferment lysate. The problem is that there's no research proving that this specific form of yeast has any anti-aging, regenerating, or gene-stimulating activity when applied to skin. You'd think that after 10 years of research, L'Oreal would publish their findings, but they haven't. Of course, there's also the issue that treating aging skin depends on more than a single ingredient or even one group of ingredients. Getting back to the bifida ferment lysate, there is limited research showing that yeast ferment filtrate (a compound different from bifida ferment lysate) reduces oxidative skin damage in the presence of UV light, but this research also showed that many other antioxidants have a similar effect (Sources: *Archives of Dermatological Research*, April 2008, pages S51–S56; and *Journal of Dermatological Science*, June 2006, pages 249–257). In the end, despite all the gene-stimulating and youth-regenerating claims, this isn't a must-have product for skin of any age, although the sunscreen is certainly capable of providing broad-spectrum protection.

☺ AVERAGE **Youth Code Day/Night Cream Moisturizer** *($24.99 for 1.7 fl. oz.)* is not a miracle formula, but in fact an average moisturizer for normal to slightly dry skin whose most intriguing ingredients will break down because of the jar packaging. See the Appendix to learn why jar packaging is a problem. L'Oreal maintains that Youth Code (just like Lancome's Genifique) took 10 years of research. Although that sounds impressive, what they came up with isn't in any way a breakthrough or worth considering over any of the moisturizers in our Best Products chapter. The crux of Youth Code is that the claim that it stimulates genes in your skin that supposedly are responsible for its regenerating power, which, as L'Oreal correctly states, slows with age and sun damage. It's critical to note that L'Oreal couches every cosmeceutical and drug-like claim for this product in cosmetic-lingo disclaimers. For example, they follow their statement "L'Oreal invents our first skincare that boosts the activity of genes" with a tiny footnote suggesting it just makes you look more youthful. So they aren't really saying anything about your genes, mainly because that would be a medical claim and would get them in trouble with the FDA. Outside of the bifida ferment lysate (discussed in the review for Youth Code Day Lotion SPF 30 above), you're getting a mix of silicones with alcohol, wax, and tiny amounts of a cell-communicating ingredient and a form of vitamin C. The rest of the formula is mostly preservatives, fragrance, and fragrance ingredients. The fragrance ingredients can cause irritation and inflammation on their own, which breaks down collagen and is counterproductive to the claims. Irritation will diminish any youth-giving qualities this formula has (which is to say, zero). The same is true for the amount of alcohol present, which is listed on the ingredient label before any of the teeny amounts of beneficial ingredients. See the Appendix to find out why alcohol is a problem for anyone who wants younger-looking, firmer skin.

☺ AVERAGE **Youth Code Serum Intense Daily Treatment** (*$24.99 for 1 fl. oz.*). Among all the Youth Code products, this serum has the most striking formulary similarity to Lancome's Genifique. Specifically, it is almost identical to their Genifique Youth Activating Concentrate, which costs three times as much as this Youth Code serum. Before we discuss the "breakthrough claims" and the technology behind this product, you need to know that it is not preferred to any of the serums on our Best Serums list. It contains some intriguing ingredients and has a silky-soft finish, but there are some problematic ingredients (such as alcohol and fragrant components) that make this a hindrance for aging skin. See the review above for Youth Code Day Lotion SPF 30 for a discussion of the gene-stimulating claims.

☺ AVERAGE **$$$ Age Perfect Hydra-Nutrition Golden Balm Eye** (*$19.99 for 0.5 fl. oz.*) has a lush, emollient texture that supplies dry skin with several restorative and smoothing ingredients. What's frustrating is that you don't need an eye cream and the most intriguing ingredient in this product won't remain stable for long because of the jar packaging. The formula contains some helpful antioxidants (and a much greater array of them than what L'Oreal typically includes), which makes the jar packaging even more disappointing. See the Appendix to learn more about the issues jar packaging presents and details on why you don't need an eye cream.

☹ POOR **Advanced Revitalift Complete Lotion SPF 15** (*$15.99 for 1.7 fl. oz.*) does not contain the UVA-protecting ingredients of titanium dioxide, zinc oxide, avobenzone, Tinosorb, or Mexoryl SX, and is not recommended. Because sun protection is a critical step in anti-aging skin care, this formula is far from advanced or complete!

☹ POOR **Age Perfect Anti-Sagging + Anti-Age Spot Hydrating Moisturizer Day Cream SPF 15** (*$15.99 for 2.5 fl. oz.*) is imperfect for skin of any age because it lacks active sunscreen agents that provide sufficient UVA protection. As you may have guessed, this is not the solution for sagging skin. It must be said that sagging skin is not an issue any skin-care products can fix, regardless of the claim or ingredients. Acknowledging this will save you a lot of time, money, and frustration (but see the Appendix to learn what you can do to help). If anything, the insufficient UVA protection in this product will make skin more prone to sagging, since sun damage is part of what causes this to happen. As for this product being a "New Menopause Innovation", that' 100% false, as nothing in this daytime moisturizer with sunscreen is unique or proven for women going through menopause nor is anything in here special for a women in her 50s. Age is not a skin type!

☹ POOR **Age Perfect for Mature Skin Hydra-Nutrition Advanced Skin Repair Daily Serum** *($19.99 for 1 fl. oz.)*. The claims for this anti-aging serum state what a well-formulated serum should do, to the extent possible, to improve signs of aging. Unfortunately, this isn't a well-formulated serum. It absolutely contains some great ingredients, including skin-smoothing silicones, soy protein, and some repairing ingredients. But it also lists alcohol as the third ingredient and contains numerous fragrance ingredients known to cause irritation. None of that is "age perfect" or "advanced," and it stops this serum from earning even a minor recommendation. Serums from Olay, Estee Lauder, Clinique, and Paula's Choice offer superior options whose formulas successfully address multiple signs of aging for all skin types. See the Appendix to learn why alcohol and a lot of fragrance aren't the least bit anti-aging.

☹ POOR **Age Perfect Hydra-Nutrition Golden Balm Face, Neck & Chest** *($19.99 for 1.7 fl. oz.)*. The concept behind this facial moisturizer for dry to very dry skin is "redensifying," which translates into making thinning skin look and feel thicker (more dense). Although this contains some ingredients that add moisture and antioxidants to stimulate healthy collagen production (which will make skin thicker to some extent), it also contains some problematic ingredients that work against this goal. Marjoram, orange peel, and the numerous fragrance ingredients in this moisturizer cause irritation that hurts skin's ability to heal and produce healthy collagen. Although marjoram is a natural source of the skin-lightening ingredient arbutin, it also contains volatile components that are known to cause inflammation, especially when used around the eyes. This inflammation is exacerbated by the other irritants, making this a moisturizer to avoid. The most intriguing ingredients in this moisturizer will not remain stable for long because of the jar packaging. See the Appendix for details on why jar packaging and excess fragrance are a problem. And, by the way, you don't need separate products for the neck and chest; there is no research anywhere showing these areas require different ingredients than facial skin.

☹ POOR **Collagen Moisture Filler Day Lotion SPF 15** *($11.49 for 2 fl. oz.)* lacks the UVA-protecting ingredients of titanium dioxide, zinc oxide, avobenzone (also known as butyl methoxydibenzoylmethane), ecamsule, or Tinosorb and is not recommended. The base formula also contains a concerning amount of alcohol, an ingredient that with continued use will break down, not restore, collagen. See the Appendix for further details on alcohol.

☹ POOR **Revitalift Complete Day Cream SPF 18** *($15.99 for 1.7 fl. oz.)* does not contain the UVA-protecting ingredients of titanium dioxide, zinc oxide, avobenzone, Tinosorb, or Mexoryl SX, and is not recommended. It is far from being a complete daytime option!

☹ POOR **Revitalift Deep-Set Wrinkle Repair SPF 15 Day Lotion** *($19.99 for 1.7 fl. oz.)* does not provide sufficient UVA protection, a topic L'Oreal is well aware of because they have a patent on a UVA-protecting ingredient. Not only are you putting your skin at risk of UVA damage (which causes wrinkles and sagging) if you choose this moisturizer as your only source of sun protection, but also the base formula contains enough alcohol to cause irritation and, potentially, free-radical damage. Sun-exposed skin needs free-radical protection, not an invitation for more damage. We could go on about other deficiencies of this formula, but let's just leave it with us stating that this isn't advanced, it won't do a thing to improve wrinkles, and it's a waste of money.

☹ POOR **Revitalift Double Lifting** *($15.99 for 1 fl. oz.)* can make skin feel tighter temporarily because of the amount of alcohol and absorbent magnesium sodium silicate it contains, but that's about drying up skin and causing irritation, which is actually wrinkle-inducing. There isn't much else to extol in this gel, and calling it advanced must be L'Oreal's idea of sarcasm.

L'OREAL PARIS SUN CARE

☺ GOOD **Sublime Bronze Pro Perfect Salon Airbrush Self-Tanning Mist, Medium Natural Tan** *($10.79 for 4.6 fl. oz.)* provides an alcohol-free formula that dries quickly and turns skin tan with dihydroxyacetone, the same ingredient in almost all self-tanners. The airbrush mist requires some practice, but once you get the hang of it this can be a quick, efficient way to apply self-tanner. This product is suitable for all skin types except sensitive. It contains fragrance ingredients known to cause irritation, so use it infrequently and avoid spraying it on your face.

☺ GOOD **Sublime Bronze ProPerfect Salon Airbrush Self-Tanning Mist** *($10.79 for 4.3 fl. oz.)* is similar to the Sublime Bronze Pro Perfect Salon Airbrush Self-Tanning Mist, Medium Natural Tan above, and the same comments apply.

☺ GOOD **Sublime Glow Daily Moisturizer, for Fair Skin Tones** *($11.07 for 8 fl. oz.)* is a lightweight moisturizer for normal to oily skin. The glow comes from the mica, while a relatively small amount of the self-tanning agent dihydroxyacetone provides a hint of tan color.

☺ GOOD **Sublime Glow Daily Moisturizer, for Medium Skin Tones** *($11.07 for 8 fl. oz.)* is nearly identical to the Sublime Glow Daily Moisturizer, for Fair Skin Tones, except this one contains more dihydroxyacetone. Otherwise, the same comments apply.

☺ GOOD **Sublime Bronze Self-Tanning Gelee, Deep, for Body** *($9.39 for 5 fl. oz.)* is nearly identical to the Sublime Bronze Self-Tanning Gelee, Medium-Deep for Body reviewed below, except this version contains more dihydroxyacetone for darker skin tones.

☺ GOOD **Sublime Bronze Self-Tanning Gelee, Medium-Deep, for Body** *($9.49 for 5 fl. oz.)* has a smooth, nearly weightless texture and thus is ideal for normal to oily, blemish-prone skin. The tan comes from dihydroxyacetone, while caramel coloring leaves a sheer tint. This can be used on the face, too!

☺ GOOD $$$ **Sublime Bronze Self-Tanning Towelettes, for Body, Medium** *($10.99 for 6 towelettes)*. Assuming you don't mind the added expense of self-tanning with disposable towelettes, these are a better option than the Sublime Bronze Self-Tanning Towelettes, for Face, Light-Medium (reviewed below). That's because they do not contain volatile fragrant components and so are much less likely to cause irritation.

☹ AVERAGE **Sublime Bronze Self-Tanning Lotion SPF 15, Deep** *($9.49 for 5 fl. oz.)* includes avobenzone for sufficient UVA protection, and is otherwise a fairly standard self-tanning lotion for normal to oily skin. The amount of alcohol poses a slight risk of irritation. Keep in mind you will need to apply this tanner liberally if it is going to be your only source of sun protection, which is why combining self-tanner (which should be applied sparingly) with sunscreen isn't the best idea.

☹ AVERAGE **Sublime Bronze Self-Tanning Lotion SPF 15, Medium Natural Tan** *($9.49 for 5 fl. oz.)* is nearly identical to the Sublime Bronze Self-Tanning Lotion SPF 15, Deep reviewed above, except this produces a lighter tan color.

☹ AVERAGE **Sublime Bronze Clear Self-Tanning Gel Medium Natural Tan** *($10.49 for 5 fl. oz.)* has a nearly weightless formula that turns skin tan from dihydroxyacetone, the ingredient used in almost every self-tanner sold. It's an option, but it comes with two caveats that make it less enticing than many other self-tanners. The first caveat is the amount of alcohol.

Most likely there's too little alcohol to cause problems for your skin, but given the number of alcohol-free self-tanners available, why take a chance? Also problematic are the numerous fragrance ingredients. Fragrance isn't skin care and a self-tanner doesn't need overpowering fragrance to work well.

☺ AVERAGE **Sublime Bronze, Gradual Self-Tanning Lotion** *($11.07 for 6.7 fl. oz.)* is an OK self-tanning lotion that would be better if it didn't contain alcohol and fragrance ingredients known to cause irritation. There are many other self-tanners that work gradually as this one does, but without the potentially troublesome ingredients.

☺ AVERAGE **Sublime Sun Advanced Sunscreen Hydra Lotion Spray, SPF 30** *($9.99 for 4.2 fl. oz.)*. A big problem with this spray-on sunscreen lotion is how forcefully it's propelled from the metal container. The lotion mist bursts with such force that it's tricky to apply this evenly to skin, not to mention it makes smooth floors slippery and can make carpets gummy with repeated use. It's great that this provides broad-spectrum sun protection and includes stabilized avobenzone for critical UVA (think anti-aging) screening, but application is an issue. This fragranced sunscreen contains a tiny amount of antioxidant grape extract, but it isn't advanced. Texture-wise, it leaves skin smooth and doesn't feel occlusive, but you may not like the somewhat greasy sheen it leaves, even after you blend really well. It's an OK option for normal to slightly dry skin.

☺ AVERAGE **Sublime Sun Advanced Sunscreen Hydra Lotion Spray, SPF 50** *($9.99 for 4.2 fl. oz.)* is nearly identical to the Sublmine Sun Advanced Hydra Lotion Spray, SPF 30 above except this contains a higher level of active ingredients necessary to reach SPF 50. Otherwise, the same review applies.

☺ AVERAGE **Sublime Sun Advanced Sunscreen, SPF 30** *($9.99 for 3 fl. oz.)* is a thin-textured lotion that provides broad-spectrum sun protection and includes stabilized avobenzone for reliable UVA (think anti-aging) screening. The water-resistant formula is silky and easy to apply, but in terms of the antioxidants L'Oreal boasts about on the label, they're barely present. It's great that this is fragrance-free and it doesn't have the thick, occlusive sunscreen feel many people (rightfully) dislike, but L'Oreal is a bit late to the game with this concept. Neutrogena did it first (and better) with their Ultra Sheer sunscreens.

☺ AVERAGE **Sublime Sun Advanced Sunscreen, SPF 50** *($10.99 for 3 fl. oz.)* is nearly identical to the Sublime Sun Advanced Sunscreen SPF 30 above, except for the higher amount of active ingredients needed to reach SPF 50. Otherwise, the same review applies.

☺ AVERAGE **Sublime Sun Advanced Sunscreen SPF 50+ Liquid Silk Sunshield for Face** *($10.99 for 1.7 fl. oz.)* is an exceptionally lightweight, silky fluid (actually, it's runny) facial sunscreen that provides broad-spectrum protection. Stabilized avobenzone provides reliable UVA protection and the formula sets to a nearly weightless finish that leaves a subtle sheen. The only issue barring a strong recommendation is the amount of alcohol the formula contains. It may be low enough that it's not cause for concern, but Neutrogena offers similar "fluid" sunscreens that are alcohol-free. This contains a tiny amount of grape extract and vitamin E (tocopherol) for a minor antioxidant boost, but not enough to qualify this formula for its "advanced" name. If you decide to try this fragrance-free sunscreen, it is best for oily or combination skin. It does not provide more than a touch of hydration.

☹ POOR **Sublime Bronze Luminous Bronzer Instant Action Self-Tanning Lotion** *($10.79 for 6.7 fl. oz.)* lists alcohol as the second ingredient, which makes it too drying and irritating for all skin types. See the Appendix for further details on alcohol in skin care.

☹ POOR **Sublime Bronze One Day Tinted Gel** *($10.79 for 6.78 fl. oz.)* isn't recommended, although we were really impressed at how well it went on and the sheer tan color it produced. Adding to our favorable impression was this bronzing gel's longevity and the fact that it didn't come off on clothing. The disappointments are that the formula lists alcohol as the third ingredient and contains several fragrance ingredients known to cause irritation that can be made worse when skin is exposed to sunlight. The alcohol can lead to dryness and incite free-radical damage, although without question it does help this bronzing gel dry quickly. Those looking for a quick tan without commitment should stick with the bronzing gels from Clinique or Bobbi Brown instead.

☹ POOR **Sublime Bronze Self-Tanning Towelettes, for Face, Light-Medium** *($10.99 for 6 towelettes)* may seem convenient, but these single-use cloths are an expensive way to self-tan! The cloths are steeped in a solution that contains the self-tanning agent dihydroxyacetone, but the number of volatile fragrant components (and the expense—six uses and you'll have to buy more) makes them not worth considering.

☹ POOR **Sublime Bronze Tinted Self-Tanning Lotion, Deep** *($10.79 for 5 fl. oz.)* isn't lotion-like at all. Instead, it's mostly water and alcohol, which lends a thin, gel-like texture. Like most self-tanning products, it turns skin brown with the ingredient dihydroxyacetone. This also contains caramel coloring for an instant sheer bronze tint. What it doesn't contain is any AHA ingredient as claimed! The amount of alcohol along with the high amount of fragrance makes this tough to recommend. See the Appendix to learn about the problems alcohol presents.

☹ POOR **Sublime Bronze Tinted Self-Tanning Lotion, Medium Natural Tan** *($10.79 for 5 fl. oz.)* is nearly identical to the Sublime Bronze Tinted Self-Tanning Lotion, Deep reviewed above and the same comments apply.

☹ POOR **Sublime Glow Moisturizing MicroFine Mist, for Medium Skin Tones** *($10.99 for 4.2 fl. oz.)* would be a slam-dunk for all skin types if it did not contain so many volatile fragrant components. The mist facilitates application, but other self-tanners offer this format without the risk of irritation. A great one to try instead is Banana Boat Summer Color Self-Tanning Mist, for All Skin Tones.

☹ POOR **Sublime Sun Advanced Sunscreen Crystal Clear Mist, SPF 30** *($10.99 for 4.2 fl. oz.)* provides broad-spectrum sun protection and includes stabilized avobenzone for critical UVA screening, but its base formula is mostly alcohol. See the Appendix to learn why alcohol is a problem in sunscreens, especially given the number of excellent options that omit this irritant.

☹ POOR **Sublime Sun Advanced Sunscreen Crystal Clear Mist, SPF 50** *($10.99 for 4.2 fl. oz.)* is nearly identical to the Sublime Sun Advanced Sunscreen Crystal Clear Mist SPF 30 above, save for a higher percentage of active ingredients required to reach SPF 50. Otherwise, the same review applies.

L'OREAL PARIS LIP CARE

✓☺ BEST **HiP Studio Secrets Professional Jelly Balm** *($9)*. Don't let the deep, dark colors fool you: This is a sheer, jelly-textured lip balm that smoothes over lips and feels decadently soft. The colors, while sheer, are still strong enough to wear on their own, or you can increase the intensity and add a patent-leather gloss shine to any lipstick. Either way, this is fantastic.

☹ POOR **Colour Riche Balm SPF 15** *($7.95)*. This tinted lip balm with sunscreen feels pleasantly light on your lips, yet delivers a surprisingly natural-looking pop of color. Unfortunately, this SPF-rated product does not provide adequate broad-spectrum protection and, therefore, can't be strongly recommended. See the Appendix to learn more about which sunscreen ingredients to look for in any SPF-rated product.

☹ POOR **Revitalift Collagen Lip Treatment Deep-Set Wrinkle Repair** *($19.99 for 0.4 fl. oz.).* L'Oreal is partly right with their statement that collagen and hydration are key to keeping lips looking young, but what they produced to address this need is abysmal. The **Lip Plumping Serum** contains lip-irritating menthol and coriander oil. The irritation that results from these ingredients causes collagen to break down, not increase. The tiny amount of the water-binding agent sodium hyaluronate isn't going to plump lips one bit, despite its association with certain lip fillers used by dermatologists. The Lip Plumping Serum is followed by the **Anti-Feathering Creme**, which is designed to keep lipstick from bleeding into lines around the mouth. The texture of this moisturizer works to temporarily fill in lines on the lips (just like most lip balms of this type), but it is too emollient to keep lipstick from traveling into lines around the mouth. Further, the small amount of collagen this contains isn't going to fuse with or shore up your lip's own collagen. You'd be better off getting collagen lip injections, although, yes, you're right, that's costly when compared with products like this—but wouldn't you rather put your money toward something that works?

L'OREAL PARIS SPECIALTY SKIN-CARE PRODUCTS

☺ AVERAGE **Youth Code Dark Spot Correcting & Illuminating Serum Corrector** *($24.99 for 1 fl. oz.)* contains two known skin-lightening ingredients, niacinamide and the vitamin C derivative ascorbyl glucoside. The problem is that other brands (including drugstore competitor Olay) did this sooner and did it better. L'Oreal's fragranced skin-lightening option doesn't bring anything new to the table, despite fancy packaging and the Youth Code name. The lightweight serum has some hydrating ability and the amount of niacinamide is impressive, but the formula also contains alcohol (the kind that causes irritation that keeps skin from being its healthy, youthful best). The amount of alcohol isn't high, but its inclusion before the vitamin C doesn't make this a must-have product. In addition to options from Olay, you'll find numerous other superior options for lightening dark spots on our Best Skin-Lightening Products list. If you decide to try this option, it is best for normal to oily skin. Note: The "10 years of gene research" claim on the box for this product sounds impressive, but what would really matter for your skin is a better formula!

L'OREAL PARIS FOUNDATIONS & PRIMERS

✓☺ BEST **True Match Super-Blendable Makeup SPF 17 Sunscreen** *($10.95)* is L'Oreal's best foundation for normal to very oily skin. It has a fluid, silky feel and blends superbly, setting to a natural matte, slightly powdery finish that is translucent enough to let your skin show through, while still providing light coverage that diffuses minor flaws and redness. The sunscreen is pure titanium dioxide, making this a gentle choice for skin (the formula is also fragrance-free). The palette of shades is not only one of the largest shade selections for a single drugstore foundation, but also one of the most neutral. Almost all the shades are excellent, and they cover a wide range of skin tones from porcelain to medium brown. Generally, the shades in the N (neutral) and W (warm) range are best. Those in the C (cool) range are hit-or-miss. The only drawback to this foundation is its drier finish. Although it does a good job of reducing oily shine and keeping skin looking polished, it tends to emphasize the slightest bit of dry skin, and can also make lines around the eye look more apparent. If you have dry areas or visible lines around the eye, it is imperative that you smooth and hydrate these areas before applying this foundation. An emollient moisturizer lightly applied around the eyes and regular use of an effective topical exfoliant should minimize this problem and make working with this foundation a better experience. All told, this is a must-try for those with normal to oily skin who don't need significant coverage and want a foundation that feels wonderfully light.

✓☺ BEST **Visible Lift Serum Absolute Advanced Age-Reversing Makeup SPF 17** *($12.48)* contains an in-part titanium dioxide sunscreen that provides reliable broad-spectrum protection. The so called skin-care ingredients amount to a mere dusting, and the small amount of vitamin C included (in the form of ascorbyl glucoside) will quickly degrade in this glass container unless you store it away from sunlight. Still, sun protection is the pinnacle of anti-aging skin care, so L'Oreal is on the right track. This slightly thick but soft-textured liquid foundation has a beautiful silkiness, exceptional blendability, and near-flawless medium coverage. Equally impressive is the neutral range of shades, although the darkest shades likely will suit only medium skin tones. Note that this foundation's finish will emphasize wrinkles if skin isn't prepped with a moisturizer or serum (you don't need a product labeled "foundation primer"). This foundation is best for normal to slightly oily skin. Someone with dry skin will find it doesn't supply nearly enough moisture.

☺ GOOD **Visible Lift Smooth Absolute Instant Age-Reversing Foundation SPF 17** *($15.95).* The only thing remotely "age-reversing" about this foundation is the built-in sunscreen, which has some benefit for improving healthy cell production, but primarily, like most sunscreens, protects against further sun damage. Keep in mind that such a benefit is hardly unique—it's true of any well-formulated sunscreen. Although the anti-aging claims for this product are exaggerated, the real headline for this liquid foundation is its performance, which is exceptional. It goes on evenly, blends seamlessly, and leaves a dewy finish that's soft and luminous, but not shiny. The formula is good for all skin types except oily. Most impressive is how completely skin-like this foundation looks, which is remarkable considering that the coverage is medium, but it can be built up to full coverage depending on how much you apply. The shades are similarly impressive, with eight mostly neutral options that run from fair to medium. The formula is tenacious, and lasts for hours without fading or turning orange. So, with all this praise, why didn't this foundation earn our top rating? The applicator. The attached synthetic-hair brush dispenses product by twisting the base. There's no way to remove the brush and there's also no way to reliably clean it (the packaging also advises against rinsing it), so you'll likely have a gunked-up brush within a couple of uses, which will mean streaky application. Although the foundation looks gorgeous when applied with a brush, the inability to clean it is hard to ignore. No matter how lovely this looks on your skin, it just isn't packaged in a way that's best for repeated applications.

☺ GOOD **Studio Secrets Professional Secret No. 1 Magic Perfecting Base** *($12.99 for 0.5 fl. oz.).* Thanks to the blend of silicones and a spackle-like texture, this light pink primer does a very good job of filling in pores and fine lines, while adding a matte, soft-focus finish to skin. The trick to keeping this from balling up is to pat the product into skin, and only where you need it. Foundations of all types smooth on nicely over top, and those with oilier skin will appreciate that the absorbents in this primer help to control oil throughout the day. As well as this performs on the skin, the jar packaging poses noteworthy problems. Primarily, it's difficult to get the right amount of product out of the small jar. Squeeze tube packaging would've made this a Best Product.

☺ AVERAGE **Infallible Advanced Never Fail Makeup SPF 20** *($14.29)* is one of the few L'Oreal foundations to feature a titanium dioxide–based sunscreen for broad-spectrum protection and it feels nearly weightless. It blends on with an undeniably silky texture. The major con is once set, the soft matte finish feels tacky and slightly uncomfortable. It lasts and lasts, but we doubt many women would want to keep this on the face for more than a few hours. Coverage-wise, this goes from light to moderate, and layering for enhanced coverage requires deft blending. The other negative issue with this foundation is that the pump applicator leaks so there's a steady stream of foundation dribbling down the side of the pump top. Very frustrating, and a constant mess. If you decide to throw caution to the wind and give this a go, it's best for those with normal to very oily skin who are seeking a long-wearing matte finish and need substantial coverage, even at the expense of looking made-up. By the way, not only do the vitamins and minerals not fight signs of facial fatigue (as L'Oreal claims), but also the amount of them in this foundation is inconsequential for providing skin with any level of benefit.

☺ AVERAGE **Infallible Never Fail Powder SPF 20** *($14.29)* is said to provide 16 hours of flawless, versatile coverage, but that is the epitome of over-promising. This compact pressed powder does indeed do a good job of controlling shine, but 16 hours just isn't possible unless you never touch your face, don't have any problem with oil, and never use a phone or hug someone. This powder foundation works better dry than wet. Dry it's a reliable, sheer powder that provides a soft matte finish to the skin. When applied wet it goes on heavy and has a cakey appearance on the skin. The included latex sponge is handy for application on the go, but you'll get a finer and more professional application with a powder brush. The number of available shades is small, but the sheerness of this powder means that most skin tones will be able to find a workable option. The SPF 20 is nice, but don't rely on this as your sole source of SPF protection because it doesn't contain sufficient UVA-protecting ingredients.

☺ AVERAGE **Magic Smooth Soufflé Makeup** *($15.95)* has a soufflé-like texture that smoothes away pores and fine lines, although only temporarily. While it does work this "magic" to a certain extent, it fails to deliver adequate coverage, and it doesn't do anything different than other foundations or primers on our Best list. Anyone looking to address anything beyond very minor imperfections will find this too sheer. Adding more to build up coverage backfires, causing it to ball up or begin to accentuate fine lines and large pores instead of concealing them. Marketed as working best with L'Oreal's Magic Perfecting Base Primer (which doesn't extend or enhance this foundation's application or wear), it leaves a soft matte finish that those with oily skin will appreciate most. In fact, this foundation's finish is so mattifying, it likely will make even slightly dry skin look worse.

☺ AVERAGE **True Match Super-Blendable Compact Makeup SPF 17 Sunscreen, Oil-Free** *($10.99)* has a creamy texture that blends easily into the skin. The included latex sponge is excellent for application of this cream-to-powder foundation. Once blended, this foundation sets to a soft matte finish that leaves skin looking more natural than made up. The creaminess of the formulation makes it best for those with normal to dry skin not prone to blemishes. True Match's large shade range is impressive and includes options for fair to dark skin tones. Despite these accolades, this doesn't provide sufficient UVA protection, which keeps it from getting a better rating and means you will need to use another product with it during the day for complete SPF protection. See the Appendix to learn which sunscreen ingredients provide the optimum UVA protection essential for anti-aging benefits.

☺ AVERAGE **Visible Lift Serum Inside Line Minimizing Makeup SPF 17 Normal to Dry Skin** *($12.29)* is still without the UVA-protecting ingredients of titanium dioxide, zinc oxide, avobenzone, Tinosorb, or Mexoryl SX. Therefore, it is not recommended for sun protection. As for the touted pro-xylane and hyaluronic acid, forget about it. Those ingredients are barely present and have no lifting effect on skin, visible or not. This foundation has a great name but is without a formula to support its most tempting claims. On the plus side, it does have a silky texture that melds with the skin and dries to a soft matte finish. You'll get light to medium coverage and, despite the fact that the target market for this is women with dry skin, the minimally moist formula is best for normal to oily skin. Out of the shades offered, watch out for those with obvious undertones of pink and peach.

☺ AVERAGE $$$ **Studio Secrets Professional Color-Correcting Primers** *($12.99)*. This series of primers is designed to offset dullness and/or redness, but these thin-textured color correctors can't really address the cause of the problem (in fact, given the amount of alcohol they contain, they could make matters worse), and the strange mix of colors doesn't correct anything. Don't count on any increased longevity to your foundation, and you'll have to correct the noticeable correcting green or pink undertones with even more powder or foundation. Note that the Light and Medium Anti-Dull shades both contain shimmer.

☺ AVERAGE $$$ **True Match Roller Perfecting Roll On Makeup SPF 25** *($14.95)*. Perhaps if your face were shaped like a living room, this roll-on foundation would work, but for most of us, this application method is neither adequate nor practical for addressing the many contours of the face, or large pores, for that matter! Furthermore, it's unlikely that the flimsy plastic applicator that comes in the compact will hold up to daily use. Also inadequate is the UVA sun protection offered by this cream-to-powder foundation, which will leave your skin vulnerable to sun damage unless you pair it with a well-formulated sunscreen. To make matters worse, the waxes in this foundation have the potential to clog pores. Should your curiosity get the best of you, here's what you can expect from this roller foundation: Full, buildable coverage that's best for normal to oily skin; a soft, matte finish; and a shade range that is neutral.

L'OREAL PARIS CONCEALERS

✓☺ BEST **True Match Concealer** *($8.95)* comes with a brush applicator (rather than the standard sponge tip), and is truly a beautiful liquid concealer thanks to its smooth, even-blending texture that feels ultra-light, yet provides fairly good coverage. It sets to a natural matte finish and does not crease, though the coverage isn't opaque enough to hide prominent dark circles. There are several shades offered, most of which are ideal neutral options for fair to medium skin tones.

✓☺ BEST **Visible Lift Serum Age-Reversing Concealer SPF 20** *($12.95)*. We're always excited when we see a mineral-based sunscreen included in concealers, because adequate broad-spectrum sun protection is essential for anti-aging benefit, and most cosmetics companies leave this crucial aspect of skin care out of eye-area products. Sun protection alone, however, does not make a great concealer, so fortunately this one also has a blendable texture, click pen–style packaging, and a tapered synthetic-hair brush applicator that works like a charm. Though there's nothing in this fragrance-free concealer that's going to visibly lift your skin, the thin liquid texture will provide lasting medium coverage of dark circles or discolorations. The shades are impressively neutral and suited for fair to medium skin tones.

☺ GOOD **Infallible 16-Hour Concealer** *($10.28)* won't really last for 16 hours without minor signs of fading or creasing (when applied to the under-eye area), but it is still a formidable stick concealer with a slightly creamy texture that doesn't have too much slip. It provides good coverage and sets to a soft powder finish that does a good job of staying in place and comes in a variety of flattering shades. This type of concealer is not recommended for use over blemishes because of the wax-like thickening agents necessary to keep it in stick form.

☺ **Magic Lumi Concealer** *($12.95)* earns its name for the subtle hint of shimmer that it imparts within the medium coverage concealer. The "lumi" effect is really understated, but it does give just a hint of luminescent glow, which, combined with the satin finish, is particularly attractive around the eye area. The liquid formula is dispensed through the click pen, which makes application a breeze. This won't be an ideal concealer for those who need a matte finish or who need to disguise acne blemishes, but it's worth a try for others.

☺ GOOD **True Match Naturale Gentle Mineral Concealer SPF 25** *($11.99)* contains 20% titanium dioxide as an active ingredient, which means this loose-powder concealer definitely provides significant sun protection, assuming you apply it evenly and liberally. Surprisingly, this has a beautiful, soft texture that doesn't look thick or chalky on skin. When applied with the cap-attached synthetic brush, you'll get smooth, medium coverage and a satin-matte finish that leaves a soft sheen. The finish feels dry but doesn't look that way on skin. Although someone with oily skin won't like the finish this powder concealer provides, it is a gentle option to use around the eyes if you don't have lines or dry skin in that area, or for concealing minor redness. The shades are flattering and neutral, but note that they go on lighter than they appear in the jar.

L'OREAL PARIS POWDERS

✓☺ BEST **Translucide Naturally Luminous Powder** *($11.79)* is a talc-free loose powder with a marvelous, powdered-sugar texture and a smooth, even finish. It feels like silk on the skin and leaves a subtle radiant finish. The amount of vitamin C this contains is negligible, and the packaging isn't the type to keep it stable anyway. The sheer shades are excellent. This fragranced powder is perfect for those with normal to dry skin.

✓☺ BEST **True Match Naturale Soft-Focus Mineral Finish** *($15.25)* is a talc-free loose powder available in translucent shades, each imparting a luminous glow that softens imperfections. The mineral part comes from the sodium-calcium-magnesium silicate base, and it lends this sheer finishing powder a soft, nearly weightless texture that perfects without looking dry or flat. This does a great job of making skin look better without making it look made-up, and the color works for most fair to medium skin tones. The built-in brush applicator, though stubby, is better than average. This could be used for evening makeup or for touching up instead of using regular powder.

✓☺ BEST **True Match Super-Blendable Powder** *($10.95)* has the distinction of offering the largest palette of shades available at the drugstore. That is to the advantage of almost all skin tones, because this is an outstanding, talc-based pressed powder. Its texture is exquisite and this is a bona-fide beauty bargain. True Match Super-Blendable Powder is suitable for all skin types, though its finish isn't as absorbent as many with oily skin will need. Still, it never looks flat or dry and in fact gives skin a natural, polished finish. Highly recommended!

☹ AVERAGE **Visible Lift Serum Absolute Advanced Age-Reversing Powder** *($12.99)*. First things first: this pressed powder is not anti-aging in the least and it absolutely does not give skin a "visible lift." It is also not "age-reversing"; no product is, but that claim would be better qualified if this fragrance-free powder at least contained a sunscreen, which it doesn't. Although this powder has a smooth, creamy texture, the talc-free formula requires deft blending to avoid looking heavy and a bit chalky on skin. Its satin finish is best for normal to dry skin, but beware that the finish can magnify dry areas if they are not sufficiently prepped with a moisturizer (or moisturizing foundation). A good anti-aging pressed powder wouldn't settle

---

🍸 Did you know alcohol in skin-care products is a big problem? See the Appendix to learn more.

into lines around the eyes yet this one does, unless you apply a very sheer layer with a brush. Unfortunately, a sheer layer isn't enough to tone down shine and set makeup, which is the main purpose of pressed powder. Turning to the shades, the range goes from Fair to Deep, but all the colors go on lighter than they appear, so the Deep shade is really best for medium to slightly tan skin tones. The anti-aging ingredients mentioned in the description for this powder likely refer to the vitamins and minerals this contains, but none of these ingredients will remain stable in a product like this because they're exposed to light and air each time you open the compact to apply.

☺ AVERAGE **Visible Lift Serum Inside Line-Minimizing Powder SPF 12** *($14.49)* lacks the UVA-protecting ingredients of titanium dioxide, zinc oxide, avobenzone, Mexoryl SX (ecamsule), or Tinosorb, which on the part of L'Oreal is just nonsense, because they absolutely know about the issue of UVA protection (in fact, they have a patent on one of the UVA-protecting ingredients). The talc-based formula glides over skin and provides a seamless, translucent finish that won't make skin look over-powdered and doesn't quickly sink into pronounced wrinkles (though no powder is impervious to eventually magnifying, rather than downplaying, wrinkles). All the shades are soft and neutral, too, which makes the insufficient sunscreen all the more disappointing.

L'OREAL PARIS BLUSHES & BRONZER

✓☺ BEST **True Match Super-Blendable Blush** *($10.95)* is a collection of silky powder blushes whose sheer colors and seamless application do indeed make them super-blendable. The palette of soft colors is beautiful and is divided into warm, cool, and neutral tones. You might find their blush groupings confusing (some of the cool shades go on more golden or peach than befits that description), but if you shop by the color itself rather than by its classification you should be satisfied. Aside from those details, this is one of the better powder blushes at the drugstore. (Note: Each shade has a subtle shine, but it gives a soft glow to the cheeks, not distracting sparkles.)

✓☺ BEST **Glam Bronze Bronzing Powder** *($12.99)* presents three shades of talc-based pressed bronzing powder. Two have a soft, radiant shine that isn't distracting, while Enchanting Sunrise is ultra-sparkly. Regardless of which shade you choose, this applies evenly and deposits soft color, though it would be nice if the shades leaned more toward tan to bronze rather than peach to copper. You may want to use this as a blush rather than a bronzer, especially if you have fair to light skin.

✓☺ BEST **Magic Smooth Soufflé Blush** *($12.95)*. This mousse-textured cream-to-powder blush smoothes on easily and blends seamlessly. The color is initially soft, but layers well for those looking to build intensity. This blush works best over clean skin or liquid foundation; those who wear powder foundation may find it appears somewhat dry. The four muted shades, all of which include luminous shimmer, lack staying power and likely will require an afternoon touch-up.

☺ AVERAGE **The One Sweep Sculpting Blush Duo** *($12.95)*. Consisting of two shades of matte and shimmer-finish powder in one pan, this duo aims to add blush and contour to cheeks in one sweep. The "one-sweep" concept comes in the form of a clever V-shaped brush that picks up a bit of each shade of powder and hugs the cheekbones nicely when applying. Although the blush color and contour do go on evenly to create a well-blended line, the powder doesn't adhere well to the brush or to skin, and it lacks enough pigment to make this truly a one-step product. What a shame, because the time-saving concept is appealing.

L'OREAL PARIS EYESHADOWS & PRIMERS

✓☺ BEST **Infallible 24 HR Eye Shadow** *($7.95)*. This cream-to-powder eyeshadow glides smoothly across skin and is easy to blend out for a smokey effect. If applied with a light hand it goes on sheer, but you can kick up the color intensity by patting it on or applying more layers. The shade range includes a mix of trendy and classic colors in luminescent shimmer and matte finishes (which are easy to identify). Better yet, it doesn't crease or fade, and it is water-resistant.

✓☺ BEST **Studio Secrets Professional Eye Shadow Singles** *($4.48)* earns accolades for its well-rounded collection of shades, smooth texture, and ability to transform from sheer to rich color by layering. The silky powder texture applies evenly and isn't the least bit "dusty." Both matte and shimmer options are available, and the shimmer does not flake, which is a major plus. Job well done, L'Oreal—and now the "secret" is out!

✓☺ BEST **HiP Studio Secrets Professional Matte Shadow Duo** *($9.99)* comes in a small collection of colors that are marketed as being complementary, but are, at best, a striking contrast. That's too bad because the slim color selection and odd combinations (green and blue together?) are the biggest disappointment here, as these shadows have a soft, dry texture with strong pigmentation. Even better, they blend well (which softens the colors nicely), and they have the stamina to last all day. Like so many other products that claim to be matte, these, too, have some subtle sparkles, but nevertheless they are very close to being matte and can possibly flatter most skin textures of the eyelid and crease area.

✓☺ BEST **HiP Studio Secrets Professional Concentrated Shadow Duo** *($7.99)* has contrasting, sometimes shocking, colors as its biggest drawback. Most of the duos have more to do with creating colorful eye designs rather than artfully shaded eyes. Application-wise, these are very smooth, so blending is effortless. They have a silky texture and moderate pigment saturation (which means that even the darkest shades may need to be layered for more intensity). Every duo has at least one shiny shade, but it clings well.

✓☺ BEST **Studio Secrets Professional Color Smokes Eye Shadow** *($5.99)*. Typically, shimmery powder eyeshadows crease throughout the day, causing eyes to look tired and older. That is not the case with these eyeshadow quads. These pressed-powder eyeshadows have a silky texture, exceptional blendability, and impressively deep pigments, which means you don't need a lot of shadow to create a gorgeous eye design, and using less helps to prevent creasing. Depending on your taste, you may find that the shades lean too much toward shimmer because each and every shade does have some degree of shine—ranging from a soft frost to flecks of glitter, and, unfortunately, the larger-flecked shadows did flake a bit. So, if you have wrinkles on your lids, they will be more noticeable. Each palette contains a generous size of at least two workable shades.

☺ AVERAGE **De-Crease Eye Shadow Base** *($8.48)* has its purpose, but doesn't replace a long-wearing, matte-finish concealer, which is essentially how this product works. It's a powdery liquid that comes in a single, pale peach-toned shade. You'll get light coverage and a solid matte finish suitable for powder eyeshadow application. The talc-based formula keeps lids matte, but again, so does a matte-finish concealer, and unlike De-Crease, your matte-finish concealer works elsewhere (such as under the eyes), too.

☺ AVERAGE **HiP Studio Secrets Professional Shocking Shadow Pigments** *($12)* come packaged in a tiny jar (with a sifter to keep things tidy) and include a small but workable eyeshadow brush for application. The colors and intense shine are way too magnified and noticeable (and not in a good way), making this best for evening makeup when you really want strong shine; in daylight it looks way too obvious and overdone. This would be rated higher if the shine had better cling; the texture is supremely smooth.

☺ AVERAGE **HiP Studio Secrets Professional Bright Eye Shadow Duo** (*$7.99*) features very colorful, bright combinations, all of which are difficult to work with if your goal is a natural eye design. These are options if you want bold colors that draw attention to themselves rather than to your eyes.

☺ AVERAGE **HiP Studio Secrets Professional Metallic Shadow Duo** (*$7.99*) has a smooth but dry powder texture that blends decently, but tends to flake during application, at least if you use more than a sheer amount. Knowing most women will go for this eyeshadow for its color payoff, which requires more product than you'd think, avoiding the flaking becomes quite the feat. The finish is more iridescent than metallic, and most of the duos are contrasting, which doesn't lend itself to the best look unless you use only one of the colors with another eyeshadow in a complementary shade.

☺ AVERAGE **Studio Secrets Professional Eye Shadow Duo** (*$5.18*) comes with instructions on the back of the compact to show where to apply each shade for a professional eye design. The pairs are composed mostly of neutral shades that work well together; most sets come with at least one matte shade and one shimmer. Although the colors are commendable, the dry, pressed-powder texture has a tendency to flake as you apply it, but it stays just fine once blended. Also, the colors go on too sheer, and in some cases must be layered for more intensity. Overall, this is just a so-so eyeshadow duo, so why bother?

☺ AVERAGE **Studio Secrets Professional Eye Shadow Quad** (*$7.15*) has the same set of pros and cons as the Studio Secrets Professional Eye Shadow Duo above, only here you get four shades in a larger compact. Otherwise, the same review applies.

☹ POOR **HiP Studio Secrets Professional The One Sweep Eye Shadow** (*$9.95*). This single flip-top container has three strips of eyeshadows arranged exactly as they would look on the eye: a neutral color for the lid, a deeper hue for the crease and a dark shade for lining. But even if they are arranged perfectly in their package, applying an entire eye design with "one sweep" just doesn't work. An all-in-one eye compact designed this way is a convenient idea, in theory, but it's impossible to use in practice. First, there's just no way to use the large curved applicator (or any applicator for that matter) to accurately apply color to three different areas of the eye at once. Every time we tried we ended up with a messy lid area that blended into one blah shade. Even with professional-size brushes, this product proved tricky to use because the strips of shadow are too narrow (and oddly wavy) to be used without transferring color from one to the other. Ultimately, this product is more frustration than it's worth, especially when you consider the waxen texture and the poor color pickup, regardless of the applicator.

L'OREAL PARIS EYE & BROW LINERS

✓☺ BEST **HiP Studio Secrets Professional Color Truth Cream Eyeliner** (*$10.19*) is a long-wearing gel eyeliner that competes favorably with those from department-store lines. It has a soft, cream-gel texture that must be applied with a brush. A mini, angled eyeliner brush is included and is workable, but most consumers will want something more elegant or capable of drawing a thinner line. Performance-wise, this applies smoothly and sets quickly to an immovable finish. Oddly, color saturation isn't as strong as for other HiP products, so you may need to layer to get more dramatic results. Still, this wears without smearing, and requires an oil- or silicone-based remover. The shades give you the option of creating a classic or trendy look.

✓☺ BEST **Lineur Intense Felt Tip Liquid Eyeliner** *($6.50)* has a felt-tip applicator that makes applying liquid eyeliner easy, and the formula dries quickly and has amazing tenacity, not to mention a resistance to smudging, smearing, or flaking.

✓☺ BEST **Voluminous Mistake-Proof Marker Eyeliner** *($7.29)* has an applicator that delivers an even, steady flow of liquid color. It works quite well, and allows better precision than you'll get from a standard, thin liquid eyeliner brush. The versatility of the slanted tip is supposed to let you draw a thin or thick line, but we couldn't get the line as thin as L'Oreal's illustration, regardless of how we held the tip or how much pressure we applied (or didn't apply, which we also tried). Still, unless you insist on a thin line, this eyeliner is definitely recommended. Application is easier than most, the formula dries quickly and doesn't smear or flake, and it removes with a water-soluble cleanser.

☺ GOOD **HiP Studio Secrets Professional Color Truth Eyeliner** *($8.79)*. This eyeliner pencil needs routine sharpening, but that's the only drawback that keeps this from earning a Best Product rating. It applies easily without skipping and the silicone-enhanced formula sets quickly to a smudgeproof powder finish.

☺ GOOD **Pencil Perfect Self-Advancing Eyeliner** *($8.48)*. This soft, creamy eyeliner goes on smooth and blends well, but it lacks the superior staying power of similarly priced long-wearing eyeliners that are also available at the drugstore. The twist-up tip is convenient, but it doesn't retract so be sure you don't expose more of the tip than is needed to draw the type of line you desire.

☺ GOOD **Telescopic Precision Liquid Eyeliner Waterproof** *($9.49)* is outfitted with the same excellent slanted-tip brush as the original version (reviewed below), and that makes it relatively easy to draw an even line following the curvature of the eye. The formula dries quickly, and once it sets, does not budge—not for water, not for tears, or for any other liquid, except makeup remover. That means you've got a truly waterproof eyeliner, but it also means that if you make a mistake, you've got to start all over (blending is not an option). Another deciding factor is that, although it lacks shimmer, this eyeliner dries to a noticeably glossy finish. That said, this is not for novice liquid eyeliner users, but if you've got a skilled hand and like the drama of a liquid liner, this is most definitely worth a try.

☺ AVERAGE **Brow Stylist Professional 3-in-1 Brow Tool** *($9.95)* offers a brow pencil, brow brush, and a mini pair of tweezers in one. The design is quite clever, and many will find the additions useful rather than gimmicky. As for the brow pencil itself, application is sheer, even, and builds well (for more intensity) without clumping. However, because the pencil is oil-based, it is prone to smearing and fading, with fading being the more obvious problem.

☺ AVERAGE **Double Extend Eye Illuminator Eyeliner** *($8.95)* is a dual-ended pencil eyeliner; one side is a traditional dark eyeliner, the other end is an ivory-toned liner meant to brighten the inside corner of the eye. This effect can be striking in photos, but in-person it can appear like you've been overzealous with the concealer, and it's gunked up in the corner of your eyes. The eyeliner itself is creamy, blends well, and sets to a soft matte finish with noticeable flecks of shimmer. The shades are designed to coordinate with your eye color, but that technique went out with the typewriter. Matching detracts from your natural eye color rather than enhancing it.

☺ AVERAGE **HiP Studio Secrets Professional Kohl Eyeliner** *($13)*. The fine point on these kohl eyeliners makes precise application a cinch. The powder texture also makes them easily blendable, and they work wonderfully to create the ever-popular smokey eye design.

Unfortunately, unless used sparingly, the powdery nature of these liners means they flake around the eye area during application, and then need to be cleaned up carefully to avoid smearing and leaving unflattering dark circles around the eye. If you can avoid this mess, and are interested in trying a kohl liner, this may be worth your while. Each of the available shades has some shimmer, making these best reserved for evening wear.

☺ AVERAGE **Le Kohl Smooth Defining Eyeliner** ($8.48) is a standard, needs-sharpening pencil. It applies smoothly without being greasy and stays in place quite well. The shade selection has been edited down to just the classics, and all of them have merit.

☺ AVERAGE **Le Kohl Duo Shadow + Liner Smooth Defining Pencil + Powder Eye Shadow** ($10.95) is a dual-sided pencil that includes a standard needs-sharpening eyeliner on one end and a pointed sponge tip on the other. The cap for the sponge-tip portion of the pencil houses a tiny disc of powder eyeshadow. Every time you replace the cap, more powder eyeshadow is deposited onto the sponge. Both sides are easy to apply and come in a range of well-coordinated colors. The pencil has a slight tendency to smudge and fade, but this is primarily a problem for those struggling with oily eyelids (in which case one of the long-wearing gel eyeliners is a much better choice). This would be rated better if not for the fact that the pencil portion needs routine sharpening.

☺ AVERAGE **MicroLinerUltra Fine Lining Pencil** ($8.79) is a needs-sharpening pencil that promises "the precision of a liquid liner." The advantage of this pencil is its slender tip that allows for a thin, discrete line, or you can build the line for more drama. Because this stays creamy, some smudging is apparent by day's end (much sooner if you have oily eyelids), but it is an option if you prefer pencil and want a very fine line.

☺ AVERAGE **Telescopic Precision Liquid Eyeliner** ($9.48) is outfitted with an excellent slanted-tip brush that makes it relatively easy to draw an even line following the curvature of the eye. The formula takes a bit longer to dry than usual, which can encourage smearing, but what's most disappointing is the color saturation runs out before you've made it to the end of the lash line, necessitating another application. This stays in place and wears quite well once set, but demands more patience than most other liquid eyeliners.

☺ AVERAGE **Wear Infinite Soft Powder Eye Liner** ($8.48) is a standard pencil with a swift, smooth application and a reliable powder finish. If you prefer pencils and don't mind routine sharpening, this is one to consider because it is less likely to smudge or fade than many others.

☹ POOR **Infallible Never Fail 16HR Eyeliner** ($8.48). Eyeliner that lasts for 16 hours is a big claim, and we wish that this one lived up to it, but we experienced smudging and smearing before lunchtime (less than 4 hours). The retractable cream pencil goes on rich and smooth, but requires a lot of effort to blend out softly (the included rubber smudger was more awkward than helpful). Most disappointing, of course, is the limited staying power, especially its tendency to run when your eyes are even slightly watery.

☹ POOR **Lineur Intense Brush Tip Liquid Eyeliner** ($8.48) is a surprisingly bad liquid liner. The main problem is the stiff brush that tends to splay and deposit color unevenly. The formula dries quickly, but remains smear-prone longer than it should, which is reason enough to leave this on the shelf.

L'OREAL PARIS LIP COLOR & LIPLINERS

✓☺ BEST **Colour Riche Lip Gloss** ($8.95) has a silky yet moisturizing texture that imparts sheer to medium color (depending on the shade) and leaves lips with a glossy finish free of stickiness. The shades are bound to please—and don't be nervous about trying the deeper hues; each goes on softer than it appears.

✓☺ BEST **HiP Studio Secrets Professional Shine Struck Liquid Lipcolor** *($12)* is an outstanding product to consider if you want the opacity of a traditional lipstick and the finish of a standard lip gloss. This cake-scented liquid lip color is applied with a traditional wand applicator, feels great, and its pigmentation ensures above-average longevity, though you may want to retouch once the emollient feel wears away. It lacks even a hint of stickiness and has a thinner, non-goopy texture that still feels moisturizing. The shade selection offers a nice mix of nude pinks and riveting reds.

✓☺ BEST **Intensely Moisturizing Lipcolor** *($10)* has a luscious, creamy texture and fully saturated colors. This has a slight tendency to bleed into lines around the mouth, but is otherwise recommended for fans of creamy lipsticks with a plush, moist finish. The shade selection is beautiful, especially if you favor bold colors.

✓☺ BEST **Colour Riche Le Gloss** *($7.95)* differs from the Colour Riche Lip Gloss above. It strikes the perfect balance of smooth texture and lasting moisture with gorgeous color and shine. The squeeze-tube, slanted-tip applicator allows you to easily control the amount of this lightly scented, thick-textured (but not at all tacky) gloss you deposit on your lips. The shiny finish left behind is understated, so those looking for strong mirror-like shine will want to look elsewhere. The large shade selection contains colors that are neither too bright nor too sheer, imparting a wash of color that's true to what you see on the packaging.

✓☺ BEST **Infallible Never Fail Lipliner** *($8.99)* is a very good automatic, retractable lip pencil. The base of the pencil's component houses a built-in sharpener for those who want a finer point before lining. The pencil glides on and imparts rich, lasting color, obviously dependent on what your lips are doing. The color selection is versatile enough that most women will find a workable shade.

☺ GOOD **Colour Juice Sheer Juicy Lip Gloss** *($8.48)* is a fragranced tube lip gloss that comes in a dazzling array of shades. As glosses go this is nothing exceptional, but the deeper shades impart longer-lasting color and the formula provides a minimally sticky, wet-look finish that leaves lips feeling moist rather than slippery.

☺ GOOD **Colour Riche Anti-Feathering Lipliner** *($8.48)* is a standard, twist-up, retractable pencil with a built-in sharpener. The sharpener part isn't really necessary given the finer point that most twist-up pencils like this one already have; plus, after one use the shavings clog the sharpener and that's that. Application is smooth and creamy, and the available colors are versatile. This does a great job of preventing lipstick from feathering into lines around the mouth!

☺ GOOD **Colour Riche Nurturing and Protective Lipcolour** *($8.95)* is rich in every way except price, which is a boon for you and your lips! This decadently creamy lipstick offers intense colors that have admirable staying power, although it is creamy enough to slip into lines around the mouth. In terms of being nurturing and protective, it is no more so than many other creamy lipsticks.

☺ GOOD **Endless Comfortable 8-Hour Lipcolour** *($9.99)* feels remarkably light and has a minimally creamy finish, yet imparts intense color that really lasts, although not for eight hours. You'll need to touch up after coffee breaks or eating (this isn't a transfer-resistant formula), but for the most part this leaves standard creamy lipsticks behind in the longevity department. With such an extensive shade range, you are bound to find a color that suits you.

☺ GOOD **Infallible Le Rouge** *($9.99)*. This long-wearing cream lipstick claims to provide 10 hours of wear, but doesn't quite hit that mark. You can potentially get through lunch before it starts to wear off and travel into the edges of your lips. It also won't feather into lines around the mouth.

☺ GOOD **Infallible Never Fail Lipstick** *($12.09).* 16-hour wear from a lipstick is a big deal, and this two-step option from L'Oreal almost reaches that goal (as long as you aren't eating anything particularly greasy). As expected, there are some caveats and trade-offs along the way. You begin by applying the lipstick to clean, dry, flake-free lips (any sign of dryness will be magnified, so be sure lips are ultra-smooth), allow it to set for one minute, and then apply the balm-style topcoat stick. The second step is a must if you want comfortable wear—the lip color makes lips feel incredibly dry as it sets, but that's part of the transfer-resistant process. Because the top coat is wax-based and less glossy than top coats on other long-wearing lip products, it tends to be more tenacious, so you use it less often to touch up—at least that's the theory. In reality, you really need to layer and reapply the top coat to keep lips feeling smooth and comfortable during the day. Once that's done Infallible Never Fail Lipstick wears and wears, with only minimal issues of color "beading" if you wait too long to touch up. L'Oreal's range of shades is impressive, favoring pinks and reds. The Zippo lighter-style packaging is a sleek way to combine both products, and is small enough to fit into any evening bag.

☺ AVERAGE **Colour Riche Anti-Aging Serum Lipstick** *($9.99)* is a very fragrant lipstick that includes a clear or tinted (depending on the shade) moisture core that supposedly contains an anti-aging serum composed of collagen and L'Oreal's sugar ingredient pro-xylane. The sticker on the side of this creamy lipstick advises users that they may feel a slight tingling sensation, and the first several minutes you have this on, that is indeed the case. Perusing the ingredient list, we saw nothing obvious that would cause the tingling we felt or that would prompt L'Oreal to issue that cautionary statement. This lipstick is oil–based and greasy enough to slip into lines around the mouth, but it's only unique ingredient is argan oil, and the formula contains only a tiny amount of it. We suspect the tingling came from the fragrance ingredients that are present, or simply from the amount of fragrance itself. In either case, the tingling is a sign that your lips are being irritated, and in no way is this lipstick head and shoulders above many other cream lipsticks. One more thing: The ingredient list does not include collagen or xylane, but that's OK because they have no anti-aging effect on lips anyway.

☺ AVERAGE **Infallible Le Gloss 8HR** *($9.99)* does last longer than a standard lip gloss, albeit not without some caveats. The look of the gloss is opaque, with flecks of shimmer throughout. The fragranced formula does have a markedly thick, sticky texture, resulting in an application that doesn't glide on smoothly. Because it's unusually viscous, it takes extra effort to move around your lips using the hollow, heart-shaped sponge applicator. While it does leave a glossy high-shine finish, it also can feel heavy on your lips, and it easily sticks to food (now that's appetizing!), long hair, and cups. As mentioned, this outlasts standard lip glosses, but at the expense of feeling uncomfortable on lips. It's your call as to whether the extra wear is worth the aesthetic and application trade-offs.

☺ AVERAGE **Infallible Never Fail Lipcolour** *($11.99)* is another lip paint/topcoat duo, although this one is packaged to resemble a Zippo lighter. The problem right off the bat is that although the base color applies sheer, it goes on unevenly, which was especially an issue with the darker shades. Application of the lighter, paler colors was better. The **Lipcolour** is, as expected, a bit drying and the color wears off unevenly, although a sheer wash of color did adhere to my lips throughout the day while eating and drinking. Reapplication of the top coat solved dryness issues, but it had to be reapplied several times during the day. Also, while the top coat is moisturizing and has a nice sheen, if you want a glossier finish for evening, you'll be disappointed with this.

L'OREAL PARIS MASCARAS

✓☺ BEST **Double Extend with Lash Boosting Serum Mascara** *($12.99)* is a two-step process that involves applying a primer followed by regular mascara. The point of difference here is pure marketing caprice. L'Oreal maintains that they've added a special lash-boosting serum to this product and it's supposed to make lashes stronger, thicker, and fuller. You'll get thicker, fuller lashes simply by applying the mascara portion of this product; however, not a single ingredient in either the primer or mascara has any effect on lash growth or natural (meaning without any mascara) thickness. The implication is that this is a unique way to boost lash appearance without resorting to a costly prescription drug, such as Allergan's Latisse, but this dual-sided product works nothing like Latisse. Although the claims are misleading (which is irksome), this mascara is another stellar option from L'Oreal. When you apply the primer followed by mascara, you'll get clean, smooth length and decent thickness without a clump or flake in sight. The mascara applied alone produces even better results, especially if your goal is lusciously thick, dramatic lashes. Note that applying the mascara without the primer results in some minor clumping, but it's easy to smooth out with the full-bristled brush. The high rating is for this product's performance as mascara, not because the lash-boosting serum actually works or because the claims tied to it have any validity.

✓☺ BEST **Double Extend Lash Fortifier & Extender Mascara** *($10.99)* is a dual-ended mascara, including a lash "Fortifier" (primer) on one end and mascara on the other. The Lash Fortifier is just clear mascara, adding extra layers that you can't really see. It's no different from adding extra layers of the black mascara on the other end of the tube, so it's a relatively unnecessary step because this mascara does magnificently well on its own, building incredible length and thickness without clumps or flakes.

✓☺ BEST **Telescopic Explosion Mascara** *($9.49)*. You may be put off by the odd shape of this mascara's applicator. Rather than a traditional, conical brush, it offers a round "Flexi-Globe" brush that looks like a medieval torture device. The Flexi-Globe applicator has spiky bristles of varying lengths and density protruding from it, and, if you can get past its scary appearance, the result is intensely thick, long lashes. After a few quick, but careful, strokes, lashes could be mistaken for falsies. This mascara can go on very heavy if you don't use restraint, but it smoothes out easily with a lash comb. It is definitely worth considering if you want to create lush, dramatic lashes quickly. As for wear, this stays on beautifully without smudging or flaking.

✓☺ BEST **Voluminous Full Definition Volume Building Mascara** *($7.29)* excels at creating long, softly fringed, and separated lashes with some thickness. It keeps lashes soft yet wears all day without smudging or flaking, and comes off easily with a water-soluble cleanser.

✓☺ BEST **Voluminous Naturale Natural-Looking Volume & Definition Mascara** *($7.29)* has a rubber-bristled brush applicator that produces prodigious length and clean definition with just a few strokes. Building thickness takes some effort, but can be done, and without leaving lashes looking heavy or spiky. True to claim, this is 100% clump-free. It stays on quite well, and removes easily with a water-soluble cleanser. Compared with L'Oreal's original Voluminous Mascara, this version provides greater thickness, but otherwise is very similar, save for the different brushes.

☺ GOOD **Double Extend Beauty Tubes Lash Extension Effect Mascara** *($10.95)*. This two-step mascara involves the typical white, wax-based primer followed by mascara. The point of difference is that the mascara forms tubes around each lash, but other than easy removal you won't gain any performance difference by choosing this concept over a traditional mascara formula. If anything, the tubes (which really do come off with water and slight agitation) can stick to your skin during the rinsing process. That's not a deal-breaker, but something to be aware of if you decide to try this mascara. Overall, the primer adds bulk and separation to lashes while the mascara extends lashes to an impressive length.

☺ GOOD **Double Extend Lash Fortifier & Extender Mascara Waterproof** *($10.99)* is a dual-ended mascara with a lash primer/conditioner on one end and mascara on the other. You apply the white "Extender" first and then sweep on the mascara. Supposedly, this pairing should bring about "lush lashes up to 60% longer," but what ends up happening is that the results with the Extender, though assuredly impressive, are the same as applying two or three coats of the mascara alone, which is exactly what we did. When we asked if the lashes on one eyelid looked longer, thicker, and more dramatic than the other, no one could tell a difference. Both the Extender and the mascara are waterproof and resistant to smudging or smearing.

☺ GOOD **Extra-Volume Collagen Mascara** *($7.95)*. Let us state from the start, just so there are no false notions about this mascara: The amount of collagen this contains is so tiny that even if it could have an impact, there isn't enough for even a minute segment of eyelashes to notice. However, collagen has nothing to do with hair growth or thickness. Collagen is a support structure in skin; it isn't related to the hair. What does plump lashes is the combination of this mascara's brush and the waxes in the formula, just like every other mascara on the market. You'll get lots of length and enhanced volume without clumps, plus near-perfect lash separation with minimal effort. This isn't much for significant thickness, but it leaves lashes softly curled and wears without flaking or smearing.

☺ GOOD **Extra-Volume Collagen Waterproof Mascara** *($7.95)* is waterproof as claimed and, after several coats, builds remarkable length and some thickness. There's a bit of clumping along the way and it smears easily while applying, so be extra careful. Otherwise, it's another good mascara from L'Oreal. As for the collagen, it is a minor part of the formula, but in any amount, collagen isn't going to plump lashes from the inside out, no more than a moisturizer with collagen will fill wrinkles.

☺ GOOD **Telescopic Mascara** *($9.48)* amounts to dramatically long, thick lashes. It uses a multi-sided comb (rather than brush) applicator and its biggest problem is immediate clumping and a too-heavy appearance. Luckily, the flipside of the comb allows for smoothing things out, but it still takes patience (and perhaps a separate lash comb or brush) to get all the clumps combed through. Although this mascara does not apply in a wink, it wears beautifully all day and keeps lashes soft.

☺ GOOD **True Match Naturale Mineral-Enriched Mascara** *($9.95)*. The only mineral of note included here is silica, which appears in countless other mascaras, including some of L'Oreal's that make no mention of being "mineral." Nevertheless, this soft-bristled mascara performs well, adding a moderate amount of length and volume (but without a lot of drama), and comes off easily with makeup remover.

☺ GOOD **Voluminous False Fiber Lashes** *($8.95)* promises long, lush lashes that deliver the same wow factor you would get with false lashes, but don't get your hopes up just yet! While it's true that you can build respectable thickness and length with this mascara, the results aren't even close to resembling false lashes. Nonetheless, this is a good, flake-free, smudge-free mascara that applies with minimal clumping. This wears well and removes easily. As for the "fiber" part of the name, this doesn't contain visible flecks of "fibers" that attach and add bulk to lashes, which is a good thing as fibers can flake off and get in your eye.

☺ GOOD **Voluminous False Fiber Lashes Waterproof** *($8.95)* is similar to the Voluminous False Fiber Lashes above, except this version is waterproof and requires an oil- or silicone-based makeup remover.

☺ GOOD **Voluminous Million Lashes Defining Volume Mascara** *($8.95)* gives lashes a clean, defined look while adding length. The large, rubbery applicator meticulously coats lashes for a clump-free and smudge-proof performance. However, if you are aiming to build thickness, you'll need to apply additional coats, and you may experience flaking as a result. The flaking is minor and not enough to keep this from earning a Good rating, but it is something to be aware of should you wish to go for all-out drama with this formidable mascara.

☺ GOOD **Voluminous Million Lashes Waterproof** *($8.95)* performs almost identically to its non-waterproof predecessor above, with the exception of its waterproofing claim, which it certainly lives up to! You will definitely need a separate eye-makeup remover to make a dent in this tenacious formula. Shower, swim, or sweat—it barely budges!

☺ GOOD **Voluminous Original Volume Building Mascara** *($7.29)* remains a superior lengthening mascara, but falters when it comes to creating noticeably thick, lush lashes. It doesn't clump or smear, however, and it does hold up beautifully throughout the day, making it a good choice if you're not expecting dramatic results as claimed.

☺ AVERAGE **Telescopic Mascara Clean Definition** *($10.59)* has a name that contradicts its uneven, too wet application that tends to stick lashes together for a look that says, "I just got out of the pool and need to take a shower." You can make lashes quite long with only minimal clumping, and the wetter formula allows darker emphasis at lash roots, which can help a bit if you can avoid smearing. With lots of effort, results from this mascara are attractive. However, lots of mascaras do all this without so much work.

☺ AVERAGE **Telescopic Explosion Waterproof Mascara** *($7.99)* is quite impressive, but this waterproof version doesn't come close to matching the performance of the original. The "spiky ball" (rather than a brush) applicator on the end affords a lot of control when applying, especially to outer and inner corner lashes. But this waterproof formula doesn't give the length, fullness, or drama of the original; it merely makes lashes look average.

☺ AVERAGE **Voluminous Waterproof Mascara** *($7.29)* won't knock your socks off with prodigious length and thickness, but it does a respectable job in both departments. The main reason to choose this is for its clump-free application and strong waterproof properties.

☹ POOR **Double Extend Eye Illuminator** *($10.95).* This dual-ended mascara is marketed as a way to play up your eye color with an illuminating topcoat that goes over a black base coat. Although the fast-drying base coat does add appreciable length and slight thickening, the sparkling top coat with a spiky ball applicator isn't the best. Each color features different shades of sparkle, but the effect is minimal compared to the risk of glitter flaking into your eye.

☹ POOR **Lash Boosting Serum** *($14.95 for 0.18 fl. oz.)* has zero effect on lash growth or thickness. This is one of those "are they kidding?" products, but sadly, the joke is on the consumer who falls for the claims. This isn't an affordable mass-market version of Latisse, the prescription lash growth product patented by Allergan. It's not remotely close to that FDA-approved proven product, although it's supposed to be applied in the same manner and the implication is all about keeping the lashes you have and enhancing their growth. The main ingredients in this dubiously named specialty product are water, alcohol, slip agent, thickener, and preservative. The amount of panthenol and amino acids (what L'Oreal touts as being able to reinforce and protect each lash) are incapable of protecting a single eyelash, and even in greater amounts these standard ingredients have no impact on the growth and shedding cycle of eyelashes, not to mention that the second ingredient is alcohol, which doesn't grow anything and is drying for lashes overall. Do not purchase this product; it is a waste of time and money.

L'OREAL PARIS FACE & BODY ILLUMINATORS

☺ GOOD **Glam Bronze All-Over Loose Powder Highlighter** *($12.99)* is a mostly impressive loose powder with shine. Designed for use on face or body, the color goes on quite different from how it looks in the jar container. You get a sheer, rosy bronze tone with a striking gold shimmer with hints of copper. The color works for most skin tones and the shine clings better than expected (loose powders with shine generally have poor cling ability). It's worth auditioning if you prefer your shine to be dusted on in powder form. Note: This contains a tiny amount of fragrance ingredients that pose a slight risk of causing irritation.

☺ GOOD **Magic Lumi Light Infusing Primer** *($12.95).* Used sparingly and strategically, this thin-textured luminizer could work as a highlighter to illuminate cheekbones or the Cupid's bow. But applied as a primer to the whole face or worn alone (as the packaging suggests), the pearlescent whitening effect will have you looking less luminous and more ghostly pale. This is similar to Lancome's Eclat Miracle Serum of Light, and remember, L'Oreal owns Lancome (and Maybelline, and Giorgio Armani Cosmetics, and Kiehl's and on and on).

L'OREAL PARIS SPECIALTY MAKEUP PRODUCTS

☺ GOOD **Clean Artiste Makeup Corrector Pen** *($10.95).* Think of this as a makeup remover in pen form and you'll have an idea of how it works. The slanted tip dispenses a mild solution capable of removing minor makeup mistakes such as flaking mascara or a too-heavy application of eyeliner. It is best for corrections in small areas—this isn't a cost-efficient or time-friendly way to remove a full face of makeup or even your eye makeup; it's just for minor repairs! The drawback is that it takes a fair amount of pressure to get this to remove eyeliner mistakes, and pressure isn't what you want in the eye area. Although this works for its intended purpose, you can get even better results with less pressure simply by dipping a cotton swab in your usual makeup remover. Consider this pen as a handy option to keep in your purse for on-the-go makeup fixes.

LA MER

Strengths: Effective cleansers (though less expensive options are available from other Lauder-owned lines); mostly good foundations; supremely good powders; the makeup brushes.

Weaknesses: Outlandish, almost mythical claims; ultra-pricey; several products contain irritants, including eucalyptus oil and lime; no AHA or BHA products; an incomplete makeup selection; one of the foundations with sunscreen does not provide sufficient UVA protection.

For more information and reviews of the latest La Mer products, visit CosmeticsCop.com.

LA MER CLEANSERS

☺ GOOD **$$$ The Cleansing Foam** *($65 for 4.2 fl. oz.)* is a foaming, water-soluble cleanser for normal to oily or normal to slightly dry skin, and it does remove makeup swiftly. The gemstones do not have a brightening effect on skin, although that's the claim you're paying dearly for; all you're getting is an ordinary cleanser.

✦ Lavender oil smells great, but fragrance isn't skin care! Find out why in the Appendix.

☺ GOOD $$$ **The Cleansing Gel** *($65 for 6.7 fl. oz.)* is an exceptionally standard, detergent-based, water-soluble cleanser that would be an option for normal to oily skin.

☺ GOOD $$$ **The Cleansing Lotion** *($65 for 6.7 fl. oz.)* supposedly derives its remarkable cleansing powers from magnetized tourmaline and declustered water, but there is no proof such water makes a cleanser any better. This is a standard, wipe-off cleanser for dry skin that is not all that different from Neutrogena's Extra Gentle Cleanser.

☺ AVERAGE $$$ **The Cleansing Fluid** *($65 for 6.7 fl. oz.)* removes makeup quickly due to its emollient ingredients. However, they're standard to most cleansing lotions and creams for dry skin, while the "extras" in this version (such as tourmaline and pearl powder) have no established benefit for skin.

LA MER TONERS

☺ AVERAGE $$$ **The Hydrating Infusion** *($95 for 4.2 fl. oz.)* has a lightweight, fluid gel texture that resembles a moisturizer but feels more like a toner; however, given that La Mer doesn't give it a typical name designation you're left guessing. But, based on the directions, which tell you to use it after cleansing and before your moisturizer, you might as well think of it as a toner hybrid. Supposedly, this is another product designed to "enhance" the fabled, near-miraculous benefits of the original Creme de la Mer, but you have to wonder: If that cream was so superior on its own, why does La Mer continue to offer product after (expensive) product to allegedly make it work better? If it's so brilliant on its own, it shouldn't need any enhancement, especially not from products that are essentially watered-down versions of the original. Aside from a potentially irritating amount of lime extract, The Hydrating Infusion is actually chock-full of seaweed-based water-binding agents and plenty of antioxidants and cell-communicating ingredients. Many of the state-of-the-art ingredients in this product are also present in products from other Lauder-owned lines, none of which have the elite price point of La Mer. The major difference between this product and other La Mer products is that they contain declustered water, gemstones, and "hydrating ferments" (whatever those are—you could describe raw sewage the same way) that La Mer claims makes them high-potency treatments. Regardless of what La Mer asserts—the Lauder company asserts myriad miraculous claims about all their products—there is no published research to support La Mer's claims. As a consumer, you're left to decide if you want to go along with the hype or bypass it in favor of less expensive options that are also well formulated. Those still considering The Hydrating Infusion should know it is best for normal to oily skin; but again, the amount of lime extract is cause for concern, especially if your skin is sensitive.

☺ AVERAGE **The Tonic** *($65 for 6.7 fl. oz.)* is an alcohol-free toner for normal to dry skin and is standard fare. It contains a minimal amount of ingredients that are beneficial for skin.

☹ POOR **The Brightening Lotion Intense** *($80 for 6.7 fl. oz.)* contains antioxidants and skin-repairing ingredients and includes vitamin C (in the form of ascorbyl glucoside) to improve skin discolorations. Unfortunately, it all turns ugly because this contains a high amount of eucalyptus oil, which can be irritating for skin (and irritation is always a problem for the health of the skin). Another concern is the fact that it also contains a generous dousing of fragrance, and fragrance is never skin care (see the Appendix to find out why). None of this is brightening; it's just irritating and overpriced.

☹ POOR **The Lifting Intensifier** *($155 for 0.5 fl. oz.)* is mostly water and alcohol with tiny amounts of plant extracts and a slip agent. The algae and gemstones are barely present, and do not have any miraculous benefits for aging skin. This product is not recommended.

☹ POOR **The Oil Absorbing Tonic** *($65 for 6.7 fl. oz.)* contains algae extract. Supposedly, the algae extract La Mer includes not only can turn back time, mend wrinkles, and heal skin, but also can reduce excess oil production for those struggling with acne. There is no research showing that algae can affect oil production. Oil production is controlled by hormones, and regular skin care products can't affect hormone production. The first ingredient is squalane, a good emollient for dry skin but a problem for oily skin. The acrylates (think hairspray) and salts have some oil-absorbing properties, but the other emollients get in the way of that. None of this will help keep oily skin matte. It contains lime and eucalyptol (also known as eucalyptus), both of which irritate skin, and as a result may stimulate oil production directly in the pore. In the end, there isn't a valid reason to try this toner; it's bound to make combination skin worse.

☹ POOR **The Radiant Infusion** *($95 for 4.2 fl. oz.)* comes with fascinating claims describing its "radical, fluid architecture" that delivers "extraordinary activity on demand," all to set in motion a "continuous wave of radiance-enhancing benefits." Quite honestly, you'd get more radiance from a brisk jog around the block than from applying this toner-like product. Considering the price, it's disheartening (and not the least bit helpful for skin) that the second ingredient is alcohol. Several of the plant extracts have benefit as water-binding agents and/or antioxidants, but the lime extract can be irritating, and nothing in this product will noticeably change skin discolorations. This should be renamed The Radiant Impediment.

LA MER MOISTURIZERS (DAYTIME & NIGHTTIME), EYE CREAMS, & SERUMS

☺ AVERAGE $$$ **The SPF 30 UV Protecting Fluid** *($70 for 1.4 fl. oz.)* is a good, though exceedingly overpriced, daytime moisturizer with sunscreen for normal to slightly dry or slightly oily skin. It has a lightweight, silky texture and contains plenty of zinc oxide for UVA protection. Although it does contain some interesting water-binding agents, antioxidants make up only a minor part of the formula, and for the price tag this carries, they should be more prominent.

☹ POOR **Creme De La Mer** *($140 for 1 fl. oz.)* is the original product created by aerospace physicist Max Huber, as described in the brand summary for La Mer on CosmeticsCop.com. As enticing as this dramatic story sounds, the reality is that this very basic cream doesn't contain anything particularly extraordinary or unique, unless you want to believe that seaweed extract (sort of like seaweed tea) can in some way heal burns and scars, but there is no research to support that claim. Even if it could, burns and scars don't have much to do with wrinkling, and this product is now being sold as a wrinkle cream. According to Susan Brawley, professor of plant biology at the University of Maine, "Seaweed extract isn't a rare, exotic, or expensive ingredient. Seaweed extract is readily available and [is] used in everything from cosmetics to food products and medical applications." So why then is this product so expensive? The price really is shocking considering that Creme de la Mer contains mostly seaweed extract, mineral oil, Vaseline, glycerin, wax-like thickening agents, lime extract, plant oils, plant seeds, minerals, vitamins, more thickeners, and preservatives. This rather standard moisturizer also contains some good antioxidants, but the jar packaging won't keep them stable during use. This also contains a skin-stressing amount of eucalyptus oil, as well as Kathon CG, a preservative blend that is recommended for use only in rinse-off products. Consumers who have a "steadfast devotion" to this product are not only wasting their money, but also hurting their skin. A good moisturizer doesn't need to cost a fortune or come in fancy packaging with legions of hype to really work.

☹ POOR **The Brightening Essence Intense** *($260 for 1 fl. oz.)*. Although the price for this product is nauseating and the claims completely ludicrous, the formula itself does have an impressive array of antioxidants and skin-repairing ingredients. None of them are miracles or unique to La Mer but the blend is definitely noteworthy. It even contains Lauder's signature use of ascorbyl glucoside (a form of vitamin C) to improve skin discolorations (La Mer is owned by Estee Lauder). Unfortunately, all this praise is for naught because eucalyptus oil is high up on the ingredient list. This fragrant oil is irritating for skin and irritation is always a problem for skin's health. Another concern is the fact that it also contains a dousing of fragrance and fragrance is never skin care (see the Appendix to find out why). One unique aspect of this product is that it contains declustered water. Trying to explain declustered water is phenomenally complex, but it is basically involves changing the molecular structure of water to a single molecule so it is more readily absorbed by cells. There is much passion about this kind of water being a miracle for the body so of course why not the skin, too? Despite the ballyhoo, there is an utter lack of research showing declustered water has any benefit whether applied topically or taken orally. websites often mention the fact that there are Nobel Prize laureates who did research on declustered water, but that wasn't about health or skin care, it was just brilliant research. Even more to the point, this synthetic water (or water of any kind) isn't the answer for skin care because the skin doesn't need more water! Instead, it needs ingredients to help skin maintain its own water balance. Moreover, if the declustered water were indeed capable of carrying skin-care ingredients into the skin in this case that would only make matters worse because you don't need the perfume and other irritating fragrant ingredients absorbing deeper into the skin.

☹ POOR **The Brightening Infusion Intense** *($95 for 4.2 fl. oz.)* contains an impressive array of antioxidants and skin-repairing ingredients. None of them are miracles or unique to La Mer but the blend is definitely noteworthy. Unfortunately, it all goes to waste because alcohol is the second ingredient. What a shame. Alcohol causes free-radical damage, irritation, dryness, and hurts the skin's ability to heal, definitely not something you want from a skin-care product (see the Appendix to find out more about alcohol on skin). This also contains fragrance, but not as much as other products from La Mer.

☹ POOR **The Concentrate** *($275 for 1 fl. oz.)* is, first and foremost, not worth even a fraction of its price. All you're getting is a nonaqueous product containing mostly silicones, seaweed extract, glycerin, film-forming agents, and several plant extracts, some of which (lime, lavender, and basil extracts, and also eucalyptus oil) are irritating to skin. The formula is rounded out by trace amounts of minerals and some additional plant extracts, but none of these, and definitely not in the amounts used here, are particularly helpful for skin, be it wrinkled or not. Seaweed (also known as algae) extract has antioxidant and anti-inflammatory properties, but it is not the magical elixir of youth La Mer makes it out to be, nor is it expensive to include in skin-care products. Bulk liquid seaweed extract costs an average of $1.50 per liter, and the amount used in this product barely amounts to a teaspoon, despite being the second ingredient listed. Like all silicone-based serums, this product will leave skin feeling incredibly smooth and silky. But knowing you can achieve this same feeling with other products that cost $250 less than La Mer's version (and that still have beneficial antioxidants) is a sobering fact, to say the least! The eucalyptus oil makes this too irritating for all skin types, and overall this serum pales in comparison to those from other Lauder-owned lines, all of which cost considerably less.

☹ POOR **The Eye Balm Intense** *($165 for 0.5 fl. oz.)*. La Mer is asking you to believe (recall that La Mer is all about believing in miracles) that the company's many ferments and its proprietary silver-tipped applicator tool are supposed to work wonders on puffy eyes, wrinkles, and uneven skin tone (think dark circles). All these claims are made for dozens of eye creams, including almost all those sold by the Estee Lauder Companies, of which La Mer is one. Regrettably, the only thing intense about this eye cream is its price. Because it's packaged in a jar, all the various "ferments," plant extracts, and the like will begin to break down the moment you open it. Jars also are unsanitary because you're dipping your fingers into them with each use, adding bacteria, which further deteriorates the beneficial ingredients. If those facts and the price aren't enough to dissuade you, consider that this eye cream also contains eucalyptus oil, which is one of the most irritating fragrant oils (Sources: *Basic and Clinical Pharmacology and Toxicology*, June 2006, pages 575–581; and naturaldatabase.com). What any potent irritant does to skin is create problems, especially in a product meant for use in the eye area. Irritation can result in collagen breakdown that will make other signs of aging more apparent anywhere on the face. The best ingredients in The Eye Balm Intense are found in lots of other moisturizers that not only cost less, but also don't expose your skin to aging irritation. See the Appendix to find out why, in truth, you don't need an eye cream.

☹ POOR **The Eye Concentrate** *($165 for 0.5 fl. oz.)* contains some incredibly helpful, state-of-the-art ingredients for creating and maintaining healthy skin. What a shame so many of them are subject to reduced potency because of jar packaging (see the Appendix for details)! Moreover, how depressing that La Mer included a troubling amount of eucalyptus oil, which only serves to irritate skin. Talk about a real burn for your money!

☹ POOR **The Moisturizing Gel Cream** *($265 for 2 fl. oz.)* is simply a lighter version of the original Creme De La Mer, and promotes a silkier finish due to the silicone it contains. Despite a light texture, this contains a lot of lime extract and enough eucalyptus to be more irritating than miraculously healing, as claimed. It is steadfastly not recommended.

☹ POOR **The Moisturizing Lotion** *($220 for 1.7 fl. oz.)* would have been a good moisturizer for normal to dry skin, but for the inclusion of lime and eucalyptus extracts, which are potentially irritating and sensitizing for all skin types. See the Appendix to learn how irritation hurts skin and makes signs of aging worse.

☹ POOR **The Oil Absorbing Lotion** *($220 for 1.7 fl. oz.)* is the lotion version of the original Creme de la Mer, and it does have a much lighter texture. However, the emollients and the lack of absorbents in this product won't keep oily skin in check. That's forgivable, but the inclusion of a significant amount of eucalyptus oil and lime is not. See the Appendix to learn how irritation hurts skin and makes signs of aging worse.

☹ POOR **The Radiant Serum** *($260 for 1 fl. oz.)* has a lot in common with other serums sold by Estee Lauder–owned brands (La Mer is owned by Estee Lauder). The difference, beyond La Mer's eyebrow-raising prices, is that there are less expensive yet similar serums that have superior formulas. This is chiefly because the superior serums omit the alcohol that is present in La Mer's The Radiant Serum, thus sparing your skin all of its potentially damaging effects (see the Appendix for more details). This water-based serum contains a very good range of plant-based antioxidants, and lesser, but still potentially helpful, amounts of skin-repairing and cell-communicating ingredients. These are the hallmarks of a great anti-aging serum, but the alcohol (coupled with this serum's price) is a deal you shouldn't get involved in. As for the claims that this serum transforms how your skin reflects light, it's all marketing wordplay. In reality, this serum's hydrating ingredients create a smooth surface that will change the way light reflects off your skin, just as any well-formulated moisturizer that costs far less will.

☹ POOR **The Regenerating Serum** *($260 for 1 fl. oz.)* seems to have taken an everything-but-the-kitchen-sink approach and then decided what the heck; let's throw in the sink, too! A cocktail approach of beneficial ingredients is definitely considered essential in any skin-care product making any claim, from moisturizing to antiwrinkle or, in this case, to regenerating. But is there a point of overkill? This serum from La Mer has one of the longest ingredient lists we've ever seen—more than 90 ingredients, including lots of fragrance and green dye! Obviously, only so much of any one ingredient can be present given that the 90 ingredients must add up to 100% of the product, and water is the largest amount of the formulation. Nonetheless, while this serum does have a silky texture and La Mer's fabled algae broth (which has never been proven to work in any regard for skin in any condition) along with several antioxidants, skin-identical ingredients, and some peptides and niacin thrown in for good measure, it isn't outstanding, especially not in comparison to less expensive Lauder products from Clinique or the Estee Lauder line itself. Many of the best ingredients in this La Mer serum show up in those other products, which have far less overwhelming price tags. Even more significant is that the best of the Clinique or Lauder versions leave out the problematic ingredients that this La Mer version contains. Shockingly, this serum is loaded with skin irritants, including lime peel extract, eucalyptus oil, and fragrant plant extracts. Irritation is always bad for skin, doing just the opposite of what you want it to do, including hurting your skin's ability to heal, causing collagen to break down, and killing skin cells.

LA MER LIP CARE

☹ POOR **The Lip Balm** *($50 for 0.32 fl. oz.)* ranks as one of the most expensive lip balms sold, and the first ingredient is Vaseline. Amazing! The seaweed and plant seeds may make this seem like more than it is, but the amount of eucalyptus oil is not lip-friendly, and it also contains the menthol derivative menthyl PCA. See the Appendix to find out how irritation hurts skin (and lips).

LA MER FOUNDATIONS

☺ GOOD $$$ **The Treatment Fluid Foundation SPF 15** *($85)*. It's a good thing this water- and silicone-based liquid foundation contains an in-part titanium dioxide sunscreen, because that's the least you should expect at this price! This has a fluid, moist texture that goes on slightly silky and sets to a satin finish replete with a glow-y shine. Although the coverage is light, this somehow doesn't look as natural on skin as it should. We've seen more natural-looking foundations from L'Oreal and Maybelline, just to give you an idea of how out of whack this foundation's price is. If you're determined to try it, you'll be pleased to know that most of the shades are impressively neutral. The Natural and Beige shades are slightly peach to peach and should be considered carefully. Consider Linen and Sand carefully, too, because they may be too yellow for some light skin tones.

☺ GOOD $$$ **The Treatment Powder Foundation SPF 15** *($95)* is a talc- and silicone-based pressed-powder foundation that includes an in-part titanium dioxide sunscreen. For the money, it doesn't rise to the top of the list of powder foundations. It's silky sheer, application feels great, and it leaves a soft, slightly dry matte finish. Coverage goes from sheer to medium, as is true for most powder foundations. La Mer's shade range excludes those with dark skin tones, but there are plenty of neutral options for light to medium skin tones. The claims about what this foundation can do for your skin are beyond exaggerated, but there's no denying it is one more good powder foundation to consider. It is best for normal to slightly dry skin.

☹ POOR **The SPF 18 Fluid Tint** *($70 for 1.7 fl. oz.)* doesn't have the same array of skin-beneficial ingredients as The Treatment Fluid Foundation SPF 15 reviewed above, nor does its sunscreen offer sufficient UVA protection. For the money, that's a real burn, and although there are some textural benefits to extol, they're not enough to make this worth considering over the tinted moisturizers with sunscreen available from Bobbi Brown, Aveda, Neutrogena, or Paula's Choice.

LA MER CONCEALER

☹ POOR **The Radiant Concealer SPF 25** *($70)* includes titanium dioxide for sunscreen protection and comes in three shades: light, medium, and dark, which isn't dark at all. The medium and dark shades are so similar that we had to ask the sales consultant which was which, and even she didn't know (not to mention that they both come in an unflattering peachy tone). This concealer has a creamy, smooth texture that sets to a fleeting matte finish, which, unfortunately, even with its matte finish, easily slips into lines and creases—not the best for making wrinkles look less noticeable and creating a radiant appearance. We also don't recommend it for covering blemishes because the emollient texture can make matters worse.

LA MER POWDER

✓☺ BEST $$$ **The Powder** *($65)* is one of the most expensive loose powders we've reviewed, yet despite the luxurious feel of this talc-based powder, the money doesn't translate into a noticeable difference worth the price. Nonetheless, it does look incredibly skin-like and creates a beautifully natural yet polished finish from each of its four sheer shades. This is bound to impress, especially if you have normal to dry skin.

LA PRAIRIE

Strengths: All the facial sunscreens include avobenzone for UVA protection; some very good serums; helpful products to smooth lines around the mouth and on lips; mostly good masks; one well-formulated AHA product; most of the makeup categories present good, though needlessly expensive, options that include foundations with reliable sun protection.

Weaknesses: Very expensive; overreliance on jar packaging; many products contain a potentially irritating amount of astringent horsetail extract; the sun products for the body are a mixed bag; no effective skin-lightening options; poor options for anyone dealing with blemishes (though La Prairie is concerned primarily with selling wrinkle creams anyway); the eyeshadow options are average, as are the pencils.

For more information and reviews of the latest La Prairie products, visit CosmeticsCop.com.

LA PRAIRIE CLEANSERS

☺ GOOD $$$ **Foam Cleanser** *($75 for 4.2 fl. oz.)* is a standard, but good, water-soluble cleanser that produces copious, soap-like foam. It's an option for normal to slightly dry or slightly oily skin, if the price doesn't make you faint. For the record, several drugstore lines offer similar cleansers for less than $10.

☺ AVERAGE $$$ **Cellular Comforting Cleansing Emulsion** *($80 for 5.2 fl. oz.)* is a very standard, very overpriced cleansing lotion for normal to dry skin. It does remove makeup but you need to use a washcloth to eliminate any residue. Some of the plant extracts can be a problem for skin if not completely removed.

☺ AVERAGE $$$ **Purifying Cream Cleanser** *($75 for 6.8 fl. oz.)* is a cold cream–style cleanser the company states can be rinsed or tissued off, but this requires effort to completely remove it. It's an OK option for very dry skin but is absurdly overpriced.

☹ POOR **Cellular Cleansing Water Face/Eyes** *($80 for 5.2 fl. oz.)* contains gentle cleansing agents to remove makeup (but not waterproof formulas) and some interesting water-binding agents. However, almost all the plant extracts can be irritating to skin, especially around the eyes, making this a poor choice at any price.

LA PRAIRIE TONERS

☹ POOR **Advanced Marine Biology Tonic** *($95 for 5 fl. oz.)* is a toner-like product that has an exceptionally long ingredient list, the lineup begins with alcohol (unbelievably, it is the first ingredient), and that instantly makes this far from advanced. Alcohol not only causes dryness and irritation, but also generates free-radical damage—none of which stimulate collagen synthesis or improve elasticity. If anything, swabbing alcohol over your skin will help break down these fundamental support elements. And the sea water and extracts are just gimmicks, meant solely to convince you that they are something special for aging skin, nothing more.

☹ POOR **Age Management Balancer** *($85 for 8.4 fl. oz.)* contains lactic acid and has a pH of 3.6, but the amount of AHA present is too low to exfoliate skin. This toner has some very good ingredients for all skin types, but the amount of horsetail can be irritating and the lavender extract isn't good news, either.

☹ POOR **Cellular Refining Lotion** *($85 for 8.4 fl. oz.)* contains irritating horsetail and ivy extracts as well as several volatile fragrant components that won't firm or hydrate skin in the least. See the Appendix to learn why irritation is a problem for everyone's skin.

☹ POOR **Cellular Softening and Balancing Lotion** *($150 for 8.4 fl. oz.)* should be brimming with ingredients that put skin in its optimum state, but La Prairie couldn't resist including the irritants horsetail, arnica, witch hazel, and eugenol, among others.

LA PRAIRIE EXFOLIANTS & SCRUBS

☺ AVERAGE $$$ **Cellular 3-Minute Peel** *($200 for 1.4 fl. oz.)* justifies its price by claiming to use professional-strength AHAs and BHA, and stating that it works without irritating skin. First, professional-strength hydroxy acids are typically used in concentrations of 20% and up, such as for facial peels. The amount of lactic acid in this product is likely around 5%, which does not distinguish this product from other 5% AHA options available at the drugstore. As far as working without irritating skin, that's not possible. This product has a pH of 2.9, which means the lactic acid will exfoliate skin. The addition of a small amount of glycolic acid and an even smaller amount of salicylic acid likely brings the total amount of exfoliating ingredients to about 7%, which is still not what any dermatologist or aesthetician would consider "professional strength." Although this product will exfoliate skin, it needs more than three minutes to do a thorough job, and the price is just insulting for what is easily exchanged for far less pricey options that are just as, if not more, effective.

☺ AVERAGE $$$ **Cellular Resurfacing Cream** *($180 for 1.4 fl. oz.)* has a beautifully emollient texture that addresses the needs of those with dry to very dry skin. However, the formula suffers from the unfortunate choice of jar packaging, which won't keep the light- and air-sensitive ingredients in this product stable during use. The amount of lactic and salicylic acids is likely enough for exfoliation, but the pH is too high for that to happen. Even if the pH were within range, you do not need to spend this much money for a well-formulated AHA or BHA product. Alpha Hydrox, Neutrogena, and Paula's Choice all have excellent, affordable options (though none of them are as emollient as this cream).

☺ AVERAGE $$$ **Essential Exfoliator** *($75 for 7 fl. oz.)* is an OK scrub for normal to dry skin, and features apricot seed powder as the abrasive agent. Plant seeds or shells are not preferred to synthetic polyethylene beads because the former typically do not have perfectly smooth surfaces, and therefore can cause tears in the skin and trigger inflammation.

☹ POOR **Cellular Microdermabrasion Cream** *($255 for 4.2 fl. oz.)* is a thick-textured yet surprisingly abrasive scrub that is too rough for most skin types, and irritating for all skin types because of the grapefruit peel oil it contains. Moreover, at this price, you might as well go for professional microdermabrasion treatments, although those are quite low-tech in terms of anti-aging benefits.

LA PRAIRIE MOISTURIZERS (DAYTIME & NIGHTTIME), EYE CREAMS, & SERUMS

☺ GOOD **$$$ Cellular Anti-Wrinkle Firming Serum** *($185 for 1 fl. oz.)* is a very good, antioxidant-rich moisturizer for normal to slightly dry skin. The truly helpful ingredients outnumber the problem-children additions, making this a contender if you prefer to spend in the upper echelon for your skin-care products.

☺ GOOD **$$$ Cellular Hydrating Serum** *($185 for 1 fl. oz.)* would rate better if it did not include more horsetail extract than it does several other ingredients that are of value for all skin types. The amount of horsetail is unlikely to be problematic, but without it, this serum would be a slam-dunk recommendation because it is loaded with antioxidants, cell-communicating ingredients, and ingredients that mimic the structure and function of healthy skin. The texture makes this best for normal to slightly dry or slightly oily skin.

☺ AVERAGE **$$$ Advanced Marine Biology Cream SPF 20** *($175 for 1.7 fl. oz.)* comes with a name that sounds more like a high school or college science course than a daytime moisturizer with sunscreen, but at least this tremendously overpriced product includes avobenzone for UVA protection. The emollient base formula for dry skin contains a smattering of marine ingredients, but there's no proof (other than from La Prairie's marketing department) that they are stellar antioxidants or have any effect on skin's firmness. What's really frustrating is that none of the plant ingredients will remain potent for long due to the jar packaging (see the Appendix for details). And, of course, you must ask yourself how liberally you'll apply this product knowing that if you apply it correctly to face and neck, you'll be replacing it every couple of months, thus spending over $1,000 per year for facial sunscreen.

☺ AVERAGE **$$$ Anti-Aging Complex** *($220 for 1.7 fl. oz.)* has over a dozen state-of-the-art ingredients for skin, but what precedes them isn't exciting, and the amount of irritating horsetail is larger than the amount of beneficial ingredients. Then, the jar packaging renders the retinol ineffective shortly after you open the product. How disappointing! See the Appendix for further details on the problems jar packaging presents.

☺ AVERAGE **$$$ Anti-Aging Day Cream SPF 30** *($200 for 1.7 fl. oz.)* is a daytime moisturizer with sunscreen, bound to discourage liberal application due to the obnoxious price, despite the fact that liberal application is essential if you are to get the amount of sun protection stated; that makes this tough to recommend even though its actives list includes avobenzone for reliable UVA (think anti-aging) protection. This product has a creamy, lush texture that those with dry skin will appreciate, and the formula contains several beneficial ingredients, plus some exotic plants with no known benefit for skin. Unfortunately, none of the plants or antioxidants will remain stable during use thanks to the jar packaging, which makes this product even more a waste of money when compared with countless other daytime moisturizers with sunscreen.

☺ AVERAGE **$$$ Anti-Aging Emulsion SPF 30** *($195 for 1.7 fl. oz.)* is a lighter version of the Anti-Aging Day Cream SPF 30 above, and the same basic comments apply.

☺ AVERAGE **$$$ Anti-Aging Longevity Serum** *($225 for 1.7 fl. oz.)* isn't a true serum, but rather a lightweight yet emollient lotion for normal to dry skin. It contains a selection of intriguing ingredients, including several plant-based antioxidants and glycoproteins that have cell-communicating properties. The disappointment is the amount of horsetail extract, which is irritating to skin. This also contains other plant extracts with dubious benefits for skin, but do have the potential to cause irritation, and that's not going to help skin's natural repair process. We wouldn't bank on this being the antiwrinkle solution any more than we consider a rice cake a satisfying meal. For the money, you're getting a substandard product that absolutely cannot keep dermal tissues from becoming rigid, as claimed. If that were true, given the basic formulation, lots of other less expensive moisturizers would be doing that, too.

☺ AVERAGE $$$ **Anti-Aging Neck Cream** *($200 for 1.7 fl. oz.)* begs the question, does neck skin age differently than the skin on your face? La Prairie seems to think so, ergo this product. The reality is that although the neck does age differently from the face, that difference cannot be addressed by skin-care ingredients, so this product is completely unnecessary. The way the neck ages is about sun damage and the fact that it has less bone structure supporting the skin, so it can sag faster than the skin on the face or chest. There are no skin-care products that can tighten the skin on your face or neck the way you want them to. The simple fact is there is no research anywhere in the world showing that neck-area skin needs ingredients different from those you use on your face. If you're using a brilliantly formulated facial moisturizer and/or serum, you can apply those products to your neck, too, as well as sun-protection ingredients, which this product sorely lacks. Other than its ludicrous price, there's nothing all that bad about the formula. It's quite rich, and will definitely feel good on dry to very dry skin, but it doesn't contain any ingredients you won't also find in numerous other facial moisturizers from La Prairie, or from other product lines that cost far less. What is pathetic given the price is that most of the beneficial ingredients this contains won't remain stable once it is opened, all thanks to jar packaging (see the Appendix for details). So, this is not only overpriced, but also a waste of money, even if you can afford to waste money!

☺ AVERAGE $$$ **Anti-Aging Night Cream** *($200 for 1.7 fl. oz.)* comes in jar packaging, so the "special" ingredients you're paying extra for won't remain stable during use (see the Appendix for details). It feels as luxurious as the image La Prairie strives to maintain, but a luxurious texture doesn't mean much if the formula isn't outstanding or if several key ingredients have their efficacy depleted due to a bad packaging decision. What a shame, because overall this is a really impressive moisturizer, although it isn't worth the price and it doesn't have special antiwrinkle abilities. This contains a small amount of fragrance ingredients known to cause irritation.

☺ AVERAGE $$$ **Anti-Aging Stress Cream** *($195 for 1.7 fl. oz.)* tries to sway consumers with the statement that the natural relaxant valerian root (which is known to have a calming effect when consumed orally) also works via topical application to relax expression lines and promote firmer, lifted skin. Even if we assume that the plant by itself has wondrous properties for wrinkles and stressed skin, La Prairie's choice of jar packaging will quickly degrade its alleged potency. Even more depressing is that there is far more alcohol in this product than there are exciting anti-aging ingredients (alcohol causes free-radical damage). At its best (which isn't that great), this is nothing more than a standard emollient moisturizer for dry skin. See the Appendix to learn more about the problems jar packaging and alcohol present.

☺ AVERAGE $$$ **Cellular Anti-Wrinkle Sun Cream SPF 30** *($140 for 1.7 fl. oz.)* protects skin from UVA radiation with its in-part avobenzone sunscreen, and has an antioxidant-laden base formula suitable for normal to dry skin. What a shame jar packaging won't keep the numerous antioxidants stable during use (see the Appendix for details). The tiny amount of lavender extract is not likely to be a problem for skin.

☺ AVERAGE $$$ **Cellular Eye Contour Cream** *($125 for 0.5 fl. oz.)* cannot help prevent more lines from forming, as claimed, because it does not contain sunscreen. This is a very standard, emollient moisturizer for dry skin anywhere on the face, although the amount of horsetail extract may prove problematic if used in the eye area. Antioxidants are in short supply, but the number of skin-identical ingredients is good. Despite this, you really don't need an eye cream (see the Appendix to find out why).

☺ AVERAGE **$$$ Cellular Night Repair Cream** *($220 for 1.7 fl. oz.)* has jar packaging that will render most of the exciting ingredients ineffective shortly after you begin using the product. Still, the peptides, oil, and silicones will make dry skin look and feel better (though for this much money every last bit of potency should be preserved).

☺ AVERAGE **$$$ Cellular Radiance Concentrate Pure Gold** *($580 for 1 fl. oz.)* is said to plump lines and wrinkles within an hour, speed exfoliation, and immediately reduce age spots, but nothing in this formula will make these claims a reality. The formula contains mostly water, silicones, alcohol, solvents, slip agents, thickener, water-binding agents, plant extracts, vitamin C, and several more plant extracts. Yes, it does indeed contain gold (it's the third to last ingredient listed), but that has no established benefit for skin, especially when it comes to turning back the hands of time. (What a waste of good metal!) Most of the plant ingredients in this serum show up in all the La Prairie moisturizers, so we suppose those can make you look younger in an instant, too. Considering that this formula cannot make good on its claims (not even a little), the price is nothing less than absurd.

☺ AVERAGE **$$$ Cellular Radiance Cream** *($580 for 1.7 fl. oz.)* is a water- and Vaseline-based moisturizer that takes an everything-but-the-kitchen-sink approach to moisturizers by including tiny amounts of dozens of plants along with gemstones and natural ingredients believed to be helpful for women experiencing skin changes due to menopause (though there is little research to support that line of thinking, at least in terms of using tiny amounts of such ingredients topically rather than orally). The price is ridiculous for what amounts to an emollient moisturizer for dry to very dry skin, and jar packaging renders the many antioxidants unstable shortly after you begin using it (refer to the Appendix for more about jar packaging). The mineral pigments in this moisturizer are what give skin a luminous finish, which is strictly cosmetic, not skin care.

☺ AVERAGE **$$$ Cellular Radiance Eye Cream** *($295 for 0.5 fl. oz.)* contains some good emollients for dry skin, but none that you won't find in hundreds of other moisturizers throughout the price spectrum. There is more mica (a mineral pigment that adds shine to skin) in this eye cream than there are state-of-the-art ingredients, and most of those will be compromised by jar packaging, which doesn't leave you with much for your money. See the Appendix to learn more about jar packaging and discover why you don't need an eye cream.

☺ AVERAGE **$$$ Cellular Time Release Moisturizer, Intensive** *($160 for 1 fl. oz.)* claims to moisturize for up to 16 hours, and has an oil-rich formula that likely lasts that long. However, time released or not, many emollient moisturizers can keep skin comfortable all day and prevent moisture loss. This overall unimpressive formula doesn't break new ground and the antioxidants won't last long due to jar packaging (see the Appendix for more on why jar packaging is a problem).

☺ AVERAGE **$$$ Essence of Skin Caviar Eye Complex** *($120 for 0.5 fl. oz.)* is a lightweight moisturizer that doesn't instantly firm skin, but will hydrate to make superficial lines less apparent. The amount of horsetail extract may cause irritation in the eye area due to its astringent properties, while the caviar extract shows up as the last ingredient on the list. See the Appendix to learn why, in truth, you don't need a special product for the eye area.

☺ AVERAGE **$$$ Extrait of Skin Caviar Firming Complex** *($130 for 1 fl. oz.)* would rate much higher and be worth the splurge if it did not contain problematic plant extracts (including horsetail and sage) along with volatile fragrant components. The amount of sunscreen agent included is odd, given that this product does not advertise an SPF rating. Taking these points into account, this is merely an average option for normal to slightly dry skin.

☺ AVERAGE $$$ **Skin Caviar Intensive Ampoule Treatment** *($570 for 6 treatments)* consists of six ampoules each of **Solvent** and **Lyophilized Substance**, which you mix together to—what else—"guard against accelerated skin aging." Neither product has an SPF rating or contains a UVA-protecting sunscreen, and since that's the best way to prevent accelerated aging with a skin-care product, right away you can tell things are bogus. The Solvent is a lightweight moisturizer that contains some slip agents, emollients, film-forming agent, plant extracts (some are irritating, while most of the others have no established benefit for skin), ceramide, and vitamin E. This also contains volatile fragrant components that may cause irritation. The Lyophilized Substance is a sugar-based powder that contains a salt form of vitamin C along with water, thickener, and the antioxidant superoxide dismutase. There's no reason those ingredients could not have been added to the Solvent, but we suppose the two-step process makes women think the set is somehow more special or customized. In the end, this isn't that exciting, and wouldn't be at even one-fourth the cost.

☺ AVERAGE $$$ **Skin Caviar Luxe Eye Lift Cream** *($295 for 0.68 fl. oz.)* has an incredibly insulting price for what amounts to mostly water, thickeners, Vaseline, and vegetable oil. Many intriguing ingredients are included in this eye cream, but all of them are listed after the pH-adjusting agent, and many won't remain stable once this jar-packaged product is opened. This isn't luxe; it's a bona fide bad beauty investment, at least if you were hoping that the cost would translate to a superior product to vanquish every eye-area woe. See the Appendix to learn why you don't need an eye cream.

☹ POOR **Anti-Aging Eye Cream SPF 15** *($155 for 0.5 fl. oz.)* is an emollient eye cream with an in-part avobenzone sunscreen that has a lot of potential; however, most of the really helpful ingredients are undermined by jar packaging (see the Appendix to learn why jar packaging is a problem and why you don't need an eye cream). The horsetail and balm mint can cause irritation (along with the many volatile fragrant components in this product), making it one to skip.

☹ POOR **Cellular Cream Platinum Rare** *($650 for 1 fl. oz.)* supposedly contains real platinum which is the justification for this moisturizer's absolutely insane price. If this really contains any discernable amount of platinum, what a waste of a good metal. What you are supposed to believe, and undoubtedly there will be those who do believe it, is that applying platinum and La Prairie's "Exclusive Smart Crystals" (now if that isn't new age mumbo jumbo lingo we don't know what is) are said to guard your skin's youthfulness. We're tempted to stop here because this doesn't really deserve a second more of our time, and definitely not yours, but just in case someone really wants to understand what kind of formulation this price tag has affixed to it, we'll finish. First, the amount of platinum powder is a mere dusting. However, even in greater amounts, platinum (despite its use in making exquisite jewelry) has no special anti-aging or any benefit for skin whatsoever. La Prairie simply chose to use it because they were banking that platinum's jewelry reputation for being prized and expensive would transfer to skin care, thus allowing them to set an extremely high price for what, in many ways, couldn't be a more basic, ordinary moisturizer for dry skin. The only possible association of platinum with skin is how it functions in some chemotherapy medications. It's included in these medications for its cytotoxic (i.e., it kills cells) capabilities when combined with other substances, but that has nothing to do with topical application or with restoring youth (Source: *Journal of Clinical Oncology*, August 2007, pages 3266–3273). That is, it has to do with killing rapidly growing cells to restore equilibrium and to shrink tumors. In all honesty, you'd be better off buying a platinum ring and rubbing that on skin than using this product. The platinum won't be helpful but at least you'll have a beautiful piece of jewelry to wear as compensation! The amount of mica in this moisturizer is enough to cast a shimmering glow on skin, but that effect is strictly cosmetic and has nothing to do with "smart crystals." Actually, it would be much smarter to use a lightweight shimmer lotion to revive the radiance of aging skin than this product! This does contain some beneficial plant extracts and antioxidants, but not nearly as much as it should, especially at this price. And the fact that they chose jar packaging is just maddening, so any beneficial ingredients won't remain stable. Even if you were undeterred by cost and overinflated claims, this product would still not be recommended because it contains silver oxide. Silver oxide is a germicide composed of silver nitrate and an alkaline hydroxide (a metallic compound bound to a metal atom). Silver nitrate is known to be caustic to skin, while silver itself can cause a permanent bluish discoloration on skin (Sources: naturaldatabase. com; and *Colloidal Silver: A Literature Review: Medical Uses, Toxicology, and Manufacture*, 2nd Edition, Clear Springs Press, LLC, John Hill).

⊗ POOR **Cellular Eye Cream Platinum Rare** (*$350 for 0.68 fl. oz.*) is a rather standard but decent combination of emollients, skin-identical ingredients, and a tiny amount of peptides. It also contains several plant extracts with the potential for irritation, including ginseng, horsetail, arnica, and fragrance, both synthetic and natural. Irritation is always a problem for skin (see the Appendix for details), but somehow it feels even more damaging when you're spending this much money. Aside from the irritation issue and the somewhat interesting formula, none of the worthwhile ingredients will remain stable because of the jar packaging. Once you open a jar the beneficial plant extracts and peptides begin to breakdown in the presence of air (see the Appendix for details on why jar packaging is a problem). Given the price of this product, you would think someone at La Prairie would know this well-documented fact. Apart from the fact that you don't need a product labeled an eye cream for the eye area (see the Appendix to learn why), there is no benefit to adding diamonds, platinum, or other precious metals to skin-care products. Platinum (despite its use in making exquisite jewelry) has no special anti-aging or any benefit for skin whatsoever, and there is no published research showing otherwise. La Prairie may have chosen platinum because they were banking that platinum's jewelry reputation for being prized and expensive would transfer to skin care, thus allowing them to set an extremely high price for this eye cream. Platinum can also be a skin sensitizer, although probably not in the minute amounts in this product. The diamond and platinum powders are supposed to brighten and add radiance. The "brightened" luminous part of the claim is tied to the sparkles the cream adds to the face, but that's makeup, not skin care. The effect can be nice, though. What is indeed adding shine to this product is a large amount of mica. Mica is a very ordinary, inexpensive ingredient used throughout the cosmetics industry to add shine. It is interesting to note that platinum powder is an industrial material used to prevent corrosion on machines and pipes. We can't address the issue of the diamond silicone blend because there is no information about its properties or its claimed benefit for skin, although we can't imagine what those benefits might be. The amount of mica in this eye cream is enough to cast a shimmering glow on skin, but that effect has nothing to do with making skin look lifted and line-free. Suffice to say, this product is a waste of money on many levels, especially when you figure it out and discover that the price is slightly more than $500 per ounce! Please avoid the seductive nature of the claims about the diamonds and platinum; those minerals are better left in the world of manufacturing, medicine, and jewelry, not skin care.

☹ POOR **Cellular Power Infusion** *($475 for 4 vials)* can be described as "outrageous," which is the first word (fit for print) that came to mind when we compared the shockingly high price of this serum to its ingredient list. For your money, you're getting mostly water, alcohol, and slip agents, some of the least expensive ingredients around, not to mention how damaging and pro-aging alcohol can be. Despite the high price, fancy vial packaging, "energy booster" claims, and the statement that you'll never look your age again, La Prairie might just be referring to looking older rather than younger, because this is really a powerful product to send skin in the wrong direction.

☹ POOR **Cellular Radiance Emulsion SPF 30** *($425 for 1.7 fl. oz.)* is so absurdly overpriced that you are not likely to apply it liberally, which is the chief danger of this product. With liberal application to face and neck, you'll be replacing this every two months, if not more frequently, which adds up to more than $2,500 per year! Without question you can get the protection this product provides for significantly less money, and better formulas, too! This could've been a decent broad-spectrum sunscreen for normal to dry skin, but the problems add up to issues for your skin that you shouldn't ignore. Though it does contain avobenzone for UVA protection, it isn't stabilized with octocrylene or any other suitable ingredient, which means it is unlikely to give you the stated level of UVA protection after you apply it. While this does contain some interesting ingredients for skin, the amounts are not impressive, especially given the cost (and that's an understatement). An additional problem is the potentially irritating amount of alcohol, along with some irritating plant extracts as well as fragrance, both natural and synthetic (see the Appendix to learn why irritation and fragrance are bad for skin). The radiance this product adds to your skin is from mica, not from gold. Mica is a very ordinary, inexpensive ingredient used throughout the cosmetics industry to add shine, but that's not skin care, it's a makeup effect. One other point: Although we often do not comment on the presence of dyes, this product contains red and yellow synthetic dyes to give it a gold cast. That's to make the cream look like it has a large amount of gold—it doesn't; there is only a trace amount. But, even if it were all gold and nothing else, that is about jewelry, not skin care.

☹ POOR **Cellular Revitalizing Eye Gel** *($155 for 0.5 fl. oz.)* contains a large amount of horsetail extract as well as lesser amounts of chemical components of the plant. Horsetail has research on its ability to relax veins when taken orally, but that does not translate to mean it can reduce puffy eyes and dark circles when applied topically. The volatile components in horsetail (including trace amounts of nicotine) can be irritating to skin. It has potential antioxidant ability, but isn't preferred to other antioxidants that provide a benefit without the potential risk (Source: naturaldatabase.com). This product also contains a preservative that is not recommended for use in leave-on products. See the Appendix to find out why you don't need a special product for the eye area.

☹ POOR **Cellular Serum Platinum Rare** *($650 for 1 fl. oz.)* is one of the most expensive products La Prairie, or any other cosmetics line for that matter, sells. You might be intrigued if you weren't so shocked by the price. Does it really contain anything that can dramatically change the face of aging skin? Of course not. For all the claims of DNA repair, Smart Crystals, and immediate firming, La Prairie's formula is mostly water, slip agents, and alcohol. This much alcohol in an anti-aging product that costs more than $600 per ounce is what should be rare. Alcohol causes cell death and free-radical damage, and that's not something you should be paying even $1 for, let alone $650. This serum-like formula also contains problematic amounts of plant extracts, including horsetail. Please refer to the review of La Prairie's Cellular Eye Cream Platinum Rare above for a discussion on platinum in skin-care products.

☹ POOR **Skin Caviar** *($175 for 1.7 fl. oz.)* is a silicone-based serum whose negatives are strong enough to make it not worth considering. In addition to some irritating plant extracts, this also contains the germicidal agent O-phenylphenol, which research has shown can cause acute skin inflammation and, potentially, ulceration (Sources: *National Toxicology Program Technical Support Series*, March 1986, pages 1–141; and *Critical Reviews in Toxicology*, 2002, pages 551–625).

☹ POOR **Skin Caviar Crystalline Concentre** *($390 for 1 fl. oz.)* is a terrible waste-of-time-and-money product. If we were working for La Prairie, we would not be able to sell this catastrophe to a single consumer without feeling like the ultimate snake oil salesperson. The concept and claim behind this serum is to create smoother, firmer skin that has increased elasticity so that wrinkles are filled out and a younger-looking visage emerges. Based on the formula, someone at La Prairie either has a cruel sense of humor or absolutely no concept of what aging skin needs to make it look and feel as good as possible. And the price goes beyond insulting! For nearly $400, you're getting mostly water, slip agents, silicones, thickener, alcohol (the drying, irritating, free radical–generating kind), and a derivative of resorcinol, which has no proven benefit for skin yet retains resorcinol's irritating properties. The peptides, caviar extract, and diamond powder may attract the cost-is-no-deterrent consumer, but none of these ingredients add up to a brilliant, elite skin-care product that provides even a modicum of antiwrinkle benefit. There are far better (and we mean much, much better) moisturizers than this available for less than $30 at the drugstore or from lines such as Paula's Choice.

☹ POOR **Skin Caviar Luxe Cream** *($390 for 1.7 fl. oz.)* may have a luxe texture, but the ingredients used to create it are commonplace and do not justify the ridiculous price. This jar-packaged moisturizer contains many antioxidants that won't remain stable once you open it, and the pH of this cream is too high for the AHA it contains to exfoliate skin. Topping things off is the inclusion of the irritants sage, arnica, and horsetail, coupled with several volatile fragrant components. Buyer beware—and see the Appendix to learn why jar packaging and irritation are bad news for your skin.

☹ POOR **White Caviar Illuminating Cream** *($450 for 1.7 fl. oz.)*. For what this moisturizer costs, it should be brimming with state-of-the-art ingredients and have the type of packaging that keeps those ingredients stable during use. This product strikes out on both counts. First, the core ingredients in this hyper-expensive moisturizer are present in numerous other moisturizers that cost a lot less, and second, many of the less expensive products are not packaged in jars (see the Appendix for details). This has a texture that is both light and emollient, in part because of the silicones it contains plus petrolatum (think Vaseline). It also contains some very good antioxidants, in particular resveratrol and vitamins C and E, as well as interesting plant extracts such as grape vine and licorice. However, it also contains several plant extracts with the potential for irritation, including ginseng and horsetail, along with fragrance, both synthetic and natural. Irritation is always a problem for skin (see the Appendix for details), but somehow it feels even more damaging when you're spending this much money. There is nothing illuminating about this product, and needless to say caviar is better on a cracker than it is on your skin. La Prairie has been touting this ingredient for years, and there still isn't a shred of published research anywhere about its claimed benefit for skin. The claims of lightening brown spots are passable given the antioxidants and licorice extracts, but those are not unique to this product and they certainly don't replace the need for sunscreen during the day. In summing up, the positives definitely don't outweigh the negatives for this moisturizer, and the price just makes it all rather ridiculous—don't you agree?

☹ POOR **White Caviar Illuminating Eye Serum** *($250 for 0.5 fl. oz.)* has a formula that is mostly water, glycerin, and alcohol. And imagine, alcohol, which causes irritation, dryness, and free-radical damage (not to mention collagen breakdown, which makes wrinkles worse), being the third ingredient in a product meant to be used around the eyes! There are some excellent beneficial ingredients in this eye serum, but all of them are listed after the alcohol, so it's all for naught. Not a single ingredient in this product is capable of lightening dark circles. If anything, the inflammation alcohol and certain irritating plant extracts this serum contains will make your eye-area woes more of a problem. La Prairie should be ashamed for creating such an inadequate formula. See the Appendix to learn why you don't need a special product for the eye area.

☹ POOR **White Caviar Illuminating Serum** *($450 for 1 fl. oz.)* contains mostly water, glycerin, and alcohol, and is a shocking waste of money! And imagine, alcohol, which causes irritation, dryness, and free-radical damage (not to mention collagen breakdown, which makes wrinkles worse), being the third ingredient in a product claiming to make your skin look and act younger! See the Appendix to learn about the problems alcohol presents for your skin. What's particularly disappointing is that there are some excellent anti-aging ingredients in this serum, but all of them are listed after the alcohol, so it's all for naught. On balance, there's an impressive, generous mix of antioxidants, anti-irritants, skin-identical ingredients, and emollients in a lotion-style serum that has a soft silky texture. The form of vitamin C (ascorbyl glucoside) included has some research indicating it can help fade brown spots, but the inflammation from the alcohol and the irritating plant extracts in this serum isn't worth the trade-off, especially not when there are effective options that don't contain irritating ingredients, which you'll find in Chapter 15, *The Best Products*, at the end of this book.

LA PRAIRIE SUN CARE

☺ AVERAGE **$$$ Sun Protection Lotion SPF 30 Body** *($85 for 6 fl. oz.)* provides broad-spectrum protection that includes avobenzone for reliable UVA protection, and it has a pleasant, smooth texture that most will find cosmetically pleasing. Unfortunately, the price is out of line for what amounts to nothing extraordinary. With any expensive sunscreen, you have to consider whether or not you'll be likely to apply it liberally each time you use it. Liberal application is essential to get the amount of sun protection stated on the label, and given the number of affordable sun-protecting options available, why overspend if you don't have to? This sunscreen doesn't contain anything that justifies its price. Formula-wise, it does have some helpful antioxidants and skin-repairing ingredients, but so do lots of other sunscreens whose prices aren't so outlandish.

☺ AVERAGE **$$$ Ultra Protection SPF 40 Eye Lip Nose** *($65 for 0.35 fl. oz.)* is an emollient, absurdly overpriced sunscreen stick (given the amount, it costs slightly more than $185 per ounce!) that provides broad-spectrum protection and includes avobenzone for reliable UVA protection, so except for the price it's off to a good start. But, speaking of price, without question you don't need to spend nearly this much to obtain great sun protection. You also must consider how the price may affect whether you'll apply this liberally or not. Liberal application is essential to get the amount of sun protection stated on the label, and given the number of affordable sun-protecting options available, why overspend if you don't have to? If you choose to indulge in this sunscreen, its thick, somewhat greasy texture limits its use to the eye, lip, and nose areas, as indicated—it's just too heavy to slather on your entire face.

LA PRAIRIE LIP CARE

☺ AVERAGE **$$$ Cellular Lip Renewal Concentrate** *($95 for 0.5 fl. oz.)* makes the odd claim of being able to revive natural lip color (which it cannot do; stick with lipstick for that!). It's essentially a lightweight moisturizer for lips that has more flavor than antioxidants or other helpful ingredients for lips.

☹ POOR **Cellular Luxe Lip Treatment SPF 15** *($50 for 0.12 fl. oz.)* has deluxe packaging, but leaves lips vulnerable to UVA damage because the sunscreen does not list titanium dioxide, zinc oxide, avobenzone, Tinosorb, or Mexoryl SX among its active ingredients. The base formula couldn't be more ordinary, and is a further insult at this price.

LA PRAIRIE SPECIALTY SKIN-CARE PRODUCTS

✔☺ BEST **$$$ Cellular Lip Line Plumper** *($130 for 0.08 fl. oz.)* contains a blend of silicones and silicone polymers that do a good job of serving as a soft spackle for lip lines. This also contains some very good water-binding agents and cell-communicating ingredients, and omits the irritants typically found in lip-plumping products. It's not as miraculous as the claims imply, but it does work temporarily to fill in lines around the mouth and makes lips look and feel noticeably smoother. For best results, use this with a semi-matte or matte finish lipstick rather than a creamy or glossy lipstick, which shortens the line-filling effect.

☺ AVERAGE **$$$ Cellular Hydralift Firming Mask** *($150 for 1.7 fl. oz.)* won't firm skin, but will reinforce its moisture barrier as claimed because of the Vaseline it contains, along with triglycerides and silicone. Several very good antioxidants are included, but their potency will be diminished due to jar packaging (see the Appendix for details).

☺ AVERAGE **$$$ Cellular Treatment Gold Illusion Line Filler** *($150 for 1 fl. oz.)*. This silicone-based product has a silky, spackle-like texture that fills in superficial winkles to a minor degree. How long the effect lasts depends on what else you apply with this product and how expressive you are. La Prairie included a large amount of the shiny mineral pigment mica and potentially irritating horsetail, which may cause irritation. Shine can make wrinkles more noticeable, so tread carefully no matter what your final thoughts about this formula. This does contain some good antioxidants, but they're joined by alcohol, fragrance, several fragrance ingredients, and pure gold, which is known to cause contact dermatitis on the face and eyelids (Sources: *Inflammation and Allergy Drug Targets*, September 2008, pages 145–162; *Dermatologic Therapy*, volume 17, 2004, pages 321–327; and *Cutis*, May 2000, pages 323–326). There isn't much gold in this product, but there isn't much of anything else helpful for skin, either. All told, the concern about the gold still exists and this isn't worth considering over better, less expensive versions of this product without the gold. An example would be Good Skin's Tri-Aktiline Instant Deep Wrinkle Filler, which costs around $40 for the same amount of product.

☺ AVERAGE **$$$ Cellular Treatment Rose Illusion Line Filler** *($115 for 1 fl. oz.)* supposedly works to make wrinkled skin look smooth and line-free, but don't get your hopes up and don't open your pocketbook. This thick but silky gel-cream is mostly silicone and has an opalescent pink tint to slightly brighten skin. Silicone primers have a softening effect—and that's it; they don't erase lines. L'Oreal's foundation primer/perfector offers similar benefits at a realistic price.

☹ POOR **Cellular Purifying Blemish Control** *($80 for 0.5 fl. oz.)* contains an unknown amount of salicylic acid as the active ingredient, but the base formula is mostly alcohol, and that's too irritating and drying for all skin types (see the Appendix for details). Further, many of the plant extracts in this product can cause inflammation.

LA PRAIRIE FOUNDATIONS & PRIMERS

☺ GOOD $$$ **Cellular Treatment Foundation Powder Finish** *($80)* is a talc-based wet/dry powder foundation that has a wonderfully smooth texture and a gorgeous silky finish. It would work best for normal to slightly dry or slightly oily skin types. Companies such as Laura Mercier, Lancome, Chanel, and M.A.C. offer even more impressive powder foundations for much less money, but if you're stuck on La Prairie, this won't disappoint. Four of the six shades are great, but avoid Rose Beige (too rose), and if you have a medium to tan skin tone, consider Soleil Beige carefully.

☺ GOOD $$$ **Cellular Treatment Foundation Satin SPF 15** *($70)* provides an in-part titanium dioxide sunscreen, which is the least you should expect from a foundation at this price. It has a fluid yet creamy texture and blends from sheer to medium coverage with a satin finish best for normal to dry skin. Among the nine shades, the four best avoided are 1.0, 3.2, 4.0, and 4.5.

☹ POOR **Anti-Aging Foundation SPF 15** *($100)* is a problem for anyone concerned with anti-aging. Not only does it lack sufficient UVA protection (i.e., it doesn't contain avobenzone, titanium dioxide, zinc oxide, ecamsule, or Tinosorb), which isn't anti-aging in the least, but also it is pro-aging because it also contains more alcohol than any state-of-the-art ingredients (and this has a very long ingredient list!). Alcohol only increases your risk of irritation, dryness, and free-radical damage. The good ingredients in this formula have to fight the alcohol as much as the environment and they are hampered by the lack of UVA protection. What a headache and absurd waste of money.

☹ POOR **Anti-Aging Hydra Tint SPF 20** *($100)*. This tinted moisturizer is not only absurdly priced, but also contains irritating fragrance and lacks the ingredients needed to shield your skin from the sun's entire range of damaging UVA rays, which is essential for anti-aging benefits (see the Appendix for details on both of these issues). Although there are some potentially beneficial antioxidants and plant extracts in this product, they don't make up for its serious shortcomings.

☹ POOR **Skin Caviar Concealer/Foundation SPF 15** *($180)* deserves credit for its convenient packaging of a liquid foundation and creamy concealer (the concealer is housed in the cap), but does not deserve your attention because its sunscreen does not contain the UVA-protecting ingredients of titanium dioxide, zinc oxide, avobenzone, Tinosorb, or Mexoryl SX. Despite its silky texture and a few bells and whistles in the base formula, we can't recommend such an expensive foundation that leaves your skin vulnerable to UVA damage—not when there are so many brilliant, markedly less expensive liquid foundations that get the sunscreen element right.

LA PRAIRIE CONCEALERS

☺ GOOD $$$ **Light Fantastic Cellular Concealing Brightening Eye Treatment** *($70)* has a silky, silicone-enhanced texture and is dispensed onto a synthetic brush via a click-pen component. The product comes with a refill cartridge, which is seemingly generous for La Prairie. In terms of camouflage, this doesn't conceal more than very minor discolorations. It works best as a subtle highlighter. The "powerful" anti-aging complex is barely present, and there is no research anywhere to support the claim that glycoproteins and plant extracts, especially in the tiny amounts here, can have an antiwrinkle effect (though they can offer general skin repair benefits). Although this has an attractive creaseless finish and comes in three good colors, we wouldn't choose it over similar, less expensive highlighters from Estee Lauder or L'Oreal.

☹ POOR **Anti-Aging Concealer SPF 20 Face/Eyes** *($70)*. This medium to full coverage concealer fails for a number of reasons. First, the liquid formula doesn't blend on smoothly and can end up looking cakey. Second, to make matters worse, the shades have a peach undertone. And third, despite its SPF 20 rating, this concealer lacks the ingredients needed to shield your skin from the sun's entire range of damaging UVA rays, which is essential for anti-aging benefits (see the Appendix for details). Don't be fooled by the "anti-aging" part of the name. The beneficial ingredients aren't present in high enough concentrations to have an anti-aging effect, and, in fact, the absence of adequate UVA protection means your skin is vulnerable to more wrinkles! One more comment: The active sunscreen ingredients in this concealer can be sensitizing if used around the eyes. Mineral actives such as titanium dioxide and/or zinc oxide are preferred for use in the eye area.

LA PRAIRIE POWDER

☺ GOOD **$$$ Cellular Treatment Loose Powder** *($80)* has an ultra-fine, talc-based texture and a sheer, minimalist finish that leaves skin looking polished and dusted with sparkles. If shiny, expensive powder is your thing, here's a good option, and both shades are translucent.

LA PRAIRIE BLUSHES & BRONZER

☺ GOOD **$$$ Cellular Radiance Cream Blush** *($70)* would be enthusiastically recommended were it not for the ridiculous price. It's a very good, nontraditional cream blush that applies and blends nicely, leaving a soft, transparent wash of color. Skin looks healthy and glowing from each of the four colors, and the shine level is almost on mute. If you're going to indulge in some La Prairie makeup and have dry skin, this would be something to seriously consider, but only for a splurge, because your cheeks won't look like you spent this kind of money on your face.

☺ AVERAGE **$$$ Cellular Treatment Bronzing Powder** *($60)* features two attractive tan colors in one compact, but this pressed bronzing powder's texture is noticeably dry, and although the shine is soft it doesn't cling well, making this a below-average option, especially for the money.

☺ AVERAGE **$$$ Cellular Treatment Powder Blush** *($55)* doesn't impress with its drier-than-usual, slightly grainy texture, though it still applies smoothly. Every shade is shiny, but the effect is closer to a soft glow than sparkles, which is a nice change of pace. Still, countless cosmetics lines offer less expensive powder blushes that have a superior texture and better array of shades, whether you want no shine, some shine, or all-out glitter.

LA PRAIRIE EYESHADOWS

☺ AVERAGE **$$$ Cellular Treatment Eye Colour Ensemble** *($70)* provides four eyeshadows in one compact, with one shade in each being dark enough to use as eyeliner. These have a smoother, silkier feel and apply better than the Cellular Treatment Eye Colour below, though still a bit unevenly. Every set has quite a bit of shine, and that's not the best for wrinkled eye-area skin; the least shiny (and most workable) set is called Les Bruns.

☹ POOR **Cellular Treatment Eye Colour** *($45)* is La Prairie's name for their powder eyeshadow singles and the name is the most enticing thing about this otherwise unremarkable product. The smooth but dry texture leads to a chunky, flake-prone application, and there are far too many pastel tones that do little to shape or shade the eye.

LA PRAIRIE EYE & BROW LINERS

☺ GOOD $$$ **Luxe Brow Liner Automatique** *($50)* is a very good retractable brow pencil that has a smooth but dry application and a soft powder finish that won't budge. The only issue (beyond the price) is that it takes some effort to get the colors to show up.

☺ GOOD $$$ **Luxe Eye Liner Automatique** *($50)* is an automatic, retractable eye pencil, but the sleek metal component is what you end up paying for. Each color goes on smoothly and leaves a slightly creamy finish that won't be impervious to smearing unless set with a powder eyeshadow. Of course, you could just line with a powder eyeshadow and be done, but this is a decent option for those who prefer pencils.

LA PRAIRIE LIP COLOR & LIPLINERS

☺ GOOD $$$ **Cellular Lip Colour Effects Luminous Transparent Glaze** *($40)* has an elegantly smooth, not-too-thick texture and a minimally sticky, sparkling finish. Featuring a brush applicator, this gloss does have movement—despite claims to the contrary—so don't expect it to not feather into lines around the mouth, just like most glosses do.

☺ GOOD $$$ **Luxe Lip Liner Automatique** *($45)* has a luxurious metal component and above-average brush on the opposite end to soften and blend the line from this automatic, retractable pencil. Because it stays creamy it can't help keep lipstick from migrating into lines around the mouth, so if that's a concern, it's best to skip this one. The Nude shade is a versatile color.

☺ AVERAGE $$$ **Cellular Luxe Lip Colour** *($55)* leans to the greasy side of creamy, which doesn't bode well for those prone to lipstick traveling into lines around the mouth. These light- to medium-coverage shimmer-laden lipsticks leave no stain, so their wear time is relatively brief. All told, there isn't a strong argument to consider these over many other creamy lipsticks, but they're not terrible either.

LA PRAIRIE MASCARAS

☺ GOOD $$$ **Cellular Treatment Mascara Instant Curl** *($40)* doesn't do anything instantly, but with patience this extends lashes to fluttering length and leaves them with a soft, fringed curl. Thickness is harder to come by, but the application is clump-free and wearability is uneventful.

☺ AVERAGE $$$ **Cellular Treatment Mascara Instant Build** *($40)* won't clump at all and leaves lashes remarkably soft, but otherwise takes a long time to produce meager lengthening. This isn't any more treatment for lashes than most mascaras, and the amount of La Prairie's Cellular Complex is minuscule compared to the standard waxes seen in this and most mascaras available today (not to mention caviar has no special benefit for lashes).

LA PRAIRIE FACE & BODY ILLUMINATORS

☺ GOOD $$$ **Cellular Treatment Illuminating Face Powder** ($60). This pressed-powder illuminator has a soft, lightweight texture that blends on smoothly, leaving a subtle shimmering glow. It comes in two sheer shades of light and medium-light, both of which are flattering and neutral, but too light for those with deeper skin tones. Are there any added benefits that make this ultra-expensive powder worth the price? In two words: No way. Even the La Prairie salespeople we talked to said that the "cellular treatment" part of the product name doesn't have any meaning. (That was a breath of honest air at the cosmetics counter, something we don't hear very often.) In the end, you're getting a pretty highlighting powder that works well, but you certainly don't need to pay this much.

LA ROCHE-POSAY (SKIN CARE ONLY)

Strengths: Very good cleansers; well-formulated, stably packaged option for those seeking products with hydroquinone or retinol or stabilized vitamin C; many fragrance-free options; a unique lip moisturizer.

Weaknesses: Some problematic, overly irritating exfoliants; several ho-hum moisturizers and sunscreens; product names that either sound convoluted or are little more than nonsense words.

For more information and reviews of the latest La Roche-Posay products, visit Cosmetics-Cop.com.

LA ROCHE-POSAY CLEANSERS

✓☺ BEST **$$$ Toleriane Dermo-Cleanser** *($22.95 for 6.76 fl. oz.)* is a very simple, fragrance-free cleansing lotion for dry skin. It poses no risk of irritating skin unless you know you're sensitive to one of the ingredients it contains, and it does a decent job of removing most types of makeup. Its value for dry, sensitive skin earns it a Best Product rating.

✓☺ BEST **$$$ Toleriane Purifying Foaming Cream** *($23.95 for 4.22 fl. oz.)* is a very good water-soluble foaming cleanser with a soft cream texture suitable for normal to slightly dry skin, and it removes makeup quickly. The detergent cleansing agents are not bad, but they're also not the best for "intolerant" skin, as La Roche-Posay asserts.

☺ GOOD **Effaclar Purifying Foaming Gel** *($22 for 6.76 fl. oz.)* is a basic, but effective, water-soluble cleanser that's best for normal to oily or combination skin. It's expensive for what you get (several options from the drugstore work just as well for less money), but this works to remove excess oil and makeup without leaving skin feeling dry. In terms of purifying skin, this cleanser does as well as any other water-soluble option.

☹ AVERAGE **$$$ Effaclar Deep Cleansing Foaming Cream** *($22.95 for 4.2 fl. oz.)* produces a foamy lather, but contains a high amount of the alkaline ingredient potassium hydroxide, making this an option only for very oily skin, and even those folks may find this too drying.

☹ AVERAGE **$$$ Physiological Micellar Solution** *($20.95 for 6.76 fl. oz.)* is just a very basic cleanser whose formula is similar to many eye-makeup removers, at its core. This contains fragrance (which skin anywhere on the face doesn't need). The claim about this respecting skin's "physiological balance" applies to any well-formulated cleanser or makeup remover; it doesn't make this a special or distinctive product. In fact, the ingredients couldn't be more ordinary.

LA ROCHE-POSAY TONER

☹ POOR **Thermal Spring Water** *($9.90 for 1.7 fl. oz.)* comes with claims of soothing, toning, refreshing, and providing antioxidant protection to skin, yet all it contains is water and nitrogen. Thermal Spring Water is just water and some extra nitrogen. This product is said to be "rich in selenium, a powerful antioxidant." Whether or not that is true (though obtaining pure selenium as an oral supplement is preferred) is irrelevant because the nitrogen used as a propellant to create a mist of water can generate free-radical damage and cause cell death (Sources: *Skin Research and Technology*, November 2011, ePublication; *Mechanisms of Ageing and Development*, April 2002, pages 1007–1019; *Toxicology and Applied Pharmacology*, July 2002, pages 84–90; and *Cellular and Molecular Biology*, April 15, 2007, pages 1–2).

LA ROCHE-POSAY EXFOLIANTS & SCRUBS

☹ AVERAGE **$$$ Physiological Ultra-Fine Scrub** *($17.95 for 1.69 fl. oz.)* is a basic, overpriced facial scrub that's an OK option for all skin types. The amount of abrasive agent is low and buffered by slip agents, so you're unlikely to overdo with this one and abrade your skin. Still, scrubs are a less elegant, less effective way to exfoliate skin compared with well-formulated AHA or BHA products. Please refer to the Best Products chapter for a list of our favorite AHA and BHA products.

☹ POOR **Effaclar Astringent Lotion Micro-Exfoliant** *($22.95 for 6.76 fl. oz.)* lists alcohol as the second ingredient, and the amount of salicylic acid is too low for exfoliation to occur. See the Appendix to learn why alcohol is a problem for all skin types.

☹ POOR **Effaclar Serum** *($42.95 for 1 fl. oz.)* is an overpriced, poorly formulated exfoliant containing about 4%–5% AHA (glycolic acid) and less than 1% BHA (salicylic acid). It's neither mild nor will it smooth your complexion. Quite the opposite is the case because the second ingredient is alcohol and that is completely problematic for all skin types. Alcohol causes free-radical damage, hurts the skin's ability to heal, and diminishes collagen. It also stimulates more oil production at the base of pores. While AHA and BHA can be excellent for removing built-up layers of dead skin cells accumulated due to sun damage or oily skin, this isn't the product to consider for this important skin-care step.

LA ROCHE-POSAY MOISTURIZERS (DAYTIME & NIGHTTIME), EYE CREAMS, & SERUMS

☺ GOOD **Anthelios SX Daily Moisturizing Cream with Sunscreen SPF 15** *($31.95 for 3.4 fl. oz.)* is noteworthy because of its combination of ecamsule with avobenzone, as stabilized by octocrylene. You can be assured of sufficient UVA protection if you apply this liberally and long enough before venturing outdoors. What's disappointing is that the excitement starts and stops right there. Nothing else about this silicone-enhanced sunscreen is that intriguing, and it doesn't contain a single antioxidant or other state-of-the-art ingredient. For the money, you should expect more. Still, it deserves a Good rating for its sunscreen alone, and the formula is suitable for normal to slightly dry or slightly oily skin. One more thing: Although Mexoryl SX is a good UVA sunscreen, it does not provide the highest level of UVA protection as claimed on the label. Titanium dioxide and zinc oxide can screen UVA rays just as well (assuming they're carefully formulated) so Mexoryl SX, while viable, is not intrinsically the best.

☺ GOOD **Hydraphase UV SPF 30** *($34.95 for 1.69 fl. oz.)* has an in-part avobenzone sunscreen which is the best part about this daytime moisturizer for normal to oily skin. The formula has a silky lotion texture but doesn't treat skin to much beyond the basics. Almost all the antioxidants are listed after the preservative, and as such don't count for much. Still, this provides great broad-spectrum sun protection and works well under makeup. The tiny amount of plant oils is unlikely to be a problem for blemish-prone skin (although those with very oily skin may want to avoid this product). Contrary to claim, the active ingredients plus the inclusion of fragrance do not make this safe for sensitive skin. Those with sensitive skin would do better using a mineral-based (titanium dioxide and/or zinc oxide) sunscreen that is fragrance-free.

☺ GOOD **Toleraine Ultra Intense Soothing Care** *($34.95 for 1.35 fl. oz.)* is designed for very sensitive skin, which explains the short ingredient list. (Generally speaking, the fewer ingredients in a product, the less likely sensitive skin is to have a reaction.) This is a thick, emollient, fragrance-free formula best for dry to very dry sensitive skin, but it's notably free of beneficial ingredients to help skin look and act younger. We can't fault La Roche-Posay for wanting to offer a rich moisturizer for very sensitive skin, but we do wonder why they didn't include some skin-repairing ingredients like ceramides or cholesterol, which are nonirritating and healing for skin, or why they didn't add soothing agents or some gentle antioxidants, although they did add shea butter for an antioxidant kick, so the formula isn't completely void of them.

This specialty moisturizer deserves consideration if your skin does not tolerate others from our Best Moisturizers list, but, based on its formula and price, it doesn't deserve our top rating.

☺ GOOD $$$ **Active C Eyes** *($40.95 for 0.5 fl. oz.)* is a silky, silicone-enriched lightweight moisturizer for slightly dry skin anywhere on the face. It contains a good amount of vitamin C (as ascorbic acid) and contains fragrance in the form of bitter orange flower extract. See the Appendix to learn why you don't need an eye cream, even one we've rated well.

☺ GOOD $$$ **Active C, for Dry Skin** *($50.50 for 1 fl. oz.)* would be an outstanding way to see if a 5% stabilized vitamin C product (packaged to ensure stability and potency) improves your skin. The silky, silicone-enhanced base with its nearly matte finish is ideal for normal to oily skin. Just to be clear, vitamin C is a very good, well-established antioxidant for skin, but it isn't the only one to consider, and in that sense you are getting a one-note product by choosing this.

☺ GOOD $$$ **Active C, for Normal to Combination Skin** *($50.50 for 1 fl. oz.)* is similar to the Active C, for Dry Skin above, and the same review applies.

☺ GOOD $$$ **Redermic + Eyes Intensive Daily Anti-Wrinkle/Firming Fill-In Care** *($43.95 for 0.5 fl. oz.)* is a fragrance-free eye cream that cannot make deep-set wrinkles vanish, nor can it help with sagging skin around the eyes or anywhere else on the face. Many skin-care products claim they can firm and lift skin, but none of them work, at least not to the extent claimed (see the Appendix for details). If you're still curious about this eye cream, it has a silky-smooth texture and contains an impressive amount of vitamin C (ascorbic acid), which has anti-aging benefits. Vitamin C isn't going to fill wrinkles or lift sagging skin, but it is among the many good anti-aging ingredients to consider. Of course, ultimately, if you're using a well-formulated facial moisturizer and serum, you don't need to add an eye cream (really). This product is a great example, as it doesn't contain a single ingredient not found in facial moisturizers, too. You have to ask why you're paying more for a teeny-tiny amount of product!

☺ GOOD $$$ **Redermic + Intensive Daily Anti-Wrinkle/Firming Fill-In Care Dry Skin** *($53.95 for 1.35 fl. oz.)* is very similar to La Roche-Posay's Redermic + Eyes Intensive Daily Anti-Wrinkle/Firming Fill-In Care above, proving once again that facial moisturizers rarely differ from their eye cream counterparts.

☺ GOOD $$$ **Redermic + Intensive Daily Anti-Wrinkle/Firming Fill-In Care Normal to Combination Skin** *($53.95 for 1.35 fl. oz.)* is very similar to La Roche-Posay's Redermic + Eyes Intensive Daily Anti-Wrinkle/Firming Fill-In Care above, proving once again that facial moisturizers rarely differ from their eye cream counterparts. This formula adds emollient shea butter and some mineral oil to the mix, so it's a better choice for dry skin (not combination skin, as this is too emollient) anywhere on the face, and it also has fragrance whereas the eye cream version is fragrance free (skin anywhere on the face does better without fragrance because fragrance isn't skin care). Otherwise, the same comments apply.

☺ GOOD $$$ **Redermic + UV SPF 25** *($53.95 for 1.35 fl. oz.)*. Two of the highlights for this product are the over-the-top claims and the over-the-top price that may discourage liberal application of this very good moisturizing sunscreen for normal to oily or combination skin. It's formulated with a decent amount of vitamin C and a novel ingredient with a minor study showing it has benefit for skin. Like any well-formulated sunscreen with avobenzone (or other UVA-protecting ingredients), this will improve wrinkling and prevent collagen and elastin breakdown. That is one of the brilliant results from wearing a well-formulated sunscreen on a daily basis. With the 5% ascorbic acid it contains you are also getting a very good dose of an inexpensive form of vitamin C, which adds excellent antioxidant protection for skin.

However, as helpful as a large amount of vitamin C can be for skin, an array of antioxidants and skin-repairing ingredients would have been better. A cocktail approach with these types of ingredients is always better than a "single shot." An interesting aspect of this formulation is that it contains an ingredient called madecassoside, a component of *Centella asiatica*, also known as the gotu kola. There is one formal study showing it to have antioxidant and cell-communicating properties, as it improved skin cell formation, but this study was all about oral consumption at high doses, not a tiny amount applied topically to skin. Still, in all likelihood it's a good antioxidant and a welcome addition to this formulation.

☺ AVERAGE **Anthelios 40 Sunscreen Cream SPF 40** *($34.90 for 1.7 fl. oz.)* is an incredibly mundane daytime moisturizer with sunscreen; the best part about this product is that the UVA range is more than covered because it contains avobenzone and ecamsule, also known as Mexoryl SX. L'Oreal continues to hold the patent on Mexoryl, which is why only their brands (of which La Roche-Posay is one) can use it. The base formula is as bland as all the company's other sunscreens with Mexoryl SX, but this is an OK option for normal to slightly dry or slightly oily skin.

☺ AVERAGE **Effaclar M Daily Mattifying Moisturizer** *($30.95 for 1.35 fl. oz.)* is a lightweight moisturizer with mattifying properties that contains a small amount of dry finish silicones, but the matte finish you'll get is short-lived due to the amount of glycerin and the thickener isocetyl stearate. The amount of alcohol in this product is borderline for causing irritation. La Roche-Posay maintains that this exfoliates skin with something they refer to as LHA, but nothing on the ingredient list matches that acronym. This contains a form of salicylic acid, but not in an amount considered effective, so don't expect any exfoliation from this merely average product. By the way, given that La Roche-Posay prides itself on being a product line for someone with sensitive skin, the number of potentially risky ingredients is embarrassing, including fragrance, acrylamide/sodium acryloyldimethyltaurate copolymer, and polymethyl methacrylate.

☺ AVERAGE **Hydraphase Intense Light Facial Moisturizer** *($32.50 for 1.69 fl. oz.)* is described as "intense" and "light" but that seems contradictory looking at the ingredient list. This water-based lotion contains a heavier ("intense") thickening agent followed by lightweight slip agents and alcohol. Unfortunately, the type of alcohol used is the kind that causes irritation that hurts skin's ability to look and act younger, but the amount is likely too low to be a serious problem. What's most disappointing is how ordinary this moisturizer is. The price isn't bad but without question you can spend less and have your choice of superior moisturizers. It's an OK option for normal to slightly dry skin, but all skin types deserve better than "OK."

☺ AVERAGE **Hydraphase Intense Riche** *($34.95 for 1.69 fl. oz.)*. The description for this product states that it reinforces "your cellular cohesion to water, so your skin stays hydrated all day long." That's an incredibly fancy way to say that this product puts a layer of emollients over skin. Shea butter, silicone, mineral oil, and urea work to prevent water loss, which is great but hardly unique to this moisturizer. Too bad the rest of the formula isn't as fancy as the claim. This adds up to a very rich moisturizer for very dry skin but it is really a basic, merely adequate cream that would have been better with antioxidants and far more skin-repairing ingredients. It would have also been helpful to leave out the fragrance, especially for compromised skin. If you have very dry skin, this is definitely worth a consideration but be sure to pair it with a serum that is loaded with state-of-the-art beneficial ingredients for the best skin care possible.

☺ AVERAGE $$$ **Rosaliac AR Intense Localized Redness Intensive Serum** *($39.95 for 1.35 fl. oz.)* is an underwhelming, utterly mundane formulation with a potentially sticky combination of water, glycerin, and film former (think hairspray). The only possibly worthwhile ingredient is a plant extract called *Tambourissa trichophylla*. There is no published research showing it has any anti-inflammatory properties whatsoever. In fact the only information comes from the ingredient manufacturer who sells lots of ingredients with all kinds of miraculous claims. Talk about believing your own fantasies! There are so many proven anti inflammatory and skin-healing ingredients those with rosacea or sensitive skin should be using, it just doesn't make sense to waste your money on a single plant extract with sketchy proof of efficacy. Skin is a complex organ and the causes of rosacea are complex, not to mention skin also needs anti-aging and cell renewal ingredients. This one-note product is off key at best.

☺ AVERAGE **Rosaliac Skin Perfecting Anti-Redness Moisturizer** (*$36.95 for 1.35 fl. oz.*) is said to neutralize redness while calming and soothing inflamed skin. It does have a mint green color, but that has minimal to no effect on reducing or covering facial redness of any kind. A sheer foundation or tinted moisturizer with real skin-tone shades would do a better job of softening skin's reddened appearance. Overall, this is a simply formulated, fragrance-free moisturizer for normal to slightly dry skin. It's just not the solution or even a great option for someone with rosacea. Anyone dealing with rosacea is likely aware that it is wise to avoid topical irritants, especially since many cases of rosacea react to various seemingly benign ingredients with no rhyme or reason. It is, therefore, best to shop for skin-care products without known irritants or potentially "active" ingredients, particularly when they're intended to be left on the skin. In the case of this product, it does not make sense to include alcohol, caffeine, and niacinamide. Alcohol and caffeine have irritant properties, while niacinamide is derived from niacin, which, although it can be beneficial, has the potential to cause facial flushing—not what someone with reddened skin needs.

☺ AVERAGE **Toleriane Fluide, Soothing Protective Non-Oily Emulsion** (*$29.95 for 1.35 fl. oz.*) is an average, fragrance-free moisturizer for normal to dry skin not prone to blemishes. Given the simplicity of the formula, this may indeed be a good option for those dealing with rosacea and the sensitivity it entails; it's just so no-frills, we couldn't rate it higher.

☺ AVERAGE **Toleriane Riche, Soothing Protective Cream** (*$27.95 for 1.35 fl. oz.*) is viewed as a simple fragrance-free formula for sensitive skin that is worth considering, but overall it is just completely ordinary and not worth the price tag in the least. There isn't one state-of-the-art ingredient and it contains aluminum starch octenylsuccinate, a drying ingredient that isn't the best for sensitive skin. For the money, the company should have at least included one antioxidant or skin-identical ingredient!

☺ AVERAGE **Toleriane Soothing Protective Skincare** (*$27.95 for 1.35 fl. oz.*) is a very basic, fragrance-free moisturizing lotion for normal to slightly dry skin. It does not contain a single anti-irritant or antioxidant, so it ends up being neither protective nor any more soothing than any other ordinary moisturizer.

☺ AVERAGE **$$$ Derm AOX Intense Anti-Wrinkle Radiance Serum** (*$59.95 for 1 fl. oz.*). This water-based serum contains some intriguing anti-aging ingredients but it cannot slow the aging process as claimed. No skin-care product can truly stop the clock, but lots of them can help your skin function in a younger, healthier manner. Overall this serum falls into the same trap many others do, which is spotlighting one or two ingredients as being the best when research doesn't show that to be the case. This time the ingredients du jour are carnosine

---

⬛ Buying skin-care products packaged in jars? See the Appendix to learn why that's a bad idea.

and pycnogenol, an antioxidant derived from a species of pine tree. Both have value for skin, but neither is the end all, be all when it comes to anti-aging. Carnosine is composed of amino acids and, when it comes to wrinkles, it is believed to help reduce glycation in skin. Glycation involves the bonding of a sugar molecule with a protein (such as collagen) or fat. When glycation occurs in our skin, the by-products it generates can weaken or destroy collagen, leading to more wrinkles. There is in vitro research showing that carnosine, when introduced to cells that generate collagen, can help mitigate the damaging effects of glycation (Sources: *Journal de la Societe de Biologie*, volume 201, 2007, pages 185-188; and *Pathologie-biologie*, September 2006, pages 396-404) due to its antioxidant action, but that would be true of any potent antioxidant that shows up in skin-care products. Given that half of the beneficial ingredients in this serum are listed after the preservative, this doesn't end up being one of the better serums available.

☺ AVERAGE $$$ **Hydraphase UV Eyes Hydrating Protective Eye Cream SPF 29** *($32.95 for 0.5 fl. oz.)* is unsuitable for sensitive skin around the eyes. The SPF rating is impressive, but the actives combine titanium dioxide (great for use around the eyes) with a synthetic sunscreen, which can be problematic when used so close to the eyes. As for the base formula, it's surprisingly bland, and the amount of alcohol is potential cause for concern because alcohol causes free-radical damage (see the Appendix for details). Given the lack of important anti-aging ingredients, such as antioxidants and barrier repair substances, this is just a boring formulation. It does contain mica for shine, but shine isn't skin care. In short, this isn't a wise choice for "fragile eyes" or for anyone with dry skin around the eyes. The formula falls short when it comes to providing the type of ingredients dry skin needs to repair itself and become more resilient. Refer to the Appendix to find out why, in truth, you don't need an eye cream.

☹ AVERAGE $$$ **Redermic [R] Anti-Aging Dermatological Treatment, Intensive** *($55.95 for 1 fl. oz.)* is a good, though fairly basic, moisturizer with retinol. Best for normal to dry skin, it contains retinol along with a fatty acid form of vitamin A (retinyl linoleate) and the cell-communicating ingredient adenoside. It isn't all that intensive and the fact that it contains fragrance isn't the best (and makes the company's "safe for sensitive skin" claim dubious). Another strike against this pricey product is that it lacks a range of antioxidants and repairing products to improve skin in multiple ways. If all you want is retinol in a moisturizing base this fits the bill, but you can find better moisturizers and serums with retinol for the same amount (or less) of money.

☺ AVERAGE $$$ **Rosaliac UV Fortifying Anti-Redness Moisturizer SPF 15** *($37.95 for 1.35 fl. oz.)* claims to be anti-redness and yet contains sunscreen actives that have sensitizing potential and that can cause redness. We have no idea why La Roche-Posay didn't formulate this daytime moisturizer with only mineral sunscreen ingredients of titanium dioxide or zinc oxide. Anyone with sensitive, reddened skin should look to those actives for sun protection because they don't cause irritation of any kind and won't make redness worse. This contains stabilized avobenzone for reliable UVA protection, which is great, but not for sensitive skin. Niacinamide and a small amount of vitamin C are on hand, but neither is noteworthy for reducing redness: Where are the proven soothing agents? And another question: Why did La Roche-Posay add coloring agents? Presumably, it was to make this product appear soothing ("Look, its soft blue tint tells me it's calming!"), but your skin will do much better with ingredients that really are soothing!

☺ AVERAGE $$$ **Substiane** *($54.95 for 1.35 fl. oz.)* makes a big deal about the amount of Pro-Xylane it contains, but what exactly is this Pro-Xylane complex? L'Oreal (La Roche-Posay's owner) includes it in several of their products as well as in their Lancome Absolue line, but not the 5% amount that's being hyped with this product. Suffice it to say, Pro Xylane is not an essential ingredient for skin, mature or not. It certainly isn't a worthy stand-in for retinoids, which is what it's often compared to! Substiane ends up being little more than a good emollient moisturizer for normal to dry skin not prone to blemishes. It does contain the amino acids serine and arginine as claimed, but not in any amount that's likely to have a specific or noticeable effect on skin.

LA ROCHE-POSAY SUN CARE

☺ GOOD **Anthelios 50 Mineral Ultra Light Sunscreen Fluid, SPF 50 Face** (*$32.95 for 1.7 fl. oz.*) lists titanium dioxide as its sole active ingredient, so it provides reliable broad-spectrum sun protection. The fact that it's also fragrance-free makes it a gentle option for those with sensitive or rosacea-affected skin, too. Sensitive or not, if you have normal to oily skin, you'll likely appreciate this product's thin, fluid texture and lightweight matte finish. It is definitely an intriguing option for those who find that most SPF-rated products feel too heavy or leave their skin shiny. We wish the formula contained more than a trace amount of vitamin E (tocopherol) for antioxidant benefits. Research is clear that combining antioxidants with sunscreen gives skin a significant environmental boost and helps further offset the damaging effects of UV light. Note: The amount of titanium dioxide in this product makes it a tricky option for those with breakout-prone skin; that is, the titanium dioxide may make matters worse. Unfortunately, the only way to know for sure is to experiment and see how your skin responds. Second note: Those who prefer a sunscreen with a sheer tint may want to consider SkinCeuticals Physical Fusion UV Defense SPF 50, whose texture and other attributes are similar to those of this La Roche-Posay product (both SkinCeuticals and La Roche-Posay are owned by L'Oreal).

☺ GOOD **Anthelios 60 Melt-In Sunscreen Lotion** (*$29.95 for 1.7 fl. oz.*) is a lightweight, matte-finish lotion claiming that it contains powerful antioxidants. It's interesting that La Roche-Posay's Anthelios 60 sunscreens do not contain Mexoryl SX (ecamsule), the UVA-protecting active ingredient that their parent company, L'Oreal, has the patent on. Instead, Anthelios 60 contains avobenzone for UVA protection. It does contain antioxidants, but only two—vitamin E and *Cassia alata* leaf—and they are barely present. This daytime moisturizer with sunscreen provides broad-spectrum protection and has a texture that those with normal to very oily skin will appreciate, but it doesn't "walk the talk" when it comes to providing a superior antioxidant boost.

☹ AVERAGE $$$ **Anthelios 60 Melt-In Sunscreen Milk** (*$35.50 for 5 fl. oz.*) is very similar to the Anthelios 60 Melt-In Sunscreen Lotion above, and the same review applies.

☹ POOR **Anthelios 45 Ultra Light Sunscreen Fluid for Body** (*$35.95 for 4.2 fl. oz.*). At one point, the Anthelios sunscreens from La Roche-Posay were all about the UVA sunscreen ecamsule, better known as Mexoryl SX. This sunscreen skips the ecamsule and provides UVA protection with avobenzone. That's fine, but what's interesting is that not too long ago, L'Oreal, the company that owns La Roche-Posay, was denigrating avobenzone in favor of Mexoryl SX! Why they're now using avobenzone is a mystery, but as far as this sunscreen is concerned, it's an overall dud. The base formula contains too much alcohol, which causes free-radical damage, dryness, and irritation, and too little of the beneficial extras (like antioxidants) you should be looking for in sunscreens. You'll get broad-spectrum sun protection, but that's about it. There are far too many sunscreens available that do not contain alcohol and that do contain antioxidants for you to consider this poor contender.

⊗ POOR **Anthelios 45 Ultra Light Sunscreen Fluid for Face** *($29.95 for 1.7 fl. oz.)* is nearly identical to the Anthelios 45 Ultra Light Sunscreen Fluid for Body above, and the same review applies.

⊗ POOR **Anthelios 60 Ultra Light Sunscreen Fluid** *($29.95 for 1.7 fl. oz.)* has the same active ingredients and percentages as the Anthelios 60 Melt-In Sunscreen Lotion above, but the base formula is different. UVA protection is assured from avobenzone, but the amount of alcohol in the base formula is cause for concern (alcohol causes free-radical damage and cell death). The big claim about this sunscreen is how its potent antioxidants provide additional protection for sun-exposed skin. Antioxidants can boost a sunscreen's effectiveness and help skin defend itself better against environmental damage, but not in the paltry amounts present in this product—and not with alcohol being so high up on the ingredient list. How disappointing!

LA ROCHE-POSAY LIP CARE

✓☺ BEST **Ceralip Lip Repair Cream** *($17.95 for 0.51 fl. oz.)* is a sufficiently creamy lip moisturizer that differs from the usual wax-based sticks or oil–based balms. It is definitely an option for dry lips, and is fragrance- and flavor-free.

⊗ POOR **Nutritic Lips** *($15.95 for 0.15 fl. oz.)* is a lip balm in stick form that contains a very good blend of emollients, waxes, and oils to protect and soften lips. Unfortunately, this also contains coriander oil, a fragrant oil that can cause contact dermatitis and photosensitivity (Source: naturaldatabase.com). Given that this lip balm doesn't contain sunscreen, it is risky to wear during daylight hours, and the potential for irritation is too high to make it worth considering over several other lip moisturizers.

LA ROCHE-POSAY SPECIALTY SKIN-CARE PRODUCTS

✓☺ BEST $$$ **Effaclar Duo Dual Action Acne Treatment** *($36.95 for 1.35 fl. oz.)* is an anti-acne product that earns its stripes, containing an effective amount of the topical disinfectant benzoyl peroxide in a fragrance-free lotion formula that contains antioxidant vitamin E and a good anti-irritant to help reduce redness from blemishes. Although pricey (there are definitely cheaper options with great formulations), it should help clear breakouts without leaving skin dry or flaky. The claims mention 0.4% micro-exfoliating LHA, which is listed as capryloyl salicylic acid. The only study on this ingredient's benefits comes from L'Oreal, the company that owns La Roche-Posay. Interestingly, their study had nothing to do with acne; rather, it compared the effects of relatively low concentrations of LHA with the effects of relatively high concentrations of AHAs (that is, the concentrations dermatologists or aestheticians use in performing AHA peels), not to the effects of AHAs at the concentrations found in skin-care products (talk about comparing apples to oranges!). There isn't any research proving LHA helps heal breakouts or somehow improves clogged pores. If you decide to try this product (keeping in mind that companies such as Clearasil, Paula's Choice, and Clinique offer less expensive, equally effective options), it is best to use it with a well-formulated BHA exfoliant, which should be applied first.

☺ GOOD $$$ **Effaclar AI Intensive Acne Spot Treatment** *($29.90 for 0.5 fl. oz.)* claims to be the first such product to blend benzoyl peroxide and salicylic acid in a single product, but that isn't what they've created. As much as we agree that it would be a convenience, there are formulary drawbacks that prevent such a marriage from being harmonious. The reasons come down to pH and stability. We know that for salicylic acid to be an effective exfoliant, the pH should be between 3-4. In contrast, according to several cosmetics chemists we've questioned, benzoyl peroxide requires a higher pH (typically around 5.5) to remain stable and maintain its efficacy. La Roche-Posay must know this, too, because the sole active ingredient in this product is 5.5% benzoyl peroxide, and the pH is just above 5. Salicylic acid is not on the active list and the form of salicylic acid they included is not the anti-acne form recognized by the FDA or Health Canada monographs. That means this is a good topical disinfectant for acne, but not a unique 2-in-1 product for those struggling with breakouts. The price ends up being absurd for what you get, as there are many well-formulated benzoyl peroxide products that cost a fraction of what this does. It is fragrance-free and it doesn't contain unneeded irritants, which is nice, but not unique.

☹ POOR **Mela-D Dark Spots SPF 15** *($51.95 for 1 fl. oz.)* includes avobenzone for UVA protection, but the base formula contains enough alcohol to cause irritation and free-radical damage for all skin types. Moreover, the amount of kojic acid is likely too low to affect skin discolorations. Daily sun protection is a key element of keeping discolorations related to sun damage from recurring or getting worse, but this product isn't a sound way to go about doing that, there are far better options for a lot less money.

☹ POOR **Mela-D Serum Anti-Dark Spot Concentrate** *($57.95 for 1 fl. oz.)* lists alcohol as the second ingredient in this serum, which makes it too drying and irritating for all skin types, not to mention the free-radical damage and cell death that alcohol causes. The amount of glycolic acid included could potentially exfoliate, but because this product contains the alkaline ingredient potassium hydroxide, the pH isn't anywhere near where it must be for efficacy. As for the kojic acid as a lightening agent, it is an option, but there are others (e.g., hydroquinone, niacinamide, and vitamin C) that have better track records. If you want to give kojic acid a try, this isn't the product to consider; instead, try Jan Marini Skin Research's Bioglycolic Lightening Gel (the Marini line is reviewed on CosmeticsCop.com). Keep in mind, however, that kojic acid is an exceptionally unstable ingredient and has some research showing it to have a negative cellular effect.

☹ POOR **Mela-D Pigment Control Concentrated Dark-Spot Correcting Serum** *($49.95 for 1.01 fl. oz.)* has the same formulary concerns as the Mela-D Serum Anti-Dark Spot Corrector above, and the same comments apply.

LANCOME

Strengths: Some good cleansers; well-formulated scrubs; almost all the sunscreens contain either avobenzone, ecamsule (Mexoryl SX), or titanium dioxide for sufficient UVA protection; large selection of self-tanning products; several excellent foundations with beautiful shades for almost every skin color; some great concealers; mostly outstanding mascaras; the Absolue powder; the liquid eyeliner; all the powder eyeshadows; some fantastic lipsticks and automatic lipliner.

Weaknesses: Expensive for what amounts to mostly mediocre to below-average skin care; no AHA or BHA products; no products to effectively treat blemishes or lighten skin discolorations; average toners; moisturizers that are short on including state-of-the-art ingredients; jar packaging; a few of the foundations with sunscreen do not provide complete UVA protection; average powder blush, eye pencils, and long-wearing lip color; relatively unimpressive makeup brushes.

For more information and reviews of the latest Lancome products, visit CosmeticsCop.com.

LANCOME CLEANSERS

☺ GOOD $$$ **Creme Mousse Confort, Comforting Creamy Foaming Cleanser** *($25 for 4.2 fl. oz.)* is a very good, creamy-feeling foaming cleanser for normal to dry skin. It works swiftly to completely remove makeup and rinses well without the need for a washcloth. This would be rated higher if it did not contain potentially irritating fragrance ingredients (of which there are many).

☺ GOOD $$$ **Galatee Confort Comforting Milky Creme Cleanser** ($48 for 6.8 fl. oz.) remains a standard, creamy cleanser for dry to very dry skin. It does not rinse without the aid of a washcloth, and is not for anyone with blemishes, however small. The amount of fragrant components demands complete removal from skin lest you risk irritation.

☺ AVERAGE $$$ **Absolue Premium Bx Advanced Creamy Foam Cleanser** ($52 for 4.3 fl. oz.) has an outrageous price, even if this cleanser's formula were "premium" as the name states; also the formula is boring and antiquated. All you're getting is a standard water-soluble foaming cleanser that is a barely passable option for normal to oily skin. This is a poor choice for dry skin because the formula lacks conditioning agents that help buffer dry skin during the cleansing process.

☹ AVERAGE $$$ **Absolue Premium Bx Advanced Replenishing Cream Cleanser** ($62 for 6.7 fl. oz.) is an absurdly expensive, completely ordinary cleansing cream that leaves us nearly speechless (well, not completely). It is beyond standard and ends up being a completely antiquated mix of water and mineral oil. Though an option for dry to very dry skin, this is just cold cream (think Pond's Cold Cream). How Lancome has the audacity to claim that it "sets a new standard in age-targeted skincare" is just obnoxious. First, if this is a new standard then so is paper. Yes, it will remove makeup, but not without leaving a greasy film, just like any cold cream. The amount of wild yam isn't enough to feed a flea at Thanksgiving, and the fragrance ingredients (which will be left on your skin because this cream doesn't rinse easily) can cause irritation.

☺ AVERAGE $$$ **Creme Radiance Clarifying Cream-to-Foam Cleanser for Normal/ Combination Skin** ($25 for 4.2 fl. oz.) is a glycerin-based cleanser with a rich, thick texture that softens and produces copious foam when mixed with water. Although the texture is luxurious, some of the ingredients that create it and supply the foam are needlessly drying for all skin types. Of particular concern is the amount of potassium hydroxide, which is typically seen in traditional soaps. Another strike against this cleanser is its intense fragrance and numerous fragrance ingredients known to cause irritation. Such ingredients are less of a risk for skin in a rinse-off product like this, but using heavily fragranced cleansers around your eyes (which you'll do if you wear eye makeup) remains a problem. Considering the price and formulary issues, this isn't a cleanser we can strongly recommend. If you prefer a foaming, creamy cleanser, you may wish to consider CeraVe Foaming Facial Cleanser, available in most major drugstores (and sold for a lot less than Lancome's version) or Paula's Choice Skin Balancing Oil-Reducing Cleanser.

☹ AVERAGE $$$ **Gel Radiance Clarifying Gel-to-Foam Cleanser Normal, Combination Skin** ($25 for 4.2 fl. oz.) is a decent, though exceedingly overpriced, water-soluble cleanser for normal to oily or combination skin. The formula's problem is the intense amount of fragrance. Much of the fragrance comes from citrus-based plant extracts that can cause irritation and that are especially a problem for use around your eyes. (Just think how much a drop of lemon or orange juice stings when you get it in your eye.) Although this removes makeup and rinses easily, your skin (and budget) will benefit more from a gentle, fragrance-free (or at least minimally fragranced) cleanser.

☺ AVERAGE $$$ **Mousse Radiance Clarifying Self-Foaming Cleanser Normal, Combination Skin** ($32 for 6.8 fl. oz.) is a standard, water-to-foam cleanser that's an OK option for normal to oily or combination skin just like in Lancome's Gel Radiance Clarifying Gel-to-Foam Cleanser.

☺ AVERAGE $$$ **Secret De Vie Precious Reviving Creme Cleanser** *($55 for 4.2 fl. oz.)* ranks as one of the most expensive cold cream–style cleansers you're likely to find. Although this is an indulgent option for dry to very dry skin and it liquefies with water to a cleansing lotion texture (and it will remove most types of makeup), it does not rinse well without the aid of a washcloth.

☹ POOR **Creme Douceur Cream-to-Oil Massage Cleanser All Skin Types** *($25 for 4.2 fl. oz.)* is a liquid cleanser that begins oily and morphs into a milky emulsion when mixed with water during the cleansing process. It removes surface debris and makeup, but the amount of alcohol and the amount of the fragrance ingredient p-anisic acid is cause for concern; this also contains other fragrance ingredients. When it's time to take off your makeup, it's much kinder to skin to use a fragrance-free silicone- or oil–based makeup remover.

☹ POOR **Gel Pure Focus, Oil Control Cleansing Gel for Oily Skin** *($26 for 4.2 fl. oz.)* is a water-soluble cleanser with too many strikes against it to make it worth considering over dozens of others, most of which cost considerably less. The alcohol content, the amount of fragrance, and the inclusion of the irritating menthol derivative menthoxypropanediol are all cause for concern and provide ample reasons to ignore this cleanser. It will not tighten or refine pores, nor does it deeply cleanse the skin.

LANCOME EYE-MAKEUP REMOVERS

☺ GOOD $$$ **Bi-Facil, Double-Action Eye Makeup Remover** *($27 for 4.2 fl. oz.)* is a good water- and silicone-based makeup remover that would be rated higher if it were fragrance-free and left out the questionable preservative quaternium-15. Still, this works well to quickly remove stubborn and waterproof makeup.

☺ AVERAGE $$$ **Effacil, Gentle Eye Makeup Remover** *($27 for 4.2 fl. oz.)* is not gentle due to the amount of detergents and fragrance it contains. It's essentially a watered-down water-soluble cleanser, and not really worth adding to your routine unless you're a soap devotee.

LANCOME TONERS

☺ GOOD $$$ **Tonique Confort, Comforting Rehydrating Toner, for Normal to Dry Skin** *($25 for 6.8 fl. oz.)* is a very good toner for its intended skin type. It contains plenty of water-binding agents, plant oil, and antioxidant vitamin E, all in stable packaging.

☺ AVERAGE $$$ **Absolue Premium Bx Advanced Replenishing Toner** *($52 for 5 fl. oz.)* is one of Lancome's better toners for normal to dry skin. However, given their track record with toners, that's not exactly high praise—especially given the price tag! For what Lancome is charging, this toner should be overflowing with beneficial ingredients such as antioxidants, skin-healing ingredients, and cell communicating ingredients. As is, you're getting an alcohol free blend of slip agents with a tiny amount of antioxidants and one cell-communicating ingredient. This toner also contains fragrance ingredients known to cause irritation, another reason to think twice before considering it. Although not present in large amounts, their potential for irritation isn't something to ignore, especially knowing that ongoing irritation hurts your skin's ability to heal and limits its ability to produce healthy collagen. Please see our list of Best Toners at the end of this book for examples of superior (and less expensive) formulas.

☺ AVERAGE $$$ **Secret De Vie Precious Reviving Toner** *($60 for 5 fl. oz.)* ends up being a very boring toner for the money, serving normal to dry skin with mostly water, slip agents, alcohol, and mineral pigments that provide shimmer to this liquid. This does not contain hyaluronic acid as claimed; rather, it contains a teeny-tiny amount of the salt form of this ingredient, which costs significantly less than pure hyaluronic acid and doesn't work quite the same (especially given the cost of this product, they should have used the real thing).

☺ AVERAGE $$$ **Tonique Douceur, Alcohol-Free Freshener** *($39.50 for 6.8 fl. oz.)* is mostly water, glycerin, and rose water. This product is basic and minimally effective for normal to dry skin, unless your only objective is to use a toner to remove the last traces of makeup (yet a really well-formulated toner can do so much more).

☹ POOR **Pure Focus Pore Tightening Toner with Matifying Powders** *($24.50 for 6.8 fl. oz.)* lists alcohol as the second ingredient and contains the potent menthol derivative menthoxypropanediol. The focus is purely on irritation here and the alcohol will stimulate oil production in the pore. See the Appendix for further details on why alcohol and irritation are so bad for oily skin.

LANCOME EXFOLIANT & SCRUBS

☺ GOOD $$$ **Exfoliance Confort Comforting Exfoliating Cream** *($25 for 3.4 fl. oz.)* is a rich, creamy topical scrub for dry to very dry skin. It contains polyethylene as the abrasive agent, which is great. The only drawback is that the emollients and silicone don't rinse well from skin, so you may need to use this with a washcloth, which exfoliates too (so why use the scrub at all?).

☺ GOOD $$$ **Pure Focus Deep Pore Refining Scrub with Purifying Micro-Beads** *($26 for 3.4 fl. oz.)* is a gel-based scrub that contains polyethylene (plastic) as the abrasive agent. The small amount of detergent cleansing agents makes this a good choice for normal to oily skin, though if breakouts are present, you should be exfoliating with a BHA product, not a scrub.

LANCOME MOISTURIZERS (DAYTIME & NIGHTTIME), EYE CREAMS, & SERUMS

☺ GOOD $$$ **Bienfait Multi-Vital SPF 30 Lotion** *($45 for 1.7 fl. oz.)* would rate higher if not for the many volatile fragrant components. Although these aren't predominant, they're a potential cause for concern and don't add anything helpful to this in-part avobenzone sunscreen. The base formula is antioxidant-rich and stably packaged, two uncommon traits for a Lancome product. This is still appropriate for normal to oily skin.

☺ AVERAGE $$$ **Nutrix, Soothing Treatment Cream, for Dry to Very Dry/Sensitive Skin** *($48 for 1.9 fl. oz.)*. First launched in 1936, this remains a very good, though basic, moisturizer for very dry skin. The fragrant components (and fragrance itself) are not suitable for sensitive skin. Two forms of lecithin are nice for skin, but skin needs more and, when you think about it, you wouldn't now be using just about anything that was made in 1936, from a washing machine to a typewriter (and TVs and microwaves weren't even invented).

☺ AVERAGE **Aqua Fusion Cream, Continuous Infusing Moisturizer** *($38.50 for 1.7 fl. oz.)* contains more coloring agent than anything exciting for skin, though at least the price isn't too out-of-line. The amino acids and minerals are but a dusting, leaving this as an average, jar-packaged moisturizer for normal to slightly dry skin.

☺ AVERAGE **Secret de Vie Night Ultimate Cellular Reviving Night Creme** *($275 for 1.7 fl. oz.)* has claims that are mere cosmetics puffery with no real meaning, and in no way does this product prompt "cellular rebirth" at night. It is nothing short of shocking that the cosmetics industry can successfully convince women to fork over almost $300 for a product like this. We suppose such grandiose claims are needed to justify this moisturizer's obnoxious price, but please don't fall for them. All you're getting for your money are standard cosmetic ingredients that show up in most other moisturizers that Lancome and parent company L'Oreal sell. Even more shocking is that it contains more coloring agents, lye, and preservatives than helpful ingredients for skin. As for the black tea, it would have antioxidant potential if Lancome hadn't packaged this moisturizer in a jar, but otherwise, this is a serious mistake, for both your skin and your budget. See the Appendix to learn why jar packaging is a problem.

☺ AVERAGE $$$ **Absolue Eye Precious Cells Advanced Regenerating and Reconstructing Eye Cream** *($108 for 0.5 fl. oz.)* contains the same basic, ordinary ingredients as most Lancome eye creams, but this one comes with a new claim, although not with a new formula. Absolue Eye Precious is being sold as having the ability to "improve the condition around stem cells." How the same ingredients can now perform such a lofty function is nothing short of marketing spin. In reality, there are more synthetic coloring agents and shiny pigments in this eye cream than ingredients that could influence stem cells, or any cells, for the better. From a formulary point of view, Lancome is using plant stem cells from a species of apple tree that is reputed to be being capable of regenerating itself when needed (and, of course, they want you to believe that if it works for a plant, then it should work for human skin). Their hypothesis is that these plant stem cells can stimulate human cells to regenerate, despite the fact there isn't a shred of research showing this to be the case. Even if there were some remote possibility that plant stem cells could affect human skin, the fact is that stem cells of any kind can have an impact only when they are alive, and if they are added to a cosmetic they will be long dead by the time the product gets to the store. Taking it a step further, this comes in jar packaging, which wouldn't keep anything stable long enough to help skin over the long term; plus, the amount of alcohol in here would kill stem cells off in a heartbeat. The only thing reconstructing about this cream is the change in the pseudo-reality Lancome is trying to spin.

☺ AVERAGE $$$ **Absolue Eye Premium Bx, Absolute Replenishing Eye Cream** *($93 for 0.5 fl. oz.)* is said to combine two advanced discoveries: Lancome's patented Pro-Xylane and their "intensely replenishing" Bio-Network. According to a report on happi.com (the Household and Personal Products Industry magazine website), Pro-Xylane is derived from xylose, a type of sugar that has water-binding properties for skin. L'Oreal Senior Vice President Alan Meyers reported that in vitro skin tests and testing on human skin showed that their Pro-Xylane complex stimulated the production of glycosaminoglycans in the skin. Glycosaminoglycans are one part of the intricate network that makes up the skin's intercellular matrix. Topical application of substances that mimic what's found in skin's intercellular matrix does help reinforce the skin's barrier function, thus allowing the intercellular matrix to function normally. L'Oreal (Lancome's parent company) may be convinced that Pro-Xylane has some wonderful effect on skin, but lots of other ingredients can do the same thing, and as it turns out, this product doesn't contain all that much Pro-Xylane. Moreover the tiny amount of Lancome's Bio-Network—consisting of soy, wild yam, sea algae, and barley—won't have the slightest rejuvenating effect on skin or counteract changes in skin that result from menopause. As is true for many of Lancome's skin-care products, this is yet another lackluster moisturizer. There's more titanium dioxide, mica, and iron oxides (all mineral pigments that are included in this product to create a radiant glow, which is strictly a cosmetic effect) than anything that could be considered innovative or of "premium" benefit for your skin, and the price for such a mundane formula has everything to do with market positioning and not real, revolutionary results.

☺ AVERAGE $$$ **Absolue Night Precious Cells Advanced Regenerating and Reconstructing Night Cream** *($155 for 1.7 fl. oz.)* costs way too much for what amounts to an average formula for normal to dry skin. The main ingredients are practically a who's who of ordinary moisturizing agents, including mineral oil, aluminum starch, synthetic coloring agents, and lye. There are more of these ingredients than anything one might think of as state-of-the-art. The price is ludicrous for what you get. See the review of Absolue Eye Precious Cells Advanced Regenerating and Reconstructing Eye Cream above for a discussion of plant stem cells in skin-care products.

☺ AVERAGE $$$ **Absolue Night Premium Bx, Absolute Night Recovery Cream** *($175 for 2.6 fl. oz.)* makes additional claims for the Pro-Xylane, such as that it restores essential moisture deep in the structure of the skin's surface. Talk about something that sounds a lot better than it is! Moreover, lots of ingredients found in other products do the same thing. Actually, there's not much of anything substantial in this moisturizer, given that alcohol, wax, and coloring agents are listed well before anything interesting or even remotely worth the money. This is one to leave on the shelf!

☺ AVERAGE $$$ **Absolue Precious Cells Advanced Regenerating and Reconstructing Cream SPF 15** *($165 for 1.7 fl. oz.)* has a slightly creamy base formula, but doesn't contain anything spectacular for skin, and absolutely nothing that justifies the price. The only anti-aging element of this daytime moisturizer for dry skin is its in-part avobenzone sunscreen. Lancome's Reconstruction Complex is built around the premise that stem cells from a certain species of apple tree can protect stem cells in human skin, thus bringing skin to "a denser quality." There isn't any convincing research proving apple stem cells are the answer for aging skin; it's just one of many so-called answers Lancome promotes given the number of products they sell claiming to be anti-aging. In reality, there are more synthetic coloring agents and Vaseline in this moisturizer than ingredients that could influence stem cells, or any cells, for the better.

☺ AVERAGE $$$ **Absolue Premium Bx, Absolute Replenishing Cream SPF 15** *($140 for 1.7 fl. oz.)* features an in-part avobenzone sunscreen that has a slightly better base formula than the Absolue Premium Bx products reviewed above, but for the money this should be brimming with state-of-the-art ingredients, and it's not. In addition, the effectiveness of the few antioxidants present in this product is diminished by the jar packaging, which is disappointing (see the Appendix for details). Last, if you're considering this for sunscreen (and that's the only anti-aging claim you can bank on), ask yourself how liberally you'll apply a sunscreen that is this expensive. And if you're still not convinced, at least put yourself in front of the Estee Lauder counter because their moisturizers with sunscreen have formulas that are way ahead of those from Lancome and many of them cost a lot less.

☺ AVERAGE $$$ **Absolue Premium Bx, Absolute Replenishing Lotion SPF 15** *($150 for 2.5 fl. oz.)* has an in-part avobenzone sunscreen, and its opaque, pump-bottle packaging will keep the vitamin E (the only antioxidant of note in this product) stable. Those are the positives. The bad news is that alcohol is the fourth ingredient. That isn't terrible, but it isn't what you want to see in a costly product meant to combat the visible signs of aging. Despite all the ballyhoo for Pro-Xylane and the Bio-Network (consisting of algae, soy, and wild yam), these ingredients are barely present. The salicylic acid in this product does not function as an exfoliant.

☺ AVERAGE $$$ **Absolue Ultimate Bx Replenishing and Restructuring Serum** *($155 for 1 fl. oz.)* promises to be a breakthrough for mature skin due to its supposed clarifying power. Those with dull, lackluster skin tones will see radiance returned, but that's due to the mica particles in this product that simply add a soft shine to skin, which is about makeup rather than skin care. Lancome never explains exactly what ingredients comprise their Pro-Xylane complex, but it is supposedly "highly concentrated" in this serum. It could be they're referring to the wild yam, soy, and algae, but these ingredients are barely present (there's much more fragrance than showcased plant extracts), so "highly concentrated" is clearly a marketing concept, not reality.

The only potentially helpful ingredient in the product for possibly "clarifying" skin is kojic acid. Lancome doesn't scrimp on this ingredient, and it is indeed known for inhibiting melanin production. However, it is not considered as efficacious as hydroquinone, especially when the latter is combined with tretinoin. Moreover, other research indicates that kojic acid is not as effective as other potential skin lightening agents (Sources: *Journal of the American Academy of Dermatology*, December 2006, pages 1048–1065; and *The Journal of Biological Chemistry*, May 2002, pages 16340–16344). Kojic acid is also prone to deterioration on exposure to light and air unless it is stably packaged, which is the case with this serum. Although it's rather one-note, this serum has the potential to lighten discolorations. But keep in mind, there are several other options (including prescription hydroquinone products) that stand a greater chance of producing superior results, and for less money. The overall formula of this serum makes it best for normal to slightly dry skin.

☺ AVERAGE $$$ **Absolue Ultimate Night Bx, Intense Night Recovery and Replenishing Serum** (*$165 for 1 fl. oz.*) has a name that is by far the best thing about this serum. Lancome just can't seem to get its anti-aging act together when it comes to creating a state-of-the-art formula that comes close (even a little) to justifying the cost. This serum contains mostly water, slip agents, thickeners, more slip agent, film-forming agents, plant extract, plant oil, and coloring agents. There are more artificial coloring agents in this product than there are the "bio-network" ingredients Lancome calls out on the label. Completely absent are noteworthy antioxidants, skin-identical ingredients, and anti-irritants. In short, anyone looking to spend in this range for a state-of-the-art serum should know that this product competes with others about as well as a rotary-dial telephone would compete with an iPhone. Just about every line surrounding Lancome at the department store offers better serums than they do, and that statement also applies to this lackluster entry.

☺ AVERAGE $$$ **Bienfait Multi-Vital Eyes SPF 28** (*$39 for 0.5 fl. oz.*) is an eye-area sunscreen that includes titanium dioxide for UVA protection, but the sunscreen ingredient octinoxate is not ideal for use in the eye area, which is where you're directed to apply this product. Even if your eye area can tolerate any sunscreen just fine, there is nothing else of benefit for your skin in here. Like many Lancome skin-care products, the really intriguing ingredients are barely present, while the standard cosmetic ingredients are front and center. The amount of mica is enough to lend a soft shimmer, but you can get that effect with other products that provide more for your money than this average mixture.

☺ AVERAGE $$$ **Bienfait Multi-Vital Night, High Potency Night Moisturizing Cream** (*$50 for 1.7 fl. oz.*) makes a big deal out of the vitamins it contains, which are said to help with skin's nightly recovery process. Don't bet on it, because the jar packaging won't keep them stable once this product is in use, and the amount of vitamins is paltry—there's actually more coloring agent. (What would you rather have, a pretty tinted moisturizer or an antioxidant-rich one?) This has the requisite silky, moist texture for normal to dry skin, but that's not enough to justify the price or jibe with the state-of-the-art claims being made for this average moisturizer.

☺ AVERAGE $$$ **Bienfait Multi-Vital SPF 30 Cream** (*$45 for 1.7 fl. oz.*) has avobenzone for sufficient UVA protection, but that's the only highlight of this daytime moisturizer for normal to oily skin. Alcohol is the fourth ingredient, which isn't great but is not abysmal, and the antioxidants are subject to deterioration due to jar packaging (see the Appendix for details). What a shame, because this moisturizer has more antioxidants than Lancome typically offers.

☺ AVERAGE $$$ **Genifique Eye Youth Activating Eye Concentrate** (*$60 for 0.5 fl. oz.*) is the addition to Lancome's Genifique serum that has been a huge hit for the company, proving that lots of women believed the marketing campaign Lancome devised for this over-priced, underwhelming serum. Popularity has never been indicative of quality; just think of how popular cigarette smoking and tanning are. Given their marketing success, however, it's hardly surprising that Lancome now has an eye-area product meant to complement the serum. The salesperson at the Lancome counter told us this is their one eye cream that "does it all," up to and including eliminating dark circles caused by heredity. As for the eye cream itself, it doesn't contain anything that can delete dark circles, whether caused by heredity or by too many sleepless nights. This has a silky texture and a formula that's remarkably similar to that of the Genifique serum, but with the eye cream, you get a smaller amount of product for more money. Also, it's packaged in a jar, so any of the good ingredients, of which there are almost none, won't remain stable. It also contains alcohol, which causes cell death and free-radical damage (see the Appendix for details and to find out why you don't need an eye cream). The sole unique ingredient in this eye cream is bifida ferment lysate, discussed in the review below for Lancome's Genifique Youth Activating Concentrate. This eye cream contains several fragrance ingredients known to cause irritation.

☺ AVERAGE $$$ **Genifique Repair Youth Activating Night Cream** ($98 for 1.7 fl. oz.) is a nighttime moisturizer that contains the same key ingredient found in the other Genifique products, but the base is more emollient and better suited for dry skin. The big question is why consider this product? Despite the gene-repairing claims, the formula for this moisturizer is about as boring as the formula of almost all others that Lancome sells (which also are supposed to renew, repair, and make your skin look younger). It is really shocking how much formulary malaise Lancome's skin-care products suffer from. There is hardly anything in here to extol, and the paltry number of beneficial ingredients will suffer due to the jar packaging because when exposed to air, these ingredients break down and become ineffective for skin (see the Appendix for details). See the review below for Genifique Youth Activating Concentrate for a discussion of the gene-repairing claim this moisturizer makes. In short, Lancome has crafted another anti-aging product whose formula doesn't support its impressive-sounding claims.

☺ AVERAGE $$$ **Genifique Youth Activating Concentrate** ($80 for 1 fl. oz.) is another "first" for Lancome and how many "firsts" can one cosmetics company have? In the case of Lancome, just like most cosmetics companies, a new "first" launches almost every month, and most consumers never notice that once the fervor subsides, there's another "first" ready to take its place. Without question, Lancome did create fervor for this product. We witnessed women lined up at the Lancome counter to try this product, and it wasn't even free-gift-with-purchase time! Aside from advertising there is no reason to be excited or even mildly amused by this lackluster formula (lackluster is the standard Lancome has maintained for some time as it's been years since they launched a truly outstanding or even interesting skin-care product). Lancome's claim for this water-based serum is that it boosts the activity of skin's genes, and by doing so, specific proteins tied to youthful skin are expressed, thus leading to younger-looking skin. Before we discuss the lack of science behind that claim, it's critical to note that Lancome couches every cosmeceutical and drug-like claim for this product in cosmetics-lingo disclaimers. For example, they follow their statement "Lancome invents our first skincare that boosts the activity of genes" with a footnote—that tiny superscript number after the statement. In this footnote at the bottom of the ad is another statement in fine print that reads "Activate skin's youthful look." So they aren't really saying anything about your genes (because that would be a medical claim and really get the ire of the FDA). The more obscure, meaningless claim of "activate skin's youthful look" is far safer, but what does that mean? It could mean whatever the company or the consumer wants it to mean. A bland moisturizer could "activate" a youthful look on dry skin by making it look moist, and that claim could appear on any product. Achieving a youthful look has nothing to do with this product or any effect on skin's genes. Back to the science (which is really complicated but bear with us). It is absolutely true that there are genes in our skin responsible for generating proteins. These proteins create antioxidant pathways that protect skin from intrinsic (internal) and external signs of aging. As we age (actually, as we accumulate more sun damage from years of exposure), these genes become less able to "express" themselves in a healthy manner. That leads to oxidation within the skin and a decreased ability for the gene-generated proteins and enzymes to handle oxidative stress. The result of these deficiencies is damaged collagen, inflammation, and unwanted changes to skin texture, such as roughness, increased sensitivity, and, yes, wrinkles (Sources: *Planta Medica*, October 2008, pages 1548–1559; *Pigment Cell & Melanoma Research*, February 2008, pages 79–88; and *Free Radical Biology & Medicine*, August 2008, pages 385–395). What is Lancome's solution to this issue? A yeast ingredient known as bifida ferment lysate. This same ingredient is the backbone of Estee Lauder's Advanced Night Repair Concentrate Recovery Boosting Treatment, which is overall a significantly better formula. The problem is that there's no research proving that this specific form of yeast has any anti-aging or gene-stimulating activity when applied to skin. There is limited research showing that yeast ferment filtrate (a compound different from bifida ferment lysate) does reduce oxidative skin damage in the presence of UV light, but this research also showed that many other antioxidants have a similar effect (Sources: *Archives of Dermatological Research*, April 2008, pages S51–S56; and *Journal of Dermatological Science*, June 2006, pages 249–257). Lancome says this product took 10 years of research, but given the formula they've created, a high school chemistry student could have done this in six days. Outside of the bifida ferment lysate, you're getting a mix of slip agents with alcohol and a tiny amount of water-binding agent. The rest of the formula is mostly preservatives, fragrance, and fragrance ingredients. The fragrance ingredients can cause irritation and inflammation on their own, which breaks down collagen and is counterproductive to the claims. Irritation will diminish any youth-giving qualities this formula has (which is to say, zero, but still …). The same is true for the amount of alcohol in this product; while the amount is likely too little to be drying or irritating, it is still capable of causing free-radical damage, something the ideal gene-assisting product should strive to reduce. What's so unfortunate is that countless women will believe the hype and go out and waste their money on this half-baked serum. Lancome could've really hit a home run by formulating this with a different type of yeast ferment and joining that with a potent cocktail of antioxidants and no alcohol. As is, you're left with a lightweight serum that will make skin feel smooth, but that offers precious little additional benefit for all skin types.

☺ AVERAGE $$$ **Genifique Youth Activating Cream Serum** ($84 for 1 fl. oz.) is similar to the Genifique Youth Activating Concentrate reviewed above, except this Cream Serum version includes a greater amount of silicone and less skin-damaging alcohol than the Concentrate. Otherwise, the same review applies.

☺ AVERAGE $$$ **High Resolution Collaser-5X Intense Collagen Anti-Wrinkle Serum** ($70 for 1 fl. oz.) is a silky textured, water-based serum with a very small amount of intriguing ingredients, and none of them are capable of pushing wrinkles "up and out" to restore a youthful bounce to aged skin. Lancome tries to impress with claims of ingredients such as coenzyme-R and vitamin C, but much like parent company L'Oreal's overused Pro-Xylane, those are just made up buzzwords. Wouldn't you rather spend your money on a serum with efficacious amounts of proven ingredients? If so, any of the serums from Olay, Paula's Choice, or, if you want to spend more, MD Skincare by Dr. Dennis Gross are distinctly preferred to this. If you're considering this serum, it's best for normal to slightly oily skin. And, of course, using this product inspired by laser technology doesn't at all equate with actually receiving laser or light-emitting treatments for your skin concerns.

☺ AVERAGE $$$ **High Resolution Eye Collaser-5X Intense Collagen Anti-Wrinkle Eye Serum** *($72 for 0.5 fl. oz.)* is a water-based serum for all skin types that doesn't contain a substantial amount of anything that can stimulate collagen production, at least no more so than your average moisturizer. When you protect your skin from sunlight and needless irritants, it is capable of generating new collagen (in a controlled manner) on its own. Lancome's blend of mostly water, silicone, glycerin, plant oil, mineral pigments for shine, and a tiny amount of antioxidant vitamins isn't what we (or modern research) consider an impressive formulation. Compared to the best serums for the eye area of your face, this is merely an average option. See the Appendix to find out why, in truth, you don't need a special serum for the eye area.

☺ AVERAGE $$$ **High Resolution Eye Refill 3X** *($60 for 0.5 fl. oz.)* is supposed to stimulate substances in skin that contribute to its support structure, but this poorly formulated product doesn't even add up to a very good moisturizer. The titanium dioxide and mica it contains lend a soft white shine to the eye area, which is what's responsible for the "luminous" appearance Lancome mentions. This has no more than a cosmetic effect on dark circles (a concealer would net far better results) and nothing in this eye cream will alleviate puffiness because the ingredient list couldn't be more ordinary; there isn't even an ingredient in here that could fake having benefit. Lancome did include a couple of novel peptides, but they're near the end of the ingredient list, which means they are barely detectable in this formula. In fact moisture-absorbing talc and nylon-66 are listed well before any of the interesting ingredients. It is also not good news that this formula includes fragrance ingredients known to cause irritation. Fragrance in any form is a problem for skin anywhere on the body, but especially around the sensitive eye area (see the Appendix for details and to find out why you don't need an eye cream). In no way, shape, or form is this eye cream akin to dermal fillers that a dermatologist administers.

☺ AVERAGE $$$ **High Resolution Refill 3X Triple Action Renewal Anti Wrinkle Night Cream** *($93 for 2.6 fl. oz.)* is an emollient moisturizer for dry skin that is a cut above what Lancome typically offers, but that doesn't say much because generally Lancome makes some of the most disappointing moisturizers and "antiwrinkle" creams available. The notion that this product has anything to do with the effects of a dermal filler or that it contains ingredients that stimulate the production of skin's supportive elements (they probably want you to think of collagen and elastin) is a joke. It won't do that anymore than will the thousands of other creams on the market. This actually contains more coloring agents than state-of-the-art ingredients, which is really depressing when you weigh the cost of this moisturizer against its limited benefits. Lancome refers to anisic acid helping to "complete the nightly cellular renewal process." Not only is there no research to support this statement, but it also ignores the fact that lots of ingredients can help skin do that, either by exfoliation (think AHA or BHA) or with antioxidants and cell-communicating ingredients, which skin needs both night and day; it doesn't go into overdrive at night and slow down in the morning. Despite fancy jar packaging and lofty claims, this is nothing more than a moisturizer.

👁 Did you know you don't need an eye cream? It's true! See the Appendix to find out why.

☺ AVERAGE $$$ **Nutrix Royal, Intense Lipid Repair Cream, for Dry to Very Dry Skin** *($58 for 1.6 fl. oz.)* contains a terrific blend of emollients to address the needs of its intended skin types. Jar packaging won't keep the tiny amount of antioxidants stable, so this ends up being a fairly expensive moisturizer whose benefits are easily obtained from other products that offer dry skin even more.

☺ AVERAGE $$$ **Platineum Eye & Lip Hydroxy(a)-Calcium, Restructuring Eye and Lip Treatment** *($85 for 0.5 fl. oz.)* is sold with claims of calcium being the key to improving aging skin, which is just silly because calcium can't fortify skin. As is the case for most Lancome moisturizers, there isn't much to extol. The majority of the formula is standard slip agents and thickeners along with a couple emollients and wax. The calcium ingredient is hydroxyapatite, and the company claims this is continuously released, working to strengthen fragile skin around the eyes and lips. Hydroxyapatite is the calcium compound found in our bones and teeth. It is also used in dermal fillers such as Radiesse, and for other types of soft tissue augmentation. It's no secret that injecting this substance in a controlled manner can have a positive effect on the appearance of wrinkles, but that is radically different from applying a small amount of it topically when it's blended into a moisturizer. There is no evidence that topically applied hydroxyapatite works even remotely like dermal fillers, yet Lancome is hoping you won't make that connection. If you're curious to see what calcium can do for your skin, try adding more calcium-rich foods to your diet and forgo this poorly formulated moisturizer (which would be far better for skin if it contained antioxidants, cell-communicating ingredients, and skin-identical ingredients).

☺ AVERAGE $$$ **Platineum Night Hydroxy(a)-Calcium Restructuring and Rein-forcing Night Cream** *($145 for 2.6 fl. oz.)* is a hyper-expensive moisturizer with Lancome's calcium complex. Of course, the fact that there's no reliable research showing calcium in any form is the way to firmer, less wrinkled skin didn't stop Lancome from creating a story around it. This is another ho-hum moisturizer that's primarily a blend of water, silicone, slip agent, thickeners, and preservative. It contains more fragrance and preservative than any beneficial or intriguing ingredients for skin, and the jar packaging won't keep key ingredients stable (see the Appendix for details). The form of calcium this contains (listed as hydroxyapatite, which is a calcium phosphate) doesn't work to restore lost facial structure to aging skin; skin showing signs of sagging or slackening must be addressed by cosmetic surgery, not sham products like this that lead women to waste their money time after time, hoping they've finally found the one product whose lifting, contouring claims are true.

☺ AVERAGE $$$ **Renergie Cream, Anti-Wrinkle and Firming Treatment** *($82 for 1.7 fl. oz.)* remains a perennial favorite of Lancome customers, but it doesn't increase skin's firmness or reduce the appearance of wrinkles better than most emollient moisturizers, which is all this product is. Maybe the women who keep buying this are holding out hope that if they use it long enough the claims will come true. It's a decent option for dry skin, but definitely leaves it wanting more for the money, and the various fragrant components pose a risk of inflamma-tion see the Appendix to find out why daily use of highly fragrant products can be pro-aging).

☺ AVERAGE $$$ **Renergie Eye, Anti-Wrinkle and Firming Eye Creme** *($62 for 0.5 fl. oz.)* is a good, fragrance-free, emollient moisturizer for dry skin anywhere on the face. Nothing in it will firm skin, but its rich texture will soften the appearance of wrinkles. Jar packaging doesn't make this an optimum choice if you want to provide skin with antioxidants. See the Appendix for more facts on jar packaging and to find out why, in truth, you don't need an eye cream.

☺ AVERAGE **$$$ Renergie Eye Multiple Action Ultimate Eye Care Duo** *($75)* is a two-piece set which consists of an eye cream and a sheer concealer (Lancome calls it a "Veil") with sunscreen rated SPF 15 (the eye cream itself does not contain sunscreen). It's a clever concept, with the eye cream housed in a jar and a portion of the product's cap housing a compact for the veil/concealer with sunscreen. Of course, the jar packaging is a problem, and the claim that it fixes six eye-area woes is more fabrication than fact. See the Appendix for details on jar packaging's problems, and why you don't need a separate product labeled an eye cream for the eye area. As for the two parts of the set: The fragranced **Eye Cream** (0.5 oz.) is a standard formula with a thick, almost waxy texture. Although it contains some state-of-the-art anti-aging ingredients, they won't remain potent for long thanks to the jar packaging. Also, there's more artificial color in this eye cream than there are ingredients that would help justify the price. Plus, there's way too much fragrance, which is not good in any product, but especially in one for use around the eyes! The **Veil** (0.14 oz.), with SPF 15, has a beautifully smooth cream-to-powder texture. It blends readily, looks natural, and provides decent coverage, although it won't replace a concealer for those with dark circles or other discolorations. Lancome offers three workable shades (Light, Medium, and Dark), each sold with the same Renergie eye cream. Regrettably, the sunscreen fails to provide reliable UVA (think anti-aging) protection because it does not contain titanium dioxide, zinc oxide, avobenzone, Mexoryl SX (ecamsule), or Tinosorb, the ingredients that cover the entire UVA spectrum. The single active sunscreen ingredient is octinoxate, a synthetic active that can cause irritation and is not best for use in the eye area. It would have been far better if this product contained titanium dioxide or zinc oxide, mineral-based sunscreen ingredients that present no risk of irritation.

☺ AVERAGE **$$$ Renergie Lift Volumetry Eye Volumetric Lifting and Reshaping Eye Cream** *($67 for 0.5 fl. oz.)* is the counterpart to Lancome's Renergie Lift Volumetry moisturizers. Of course, you don't need an eye cream because there is no research showing that eye-area skin needs something different from skin elsewhere on the face; if there is a difference, we're not aware of what it is because no one anywhere in the world has ever explained what those ingredients are. This particular eye cream illustrates that point beautifully. It does not contain a single ingredient you won't find in lots of Lancome facial moisturizers, which means the difference comes down to marketing and little else. And, like most Lancome moisturizers, this is an ordinary formula whose price is an insult considering what it doesn't contain. This pink shimmer-tinged eye cream contains some skin-silkening ingredients, but the amount of alcohol is cause for concern, as is the fact that this contains more wax and coloring agents than state-of-the-art anti-aging ingredients. The pink shimmer adds a brightening effect around the eyes, but you can achieve that with makeup (shimmer isn't skin care). Reading the claims, the intent behind this product is cell communication, telling skin cells to act younger. That's an excellent idea, but this formula contains too small an amount of the kinds of ingredients that can do that. Moreover, what little good ingredients are in here will break down thanks to the jar packaging (see the Appendix for details).

☺ AVERAGE **$$$ Renergie Lift Volumetry Night Volumetric Lifting and Reshaping Night Cream** *($110 for 2.6 fl. oz.)* is touted to have cell communicating properties and, in essence, Lancome wants you to believe that the tiny amounts of cell-communicating ingredients in this product can somehow "talk" to your sagging jawline, "telling" it to go back to its original, taut position and somehow stay there. Of course, that isn't possible, in any way, shape, or form, because where would the excess loose skin go? Many skin-care products claim they can firm and lift skin, but none of them work, at least not to the extent claimed. See the Appendix for news on what you can do to help sagging skin. After all is said and done, this product can be a good moisturizer for normal to very dry skin, but, for the money, the formula is disappointing. The small amount of beneficial ingredients (and mind you, there's more alcohol and synthetic coloring agents in here than anti-aging ingredients) will deteriorate thanks to the jar packaging, which won't keep the good ingredients stable.

☺ AVERAGE $$$ **Renergie Lift Volumetry Volumetric Lifting and Reshaping Cream SPF 15 Normal/Combination Skin** *($90 for 1.7 fl. oz.)* is an in-part avobenzone sunscreen that is said to have a formula that communicates with your cells. In essence, Lancome wants you to believe that the tiny amount of cell-communicating ingredients in this product can somehow "talk" to your sagging jawline, "telling" it to go back to its original, taut position and somehow stay there. Of course, that isn't possible, and the question of where the excess (loose) skin will go remains unanswered. There's also the issue that what causes skin to sag and your face to lose volume is a complex process that skin-care products cannot fix. That's why dermal fillers and cosmetic surgery are so integral to improving one's appearance when facial contours shift with age and due to other factors, such as genetics, estrogen depletion, and cumulative sun damage. This product can provide broad-spectrum sun protection, but, for the money, the formula is a resounding disappointment. The small amount of beneficial ingredients (shockingly, there's more coloring agent than anti-aging ingredients in this product) will deteriorate thanks to the jar packaging, and, as mentioned, this cannot re-contour a sagging jawline. Given these facts, the cost is an insult. If you choose to purchase this anyway, its formula is best for normal to slightly dry skin.

☺ AVERAGE $$$ **Renergie Lift Volumetry Volumetric Lifting and Reshaping Cream SPF 15 Normal to Dry Skin** *($90 for 1.7 fl. oz.)* is nearly identical to Lancome's Renergie Lift Volumetry Volumetric Lifting and Reshaping Cream SPF 15 Normal/Combination Skin. The texture is slightly thicker, but that's about it. As such, the same review applies.

☺ AVERAGE $$$ **Renergie Microlift Eye R.A.R.E., Superior Lifting Eye Cream** *($60 for 0.5 fl. oz.)* has aspirations to defy gravity's pull on skin, and is said to be inspired by "the latest vertical surgery techniques" which grant this cream "exceptional lifting power." Such claims may make you think twice about booking a consultation with a cosmetic surgeon, but we assure you such an appointment would be time well spent compared to using this inferior product. Apparently a "breakthrough" oligopeptide in this product is able to double the synthesis of protein linked to shoring up collagen. If that were true, the result would be smoother, less lined, plumped skin. The only peptide in this product is acetyl tetrapeptide-9, and it is barely present. In fact, there are far more preservatives and volatile fragrant components in this jar-packaged cream than peptide (and the amount of alcohol, while not likely irritating, is still disappointing). Acetyl tetrapeptide-9 is part of a trademarked complex known as Dermican manufactured by Laboratoires Serobiologiques. That company's research shows that this peptide acts on a certain proteoglycan (a sugar molecule that forms the ground substance of connective tissues such as collagen) known as lumican, which is said to play an important role in the synthesis and organization of collagen fibers in skin. The kicker is twofold: The company's research is not substantiated, and the usage level they recommend (1%-3% Dermican) is not even remotely close to what Lancome chose to use. Even if Dermican could work as claimed, you're barely getting any of it in this product, which leaves you with another mundane moisturizer for normal to slightly dry skin. One last note regarding lumican: there is research showing that this proteoglycan's deterioration in skin over time likely plays a role in skin's aged appearance. In addition, animal research suggests that lumican expression is reduced as estrogen levels decrease, such as occurs after menopause (estrogen plays a role in collagen synthesis and organization). (Sources for the above: *Journal of Dermatological Science*, September 2007, pages 217–226; *Molecular and Cellular Biochemistry*, September 2005, pages 63–72; and *Glycoconjugate Journal*, May-June 2002, pages 287–293). Check out the Appendix to learn more about the problems jar packaging presents and to find out why you don't need an eye cream.

☺ AVERAGE $$$ **Renergie Microlift Neck R.A.R.E., Superior Lifting Neck Cream** *($82 for 1.7 fl. oz.)* is said to be the answer for the "thin, delicate skin" on the neck and chest when these areas begin to show a lack of firmness; at least that's what Lancome wants you to believe. To that end, they've developed what they refer to as Bio-Stimulating Technology that, are you ready for this, sends a "dynamic impulse" that spreads throughout the layers of skin. First of all, this product is not a defibrillator for aging skin; second, what exactly is a "dynamic impulse"? A dynamic impulse could be the urge to eat chocolate cake or to drink a glass of water. In this case, "dynamic impulse" is mere marketing chicanery. Most important is the fact that this moisturizer is another in Lancome's endless parade of ordinary formulas with claims that are far more elaborate than the ingredients inside. For as much money as they're charging, it's disheartening to realize you're getting mostly water, slip agents, Vaseline, emollient thickeners, wax, silicone, and coloring agents. The jar packaging won't keep the minimal amounts of intriguing ingredients stable during use (see the Appendix for details), and this also contains fragrance ingredients that can cause irritation, especially on "thin, delicate skin." Labeling this product as a superior lift for sagging neck skin is an affront to all cosmetic surgeons, whose skilled handiwork really can make a beautiful difference when skin becomes lax due to a combination of age and sun damage. They, not Lancome, deserve your anti-aging dollars when skin on the neck becomes lax.

☺ AVERAGE $$$ **Renergie Microlift Night R.A.R.E, Superior Firming Night Cream** *($98 for 2.5 fl. oz.)* is an average moisturizer with an absurd price tag. Reading the claims for this moisturizer, you can't help but think it is essentially shock therapy for skin that has lost its firmness and youthful contours! But, this is a Lancome moisturizer and, therefore, you shouldn't expect much because Lancome makes some of the most ordinary, poorly formulated moisturizers around. The amount of intriguing ingredients pales in comparison to the amount of those that Lancome deems more important for a product's appeal, namely fragrance, coloring agents, and mica, the latter of which lends a soft glow to skin. This is a mundane option for dry to very dry skin, but there is nothing rare, lifting, or superior about it, and your skin truly deserves better.

☺ AVERAGE $$$ **Renergie Microlift R.A.R.E., Intense Targeted Repositioning Lifter** *($115 for 0.8 fl. oz.)* essentially promises to lift, firm, and reposition sagging skin. We ask you: What are all the other products Lancome sells doing on the shelf with the same claims if this one is the best? The effect is supposed to last all day, with notable redefining of contours appearing after only 4 weeks. Wow! Should you cancel that face-lift? Hardly. There's no reason to invest in this waste-of-time-and-money product. The backbone of the formula is water, slip agent, silicone, soy protein, and preservative; it actually contains more preservative than anything really helpful for skin, except the soy protein, which is hardly a stellar, miracle ingredient. Even if it were, Aveeno includes the same ingredient in its products and charges a lot less. None of these ingredients can lift sagging skin or redefine facial contours (see the Appendix to find out what you can do to improve this). This contains a small amount of film-forming agents that may make skin feel tighter, but that sensation isn't the equivalent of skin being lifted back into place. Several fragrance ingredients that cause irritation only make matters worse for aging skin. See the Appendix to find out why routine use of fragrant products is bad for everyone's skin—even if you cannot see the damage taking place.

☺ AVERAGE **$$$ Renergie Night, Night Treatment** *($98 for 2.5 fl. oz.)* claims to accelerate surface cell renewal so that skin is "re-energized" and "looks well-rested." Sounds great, but those benign claims can be made for just about any moisturizer no matter what it contains. All in all, Renergie Night is a very expensive basic moisturizer whose jar packaging won't keep the good ingredients (which there are woefully little of) stable. The formula may be exclusive to Lancome, but no one else would want it anyway.

☺ AVERAGE **$$$ Renergie Oil-Free Lotion, Anti-Wrinkle and Firming Treatment** *($82 for 1.7 fl. oz.)* is a silicone-enhanced lightweight lotion for normal to slightly oily skin. Although the packaging will keep the vitamin E stable, there's barely a drop of it in here. This is very expensive for nothing special beyond Lancome's marketing mystique.

☺ AVERAGE **$$$ Secret De Vie, Ultimate Cellular Reviving Creme** *($250 for 1.7 fl. oz.)* is described as "Lancome's ultimate luxury." Secret De Vie asks you to believe that its key ingredient complex, Extrait de Vie (extract of life), "delivers intense restorative action to six major cell types for instant, visible, exceptional results." Notice that Lancome is trying very hard in this seductive wordplay to attempt to convince consumers that spending this much on a special formula (one that is shockingly similar to almost every other Lancome cream being sold) is somehow worth the extra expense. The company didn't even bother to use stable packaging, instead choosing a futuristic, orb-like jar. Extrait de Vie does sound romantic and exotic, but there is nothing in this product that is in any way unique or even moderately interesting. The majority of the product consists of water, silicones, glycerin, thickener, silicone polymer, aluminum starch, wax, vitamin E, and several plant extracts, including peppermint leaf (though the amount is likely too small to cause irritation). Paying significantly more for this versus almost any of Lancome's other moisturizers, none of which are as impressive as what most other Lauder-owned companies are offering, is not good skin care.

☺ AVERAGE **$$$ Secret De Vie Eye, Ultimate Cellular Reviving Eye Creme** *($150 for 0.5 fl. oz.)* is an emollient moisturizer for dry skin anywhere on the face, but the price is outrageous for what you get. Here, there's no reason to comment on the jar packaging because there are no light- or air-sensitive ingredients in this far-from-ultimate eye cream. You don't need an eye cream at all (see the Appendix to find out why) and definitely not an overpriced one like this.

☺ AVERAGE **$$$ Soleil Ultra Expert Sun Care SPF 50 Sunscreen Face Cream, for Sensitive Skin** *($31.50 for 1.7 fl. oz.)* features an in-part titanium dioxide sunscreen, and contains fragrance. Another point of contention for those with sensitive skin is the amount of alcohol in this product, not to mention the amount of preservatives, listed well before any type of soothing agent. What a shame, as this has a beautifully lightweight texture.

☹ POOR **Bienfait Aqua Vital Continuous Infusing Moisturizer Cream** *($45 for 1.7 fl. oz.)* is a lightweight moisturizer that is oil-free and has a silky texture, but the overall formula leaves much to be desired. There's more alcohol and artificial coloring agent in this cream than there is the state-of-the-art ingredients that all skin types need to repair and promote a younger appearance. Also in the formula are a lot of fragrance ingredients, but fragrance isn't skin care. See the Appendix to learn more about fragrant skin-care products and how alcohol damages skin.

☹ POOR **Bienfait Aqua Vital Continuous Infusing Moisturizer Lotion** *($45 for 1.7 fl. oz.)* is a lightweight, lotion version of the Bienfait Aqua Vital Continuous Infusing Moisturizer Cream above, and the same review applies.

☹ POOR **Bienfait Multi-Vital Glow SPF 15** *($46 for 1.7 fl. oz.)* is a product that is infuriating to us; despite L'Oreal's media blitz for their UVA-protecting sunscreen ingredient Mexoryl SX, also called ecamsule, Lancome (L'Oreal owns Lancome) is still launching sunscreens that leave skin vulnerable to UVA damage! That is just shocking! Can you imagine?!! A company knows about UVA protection, it advertises in the media how important it is for skin, and then it goes and offers sunscreen products that not only leave out their pivotal ingredient, but also do not include any other viable option such as titanium dioxide, zinc oxide, or avobenzone (the latter also called butyl methoxydibenzoylmethane). There are numerous UVA-protecting products available, including from Lancome. Really, at this point in the sunscreen game, Lancome should be hanging their heads in shame.

☹ POOR **High Resolution Refill 3x Triple Action Renewal Anti-Wrinkle Cream SPF 15 Sunscreen** *($78 for 1.7 fl. oz.)* leaves skin vulnerable to UVA damage because the active ingredients it contains don't protect across the entire UVA spectrum. Amazing and endlessly frustrating, because Lancome owns the patent on Mexoryl SX, an ingredient that does provide protection across the a key part of the UVA spectrum. How does that make sense? When people ask us why cosmetics companies do what they do, we can often surmise the marketing logic (like jar packaging, because women like using jars), but when it comes to protecting your skin from UVA rays from the sun, which are responsible for serious skin damage and wrinkling, we can't fathom why a company like Lancome, given their ingredient resources, would ignore this. It makes us want to scream (and sometimes we do). As usual for Lancome's daytime moisturizers with sunscreen, the base formula has an elegant silky texture, but it offers skin little in the way of exciting, helpful ingredients. You won't even get single-action antiwrinkle power by using this product.

☹ POOR **Pure Focus Matifying Moisturizing Lotion** *($38 for 1.7 fl. oz.)* barely moisturizes thanks to its alcohol content, and irritates with the menthol derivative menthoxypropanediol. Skin does not need to tingle or be irritated to look matte! The alcohol in this product will make oily skin worse by stimulating oil production in the pore; see the Appendix for further details and to learn about the problems alcohol presents.

☹ POOR **Renergie Lift Volumetry Neck Volumetric Lifting and Reshaping Neck Cream** *($90 for 1.7 fl. oz.)* is a waste of money, like all neck creams, and this one is no exception. It is a stunningly basic moisturizer formula that's designed for dry skin and it doesn't contain a single ingredient that's unique for skin on your neck. The neck area doesn't require special ingredients over and above what your face needs, and there isn't a shred of research proving otherwise.

☹ POOR **Renergie Microlift Eye R.A.R.E. Intense Repositioning Eye Lifter** *($72 for 0.5 fl. oz.)* is an exceptionally poor formula that cannot lift or reposition sagging eye-area skin in any way, shape, or form. With alcohol as the second ingredient, this product can't hydrate your skin, but it will cause dryness, free-radical damage, and irritation that leads to collagen breakdown and hurts your skin's healing process: That's what alcohol does to skin! Lancome maintains that the peptide in this eye-area product helps "rebundle" collagen, but even if that were the case (which it isn't, and there is no published research showing otherwise), the alcohol works against such anti-aging action. Although we wish it were not the case, the truth is that skin-care products cannot take sagging skin and lift it back into its youthful position. The numerous factors that lead to sagging (sun damage, muscle laxity, bone loss, fat pads shifting, and gravity) cannot be addressed by skin-care products; you need cosmetic corrective procedures for genuine improvement. Besides, if products like this really worked as claimed, you have to wonder: Where does all the loose skin go? Lifting excess, sagging skin without accounting for the excess would look strange, not youthful! This product is not even close to a surgical eye-lift. See the Appendix to learn why you don't need an eye cream, and definitely not one like this!

☹ POOR **Secret de Vie, Ultimate Cellular Reviving Life Source Serum** *($275 for 1 fl. oz.)* is a poorly formulated, inadequate, and absolutely pathetic water-based serum. Calling this an "awesome discovery" for skin is marketing hubris. For the money, you should know up front that the core ingredients in this product are extremely common and mundane. In fact, several L'Oreal products offer similar formulations. However, L'Oreal's status as a mass market brand means they'd never charge this much money for anything, even when almost identical to its expensive counterpart. Because this is a premium product (in price and claims only), Lancome had to devise a story to convince consumers that it's worth the splurge. This time the fabled Extrait de Vie (extract of life) is said to be made super potent because Lancome combines marine ingredients from bodies of water with different temperatures (as in hot and cold). There is no published research anywhere proving these sea extracts (listed as algae and various ferments, the same ingredients that show up in Biotherm products, another L'Oreal-owned company) are capable of prolonging the life of skin cells. Even if they did, merely allowing skin cells to live longer doesn't mean that skin gets firmer or that wrinkles diminish. If the skin cells are damaged (such as from sun exposure), they'll still be damaged. It's just that they'll hang on longer before dying out—and how is that helpful or healthy for skin? It isn't, and it's one of many reasons why this serum is a complete waste of time and money.

☹ POOR **Visionnaire LR 2412 4% Advanced Skin Corrector** *($84 for 1 fl. oz.)* is said to be "Much more than a wrinkle corrector" because it also addresses the concerns of large pores, red marks, and uneven skin tone. The claims are enticing, but the reality is this is not an advanced product in the least; it's more skin-corrupting than skin-correcting thanks to the amount of alcohol and the fact that its LR 2412 ingredient (discussed below) isn't the miracle antiwrinkle breakthrough it's made out to be. This has a silky texture just like most serums, but the amount of alcohol is cause for concern. Not only is there more alcohol than there are state-of-the-art anti-aging ingredients, given the amount of alcohol present, your skin faces potential free-radical damage and collagen breakdown with daily use—even if you cannot see or feel the irritation taking place. It's important to note that all the marketing language Lancome uses in their ads and on their website for this product never directly states what this product does for your skin. Like thousands of products, it claims to have clinical results of happy women who thought their skin looked better, but that's not science because we have no idea what these women were basing their results on, or what questions were part of the questionnaire. Often these types of cosmetic clinical studies don't allow a woman to make a negative comment of any kind. When you read between the lines, the language in the ads is all smoke and mirrors. So, what is Lancome's LR 2412 ingredient (allegedly being used at a 4% concentration)? LR 2412 is derived from the jasmine plant. Lancome maintains that this ingredient is a molecule "designed to propel through skin layers." As it does so, it "triggers a cascading series of micro-transformations." Sounds like a magic wand for your skin, doesn't it? And Lancome's constant reminder that this ingredient is protected by 20 patents makes it seem even more remarkable—but a patent has nothing to do with efficacy; it is only about a unique way to use any ingredient. A patent can be obtained simply by presenting an idea, not proof that the idea actually works. Plus, the way Lancome presents this in their ads, it doesn't actually say the 20 patents have anything to do with this product. As it turns out, simply "propelling" an ingredient through skin is not a guarantee of anything beneficial happening, and it may even make matters worse. For example, many ingredients, such as sunscreen actives, are meant for and should stay on the skin's surface; you don't want them to penetrate through multiple layers of skin because they need to protect the skin's surface. Also, lots of ingredients can "propel" through skin and cause beneficial changes along the way, such as most antioxidants, glycerin, sodium hyaluronate, ceramides, retinol, and numerous other repairing ingredients whose daily use helps improve skin's appearance and healthy functioning. In essence, Lancome's claim makes LR 2412 sound innovative, when it's really nothing new or all that exciting. But the ballyhoo sure makes it tempting! On the ingredient list for Visionnaire, LR 2412 is listed as sodium tetrahydrojasmonate, which, as mentioned, is derived from the jasmine plant. Also listed is tetrahydrojasmonic acid. Both of these ingredients, in their natural state, are lipids (fats) that help the jasmine plant signal when repair is needed and that control the life cycle of the plant's cells (Sources: *Plant Physiology*, April 2010, pages 1940–1950; and *PLoS Biology*, September 2008, page e320). Lancome wants you to believe that these lipids, which in the jasmine plant repair environmental damage and control cell behavior, can somehow have similar effects on your skin, such as improving wrinkles, large pores, and red marks when applied to skin via their bioengineered LR 2412 molecule. Unfortunately, there isn't a shred of published research to support their assertion. More to the point, even if these jasmine-derived ingredients were miracle workers for wrinkles, large pores, and red marks from acne, the amount of alcohol in the formula likely will harm your skin in the process, so any potential benefit is muted. Of course, you also have to ask yourself: If LR 2412 is able to tackle the major concerns mentioned, why is Lancome selling so many other antiwrinkle products that don't have this ingredient? Shouldn't they just admit that LR 2412 is the best and stop selling their antiwrinkle products that don't include it? Not too long ago, Genifique was Lancome's new darling, but now it appears that Visionnaire is the answer. We wish the people at Lancome would make up their minds. There really isn't much else of note in Visionnaire. It contains a small amount of the cell-communicating ingredient adenosine, but so do many other products, although many of those other products also provide a range of anti-aging ingredients, which is what skin really needs. Skin is a complex organ (the body's largest) that requires a range of beneficial ingredients to be at its healthy, youthful best, not just a derivative of jasmine or adenosine, especially not for this amount of money. In the end, for all its promotion, Visionnaire isn't all that visionary, though it will make skin feel silky

LANCOME SUN CARE

☺ AVERAGE $$$ **Bienfait UV SPF 50+** *($35 for 1.7 fl. oz.)* is a fragrant, thin-textured lotion which provides UVA protection with stabilized avobenzone. It feels lightweight and silky so it's compatible with normal to oily skin, but the amount of alcohol is cause for concern because it causes free-radical damage, irritation, and dryness. Even more disappointing, given the price and size of this sunscreen, is that it contains zero of the beneficial extras that all skin types need to look and function in a younger, healthier manner. For the money, it is an understatement to say there are far better formulations than this one, and for less money.

☺ AVERAGE $$$ **Flash Bronzer Anti-Age Tinted Anti-Age Self-Tanning Face Lotion SPF 15 Sunscreen** *($40 for 1.7 fl. oz.)* has a combination of sunscreen and self-tanning lotion, but these two products aren't ideal when combined. Why? It comes down to how much is needed: Sunscreen must be applied liberally to attain the level of protection stated on the label, while most people do best with a self-tanner when they apply it sparingly in thin layers. If you use this self-tanner with sunscreen as your sole source of sun protection, you're likely not applying enough, but applying the right amount for reliable sun protection may make your self-tan too dark or blotchy. Self-tanners with sunscreen are an OK adjunct to your regular sunscreen or foundation with sunscreen. As for this product, it is an OK option for normal to oily skin, but it does contain fragrance ingredients known to cause irritation. The amount of alcohol is likely too low to be cause for concern.

☺ AVERAGE **$$$ Soleil Ultra Expert Sun Care SPF 50 Sunscreen Face and Body Lotion, for Sensitive Skin** *($34.50 for 5 fl. oz.)* contains too many sunscreen actives to be considered a viable option for sensitive skin, and the propylene glycol can enhance their penetration into skin, another minus for sensitive skin. And why add fragrance? Someone at Lancome must have missed Skin Care 101 if they thought that would be good for sensitive skin! An in-part titanium dioxide sunscreen helps provide broad-spectrum protection, but the base formula is mundane, not "expert" and not worth the expense.

☹ POOR **Flash Bronzer Oil-Free Tinted Self-Tanning Face Lotion with Pure Vitamin E** *($37 for 1.7 fl. oz.)* has a great lightweight texture and it's tinted with natural and synthetic coloring agents for instant bronze gratification. Lancome also includes light-reflecting minerals for shine, assuming you want a shiny tan. The problem? This self-tanning lotion contains a potentially irritating amount of several fragrance ingredients, including the troublemaker eugenol. Given the number of self-tanners available that work just as well as this but without the risk of irritation, why take your chances (and spend too much money) on this one?

☹ POOR **Flash Bronzer Tinted Self-Tanning Body Gel** *($34.50 for 4.2 fl. oz.)* contains a lot of alcohol and that is the reason this self-tanner dries in a flash. The gel texture feels ultra-light, but between the alcohol and the fragrance, you're subjecting your skin to needless irritation in exchange for a sunless tan. Given the number of self-tanning gels that work beautifully but omit the needless irritants, why settle for this expensive, overly fragranced mistake?

☹ POOR **Flash Bronzer Tinted Self-Tanning Leg Gel with Pure Vitamin E** *($37 for 4.2 fl. oz.)* contains the same ingredient (dihydroxyacetone) found in almost every self-tanner sold today. Knowing this, there's no compelling reason to consider spending this much money on a self-tanner, especially not once you learn that it also contains a potentially skin-damaging amount of alcohol and numerous irritating fragrance ingredients. By the way, there is nothing about this formula that makes it unique for the legs; like most Lancome self-tanners, the formula is tinted for instant color and it contains shiny mineral pigments to give skin a shimmer finish.

LANCOME LIP CARE

☹ POOR **L'Absolu Rouge La Base Revitalizing Lip Treatment Highlighting Effect Pro-Xylane SPF 10 Sunscreen** *($29)* loses points immediately for failing to provide sufficient UVA protection. Your lips remain vulnerable to the sun's UVA rays if the product doesn't include one or more of the following active ingredients to cover the entire UVA spectrum: titanium dioxide, zinc oxide, avobenzone, Mexoryl SX (ecamsule), or Tinosorb. This product also is a problem for your lips because the SPF rating of 10 is below the standard recommended by most medical boards around the world: SPF 15 or greater. As a lip balm, this has a very greasy texture that, when paired with lipstick, causes the color to practically slide right off. It's a terrible base for lipstick and there are better lips balms.

LANCOME SPECIALTY SKIN-CARE PRODUCTS

☺ AVERAGE **$$$ Bright Expert Dark Spot Corrector** *($65 for 1 fl. oz.)* is Lancome's try at lighteners. Just like Clinique's Even Better Clinical Dark Spot Corrector claims to rival "the leading prescription ingredient" (which is the gold standard, hydroquinone), this entry from Lancome makes the same boast. The difference is that Clinique uses a mix of ingredients with some promising research behind them, while Lancome defaults to little more than enticing marketing copy and limited research for a less impressive formula. However, neither formula is going to be as effective as prescription-strength hydroquinone (4% strength), a fact with which almost any dermatologist familiar with the research behind that active ingredient would agree. Bright Expert Dark Spot Corrector has a lightweight, gel-like texture that slips easily over skin, but doesn't contain much that can significantly lighten sun-induced brown skin discolorations. Lancome maintains this product is clinically proven, but the results of their study were not peer-reviewed or published, so you're left to take their word for it. The ingredients in this product that may have some skin-lightening ability (though research is limited) include yeast extract and ellagic acid. Of these two, the research on ellagic acid is more compelling, especially because we don't know what type of yeast Lancome includes in this product. Certain strains of yeast have some intriguing research pertaining to skin discolorations, while generic "yeast extract," which is what Lancome lists on the ingredient list, does not. Studies have shown that ellagic acid (a polyphenol antioxidant that may be natural or synthetic; a natural source is pomegranate rind) works as well as the skin-lightening ingredient arbutin on patients with brown discolorations. The problem? There's only one small study that examined topical application. The other studies have shown oral administration of ellagic acid has the same effect, but made no mention of its use in skin-care products (Sources: *The Journal of Dermatology*, September 2008, pages 570–574; *Journal of Nutritional Science and Vitaminology*, October 2006, pages 383–388; and *Bioscience, Biotechnology, and Biochemistry*, December 2005, pages 2368–2373). Given the lack of substantial research on ellagic acid, it's surprising Lancome chose it over more thoroughly researched options such as various licorice extracts, arbutin, kojic acid, or even over-the-counter strengths of hydroquinone. What we don't know is how much ellagic acid is needed to produce a result on brown spots, but the amount of it in this product is likely less than 1%, so who knows what results, if any, you may see. Beyond the paltry potential for skin lightening, the amount of fragrance ingredients in this highly fragrant product is likely to cause irritation, even if you cannot see it, and that's detrimental to your skin. Please see the Appendix for details on why fragrance ingredients almost always spell trouble.

☹ POOR **Hydra-Intense Masque Hydrating Gel Mask with Botanical Extract** *($32 for 3.4 fl. oz.)* lists alcohol as the second ingredient, which doesn't make this mask the least bit hydrating. This is about as do-nothing (except irritate) as do-nothing products get! See the Appendix to learn why alcohol is bad for everyone's skin.

☹ POOR **Pure Empreinte Masque Purifying Mineral Mask with White Clay** *($32 for 3.4 fl. oz.)* has the makings of a very good clay mask for oily skin, but the inclusion of potent skin-irritant camphor was unwise and makes this not preferred to almost any other clay mask being sold.

LANCOME FOUNDATIONS & PRIMERS

✓☺ $$$ **Dual Finish Versatile Powder Makeup** *($36.50)* has been part of Lancome's foundation lineup for years and has deservedly attained classic status. This talc-based wet/dry powder foundation offers a soft matte finish and a selection of beautiful colors for fair to very dark skin. The application is smooth with a silky, almost creamy-feeling texture that's best for normal to dry skin. The squalane and mineral oil in the formula are not the best ingredients to temper shine, but they keep this powder from looking too dry or chalky. It is best applied with a brush for sheer coverage or a makeup sponge for medium coverage. Also available is **Dual Finish Fragrance Free Versatile Powder Makeup**, which costs the same but omits the fragrance, and that's the best way to go for the health of your skin!

☺ GOOD $$$ **Ageless Minerale Skin-Transforming Mineral Powder Foundation with White Sapphire Complex SPF 21** *($42)* is Lancome's contribution to the mineral makeup craze, and it's fairly impressive. With titanium dioxide as the sole active ingredient, broad-spectrum protection is assured. This loose-powder foundation has an almost creamy texture that is easy to buff on skin, though it must be done quickly and not over a surface that's too moist or it will grab and change color almost immediately. This provides light to medium coverage with a single application, or can be layered for additional coverage, although doing so can create a too heavy appearance, so use restraint. The sifter comes equipped with a closure to keep mess to a minimum, which is great. This powder's finish on skin is best described as "glowing matte" because the overall effect is matte, but it contains shiny pigments that give skin a dimensional glow, which is not the best for those with oily skin who are trying to suppress shine. By the way, despite the name, this foundation doesn't contain any white sapphire. This is best for normal to slightly dry skin. Contrary to claims, it will settle into lines, so it's not a foundation to try if wrinkles are prominent.

☺ GOOD $$$ **Bienfait Multi-Vital Teinte High Potency Tinted Moisturizer SPF 30** *($45)* is one of the few tinted moisturizers with a high SPF rating and sufficient UVA protection, thanks to its in-part titanium dioxide sunscreen. Although closer to a light-coverage foundation than a tinted moisturizer (it isn't as sheer as you might think given the name), it has a light lotion texture that blends easily and would be suitable for normal to slightly dry skin. It has a soft, dewy finish and blurs minor flaws nicely. The main issue is that most of the shades lean toward the peachy side, and this isn't sheer enough to accommodate for the color shift. This is definitely one to test at the counter. By the way, Lancome's claim that this product is vitamin-enriched makes it sound like it's bursting with antioxidants, and it isn't. They're in here, but not in amounts that will make a discernible difference.

☺ GOOD $$$ **Photogenic Lumessence Compact Light-Mastering & Line-Smoothing Makeup SPF 18** *($42)* is a very good, modern cream-to-powder makeup that provides sufficient UVA protection thanks to its pure titanium dioxide sunscreen. This smoothes over skin easily and blends to a soft powder finish that leaves a subtle glow. Best for normal to slightly dry skin not prone to breakouts, this foundation provides sheer to medium coverage, although medium coverage requires layering and diminishes this makeup's natural look. It poses a slight risk of creasing into lines around the eye and isn't the best for those with large pores because after a few hours it slips into them and magnifies their appearance. As for the shade selection, it is mostly excellent and includes options for light to dark, but not very dark, skin tones.

☺ GOOD $$$ **Renergie Lift Makeup SPF 20** *($44)* is positioned as Lancome's anti-aging makeup (which it isn't), but thankfully it does have excellent sun protection and that goes a long way toward reducing the development of wrinkles and skin discolorations when worn daily! All the anti-aging claims and statistics in the world don't mean a thing without a sufficient sunscreen in your daily routine, and this in-part titanium dioxide foundation is a great way to get it. This silky liquid foundation is smooth and a pleasure to blend. The finish is natural and slightly moist, and provides medium coverage without creasing into lines. You

---

♦ Irritating ingredients are a problem for all skin types. Find out why in the Appendix.

probably guessed that this won't lift the skin anywhere, but by creating the illusion of smoother, even-toned skin it can make wrinkles (we're talking superficial lines, not pronounced wrinkles) look less apparent; silicone technology comes through again! Of the shades available, the only missteps are a couple with a slightly peach or slightly orange undertones. If you have normal to dry skin and want to experience a state-of-the-art foundation with effective sun protection, this is highly recommended.

☺ AVERAGE $$$ **Absolue BX Makeup Absolute Replenishing Radiant Makeup SPF 18** *($60)* is one of Lancome's most expensive foundations, and has been reformulated for the worse, at least in terms of the sunscreen. Whereas this once had an in-part titanium dioxide sunscreen, that UVA-protecting ingredient has been dropped in favor of octinoxate, which doesn't provide enough UVA protection (something Lancome knows about, so the change is really frustrating). Positioned as anti-aging makeup for mature skin, the only legitimate anti-aging element (sunscreen) is now inadequate. The "Bio-Network" of wild yam, sea algae, and other plant extracts cannot rejuvenate skin or increase its firmness. Even if these plants were the answer to forestalling that face-lift, the amount of them in this foundation is paltry. Taken on its merit of foundation alone, this has an exquisite, fluid texture that glides over skin. It provides almost full coverage and sets to an attractive satin-matte finish that won't make dry skin look dull (that's assuming you've taken pre-makeup steps to smooth over dry patches). Lancome claims this will not settle into lines, and for the most part, that's true. Deep wrinkles will see some settling, but this does a good job of smoothing over superficial to moderate lines. Almost all the shades are impressive, and there are options for fair to dark (but not very dark) skin tones. This makeup doesn't provide much anti-aging benefit, but as a foundation for normal to dry skin it has its strong points.

☺ AVERAGE $$$ **Absolue Makeup Absolute Replenishing Cream Makeup SPF 20** *($60)* is one of Lancome's most expensive foundations. Is it worth it? The disappointing lack of sufficient UVA protection doesn't get this foundation off to a good start. However, its creamy application and silky, slightly moist finish are bound to please those with dry skin. Ironically, for a creamy foundation this isn't an ideal formula for someone with very dry skin. That's because it contains silicone and water-binding agents rather than the oils or emollient ingredients that would provide the extra moisturizing necessary to make very dry skin feel smooth and comfortable. The real reason to consider this foundation is that it provides full coverage without looking heavy or too thick. It conceals without looking too conspicuous, so if you need significant coverage, have dry skin, and are willing to pair this with a broad-spectrum sunscreen, it is an option. Most of the shades are flattering and neutral, but watch out for any slightly peach or pink undertones. One last comment: Lancome's justification for this foundation's high price is its claim that the product's "exclusive bio-network" (featuring wild yam and algae) helps "revitalize and restore skin elasticity." Unfortunately, there's no proof anywhere that those ingredients can do that. Just as their Absolue skin-care products are ineffective for this purpose, so is this foundation that shares the Absolue name and over-hyped ingredients. There's more fragrance in this makeup than yam or algae.

☺ AVERAGE $$$ **La Base Pro Perfecting Makeup Primer Smoothing Effect, Oil Free** *($42)* isn't anything new under the sun. The "exclusive" formula is nothing more than silicone and a silicone polymer. You'd think for the cost they could have at least added some vitamin E or a soothing agent, though they thankfully omitted fragrance. This clear primer has a thick, slight gel texture that instantly transforms into a weightless silky feel which smoothes skin. Applying a sheer layer of dry-finish silicones to skin can help enhance makeup application, but you don't need to seek out a special primer to find these traits. Instead, look for an antioxidant-laden silicone serum that also contains some other helpful ingredients. You're simply not getting your money's worth with this no-frills primer from Lancome.

☺ AVERAGE $$$ **Oscillation Powerfoundation SPF 21** *($48)* is a loose powder with a pure titanium dioxide sunscreen housed in a component that has the powder sitting at the bottom of the base. A sifter unit is attached between the base and the product's top. When you uncap it, you'll find the applicator, which consists of a soft sponge attached to a short handle. There's a tiny button on the handle, that, when pressed, causes the sponge to vibrate. You shake some powder out of the sifter, and dip the sponge in to pick up the powder. From there, you're directed to press the button to start the sponge vibrating as you stroke the powder in one smooth motion over your face. According to Lancome, this vibrating powder foundation is supposed to provide a flawless complexion that also improves skin with each use. The only aspect of this product that can improve skin is the sunscreen, but that is hardly unique to this product; there is nothing else it contains that can remotely be construed as skin care. In terms of appearance, it works as well as any good loose-powder foundation. The trick with this is how you apply it, which is not foolproof. You need to apply it in smooth downward strokes instead of circular motions and then you can get a fairly soft matte finish with light to medium coverage. This is not a full-coverage makeup, though Lancome sells it as such. You can get close to full coverage, but the trade-off is a powdery finish that looks dry, cakey, and heavy. Lancome also claims this is a non-messy way to apply mineral makeup, but that is absolutely not the case. Loose powder gets all over the place inside and outside the packaging, even with careful use. The powder has a smooth, finely milled texture and the sponge applicator is soft and relatively durable. All told, this is neither revolutionary makeup nor worth the price. The vibrating concept isn't all that helpful, either, and most people will find that they need to stop the vibration and use the sponge for precise blending. You will probably find that the powder looks much better when applied with a regular sponge and then buffed with a powder brush. Most of the shades are excellent, and there are options for fair to dark, but not very dark, skin. This is best for normal to slightly oily skin, but it's not really worth the cost or frustrations.

☺ AVERAGE $$$ **Photogenic Lumessence Light-Mastering & Line-Smoothing Makeup SPF 15** *($42)* has a lot going for it until you realize that it doesn't provide sufficient UVA protection because it doesn't contain avobenzone, titanium dioxide, zinc oxide, Mexoryl SX (ecamsule), or Tinosorb. Lancome knows better because they have the patent on the UVA-protecting ingredient ecamsule, and they have for years. So, the fact that they keep launching foundations whose sunscreens fall short is maddening. If you're willing to pair this foundation with a daytime moisturizer that contains the right UVA-protecting ingredients it is an option, but considering there are lots of foundations that get this aspect of the formula right, why bother with this one? As a foundation this has a fluid, very silky texture that feels amazing and blends easily. It provides light to medium coverage and has a marvelously skin-like finish. The formula is best for normal to slightly dry or slightly oily skin. As usual for Lancome, the shade range is excellent, especially for those with fair to light skin tones. The dark shades don't do as well, with some being too orange and copper. What about the light-mastering claims? You won't see any refraction going on, but the pigments in this foundation look quite natural, although it absolutely will not make lines, wrinkles, and pores vanish. Despite the lofty claims, this foundation would be rated a Best Product if not for the deficient sunscreen.

☹ POOR **Rénergie Éclat Multi-Lift Tinted Skincare** *($75)* is an overpriced tinted moisturizer that fails to meet our standards for a number of reasons. First, from an aesthetic perspective, the thick, emollient texture blends on unevenly and leaves a tacky, shiny finish (something that those with oily skin will particularly dislike). It feels good on dry skin, but the texture and finish are just not pretty. Another issue is that the shade selection is small and some of the shades have unflattering orange to copper undertones. From a formulary standpoint there is no way you are going to see any lifting effect with this product; there just aren't ingredients that can do that (see the Appendix to find out what you can do). Although this contains some beneficial ingredients, it also contains skin irritants like linalool, limonene, citronellol and fragrance which are bad news for everyone's skin (see the Appendix for details). There are numerous tinted moisturizers that out-perform this and cost significantly less.

⊗ POOR **Teint Idole Ultra 24H Wear & Comfort Retouch-Free Divine Perfection SPF 15 Sunscreen** *($44)*. Talk about the yin and yang! This fragrance-free liquid foundation with an extraordinarily long name ping-pongs from strong positives to not-good-for-skin negatives, adding up to a product that we simply cannot recommend (though we really struggled with this, as its strong points are really wonderful). Let's get the negatives out of the way first: This foundation's sunscreen fails to provide reliable UVA protection, which is essential for anti-aging benefits. Therefore, if you decide to use this, you'll need to apply a broad-spectrum daytime moisturizer with sunscreen beforehand (not the best for those with very oily skin and who don't want to layer products). See the Appendix to learn which active ingredients to look for in any SPF-rated product. The other issue is the inclusion of alcohol. It's the third ingredient and this foundation definitely has alcohol's telltale odor. Although the alcohol contributes to this foundation's texture and setting time, it is present in an amount that has the potential to be irritating. Given the number of great foundations that don't contain alcohol, there's no compelling reason to choose one that does; why risk the irritation and problems (like collagen breakdown)? See the Appendix for further details on the problems alcohol causes. OK, now for the positives: This has a supremely silky yet light texture that provides enough playtime for you to blend before it sets to a (very) long-wearing matte finish. The matte finish is beautiful; it makes skin look refined and dimensional rather than flat and drab. There's almost a hint of satin, yet the feel is decidedly matte. It's best for normal to oily or combination skin. Coverage-wise, this layers well, so it hides most imperfections and does so without looking heavy (though it does look like makeup—it's not that perfect). Best of all are the shades, which are plentiful and offer beautiful options for skin tones ranging from porcelain to ebony. We wish the formula didn't have the drawbacks it does, because Lancome did a brilliant job with the shades. If you decide to try this (despite the positives, there are strong reasons not to), the shades to avoid due to peach overtones are 350 Bisque C and 430 Bisque C. Shades to consider carefully include 260 Bisque N and 320 Bisque W.

⊗ POOR **Teint Idole Fresh Wear 18 Hour Shine-Free Makeup SPF 15 Sunscreen** *($34)* claims 18-hour shine-free wear, and who wouldn't be anxious to check this out, especially if you have oily skin? Regrettably, there are two major drawbacks that keep this from living up to the hype. First, the sunscreen fails to supply adequate UVA protection, an issue that Lancome knows all about because they happen to own a patent on the UVA-protecting ingredient ecamsule. Their constant mistakes in this regard infuriates us. Second, one of the main ingredients is alcohol—the kind that causes free-radical damage, irritation, and enhanced oil production. What a letdown, especially when you consider that this has a wonderfully silky, weightless texture that looks like a second skin. It provides a lasting matte finish, but in terms of shine, you will see some in a few hours or sooner—this doesn't make good on its promise of matte skin for 18 hours. Most of the shades are very good, but it really doesn't matter because this liquid foundation with sunscreen is not recommended.

☹ POOR **Teint Miracle Lit-From-Within Makeup Natural Skin Perfection SPF 15 Sunscreen** *($39)* lacks sufficient UVA protection, which is one of the biggest disappointments with this liquid foundation; and something Lancome knows a lot about because nearly every product they sell outside of the United States is loaded with UVA-protecting ingredients, including one for which they own the patent! Another disappointment is the amount of alcohol; it's actually strong enough that you can smell it. No liquid foundation with alcohol as its third ingredient can hydrate your skin for 18 hours as claimed. Alcohol causes free-radical damage, irritation, and dryness, none of which is good for your skin. Whatever "instrumental test" Lancome used to justify their hydration claim sounds convincing, but they wouldn't tell us how the test was done or exactly what instrument they used. Without that information, this is a marketing study, not a real scientific analysis. There are some good aspects of this foundation. It has a thin, fluid, exceptionally silky texture that's easy to blend. It sets to a finish that feels matte, but leaves skin with a subtle, luminous glow that's quite skin-like. Lancome refers to the glow as Aura-Inside technology, but it's just shine, the result of the same shiny particles that many foundations and powders contain; it isn't a miracle breakthrough. In terms of the shades, as usual, Lancome produced mostly stellar colors, though there are some pink, peach, red, or gold undertones in a few of the shades that should be avoided. On balance, this could have been an exemplary foundation for normal to slightly dry or slightly oily skin, but its drawbacks are not to be overlooked.

LANCOME CONCEALERS

✓☺ BEST **$$$ Maquicomplet Complete Coverage Concealer** *($29.50)* is a smooth, liquidy concealer with excellent, crease-free, medium to full coverage, and a soft matte finish. The shades are mostly neutral shades for fair to dark skin tones.

☺ GOOD **$$$ Effacernes Waterproof Protective Under-eye Concealer** *($29.50)* has a creamy texture that provides significant coverage and allows for smooth blending. The squeeze tube takes some getting used to (it's easy to dispense too much product), but once you acclimate, this concealer is aces, and it doesn't crease! Contrary to the name, this concealer is not waterproof.

☺ GOOD **$$$ Teint Miracle Instant Retouch Pen Lit-From-Within Perfector** *($29.50)* has a silky, lightweight texture and a soft matte (in feel) finish that provides subtle illumination without quickly creasing into lines. Many cosmetics lines offer a brush-on highlighter to help brighten shadowed areas while also offering some coverage (like a concealer). Lancome's contribution comes packaged in a pen, which you click to distribute the product onto the brush. Because this doesn't provide considerable coverage, it works best as a highlighter applied after concealer. You can use it to help brighten dark circles or on your eyelids as a base for eyeshadow. The shade range present options for fair to tan skin tones.

LANCOME POWDERS

✓☺ BEST **$$$ Absolue Powder Radiant Smoothing Powder** *($56)* carries a price that may make you look anything but radiant, but wait until you feel its ultra-silky, otherworldly texture. This is one of the most elegant loose powders available. Although the talc-based formula isn't too different from many other powders, the milling process does create a slight difference. This has a non-drying sheer finish suitable for normal to dry skin. All the shades resemble real skin tones.

✓☺ BEST **$$$ Ageless Minerale Perfecting and Setting Mineral Powder with White Sapphire Complex** *($36)* is a very silky, sheer setting powder that leaves an attractive satin finish on skin. The pale flesh tone is supposed to be translucent, but is too white for tan to dark skin tones. If you have a light skin tone and normal to dry skin, this is a very good setting powder to consider.

✓☺ BEST **$$$ Translucence Mattifying Silky Matte Powder** *($29)* is magnificent in every respect, though it should be stated that you don't need to spend this much to get a great pressed powder. The texture is disarmingly silky, so this applies and blends smoothly, looking very skin-like and not the least bit dry or powdery. As with the best pressed powders, skin is left looking polished and refined with a soft, lasting matte finish. Those with oily skin will find touch-ups will be needed, but you can layer or reapply this powder without it looking thick or cakey. This provides sheer coverage (it's not a powder foundation) and the shade range is marvelous, with options for fair to slightly dark skin tones. The darkest shades (in the "Suede" range) can look ever-so-slightly ash, but if applied with a brush instead of the included sponge they're perfect.

LANCOME BLUSHES & BRONZERS

☺ GOOD **$$$ Tropiques Minerale Mineral Smoothing Loose Bronzer** *($39.50)* produces an attractive bronze sheen that includes a hint of sparkles. Applying this powder bronzer in loose form isn't the tidiest way to fake a tan, but with the right brush it can produce a nice glow. Of the two shades, Natural Ambre is the most convincing.

☺ AVERAGE **$$$ Blush Subtil Delicate Oil-Free Powder Blush** *($30)* hasn't kept pace with the latest and greatest powder blushes from Estee Lauder due to the dry texture and slightly choppy application. If you decide to try this, it includes mostly matte options and each of the colors goes on quite sheer.

☺ AVERAGE **$$$ Blush Subtil Shimmer Delicate Oil-Free Powder Blush** *($30)* has the same texture as the original Blush Subtil, but each shade is imbued with sparkles (this isn't a low-glow shimmer). The good news is the sparkles cling well and the colors apply softly, but this isn't enough to make it worth choosing over better blushes that cost less.

☺ AVERAGE **$$$ Star Bronzer Long Lasting Bronzing Powder Natural Glow** *($35)* is a decent bronzer that goes on sheer and smooth and layers well if you need more intensity. The colors range from light to medium-dark and each has a flattering bronze hue. The "Glow" part of this bronzer's name comes from the tiny speckles of glitter that are included in the pressed powder. Although it's a minor part of the formula, glitter isn't exactly the most natural-looking way to fake a sun-kissed glow.

LANCOME EYESHADOWS & PRIMERS

☺ GOOD **$$$ Color Design Sensational Effects Eye Shadow Quad Smooth Hold** *($43)* is an expensive way to assemble an eyeshadow collection; however, every quad has well-coordinated colors that apply smoothly, if a bit soft, and have a suede-smooth texture. At first glance, some of the quads appear contrasting, but the colors blend together well, with most imparting a soft shimmer finish. The effect of any of the quads isn't necessarily sensational, but definitely versatile, and the shine doesn't flake.

☺ GOOD **Color Design Sensational Effects Eye Shadow Smooth Hold** *($18)* feels quite silky and applies smoothly without flaking or skipping. Medium to deep shades are easy to soften, and overall this eyeshadow takes full advantage of advances in powder technology. The shades and finishes are divided into matte, sheen, shimmer, metallic, lustrous, and intense.

The matte shades are our preference (no surprise there). The sheens have a low-luster finish, appropriate unless your eyelid skin is noticeably wrinkled. Shimmer and Metallic are the shiniest group, while the Intense group is primarily deep shades best for eye lining. Lustrous shades have a sparkling shimmer and softer colors, and those who crave shine will find some beautiful colors in this group.

☺ AVERAGE $$$ **Color Design Eye Brightening All-in-One 5 Shadow & Liner Palette** *($49)* includes four eyeshadows and a powder line in one sleek compact. You should toss out the sponge-tip applicators Lancome includes because they are poor substitutes for professional eyeshadow brushes. Designed to be applied wet or dry, the shadows have a smooth, almost creamy texture and even application. Applied dry, the color impact is surprisingly soft; used wet, the colors go on true and allow for dramatic shading (or pops of bright color, if that's what you're after). The liner shade in each set is the darkest color and is best used wet for maximum effect. The downside is that all the palettes have moderate to intense shine; the shiniest shades (those with visible flecks of finely milled glitter) tend to flake.

☹ POOR **Aquatique Waterproof EyeColour Base** *($25.50)* is still around and that means Lancome is succeeding at convincing some women to use a separate product (beyond foundation or concealer) to even out the skin tone on their eyelids and to prevent eyeshadows from creasing. The opaque, thick formula creases, and what's worse is that the shades are not neutral enough to work on a variety of skin tones.

LANCOME EYE & BROW LINERS

✓☺ BEST $$$ **Artliner Precision Point EyeLiner** *($29.50)* remains one of the best liquid eyeliners around thanks to its easy-to-apply, quick-drying, long-lasting formula and superior brush.

☺ GOOD $$$ **Modele Sourcils Brow Groomer** *($24)* is a brow mascara available in clear or with a tint. The lightweight formula keeps the brow groomed without being sticky, and the densely bristled brush is best for thicker, unruly brows.

☺ AVERAGE $$$ **Le Crayon Kohl** *($25.50)* needs routine sharpening, which is why it is not rated higher, but for those willing to tolerate that drawback this is a very good eye pencil. It applies smoothly and is minimally prone to smudging or smearing. There are some wild colors that do little to emphasize eyes, but the classics are there as well.

☺ AVERAGE $$$ **Le Crayon Poudre Powder Pencil for the Brows** *($25.50)* is one of the best needs-sharpening brow pencils. It goes on easily, if a bit creamy, and the colors (with options for all but black brows) are matte and soft. There's even a good brush at one end for softening and blending the color. This would be rated better if not for the need to keep it sharpened, which isn't convenient.

☺ AVERAGE $$$ **Le Style Waterproof Long Lasting EyeLiner** *($25.50)* is a smooth-textured, automatic, nonretractable eye pencil with mostly shiny colors that all tend to smudge, though no more so than most creamy pencils. This is fine for a smoky look, but it breaks down readily when wet.

LANCOME LIP COLOR & LIPLINERS

✓☺ BEST $$$ **Color Design Sensational Effects Lipcolor** *($22)* has a smooth, creamy texture that hydrates lips without feeling too thick or greasy. Lancome offers an extensive range of gorgeous shades, divided by finish (though all except the Mattes have the same creamy feel). Shimmer shades impart soft shine, Sheens impart a metallic iridescence, Metallics offer a strong metallic finish, and Creams have a soft, semi-gloss finish. The small collection of Mattes is very good and provides a true matte finish that feels comfortable rather than dry. Regardless of finish, each shade, particularly the reds, has a great stain so these last longer than standard cream lipsticks (the Mattes have even more impressive longevity). Quite simply, this is Lancome's most impressive lipstick, and at this price it should impress!

✓☺ BEST $$$ **Le Crayon Lip Contour** *($23.50)* is an above-average automatic, retractable lip pencil with good colors and a smooth application. This lipliner really stays put and is an ideal choice for those prone to having lipstick feather into lines around the mouth.

☺ GOOD $$$ **Color Fever Gloss** *($26)* is billed as a lip gloss, but is closer to a liquid lipstick thanks to its smooth, moist feel and pigment level. A glossy, non-sticky finish is part of the deal, and most of the colors are striking. Paying this much for gloss is definitely not necessary, but at least Lancome provided exquisite packaging and a cleverly angled sponge-tip applicator that lets you apply more color in less time.

☺ GOOD $$$ **Juicy Tubes Ultra Shiny Lip Gloss** *($18)* has a thick, syrupy texture and each translucent color leaves lips with a wet-look shine and a slightly sticky feel. The shades tend to rotate seasonally and sometimes have special "artist-inspired" packaging even though the formula remains the same. This lip gloss contains fragrance.

☺ GOOD $$$ **L'Absolu Nu Replenishing & Enhancing Lipcolor-Bare Lip Sensation** *($29.50)* has a smooth, creamy texture that imparts sheer color and leaves a glossy finish, but it doesn't offer anything special or unique beyond its gorgeous packaging. Think of this as lip gloss in stick form, except you get a bit more color than you get with a standard sheer gloss. Longevity-wise, you'll be touching up often with this lipstick—and it isn't for anyone with lines around the mouth because the color moves there quickly.

☺ GOOD $$$ **Rouge in Love High Potency Lipcolor 6 Hour Wear** *($25)* claims six hours of wear and that is a refreshingly honest and mostly realistic claim for this unusual lipstick. Unlike traditional lipsticks, the formula is silicone-based rather than relying on oils and waxes as the predominant ingredients (those are present in lesser amounts). Lancome's blend of silicones with the aforementioned ingredients has produced a lipstick that's feels creamy yet is also lightweight and beautifully silky. This also has a glossy finish that isn't too slippery and doesn't feel greasy. It's a hybrid of a creamy and semi-matte lipstick and as a result you get an impressive amount of staying power. Helping to enhance this lipstick's staying power is the richly pigmented shades. Each saturates lips with rich color and the shade range caters to most tastes, from subdued to bold (though because each shade goes on opaque, this isn't for fans of a sheer lip look). The only drawback, besides the price, is that the formula contains fragrance and fragrance ingredients known to cause irritation. This isn't a deal-breaker, but no question there would be more to love about Rouge in Love if it were fragrance-free.

☹ AVERAGE $$$ **La Laque Fever Lip Shine** *($26.50)* claims that it provides high-potency color and shine that lasts for six hours. Don't count on it! Even though this gloss is more pigmented than most, its slick texture tends to fade quickly, necessitating frequent touch-ups. It isn't the least bit goopy or sticky, and the wet-looking, prismatic shine is attractive—but at best you'll get slightly longer wear time than what you get from a standard lip gloss. The applicator for this gloss is unique and won't be to everyone's liking, so be sure to test it before purchasing. (Swatch some gloss on your hand so you get an idea of how the applicator deposits product.)

☺ AVERAGE $$$ **Le Lipstique LipColouring Stick with Brush** *($24.50)* is a standard pencil with a tapered blending brush at the other end. That's convenient, but not worth the price. This does have some staying power, leaving a slight stain on the lips, and the shade selection is plentiful.

☺ AVERAGE $$$ **Color Fever Plumper Plumping Vibrant Lip Shine** *($29)* is Lancome's version of Maybelline New York's Lip Plumper XL (Lancome and Maybelline are both owned by L'Oreal). The formulas are nearly identical, and both contain a potent menthol derivative (ethyl menthane carboxamide, to be exact) that makes lips tingle (as claimed) and enlarge slightly from the resulting irritation. This plumper is too irritating for daily use, but is an OK option for special occasions when you'd like a sheer, sparkling lip gloss that adds a little something extra to lips.

☹ POOR **L'Absolu Rouge Advanced Replenishing & Reshaping Lipcolor Pro Xylane SPF 12 Sunscreen** *($29.50)* lacks the right UVA-protecting ingredients to protect lips (which get sun damage, too) from the entire UVA spectrum, which is an insult at this price. Labeling this "advanced" is a joke, and the formula doesn't contain anything called Pro Xylane—even Lancome's staff couldn't explain what it was; they simply read from their sales training manual. This cream lipstick does have a unique texture that is light yet substantially moisturizing (it contains a lot of nut oil) and the colors plus the dimensional shimmer most of them have are riveting, as it the magnetic closure of the case. But to go as far as stating this lipstick can reshape lips is a joke. Any shimmer lipstick applied well can make lips look slightly fuller due to its reflective quality, and smoother due to its combination of lip line-filling waxes and polymers. Such technology isn't unique to Lancome, and this lipstick doesn't deserve your attention.

LANCOME MASCARAS

✓☺ BEST $$$ **Definicils High Definition Mascara** *($26)* is an extraordinary lengthening mascara that builds some thickness with minimal to no chance of clumping. The only drawback, and this is a minor complaint, is it can go on a bit too wet, which increases the chance of it smearing before your lashes dry. Still, that's a minor quibble; this is a longstanding favorite for good reason!

✓☺ BEST $$$ **Definicils Waterproof High Definition Mascara** *($26)* does everything Lancome's regular Definicils mascara does to lengthen, lightly thicken, and separate the lashes, but with a waterproof formula that wears and wears. It is Lancome's premiere waterproof mascara, and the formula leaves lashes feeling soft (an uncommon trait for waterproof mascaras).

✓☺ BEST $$$ **L'Extreme Instant Extensions Lengthening Mascara** *($26)* is positioned as a lengthening mascara, and it does just that. With a brush similar to mascara hall-of-famer Definicils, L'Extreme quickly elongates lashes with barely a clump. It allows you to create long, fringed lashes with subtle thickness and wears well throughout the day. As impressive as this mascara is, you don't have to spend this much for such results, but that doesn't mean this entry from Lancome is undeserving of a Best Product rating!

☺ GOOD $$$ **Cils Booster XL Super-Enhancing Mascara Base** *($23)* is a lash primer that really works. Pre-mascara, it adds bulk and length to lashes, allowing the actual color-enhancing mascara to cling better and apply evenly. What you'll notice is more thickness and oomph to lashes than using just mascara alone. This type of product isn't for everyone (most women won't want to bother with two steps), but those with short or sparse lashes should give this a try and see for themselves what a difference it makes.

☺ GOOD $$$ **Hypnose Custom Volume Mascara** *($26)* doesn't perform as claimed. This is far from being a poor mascara because it does do a reasonably good job of separating, lengthening, and slightly thickening lashes without a single clump, leaving lashes soft rather than brittle. It also removes well with a water-soluble cleanser. But if you were expecting impossibly long, voluminous lashes, this isn't the mascara for you.

☺ GOOD **$$$ Hypnose Drama Waterproof Mascara** *($26)* does a good job of lengthening lashes and holding curl, and it lives up to its waterproof name. You will need an eye-makeup remover for this one! It also adds volume, but does so at the expense of slightly clumpy lashes, but nothing that a lash comb can't fix. Overall, it's a good waterproof mascara that doesn't flake or smudge.

☺ GOOD **$$$ Oscillation Intensity Vibrating Intensifying Powermascara** *($35)* comes with alluring claims of "high voltage lash transformation." The voltage analogy is strange because the only electrical feature is that the battery makes the brush vibrate. In fact, the vibration feature can be a bit cumbersome because you have to hold the button on the cap down as you apply, making application rather awkward. Although the vibrating effect is "kinda cool," at best it just helps this heavy mascara go on somewhat more evenly. Whether the vibration feature is turned on or off, the full, rubber-bristled brush allows you to create dramatically long, thick lashes without flaking. This isn't a mascara for those who want a natural lash look, but if big, bold lashes are your goal, this makes it happen! It also removes easily with a water-soluble cleanser. Drawbacks include some clumping, minor smearing upon application (this can be remedied by keeping the vibration turned off), and the fact that this goes on a bit wet, necessitating some comb-through for defined, fringed lashes.

☺ GOOD **$$$ Oscillation Powerbooster Vibrating Amplifying Primer** *($39.50)* comes with claims intended to make this sound like several of the expensive lash growth products being sold, including prescription-only Lastisse. However, Lancome words the claims very carefully so that the claims remain cosmetic. After all, "amplifying lashes" could mean several things or nothing at all. As it turns out, this product is little more than an expensive way to add bulk to lashes before applying mascara. The formula contains standard thickeners and waxes, and absolutely nothing that can impact lash growth or thickness, at least nothing beyond a cosmetic effect that will be gone as soon as you remove the product from your lashes. The vibration element is more gimmicky than helpful (it's difficult to keep the button depressed, which is what turns on the vibration), but this primer does add extra oomph to lashes and enhances mascara application. This isn't a necessary product if you're already using a great mascara (Lancome offers several), but this primer does make a difference when used with less impressive mascaras.

☺ GOOD **$$$ Oscillation Vibrating Infinite Powermascara** *($35)* is not an ingenious, futuristic way to get a better, cleaner application of mascara, even though we wish it could be. Activating the brush drenched lashes in mascara and caused wet clumps that were tricky to smooth out. Ironically, taking the brush off vibration mode allowed for better smoothing, lash separation, and dramatic length. Lots of mascara gets deposited at lash roots, so the effect when you're done cleaning things up is startling, especially if your lashes are already longer than average. Although we can't recommend this mascara for its special features (and the price is sticker shock given great or even better mascaras that are available for one-third the price), we cannot deny its impressive lengthening ability, either. Note: This mascara has a pervasive rose fragrance and is not recommended for sensitive/teary eyes.

☺ AVERAGE **$$$ Hypnose Doll Lashes Mascara** *($26)* gives you a decent amount of lengthening and separation, but very little volume or thickness. Multiple coats tend to make lashes appear more spidery than full, though one could argue that this is the intended "doll lash" effect. The tapered brush is dense with thin plastic bristles that can make the already wet, rose-scented formula appear extra goopy on lashes. Bottom line: This isn't one of Lancome's better mascaras.

☺ AVERAGE **$$$ Hypnose Drama Instant Full Body Volume Mascara** *($26)* is disappointing. The problems begin with a very large, unwieldy brush that practically guarantees you'll get mascara where you don't want it, like on the eyelid and the skin along the lower lash line. Application is uneven to the point of being messy, but with patience you can smooth things out and avoid a clumpy, spiked appearance. With proper cleanup (have a clean lash brush or comb handy) the result is very long, dark, and slightly thickened lashes.

☺ AVERAGE $$$ **Hypnôse Waterproof Custom Volume Mascara** *($26)* disappoints compared to its non-waterproof counterpart, but is nevertheless a respectable mascara for length and clean lash separation. Thickness (referred to in the name as "volume") is fairly scarce, but at least this holds up well under water or during a good cry.

☺ AVERAGE $$$ **L'Extreme Waterproof Instant Extensions Lengthening Mascara** *($26)* withstands tears and swimming (actually, it's so tenacious that it takes more effort than usual to remove it); however, it builds minimal length and thickness. At best you'll achieve moderate length and a smidgen of thickness with lots of effort, and for this price (and Lancome's reputation as a mascara leader), that's disappointing.

☺ AVERAGE $$$ **Oscillation Water-Resistant Vibrating Infinite Powermascara** *($35)* is another battery-powered mascara from Lancome and it works in a similar fashion to Lancome's Oscillation Vibrating Infinite Powermascara. On the downside, once set this breaks down readily with water. In fact, we were able to remove most of it by splashing my face with water, so don't count on the water-resistant claim even a little.

☹ POOR **Definicils Precious Cells High Definition Amplifying Mascara** *($29.50)* contains no "precious cells" of any kind (at least not our definition of precious), but given the price, you'd think there would be. This mascara is said to regenerate the condition of lashes in four weeks, with subtle claims that may lead some consumers to think the formula can grow lashes or reduce eyelash loss. It can't. In fact, the waxes and thickeners in this mascara are the same ones found in hundreds of other mascaras, including most that cost less than $10, like those sold by Lancome's parent company L'Oreal. This product contains a tiny amount of plant oils and a teeny amount of stem cells from apples, but none of these ingredients have been shown to promote lash growth of any kind. (Stem cells from apples would increase apple cell growth, not human cell growth, right?) Even if this were somehow a regenerative formula, performance-wise, this isn't one of Lancome's better mascaras. Application is overly wet, creating a slightly uneven look with clumps that need smoothing. What surprised us most was that this mascara flaked slightly within seconds of drying. It also is overly fragranced—hours later, the potent scent is still noticeable. Lancome doesn't list fragrance, but this does contain phenethyl alcohol, an ingredient whose primary function is fragrance.

LANCOME FACE & BODY ILLUMINATORS

☺ GOOD $$$ **Eclat Miracle Serum of Light Complexion Illuminator** *($37)* is a sheer, water-based, fragrance-free liquid shine product for your face. It is supposed to contain "liquid mirror" particles that work to provide a continuous illuminated effect. Sounds interesting, but it's really just a roundabout way to tell you that this product leaves a shiny finish. The amount of shine is sheer to moderate, depending on how much you apply. A dab produces a soft, luminous finish without obvious sparkles; add more and the shine factor increases but never becomes glittery or glaring. This is surprisingly easy to blend and can be applied under or over your makeup. Because the translucent white color and shine of this product is meant to highlight, it is best used on the high points of your face or on the brow bone. The alcohol this contains is slight cause for concern. Although it's not present in a high amount, there's enough that you'll smell it before this illuminating product sets. It is best to avoid applying this close to your eyes. Eclat Miracle's formula is best for normal to oily skin (though note products like this make oily areas look oilier).

LANCOME BRUSHES

✓☺ BEST **Mineral Powder Foundation Brush** *($37.50)* is phenomenally soft and perfectly shaped for expert application of loose or pressed powder. It is one of Lancome's better brushes and definitely worth considering for its performance and price.

☺ GOOD $$$ **Lancome Brushes** *($20–$56.50)* tend to be a good option but, although many of them are worthwhile, the overall collection is disappointing compared to those from Bobbi Brown, Stila, Laura Mercier, M.A.C., or Paula's Choice. A consistent issue is the overall size of the brush, with an overriding tendency to be either too small or too large for the intended area. Still, there are some winners here, including the **Foundation Brush #2** ($34.50), **Concealer Brush #8** ($26.50), **Retractable Lip Brush #9** ($25.50), and **Angle Shadow Brush #13** ($26.50).

LAURA GELLER (MAKEUP ONLY)

Strengths: Liquid foundation and concealer; lots of products to add shine to skin; good selection of pressed powders; the cream and liquid blush; enviable lip gloss; the sugar-themed eyeshadows; great brow tint; one remarkable mascara; original Spackle.

Weaknesses: Limited complexion products; no foundations, concealers, or powder shades for dark skin tones; contour powder is way too shiny; several average powder eyeshadows; disappointing long-wearing lip paint; incomplete and often not well-made assortment of brushes; claims that products do not contain parabens or mineral oil, but they do (yet neither ingredient is harmful).

For more information and reviews of the latest Laura Geller products, visit CosmeticsCop.com.

LAURA GELLER FOUNDATIONS & PRIMERS

✓☺ BEST **Barely There Tinted Moisturizer SPF 20** *($30)* is a superb tinted moisturizer that includes the mineral sunscreens titanium dioxide and zinc oxide as active ingredients. It has a silky, lightweight texture that's a pleasure to blend. This sets to a delicate satin matte finish and provides sheer to light coverage that diffuses minor flaws and redness. The formula contains several antioxidants, but the choice of clear tube packaging means they won't remain effective for long unless you're diligent about keeping it protected from light. Otherwise, this is recommended for normal to dry or slightly oily skin, and is suitable for sensitive skin provided you're not sensitive to the plant extracts this contains. Those looking for a similar, less expensive product in better packaging should consider Paula's Choice Barely There Sheer Matte Tint SPF 20. If you opt for Geller's version, all the shades are workable, though Deep is slightly orange and the trickiest to use.

☺ GOOD $$$ **Phenomenal Foundation** *($36.50)*. Claiming that this liquid foundation is "phenomenal" is pushing things a bit because it automatically implies this is the ultimate foundation—it isn't. We are not, however, saying that it isn't worth considering, because it is in fact a very good option; it's just not the best of the best. Dispensed from a pump, it has a creamy texture that applies light and silky, setting to a satin-matte finish that remains slightly moist. It is best for normal to slightly dry skin (oily areas will show shine in short order). Coverage is in the medium range and this does a reasonably good job of not magnifying pores and lines (it works much better if you apply Geller's Spackle primer first, but there are other foundations that look better on skin and that don't need a primer). Among the small selection of shades, Medium is slightly peach and should be considered carefully. Deep is not that dark and is best for tan skin tones.

☺ GOOD $$$ **Spackle Tinted Under Make-Up Primer** *($27.50 for 2 fl. oz.)* is nearly identical to Laura Geller's original Spackle Under Make Up Primer below, except for its sheer tint (Bronze, Champagne, or Ethereal) that leaves skin with a subtle radiant glow.

☺ GOOD **Spackle Under Makeup Primer** *($25)* is by far Geller's most popular product and the one from her line we're asked about most often. And it's no wonder: This pump-dispensed primer is sold as the ideal undercoat to perfect skin's texture. Most primers contain a lot of silicone to smooth skin and provide a silky canvas for foundation (and, to some extent, help to temporarily fill in large pores and superficial lines). Spackle is mostly water and film-forming agent with lesser amounts of silicone. It feels very light and has a smooth finish that is ever-so-slightly tacky at dry-down. This is easy to apply, sets quickly, and contains shiny pigments to lend a subtle glow to skin (this glow may be why so many women feel their skin looks better with this product; if you have a dull complexion, applying any slightly shimmery product will help, but it's more effective to deal with dullness during your skin-care routine than with makeup effects). We sampled Spackle both with and without Geller's foundation, and found that the Spackle did enhance the effect of the foundation. It was easier to apply and it looked better because it didn't show signs of sinking into pores and lines. Does that mean Spackle is a must-have? Absolutely not. There's nothing wrong with adding this product to your routine, but your skin would be better off using a weightless matte- or satin-finish serum loaded with beneficial ingredients (the botanicals in Spackle don't quite cut it, and some, such as witch hazel, are irritating). Moreover, almost all of today's best foundations can make skin look smooth, even without the need for a primer. If your foundation isn't making your skin look the way you want it to, consider trying a new foundation before trying a primer. Those who remain intrigued by this product should know it is suitable for all skin types except sensitive.

☺ GOOD $$$ **Welcome Matte Skin Enhancer** *($23.50)*. We're surprised this product isn't named Spackle, like others from Laura Geller, because this nonaqueous silicone-based gel really does have a spackle-like texture. It feels very silky and works to a minor extent to temporarily fill in large pores and smooth superficial lines. The weightless finish is ideal for oily skin and facilitates makeup application. Because this isn't super-absorbent, those with very oily skin should explore Smashbox's Anti-Shine or Paula's Choice Shine Stopper before this.

LAURA GELLER CONCEALERS

☺ GOOD $$$ **Crease-Less Concealer** *($23.50)* is packaged in a pen-style component that includes a built-in synthetic brush applicator. The fluid, silky texture has an excellent, weight-less application that sets to a matte finish with a hint of shine. You'll get moderate coverage, so this is best for minor flaws and slight darkness under the eyes (those with pronounced dark circles will need better camouflage). Two of the three shades are great; avoid Deep, which is too peachy rose to look convincing.

☺ AVERAGE $$$ **Caulk Pencil & Sharpener** *($24.50)*. What a name! Who would want to use a concealer with a name reminiscent of that goop that comes in a tube and that you use to seal holes and prevent water damage? Apparently someone does, because this is sup-posedly one of Geller's bestsellers. The good news is that this isn't really caulk. It is a chunky, needs-sharpening pencil outfitted with a sponge tip on one end for blending. The "caulk" end has a silicone-based texture that glides on and blends superbly, while the texture feels lighter than you'd expect. Dotting this on skin provides instant full coverage that can look heavy, but it softens well during blending and winds up being a good option for those who need ample coverage that doesn't appear too opaque. The problem is that among the three shades, two (Medium and Dark) are very peach. The peachiness softens as you blend, but it will still look odd on many skin tones. The best shade to try, if you don't mind sharpening, is Light. It will crease into lines around the eyes unless carefully set with powder, which can make lines look more obvious. All in all, there are better concealer options.

☺ AVERAGE $$$ Hide-N-Shine *($20.50)* comes in a compact with two colors, one of which is too peach or orange to use regardless of the duo you're considering. Mixing the shades to get a better color is an option, but one that's not really necessary given the plethora of good neutral-toned concealers available in many formats (e.g., liquid or cream). We wish the colors were better because this applies, blends, and covers beautifully, setting to a soft matte finish with a hint of shine. It is minimally prone to creasing into lines around the eye. All told, this is recommended only if you're OK with mixing two shades for a result that's not as good as it should be.

☺ AVERAGE $$$ **The Real Deal Concealer Serious Coverage** *($20)*. Housed in a flat, small tube this is a slightly thick, creamy concealer that really does provide serious coverage. It's the type of coverage that can conceal dark circles and dark spots, including birthmarks (although most port wine stains will need something more for complete camouflage). This is surprisingly easy to blend due to its inherent silky texture, and it's a plus that thinning this out during blending doesn't significantly decrease coverage. What will be a deal-breaker for many people, however, is the fact that this never really sets to a long-wearing finish; it remains moist and slick, and as such is prone to creasing, fading, and smearing unless set with a lot of powder. Of course, setting it with powder can make such opaque coverage more obvious, so it isn't the best look unless you have something major to hide. If you're willing to accept the trade-off, this concealer is an option, but test it before buying. Among the four shades, Light and Medium are best. Medium Deep tends to be too orange, and Deep is workable but will be too dark for those with tan to light brown skin.

LAURA GELLER POWDERS

☺ GOOD $$$ **Matte Maker** *($22)* contains a high amount of the very absorbent ingredient calcium carbonate. As such, it is effective at keeping excess shine in check and is best for oily to very oily skin. The smooth, drier-than-usual powder can be difficult to pick up with a brush, but you don't need much to achieve a mattifying effect. Best for blotting, only one color is available and it applies transparently.

☺ AVERAGE $$$ **Shade-N-Sculpt Contouring Powder with Brush** *($39.50)*. Housed in one compact without a divider is a muted brown pressed powder and a pale beige-gold highlighting powder. The brown shade is acceptable for contouring medium to tan skin tones, but the effect will be anything but subtle thanks to the large flecks of gold shine that were added. The highlighting powder's shine is subtle and much more workable. Contouring is never about adding shine to skin, and should be a deal-breaker for most professional makeup artists; but of course, there are always exceptions to every rule in the world of makeup application. The full-size brush that comes with the kit is an acceptable option, so you don't need to purchase an additional brush.

🌹 Highly fragranced products smell good, but won't help your skin! See the Appendix for details.

Laura Geller Blushes & Bronzers

✓☺ BEST **$$$ Air Whipped Blush** *($26)* has a sponge-like silky texture and is really easy to apply. A tiny dab produces a soft flush of translucent color to enliven your cheeks. The shade selection is bare bones, but what's available is good (though the Whisper Petal shade is infused with obvious flecks of shine). Although this blush is fine for all skin types, it's expensive for what you get. The company plays up the antioxidants, but because this blush is packaged in a jar, they won't remain stable once the product is opened.

☺ GOOD **$$$ Blush-N-Brighten** *($31)*. This marbled pressed powder presents a blend of colors in one compact. Swirling a brush over the tablet blends the hues together to create one shade that enlivens cheeks with color and a strong shimmer finish. The texture is smooth yet dry and application is sheer and even. You don't have to spend this much money for shiny blush, but it is an option, and all the colors are workable.

☺ GOOD **$$$ Balance-N-Bronze** *($31)* has a marbled pattern that blends several colors together. Once you swirl a brush over the melange of colors and apply it to your skin, the effect is a soft rosy tan that looks best on fair to medium skin tones. The powder has a smooth, dry texture that applies sheer and builds well for additional depth. Its finish is matte (in feel), but it leaves a soft glow on skin. Less expensive versions of this product are readily available from Physician's Formula, but this is still an option.

☺ GOOD **$$$ Bronze-N-Brighten** *($31)* is similar to the Balance-N-Bronze above, except here you get a muted bronze shade with rose undertones that's best for light to medium skin tones. Otherwise, the same comments apply.

☹ AVERAGE **$$$ The Real Deal Blush Stick SPF 15** *($26)*. This cream-to-powder twist-up stick blush comes in two shades, both of which impart sheer, natural-looking color with a good amount of shine yet a dry finish. Application isn't as easy as you might expect from a cream-to-powder blush, and you'll need to layer and blend more than usual. Dabbing this blush on cheeks and then blending upward with fingertips yielded the best results. This blush also has the novelty of an SPF rating that includes adequate broad-spectrum protection. While it's nice to boost your sun protection when you can, you need a lot more coverage than a blended-out application of blush to protect against sun damage, and you need to cover more of your face than just a swatch of blush.

Laura Geller Eyeshadows & Eye Primers

☺ GOOD **$$$ Marble Cakes Baked Eyeshadow & Liner Duo** *($23)* is a circular 2-in-1 powder compact that offers a cake eyeliner and shimmery coordinating powder shadow, and comes with a dual-ended synthetic brush for blending and lining. Available in only two shade options (Blue or Brown), the eyeliner is exceptional, with rich, lasting color that performs best when applied wet and that won't budge once dry. The shadow is too shimmery for wide appeal, but it does compliment the liner nicely, and could work in addition to a more deeply pigmented contour shadow. The real star here is the multi-functional full-size brush, which has the density to capture and distribute powder nicely, while the angled liner end delivers precision results.

☺ GOOD **$$$ Sugar Free Matte Baked Eyeshadow Duo** *($23)* is a standard, but good, powder eyeshadow whose name makes it sound like something to snack on if you're concerned about carbs. The "baked" concept refers to the fact that these eyeshadows begin in liquid form and then are cooked at high heat in terracotta pots until they solidify. There's really no benefit to making eyeshadows this way (though it sounds good in marketing materials), and in the case of this product, the result is the same smooth texture and even application of many good eyeshadows. The duos are nearly matte—only a soft shine is visible—and the shades work well together.

☺ GOOD **$$$ Sugared Baked Pearl Eyeshadow** *($23)* is just a shiny powder eyeshadow with a very smooth texture and even, flake-free application (unless you overdo it). The small selection of shades has a strong shimmer and works best for highlighting the brow bone.

☺ GOOD **$$$ Wonder Wand** *($19.50)*. We wish Geller would parlay this loose-powder eyeshadow into a pressed eyeshadow because it has an otherworldly smooth texture that clings like a second skin and imparts sheer, buildable color with an attractive, though none-too-subtle, shimmer. As a loose powder, however, it's hard to blend on as eyeshadow. At least the packaging minimizes mess and the pointed sponge-tip applicator (while not preferred to a good eyeshadow brush) allows for greater versatility than standard sponge applicators. If used sparingly, this is a very good way to highlight the brow bone or under-eye area for evening glamour.

☹ AVERAGE **$$$ Baked Marble Eyeshadow** *($23)* contains large particles of shine that not only distract from the result once applied, but also give this powder eyeshadow a slight grainy feel. Color deposit is good and the shine clings decently, so this is still an OK option if you want impact accompanied by large flecks of shine for your eyeshadow look.

☹ AVERAGE **$$$ Eye Rimz Baked Wet/Dry Eye Accents** *($26)* is marbleized and flecked with two colors in one compact. As described, the dominant color is black and you swirl it with another color to achieve a dimensional, metallic effect. This comes with a good brush and applies smoothly, but you have to be careful to not pick up too much on the brush or it will flake. As with most powder eyeshadows, this may be used wet or dry. Note that the emollients in this powder lead to some fading and smearing after several hours of wear.

☹ AVERAGE **$$$ Eye Spackle** *($24)* is sold as a prep product to apply to the eyelid and under-brow area pre-eyeshadow, but is nothing more than a cream concealer whose opaque and whitish finish brightens the eye area, but also leaves an unattractive, heavy look unless applied sparingly. The creamy finish is crease-prone, and this is not preferred to numerous matte-finish concealers that work beautifully as a base for eyeshadows.

LAURA GELLER EYE & BROW LINERS

✓☺ BEST **$$$ Eyebrow Tint & Tamer** *($21.50)*. Housed in one dual-sided package are a clear brow gel and a brow tint. Both are applied with built-in mascara brushes, and each has a clean, smooth application that sets unruly brows without feeling tacky or gummy. The brow tint is sheer yet does its part to define. There are two good colors (but no options for black or auburn/red brows).

☹ AVERAGE **$$$ Baby Cakes Baked Eyeliner Palette** *($34)*. A flip-top palette houses four shades of super-smooth powder eyeliner made for wet or dry application, the former being preferable because it yields more intense and lasting results without flaking. The included synthetic eyeliner brush is tiny and unsuitable for dry application, but when wet it creates a pencil-thin line that lasts. The major drawback is the shades, all of which contain noticeable shine, with Blue Sugar wearing far more like a stripe of glitter than eyeliner. Dutch Chocolate is vibrant and gorgeous, but as a whole the palette is hardly worth the price for one or two viable shades. Consider cherry-picking shades you'll actually use, as Laura Geller offers larger sizes of this product in workable duos of colors for nearly half the price—and with a larger brush to boot!

☹ AVERAGE **$$$ Baked Cake Eyeliner Duo** *($26.50)*. Housed in a flip-top compact are two shades of pressed-powder eyeliner designed to be applied wet or dry. Dry application is sheer and slightly flake-prone, even when used sparingly. Wet application is preferred because the immediate result is an intense line that works well to define the eyes without any mess or flaking. The included synthetic eyeliner brush is ideal. Both shades (one is distinctively dark and the other is a colorful, medium tone) contain noticeable shine. Those hoping for longevity won't be disappointed, but should know that gel eyeliners last even longer and aren't prone to fading.

☺ AVERAGE **Powder Pencil Eyeliner** *($15.50)* would be rated a Best Product were it not for the fact that it needs routine sharpening. Once set to its powder finish, this is minimally prone to smudging and wears beautifully. Application, while smooth, is sheer, so you must layer it to truly define your eyes. The silver and green shades have shine, and are alternatives only for special occasion makeup.

☺ AVERAGE $$$ **Brow Marker Long-Lasting Brow Color** *($23)* is a liquid brow color housed in a felt-tip pen-style applicator. The thin, precision brush allows you to get in between brow hairs to create the illusion of a fuller brow, and it's surprisingly easy to apply. The problem is that the amount of alcohol in this formula and the film-forming agent can make brow hairs feel dry and slightly sticky at the same time. Although the application and concept are admirable, the formula itself needs work.

☹ POOR **Double Eye Appeal & Sharpener** *($21)*. The appeal of this needs-sharpening pencil sounds good on paper, but in practice you'll be left wondering why you wasted your money. Designed to highlight and clarify skin with its dual-sided nude cream and pale gold colors, this pencil's texture is too thick and creamy to last, so the minor results are short lived and look sloppy in no time. The promises this pencil makes are a better bet (and more easily attainable) from liquid or powder shine products than from a pencil.

LAURA GELLER LIP COLOR & LIPLINERS

✓☺ BEST $$$ **Creme Couture Soft Touch Matte Lipstick** *($18)*. Much more unique than Geller's regular Lipstick reviewed below, Creme Couture Soft Touch Matte Lipstick feels creamy and light at the same time. Its rich cream finish with a low shine helps spotlight this lipstick's bold opacity. It is recommended for fans of semi-matte lipstick, and the formula allows it to wear longer than standard cream lipsticks.

✓☺ BEST $$$ **Shine & Shield SPF 15 Lip Gloss** *($18)*. Boasting excellent broadspectrum sun protection thanks to the inclusion of zinc oxide, this squeeze-tube gloss has a thick texture that's easy to apply and doesn't feel sticky or look overly shiny. In fact, it's more like a lip balm than a gloss, one that imparts a splash of cocoa butter–scented color without looking overdone. The three shades—nude, coral, and berry—are quite versatile, with only a hint of subtle shimmer. Like many moisturizing lip products, this one wears away quickly, so you'll need to reapply often, especially if you're out in the sun.

☺ GOOD $$$ **Lipstick** *($15.50)* is a standard, lightweight cream lipstick with a creamy finish plus shimmer. It provides moderate coverage and comes in an acceptable range of shades, though non-shimmer and darker colors are lacking.

☺ AVERAGE **Lip Liner** *($15.50)* is typical in every respect, right down to the range of safe yet versatile nude and pink-brown colors. The finish is creamy, but it stays in place reasonably well.

☺ AVERAGE **Lip Parfaits** *($14)* may be visually appealing in its container due to the swirled, intertwining colors, but in the end, it's just a standard lip gloss with a moderately thick texture and slightly sticky but glossy finish.

☺ AVERAGE **Lip Stay** *($14.50)* is Geller's contribution to the two-step, long-wearing lip paints. This begins well, with a silky-textured coat of color that applies evenly and allows for full coverage. It sets in 30 seconds, and then you can apply the glossy top coat. Actually, you need to apply this top coat, because without it the lip paint makes your lips feel progressively drier. After less than an hour of wearing this and with one gloss touch-up, we began to notice problems. The color was peeling and fading toward the center of our mouths, the smooth gloss feeling was wearing off too soon, and the gloss itself was, if you can believe it, difficult to apply. Let's chalk this up to "nice try but no cigar," and stick with companies that offer better versions of such products, including Cover Girl, M.A.C., Estee Lauder, and Maybelline.

☹ POOR **Lip Heal & Seal Lip Gloss** *($20)*. Packaged in one tube are two separate products for lips. The **Lip Heal** portion is housed in a separate inner tube (a tube within a tube) and dispenses with the **Lip Seal** portion of the product. Although this has a great smooth feel and glossy finish, it is not recommended because it contains the irritating menthol derivatives menthyl lactate and menthoxypropanediol—neither of which is the least bit healing for lips. See the Appendix to find out how irritation hurts everyone's skin (and lips)!

LAURA GELLER MASCARA

☺ GOOD $$$ **Mighty Mascara & Fortifier** *($21.50)* features a regular mascara on one end and a lash primer on the other. Both products have the same ingredient list, and there is nothing fortifying about it. Including a tiny amount of panthenol and elastin in a lash product isn't going to produce stronger lashes. The **Mascara** builds equal parts length and thickness without clumping or smearing (but be sure to let it dry completely before blinking too much), while the **Fortifier**, if applied before the Mascara, allows you to add a bit more thickness at the expense of some clumping and a less-even application. Used alone or together, this duo is workable, but L'Oreal and Maybelline sell similar products that perform better at one-third the price.

LAURA GELLER FACE & BODY ILLUMINATORS

☺ GOOD $$$ **Baked Body Frosting** *($45)*. Given this product's name, you may be envisioning a whipped cream–textured product. However, the "frost" refers to the shine of this pressed shimmer powder. The mica- and talc-based formula goes on smooth and dry and isn't too powdery, and it finishes to a satin shine that works best for fair to medium skin tones. Dusted on with a brush or applied with a sponge, this is an attractive way to highlight skin from the neck down (though it can certainly be used on the face, too). Caution: The shine and some color will come off on clothing.

☺ AVERAGE **Liquid Candlelight Face & Body Glow** *($23.50)* imparts sheer shine. Its application has a lot of slip, which makes blending over large areas easier, though it does take time to set. The problem is that the shine is mostly from obvious gold particles rather than from finely milled shimmer pigment. Therefore, the effect is showy instead of "glow-y," and not something to consider if your objective is to re-create the soft, alluring glow that real candlelight has on skin; Lorac, Chanel, and Stila have better options in that regard.

LAURA GELLER BRUSHES

☺ AVERAGE **Professional Brush Collection** *($45)* is a seven-piece brush set that has an attractive price and even comes with its own brush holder (not a brush roll or bag; instead it's a cup like what you'd use to store pencils on your desk). The set turns out to be not the value it could've been because half of the brushes are either not needed or are poorly made. The worthwhile brushes in this set include the Angled Powder Brush, Eyeshadow Brush, and

Eyeliner/Eyebrow Brush. The others just don't pass muster for professional makeup tools, and the flat, fan-like Blush and Highlighter Brush is no substitute for a traditional domed powder blush brush.

LAURA GELLER SPECIALTY MAKEUP PRODUCTS

☺ GOOD $$$ **Line & Define** *($20)* is sold as "a careful pairing of color-coordinated eyeliner and mascara." The duo is a good option if you don't mind shiny eyeliner. The mascara lengthens and separates lashes quickly without clumping, but doesn't do much to build thickness. The liquid liner's thin brush applies well and the liner goes on evenly and dries fast, which is a plus. Liquid liner wearability is generally good, save for some minor fading (but no flaking).

☺ GOOD $$$ **Waterproof Eye Spackle** *($22)*. This click-pen–style liquid eye-area primer claims that it can make any Laura Geller powder eyeshadow or eyeliner waterproof. We were pleased to discover that it worked beautifully, not only with Geller's eye makeup, but also with every other brand we tried! A thin layer of this product helped powder eyeshadow adhere and stay put, even when rubbed under water. You do need to give this product ample time to set before you layer powder eyeshadow on top. Depending on the shadow you use, you may see some darkening of the shade or dulling of the shimmer finish (which might not be a bad thing). The main drawback of this product is that it tends to ball up if you apply too much or blend too vigorously. Given the "spackle" name, one might think you need a generous amount, but a thin layer patted over your eyelids works best. The two shade options are flesh-toned peach and pale pink, both of which are suitable for fair to medium skin tones.

☹ AVERAGE $$$ **Lip Spackle** *($24)* is sold as a base for lipstick and for filling in lines on lips for smoother application of lipstick and gloss. It feels light and has a soft, sheer powder finish that doesn't impede lipstick application. Lipstick appearance is another thing: Unless you apply your lipstick very carefully and don't push lips together to blend (as many women do), this product can make lipstick look oddly colored and uneven. It is definitely not recommended for use with sheer lipsticks or glosses. If you're curious to try it, this functions best with opaque matte or semi-matte lipsticks.

LAURA MERCIER

Strengths: Many fragrance-free products; top-notch water-soluble cleansers; the serum and serum-type moisturizers are worth a look; some extraordinary foundation and powder products; great powder blush, cream blush, and powder eyeshadows; a couple impressive mascaras; mostly great shimmer products; the makeup brushes; the Bronzing Gel.

Weaknesses: Expensive; some of the products with sunscreen lack sufficient UVA-protecting ingredients; no products to treat acne or lighten skin discolorations; jar packaging; none of the makeup products with sunscreen contain the right UVA-protecting actives; the various Primers are merely OK; average eye pencil, brow-enhancing, and lip pencil options.

For more information and reviews of the latest Laura Mercier products, visit CosmeticsCop.com.

LAURA MERCIER CLEANSERS

✓☺ BEST $$$ **Flawless Skin Oil-Free Foaming One-Step Cleanser** *($35 for 6.8 fl. oz.)* is a liquid-to-foam, water-soluble cleanser that's an excellent option for normal to dry skin. It removes makeup and rinses easily, and is fragrance-free. Of course, you don't need to spend this much for a great cleanser, but if you're determined to do so, you may as well buy one that's beautifully formulated and fragrance-free, and this one fits the bill.

✓☺ BEST **$$$ Flawless Skin One-Step Cleanser** *($35 for 6.8 fl. oz.)* is a very good, though overpriced, fragrance-free cleanser for normal to oily or combination skin. It is water-soluble and rinses without a residue, plus it removes makeup easily (though for waterproof formulas you'll need a separate remover). The tiny amount of witch hazel extract is not cause for concern.

☺ AVERAGE **$$$ Flawless Skin Purifying Cleansing Oil** *($40 for 6.8 fl. oz.)* is an oil–based cleanser and makeup remover for dry to very dry skin. The main ingredients are not "light," and this should not be used by anyone with oily skin. Mercier claims this "leaves less oil molecules on the surface of skin," but that's impossible. The mineral oil base doesn't rinse easily without a washcloth, and no matter how you slice it, more oil molecules will be left on your skin than when you began.

LAURA MERCIER EYE-MAKEUP REMOVER

✓☺ BEST **$$$ Flawless Skin Dual Action Eye Makeup Remover Oil-Free** *($22 for 3.4 fl. oz.)* is an excellent fragrance-free eye-makeup remover that works swiftly to remove all types of eye makeup. The gentle formula's only drawback is its price; without question, you can find less expensive eye-makeup removers from. But, if you don't mind spending more than neces- sary, this does the job beautifully!

LAURA MERCIER MOISTURIZERS (DAYTIME & NIGHTTIME), EYE CREAMS, & SERUMS

☺ GOOD **$$$ Flawless Skin Daily Face Shield SPF 40** *($45 for 1 fl. oz.)* is a thin-textured, surprisingly fluid lotion that contains an in-part titanium dioxide sunscreen in a silky formula best for normal to oily skin. The lightweight texture and soft matte finish work great under makeup, which was likely Mercier's intention. This would earn a higher rating if the antioxidants were more prominent. Still, if you're looking for a sheer, fragrance-free daytime moisturizer that provides ample sun protection, here's a good option!

☺ GOOD **$$$ Multi-Vitamin Serum** *($70 for 0.6 fl. oz.)* is a two-part product consisting of water-based **Phase 1** and silicone-based **Phase 2**. Both contain ingredients that will smooth and hydrate skin, and both contain several antioxidants, although Phase 2 has slightly more. From a formulary standpoint, there was no need for this product to be split into two phases. The explanation given by a Mercier salesperson was that the water in Phase 1 doesn't mix with the plant oils in Phase 2, but that is an issue that any cosmetics chemist could overcome by choosing the correct ingredients to keep them blended together. We suppose Mercier simply wanted her serum to seem different and more scientific, and so consumers are directed to mix several drops from both phases before applying it to the skin. If the mixing step doesn't bother you, this is a very well-formulated, antioxidant-rich serum that is recommended for all but blemish-prone skin. Its packaging ensures the antioxidants will remain stable during use. The firming sensation you get from this product comes from the film-forming agent in Phase 1, which can temporarily make skin feel taut and look smoother. This product does not contain fragrance per se, but does contain a small amount of orange oil, which imparts a scent (and may cause irritation, the only misstep in an otherwise superb product).

☺ AVERAGE **$$$ Flawless Skin Mega Moisturizer SPF 15 Normal/Combination Skin** *($45 for 2 fl. oz.)* includes avobenzone for UVA protection, and wraps it in a decently emollient base for normal to dry skin. The antioxidant vitamins will be subject to deterioration shortly after this jar-packaged product is opened (see the Appendix for details), which is why this isn't recommended over many other daytime moisturizers with sunscreen, including many that cost less. If you decide to overlook the concerns about jar packaging, this is best for normal to dry skin.

☺ AVERAGE $$$ **Flawless Skin Mega Moisturizer SPF 15 Normal/Dry Skin** *($50 for 2 fl. oz.)* is a silky moisturizer that features an in-part avobenzone sunscreen. The silicones are suitable for normal to oily skin, but the emu oil and the amount of castor oil are not for anyone prone to breakouts. Unfortunately, jar packaging undermines the effectiveness of the antioxidant vitamins this contains—and that's very disappointing considering this product's price! See the Appendix to learn why jar packaging is a problem.

☺ AVERAGE $$$ **Flawless Skin Repair Creme** *($95 for 1.7 fl. oz.)* has a great name—is there any doubt what this product promises? Yet the miracle ingredient is "deep sea water." Regardless of depth, water of any kind is not the key to flawless skin. The majority of ingredients in this product appear in hundreds of other moisturizers, which is all this "treatment" really is: a basic moisturizer. What's particularly dismaying is that the many antioxidants and cell-communicating ingredients won't stay potent for long because of jar packaging. Spending this much for what amounts to a letdown isn't advised, but it still has potential for normal to dry skin. In better packaging, this would be an excellent, though overpriced, moisturizer for normal to dry skin.

☺ AVERAGE $$$ **Flawless Skin Repair Day Creme SPF 15** *($95 for 1.7 fl. oz.)* is best suited for normal to slightly dry skin, but lacks adequate UVA protection which is essential for anti-aging benefit. Beyond the sunscreens, the base formula is quite good, even assuming that you know the powerful Deep Sea Water claim is just plain hokey. What's not so good is that several state-of-the-art ingredients in this daytime moisturizer are going to lose potency due to the jar packaging, which is really unsettling given how much this product costs. See the Appendix for further details about jar packaging.

☺ AVERAGE $$$ **Flawless Skin Repair Serum** *($95 for 1 fl. oz.)* costs way too much for a formula that doesn't give your skin as much of the good stuff (antioxidants, skin-repairing ingredients) as it should. It is truly embarrassing that for $95 you're getting mostly water, glycerin, slip agents, and thickeners! We're concerned that the amount of benzyl alcohol is greater than several state-of-the-art ingredients (which are present in tiny amounts when your skin deserves oodles of these). Benzyl alcohol can be irritating when used in high amounts, and its prominence in this serum is cause for concern.

☺ AVERAGE $$$ **Secret Finish** *($27 for 1 fl. oz.)* is just an overpriced lightweight moisturizer that won't make a discernible difference in how your makeup wears. It is merely water, slip agent, thickener, rice starch (for a soft matte finish), plant extracts (including witch hazel, an irritant), vitamins, preservatives, more silicone, fragrance, and coloring agents.

☹ POOR **Flawless Skin Repair Eye Serum** *($80 for 0.5 fl. oz.)* is a water-based serum that lists most of its really intriguing ingredients after the mineral pigment mica, which lends a shimmer finish to the eye area. How disappointing, but the deal-breaker is the inclusion of geranium and arnica in amounts bound to be troublesome for the skin around the eyes or anywhere on the face for that matter. See the Appendix to learn more about the issues irritation presents and to find out why you don't need a special serum for the eye area.

☹ POOR **Flawless Skin Repair Oil-Free Day Lotion SPF 15** *($95 for 1.7 fl. oz.)* is loaded with beneficial ingredients like antioxidants and cell-communicating peptides. Its lightweight, silky texture is ideal under makeup, too. Unfortunately, the sunscreen does not provide sufficient UVA protection, which means your skin is left vulnerable to the sun's most aging, wrinkle-causing rays. The active ingredient this product contains provides some UVA protection, but "some" doesn't cut it if your goal is keeping skin young and healthy-looking as long as possible.

⊗ POOR **Flawless Skin Tone Perfecting Creme** *($95 for 1.7 fl. oz.)*. Considering this product's price and antioxidant-rich formula, it's a shame that it comes in jar packaging. This moisturizer has great potential for dry skin, and its texture is lush, emollient, and notably silky. However, because jar packaging allows air into the product with each use, you're diminishing the potency of the plant oils and antioxidants, including the potency of the quercetin (see the Appendix for details). Another disappointment is that many of the state-of-the-art beneficial ingredients are listed after the preservative, which means there isn't much of them in here anyway. By the way, there's some intriguing research indicating that quercetin can diminish skin discolorations, but it's not going to do that for long if it's packaged in a jar and routinely exposed to light and air. The illuminating effect is courtesy of the mineral pigment mica, an ingredient that's not unique to this product.

LAURA MERCIER LIP CARE

☺ GOOD $$$ **Lip Silk** *($22 for 0.4 fl. oz.)* is a very good, Vaseline-based lip balm that contains silicone for a silky finish and lighter texture. This also contains vitamin E and a cell-communicating ingredient. The glycolic and salicylic acids do not function as exfoliants.

☹ AVERAGE $$$ **Lip Plumper** *($30)* contains a flavoring agent that works with other ingredients in the gloss to build a progressive cooling sensation. Within several minutes of applying this lip gloss-like product (which comes in pleasing range of sheer to clear shades), your lips will be tingling like church bells on Sunday and may be a bit plumper as a result. Of course, that tingling and any increased fullness is the result of irritation, and that's not the best thing to do to lips on a routine basis. For occasional use (or applied over lipstick, which blocks most of the active minty flavor from causing irritation) this is an option, and it does have a rich, glossy finish that feels smooth and surprisingly light, though the subtle difference isn't really worth the money.

⊗ POOR **Lip Balm SPF 15** *($20 for 0.12 fl. oz.)* does not contain the UVA-protecting ingredients of titanium dioxide, zinc oxide, avobenzone, Tinosorb, or Mexoryl SX, and is not recommended. What a shame, because this is otherwise a stellar lip balm.

LAURA MERCIER FOUNDATION & PRIMERS

✓☺ BEST $$$ **Illuminating Tinted Moisturizer SPF 20** *($42 for 1.7 fl. oz.)* is an awesome tinted moisturizer if you have normal to dry skin and want an attractive glow finish that is sophisticated without being sparkly. Unlike Mercier's other tinted moisturizers, this one gets the UVA issue right by including avobenzone. The silicone-enhanced formula contains several antioxidants, is fragrance-free, and comes in five versatile sheer shades ideal for fair to medium skin tones. Unless your skin is sensitive to synthetic sunscreen actives or you want more coverage, there is every reason to consider this formidable tinted moisturizer. You also can blend it with a foundation if you need more coverage, but keep in mind that doing so will diminish the amount of sun protection you get (unless your foundation also includes sunscreen).

✓☺ BEST $$$ **Mineral Powder SPF 15** *($35 for 0.34 fl. oz.)*. The drawbacks of mineral makeup (potential discoloring over oily areas, making dry skin or dry areas look and feel even drier, messy application—after all, it is loose powder) do apply here to some extent. However, this product's overall excellent attributes balance those negatives and make this a mineral makeup worth exploring. The broad-spectrum sunscreen is provided by 20% zinc oxide, an amount that also lends this powder its opacity and ability to provide nearly full coverage and an absorbent finish. The zinc oxide is joined by pearl powder and lesser amounts of other ingredients common to mineral makeup, including mica and bismuth oxychloride. Together they create a silky, dry texture that blends better on skin than any other mineral makeup we've tested (and we've tested them all!). Its finish is matte in feel, but the pearl powder lends an attractive, non-sparkling, dimensional glow to skin that keeps it from looking too dull or flat. All the shades available (with no options for tan to dark skin tones) demand careful testing because they apply either lighter or darker than they appear in the container. Speaking of the container, the sifter has a clever closure that keeps the powder from spilling out during travel, a thoughtful touch. Applying this with a brush nets the most natural results; applying it with a sponge provides a noticeably opaque finish.

✓☺ BEST **$$$ Powder Foundation** *($40)* is a superior and comes in gorgeous shades, including options for light and dark (but not very dark) skin tones. This talc-based powder offers a suede-smooth texture, even application, and light to medium coverage when used dry. If you use it wet it provides fuller coverage, but you also run the risk of streaking if you're not careful. If the price isn't too off-putting and you have normal to oily or combination skin, this is a must-try and it's on the very short list of today's best pressed-powder foundations. One caution: Each shade has a hint of shine. While the shine isn't distracting, you should be aware of it if you're looking for a completely matte finish.

✓☺ BEST **$$$ Silk Creme Foundation** *($42)* has a name that's 100% accurate. One of the hallmarks of Mercier's foundations is how well they mesh with skin. Her formulas, even this one that provides significant coverage, somehow manage to look very skin-like, primarily because they don't settle into lines, pores, and minor crevices. Silk Creme Foundation's silicone base blends expertly and sets to a silky matte finish. It is one of the few almost-full-coverage foundations that doesn't look too thick and that doesn't dull down healthy skin's natural luminosity. Granted, as exceptional as these qualities are, this foundation still looks like makeup—no one will believe you're sporting a sheer look—but if that's the kind of coverage you're looking for, this deserves serious consideration by those with normal to oily skin. Each of the shades are impeccable.

☺ GOOD **$$$ Foundation Primer-Radiance** *($30)* has a pearlescent, luminous quality that is quite noticeable upon initial application, but becomes sheer and ends up having a subtle glow. When worn alone, this primer does indeed leave skin looking more radiant, and under makeup the glow only slightly peeks through, depending on how much foundation, powder, or tinted moisturizer you apply over it. The silky formula smoothes over skin and provides an excellent base for foundation. As an added bonus, the formula includes some antioxidants and nonfragrant plant oils that are helpful for normal to dry skin, but the antioxidants aren't present in amounts worth getting excited about. Still, it's nice to see them in a primer, as these products tend to omit helpful extras. Primers aren't a necessary step to your makeup routine, but if you want to give this extra step a try, this is a great option!

☺ GOOD **$$$ Mineral Pressed Powder SPF 15** *($35)* happens to be a very good powder foundation. Packaged in a sturdy compact, the texture is creamy-smooth, allowing it to seamlessly blend with skin. Mineral makeup devotees will surely appreciate that the pressed-powder format significantly cuts down on the mess involved with most loose-mineral makeups. That said, it's still all too easy to pick up more mineral powder with your brush than you need (the included sponge is not recommended), so start small and work up from there. Even in small quantities, the coverage is far from sheer, making this a very good choice for those looking for medium to full coverage from a powder. The SPF rating comes from zinc oxide, so this provides very good broad-spectrum sun protection. Zinc oxide also lends a great deal of opacity, which is great for building coverage, but also poses the risk of appearing heavy or ashy, even though this powder manages to feel quite light on the skin. Of the seven shades, there are workable options for fair to medium skin tones, but the deepest shade, Rich Chestnut, is too orange by far. All the shades have a subtle sheen to their finish, but nothing that could be considered truly shimmery. It's worth noting that though they share the same names, the shades are not identical to those of Laura Mercier's loose Mineral Powder SPF 15.

☺ GOOD $$$ **Oil-Free Supreme Foundation** *($42)* is a slightly tweaked version of Mercier's longstanding Oil-Free Foundation. There are very few differences between the formulas. The Supreme version still has a lot going for it, but as foundation technology has improved we're surprised that this liquid foundation has mostly stayed the same. It simply isn't as silky or elegant as many other liquid foundations designed for oily skin. But it remains worthy of consideration by anyone with normal to oily skin. The fluid, densely pigmented texture is dispensed from a pump and blends out to a seamless, soft matte finish with medium coverage that can appear thick unless you blend it meticulously. Twelve shades are on hand, with options for very light but not for very dark skin tones. The only shades to consider avoiding are Shell Beige (slightly pink) and Suntan Beige (slightly peach). Porcelain Ivory is a very good shade for fair skin. Use caution with the darkest shades, as once these set they can look a bit ashen. Note: This foundation contains a high amount of the sunscreen ingredient ethylhexyl methoxycinnamate. Although this isn't a bad ingredient, some will find it sensitizing when applied around the eye area. If you notice stinging or burning around the eyes with this foundation, the sunscreen ingredient is the likely culprit.

☹ AVERAGE $$$ **Creme Smooth Foundation** *($50)* is one of the few foundations available emollient enough for those with dry skin. That's because the ingredients necessary to create a rich, moisturizing texture tend to have an oxidizing effect on the pigments in the formula. That in turn means that the shade you applied in the morning may begin looking more orange or peach as the day goes on, especially if you have oily areas (such as on or near the nose). The other reasons are that the formulas tend to separate in the package and it's tricky to blend powder-based products over a foundation with a notably moist finish. Creme Smooth Foundation appears to have avoided these pitfalls. This thick foundation is packaged in a large, heavy jar. Although Mercier added some antioxidants to the formula, the fact that it's packaged in a jar means the beneficial ingredients won't remain stable once it is opened (see the Appendix for details). Texture-wise, this leans toward the greasy side of creamy, and it has moderate slip during blending. You'll find this sets to a satin matte finish that doesn't mesh with skin as well as some of Mercier's other foundations, at least not without diligent blending. Coverage goes from medium to full; in fact, even if you try to apply this makeup sheer, it's difficult to get less than medium coverage. Not surprisingly, the formula is best for dry skin not prone to breakouts. The shade range is mostly excellent with good options for light to dark (but not very dark) skin tones. Consider the slightly peach Tawny Beige carefully and avoid the orange-toned Honey Beige.

☹ AVERAGE $$$ **Foundation Primer-Hydrating** *($30 for 1.7 fl. oz.)* contains a minimal amount of hydrating ingredients and more witch hazel than should be applied to normal to dry skin, though overall the amount and water form are unlikely to cause irritation. All the antioxidants and other intriguing ingredients are listed well after the preservatives. At best, this water- and silicone-based lotion will create a silky-smooth surface for makeup application, but so will many other serums and moisturizers that, while not officially sold as primers, will perform the same function while providing greater benefit.

☺ AVERAGE **$$$ Foundation Primer-Mineral** *($30)* is a silky, lightweight lotion whose main mineral is absorbent silica. It leaves a radiant finish that doesn't feel the least bit greasy, likely because alcohol is the fifth ingredient. Even if you have oily skin and want a matte finish primer, there are better options than this.

☹ AVERAGE **$$$ Foundation Primer Oil-Free** *($30 for 1.7 fl. oz.)* has a thinner, less silky texture than Mercier's other primers, and it omits the problematic fragrant extracts and oils. It is oil-free, but it lacks absorbent ingredients and contains too many thickeners to make someone with oily skin happy. It is best viewed as an ordinary, lightweight moisturizer to remedy slightly dry skin. There are lots of better products to consider applying before foundation, and most of these aren't labeled or sold as primers.

☺ AVERAGE **$$$ Moisture Supreme Foundation** *($42)* is expensive and for what this fragrance-free foundation costs, it should perform better than it does. On the plus side, this is indeed a moisturizing foundation suitable for dry skin. It leaves a moist, satin finish and contains some notable plant oils to keep skin smoothed and hydrated. The light cream texture smoothes easily over skin, providing medium to almost full coverage from only a small amount of product. The major drawback is that once set, this tends to look heavy and very much like makeup sitting on the skin as opposed to meshing with it for a more natural, yet refined, appearance. The finish also tends to sink into and magnify wrinkles and definitely highlights areas with enlarged pores (though large pores are typically not a complaint for women with dry skin). Turning to the shades, there are some beautiful options for fair to dark skin tones, along with some that are a must to avoid. Porcelain Ivory is excellent for very light skin, assuming you're willing to tolerate that this foundation really looks like makeup. Colors to avoid include the rosy-pink Shell Beige, slightly orange Honey Beige, and coppery Toffee Bronze (though this may work for certain dark skin tones). Note: This foundation contains the sunscreen ingredient ethylhexyl methoxycinnamate. Although it is not rated with an SPF and should not be relied on for sun protection, this sunscreen ingredient can be a problem when used around the eyes (such as on the eyelid area). If you notice signs of stinging or eye irritation, this ingredient is the likely culprit.

☺ AVERAGE **$$$ Tinted Moisturizer SPF 20** *($42 for 1.5 fl. oz.)* is a star product for Laura Mercier, and is often featured in fashion magazine "best of beauty" lists. There's good reason for the accolades, because this tinted moisturizer has a beautifully smooth texture and silky application that results in an elegant tinted moisturizer with a soft satin finish. It does a good job of blurring minor imperfections and promoting a more even skin tone. The major letdown is the lack of sufficient UVA protection. Well, that and many of the shades tend to be too peach or pink, though most are too sheer for these off-tones to be considered a problem. In early 2010, Mercier launched three new shades (Bisque, Caramel, and Mocha) and these have a different formula than the original. The newest shades include avobenzone for reliable UVA protection. The Mercier counterperson we spoke with did not know if the other shades would be transferring to this improved sunscreen formula or not. For now, the Bisque, Caramel, and Mocha shades are worth considering and earn a Good rating. Both formulas are best for normal to dry skin.

☹ POOR **Foundation Primer** *($30 for 1.7 fl. oz.)* is a thin, lightweight cream-gel that contains some antioxidants whose effects are counteracted by too many fragrant extracts and

---

⚕ Exposing oily skin to irritating ingredients makes it worse! See the Appendix to learn more.

oils, all of which damage skin. It's supposed to contain light-reflecting ingredients that protect the skin, but it doesn't (unless you consider the emollient shine from the finish protecting). The formula won't help skin in the least. Although Mercier was one of the first to popularize the concept of makeup primers, her original formula is far from the best.

☹ POOR **Tinted Moisturizer Oil-Free SPF 20** *($42 for 1.7 fl. oz.)* is oil-free but is also unfortunately free of the UVA-protecting ingredients of titanium dioxide, zinc oxide, avobenzone, Tinosorb, or Mexoryl SX, and is not recommended. There are plenty of tinted moisturizers that get the critical issue of UVA protection right, so no need to focus on this one.

LAURA MERCIER CONCEALERS

☺ GOOD **$$$ Secret Concealer** *($22)* is meant for the eye area and is far more user-friendly than the Secret Camouflage reviewed below. It comes in a small pot and offers decent shades, each with a very creamy-smooth, petrolatum-based texture. It covers well but does tend to crease during the day. Give this a test run before you decide to purchase, and be sure to set it with powder.

☺ GOOD **$$$ Undercover Pot** *($34 for 0.2 fl. oz.)* combines two of Mercier's concealers and her Loose Setting Powder in one stacked package. The concealers are in a flip-top compact while the loose powder rests in a jar underneath. It's difficult to rate this trio because the **Secret Camouflage** received an Average rating on its own, the **Secret Concealer** earned a Good rating, and the loose powder remains a Best Product for its many wonderful attributes. If you're not familiar with Mercier's products, please read the individual reviews for the products in this set. The Secret Concealer and Loose Setting Powder combination is great; the Secret Camouflage is a heavy duty, thick-textured concealer that can be mixed with Secret Concealer to aid application or soften the coverage a bit. There are four pairs of shades offered, all of which can be mixed to work for light to medium skin tones. The loose powder is the same translucent shade regardless of which set you choose. Be sure to test this at the counter before purchasing; blending your own concealer shades isn't the easiest way to go, and some will find the texture of both too much.

☺ AVERAGE **$$$ Secret Camouflage** *($28)* is a two-sided compact concealer with a thick, dry texture and truly opaque camouflage coverage. All the duos have yellow to beige or peach to copper colors that can work if mixed in the right proportions, but why would you want to do that when there are so many excellent one-step concealers available? Still, this concealer has its appeal and there's no denying it provides formidable coverage, especially for dark circles. Secret Camouflage was reformulated in mid-2011, with the goal being to make it easier to blend. Although the texture is slightly creamier and more pliable, this is still a tricky product to work with, mostly because its success depends on how adept you are at mixing two shades to create a custom color that looks convincing. With the reformulation, all the shades remained the same. The best sets are for those with fair to light-medium skin tones; SC4 and SC6 are too peach or copper to recommend, and SC3 is the most neutral duo. This is an option for all skin types, but the texture of this concealer makes it an iffy proposition for use on breakouts.

LAURA MERCIER POWDERS

✓☺ BEST **$$$ Loose Setting Powder** *($34)* has an out-of-this-world silky texture that blends beautifully over the skin and leaves a satiny-smooth, dry finish. The formula is talc-based and also includes a small amount of cornstarch for extra absorbency without a heavy feel. The single shade (Translucent) is best for fair to light skin tones, though it can work for medium skin tones if brushed on sheer.

✓☺ BEST **$$$ Pressed Setting Powder** *($30)* has many of the same qualities as Laura Mercier's Loose Setting Powder above. The formula is talc-based and also includes a small amount of cornstarch for a more absorbent finish. While the texture is smooth and dry, the sole Translucent shade is recommended only for fair to medium skin tones.

☺ GOOD **$$$ Invisible Loose Setting Powder** *($34)*. This talc free, colorless loose powder offers a soft, refined finish that helps make normal to oily or combination skin look polished while temporarily minimizing the appearance of large pores.

☺ GOOD **$$$ Mineral Primer** *($30)* is a silky loose powder with a natural affinity for skin. Although the color is pure white, it applies sheer and creates a slight brightening effect without looking chalky or too shiny. Despite this, it's not for everyone and is definitely something you'll want to test before purchasing. This mica-based powder is said to boost the effectiveness of the sunscreen(s) in other mineral formulas, but it cannot do that. In fact, that's a sketchy claim to make since this powder does not sport an SPF rating or active sunscreen ingredients.

☺ GOOD **$$$ Secret Brightening Powder** *($22)* is a weightless, talc-based loose powder that is meant for (and does a great job of) highlighting skin, especially under the eyes—but again, the effect is subtle. There is no reason a similar effect cannot be created by the artful use of a standard concealer and powder, but for those inclined to experiment (and especially for makeup artists), this product, though pricey, may be worth it.

☺ GOOD **$$$ Smooth Focus Pressed Setting Powder** *($32)* comes with a mint-green tint, but don't worry, it won't show on skin and, in fact, it brushes on almost colorless (and green doesn't counteract redness anyway; if it did remain on skin it would just be reminiscent of Kermit the frog). It is workable for all skin tones except very dark. The sheer, silky texture is finely milled and provides a beautiful non-drying matte finish without any coverage. This talc-free powder is great for touching up oily shine, but for the best results you'll still want to blot excess shine before powdering. The anti-irritants in this powder are there for appearance only, as they don't have much, if any, benefit in a powder exposed to air and pressed into powder form.

☹ POOR **Mineral Finishing Powder** *($32)* is designed to "set" other mineral powders, which is a ridiculous notion—on a par with stating you need to set your liquid foundation with another liquid foundation because somehow your usual foundation just isn't setting well on its own. As it turns out, this sheer powder has a very dry texture that feels scratchy and effectively dulls the complexion. It also contains silver, a metal that can cause problems for skin, including discoloration. This is a must to avoid and one of Mercier's only resounding disappointments.

LAURA MERCIER BLUSHES & BRONZERS

✓☺ BEST **$$$ Creme Cheek Colour** *($22)* ranks as an outstanding cream blush for normal to dry skin. It's creamy without being greasy, has enough slip to blend evenly, and offers a smooth satin finish from each of its four sheer colors. Those who find this type of blush appealing may wish there were more shades available, but each one is excellent.

✓☺ BEST **$$$ Second Skin Cheek Colour** *($24)* is an amazingly good powder blush. It feels beautifully smooth and application is soft with even results. Best of all, the finish is almost matte and the amount of shine is completely suitable for daytime wear. The attractive range of shades is tailored to those with fair to medium skin tones. The company claims this blush makes skin look "naturally blushed" and, thanks to this product's affinity for skin and seamless application, it does!

☺ GOOD **$$$ Bronzing Duo** *($32)* combines a pressed bronzing powder and powder blush in one compact. The colors are not separated by a divider, so it's best to swirl your brush over both. Doing so results in a soft bronze color with a hint of pink, peach, or muted rose, depending on which duo you choose. The texture is soft and slightly powdery and application is good. You'll get a strong color payoff and the finish is laced with shine, but it's soft.

☺ GOOD $$$ **Bronzing Pressed Powder** *($32)* has a silky, non-flaky texture that applies evenly, imparting a soft shimmer finish and healthy, natural bronze color.

☺ GOOD $$$ **Bronzing Gel** *($32 for 1.69 fl. oz.)* is a standard, sheer gel bronzer that's infused with particles of shine that call attention only to themselves in daylight. If you're a fan of shine you'll find this a tempting option, and the color is utterly believable, even on fair skin tones. It has just enough copper-red pigment to closely mimic a natural tan, but the consistency makes it best for use over bare or lightly moisturized skin rather than blended over foundation (especially matte-finish foundation, which causes the gel to grab and look dotted on the skin).

LAURA MERCIER EYESHADOWS

✓☺ BEST $$$ **Luster Eye Colour** *($22)* is a smooth-textured, highly blendable eyeshadow that goes on soft and requires layering for shading and detail. The "luster" part of the name refers to this powder eyeshadow's satin sheen.

✓☺ BEST $$$ **Matte Eye Colour** *($22).* Mercier has crafted a powder eyeshadow with unbelievably smooth texture and near-perfect application, even for the darkest shades. The finish on each shade isn't true matte, but it comes very close, with only a hint of sparkle. The shade range is good, but would be better if it had more mid-toned shades. There are plenty of options for those seeking lighter colors.

☺ GOOD $$$ **Caviar Stick Eye Colour** *($24)* is a twist-up stick eyeshadow with a cream-to-powder texture that glides on easily, blends beautifully, and deposits rich, dramatic color with a single swipe. Despite the powder finish, the formula retains a slight amount of movement after it sets, so those with oily eyelids will experience some smearing and fading during wear. As usual for Mercier, most of the shades are gorgeous, especially if you want to create a deep, smoky eye design. Amethyst, Cocoa, and Khaki are the standouts but Smoke is beautiful, too. Each shade has some degree of shine, from a subtle metallic sheen to noticeable shimmer. Because of this, Caviar Stick Eye Color isn't the best choice if you have a crepey or wrinkled eyelid (and the colors are too dark to work well on the typically smooth brow bone area).

☺ GOOD $$$ **Eye Basics** *($24)* are liquid eyeshadows that come in a tube with a sponge-tip applicator. Each shade has a lightly creamy, sheer texture that blends easily and dries to a natural matte (in feel) finish. This works almost as well as a matte-finish concealer over the eyelids.

☺ GOOD $$$ **Metallic Creme Eye Colour** *($22)* is the one to choose if you want strong colors with a metallic finish but don't want to get it from a powder eyeshadow. This silky cream blends seamlessly, with just the right amount of slip. Its powdery (in feel) finish doesn't hold up all day, so expect some movement and a bit of creasing, though blending it with a powder eyeshadow all but eliminates this side effect.

☺ GOOD $$$ **Sateen Eye Colour** *($22)* is a high-shine powder eyeshadow with a supremely smooth texture that blends with ease. Each shade applies softer than it appears (by about 50%), so layering is required for a notable color payoff. Still, there are some excellent colors if you want sparkling shine.

☺ GOOD $$$ **Satinee Creme Eye Colour** *($22)* is a pearlescent cream shadow. The shimmer factor is pretty high, so if you have any lines or less-than-taut skin around the eye area, this is not for you. However, if you don't have those issues, these cream shadows have a lot going for them. The available shades range from sheer to strong; with each, a little goes a long way. These shadows layer well and blend easily (though you have to be quick), allowing you to customize the shade and depth you want. Once on, these shadows wear for hours with minimal fading or creasing.

☺ AVERAGE **$$$ Mineral Eye Powder** *($20)* is a loose powder packaged in a pot with a sifter to control how much is dispensed. The sifter consists of one hole in the center, which keeps this from being too messy, but it still dispenses too much powder at once, and this is concentrated, pigment-rich stuff! The shine is intense and clings reasonably well, though is way too much for aging eyelids or use near wrinkles. If that's not a problem for you, this is worth a look.

☹ POOR **Baked Eye Colour** *($22)* is overdone. Whether an eyeshadow is "baked" (essentially, the pressed-powder formula is exposed to high heat in an oven so it sets to a specific domed shape) or not, what matters most is its texture and application. The texture is smooth, but notably dry, making for average application that isn't as smooth or foolproof as Mercier's regular unbaked powder eyeshadows.

☹ POOR **Sequin Eye Colour** *($22)* has a sheer, dry texture with an average application that goes on softly. Unfortunately, the shimmer particles and flecks of glitter don't cling well, so this shadow begins flaking almost immediately and keeps flaking throughout the day.

LAURA MERCIER EYE & BROW LINERS

☺ GOOD **$$$ Eye Brow Gel** *($20)* is a basic, efficient, clear brow gel. It's a great way to keep unruly brows in place, but there is no reason to spend this much when there are equally good options available from several drugstore lines.

☺ AVERAGE **$$$ Brow Definer** *($20)* is sold in tiny glass pots and is accurately described as a wax/gel formula. The wax content lends a stiff texture to this product and also makes for a less-than-smooth application. However, with a good brush and some patience, this is an option to fill in, groom, and define brows with soft color and a non-sticky finish. All shades are recommended but are best for brunettes.

☺ AVERAGE **$$$ Brow Powder Duo** *($24)* features two dry-textured brow powders in one compact. The color combinations are quite good, and there are suitable options for redheads and blondes, along with traditional options for brunettes—but all the colors are sparkly. Why the eyebrows need to shine is beyond us, but if this appeals to you, these brow powders apply and blend well.

☺ AVERAGE **$$$ Caviar Eye Liner** *($22)* is sort of like a soft-textured kohl pencil in compact form. It begins slightly creamy and sets to a dry finish. Application is smooth but sheer, so you'll need to layer for the best definition. A matte powder eyeshadow or one of the cream-gel eyeliners produces longer-lasting results with less effort.

LAURA MERCIER LIP COLOR & LIPLINERS

☺ GOOD **$$$ Creme Lip Colour** *($24)* is pricey for a standard cream lipstick with a slightly glossy finish. However, the colors are beautiful and it isn't slippery or greasy, so it's unlikely to migrate into lines around the mouth. **Shimmer Lip Colour** ($24) has the same texture as the Creme Lip Colour, though each shade has a soft to moderate shimmer finish and the colors aren't as rich.

☺ GOOD **$$$ Lip Stain** *($20)* is said to provide the visual effect of a stain along with the comfort and sheen of a gloss. A pot-packaged lip gloss is what this is; the stain effect is minimal yet the sheer colors are great and bound to please those looking for a softer lip color to wear alone or over lipstick. It has a slightly sticky yet glossy finish.

☺ GOOD **$$$ Sheer Lip Colour** *($22)* is exactly that, a sheer lip color with a glossy finish and marvelous, versatile colors that all have a slight stain.

☺ AVERAGE **$$$ Lip Glace** *($24)* costs too much to make it worth strong consideration over many other standard lip glosses, but if you decide to indulge, this is a moderately sticky, sparkling wet gloss applied with a sponge tip.

☺ AVERAGE **$$$ Lip Pencil** *($20)* has a standard creamy texture and a dry finish. The expansive color range includes options that coordinate well with Mercier's lipsticks. Less expensive pencils abound, but these work well if you don't mind routine sharpening.

LAURA MERCIER MASCARAS

✓☺ BEST **$$$ Long Lash Mascara** *($24)* is a beautifully done mascara whose tiny brush makes creating long, separated lashes easy. This goes on smoothly with only a slight tendency to clump, but is easily smoothed out as you continue to brush through lashes. Pigmentation is intense, so the overall effect is quite dramatic. Long Lash Mascara removes with a water-soluble cleanser and wears all day without flaking or smearing.

✓☺ BEST **$$$ Thickening and Building Mascara** *($20)* is a pleasure to apply, and it builds impressively long, lifted lashes with a fair amount of thickness. Lashes look full, soft, and fringed—all without clumping or smearing.

☺ GOOD **$$$ Waterproof Mascara** *($20)* has a formula that is easy to apply, makes it through the day without flaking, and really is waterproof (though you may notice slight smearing). It takes some effort to build long, thick lashes, but the result is worth it and your lashes aren't left feeling stiff or brittle.

☺ AVERAGE **$$$ Full Blown Volume Lash Building Mascara** *($24)* is merely average in regard to its ability to lengthen and thicken lashes. On the plus side, it does create nice definition without clumping or flaking, and leaves lashes feeling soft instead of stiff or brittle, but the overall result is not as dramatic as one would hope. You can find less expensive mascaras at the drugstore that add dramatic flair to lashes.

LAURA MERCIER FACE & BODY ILLUMINATORS

✓☺ BEST **$$$ Shimmer Bloc** *($38)* deserves consideration if you're looking for a shiny pressed powder to highlight or add a glow to your skin. You get four colors in one compact, and the tightly pressed formula is not flyaway, which makes application that much easier. Even better, the prismatic shine clings well and tends to not flake. If you want shimmer from a powder, it doesn't get much better than this!

☺ GOOD **$$$ Illuminating Powder** *($35)* presents four squares of color in one compact, without dividers between them. The result from either of the two quads is akin to a shimmery blush, with the shine level being moderate and best for evening.

☺ AVERAGE **$$$ Loose Shimmer Powder** *($34)* has a sheer, silky texture and sparkling, dimensional finish. The formula doesn't cling as well as it should, so you'll get some flaking, but if you're going for all-over shine, that's not such a big deal.

☺ AVERAGE **$$$ Mineral Illuminating Powder** *($32)* is a mica- and talc-based loose powder that creates a multidimensional shine from its pearl and diamond powders. Unfortunately, the shine clings poorly. You'll get illumination from this silky, weightless powder, but there are other ways to get there that don't involve the mess and that don't leave you with short-lived results. A great example would be Mercier's Illuminating Tinted Moisturizer with sunscreen.

LAURA MERCIER BRUSHES

☺ GOOD $$$ **Laura Mercier Brushes** *($10–$52).* Mercier has done her homework when it comes to brushes. Most of these are masterfully shaped and are dense enough to hold and deposit color evenly on the skin. Almost every brush is available with a long or short handle, which is an attractive option. The best among this collection of either natural or synthetic hairs are the **Powder Brush** ($52); the synthetic hair **Camouflage Powder Brush** ($28), which is more appropriate for eyeshadows; **Bronzer Brush** ($45); and the **Cheek Colour Brush** ($45). Almost all the **Eyeshadow Brushes** ($24–$34) are worth a closer look, particularly the **Eye Crease Brush** ($29), **Smudge Brush** ($24), and **Corner Eye Colour Brush** ($25). All told, you should be quite pleased with the versatility and performance of most Mercier brushes.

LAURA MERCIER SPECIALTY MAKEUP PRODUCTS

✓☺ BEST $$$ **Secret Finish Mattifying** *($27 for 1 fl. oz.)* has a thick, translucent texture that quickly softens to a silky-smooth matte finish. The absorbent silicones work briefly to control excess shine, but this isn't going to last for hours, so it's not the best for those with seriously oily skin. However, the fragrance-free formula works to temporarily fill in large pores and allows foundation to apply smoothly and evenly. Mercier touts this as being "primarily for touch-ups throughout the day," which means you're supposed to dab this on over makeup. That's doable, as long as you spread the product over clean fingers to thin it out before dabbing it on shine-prone areas. Secret Finish Mattifying is elevated to Best Product status due to its antioxidant-rich formula and its value for those with sensitive skin that's also oily.

☹ POOR **Under Eye Perfecter** *($22)* is supposed to conceal dark circles with its unique Orange/Yellow formula for light skin tones and Mauve/Rose formula for fair/medium skin tones. The Mauve/Rose allegedly hides pink-to-purple dark circles. In reality, all this product does is make your under-eye area look very rosy, which is not flattering, to say the least. The recommendation to use this under your concealer is a problem because you'll just be piling on more makeup, risking slippage into lines during the day. This is an unnecessary product in your makeup routine because your dark circles will be no more hidden than if you used concealer alone, and in fact they'll likely look worse, especially as you try to figure out how to meld the color corrector with your regular concealer, a process that can create a third, odd-toned shade.

M.A.C.

Strengths: A Lauder-owned company, with some impressive moisturizers; all the daytime moisturizers with sunscreen include sufficient UVA protection; excellent lip balm; excellent foundations (some whose sunscreen includes the right UVA-protecting ingredients) in a mostly gorgeous range of shades; great concealers; the Select Sheer and Mineralized powders; the Sheertone Blush and traditional cream blush; wide selection of powder eyeshadows in various finishes; Fluidline and Technakohl Liner; dizzying array of lipstick shades in mostly sumptuous formulas; all the Pro Longwear Lipcolour options; several very good mascaras (regular and waterproof); the makeup brushes; most of the Prep + Prime products work as claimed.

Weaknesses: A few products with uncomfortably high levels of known or potential skin irritants; no effective AHA or BHA products; no anti-blemish products; some of the foundations were downgraded because their sunscreen did not offer sufficient UVA protection; several average pressed and loose powders; Cream Colour Base; the Lustre and Velvet eyeshadows; the traditional eye pencils (that need sharpening); Brow Set and Brow Finisher; Lipglass and Plushglass; the Brush Cleanser.

M.A.C. CLEANSERS

✓☺ BEST **$$$ Wipes** *($15 for 30 sheets)* are sturdy yet soft cloths that easily and quickly remove all types of makeup, including long-wearing lip stains and waterproof mascara. The formula combines gentle cleansing agents with a solvent and silicones to accomplish this, and most will find it a soothing experience. Wipes are convenient, but keep in mind that a water-soluble cleanser with a washcloth is just as effective (and costs less per use).

☺ AVERAGE **$$$ Cremewash** *($20 for 3.4 fl. oz.)* is a water-soluble cleanser that produces copious foam. The main cleansing agent is the soap constituent potassium myristate, which means this cleanser can be drying for some skin types, rather than "super-hydrating" as claimed. It is an OK option for normal to oily skin, and removes makeup easily.

☺ AVERAGE **$$$ Green Gel Cleanser** *($20 for 5 fl. oz.)* is an OK, water-soluble cleanser for normal to very oily skin. The drying TEA-lauryl sulfate cleanser is third on the ingredient list, which doesn't make this preferred to several other (less expensive) gel cleansers.

☹ POOR **Cleanse Off Oil** *($26 for 5 fl. oz.)* isn't any better than removing makeup with a gentle cleansing lotion or even plain olive oil because it contains irritating bitter orange and lavender oils. This is not recommended for any skin type, and would be a problem for eye-area use.

☹ POOR **Lightful Cleanser** *($25 for 3.4 fl. oz.)* has a cleansing formula that contains too many drying, soap-like ingredients. As such, it is not recommended or preferred over lots of other cleansers, including dozens that cost less. It removes makeup easily and contains some plant extracts with research pertaining to their skin-lightening ability; however, in a cleanser these ingredients are rinsed down the drain before they can affect discolorations.

M.A.C. EYE-MAKEUP REMOVERS

☺ GOOD **$$$ Pro Eye Makeup Remover** *($19 for 3.4 fl. oz.)* is a standard, detergent-based eye-makeup remover that works as well as any, and is fragrance-free. The formula claims to be pro-quality, but isn't different from what most other lines offer for less money.

☺ AVERAGE **$$$ Gently Off Eye and Lip Makeup Remover** *($19 for 3.4 fl. oz.)* is a standard, but effective, dual-phase makeup remover with silicone. The plant extracts are a mix of fragrant rose and soothing cucumber, with rose extract not being the best for use around the eyes. Although this works very well, it doesn't best less expensive options from Almay or Neutrogena that are available at the drugstore.

M.A.C. TONERS

✓☺ BEST **Lightful Softening Lotion** *($30 for 6 fl. oz.)* is an excellent toner for all skin types, particularly normal to dry skin. Its formula contains an impressive mix of antioxidants, repairing ingredients, and soothing agents designed to calm redness and reinforce skin's healthy barrier function. Along with any of the toners from Paula's Choice, this is a rare example of what a well-formulated toner should contain! The amount of vitamin C (ascorbyl glucoside) in this toner may help improve skin discolorations, but ideally you'll want to pair it with other products (including a sunscreen rated SPF 15 or greater) that also contain ingredients that fight discolorations.

☺ AVERAGE **$$$ Fix +** *($20 for 3.4 fl. oz.)* is a standard, but good, alcohol-free toner for normal to dry or slightly oily skin. The mist application is convenient, but don't mist this over your makeup—nothing in the formula will "finish" it or prolong wear. Quite the opposite is true!

M.A.C. MOISTURIZERS (DAYTIME, NIGHTTIME), EYE CREAMS, & SERUMS

✓☺ BEST **$$$ Prep+Prime Skin Brightening Serum** *($40 for 1 fl. oz.).* This thin-textured, lightweight serum is an excellent choice for those with normal to oily skin. It provides a good complement of ingredients all skin types need to look and feel healthy, but without any heavy or occlusive ingredients that oily skin doesn't need. The brightening aspect comes from the form of vitamin C (ascorbyl glucoside) this serum contains. Although "brightening" isn't the same as "lightening" (the latter being a term associated with active skin-lightening ingredients such as hydroquinone), you may see discolorations improve due to any form of stabilized vitamin C. Even if your discolorations don't budge, the vitamin C offers multiple benefits for skin, and it is joined by several other antioxidants. Ignore the "charged water" claim; there's no proof that charging water with minerals makes water more hydrating. Besides, skin needs much more than water to be hydrated; for example, it needs barrier repair ingredients to help maintain its water balance (and too much water is detrimental for skin). The only drawback of this serum is the inclusion of fragrant tuberose extract; however, it's not a deal-breaker unless you have sensitive skin.

✓☺ BEST **$$$ Prep + Prime Vibrancy Eye Primer** *($30 for 0.5 fl. oz.)* is a lightweight eye cream that has a moist feel and shiny finish thanks to the shimmering pigments it contains. By combining pigments normally used in makeup, M.A.C. has created an eye-area product that smoothes and brightens, so in that sense it can improve the appearance of dark circles. The improvement is subtle (a concealer goes a lot further), but this can help. Even better, this contains a good range of antioxidants and water-binding agents along with a range of cell-communicating ingredients to help improve signs of aging. Despite all this praise, the fact remains that you don't need an eye cream or special eye-area product, even one that's supposed to prep skin for makeup. A well-formulated facial moisturizer or serum loaded with beneficial ingredients works just as well, no need for a separate product! Still, if you're curious to try an eye cream with "primer" benefits, this is a good option. Its smooth finish isn't greasy so it won't cause concealers to slip into lines or eyeliner to smear.

✓☺ BEST **Strobe Cream** *($15 for 1 fl. oz.)* contains mineral pigments to optically "brighten" skin, which basically means particles of shine to make skin look radiant rather than dull. Looking beyond the light show reveals a well-formulated moisturizer brimming with the essential elements normal to dry skin needs to look and feel its best. Almost all the antioxidants included have considerable research documenting their topical benefit for skin.

✓☺ BEST **Studio Moisture Fix SPF 15** *($30 for 1.7 fl. oz.)* has an in-part zinc oxide sunscreen with a beautiful silky texture, provides a soft matte finish, and is loaded with anti-oxidants, skin-identical substances, and anti-irritants. It is a brilliant option for normal to oily skin, although the amount of zinc oxide (and its slight whitening effect) may prove tricky to work with on darker skin tones. This product does contain fragrance.

☺ GOOD **$$$ Lightful Essence** *($40 for 1 fl. oz.)* is a good vitamin C serum, whose form of vitamin C (ascorbyl glucoside) has a decent amount of research pertaining to its ability to improve brown discolorations. Other forms of vitamin C have more research behind them, but this serum also contains a great range of antioxidants and other ingredients all skin types need to look and act younger. The texture of this serum is fluid and its finish can feel a bit tacky, so it's best used at night rather than under makeup during the day. The lack of cell-communicating ingredients and inclusion of fragrance kept this from earning our top rating, but it's still worth considering and the price isn't too out of line for what you get.

☺ GOOD **Strobe Liquid** *($30 for 1.7 fl. oz.)* is the fluid version of M.A.C.'s popular Strobe Cream. Strobe Cream is one of the better moisturizers M.A.C. offers, and Strobe Liquid follows suit by treating normal to oily skin to an impressive mix of antioxidants and water-binding agents. Although not as well rounded as Strobe Cream, this is still worth considering as long as you're OK with the obvious opalescent pink shimmer that it leaves. Strobe Cream's shimmer is subtle, giving your skin a well-rested glow, while Strobe Liquid tosses subtlety out the door and turns the shine dial to "loud," which won't please someone with oily skin.

☺ GOOD **$$$ Oil Control Lotion** *($30 for 1.7 fl. oz.)* doesn't control oil as much as it just leaves a smooth matte finish. This is a good moisturizer for oily skin types with dry patches. It contains a few antioxidants and cell-communicating ingredients in stable packaging.

☹ AVERAGE **Complete Comfort Creme** *($32 for 1.7 fl. oz.)* contains some excellent ingredients for dry skin; the fact that it's packaged in a jar is disappointing. The antioxidants in this formula won't remain potent once this is opened and dry, sensitive skin needs these vital ingredients. Please see the Appendix to learn more about the problems jar packaging presents. This moisturizer is supposed to be great for sensitive, reddened skin, but it contains fragrance and some fragrant plant extracts that won't improve the issues that come with having sensitive skin. What a shame, because the formula also contains some great soothing agents, including soothing plant extracts.

☹ AVERAGE **$$$ Fast Response Eye Cream** *($30 for 0.5 fl. oz.)* is a silicone-based moisturizer that contains several antioxidants, but also enough caffeine to make it problematic for use around the eyes due to its irritant potential. This contains fragrance in the form of methyldihydrojasmonate. See the Appendix to learn why, in truth, you don't need an eye cream.

☹ AVERAGE **$$$ Lightful Moisture Creme** *($40 for 1.7 fl. oz.)* is a lightweight, but substantially hydrating, moisturizer for normal to slightly dry or dry skin, and it is jam-packed with cell-communicating ingredients, antioxidants, and beneficial plant extracts. How frustrating that all these ingredients will quickly become less effective due to jar packaging that doesn't keep air-sensitive ingredients stable during use. In better packaging, this would be highly recommended! See the Appendix to learn more about the problems jar packaging presents.

☹ POOR **Studio Moisture Cream** *($32 for 1.7 fl. oz.)* contains a large amount of *Aleurites moluccana* oil. Also known as tung seed oil, it is known to cause sweating on contact and can cause acute contact dermatitis. It is also a good source of linolenic and linoleic acids, but so is evening primrose oil, without the negatives (Source: naturaldatabase.com). What a shame, because this moisturizer for normal to dry skin contains some very helpful ingredients.

M.A.C. LIP CARE

✓☺ BEST **$$$ Lip Conditioner** *($15 for 0.5 fl. oz.)* is an exemplary, stably packaged lip balm that's based around Vaseline, but contains appreciable amounts of several antioxidants and skin-identical substances. It is highly recommended for dry, chapped lips, and the tube applicator is convenient when you're on the go.

☹ AVERAGE **$$$ Lip Conditioner Stick SPF 15** *($15)* contains 1% titanium dioxide, which is decent, but not great, UVA protection. A higher percentage would be far better for your lips. The balm itself is basic and will shield your lips against moisture loss while providing a smooth finish.

☹ POOR **Lip Conditioner SPF 15** *($15 for 0.5 fl. oz.)* leaves lips vulnerable to UVA damage because it does not contain titanium dioxide, zinc oxide, avobenzone, Tinosorb, or Mexoryl SX (ecamsule). Its formula is also not nearly as elegant as that of the regular Lip Conditioner. The same review applies for M.A.C.'s **Tinted Lip Conditioner SPF 15** ($15 for 0.5 oz.).

☹ POOR **Plushglass** *($19.50)* is similar to Clinique's Full Potential Lips Plump and Shine, but omits the peppermint oil. Still around to irritate lips into a plump state are ginger root and capsicum (pepper) oils, neither of which are great to use consistently. This is otherwise a standard sheer lip gloss with a smooth feel and minimally sticky finish (it does feel nicer than Clinique's version). Compared to Clinique's plumping option, the omission of peppermint oil makes this the lesser of two evils, though it's still difficult to recommend for anything but occasional use.

M.A.C. SPECIALTY SKIN-CARE PRODUCT

☺ GOOD **$$$ Blot Film** *($15 for 30 sheets)* is a set of 30 uncoated sheets of thin plastic material with absorbent properties. They work well to soak up excess shine and perspiration. Whether you choose them over tissue paper–style blotting papers comes down to personal preference.

M.A.C. FOUNDATIONS & PRIMERS

✓☺ BEST **$$$ Matchmaster SPF 15 Foundation** *($33)*. The selling point for this liquid foundation with reliable broad-spectrum sunscreen is the "translucent pigments" that are said to offer a "personalized finish" influenced by your skin's undertone. M.A.C. may well be using translucent pigments, but we suspect many other companies are as well, given how much better foundations look today than they did even five years ago. M.A.C.'s claim is really just stating what any good foundation does when you find the right shade: It looks natural, melds with your skin, and matches your skin's undertone (which is typically yellow-based), rather than masking it or playing up what you see on the surface (i.e., redness or a pink cast). Claims aside, this is an excellent option. It has a fluid, silky texture and a smooth creaminess that is a pleasure to blend. The finish is natural matte and it gives skin a dimensional rather than flat quality—very attractive. Coverage is in the medium range, but as with other foundations that provide this level of coverage, it can be blended sheer; keep in mind that the more sheer it is, the less sun protection you get. The formula is best for normal to slightly oily or combination skin, and it is fine for breakout-prone skin. The shades are quite good, especially those for fair to light and dark skin tones. In fact, the darker shades here are some of the best we've seen from M.A.C. Watch out for shade 6, which has a strong gold tone that won't work for most medium skin tones, and shade 7, which is very peach. The other shades are recommended.

✓☺ BEST **Prep + Prime Line Filler** *($20 for 0.5 fl. oz.)*. Now this is what we mean by a well-formulated primer! Rather than just being a mix of silicones and fragrance, this combines a dry-finish silicone polymer with emollients, film-forming agents, and copious antioxidants to help smooth skin, temporarily fill in superficial lines, and create an even canvas for foundation. It is similar to any well-formulated serum because it leaves skin feeling silky while imparting lots of beneficial extras that go beyond just prepping skin for makeup. As mentioned, the line-filling ability of this Prep + Prime product is minor and short-lived, but it will make a subtle difference. The matte finish of this product makes it suitable for all skin types, but those of you who tend to break out may want to choose a serum that doesn't contain emollients. The good news is there are plenty of serums that meet that description.

✓☺ BEST **Studio Fix Powder Plus Foundation** *($27)* remains one of the top pressed-powder foundations available, despite several impressive entries from other companies. It has an exceptionally silky, talc-based texture that applies and blends like a dream. As usual, wet or dry application is possible, but using this wet poses the risk of streaking. Dry application provides light to medium-full coverage. If you prefer this type of foundation and have normal to slightly dry or slightly oily skin, it is highly recommended. Almost all the colors are impressive (albeit repetitive) for a broad range of skin tones, but the following shades are best avoided due to pink, orange, or peach overtones: C6, NC42, NW25, NW30, NW40, and NC40.

✓☺ BEST $$$ **Studio Sculpt SPF 15 Foundation** *($30)*. This creamy liquid foundation with an in-part titanium dioxide sunscreen doesn't offer the user any greater sculpting abilities than any other foundation. Besides, it isn't foundation that plays a large role in sculpting the face via makeup; that type of detailing is done with contouring, blush, and eyeshadow placement (plus proper blending). Aside from the name, as a foundation with sunscreen, this is a workable option for those with normal to slightly dry or oily skin. It dispenses somewhat thick at first, but softens as it warms to skin temperature. Application is smooth and even, and this provides no less than medium coverage (you can get nearly full coverage if needed). It finishes satin matte with a powdery feel, and does a reasonable job of keeping shine in check. Another attribute of this foundation is its long-wearing, tenacious nature. It holds up really well if you perspire (those in humid climates, take note) and requires more than a water-soluble cleanser when you're ready to remove it. As usual, M.A.C's shade range is extensive and mostly impeccable; there are equally good options for fair to dark skin tones. The shades to avoid due to overtones of orange, peach, or copper are NC45, NW30, NW35, and NW45. The NC35 shade is slightly peach but workable for medium skin tones.

☺ GOOD $$$ **Mineralize Foundation Loose** *($30)*. We had to stifle a chuckle as we watched the M.A.C. salesperson bring out the testers for this loose-powder "mineral" foundation. They were in a black plastic bag, which was dusty with powder. As she removed each shade, even though all were capped, powder was everywhere. Therein is one of my major gripes about this type of makeup: It is incredibly messy unless it comes in a component that minimizes powder spill. M.A.C's packaging doesn't quite cut it, but we've seen worse. In terms of performance, this wins points for its feather-light, mica-based texture that feels lighter than most loose mineral powders. Although this provides light to barely medium coverage, it feels like you're wearing nothing at all. Shine is there, but definitely on the subtle side. This has a dry matte finish but still casts a soft glow on skin. Among the nine shades, Light, Light Medium, and Medium are excellent. The middle range of colors—Medium Plus, Medium Deep, and Dark—tends to be slightly peach to orange, and should be considered carefully. The Deeper Dark shade is a very good bronze tone for those who want a loose bronzing powder without a rosy cast. The cap for this foundation features a sponge for applying the makeup. It works decently, but a larger sponge or full (meaning dense) powder brush is preferred. All told, this is a fairly impressive entry into the ever-expanding category of mineral makeup.

☺ GOOD $$$ **Prep + Prime Face Protect SPF 50** *($30 for 1 fl. oz.)* is disappointing due to the shortage of antioxidants. It is otherwise a very good in-part zinc oxide sunscreen in a silicone-enriched base that is ideal for use under makeup. The amount of zinc oxide leaves a slightly white cast, but this is a non-issue if you're going to follow with foundation. Unless you are prone to breakouts from zinc oxide, this is an excellent, fragrance-free daytime moisturizer (or primer, if you prefer) for normal to very oily skin.

☺ GOOD $$$ **Prep + Prime Fortified Skin Enhancer SPF 35** *($30)*. A tinted foundation primer with sunscreen, this is a fairly unusual product with a mixed bag of pros and cons. This has a lightweight, slightly creamy texture that blends easily and sets to a soft matte finish that also imparts a subtle, healthy glow on skin. The sunscreen provides broad-spectrum protection thanks to the inclusion of titanium dioxide and zinc oxide, among other actives, and, unlike most foundation primers, this contains an assortment of soothing and repairing ingredients. In the negatives column is the fact that this shouldn't be used as your sole source of sun protection. Why? Because most people aren't going to apply this liberally enough to achieve the amount of sun protection stated on the label. Even if you did that, applying this liberally causes it to look and feel heavy on your skin, magnifying large pores and shiny areas. The shades offer mixed results, too, with Adjust being the only flesh-toned option (best for light to light-medium skin tones). The remaining shades include soft yellow, pale pink, and soft peach, all of which are designed as color-correcting options to wear beneath your foundation. The problem is that the color-correcting shades tend to turn your foundation a strange color unless you apply this primer sparingly (but, as mentioned above, that means sun protection will be compromised). On balance, this product deserves its rating based on the overall formula and its somewhat unique attributes. If you decide to test this, make sure you combine it with a moisturizer or foundation with sunscreen rated SPF 15 or greater to ensure you're getting adequate sun protection. This Prep + Prime product is best for normal to combination skin, but be aware that its finish can make oily areas appear shinier within a couple of hours (be sure to finish with powder).

☺ GOOD $$$ **Prep + Prime Skin** *($28)* is an ultra-light, fragrance-free lotion meant to be applied to skin before foundation. This product doesn't necessarily prime skin better than similar products labeled as moisturizers, gels, or serums, but it does indeed create a silky-smooth, non-greasy surface that facilitates makeup application. Whether it's for you depends strictly on whether your skin needs help in this regard. Compared with other products sold as primers, this formula goes a bit further by being more than a mixture of silicones and water. Prep + Prime Skin contains appreciable amounts of plant extracts that serve as antioxidants and anti-inflammatory agents. It is a suitable formulation for normal to slightly dry or slightly oily skin, but has one potential drawback: shine. This M.A.C. product's shine is more obvious and more glittery than shimmery. If you don't mind added shine under your makeup (or on bare skin), this won't be an obstacle.

☺ GOOD **Prep + Prime Skin Refined Zone Treatment** *($20 for 0.5 fl. oz.)* is a good, lightweight mattifier for oily to very oily skin. It may be applied under or over makeup (pat it on oily areas to touch up and be careful not to rub) and helps keep skin shine-free. This does not contain ingredients capable of exfoliating skin, so that part of the claim is inaccurate. Sodium salicylate cannot exfoliate like salicylic acid does, and the pH of this product isn't within range for exfoliation anyway.

☺ GOOD $$$ **Studio Fix Fluid SPF 15** *($27)* has a beautifully silky texture and ultra-smooth application that sets to a natural matte finish. Best for normal to oily skin, it provides medium coverage and comes in a wide range of shades, of which only four are poor contenders. NC55 is too ash, NW30 and NW35 too peach, and NW45 has a copper overtone that makes it a tough match for darker skin tones. NW50 and NW55 are ideal shades for dark skin, and there are options for very light skin, too. As for sunscreen, the combined amount of active ingredients is low enough that we would not advise relying on this foundation as your sole source of sun protection. For best results, apply a lightweight moisturizer rated SPF 15 or greater first.

☺ GOOD $$$ **Studio Tech Foundation** *($30)* is a next-generation cream-to-powder foundation that offers a lighter, almost weightless texture, smooth application, and a soft satin finish that tends not to grab onto dry areas. It combines the super-light feel of a water-to-powder makeup with the slip and smoothness of silicone-based cream-to-powder makeups. Studio Tech applies easily and provides light to medium coverage. A staggering range of shades is available, with suitable options for very light (NC15, NW15) and darker (NW50, NW55) skin tones. Although the majority of the shades lean toward neutral, six of them are too orange or peach for their intended skin tones: NC40, NC45, NC55, NW25, NW30, and NW40. This formula is best for normal to slightly dry and dry skin—the non-matte, non-powdery finish won't do much to temper shine, and even though this is not traditional cream-to-powder makeup, enough waxes and thickeners are present to make it problematic for those battling blemishes. If your skin fills the bill for this makeup, it's certainly worth checking out.

☺ AVERAGE **$$$ Mineralize Satinfinish SPF 15** *($30)* has so much going for it, yet the sunscreen lacks sufficient UVA protection. Surprisingly for this mineral-themed foundation, M.A.C. did not opt to use titanium dioxide or zinc oxide for the sunscreen, a typical standard in this category of makeup. This fluid foundation dispenses from a pump and has a beautifully smooth texture and soft matte finish that gives a good dimensional (rather than flat) quality to skin. Achieving medium coverage is easy; in fact, this is difficult to make sheer. It has a hint of shine and of the available shades, the following should be considered carefully due to their peachy casts: NW30, NW35 (way too peach for most), NW43 (also quite peach), and NW45. This is a product to consider if you have normal to slightly dry or slightly oily skin and are willing to pair it with a separate product during the day that contains the UVA-protecting ingredients of zinc oxide, titanium dioxide, avobenzone, Tinosorb, or Mexoryl SX.

☺ AVERAGE **$$$ Mineralize SPF 15 Foundation** *($33)*. Sadly, this mineral attempt fell off the bandwagon, primarily because the SPF doesn't include the UVA-protecting ingredients of titanium dioxide, zinc oxide, avobenzone, ecamsule, Tinosorb, or Mexoryl SX. As a foundation it has a creamy texture with minimal slip that still manages to blend quite well. The finish isn't powdery (the M.A.C. artist was quick to point out that this is not a cream-to-powder foundation, and she was right) and looks surprisingly skin-like, especially if blended down a bit. As for coverage, it's within the light to medium range, while the formula is best for normal to dry skin not prone to breakouts. There are over 20 shades available, with options for fair to dark (but not very dark) skin. Most of them are beautiful, but there are some to avoid, including the markedly peach NW35, NW40, NW43, and NC45. Shades to consider carefully include NC40, NC50, and NW45. Despite some strong positives, this foundation's lack of sufficient sun protection keeps it from earning a Good rating.

☺ AVERAGE **$$$ Pro Longwear SPF 10 Foundation** *($30)*. A foundation that promises to wear for 15 hours is bound to prompt some curiosity, but does Pro Longwear deliver on its promise? Well, in the sense that it stays on your skin, yes. However, someone with oily skin won't find this leaves them looking fresh-faced and matte all day, or even for a few hours. Still, this is a silky liquid foundation that provides medium coverage from the get-go. It's difficult to get light coverage from this foundation, so you have to be okay with medium coverage. It does go on silky and is easy to blend, but the matte finish feels a bit tacky. This foundation tends to sit on top of skin rather than mesh with it as today's best foundations do. As a result, lines, large pores, and crevices are magnified rather than downplayed, especially if you're not adept at blending. Also disappointing is the SPF rating. If you want your foundation to be your main source of sun protection, SPF 15 is the minimum, although it's nice to see that M.A.C. opted for pure titanium dioxide to provide broad-spectrum protection. Given this foundation's mixed bag of pros and cons, it isn't your best option. On a positive note, M.A.C. created

☀ Sunscreens must provide reliable UVA (anti-aging) protection. See the Appendix for details.

options for fair to dark skin tones, and most of the colors are excellent. The ones to avoid, or at least to consider carefully, include NW25 (peach), NC42 (too gold for most medium skin tones), NC45 (orange), NW30 (slightly peach), NW40 (very peach), and NW50 (consider with caution because it turns slightly ash).

☹ AVERAGE **$$$ Select SPF 15** *($27)* has a formula very similar to the Studio Fix Fluid SPF 15, and is another M.A.C. foundation whose sunscreen lacks sufficient UVA-protecting ingredients. If you're already using a separate sunscreen rated SPF 15 or higher and want to give this a try, it has a fluid, lightweight texture that blends easily and sets to a silky matte finish. This offers slightly less coverage than the Studio Fix Fluid and is preferred for normal to slightly dry or slightly oily skin. Among the mostly excellent shades are a few duds: NC45 is slightly orange, NW25 is slightly peach, NW35 is very peach, NW45 is a bit too coppery, and NW50 is slightly ash.

☺ AVERAGE **$$$ Studio Moisture Tint SPF 15** *($30)* is not recommended over many others. The reason is the lack of sufficient UVA-protecting ingredients of avobenzone, zinc oxide, titanium dioxide, ecamsule, Mexoryl SX, or Tinosorb. The convenience of a tinted moisturizer with sunscreen is lost if you need to double-up and use another product that provides better UVA protection. If you still want to try this, it has a fluid, weightless texture with just enough slip to make blending easy. It provides sheer coverage, comes in a great shade range, and sets to a satin matte finish best for normal to slightly dry skin. This contains fragrance in the form of methyldihydrojasmonate.

M.A.C. CONCEALERS

✓☺ BEST **Select Cover-Up** *($17)* is a great concealer. Lightly creamy with a natural matte finish, this liquid concealer provides good camouflage with minimal risk of creasing. Thirteen mostly neutral shades are available, plus four color correctors, of which Colour Corrector Peach is an OK option. Colour Corrector Pink may work for some porcelain skin tones, though it has an opalescent finish. Of the regular shades, the ones to be cautious with are NC45, NW35, and NW45.

☺ GOOD **Select Moisturecover** *($17)* is another great liquid concealer, though this definitely has a creamy feel. Easy to control during application and providing medium to full coverage, this sets to a smooth finish that's minimally prone to creasing. The palette of shades is practically a case study in neutral to yellow tones for fair to dark skin, and the only color to consider carefully is the slightly peach NW30.

☺ GOOD **Studio Finish Concealer SPF 35** *($17)* has a formidable sunscreen that's in-part titanium dioxide, and the creamy texture is smoother and thus easier to blend. This is still a full-coverage concealer, and it takes practice to achieve the level of coverage you want without using too much product. It is excellent for concealing redness, dark circles, and other discolorations, but too emollient to use over blemishes. A wide range of shades are available, and almost all of them are exceptional. NC42 is too yellow for most skin tones, while NC45, NW35, and NW40 suffer from peach overtones. NW45 is too coppery for most dark skin tones, but the deeper NW50 is ideal. Fair to light skin tones will find more than one suitable shade, so be sure to test this at the counter before making a purchase.

☺ GOOD **$$$ Prep + Prime Highlighter** *($23)* is packaged in a click pen–style component outfitted with a built-in synthetic brush. As you click the base of the component, the fluid highlighter is fed onto the brush, ready for application. Applying this with the brush or your finger is easy thanks to its excellent silky texture. You have to blend quickly though, because this sets to a soft matte finish within seconds. Coverage is in the light to medium range, less than what you'd get from a regular concealer. Used as a highlighter under the eyes, on the brow bone, or along the bridge of the nose, this comes in three workable shades: Bright Forecast is best for medium skin tones and is trickiest to use due to a slight peach cast; Light Boost is a soft, champagne gold that's best for light to medium skin tones; and Radiant Rose is a pale, opalescent pink that is the most "brightening" of the shades, best on fair to light skin tones. One caution: The finish and the lack of hydrating ingredients in this product mean it will emphasize fine lines and wrinkles if you don't first prep with a moisturizer.

☺ GOOD $$$ **Pro Longwear Concealer** *($17).* The one thing we don't like about this concealer packaged in a glass bottle is its pump applicator, which makes it really tricky to dispense only what you need. Inevitably, you end up getting much more than you need, and trying to put it back in is a chore, which adds up to a waste of money. It also requires a bit more time than usual to blend, but does provide impressive coverage and has a smooth finish, with only a slight tendency to crease into lines around the eyes. It holds up really well, and is definitely one to consider if you're trying to camouflage dark circles or minor pigmentation issues, such as those from sun damage or acne. The shade range is extensive for a concealer, and most of the shades are excellent. Consider shades NW25, NW35, and NC42 carefully due to their peachy tones, and avoid shade NW40 due to rose overtones. Otherwise, those with fair to dark skin should be pleased with what M.A.C. provides. Despite the pump dispenser, which takes practice to get just the right amount with each use, this is worth considering.

☺ AVERAGE $$$ **Mineralize Concealer** *($19)* doesn't contain any "mineral" ingredients beyond the standard cosmetic pigments (mica, iron oxides) that show up in thousands of makeup products. Otherwise, this liquid concealer with a brush applicator has a fairly even mix of pros and cons. On the plus side is a long-wearing matte finish that's minimally prone to creasing. Another gold star goes to the shades, as most are wonderfully neutral and include options for fair to dark (but not very dark) skin tones. The only shades to avoid include the peachy NW30 and orange-ish NC60, and you should consider NW35 carefully, if at all. On the minus side, this has so little slip that blending must be quick—even then, it can be tricky because the formula tends to drag over skin, even if applied over a smooth foundation. Also an issue is the coverage, which tends to be spotty, while the finish is on the dry side, so this magnifies fine lines (it isn't even a little bit creamy). It's an OK concealer for use on breakouts or minor redness, but isn't one of M.A.C.'s best options for use around the eyes or to conceal dark discolorations.

☺ AVERAGE $$$ **Studio Sculpt Concealer** *($17)* has just enough slip to make blending a non-issue, but it remains creamy and is crease-prone unless set with powder. Even when you use powder, this thick concealer's finish doesn't hold up nearly as well as its partner product, Studio Sculpt SPF 15 Foundation. Still, it provides good coverage without looking heavy and the shade range is impressive. You'll find colors for fair to dark skin tones and only a few to avoid. Those to avoid are the peachy NW30 and the orange-ish NC50, and consider NC42 carefully. One other comment: This concealer is packaged in a heavy glass jar that some will find cumbersome, especially for travel.

M.A.C. POWDERS

✓☺ BEST $$$ **Mineralize Skinfinish** *($29)* is a sheer, talc-based pressed powder that looks wonderfully natural on skin. It's almost impossible to make this powder look heavy, thick, or dry. Those with normal to dry skin will appreciate the slight sheen this leaves behind (and remember, talc is a mineral, too, so M.A.C.'s name for this product is accurate). All four shades are neutral and highly recommended, but there are no options for very dark skin tones. For those with oily skin, note that the sheen this powder leaves can make oily areas appear shinier.

✓☺ BEST $$$ **Select Sheer Loose Powder** *($23)* sets a new powder precedent by offering an ultra-light texture that seems to disappear into the skin, yet provides a smooth, dimensional, polished finish. The talc-based formula has an understated shine that is visible, but that doesn't detract from this powder's incredibly light texture and fine finish. The shades are typically M.A.C., meaning there are many noteworthy neutral tones. Each shade goes on very sheer and imparts just a hint of color, so getting an exact match isn't essential, and the choices are plentiful. NW35 is a beautiful option for bronzing powder, and shade NC5 is for the most porcelain skin tone.

✓☺ BEST $$$ **Select Sheer Pressed Powder** *($23)* is basically a pressed version of the Select Sheer Loose Powder, except that this powder does not have any shine and, as is true for most pressed powders when compared to loose powders, it offers more coverage. Most of the shades are exceptional, although NW43 may be a touch too copper for some dark skin tones and NW50 is slightly ash. Shade NC55 makes an excellent bronzing powder color. Overall, this is a wonderful pressed powder, especially if you want a finished look but aren't a fan of traditional powders. Those with oily skin may find this not absorbent enough, but it's still worth auditioning.

✓☺ BEST $$$ **Studio Careblend/Pressed Powder** *($23)*. "Marvelous all around" is a great way to describe this ultra-smooth, talc-based pressed powder that's best for normal to dry skin. M.A.C.'s claims about this powder are 100% accurate: It blends superbly and leaves a sheer, natural matte finish that doesn't look the least bit powdery.

☺ GOOD $$$ **Mineralize Skinfinish/Natural** *($29)* has a smooth, dry texture that applies sheer and even, making it easy to blend. The finish is soft matte with a hint of sparkle, which M.A.C. describes as "dimensional," but in reality, it's just shine. This is a good option if you want light coverage from a pressed powder and have normal to oily skin. The shade range is mostly neutral with a slight emphasis toward warm (yellow) tones. The only shade to avoid is the peachy Medium Dark.

☹ AVERAGE $$$ **Magically Cool Liquid Powder** *($30)*. Fans of Prescriptives' former Magic Liquid Powder will recognize the unique formula of this "fluid" loose powder. The water-based formula doesn't contain typical powder ingredients like talc or a high amount of mica; instead, it contains ingredients typically seen in oil-free moisturizers, but this looks, and in many respects performs, like a powder. Now that's magic! The drawback of this powder is the amount of shine in each shade. There are options for fair to dark skin tones, and although the color of each goes on almost translucent, the shine is laid on thick, even when you apply it lightly with a brush. If you decide to try this, we don't recommend using it all over your face (this won't replace your regular loose or pressed powder). Upon application, it feels wet and a bit cooling (as the water evaporates from your skin), and the finish, besides being shiny, is also slightly damp. It's an OK option as a shiny highlighting powder with a unique feel, but that's about it.

☹ AVERAGE $$$ **Prep + Prime Transparent Finishing Powder** *($23)* is an expensive loose powder when you consider you're getting less than a quarter ounce and the effect this provides isn't anything special or extraordinary. It's just a good, sheer, absorbent loose powder. Considering the powder is pure white, the sheer application saves it from making your complexion look ghostly—but it's worth noting this doesn't go on colorless. We tried this as a touch-up on fair skin and noted a slightly discernible white cast and tinge of a washed-out look that had us reaching for more blush. This fragrance-free powder's absorbent, refining finish helps reduce the appearance of pores. M.A.C. claims this also reduces wrinkles, but it has minimal effect and, if you apply too much, its dry finish will make wrinkles more apparent. In the end, this is merely an OK yet overpriced option for oily skin.

M.A.C. BLUSHES & BRONZER

✓☺ BEST **$$$ Bronzing Powder** *($23)* is a talc-based, pressed-powder bronzer with an extremely smooth texture and dry finish. It comes in five believable tan shades, three of which have a very shiny finish. Matte Bronze is truly matte and Bronze is almost matte. Looking to spend less money for similar results? Try Wet 'n Wild's Bronzer ($2.99).

☺ GOOD **$$$ Mineralize Blush** *($23.50)*. This shine-infused pressed-powder blush has a silky, slightly dry texture and reliable application with an even color deposit. The marbleized pattern of each shade is infused with sparkles that give this blush its shiny finish, and they tend to cling well. This is a very good blush for those looking to color and add shine to their cheeks.

☺ GOOD **$$$ Powder Blush** *($20)*. Powder Blush presents almost 50 shades, from the palest pinks and peaches to the deepest browns and plums. The vast palette is divided into five finishes and two formulas. The Satins feel silkier than the Mattes or Frosts and have good pigmentation with less tendency to grab. All of them are worth checking out.

☺ GOOD **$$$ Powder Blush - Sheertone/Sheertone Shimmer** *($20)*. Best among M.A.C.'s powder blushes are the Sheertone and Sheertone Shimmer shades. Although both lack the pigmentation of the other M.A.C. blushes, they apply extremely well, have a super-silky texture, and the regular Sheertone comes in a beautiful range of true matte colors. The Sheertone Shimmer version is just that, sheer colors with a soft shimmer finish. They work well for evening makeup, but most have too much shine for daytime, at least if you work in a professional environment. Both Sheertone formulas have limited options for darker skin tones, but fair to medium skin tones are well served.

☹ AVERAGE **$$$ Cream Colour Base** *($17.50)* has been around for years, and the color collection keeps expanding, so there must be a lot of people buying these somewhat slick, crease-prone (when used as eyeshadow) colors. The shade range offers options for eyes, lips, and cheeks, and their intensity varies, so this is definitely a product to test at the counter before purchasing. The creamy base is ill-advised for blemish-prone skin, but normal to dry skin looking to add a soft, radiant (or iridescent, depending on the shade) glow may want to give this a try.

☹ POOR **Cremeblend Blush** *($20)*. M.A.C. positions this cream blush as being versatile and a cheek color for the perfectionist. The problem is that it's neither: This goes on creamy and stays that way, whereas a versatile blush would set to a soft powder finish for longevity that would keep it from moving into pores or slipping during the day. If you're a perfectionist you most likely will be disappointed by how poorly this applies—and how bad it can look on your skin.

M.A.C. EYESHADOWS & EYE PRIMERS

✓☺ BEST **Eye Shadows - Veluxe** *($15)*. Veluxe shades (don't ask us what Veluxe means; we assume it's a combination of velvet and luxurious) have the most beautifully silky texture and even application of all M.A.C.'s powder shadows. We wish there were more shades, but the following shades are excellent: Samoa Silk and Brown Down.

✓☺ BEST **Matte2 Eye Shadow** *($15)* has a true matte finish that is great! This time around the emphasis is on creating a dimensional rather than a flat matte finish, courtesy of improved pigment technology. The result is definitely matte, but more skin-like than the many chalky matte eyeshadows from years ago. However, there have always been exemplary matte eyeshadows to be found; it was just difficult to locate them in a sea of shiny eyeshadows (which have also come a long way over the years). M.A.C. has produced a pressed-powder eyeshadow with a luxuriously smooth, almost creamy-feeling texture that, as expected, blends easily. That fact is a plus because all the shades are pigment-rich. You'll get excellent coverage with these shadows, and they have a silky-smooth finish with staying power.

✓☺ BEST **$$$ Paint Pot** *($17.50)* comes in, you guessed it, a pot. These have a soft, buttery texture that leads to a smooth, even application, whether applied with a natural-hair or synthetic brush (the synthetic brush produces a stronger color, while natural-hair brushes net a softer color deposit). These set quickly to a long-wearing, waterproof powder finish, so be sure blending is quick and precise. Once set, these absolutely do not crease, fade, or smudge, which is very impressive. All the colors are workable, though some are a bit too colorful. The matte options include Soft Ochre, Quite Natural, and Painterly, which works as a great base color for the eyelid. The others have a soft to brazen shine. Because of Paint Pot's finish, you can apply other shadows or pencil liner over it without disruption.

✓☺ BEST **Prep + Prime Eye** *($17)* works well as a cream-to-powder concealer for the eye area as well as for other discolorations. Its creamy texture quickly morphs into a silky, weightless matte finish that is minimally prone to creasing. The finish can look slightly powdery, but the effect is canceled once eyeshadow is blended over it. The five shades present options for light to dark skin tones, but nothing for someone with porcelain to fair skin.

☺ GOOD **Eye Shadows** *($15)* maintain the same almost-smooth, dry texture they've had for the past several years. The only real difference this time around is that many of the colors go on softer and more sheer. You'll notice less of this with the medium to dark shades, which tend to go on grainier and deeper than they look and don't blend as evenly as the best eyeshadows, but there is minimal flaking. These are not the smoothest shadows in town, but they do the job. Although the shades are labeled **Satin**, **Frost**, **Lustre**, **Matte**, **Velvet**, **Veluxe**, and **Veluxe Pearl**, they are arranged by color, not formula or finish, on the tester unit. The large number of Matte (most of the shades are indeed matte) and Satin shades apply much better, though the darker Matte shades drag a bit, so blending must be precise. Skip the Veluxe Pearl shades and avoid the Lustre and Velvet finishes due to their grainier texture and tendency to flake. The Satin and Matte finishes work best and offer the widest range of shades, too.

☺ GOOD **$$$ Paint** *($17.50)* is essentially a cleverly named and packaged cream-to-powder eyeshadow. Dispensed from a tube (don't apply too much pressure because you'll end up wasting product), the concentrated formula blends very well and has a natural opacity that can almost take the place of your foundation or concealer as a means for evening-out skin on the eyelid and under-brow area. Most of the colors are neutral and workable yet supply intense shine. There are a few softer shades that can work for a mildly shiny look. Paints can be used alone or mixed with other products, and they sheer out well if you prefer a subtle wash of color. Regardless of color or shine intensity, these tend not to crease and last all day without fading or smearing.

☺ GOOD **$$$ Pro Longwear Eye Shadow** *($20)* has a silky and slightly creamy pressed-powder texture that blends effortlessly on skin and offers flake-free application. The shade range contains a mixture of classic and trendy colors, all of which have a subtle, iridescent shimmer. Colors go on semi-sheer, but can easily be layered for more intensity. There's nothing especially "longwear" about this when compared with an average pressed-powder shadow, nor is it more "pro" than M.A.C.'s other powder eyeshadows. This is just one more eyeshadow to consider.

M.A.C. EYE & BROW LINERS

✔☺ BEST **Eye Brow Pencils** *($15)* are automatic, nonretractable, ultra-sleek pencils that apply easily and impart soft color without being greasy or smudging. The colors are brow-perfect, but don't ask me to explain the sexually charged names such as Stud, Lingering, and Fling!

✔☺ BEST **Fluidline** *($15)* is nearly identical to Bobbi Brown's Long-Wear Gel Eyeliner, a once-unique product that we love because of its remarkably easy application and tenacious wear. Long Wear Gel Eyeliner, M.A.C. Fluidline, and Stila's Smudge Pots are among the only eyeliners that can stand up to oily eyelids without fading, smearing, or running. All these have a slightly moist application that sets to a long-wearing matte finish. Fluidline is every bit as tenacious as Brown's Long-Wear Gel Eyeliner, but the colors are mostly … well, they're odd. Yes, classic browns and black are available, but most of the shades are not meant to define the eye so much as to add a shock of color. Peacock blue and bright purple are indeed eye-catching, but neither fulfills the main purpose of eyeliner, which is to define and accent the eye and enhance the depth of eyelashes. Rich Ground, Dipdown, and Blacktrack are the most versatile choices.

✔☺ BEST **Technakohl Liner** *($15)* is the eyeliner pencil to choose if you want a smooth application that doesn't drag or skip while imparting rich color. Initially creamy, this automatic, retractable pencil's formula sets to a soft powder finish that remains smudge-resistant. All but one of the shades is laced with shine, so if that's not on your must list, stick with Brownborder. And unless your eyelining goal is to draw attention to the liner rather than to your eyes, skip Jade Way, Auto-de-blu, and Smoothblue.

✔☺ BEST **$$$ Penultimate Eyeliner** *($18.50)*. What a great name for a liquid eyeliner! The precision brush allows one to draw an extremely thin line that can be easily thickened with a successive coat. Application is even, it dries fast (which is desirable because it minimizes the chance of smearing), and, once set, it lasts quite well. Those with moderately oily to oily eyelids will find this a bit smudge-prone and not preferred to silicone-enhanced gel liners (such as M.A.C. Fluidline). If oily eyelids aren't a concern and you prefer liquid liners, this is a terrific choice. It is available only in Rapidblack, which is a rich and dramatic.

☺ GOOD **$$$ Liquidlast Liner** *($18.50)* has a thin, flexible brush to ensure even application (assuming you have a steady hand). Dry time is average, so this isn't a liquid liner for anyone who flinches easily. Once set, it wears quite well, fading only slightly, and without smearing or flaking. Coco Bar and Point Black are the classic colors for a variety of eye-makeup designs. The remaining shades have a strong shimmer or metallic finish that is best for evening makeup and not appropriate for wrinkled eyelids.

☺ GOOD **$$$ Superslick Liquid Eye Liner** *($18.50)* is a good option for a smudge-proof liner that doesn't flake as the day wears on. True to claim, this liner dries within 15 seconds, and the flexible felt-tip brush allows for smooth application whether you desire a thick or thin line. We'd suggest steering clear of Pure Show (bright, golden yellow) and Nocturnal (very bright silver), but other shades in this line are worth experimenting with and offer good color payoff with a metallic finish, which is best reserved for evening use.

☹ AVERAGE **Brow Set** *($15)* is a basic brow gel formula that comes with a very good brush and has a minimally sticky finish. The Clear option is best; the others imbue brows or lashes with noticeable shimmer and have a tacky finish that can feel strange.

☹ AVERAGE **Eye Pencils** *($14)* are utterly standard (right down to the commonplace colors) and comparable to most of the other pencils out there. The same comments apply to M.A.C.'s **Eye Kohl** ($15). For lining the eyes, M.A.C.'s matte eyeshadows or Fluidline shades are a better alternative.

☻ AVERAGE **Powerpoint Eye Pencil** *($15)* glides on with no tugging or skipping, but smears easily before it sets. Allow a minute or two for this to set, and you will be treated to several hours of fail-safe wear. As usual, M.A.C.'s shade selection is a mix of classic (brown and black) shades with trendy and unusual shades (jade green) meant to satisfy a wide variety of tastes. The soft, creamy texture of this pencil means it is difficult to create a fine, thin line, but it works great for thicker or smokier lines. The only other drawback? It needs to be sharpened, which keeps it from earning a Good rating.

☹ AVERAGE $$$ **Penultimate Brow Marker** *($18.50)*. If the single, reddish-brown shade M.A.C. offers for this liquid brow marker-like product works for you, then it's worth considering. The felt tip–style brush allows you to "paint" between your brow hairs, resulting in a natural, but filled in, look that is easy to apply and that lasts. It takes several seconds to set so watch out for smearing, but once it dries you can continue to groom your brows without worry. The color demands careful testing at the counter before making a purchase, and it obviously isn't for those with blonde or black eyebrows. If you're looking for more shades from the same type of brow "marker," consider Paula's Choice Browlistic Long-Wearing Precision Brow Color.

☻ POOR **Brow Finisher** *($15)* is a twist-up, waxy, tinted stick that's packaged like a brow pencil. The texture is so waxy that application is difficult and it tends to stick brow hairs together, not to mention the waxy smell (all the testers we played with had an "off" odor). This also feels tacky on brows and isn't something most women would want to tolerate given the variety of other options (including clear and tinted brow gels) that groom and define while being almost imperceptible.

M.A.C. LIP COLOR & LIPLINERS

✓☺ BEST **Lipsticks** *($14.50)*. M.A.C.'s Lipsticks remain one of the major attractions of this line. The majority of the formulas provide lush textures and feel comfortable, and the color range is nearly unparalleled. The **Amplified Cremes** have an overall texture and application very close to the Satin Lipsticks, but these offer enhanced opaqueness and a touch more gloss. The **Mattes** are not true mattes, but come pretty close with their deeply pigmented, full-coverage colors and non-glossy finish. The **Satins** are softly creamy with a rich, opaque texture and moist finish, and offer the best compromise of long wear and desirable creaminess. Less impressive but still recommended are the **Frosts**, which are creamy with medium coverage and a soft shimmer to true frost finish. The **Glazes** present a much smaller shade selection with colors that are more sheer and less glossy than the **Lustres**, which comprise M.A.C.'s largest collection of sheer lipsticks. Each has a glossy finish and enough slip to easily make its way into any lines around the mouth. If that's not an issue for you, these are worth checking out.

✓☺ BEST $$$ **Cremesheen Glass** *($19.50)* is a unique lip gloss. Think of it as a cross between a standard brush-on gloss and a lip balm and you'll have a good idea of how it feels and looks on lips. In a word, the effect is beautiful. The texture is very smooth and it leaves lips with a balm-like sheen that fills in superficial lip lines. The shade range is pleasing, and tends to favor sheer pastels and brighter tones.

✓☺ BEST $$$ **Pro Longwear Lipcolour** *($22)* is a dual-sided product, one end holding the lip color and the other a brush-on, glossy top coat. Although the concept is the same as Outlast from Cover Girl and all the other imitators, M.A.C.'s version excels because the colors go on so easily and evenly with a single application and, more important, because the top coat feels better than those of competing products. It actually goes a long way not only keeping lips glossy, but also in preventing the color beneath from chipping or peeling as the top coat wears off. As a result, you get amazingly long-lasting lip color combined with a superior top coat that keeps up appearances, and that makes this option from M.A.C. a must-try.

✓☺ BEST **$$$ Pro Longwear Lustre Lipcolour** *($22)* is a departure from the original Pro Longwear in two ways: the colors (they're less opaque, though not sheer) and the accompanying top coat, called **Mirror** (which is infused with mutlicolored glitter rather than being clear and glossy). The application process and impressive wear time are the same, but we're not fans of the glittery top coat because it limits the use of the striking but soft colors of the Pro Longwear Lustre Lipcolour. The good news is you can purchase one of M.A.C.'s other top coats to accompany the Lustre shade you like—the bad news is it must be purchased separately (it screws onto the color-base component so you can alternate top coats as needed). See if you like the glittery top coat before committing to this. Otherwise, this product is highly recommended.

☺ GOOD **Cremesheen Lipstick** *($14.50)* is greasier than M.A.C.'s Satin Lipstick formula reviewed above, but it imparts slightly more color. This slips on easily and feels comfortably emollient, while leaving a slightly glossy finish. It provides full coverage and the shade range presents many enticing options, including Dare You and Party Line for those tempted by luscious reds.

☺ GOOD **Lustreglass** *($14.50)* has the same wet-look shine as M.A.C.'s original Lipglass, but the Lustre version kicks up the color, so this is more of a lipstick/gloss hybrid than standard gloss. The brush applicator helps the gloss glide on, and considering this gloss's thicker texture, it is comparably non-sticky. The shimmer-infused shades feature mostly soft choices that should please most gloss fans, especially if applied over a regular lipstick.

☺ GOOD **$$$ Dazzleglass Lipcolour** *($19.50)*. Due to its popularity, this limited-edition gloss has become a stable part of M.A.C.'s line. The sheer- to light-coverage shades are infused with crystalline-like sparkles that cast a sultry multidimensional shine to lips. Unlike many sparkle-infused lip glosses, the sparkle particles are very tiny, so they look sophisticated rather than showy, and they don't feel grainy as the moisturizing feel of the gloss wears away. The slightly thick texture isn't as uncomfortably sticky as M.A.C.'s Lipglass.

☺ GOOD **$$$ Pro Longwear Lip Pencil** *($18)* has a slightly creamy texture that blends on evenly to line lips with matte color. True to its name, this sets to a stay-put finish that lasts throughout the day. The shade range includes various tones of nude, brown, red, mauve, plum, and pink. The only negative is that this pencil requires routine sharpening versus the more convenient, retractable lip pencils on the market. Normally, we don't give this type of lip pencil a positive rating, but in this case we made an exception because of its impressive staying power.

☺ GOOD **$$$ Sheen Supreme Lipglass** *($19)* is a fairly standard, but good, lip gloss housed in a click pen–style component outfitted with a synthetic brush applicator. The somewhat thick gloss is fed onto the brush tip, ready for application. A problem, at least for the first few uses, is that the brush remains noticeably stiff and inflexible, which hinders an even application. This isn't a deal-breaker, but before you begin clicking to feed the gloss onto the brush, use clean fingers to play with the brush a bit so it becomes flexible enough to smoothly apply the gloss. Once on, this feels moist but not sticky, and imparts bright yet sheer color along with a shimmer-spiked glossy sheen. M.A.C. offers a mix of pastel, nude, and fruit-colored shades, each of which goes on softer than you might suspect. As with most glosses, the color and finish are fleeting, but it's great that this doesn't feel goopy or too slick; it tends to stay in place decently well!

☺ AVERAGE **Cremestick Liner** *($14.50)* is too creamy for its own good. The creaminess enhances application, but because it stays creamy, you'll find it fades and is definitely capable of traveling into lines around the mouth. One other point: This applies sheer, so if you want to define your mouth you need to layer quite a bit, which only makes the creamy finish more fleeting.

☺ AVERAGE **Lipglass, Clear and Tinted** *($14.50)* is a very thick, tenacious gloss whose heavy, syrupy texture is not for everyone. The tinted version has a slightly thinner texture and comes in a tube with a wand applicator; original Lipglass is packaged in a squeeze tube. The extensive shade range for Tinted Lipglass goes from sheer to dramatic.

☹ AVERAGE **Lip Pencils** *($13)* have a superior color selection, but that's the only thing that separates these standard, needs-sharpening pencils from nearly identical pencils found in almost every other line.

☺ AVERAGE $$$ **Pro Longwear Lip Creme** *($17)* attempts to eliminate the lip paint/glossy top coat process by presenting an all-in-one transfer-resistant lipstick. Unfortunately, the results are less than pleasant. This lipstick has a dry, slightly uneven application. The minimally creamy texture feels very light and has little movement once set to a soft gloss finish. In terms of long wear, each shade has a considerable stain that keeps color impact on your lips (even though the slight creamy feel is fleeting). Definitely a lipstick to try before you buy, and definitely not as highly recommended as M.A.C.'s original Pro Longwear Lipcolour.

☺ AVERAGE $$$ **Pro Longwear Lipglass** *($19.50)*. Longwearing? Yes. Comfortable? Not so much. The thick, gooey texture of this lip gloss drags across your lips and requires extra effort to achieve even application. Once set, this gloss feels heavy and tacky and has the tendency to catch any stray hairs blowing its way. Expect to be annoyed! On the plus side, the colors go on with impressive opacity and a moderate amount of shine in shades of pink, plum, nude, brown, red, and coral. Although this lip gloss may stay put longer than most, we suspect that most women will find the uneven application and unpleasant texture aren't worth it.

☺ AVERAGE $$$ **Sheen Supreme Lipstick** *($14.50)* is best thought of as a lip gloss in lipstick form, although it has drawbacks that don't make it preferred to a regular lip gloss. The thick, emollient texture feels greasy and, surprisingly, applies unevenly. M.A.C.'s shade range presents classic nude, pink, and rose tones alongside some shockingly bright colors, such as fusions of purple and fuchsia and vivid orange.

M.A.C. MASCARAS

✓☺ BEST $$$ **Haute & Naughty Lash** *($19)* has exceptionally clever packaging that allows the single brush to produce completely different results. It works because the mascara container has two different wipers. Inside any mascara tube, the wiper is what cleans the brush and controls how much mascara is deposited when you remove the wand prior to application. With Haute & Naughty Lash, you can remove the wand in one of two ways, depending on which part of the cap you unwind. The pink-topped portion allows a medium amount of mascara to be deposited onto the brush, which allows for clump-free length and lash separation with just a few strokes. Your lashes will be dramatically longer and you'll see subtle thickness. Using the sparkling purple top deposits a more generous amount of mascara onto the wand, which increases the intensity. From the first stroke, lashes are substantially thickened and defined. All in all, this is a versatile (and, quite frankly, ingenious) 2-in-1 mascara that really does give you two different, equally distinctive looks. It costs a bit more than M.A.C.'s other mascaras, but if you can see yourself using both wipers for the different results each provides, it is a worthy splurge.

✓☺ BEST **Studio Fix Lash** *($15)* is an excellent choice for mascara wearers who may not have the expertise or desire to deal with more dramatic or difficult-to-control mascaras. This is a mascara that anyone can get right with one coat! The formula feels extremely lightweight and it goes on lashes easily and evenly thanks to its fool-proof brush with short rubber bristles. The mascara volumizes and lengthens in equal measure; holds a curl; and doesn't smear, flake, or clump. Better still, lashes stay soft. The only drawback is that it's slightly stubborn to remove; otherwise, it's an outstanding mascara. Color us impressed M.A.C.! Identical to this mascara but available in an inky-black color is their **Studio Fix Boldblack Lash** ($15).

✓☺ BEST **Zoom Lash Mascara** *($15)* can go on a bit too heavily (especially if you're too zealous while applying it), but it builds impressive thickness with minimal effort and does so without bothersome clumps or smudges. This is also supposed to curl lashes, but the effect is subtle; you'll still need your eyelash curler (assuming you ordinarily use one). This mascara is best for those who want lash drama, not demureness, and ranks among M.A.C.'s best. For even more drama and super-dark lashes, go for **Zoom Fast Black Lash Mascara** (identical to original Zoom Lash except the black color is darker and inkier).

✓☺ BEST **Zoom Waterfast Lash** *($15)* is not only tenaciously waterproof, it's also very good at lengthening and defining lashes while building some thickness and leaving lashes with a soft, fringed curl. Some minor clumping occurs with each use, but the brush allows for quick smoothing. Once set, this wears without flaking or smearing—and even if you're completely submerged in water this will not budge. Removing it requires an oil- or silicone-based makeup remover; water soluble cleansers won't make the slightest dent! A nice extra is that this won't make your lashes feel dry and brittle.

☺ GOOD **Opulash Mascara Volume** *($15)* separates lashes well while producing good (but not prodigious) length. Surprisingly, thickness is minimal, and adding successive coats doesn't do much to change that. For lack of a better word, lashes are left looking fluffy and they have a soft curl. This mascara removes easily with a water-soluble cleanser and it did not exhibit any flaking or smearing throughout the day.

☺ GOOD **Plush Lash** *($15)* doesn't, despite its name, leave lashes feeling or looking all that plush. The oversized brush is difficult to work with, but with practice, the results can be evenly defined, long, and slightly curled lashes. Thickness doesn't come easily to this mascara, even with successive coats—though you can apply a lot of this without a hint of clumping.

☺ GOOD **Splashproof Lash Waterproof Mascara** *($15)* allows you to create lasting thickness and length with minimal effort, though it can clump slightly as it builds. This is also tenaciously waterproof, and a bit difficult to remove (have a silicone- or oil–based makeup remover handy). This mascara competes nicely with the top choices from drugstore lines Maybelline, L'Oreal, and Cover Girl, and is only a bit more expensive.

☺ GOOD $$$ **False Lashes Mascara Volume** *($19)* is supposed to replicate the dramatic look of false eyelashes, and it almost succeeds. The nimble brush features densely packed bristles that do a good job of adding thickness and impressive length, with only minor clumping that's easily smoothed out. Consider this a building mascara, which means you'll need several coats to come close to the effect you get with false eyelashes. The formula wears well throughout the day and comes off easily with a water-soluble cleanser.

☺ AVERAGE **Prep + Prime Lash** *($15)* is meant to smooth and condition lashes, but doesn't do much better in this regard than most mascaras—there is nothing in this product that is all that conditioning for lashes, though it does make them feel soft. It is also supposed to intensify "the build and lengthening quality of all [mascara] formulas," but that didn't happen. Side-by-side testing confirmed what is true of almost all lash primers: They tend to make mascara trickier to apply and don't help lengthen or thicken lashes any more than simply applying two or three coats of regular mascara. We suppose this is an OK option if you're using a lackluster mascara, but the bigger question is why you're not using a superior mascara, given how many there are! This does make a noticeable difference with average mascaras.

M.A.C. FACE & BODY ILLUMINATOR

☺ GOOD $$$ **Pigment** *($20)* comes in small jars of shiny loose powder, available in almost every color imaginable and with a shininess scale that goes from sheer to POW! Most of the colors cling surprisingly well and allow you to create an array of effects. The shades labeled Glitter cling terribly and flake everywhere. Although Pigments can be messy to use, they add some kick to evening or special-occasion makeup. The best colors include Naked, Dark Soul, Melon, Tan, Vanilla, and Chocolate Brown.

☺ GOOD $$$ **Lustre Drop** *($20)* is a simple way to add subtle radiance to your skin without making your moisturizer or foundation feel heavy or sticky. The silky, sheer texture of this water-based bronzer is more like a liquid shimmer highlighter than a true liquid bronzer. It's easy to blend with fingertips or a brush and, with the bottle's tiny dispenser tip, you don't have to worry about squeezing too much product at once. Both shades are flattering and would work well for light to dark skin tones. Sun Rush has a soft golden color and Pink Rebel a rosy tan.

M.A.C. BRUSHES

✓☺ BEST **M.A.C. Brushes** *($11–$71)*. M.A.C. has one of the best selections of brushes you'll find anywhere (over 40 different brushes). The big brushes are a little pricey, but they last forever if you take care of them. Though there are indeed good, inexpensive brushes to be found, if you're going to splurge, this is one area where the extra expense won't be wasted. Be sure to check out M.A.C.'s variety of eyeshadow brushes, particularly the **#275 Medium Angled Shading Brush** ($24.50), an excellent, versatile eyeshadow brush. Also, test the **#217 Blending Brush** ($22.50). Other top choices include the **#168 Large Angled Contour Brush** ($34), **#195 Concealer Brush** ($22.50), **#208 Small Angled Brow Brush** ($19.50), **#219 Pencil Brush** ($24.50), **#239 Eye Shading Brush** ($24.50), **#242 Shader Brush** ($24.50), **#249 Large Shader Brush** ($30), and all the various **Angled Shader Brushes** ($19.50–$32.00). Avoid the **#204 Lash Brush** ($11), which is easily duplicated by washing off an old mascara wand.

☹ AVERAGE **Brush Cleanser** *($13)* is an alcohol-based solution that does remove makeup and excess oil from brushes, but will eventually make natural hair dry and stiff. Although it's OK for occasional quick clean-ups, washing your brushes with a gentle shampoo and water is preferred.

M.A.C. SPECIALTY MAKEUP PRODUCTS

✓☺ BEST **Prep + Prime Lip** *($15)* is a base that is applied before lipstick to facilitate application and prevent it from feathering into lines around the mouth. Guess what? It works! The silicone- and wax-based stick forms a great barrier to keep color in place, in a way similar to long-discontinued products such as The Body Shop's No Wander and Coty's Stop It! As good as this product is, keep in mind that it won't prevent greasy, slippery lip glosses from migrating into lines around the mouth. It works best with moderately creamy or satin matte lipstick formulas, of which M.A.C. has plenty!

MAKE UP FOR EVER

Strengths: A couple of good cleansers and makeup removers; one good lip balm; the newer foundations have many wonderful qualities; impressive options (and shade ranges) for powders, powder blush, and powder eyeshadow; some extraordinary lip glosses and lipstick/lip color options (and again, the shade ranges are remarkable); a few formidable mascaras; good shimmer options; the huge selection of makeup brushes.

Weaknesses: Expensive; a few products suffer from needlessly irritating ingredients; average toner; the foundations and concealers that have been in this line longest are behind the times; mostly average eye and lip pencils; the Diamond Powder; mostly lackluster specialty products.

For more information and reviews of the latest Make Up For Ever products, visit CosmeticsCop.com.

MAKE UP FOR EVER CLEANSERS

☺ GOOD **$$$ Gentle Milk, Moisturizing Cleansing Milk** *($43 for 16.9 fl. oz.)* is an OK option for normal to slightly dry skin not prone to blemishes. The milky cleanser removes makeup easily and leaves minimal residue. It would be better without the volatile fragrant components, but their presence is minor.

☹ AVERAGE **$$$ So Divine, Moisturizing Cleansing Cream** *($27 for 4.4 fl. oz.)* is a cold cream–style cleanser for very dry skin, and requires a washcloth for complete removal. The tiny amount of plant extracts either have a soothing quality or impart subtle fragrance.

☹ POOR **Extreme Cleanser, Balancing Cleansing Dry Oil** *($30 for 6.76 fl. oz.)* is a lotion-textured creamy cleanser that contains a dry skin–compatible amount of oil, which also helps dissolve makeup. Despite this, it is not recommended for any skin type because it contains rosemary oil, pepper extract, and volatile fragrant components that can cause irritation.

MAKE UP FOR EVER EYE-MAKEUP REMOVER

☺ GOOD **$$$ Sens'Eyes, Waterproof Sensitive Eye Cleanser** *($23 for 3.38 fl. oz.)* works well to remove waterproof eye makeup, but isn't preferred for sensitive eyes over similar but less expensive options from Almay, Neutrogena, or Paula's Choice. This product is fragrance-free.

MAKE UP FOR EVER TONERS

☹ AVERAGE **$$$ Cool Lotion, Moisturizing Soothing Lotion** *($43 for 16.9 fl. oz.)* costs a lot for what amounts to an average toner that's primarily water, grape water, solvent, and slip agent. It's a mediocre option for normal to dry skin.

☹ AVERAGE **$$$ Mist & Fix** *($27 for 4.22 fl. oz.)* is supposed to be used not only to touch up makeup, but also to protect skin against external damage. This spray-on product consists primarily of water, slip agent (methylpropanediol, which absolutely won't refresh makeup), and film-forming agent, similar to what's used in hairsprays. This has a slightly sticky finish that can feel odd, but we suppose it does provide some protection from makeup fading and slipping. Overall, this is a gimmicky product that's a poor solution for those looking to reinforce or touch up makeup on-the-go. A good oil-blotting paper and quick dusting of pressed powder (and lipstick touch-up, of course) are much better.

MAKE UP FOR EVER MOISTURIZER

☹ AVERAGE **$$$ HD Elixir** *($38 for 0.4 fl. oz.)* is a lightweight moisturizer with a toner-like consistency. Its main ingredients are as ordinary and mundane as it gets: water, glycerin, slip agents, and a couple of emollient thickeners. Marketing this as a "breakthrough formula" is just silly; it's akin to suggesting a skateboard is a breakthrough vehicle. This contains a smattering of impressive ingredients, but the amounts are too small for your skin to notice. As for the hydration boost claim—"520% increase after 15 minutes"—it's just an over-hyped and trivial skin effect. For example, simply sitting in the bathtub for several minutes can boost skin's hydration (water content) that much and more, but that's not good for skin. Too much water can disrupt skin's barrier function, leading to a loss of the critical substances skin needs to stay intact and healthy. In the end, you don't want this product to work as claimed. Thankfully, it doesn't.

MAKE UP FOR EVER LIP CARE

☺ GOOD **$$$ Moisturizing Lip Balm** *($18)* is a colorless, emollient, glossy lip balm that works well to remedy and prevent dry, chapped lips. It does not contain any irritants and it does not feel too thick or waxy.

MAKE UP FOR EVER SPECIALTY SKIN-CARE PRODUCTS

☹ AVERAGE **$$$ Stop Shining +** *($16)* is a thick, nonaqueous, silicone gel with absorbent properties meant for use over oily areas. It doesn't hold up all day, nor is it as effective as similar products from Clinique, Paula's Choice, and Smashbox that combine silicones with absorbents, but it may be worth a try if your oily areas aren't too out of control.

MAKE UP FOR EVER FOUNDATIONS & PRIMERS

✓☺ BEST **$$$ Duo Mat Powder Foundation** *($32)* provides everything a pressed-powder foundation should, and excels in each area. The talc- and silicone-based formula feels buttery smooth and blends on like a second skin. The slightly dry, non-chalky matte finish is ideal for normal to very oily skin, and this provides light to medium coverage that doesn't mask skin, but does make it look refined and polished. The selection of shades is first-rate; the only questionable colors are the slightly orange 209 Warm Beige and the slightly peach 214 Dark Beige. Shades 216 Caramel and 218 Chocolate are beautiful for darker skin tones or used as matte bronzing powders. Shade 200 Beige Opalescent has a soft shine that will magnify oily areas. This powder foundation does contain fragrance.

✓☺ BEST **$$$ HD Invisible Cover Foundation** *($40)*. This water- and silicone-based liquid foundation is among the best of the best, assuming your preferences mesh with what it provides. The creamy, fluid texture has great slip, but not so much that blending is a problem. It sets to a natural matte finish that looks incredibly skin-like, while offering medium to almost full coverage. The pigment technology behind this makeup, like many of today's best foundations, allows it to blur imperfections and improve skin tone without feeling or looking like a mask. The selection of shades is staggering, and staggeringly good, too. The range offers options for fair to very dark skin tones, and the pump-bottle packaging is sleek and easy to use. As is often the case when a product has more than two dozen shades, not all of them are slam-dunks. The following shades are not recommended because they are too rose, pink, orange, or peach: 135 Vanilla, 145 Neutral, 150 Pink Beige, 160 Golden Beige, 170 Caramel, and 165 Honey Beige. The shades 177 Cognac, 178 Chestnut, and 180 Brown are beautiful dark tones; 125 Sand is slightly peach, but still worth considering; and 130 Warm Ivory is slightly pink, but may work for some light skin tones. Whether you choose this for day-to-day or on-camera use, its skin-perfecting qualities are exemplary. The formula makes it best for normal to very oily skin.

☺ GOOD **$$$ Face and Body Liquid Makeup** *($38)* is a liquidy, water-based foundation that also contains a blend of silicone and plant oil, so this has a good amount of slip on the skin, yet blends readily to a natural matte finish. Coverage can go from sheer to medium, and allows you to build coverage without it looking thick. The large shade range is deceiving because many shades look too peach, orange, or pink in the bottle, yet almost all of them end up being soft and neutral on the skin—plus there are equally good options for fair and dark skin tones with plenty of great shades in between this spectrum. Consider Natural Beige 3 and Honey 42 carefully, as both finish slightly peach. This can be used on the body if desired, but it isn't as tenacious or clingy as products like DermaBlend, so the results can be mixed. This lightweight formula works best for normal to slightly dry or slightly oily skin.

☺ GOOD $$$ **HD Microperfecting Primer** *($32 for 1.01 fl. oz.).* As a makeup primer this works fine, but the inclusion of color-correcting pigments (something almost all other primers don't include) is a twist worth ignoring. The biggest offenders in this group are the Green and Mauve shades, both of which are sheer, but add an odd tone to skin that doesn't mesh well with foundation. The Blue color is barely blue (which is good) and applies like an ethereal white. As such, it is an acceptable option for very fair skin tones with a pink cast that needs neutralizing. The Neutral shade adds a soft luminescence to skin, while Caramel and Yellow (which isn't pure yellow, rather more of a neutral putty color) also are workable options. The silky, lightweight texture of this primer helps smooth and enhance skin texture while adding a subtle shine that can boost dull or sallow complexions. The "nourishing" ingredients mentioned in the claims for this primer are present in such tiny amounts that your skin won't notice, so this isn't preferred to prepping your skin with a silky serum that contains beneficial ingredients. Still, this is worth a try if you need to brighten your complexion or tone down (in a subtle manner) an uneven skin tone. Be sure to test this in natural light before purchasing—something Sephora stores (where this product is exclusive) readily allow.

☺ GOOD $$$ **Mat Velvet + Mattifying Foundation** *($34)* has a thin fluid texture with enough slip to allow smooth blending before setting to a strong matte finish. Coverage goes from medium to almost full, and this foundation camouflages redness on skin quite well. The absorbent formula is ideal for oily to very oily skin, with the only caveat being the fact that this contains a small amount of fragrance ingredients known to cause irritation. The likelihood these ingredients will cause a problem is low, but this no longer earns our top rating because there are plenty of outstanding foundations that are fragrance-free, which is always the better way to go. Sixteen mostly impressive shades are available. The ones to avoid due to obvious peach or orange tones are Sand, Neutral Beige, and Golden Beige. Soft Beige and Honey Beige may be too peach for some skin tones, but are worth a look. Alabaster is a superb shade for very fair skin, while the Brown and Chocolate shades are gorgeous, non-ashy shades for ebony skin tones.

☺ GOOD $$$ **UV Prime SPF 50/PA +++** *($30)* straddles the line between a primer (which usually is silicone-based and nearly weightless) and a lightweight moisturizer with sunscreen. The sun protection is plentiful and powered by titanium dioxide for sufficient UVA protection. The silky texture and finish of this formula gets progressively matte as it sets; however, it doesn't make skin look flat or dull, although it does leave a soft white cast. You get what can only be described as a matte glow. This works great under makeup, especially for those with normal to oily skin. It would be rated a Best Product if the formula contained a more substantial amount or range of antioxidants and it was formulated without potentially irritating fragrance ingredients.

☹ AVERAGE $$$ **All Mat, Face Matifying Primer** *($45 for 1.01 fl. oz.)* creates a smooth matte finish thanks to its formula of silicone, slip agent, silicone polymers, and mineral-based absorbents. It is an option for normal to very oily skin looking to prolong a matte finish, but what a shame this pricey product lacks truly helpful ingredients for skin. If anything, the fragrance ingredients in this primer put skin at risk for irritation.

☺ AVERAGE **$$$ Liquid Lift Foundation** *($41)* is overpriced for what amounts to a very basic formula that absolutely cannot lift skin or impart a tightening effect. It has a fluid, silky texture and nice slip, which makes blending easy. Coverage is medium and it leaves a slightly dewy finish suitable for someone with normal to dry skin. Among the six shades (best for fair to medium skin), only Golden Beige 5 stands out as too peach.

MAKE UP FOR EVER CONCEALER

✓☺ BEST **$$$ Full Cover Concealer** *($30)*. Take the name for this concealer seriously, because Make Up For Ever certainly did! This fairly thick concealer softens on contact with skin and provides superior coverage for all manner of discolorations and flaws. It has minimal slip, so is best dotted on small areas and blended quickly. It sets to a long-wearing matte finish that resists creasing, but the texture and drier finish of the product is capable of exacerbating lines around the eye, which is true for concealers in general. Most of the shades are remarkable and there are options for fair to dark skin tones. Beige 8 and Dark Beige 12 are slightly peach, but still worth considering; avoid Fawn 14, which is decidedly orange. Ebony 20 is very dark and has a slightly ash finish, so consider it carefully if your skin tone is dark enough to warrant using this color. Full Cover Concealer is excellent to use over blemishes and to cover the pink to red marks that linger after a blemish has healed.

☺ GOOD **$$$ Lift Concealer** *($22)* begins liquidy, but dries quickly to a long-lasting, powdery matte finish. It provides good coverage that you can build to move up from light to medium coverage. This water-, talc-, and silicone-based formula comes in a tube and is best for oily skin or for use over oily areas. Five shades are available, with the best ones being Medium Beige 2, Neutral Beige 3, and Matte Beige 4. By the way, this won't lift skin in the least, so don't bank on that benefit.

☺ AVERAGE **$$$ 5-Camouflage Cream Palette** *($36)* comes in a palette with four flesh-toned colors along with a color corrector. You can blend the shades together to create a custom match, but unless you need significant coverage and are willing to put up with this product's difficult texture, this is easy to pass up. The waxes in this concealer are a poor choice for use over blemishes, but do lend an opacity that helps conceal red marks, dark circles, or flat scars. There are a handful of palettes, with No1 and No2 being the best, save for their color-correcting shades. The darkest palette is workable, but they're more work than you should have to put up with from a concealer!

☺ AVERAGE **$$$ Camouflage Cream** *($18)* is a range of cream concealers that are identical to those in Make Up For Ever's Camouflage Cream Palettes reviewed above. The shades to avoid include Yellow Green 16, Green 17, Mauve 18, Pink 19, and Orange 20.

☺ AVERAGE **$$$ HD Invisible Cover Concealer** *($28)* is housed in a pen-style applicator with an angled silicone rubber tip. You click the base of the component to dispense this slightly thick liquid. It has minimal slip and is concentrated, so just a dot provides moderate to full coverage that doesn't crease. Definitely a matte-finish concealer, this suffers in comparison with the line's Full Cover Concealer because it has a tendency to look too opaque and chalky. Softening this effect isn't all that easy, and doing so lessens its impressive coverage. If you decide to test this, the shade range is unusually extensive. That said, there are some colors to avoid. The following shades are too pink or peach: 320 Pink Beige and 350 Apricot Beige. Shade 370 Ebony is great for dark skin tones.

☹ POOR **Concealer Pencil** *($18)*. Concealer Pencil is a dual-sided pencil that comes in two different skin tones, one for lighter skin and one for medium skin. It's greasy, looks heavy, and is unsuitable for use over blemishes.

MAKE UP FOR EVER POWDERS

✓☺ BEST **$$$ Super Matte Loose Powder** *($24)* has a super-fine, ultra-light texture and a soft, dry finish that's ideal for oily skin. This talc- and silica-based loose powder looks beautiful on skin, and each shade is great.

✓☺ BEST **$$$ Multi Loose Powder** *($34)* is identical to Make Up For Ever's Super Matte Loose Powder above except with the Multi option you get four shades of loose powder stacked together (each shade comes in its own clear plastic jar). Watch out for the 02 Corrective shade set, as these are very pale and can make skin look ghostly unless applied very sheer. Of course, ultimately most women won't need four shades of loose powder for daily use. However, these can come in handy for makeup artists and the stackable colors travel well.

☺ GOOD **$$$ Velvet Finish Compact Powder** *($29)* has a talc- and kaolin (clay)-based texture that feels slightly thick and dry, but it applies smoothly, leaving a velvety matte finish. Failing to blend carefully or brushing on too much of this powder results in a chalky appearance, so use restraint. Each of the eight shades applies lighter than they appear in the compact, but all of them are very good. Caramel and Chocolate are great for dark skin tones or for use as bronzing powder on medium to tan skin tones.

☹ AVERAGE **$$$ HD High Definition Powder Microfinish Powder** *($30)*. The sole ingredient in this one-shade-fits-all loose powder is silica. This dry-finish mineral is engineered to have a very unusual texture, which it does. A simple touch and you'll know that it is truly unusual. It has a strange sensation of movement and feels unbelievably and immeasurably silky. Although touching it may feel good, wearing it is an entirely different issue and one you won't find as interesting. Although this is designed to be "universally flattering," it won't flatter anyone. The silica will exaggerate even the slightest amount of dry skin, while the whiteness of this powder can make even fair skin tones look artificially pale. Moreover, this is simply too sheer to completely even-out all skin tones as claimed. High definition may be akin to high-tech, but this powder doesn't give you a visage that will have you ready for an extreme close-up. If anything, even when applied sheer, this can leave skin looking artificially pale and somehow also manages to make your foundation look uneven.

MAKE UP FOR EVER BLUSHES & BRONZER

✓☺ BEST **$$$ HD Microfinish Blush** *($25)* is, in a word, fantastic. More of a lightweight lotion than a liquid, this has a silky texture and concentrated formula that imparts soft color only if you're really careful to apply sparingly. Initially we were dismayed by the tiny amount of product, but believe us, a little goes a very long way! A couple of dots of this and you'll find cheeks are sufficiently blushed with an amazingly skin-like soft matte finish, complete with just a hint of glow, which keeps this blush from looking flat. This melds with skin and doesn't magnify imperfections, which is brilliant. The shades range from soft pastels to vivid brights, which look gorgeous on darker skin tones. If you're bored with powder blush or in the mood to explore a novel approach to blush, you simply have to check this out!

☺ GOOD **$$$ Mat Bronze** *($30)* is a good talc-based bronzing powder whose smooth texture prompts a noticeable color payoff and even application. All the shades are matte, which is a real find in this age of shimmering bronzing powders. We wish the shade range was more bronze-like. As is, the best shade is Earth 6. Dark Bronze 4 is good, too, but for some reason tends to grab on skin more than the other colors. Light Bronze 0 and Medium Bronze 2 are too fleshy or peachy to approximate a tan.

☺ GOOD **$$$ Powder Blush** *($24)* comes in a bountiful array of shades, from the pinkest pinks to the most understated neutrals. These are strongly pigmented shades, and without careful, sheer application they tend to grab on the skin, which is a side effect of this blush's drier texture. Use restraint and you likely will be pleased with the results and the long wear. Several shiny shades are also available, and the good news is the shine clings well and applies evenly.

☺ GOOD **$$$ Sculpting Blush** *($24)* doesn't allow you to "sculpt" your face because blush doesn't really do that. Sculpting is best done with a combination of tan to brown and cream (light) colors because the goal is creating shape and definition via highlights and shadows. Such an effect cannot be achieved with pink, rose, and peach blush colors, and that's mostly what you're getting here. Despite the odd name, this pressed-powder blush comes in a sleek, slim compact. Its texture is smooth and on the dry side, but it applies evenly and provides fairly strong color. For best results, apply sparingly with a good blush brush and build as needed. Women with darker skin tones will appreciate the pigmentation this blush has! Almost all the shades fall into the pastel range, and most have a hint of shine, but it's soft and flattering rather than glittery—and it doesn't flake. All told, a well-done though pricey powder blush that's suitable for all skin types.

MAKE UP FOR EVER EYESHADOWS

☺ GOOD **$$$ Aqua Cream Waterproof Cream Color** *($22)* is a long-wear, highly pigmented cream that can be used as an eyeshadow, blush, or lip color. In each of those functions, Aqua Cream sets to a matte finish and is resistant to water, moisture, and perspiration (so much so, you'll likely need an oil- or silicone-based makeup remover to take it off). True to claims, you won't have to worry about smudging or creasing, but no matter where you apply it, it's important to instantly blend the product because it sets quickly once applied. The shade range is a bit on the wild theatrical side with a mixture of neutral and bright tones, but out of the 22 colors, there are some beautiful options to consider in a variety of intensities and finishes (shimmer, matte, and metallic). Although you can use Aqua Cream on the eyes, lips, or cheeks, we found it most ideal as a cream eyeshadow because it is resistant to creasing and smudging and it won't flake. There are some over-the-top shades you might want to avoid, such as Intense Blue, but others such as the shimmer-finish Pink Beige and Taupe are quite stunning. This product works OK as a stay-put cheek color, but avoid the extremely bright colors such as Fuchsia and Orange, which not only look unnatural, but also have a tendency to seep into pores, bringing more attention to them. In terms of using this as a lip product, the texture is a bit more mattifying than what's comfortable for use on the lips, making them look overly dry or cakey.

☺ GOOD **$$$ Eyeshadow** *($19)* has a texture, application, and intensity that is nearly identical to that of the Powder Blush reviewed above. The range of shades is staggering (though most Sephora boutiques only stock a fraction of them), with some of the most imaginative (and largely unnecessary) shades right next to the earth and neutral tones that are universally flattering. These apply evenly, and most of the shades provide opaque coverage, which lets them last without creasing or fading.

☺ GOOD **$$$ Matte Eye Shadow** *($19)* has a dry but reasonably smooth texture that applies somewhat unevenly due to each shade's strong pigmentation. The best approach is to apply in sheer layers with a brush until the desired effect is achieved. The shade range is quite broad and includes many bold colors that work better for shock value than shaping and shading the eyes. Still, if you're looking for bright blue, green, fuchsia, and red powder eyeshadows, you'll find them here! We urge you to stick with the numerous flesh-toned and neutral to brown shades that round out this collection. Examples include Beige, Cafe Latte, Cinnamon, Beige Brown, Chocolate, Coffee, True Brown, Fawn, Earth, and Grey Beige.

☺ AVERAGE **$$$ Diamond Shadow** *($20)* is positioned as a long-wearing iridescent eyeshadow, but the large particles of holographic glitter don't cling well—you'll notice them on cheeks and clothing shortly after application. Although these shadows have a dry, almost grainy texture, they blend smoothly, which is a positive. The shade range presents mostly unworkable options unless you want strong, contrasting colors to make more of a statement than your eyes do.

☺ AVERAGE **$$$ Pearly Waterproof Eyeshadow Pencil** *($18)* is a standard chubby pencil with a creamy texture that glides over the skin and imparts sheer, shimmering color. This pencil is not preferred to the Eyeshadow, but some will undoubtedly find it intriguing, and the formula is waterproof.

MAKE UP FOR EVER EYE & BROW LINERS

☺ GOOD **$$$ Aqua Creamliner** *($20)* is similar to the many long-wearing gel eyeliners being sold at department stores. Make Up For Ever's point of difference is a creamier formula that contains some oil, so don't expect this to last as long as the competition. Still, application is swift and pigmented and it sets quickly and won't budge, at least not for several hours. Those with oily eyelids may find this breaks down before they'd like; others without that problem may want to give this an audition.

☺ GOOD **$$$ Cake Eyeliner** *($16)* is a very standard cake eyeliner that must be used with damp brush. Available in two classic shade (black or brown), this is an old-fashioned yet still effective method for lining your eyes. Eyeliner Cake lasts longer than most eye pencils, but cannot outlast a silicone-based gel eyeliner.

☺ GOOD **$$$ Color Liner** *($19)* is a good liquid eyeliner that features a soft but firm-textured brush and a formula that applies easily and dries quickly. All the colors have a strong iridescent finish, making them best for evening makeup on unwrinkled eyelids. Best of all, once dry, the formula holds up remarkably well.

☺ AVERAGE **$$$ Aqua Eyes Waterproof Eyeliner Pencil** *($18)* needs sharpening and has an unusual base of cottonseed and jojoba oils, neither of which are as waterproof as silicone-based pencils, though it does hold up to minimal water exposure (think crying versus swimming). Although the application is creamy, this sets to a tacky finish that stays put. All the shades are laced with shine, so choose carefully.

☺ AVERAGE **$$$ Aqua Liner** *($23)* has an ultra-thin brush that applies the slow-drying liquid liner well. It is reasonably waterproof once set, but has a tendency to fade, making it an average choice and not really worth its price.

☺ AVERAGE **$$$ Eyebrow Pencil** *($18)* has to be sharpened, which is a pain, but it applies very smooth and has a lightweight, non-waxy texture and a soft powder finish that won't smear or smudge. All the colors are workable (and matte), making this an easy recommendation if you don't mind sharpening.

☹ POOR **Kohl Eye Pencil** *($17)* is a substandard pencil that applies too thick, flakes a bit, and is very prone to smearing. Avoid it unless you like eye makeup that demands constant upkeep!

MAKE UP FOR EVER LIP COLOR & LIPLINERS

✓☺ BEST **$$$ Liquid Lip Color** *($20)* remains a favorite. The ultra-smooth texture imparts intense, opaque color and a completely non-sticky, high-gloss finish. This lipstick/gloss hybrid comes in a tube with a brush applicator, and the opening of the tube is large enough to prevent the brush from splaying—a major plus. Consider this a must-try if you like the opacity of lipstick with the finish of a lip gloss.

✓☺ BEST **$$$ Rouge Artist Intense** *($19)* is a lipstick lover's dream in terms of selection, but before you dive in to the 50 shades offered, you'll want to arm yourself with this vital info: The lipstick is offered in four finishes: **Matte**, **Cream**, **Pearl**, and **Satin**. We're sad to report that the Matte is terrible with a capital "T." This is the type of matte lipstick that causes women to never want to try another matte formula again. It's dry, difficult to apply evenly, and stubborn when it comes time to remove it because, basically, it stains your lips. The Cream and Satin formulas fare much better. Each has a classic creamy texture that's slightly on the dry side, but they still have good movement during application. Once on, you'll enjoy full coverage and lasting color with a cream finish. The Pearl formula is nearly identical to that of the Cream, but each Pearl shade has a glittering shine rather than a glossy or dimensional finish. The big deal with all these finishes is the intense pigmentation—and the colors really do have impressive staying power. The shade selection runs the gamut and offers several winners, especially for pinks, reds, and all manner of coral. The Best Product rating applies to the Cream and Pearl finishes only; we do not recommend the Matte formula.

✓☺ BEST **$$$ Super Lip Gloss** *($16)* is one of the smoothest, least sticky glosses you're likely to find. It comes in a tube and is silicone-based, so it can feel slippery (and can encourage lipstick feathering if you're prone to that), but women who have a problem with bleeding lipstick should stay away from glosses in the first place. The available shades are beautiful and include some unconventional (but sheer) options.

☺ GOOD **$$$ Lab Shine Lip Gloss** *($18)*. This fragranced lip gloss with a brush applicator is offered in three different finishes (though all are glossy): **Diamond** has a sparkling shine and the colors tend to be quite sheer; **Star** provides a pearlized, less sparkling finish and the shades have more depth; and **Metal** has a metallic, chrome-like sheen and its shades have heavier coverage, almost approaching a standard lipstick. Regardless of which finish and level of coverage you prefer, each Lab Shine gloss has a thick, slightly syrupy texture with a slight sticky finish that's tolerable. The look is high gloss and, as usual with Make Up For Ever, the shades are excellent, whether you want soft or bold color. Although this is a very good gloss, its slight stickiness and lingering fragrance prevent it from earning our top rating.

☺ GOOD **$$$ Rouge Artist Natural** *($19)* isn't quite as nice as the Rouge Artist Intense lipstick above, but is a worthy choice if you prefer a creamy lipstick that's not too slippery and leaves a cream-gloss finish from colors that announce their presence without being opaque. Because the creamy texture veers toward being a bit greasy, this isn't a lipstick for those with lines around the mouth. It applies easily and feels great, not to mention the shades are plentiful and should have wide appeal. Each color, even the dark ones, has minimal stain, one more reason this isn't rated as high as Rouge Artist Intense.

☹ AVERAGE **$$$ Aqua Lip Waterproof Lipliner Pencil** *($18)* is a standard, needs-sharpening lip pencil that glides on swiftly for quick application, but remains creamy until it has set (which takes a few minutes); after it sets it feels a bit tacky. This is waterproof, yet comes off easily with a water- and detergent-based makeup remover. The shade range is quite good, with no oddities and plenty of pink-brown and red tones.

☹ AVERAGE **$$$ Matte Lip** *($20)* is designed to be used over lipstick to minimize a glossy or creamy finish. It's somewhat odd given that you can achieve this finish by simply choosing a demi-matte or regular matte lipstick. Dabbing this colorless, cornstarch-based cream over lipstick can be a messy task, but it does mattify and is an option if applied very carefully.

☹ POOR **Glossy Full Couleur** *($19)* adds a striking vinyl sheen to lips when applied over any lipstick. Essentially a colorless lip gloss, this product loses points for its undeniable mint flavor and for containing fragrant components that can be irritating to lips. The amount of peptide won't plump lips even a little.

MAKE UP FOR EVER MASCARA

✓☺ BEST **$$$ Lengthening Waterproof Mascara** *($23)* has been improved and is an excellent lengthening mascara that is indeed waterproof. The tiny, tailored brush allows easy access to every lash, extending them beautifully, but building little in the way of thickness. Clumps are absent though, so if length and waterproofing are what you're after, this works beautifully.

☺ GOOD **$$$ Lash Fibers Volume and Length Lash Primer** *($20)* is essentially a mascara without pigment. The well-designed, slightly curved brush makes it easy to reach every lash, so you can add bulk and some thickness to your lashes before applying mascara. Although this makes a nice difference (lashes are noticeably longer with enhanced volume), you can achieve the same results from a great mascara alone. However, those who don't ordinarily use a mascara that lengthens and thickens to a dramatic degree may want to use a primer like this for times when more lash impact is desired. This primer leaves lashes soft and doesn't cause mascara to clump or skip when it's applied immediately afterward.

☻ AVERAGE **$$$ Smoky Lash Extra Black Mascara** *($22)*. This very black mascara makes eyes noticeably more dramatic, especially if you have fair to light skin and light-colored eyes. It goes on a bit heavy, but builds considerable length and separates lashes well. Unless you wipe down the wand before applying, you will notice some slight flaking, which is not great news for any mascara, especially one in this price range. However, the flaking doesn't occur throughout the day, so if you're craving very dark, long lashes, this may be worth auditioning.

☹ POOR **Aqua Smoky Lash Waterproof Extra Black Mascara** *($22)* definitely makes lashes dramatically dark, but its messy, uneven application smears from the beginning and doesn't let up. Within moments we noticed flaking and by midday the entire upper lash line was splotched with smeary mascara. All this for average length and a formula that is moderately waterproof. Even though much of it comes off before you want it to, removing the rest of it is no easy feat—the ultimate irony for one of the worst waterproof mascaras in recent memory.

MAKE UP FOR EVER FACE & BODY ILLUMINATORS

☺ GOOD **$$$ Compact Shine On** *($29)* is a smooth-textured, talc-based pressed powder with a shine that has elements of subtle glow (finely milled shimmer pigments) and visible sparkles (which, while visible, aren't gaudy). The shine clings better than you'd expect, and all three shades are soft, sheer options for highlighting areas of the face or body.

☺ GOOD **$$$ Diamond Cream** *($36)* presents shimmer in lotion form and it's another concentrated product, so apply sparingly until you get the desired effect. It does have a slightly tacky finish, but the shine doesn't flake. It actually works best mixed with a standard body lotion for a soft glow.

☺ GOOD **$$$ Shine-On Powder** *($26)* has an honest name, as most powders with shine also claim to keep skin matte while concurrently adding sparkles to the skin. This talc-based loose powder has a pleasant texture and its finely milled shiny shades work well for a low-key evening look.

☺ GOOD **$$$ Uplight Face Luminizer Gel** *($29)* is packaged in a bottle with a pump applicator, so you need to be careful about how much you dispense so as not to waste product.

Only a small amount of this lightweight cream is needed to highlight skin. Three different finishes are available from the selection of eight shades; those with a dewy or pearlized finish are best. The sparkling shades are more suitable for evening makeup unless you want glitter on your face during the day. All the colors go on softly and offer attractive options for highlighting, whether you want soft ivory, pink, gold, and peach. This product contains fragrance and is suitable for all skin types except sensitive. It works well whether applied over or under foundation.

☹ POOR **Diamond Powder** *($24)* offers truly diamond-like shine in the form of another messy loose powder. Unfortunately, although the effect is very cool, the powder flakes endlessly and feels slightly grainy.

MAKE UP FOR EVER BRUSHES

✔☺ BEST **Make Up For Ever Brushes** *($13-$54)*. You will find that Make Up For Ever's Brushes have something to offer everyone, whether you're a makeup brush neophyte or connoisseur. The brushes include both natural and synthetic hair options, and the majority are expertly shaped and sized appropriately for their intended purpose. There are some superfluous ones to consider carefully, but that chiefly depends on what your needs are. All in all, the choices are plentiful and the prices are comparatively reasonable. The only unfortunate element is that most Sephora stores sell only a small portion of this company's brushes. To view the entire collection, you need to find a Make Up For Ever counter in a department store or visit their flagship store in New York.

MAKE UP FOR EVER SPECIALTY MAKEUP PRODUCTS

☺ GOOD **$$$ Sculpting Kit** *($45)*. Housed in one slim compact are two shades of silky, fragrance-free pressed powder: a light shade for highlighting and a dark shade for contouring and creating depth/shadows. Used with the appropriate angled contour brush (Make Up For Ever sells these, as do M.A.C. and Sephora), the two powders work beautifully to sculpt your face and define your features. The process of contouring is an art and requires practice to look right (and be convincing). It may not be something you do daily, but for special occasion makeup it can make a big difference (especially if you're going to be photographed). Almost without exception the covers of fashion magazines show models and actresses whose features have been softly contoured and highlighted to a flattering degree. You can do this, too, but again, it takes practice. The shade options in Sculpting Kit are a mixed bag; the darker shade in 02 Neutral Light is too warm (orange-ish) for light skin tones, while 01 Light Pink isn't pink at all and is actually soft and neutral (a much better choice for fair to light skin tones). Shade 04 Dark is great for tan skin tones while 03 Gold is the trickiest to work with unless you blend the two shades together and use them for bronzing powder rather than for contouring and highlighting. Regardless of which set you choose, these go on smoothly and impart soft color that's easy to build—and the color lasts. This is worth seeking out if you don't mind the expense and want to try your hand at contouring/highlighting.

☺ GOOD **$$$ Waterproof Eyebrow Corrector** *($19)* is a creamy liquid eyebrow tint packaged in a squeeze tube. The idea is to dispense a small amount on your brow brush and then fill in and shade the brows. It's an intriguing way to experiment with brow color and, with practice, you can create defined brows that look natural. All the shades are workable and best for dark blonde to dark brown brows. If you need your brow color to be waterproof, this fits the bill, and once set, it doesn't smudge or smear.

☺ AVERAGE **$$$ Eye Seal** *($21).* This liquid is meant to turn any powder-based eye makeup into a waterproof formula. The alcohol-free formula contains quick-drying solvents and film-forming agents that are water-resistant, but application is an issue. For example, when you use a brush to apply Eye Seal over, say, a powder eyeshadow, the fluid removes the makeup. We couldn't figure out a way around this, but the Sephora salesperson had a solution: Apply the powder product to your hand, then add a drop of Eye Seal and mix it together with the brush. That worked better, but it's messy and the results can still be uneven. In short, the formula contains ingredients typically seen in eye-makeup removers, although it's intended to enhance the longevity of makeup. I'd advise you to leave this on the shelf and use almost any other way to line your eyes.

☹ POOR **Glitter** *($13).* Glitter is glitter, and in this case, just like in kindergarten art class, these tiny pots spread sparkles anywhere you want them to go as well as places where you don't want them. The problem is with the product's extremely poor cling factor. It gets everywhere without staying where you originally placed it.

MARY KAY

Strengths: Most products are fragrance-free; some noteworthy cleansers and sunscreens; every sunscreen offers sufficient UVA protection; packaging that keeps light- and air-sensitive ingredients stable during use; very good eye-makeup remover and topical disinfectant with benzoyl peroxide; two good foundations.

Weaknesses: The overall collection is a mixed bag of exciting and disappointing products; several outdated moisturizers and greasy cleansers; no AHA or acceptable BHA products; unexceptional topical scrub; irritating lip balms; the Medium Coverage Foundation, the Waterproof Mascara, and the Eye Primer aren't necessary.

For more information and reviews of the latest Mary Kay products, visit CosmeticsCop.com.

MARY KAY CLEANSERS

✓☺ BEST **Deep Cleanser Formula 3** *($12 for 6.5 fl. oz.)* is a very good water-soluble cleansing lotion for normal to slightly oily skin. It rinses cleanly, removes makeup, and does not contain fragrance.

☺ GOOD **$$$ Facial Cleansing Cloths** *($15 for 30 cloths)* are a convenient way to refresh your face on the go. The mild formula is fragrance-free and it contains soothing plant extracts that don't pose even a slight risk of irritation; that is, unless you're allergic to them. The cloths don't work well to remove most types of makeup, including waterproof mascara, but they're great for freshening up post-workout or while traveling.

☺ AVERAGE **$$$ Botanical Effects Cleanse 1** *($14 for 4 fl. oz.).* Given the plant-sourced ingredients are few and far between, the only thing really botanical about this product is its name. While the claims aren't over the top, labeling this hypoallergenic and antioxidant-rich is a bit like calling a typewriter a good way to quickly communicate. The preservative base alone puts that claim in question, as does the milk thistle. Even though it can have antioxidant properties, milk thistle can also cause an allergic or sensitizing reaction for those prone to hay fever (Source: naturaldatabase.com). At least in a cleanser these wouldn't be left on the skin for very long, but why are they in here at all? Given the size of this cleanser, it veers toward being overpriced for what you get which is simply an emollient, cold cream–style cleanser with a blend of mostly water, Vaseline, and emollients. That's not bad for skin, just greasy, requiring a lot of wiping and pulling to get it off. If you have very dry skin this would work just fine, but think twice about spending this kind of money for what ends up being just an ordinary cleanser with a couple of questionable aspects of the formulation that aren't the best for sensitive skin.

☺ AVERAGE $$$ **Botanical Effects Cleanse 2** *($14 for 4 fl. oz.)* is a rather simplistic though emollient plant oil–based cleanser would be appropriate for someone with normal to dry skin. It doesn't rinse all that easily and would be better if used with a soft washcloth to be sure it was removed completely. It claims to be suitable for sensitive skin, but the ingredient list doesn't quite support that notion. It does contain a *Momordica grosvenorii* fruit extract that has some research showing it has benefit when taken orally to treat diabetes, but that has little relationship to skin. It also contains two fragrant plant extracts, including *Plumeria alba* and the giant water lily. Both of these can be potentially irritating when they come in contact with skin; however, in a cleanser everything is removed from skin, so the irritation from those plants is less of an issue, though ideally they shouldn't be in here at all. Overall, this isn't a bad cleanser but definitely questionable for sensitive skin. For the money there are better options out there.

☺ AVERAGE $$$ **TimeWise 3-in-1 Cleanser, for Normal to Dry Skin** *($18 for 4.5 fl. oz.)* is a very standard and somewhat greasy cleansing lotion for dry to very dry skin. The mineral oil, Vaseline, and clay make this difficult to remove with a washcloth, and this should be avoided if you have dry skin with blemishes.

☹ POOR **Botanical Effects Cleanse 3** *($14 for 4 fl. oz.)*. The only thing botanical about this cleanser is its name, as it contains far more synthetic ingredients than plants. That's not necessarily bad for skin, but it does speak to this product's misleading claims as there is nothing purifying or hypoallergenic about it. See the Appendix to learn why the hypoallergenic claim cannot be relied on. The first ingredient after water is TEA-lauryl sulfate, a cleansing agent known for its irritating properties. The other detergent cleansing agents are gentle enough, but they should have come first in this formula to truly be appropriate for sensitive skin as claimed. The small amount of plant extracts in here include *Kunzea ericoides*, an Australian plant that has some antibacterial properties, but in a cleanser they would just be rinsed down the drain so the benefit for blemishes is minimal (and this doesn't have the research behind it that antibacterial agents like triclosan do). This also contains milk thistle, which is can be a good antioxidant, but is also problematic for those with hay fever. However, in a cleanser it poses less of a problem than if it was left on the skin. *Psidium guajava* is another plant extract included which has a tiny amount of research showing it can be an antioxidant, which is nice but useless in a cleanser that is rinsed down the drain.

☹ POOR **TimeWise 3-in-1 Cleansing Bar** *($18 for a 5 ounce bar)* is a standard, drying bar soap that does not contain a single ingredient capable of exfoliating skin as claimed. On that same note, this soap cannot "reduce the visible signs of aging." What a ridiculous claim for a product that's basically a bar of Dove Soap!

☹ POOR **TimeWise 3-In-1 Cleanser, for Combination to Oily Skin** *($18 for 4.5 fl. oz.)* lists the drying detergent cleansing agent TEA-lauryl sulfate as the second ingredient and also contains a couple of irritating plant extracts, making this expensive cleanser a poor choice for anyone.

MARY KAY EYE-MAKEUP REMOVER

✓☺ BEST **Oil-Free Eye Makeup Remover** *($15 for 3.75 fl. oz.)* works quickly and beautifully to remove all types of makeup. The silicone-enhanced, fragrance-free formula may be used before or after cleansing and must be shaken well before each use.

MARY KAY TONERS

☺ GOOD **Botanical Effects Freshen 1** *($14 for 5 fl. oz.)*. In some ways this is one of those rare products in the world of skin care: A very good toner that actually has some helpful ingredients for skin. Although it's not loaded with beneficial ingredients and isn't all natural, the formula has possibilities for someone with normal to dry skin. The possible misstep is the milk thistle extract this contains. Although it does have antioxidant properties, it can also cause allergic or sensitizing reactions for those with hay fever (Source: naturaldatabase.com). That isn't the best for someone with sensitive skin, but in the category of toners this is definitely one of the better ones out there.

☺ AVERAGE **Botanical Effects Freshen 3** *($14 for 5 fl. oz.)*. This very simple toner formula uses several synthetic, fluid ingredients to suspend a few plant extracts that are supposed to help oily, blemish-prone skin, yet the results you're hoping for aren't likely to happen. The small amount of plant extracts in here include *Kunzea ericoides*, an Australian plant that has some antibacterial properties, but it has never been studied to determine if (or how) it effects breakouts. This also contains milk thistle, which can be a good antioxidant, but is also problematic as a sensitizer for those with hay fever (Source: naturaldatabase.com). *Psidium guajava* is another plant extract included that has a tiny amount of research showing it can be an antioxidant. That's nice, but the amount this toner contains is too small to be of much consequence for your skin. At best, this is an OK option for normal to oily or combination skin.

☹ POOR **Blemish Control Toner Formula 3** *($13 for 6.5 fl. oz.)* won't control blemishes, but will instead cause irritation and redness due to the alcohol, eucalyptus oil, and menthol it contains. See the Appendix to learn why irritation is so bad for oily, blemish-prone skin.

☹ POOR **Botanical Effects Freshen 2** *($14 for 5 fl. oz.)* is a simplistic toner that could have been so much more than what it is. The few plant extracts are placed around several synthetic ingredients, so the main botanical aspect of this toner is really just its name. It could have been a decent formula appropriate for normal to slightly dry or slightly oily skin, but three of the plant extracts have potential for irritation: Giant water lily extract, the *Momordica grosvenorii* extract, and the milk thistle extract (the latter is particularly a problem for those with hay fever though it is a very good antioxidant).

MARY KAY SCRUBS

☺ AVERAGE **$$$ TimeWise Microdermabrasion Set** *($55)* is Mary Kay's contribution to at-home microdermabrasion kits. This two-part product features a topical scrub and post-treatment moisturizer. **Step 1: Refine** ($30 for 2 ounces; may be purchased separately) contains alumina crystals as the abrasive agent, and yes, this is the same ingredient used in professionally administered microdermabrasion treatments. But there's a difference between massaging a scrub on your skin and how the microdermabrasion machine works (and the way it's operated). Further, recent research has shown that microdermabrasion doesn't appear to have a cumulative benefit. Either way, products like this (when used gently) are indeed viable topical scrubs. What we like is that Mary Kay's version is free of added irritants and that it rinses easily (many microdermabrasion scrubs are difficult to remove with water). **Step 2: Replenish** ($25 for 1 oz.; may be purchased separately) is to be applied after Step 1-Refine, though we can think of many other serum-type moisturizers that have formulas superior to this, including those from

The Reviews M

Aveda, Clinique, Estee Lauder, Olay, and Paula's Choice. Rather than create a product brimming with antioxidants, anti-irritants, and cell-communicating ingredients, Mary Kay created a functional but ordinary product that is just an OK option for normal to slightly oily skin. It's being marketed for dry or oily skin, but if you have dry skin, Replenish will leave your skin wanting more, and for oily skin it may prove too emollient. It has some good antioxidants and the packaging will keep them stable, but the amounts are likely too small to bring much benefit to your skin. Overall, there is nothing about the scrub in this kit that can't be replaced by a washcloth, and there are better moisturizers than this.

MARY KAY MOISTURIZERS (DAYTIME & NIGHTTIME), EYE CREAMS, & SERUMS

✓☺ BEST $$$ **Timewise Night Restore & Recover Complex-Combination/Oily** *($40 for 1.7 fl. oz.)* is a very good, lightweight, fragrance-free moisturizer that is best for normal to slightly dry or slightly oily skin. Those with oily skin will likely find this feels too heavy, despite its lotion-like texture. The formula does not contain anything special or unique to skin's needs at night. The notion that skin need special ingredients at certain times of the day really only applies to sun protection during daylight hours; otherwise, skin needs the same types of ingredients (such as antioxidants and repairing substances) every second of the day, not only at night. This moisturizer contains a nice mix of antioxidants, cell-communicating ingredients, and skin-identical substances that work to repair skin's surface and help prevent moisture loss. When skin is fortified with these ingredients and protected from daily sun damage, it will do what it loves to do when in top shape: generate healthy collagen. So although Mary Kay's collagen-building claim is accurate, this is far from the only moisturizer to offer that benefit. Ultimately, the one reason to think twice about this is the price. While it's not outrageous, you can find less expensive moisturizers that provide your skin with an equally good mix of beneficial ingredients.

✓☺ BEST $$$ **Timewise Night Restore & Recover Complex-Normal/Dry** *($40 for 1.7 fl. oz.)* is a more emollient version of the Timewise Night Restore & Recover Complex-Combination/Oily above, and the same review applies.

✓☺ BEST $$$ **TimeWise Targeted-Action Line Reducer** *($40 for 0.13 fl. oz.)* deserves a Best Product rating for its elegant formula laced with several antioxidants, soothing agent, and a cell-communicating ingredient. The antiwrinkle claims for this product are far-fetched because this click pen–dispensed product works poorly and doesn't really act like spackle, especially if you smile. This will not fill in deep, etched lines like those that occur along the naso-labial folds. Wrinkles aside, the formula as a whole is very good for normal to dry skin, whether around the eyes or on other areas that need temporary smoothing. And thank you, Mary Kay, for not implying in the least that this product is better than Botox or dermal injections!

☺ GOOD **Botanical Effects Hydrate 1** *($16 for 3 fl. oz.)* is a good, basic moisturizer for dry skin. It claims to contain an antioxidant-rich botanical complex, but the ingredient list doesn't reflect that statement. The blend of emollients, plant oil, and Vaseline is definitely something dry skin will appreciate and the small amount of plant based anti-irritants and vitamin E is nice, just not exciting. Given the price, someone on a budget with dry skin won't be disappointed. One potential problem to keep in mind is that this contains milk thistle, which can be a good antioxidant, but can also be sensitizing for someone with hay fever (Source: naturaldatabase.com).

☺ GOOD **TimeWise Day Solution Sunscreen Broad Spectrum SPF 35** *($30 for 1 fl. oz.)* is an in-part zinc oxide sunscreen that provides sufficient UVA protection, while the fluid, lightweight formula contains a decent selection of antioxidants, skin-identical ingredients, and hydrating ingredients for normal to slightly dry skin. This also has a silky finish that wears beautifully under makeup. On balance, there are better daytime moisturizers with sunscreen, but this certainly isn't a bad option to consider if you're a fan of Mary Kay products.

☺ GOOD **$$$ TimeWise Firming Eye Cream** *($30 for 0.5 fl. oz.)* is a very emollient, Vaseline-based moisturizer for dry to very dry skin anywhere on the face. Lots of thickening agents combine with smaller amounts of peptides and a few antioxidants to round out the skin-beneficial traits of this product (but, regrettably, it won't firm skin). Despite the positives, the truth is you don't need an eye cream (see the Appendix to find out why).

☺ AVERAGE **Botanical Effects Hydrate 2** *($16 for 3 fl. oz.)* is a basic, lightweight moisturizer for normal to slightly dry or combination skin. It contains some helpful ingredients to improve dry skin, but lacks state-of-the-art ingredients all skin types need to look and act younger. The botanical name and claims don't jibe with a formula that contains a good deal of synthetic ingredients, but as with many skin-care products, sometimes a blend of synthetic and natural ingredients works best. Where this goes astray is with some of the fragrant plant extracts, as these can be sensitizing. The milk thistle this contains could have some interesting antioxidant properties, but it can also be a potent allergen or sensitizer for those prone to hay fever (Source: naturaldatabase.com. This isn't among Mary Kay's best moisturizers, but it can be an OK option for those on a budget.

☹ AVERAGE **Botanical Effects Hydrate 3** *($16 for 3 fl. oz.)*. This lightweight, silky moisturizer is about as "botanical" as polyester. That doesn't make it bad, it just makes the name and accompanying claims misleading, though it does contain a few plant extracts tucked in between several synthetic ingredients. *Kunzea ericoides,* a plant extract that may have antibacterial properties, has never been studied for its impact on acne; the guava extract has a small amount of research showing it to be effective as an anti-irritant. That's good but the amount in here is comparatively small to have much of an effect. This also contains milk thistle, which does have antioxidant properties, but it can also be a potent sensitizer for those prone to hay fever (Source: naturaldatabase.com). Given the vast selection of plant extracts with proven properties for oily skin, why bother with those that have a big question mark as to their benefit or problems?

☺ AVERAGE **Intense Moisturizing Cream** *($30 for 1.8 fl. oz.)* is a very standard, humdrum moisturizer that is primarily water, mineral oil, Vaseline, and waxes with little to no antioxidants or water-binding agents. In the end, this is an OK moisturizer for dry to very dry skin. However, in this price range, far better options are readily available.

☺ AVERAGE **Oil-Free Hydrating Gel** *($30 for 1.8 fl. oz.)* is considerably more modern than the Intense Moisturizing Cream above, and has a wonderfully silky, lightweight texture for normal to oily or combination skin. The drawback is jar packaging, which won't keep the antioxidants in this product stable once it's opened (see the Appendix for details).

☺ AVERAGE **TimeWise Age-Fighting Moisturizer, for Combination/Oily Skin** *($22 for 3 fl. oz.)* has a fluid texture and silky feel. It's a suitably light moisturizer for its intended skin types, and leaves a soft matte finish. Regrettably, it lacks a good selection of antioxidants and ingredients that mimic the structure of healthy skin. And, of course, without a sunscreen, this product cannot fight aging any more than an ant can drive a car.

☺ AVERAGE **TimeWise Age-Fighting Moisturizer, for Normal/Dry Skin** *($22 for 3 fl. oz.)* has a creamy but light texture and contains some helpful ingredients for normal to dry skin, but most of the impressive ingredients are listed after the preservatives, so they're barely functional. Moreover, antioxidants are in very short supply, so this doesn't put up much of a fight against signs of aging.

☺ AVERAGE **TimeWise Age-Fighting Moisturizer Sunscreen Broad Spectrum SPF 30** *($22 for 3 fl. oz.)* deserves kudos for its in-part avobenzone sunscreen (the sunscreen is the most anti-aging part of this product), but the base formula for normal to slightly dry skin is rather boring, with insignificant amounts of antioxidants and other skin-repairing ingredients that take anti-aging beyond daily sun protection. In short, your skin needs more than this provides. It contains fragrance in the form of ethylene brassylate and methyldihydrojasmonate.

☺ AVERAGE **$$$ TimeWise Age-Fighting Eye Cream** *($26 for 0.65 fl. oz.)* is a decent, lightweight moisturizer for slightly dry skin anywhere on the face. The lack of antioxidants and skin-identical ingredients is disappointing, but this contains peptides, which theoretically function as cell-communicating ingredients. Still, you don't need an eye cream and we urge you to reference the Appendix to find out why.

☹ AVERAGE **$$$ TimeWise Replenishing Serum+C** *($55 for 1.5 fl. oz.)* is separated into four vials, with the contents of each said to last one week. After four weeks, you're supposed to see amazing results. On seeing the ingredient list, we were disappointed. Not only does the formula contain more alcohol and film-forming agent than superstar, beneficial anti-aging ingredients, but also it doesn't list a single form of vitamin C. We called the company to inquire about this, and they reported that the vitamin C is coming from the *Myrciaria dubia* and *Terminalia ferdinandiana* fruit extracts. The former is said to have the highest potency of vitamin C, which is an impressive claim. As it turns out, *Myrciaria dubia* (also known as camu-camu) is a potent source of vitamin C, although the amount in this serum is proportionately low, so it comes down to a "who cares?" ingredient, at least in the manner Mary Kay chose to include it. (Why not just use vitamin C itself in a potent stable form rather than deliver it through a plant?) Despite the medicinal vials of serum and collagen-protecting claims, this isn't a serum to get even mildly excited about. Lots of companies offer products with vitamin C along with other beneficial ingredients and no irritants. Skip this Mary Kay problematic formula and consider the vitamin C-loaded serums from MD Skincare by Dr. Dennis Gross, Dr. Denese New York, SkinCeuticals, Cellex-C, or Paula's Choice (RESIST Super Antioxidant Concentrate).

☹ POOR **TimeWise Night Solution** *($30 for 1 fl. oz.)* is a clear, slightly tacky serum that's loaded with antioxidants and peptides. The Poor rating is because these ingredients are joined by several fragrant plant extracts that cause irritation, including geranium, wild mint, rose, orange, and jasmine. The tingling sensation this causes is not good news for aging skin. See the Appendix to learn why irritation is a problem for all skin types.

☹ POOR **TimeWise Targeted-Action Eye Revitalizer** *($35 for 0.34 fl. oz.)* asks you to "imagine a product so powerful, it can reduce the appearance of both dark circles and under-eye puffiness in just two weeks." That's something many people would love to achieve given how common these eye-area skin conditions are. But this product and its roller-ball applicator cannot produce such results. The water- and film-forming agent–based fluid contains some state-of-the-art ingredients, but neither they nor the numerous plant extracts (some of which are irritating) have been proven to lighten dark circles and make puffiness recede. This is actually more of a problem for skin around the eyes because it contains the irritating menthol derivative menthyl lactate (for the cooling sensation mentioned in the claims). See the Appendix to learn of the problems irritation presents and to find out why you don't need an eye cream.

MARY KAY SUNSCREEN & SELF-TANNER

✓☺ BEST **SPF 30 Sunscreen** *($14 for 4 fl. oz.)* is a water-resistant sunscreen for normal to oily skin. It includes avobenzone for UVA protection and contains a nice selection of vitamin-based antioxidants (plus green tea) known to help skin defend itself better from sun exposure. This is an outstanding sunscreen formulation that's priced right; it does contain fragrance.

☺ GOOD **Subtle Tanning Lotion** *($16 for 4 fl. oz.)* is labeled a "subtle" self-tanner because it contains less dihydroxyacetone, the ingredient that turns skin a tan color. That's nice, but nothing special that cannot be found at the drugstore from lines such as L'Oreal, Neutrogena, and Jergens for less money. If you're considering this product, it's best for normal to dry skin, but it contains too much fragrance to be suitable for sensitive skin.

MARY KAY LIP CARE

✓☺ BEST **Lip Protector Sunscreen SPF 15** *($7.50 for 0.16 fl. oz.)* combines an in-part zinc oxide sunscreen with petrolatum and other lip-smoothing emollients and antioxidant soybean oil along with vitamin E. This smart lip balm is a beautiful option for keeping lips smooth and protected year-round. The addition of yellow coloring agents helps offset the slight white cast from the zinc oxide, a thoughtful touch.

✓☺ BEST **$$$ Timewise Age-Fighting Lip Primer** *($22.50 for 0.5 ounce)* is a silicone- and wax-based spackle for filling in lines on the lips and around the mouth. It works to a minor extent, but the effect is temporary and diminishes faster if you wear greasy or overly glossy lipsticks. What's particularly impressive is the amount of antioxidants and cell-communicating ingredients this contains. Those help skin repair itself while reducing inflammation, and earn this product a Best Product rating.

☹ POOR **Satin Lips Lip Balm** *($9.50 for 0.3 fl. oz.)*. Your lips will thank you if you skip this menthol-laced balm in favor of plain Vaseline, which is the main ingredient in this pricey product.

☹ POOR **Satin Lips Lip Mask** *($9.50 for 0.3 fl. oz.)* isn't satiny in the least and lips don't need a clay mask with the kind of aggressive exfoliation this causes when massaged over the mouth. Furthermore, the menthol in here isn't the least bit helpful, and may make chapped lips worse.

MARY KAY SPECIALTY SKIN-CARE PRODUCTS

✓☺ BEST **Acne Treatment Gel** *($7 for 1 fl. oz.)* lists 5% benzoyl peroxide as the active ingredient, and is a very good, gel-based topical disinfectant for those battling blemishes. It contains soothing anti-irritants that help reduce redness while disinfecting your skin.

✓☺ BEST **$$$ TimeWise Even Complexion Essence** *($35 for 1 fl. oz.)* promises to restore a natural, even tone to skin while helping to reverse skin discolorations. Eschewing the established skin-lightening agent hydroquinone, this water-based serum contains niacinamide, ascorbyl glucoside (a form of vitamin C), and undecylenoyl phenylalanine instead. There is some research showing that niacinamide can interrupt the transfer of melanocytes (pigmented skin cells) to keratinocytes (regular skin cells that make the protein keratin), which would essentially cut the discoloration process off at the pass. However, these studies were done in vitro (test tube) rather than on human skin. Moreover, while the researchers pointed out that a positive outcome was dose-dependent, the dosage was not revealed (Source: *Experimental Dermatology*, July 2005, pages 498–508). A smaller study done on human skin revealed that a 5% concentration of niacinamide produced a noticeable effect on discolorations after four weeks of use (Source: *British Journal of Dermatology*, July 2002, pages 20–31). There is minimal substantiated research concerning the ability of the vitamin C derivative ascorbyl glucoside to lighten skin, although it has shown potential. And emerging research is showing that the novel ingredient undecylenoyl phenylalanine is an exciting option, especially when combined with niacinamide, as is the case here. Ultimately, this is a potentially good alternative skin-lightening product, though Mary Kay is definitely not using 5% niacinamide. Nonetheless, this product is worth considering by all skin types as a lightweight serum that contains several vitamin- and plant-based antioxidants as well as water-binding agents, including peptides. It stands a fairly good chance of improving brown spots, too.

☺ GOOD **Beauty Blotters Oil Absorbing Tissues** *($6 for 75 sheets)* are non-powdered thin sheets of linen-type material that do their job to absorb excess oil and perspiration. The price is good, too.

☺ GOOD **Botanical Effects Mask 1** *($14 for 4 fl. oz.)* is a good, though unexciting, moisturizing mask for normal to dry skin, but that's about it. The formula isn't ideal for sensitive skin because it contains one potentially troublesome plant extract and lacks a good range of proven soothing ingredients. One possible problem to consider is that it contains milk thistle, which can cause allergic or sensitizing reactions for someone with hay fever (Source: naturaldatabase. com), making it somewhat questionable for those with sensitive skin as claimed.

☺ AVERAGE **Botanical Effects Mask 3** *($14 for 4 fl. oz.)*. This completely ordinary clay mask contains several problematic ingredients that won't help skin and are definitely contraindicated for sensitive skin. Although this contains standard absorbents found in many masks for oily skin, it also contains irritants that can actually trigger oil production directly in the pore, making oily skin worse. The TEA-lauryl sulfate in here is known for its irritating properties and the bitter melon and milk thistle extracts can cause allergic or sensitizing reactions (Source: naturaldatabase.com). Given these questionable ingredients (and your skin only deserves the best ingredients), this is not the best for sensitive, oily skin (or any skin type).

☺ AVERAGE **Clarifying Mask Formula 3** *($14 for 4 fl. oz.)* is a standard clay mask that is an OK option for oily to very oily skin, but contains potentially problematic lavender along with a tiny amount of TEA-lauryl sulfate. It's not terrible, but better clay masks abound.

☺ AVERAGE **Oil Control Lotion Formula 3** *($18 for 4 fl. oz.)* doesn't carry a high price, which it shouldn't, because this is a very ordinary mix of water, silicone, slip agent, thickener, and film-forming agent. It is a substandard option for normal to oily skin, and does not do a remarkable job at keeping skin shine-free.

☺ AVERAGE **Oil Mattifier** *($15 for 0.6 fl. oz.)* is much better at curtailing surface shine (oiliness) than the Oil Control Lotion Formula 3 reviewed above. The tiny amount of alcohol isn't cause for concern. The solvent isododecane and the silicones help promote and maintain a lightweight matte finish. It would have earned a higher rating had it included antioxidants, cell-communicating ingredients, or skin-identical ingredients, something all skin types can benefit from immensely.

☺ AVERAGE **$$$ TimeWise Even Complexion Mask** *($20 for 3 fl. oz.)* is a very basic, out-of-date formula (think typewriter versus computer) In the form of a lightweight gel mask. It is meant to enliven tired, dull skin. It does provide some minor hydrating benefit, but actually has more problems than benefits. This mask consists mostly of water, slip agent, gum-based thickener, and film-forming agent (think hairspray). You may notice a slight tightening effect, but that's temporary and incapable of making skin look less dull. Mary Kay included a few intriguing plant extracts, but their meager presence isn't going to make a difference for your skin. The formaldehyde-releasing preservative high up on the ingredient list, along with triethanolamine, is really a problem for skin.

☹ POOR **Botanical Effects Mask 2** *($14 for 4 fl. oz.)* is a clay mask with gritty particles of lime peel powder, magnesium aluminum silicate, and apricot seed powder along with a couple of problematic plant extracts. The clay in here will definitely absorb oil but, depending on how oily your skin is, this result can be short-lived. The scrub particles can be too abrasive and leaving them on the skin until the mask dries presents a risk of irritation that isn't good for anyone's skin. The formula also includes a potentially irritating amount of the cleansing agent TEA-lauryl sulfate, as well as two plant extracts (*Plumeria alba* and the giant water lily) known to be irritating. None of that is helpful for any skin type. The milk thistle this contains could have some interesting antioxidant properties but it can also be a potent allergen or sensitizer for those prone to hay fever (Source: naturaldatabase.com).

☹ POOR **TimeWise Moisture Renewing Gel Mask** *($20 for 3 fl. oz.)*. Moisture-renewing is something this mask is incapable of doing because alcohol is the second ingredient. What were the folks at Mary Kay thinking? Alcohol in this amount causes, not helps, dryness and it also damages healthy collagen production and incites free-radical damage. None of this is good for skin, so this mask is not recommended.

MARY KAY FOUNDATIONS & PRIMERS

✔☺ BEST **Mineral Powder Foundation** *($18)* is technically not on a par with "standard" mineral makeup because the main ingredient is talc. The irony is that talc is a mineral, yet that doesn't stop most mineral makeup brands from avoiding its use due to unfounded health concerns. Mary Kay has crafted a fragrance-free loose-powder foundation with a superior smooth texture that feels almost creamy and blends beautifully. What you will get with this foundation is an initially sheer application with light to medium coverage (depending on how you layer it) that's not nearly as heavy as that from several other mineral foundations. It also won't give your face that "glow" or sparkling shine that mineral foundations are well known for (which may not be the best for someone with oily skin who might want a more a matte appearance from their powder application). The application brush (sold separately) does a respectable job, although the bristles are a bit stiff and we suspect many women will prefer a softer powder brush, which works far better for applying foundations like this one. The variety of shades includes mostly impressive, neutral options. Bronze 1 will be too peach for most medium to tan skin tones, but Bronze 2 is a winner. If you're curious to try a mineral foundation and don't mind the mess they can cause (it is loose powder, after all, and Mary Kay doesn't offer a tidy component), this is highly recommended as one of the best available, most notably for how great it looks on skin. As is the case with all mineral-type foundations, it can make dry skin or dry spots look worse unless they're sufficiently prepped with moisturizer (and you must allow the moisturizer to absorb, or the powder will grab in spots and look uneven).

☺ GOOD **Creme-to-Powder Foundation** *($14)* is smooth without feeling greasy or too thick, and provides medium coverage with an effect that's not too powdery or too creamy. This is more akin to traditional cream-to-powder foundation, which means it is best for normal to slightly oily skin without dry patches—which this foundation's finish exaggerates. Ten shades are available; among them, Ivory 2, Beige 2, Bronze 1, and Bronze 2 are best avoided due to overtones of rose or orange.

☺ GOOD **Foundation Primer Sunscreen Broad Spectrum SPF 15** *($16 for 1 fl. oz.)* has a silky texture that slips over skin easily and leaves a matte finish, which is a good prep for a smooth and lasting foundation application. As a bonus, it contains sunscreen that includes stabilized avobenzone for reliable UVA (think anti-aging) protection. The formula does not include fragrance or other irritants, but unfortunately, it also lacks skin-beneficial ingredients. To be considered a Best Product, a foundation primer should offer added benefit for the skin in the form of cell-communicating ingredients, antioxidants, or skin-identical ingredients.

☺ GOOD **TimeWise Matte-Wear Liquid Foundation** *($20)* is a great liquid foundation whose true matte finish is especially well suited for those with oily skin. Just a small amount provides medium to full coverage and this has a lightweight, fluid texture that goes on silky-smooth. The only downside is that the matte finish has a tendency to accentuate fine lines and dry patches of skin (including those you may not have known were there). It is essential to prep skin with a moisturizer (preferably one with sunscreen) before applying this foundation. The shade range is stunning with some beautiful options for all skin tones.

☺ GOOD **Tinted Moisturizer with Sunscreen SPF 20** *($18)* has a fluid, beautifully smooth texture that blends easily, providing sheer to light coverage and a satin matte finish. The in-part zinc oxide sunscreen makes this a smart choice for daytime use by those with normal to slightly dry or slightly oily skin. The shades could have been more neutral (the overtones of pink and peach are odd), but this is sheer enough so that the lesser shades (which would be Beige 1 and Bronze 1) are still options if one of the other colors doesn't work for you.

☺ AVERAGE **TimeWise Luminous-Wear Liquid Foundation** *($20)* delivers a luminescent finish that leaves skin with a soft glow and provides enough moisture to please those with dry skin. Unfortunately, on initial application, it doesn't go on as evenly and smoothly as it should, which requires extra effort to avoid a streaky appearance. This foundation ends up being a mixed bag of both strengths and weaknesses.

☹ POOR **Medium Coverage Foundation** *($15)* feels (and looks) like a giant step backward compared to the marvelous foundations from the Lauder companies, L'Oreal, Cover Girl, and many others. It is a fairly smooth liquid foundation, but it doesn't blend all that well and ends up having a dry, slightly chalky, flat finish that can look artificial and masklike on skin. Rather than floating over or merging with the skin, the pigments in this foundation tend to creep into every crevice, which magnifies dry areas and can make skin look tired and older than it is. Twenty shades are available; although most of them are just fine, the overall look of this foundation isn't one we'd encourage you to explore.

MARY KAY CONCEALERS

✔☺ BEST **Concealer** *($10)* comes in a squeeze tube and is very concentrated. This has an excellent, silicone-enhanced texture that blends without slip-sliding all over your face or creasing into lines. It provides almost full coverage without looking thick or creasing, so it's a top choice if you have very dark circles. Note that this concealer's finish magnifies dry, flaky skin, so be sure to apply moisturizer or serum first. The seven colors are fairly good, with the best ones being Ivory 1, Beige 1, Beige 2, and Bronze 1. The Bronze 2 shade is not recommended due to its strong copper cast. The Yellow shade should be considered carefully; most will find it too yellow, and it is best applied before rather than after foundation to help minimize its yellow overtone.

☺ AVERAGE **$$$ Facial Highlighting Pen** *($18)* has a built-in synthetic brush applicator. Although labeled a highlighter, its finish and coverage on skin are closer to that of a true concealer, as are the four shades. Among those, shades 1 and 3 have a peach cast that's tricky to soften. Estee Lauder's Ideal Light Brush-On Illuminator costs slightly more, but is an overall much better product if your goal is to highlight skin and reflect light to make shadowy areas brighter.

MARY KAY POWDERS

✔☺ BEST **$$$ Sheer Mineral Pressed Powder** *($16)* is an outstanding, super-smooth pressed powder. The talc-free formula feels creamy and is a pleasure to apply. It produces a natural finish that looks beautiful on normal to dry skin. The formula contains emollients that those with oily skin don't need, not to mention that they hinder this powder's absorbency. Minerals are included in token amounts for marketing purposes, but that doesn't keep this powder from earning our top rating. All the shades are recommended and each goes on softer and more sheer than it appears. There are shades for fair to tan skin tones.

☺ GOOD **Loose Powder** *($14)* is a talc-based powder with a soft, dry consistency and sheer finish. Six colors are quite good—only Bronze 1 can be too peach for most skin tones.

☺ GOOD **Mineral Highlighting Powder** *($12)* has a smooth, dry texture that offers a soft, even color deposit. Both the shimmer and matte options are attractive and best for highlighting fair to light skin tones (and the highlighting will be subtle, which is what you want for artfully applied makeup). Purchased individually, the powder tablet arrives enclosed in a handy plastic case. If you opt to purchase the Mary Kay Compact, it can house two Mineral Highlighting Powders.

☺ AVERAGE **Mineral Bronzing Powder** *($12)*. This creamy-smooth, pressed-powder bronzer's main mineral is talc, which is fine because talc is a mineral, despite being maligned by many mineral makeup–only companies. Although Mary Kay offers matte and shimmer duos (each featuring a tan to bronze tone alongside a complementary lighter shade), the color deposit is minimal even if you apply a lot of it. The shimmer options impart more shine than color, while the matte options may leave you wondering why you bothered. This just goes to show that a sublime texture is not enough if it doesn't apply and build well. Still, this is worth considering if you want really sheer color or hints of shimmer. Purchased individually, the powder tablet arrives enclosed in a handy plastic case. If you opt to purchase the Mary Kay Compact, it can house two Mineral Bronzing Powders.

MARY KAY BLUSHES

✓☺ BEST **Cream Blush** *($13)* is an exemplary, modern-day way for those with normal to dry skin (and invisible to small pores) to wear this type of blush. The initially slick texture glides over the cheek area, but is surprisingly easy to control while blending. A tiny dab is all that's needed for a soft, translucent flush and finish that adds a soft glow without resorting to sparkles. Mary Kay describes the finish as "powdery" and it is, though just slightly. It feels more powdery than it looks, which is why those with oily skin most likely won't appreciate how this blush looks or wears. Only two shades are available but both are great: Sheer Bliss is best for fair to light skin while Cranberry is beautiful on medium to tan skin (or lighter skin tones if you want a stronger pop of color). This has impressive staying power, too. Note: Although this does not have a detectable scent, it does contain a fragrant plant extract (but only a tiny amount).

☺ GOOD **Mineral Cheek Color** *($10)* acquits itself nicely for those seeking a smooth, sheer, dry pressed-powder blush. The matte shades include Berry Brown and Cinnamon Stick. If you prefer a subtle shine, consider Cherry Blossom, Shy Blush, Strawberry Cream, or Sparkling Cider. The remaining shades are noticeably shiny and really too much for daytime wear (plus the colors are the least appealing even if they didn't have shine). This is suitable for all skin types and is fragrance-free. Purchased individually, these powder tablets arrive enclosed in a handy plastic case. If you opt to purchase the Mary Kay Compact, it can house two blushes.

MARY KAY EYESHADOWS & EYE PRIMERS

✓☺ BEST **Mineral Eye Color** *($6.50)*. Talc is the main mineral in these sold-singly powder eyeshadows. Talc is not a bad thing—quite the contrary—most other minerals have a drier texture that hinders smooth application, and that's not the case here. Their previous powder eyeshadows (which these are very similar to) were also enviably silky. The matte shades include Hazelnut, Silky Caramel, Coal, Espresso, and Cinnabar; soft shine shades include Spun Silk and Ivy Garden. The remaining shades are very shiny, though the shine does cling well. Avoid the too-purple Iris and too-blue Denim Frost, and watch out for the very shiny shades if your eyelid is wrinkled. Purchased individually, these powder tablets arrive enclosed in a handy plastic case. If you opt to purchase the Mary Kay Compact, it can house up to six eyeshadows.

✓☺ BEST **Mineral Eye Color Bundle** *($19.50)*. Mary Kay has taken their outstanding Mineral Eye Color powder eyeshadows and packaged three shades in one box. The shades are singles grouped together, but each shade comes in its own plastic case (so this isn't like your standard powder eyeshadow trio). The shade groupings are meant to emphasize eye color; for example, the trio for hazel eyes has a medium and deep cool brown with a soft shimmering gold and the trio for blue eyes has warmer brown colors. For the most part, the shades selected to bring out each eye color (there are trios for green and brown eyes, too) are workable and it's nice that Mary Kay didn't go the matchy-matchy route because matching your eyeshadow and eye color won't make your eye color stand out. All told, this is well done, though with each set there's at least one shiny shade.

☺ GOOD **Cream Eye Color** *($13)* is a very good cream-to-powder eyeshadow whose light-weight, silky texture is easy to apply and blend. You get a fair amount of "playtime" before the formula sets in place, which is helpful because one of the drawbacks of this type of eyeshadow is how quickly it must be blended. Once set, this stays locked in place and only shows slight signs of creasing after a long day. The shade range is small but well edited, though each one is loaded with shine. Whether applied sheer or layered (and the formula layers beautifully), each shade has an intense, semi-metallic sheen. If shine is what you want, go for it—but keep in mind this much shine magnifies wrinkles or less-than-taut eyelids. Be sure to recap this product tightly after each use. Leaving the cap off or not putting it on securely can cause the formula to dry out.

☹ AVERAGE **Eye Primer** *($12 for 0.3 fl. oz.)* is a slightly thick, water- and talc-based white cream meant to prevent eyeshadows from creasing or smudging. Despite the prominence of talc, this remains slightly moist and doesn't work as well for its intended purpose as a flesh-toned matte finish concealer. It's OK, but not suitable for anyone who has trouble getting eyeshadows to stay put.

MARY KAY EYE & BROW LINERS

☺ GOOD **Brow Gel** *($10)* is a basic, workable option whose lightweight, clear formula helps groom brows and keep them in place. It's pretty much what a good brow gel should do, and it does its job without flaking or feeling sticky. The holding agent in this gel is stronger than many others, so it's a good choice if your brows are best described as "unruly." This does contain fragrant plant extracts.

☺ GOOD **Liquid Eyeliner** *($11)* sports a brush that's easy to control and a formula that dries fast and lasts. This liner is water-resistant as claimed, but note that if you swim with this and then rub your eye, it comes off immediately.

☺ GOOD **Mechanical Brow Liner** *($10)*. This automatic (doesn't need sharpening), retractable brow pencil is available in one color, a soft blonde shade that's best for blonde to light brown brows. It applies smoothly and evenly and sets to a long-wearing finish. We disagree with the versatility Mary Kay claims this single shade has, as it certainly won't look convincing if you brows are medium to dark brown, black, or any shade of red or auburn. However, it's a good, basic brow pencil.

☺ AVERAGE **Brow Definer Pencil** *($10)* is a standard brow pencil that needs routine sharpening, but if you're OK with that, the results are great, as is the soft powder finish. Application and color deposit are good, and in fact the shades themselves are impressive with options for blondes and redheads. This would get a higher rating if sharpening wasn't a requirement.

☹ AVERAGE **Eyeliner** *($12)* doesn't need sharpening (it's a twist-up pencil), but isn't retractable. The amount of pencil that sticks up past the opening is long enough to break off if you apply too much pressure, so that's caution number one. Caution number two is that this applies somewhat unevenly and the tip of the pencil tends to crumble a bit. Once set, this remains a bit creamy to the touch, but it stays in place surprisingly well. If you're willing to tolerate this pencil's shortcomings it's worth exploring, and the shades offer classic and trendy colors.

MARY KAY LIP COLOR & LIPLINERS

✓☺ BEST **Creme Lipstick** *($13)* feels creamy without a hint of greasiness, and imparts rich, riveting color that really lasts. The range of shades is divided into color groups, and it's a logical system that makes it easy to focus on the types of shades you prefer. This offers a soft gloss finish without feeling slick, and doesn't fade into lines around the mouth as quickly as many creamy lipsticks do. We have a winner!

✓☺ BEST **Lip Liner** *($12)* is an automatic, retractable pencil that glides on with ease and leaves a silky, long-wearing finish that keeps lips defined for hours. The finish helps keep lipstick from bleeding into lines around the mouth, which is a great feare if you struggle with this issue (but note that no lip pencil will stop a greasy or glossy lipsk from migrating to those pesky lines, so be careful about which lipstick you choose). Thade selection includes a colorless option (Clear) as well as a few soft, versatile shades. Be cl with the darker shades (Chocolate, Plum, Caramel, and Cappuccino) as these go on quong and are really best for women of color who have naturally darker lips (but even on an with ebony skin the Chocolate shade can look alarmingly dark). Mary Kay claims thisr contains anti-aging ingredients to help protect against elastin loss and environmental, but the teeny-tiny amounts used aren't likely to deliver the intended benefits

✓☺ BEST **Nourishine Plus Lip Gloss** *($14)* is a standard, buy good, lips gloss that comes in an enticing range of shades, several of which are imbued wsoft to glittering shimmer. The semi-thick texture applies smoothly and is just slightly sticknaking for comfortable wear that keeps lips soft.

☺ GOOD **Liquid Lip Color** *($13)* comes in packaging that incldes an applicator highly reminiscent of lip gloss, but it has more in common with lipstick.he lightweight, creamy texture imparts moderate color and a non-sticky, soft gloss finish. Thmoisture you get from this liquid lipstick doesn't last long, which means you will need to reapply often to maintain a comfortable feel. Mary Kay describes the shades as "rich" but they don't apply as intense as they appear, which actually makes them more wearable for a variety of women. Still, we wouldn't describe the color as "sheer"! Note: Upon application you may notice a slight minty flavor and brief tingling sensation. That's not the best news, but at least Mary Kay's formula doesn't include menthol or peppermint oil.

MARY KAY MASCARAS

✓☺ BEST **Lash Love Mascara** *($15)* gets the official title of Mary Kay's best mascara, at least if your preference is for mascara to quickly lengthen and softly thicken lashes without looking overdone. The rubber-bristled brush produces long lashes quickly; a couple of strokes take lashes from barely there to "out to there," and although there's some clumping along the way, it's minor and easily remedied with a lash brush. Subsequent coats add to the thickness this provides, but length and definition are what Lash Love Mascara does best. The formula holds up well during the day yet is easy to remove with a water-soluble cleanser.

☺ GOOD **Lash Lengthening Mascara** *($10)* does just what the name says, and accomplishes its task without clumping, flaking, or smearing. You won't notice any thickness, but if longer lashes are all you're after, this is one to try.

☺ GOOD **Ultimate Mascara** *($15)* doesn't reach the status of being worthy of its "ultimate" name, but it's nevertheless a good mascara that builds length and thickness quickly and in equal measure. Subsequent applications yield diminishing returns, which is why this isn't the one to choose if your objective is "ultimate" lashes.

☹ AVERAGE **Waterproof Mascara** *($10)* works just as most waterproof mascaras do, meaning it lengthens lashes, doesn't do much to thicken, yet holds up when lashes get wet. The average aspect of this mascara is that it takes longer than it should to provide any noticeable difference in your lashes.

MARY KAY BRUSHES

☺ GOOD **Brush Collection** *($48)* includes five brushes in a well-constructed synthetic leather case that includes extra pouches so you can add more brushes in the future. The **Powder Brush** and **Blush Brush** are quite soft and appropriately dense, though the Blush Brush would work better if its head were larger. The **Eye Definer Brush** and **Eye Crease Brush** don't fare as well, but aren't terrible, while the dual-sided **Eyeliner/Eyebrow Brush** is practical and functional (though the Eyebrow Brush is a bit too stiff). It's an overall worthwhile brush set that is priced fairly for what you get. Some Mary Kay brushes are sold individually, too, and those we recommend and rate ☺ GOOD include the **Cream Eye Color/Concealer Brush** ($10), **Liquid Foundation Brush** ($10), and **Mineral Foundation Brush** ($10). Avoid the **Compact Cheek Brush** ($2.50) as it does not even begin to compare to a regular, full blush brush.

MAYBELLINE NEW YORK

Strengths: The line earned Best ratings for products in almost every category; many excellent foundations; superior mascaras; inexpensive makeup brushes; some terrific concealers, powders, blush, eyeshadow, eyeliner, lipstick, and bronzer options.

Weaknesses: The makeup removers; most of the foundations with sunscreen lack the right UVA-protecting ingredients; disappointing lipliners; average lip gloss; the loose powder eyeshadow; Great Lash mascaras have an undeserved reputation.

For more information and reviews of the latest Maybelline New York products, visit CosmeticsCop.com.

MAYBELLINE NEW YORK EYE-MAKEUP REMOVERS

☺ GOOD **Expert Eyes Eye Makeup Remover Towelettes** *($6.98 for 50 towelettes)* are small cloths packaged in a resealable pouch. The simple, gentle formula works well to remove makeup unless the formula is long-wearing or waterproof, in which case too much "elbow grease" is needed, and that's not great for skin around the eyes. The tiny amount of lavender extract is not cause for concern.

✝ Lavender oil smells great, but fragrance isn't skin care! Find out why in the Appendix.

☹ POOR **Expert Eyes 100% Oil-Free Eye Makeup Remover** *($4.65 for 2.3 fl. oz.)* is an antiquated eye-makeup remover with too much boric acid and isopropyl alcohol to use it around the eyes. It is not recommended.

MAYBELLINE NEW YORK LIP CARE

☺ AVERAGE **Baby Lips Moisturizing Lip Balm SPF 20** *($3.99)* keeps lips feeling soft and delivers a substantial splash of color in a variety of fun, flattering shades (plus a colorless option). Unfortunately, for an SPF-rated lip balm, it doesn't deliver adequate UVA (think anti-aging) protection, making this impossible for us to recommend. Even if this contained the right active ingredients for reliable UVA protection (see the Appendix for details), this lip balm contains several fragrance ingredients known to cause irritation—and that will only make dry, chapped lips worse.

☺ AVERAGE **VolumeXL Seduction Xtreme Lip Plumper** *($8.99)* contains a potent menthol derivative (ethyl menthanecarboxamide, to be exact) that makes lips tingle (as claimed) and enlarge slightly from the resulting irritation. The plumping effect won't cause people who know you to do a double-take over your inflated mouth, but this is an inexpensive option for occasional use because irritating lips like this daily can cause chapped lips. Maybelline offers a clear shade along with several sheer colors (they look much darker in the container than they apply). The texture of each is akin to traditional lip gloss, meaning slightly thick and sticky with a glossy finish. All in all this is an OK option for special occasions and the dispensing method from the sleek component is better than that of many other lip plumpers.

MAYBELLINE NEW YORK FOUNDATIONS & PRIMERS

✓☺ BEST **Dream Liquid Mousse Airbrush Finish** *($9.79)* is a liquid foundation dispensed via an elegant pump. It has a luxuriously silky texture that meshes so well with skin it looks like a second skin. In that sense, and because this offers light to medium coverage, it's not going to conceal moderate to glaring flaws. However, it will blur minor flaws and discolorations and leave your skin with a luminous matte finish that's very attractive. The formula is best for normal to oily skin, but those with dry areas will do fine with this foundation as long as they prep their skin with a moisturizer (preferably one that contains sunscreen). The range of shades is commendable and includes options for fair to dark (but not very dark) skin tones. Avoid Honey Beige and Pure Beige because both lean toward being too peach for medium skin tones.

✓☺ BEST **Dream Smooth Mousse Foundation** *($9.79)* is outstanding and an exceptional value. Although the texture of this cream-to-powder foundation isn't as fluffy as other products in the Dream Mousse line, application is still even, smooth, and effortless. What's most impressive (and surprising, given this product's claims that it's "ultra-hydrating," which it isn't) is the smooth, powdery matte finish that looks amazingly natural. This foundation isn't one that those with dry skin should avoid; however, they should prep their skin first with a moisturizing broad-spectrum sunscreen rated SPF 15 or greater. (Maybelline didn't include sunscreen in this foundation, but that's not a deal-breaker by any means.) The blend of silicones in this foundation means that it will stay put on skin and will even withstand moderate moisture, like a light sweat. Of the 10 shades available, there are options for fair to medium (but not dark) skin tones, with Pure Beige standing out as the only iffy shade because it has noticeably peach undertones.

✓☺ BEST **Dream Matte Mousse Foundation** *($9.79)* has a smooth, whipped texture that feels wonderfully light on the skin and blends impeccably, setting to a slightly powdery matte finish. Coverage can go from sheer to medium, and this foundation layers well for additional coverage without a heavy or caked appearance. The nonaqueous silicone formula's main drawback is that it exaggerates any degree of dry skin. Therefore, either exfoliate your skin before using it or make sure your skin is prepped by applying a moisturizing sunscreen. Of course, applying a moisturizer negates this matte makeup's benefit for oily skin, but someone with very oily skin (who is unlikely to have any dry patches) can skip this step. Of the shades available, there are options for light and dark (but not very dark) skin tones. The only shades to steer clear of due to strong overtones of pink or peach are Creamy Natural, Pure Beige, Medium Beige, and Tan. Porcelain Ivory is a good shade for fair skin tones, while Cocoa is a deep brown shade that doesn't turn ashy on skin, always a plus! Classic Ivory may be too peach for some light skin tones.

✓☺ BEST **Superstay Makeup 24HR** *($10.99)* boasts of its 24-hour wear time, but that begs the question of why you'd want to wear your makeup for that long. At some point during the day, you should remove your makeup (and whatever was applied underneath) to treat your skin to other products that don't involve color or camouflage. That said, Superstay Makeup has a formula that all but guarantees long wear. It has a smooth, semi-fluid texture that blends well and sets to a strong matte finish that feels and looks powdery. We wish this foundation looked better on skin, but as is, it casts a somewhat dull finish that isn't as good as, say, L'Oreal's True Match Super Blendable Makeup, or, for oily skin, Clarins Truly Matte Foundation SPF 15. The finish isn't a deal-breaker, but many of the shades look neutral in the bottle and then set to an unattractive peach, rose, or pink tone. Avoid any shades ending in "Beige" (e.g., Pure Beige, Honey Beige) and consider the medium tones carefully. The lightest and darkest shades are best. Back to wearability, this foundation stays on so well it practically stains the skin. A water-soluble cleanser won't work; you need an oil- or silicone-based makeup remover or plain cold cream to take this off. This foundation is best for oily skin in humid climates; it is not recommended for dry skin or skin with signs of dryness.

☺ GOOD **Mineral Power Natural Perfecting Powder Foundation SPF 18** *($9.99)* is a refined loose-powder foundation that's based around mica and zinc oxide, so it has a dry finish and provides adequate coverage for minor flaws or redness and a moderate glow (but no shimmer). It blends on smoothly and has the added benefit of providing adequate broad-spectrum sun protection, thanks to the inclusion of titanium dioxide. The claim that the minerals are "triple-refined" means an improved texture, but mineral makeup options from L'Oreal, Laura Mercier, and Revlon among others have comparable textures. Application can still be a messy proposition, and the included "kabuki" brush is too small to be practical, not to mention it should be softer. For those who think loose-powder foundation is the way to go, this lends a dry matte finish that will do a good job of controlling oil, but the finish will look and feel too dry for anyone with dry areas. As with most mineral makeups, you may notice some deepening of the shade over oily areas (this tends to happen after several hours of wear). Maybelline offers eight shades, most of which go on more neutral than they appear in the container. The only one to consider carefully is the slightly rose Creamy Natural; avoid Sandy Beige, as this is too peach for most medium skin tones. The Good rating pertains to this product's value for those seeking mineral makeup. We maintain that a liquid or compact foundation bests such makeup in most respects, and is easier to work with.

☺ AVERAGE **Fit Me! Foundation SPF 18** *($7.99)* has many good qualities, but the sunscreen doesn't include adequate UVA protection (see the Appendix for details). For a sheer foundation it performs very well, with plenty of slip to make blending easy, but although it provides very natural-looking coverage, it will cover only minor skin imperfections. Once this sets, the finish is best described as matte with only a slight sheen, but no shimmer. The shades are divided into colors for Light, Medium, and Deep skin tones, with corresponding numbers for Maybelline's Fit Me! Pressed Powder shades, along with skin-tone matches for Maybelline's Fit Me! Concealer. One warning: Fit Me! Foundation tends to change color a bit once it's on your skin for a few minutes, so you want to spend plenty of time with the testers before you decide on a shade. Many Light shades veer toward orange and peach tones after setting, while Medium shades look quite yellow. There isn't any single shade to definitely avoid, but picking the best one is more of a gamble than usual.

☺ AVERAGE **Instant Age Rewind Eraser Treatment Makeup SPF 18 Sunscreen** (*$12.99*). It's always disheartening to discover that a foundation claiming to make skin look younger doesn't get its UVA sunscreen ingredients right. With the sole active ingredient being octinoxate, this doesn't provide sufficient UVA protection, which is a key element in keeping wrinkles and loss of firmness to a minimum. This liquid foundation includes a built-in rounded sponge applicator, which is unusual and not exactly helpful. You twist the neck of the bottle until you hear a click, which signals foundation is being dispensed onto the white sponge applicator. As mentioned, the sponge isn't helpful, the main reason being that in order to keep this foundation from settling into pores and wrinkles, you absolutely need to blend it with your fingers or another sponge. The attached sponge does a decent job, but that's in large part because of this foundation's exceptionally silky texture. You'll surprised at how much better this looks when blended with your fingers (something we ordinarily discourage) instead of with the included sponge. Using fingers allows this foundation to mesh with skin rather than look like it was sitting on top of it, waiting to creep into wrinkles. Coverage is in the light to medium range, and this has a satin-smooth finish. By the way, the anti-aging ingredients Maybelline touts on the label are present in amounts too small for your skin to notice, let alone improve. Turning to the selection of shades, they're deceptively disappointing. Many appear neutral in the bottle, but when blended on skin they take on an unattractive peach cast that's difficult to soften. The only shades to consider are Nude, Buff Beige, Buff, and Tan. But rather than settle for this foundation's weaknesses, why not consider L'Oreal's True Match Super Blendable Makeup SPF 17? You'll get better sun protection and a much improved range of shades.

☺ AVERAGE **Instant Age Rewind Radiant Firming Makeup SPF 18** (*$9.99*). No one's skin will be any firmer or "look younger instantly" with this water- and silicone-based foundation. Plus, any age-rewinding credibility this foundation hoped to have is lost in advance—its sunscreen does not provide complete UVA protection because it doesn't contain avobenzone, titanium dioxide, zinc oxide, Mexoryl SX (ecamsule), or Tinosorb. The lack of UVA protection is disappointing, because this foundation's texture and application are beautiful. It provides medium coverage and sets to a smooth matte finish enhanced with shiny particles (be careful, because the shine can enhance your wrinkles). The selection of 12 shades includes some excellent options for all skin tones, but especially darker skin tones, which will appreciate Tan, Caramel, and Cocoa (one of the best dark shades you'll find at the drugstore). This foundation has more pros than cons, but is an option for normal to slightly dry or slightly oily skin only if you're willing to pair it with a sunscreen that provides better UVA protection.

☺ AVERAGE **Instant Age Rewind The Primer Skin Transformer** (*$9.99*). This thick primer owes its silky texture and powder-like finish to the silicones it contains. Age won't be rewound one second because this formula lacks any anti-aging ingredients. Instead, you get a soft pink tint that subtly enlivens the complexion. This primer isn't enough to make wrinkles or large pores vanish (a claim that's definitely implied), but it does create a smooth, even surface to enhance makeup application. That's great, but this becomes less appealing when you consider the number of moisturizers and silicone-based serums that provide the same smoothing benefit, and give your skin an array of beneficial ingredients that help it look younger.

☺ AVERAGE **Mineral Power Natural Perfecting Foundation SPF 18** *($9.99)* disappoints in name and for the lack of sufficient UVA-protecting ingredients. This isn't a mineral foundation in the true sense of the word because none of the traditional mineral-type ingredients are in this liquid foundation. Although it could be argued that the silicones are derived from the mineral silica, they don't resemble this mineral by the time the finished ingredient (such as dimethicone) is added to the product. Despite the misleading name, this foundation has many good qualities. Of course, that makes it all the more disheartening that the sunscreen comes up short. With reliable sun protection this silky foundation that provides medium coverage and a smooth matte finish would have been ideal for normal to oily skin. Its finish is beautiful and doesn't feel the least bit thick or make skin look pasty. The range of 16 shades is one of the best Maybelline has ever produced; only Creamy Natural suffers from being more than slightly peach. There are suitable shades for fair and dark skin, too, so if you're willing to pair this with a broad-spectrum sunscreen with UVA-protecting ingredients, it's worth auditioning. See the Appendix to find out the UVA-protecting ingredients to look for in any SPF-rated product. It really is critical to get this right!

☹ POOR **Dream Nude Airfoam Foundation SPF 17** *($10.99)* is a shockingly poor foundation. From the packaging and dispenser (which resembles a can of spray paint), to the texture (watery) and finish (shiny and streaky), we just can't help but wonder what Maybelline was thinking! There's just no way to make your foundation look polished and blended when you're dealing with a goopy pile of foam-like bubbles that refuse to stick to a brush, fingertips, or skin. The high water content means that this foundation takes a long time to set, and once dry it runs and streaks at the slightest bit of moisture (including perspiration). Performance aside, even on the formulary level, there's nothing redeeming about this foundation, which includes the skin-irritant alcohol; it also fails to provide adequate UVA sun protection (see the Appendix for details).

MAYBELLINE NEW YORK CONCEALERS

✓☺ BEST **Dream Lumi Touch Highlighting Concealer** *($7.99)*. This thin-textured concealer/highlighter hybrid is an outstanding option for those looking for light coverage to even-out discolorations and add a bit of subtle shine to their complexion. It's not recommended for concealing blemishes because the illuminating effect will draw attention to them, especially if they are raised. However, this works beautifully to cover dark circles and add luminosity to the top of the cheekbones or down the bridge of the nose. Housed in a click-pen with a synthetic-brush applicator, the fluid texture applies and blends easily, and the six shades (a generous range for this type of product) offer luminous options for fair to medium skin tones. Though this product adds radiance, it's still opaque enough to provide some coverage without appearing too shiny or too sheer. Set with powder, this concealer won't crease or settle into lines, though coverage has a tendency to dissipate after several hours.

☺ GOOD **Fit Me! Concealer** *($6.49)* has a light texture that makes application and blending very easy, setting to a soft matte finish that appears skin-like without any creasing. Although the shade range is impressive and neutral, what prevents this concealer from earning our top rating is the sheerness of the coverage. It definitely will help conceal mild dark circles and discolorations, but that's about the extent of what this product can cover up. This coverage limitation is a shame—it was almost a perfect fit!

☺ GOOD **Mineral Power Liquid Concealer** *($8.03)* beckons you to replace artificial colorants with mineral pigments for natural coverage. Such a claim may make you think this concealer is different from the norm, but it isn't. The minerals in question (iron oxides, mica, and titanium dioxide) are present in almost every foundation or concealer being sold today. Besides, what good are mineral pigments if what they're mixed with doesn't create a pleasing texture and long-wearing finish? Luckily, Maybelline succeeded with that task. This concealer has a smooth, lightweight texture, and just enough slip. It provides good coverage and a solid matte finish with a hint of shine. Creasing should not be an issue, but this concealer's finish can magnify the look of wrinkles around the eye. Each of the six shades is worth considering, particularly the lighter colors. Beige Medium may be too peach for some medium skin tones, but isn't terrible.

☺ AVERAGE **Instant Age Rewind Eraser Dark Circles Treatment Concealer** *($9.99)* provides good coverage for dark circles and the matte finish is acceptable at first, but within an hour or two this creases, making fine lines under the eyes look dry and tired. If you prep the eye area with a good moisturizer and are diligent about blending and setting with a powder, you can minimize the product's tendency to crease, but that's a lot of work, especially when there are many concealers that provide smooth, creaseless coverage with less effort. The unique, oversized rounded sponge-top applicator is tricky, because once you've twisted the product up to dispense onto the sponge, it's difficult to tell exactly how much concealer is being applied—and with a product this concentrated, you don't need a lot before it starts looking too heavy.

☹ POOR **Coverstick Corrector Concealer** *($5.82)* is a dated oil- and wax-based formula that is too greasy to stay put for long, and it creases easily. It also tends to look too thick and heavy on skin, even when blended thoroughly. Maybelline claims this is their #1-selling concealer, and while that may be true in volume, it is not so in performance, especially when compared to their other concealers.

☹ POOR **Superstay Concealer 24HR** *($7.99)* promises to wear for 24 hours without transferring. It contains ingredients that can definitely go the distance in terms of long wear, but the bigger concern is why you'd be wearing makeup for 24 hours straight. This certainly won't hold up well if you sleep in it, and at some point in the day, makeup needs to be removed so that your skin can be treated with other products. We have no complaints about the minimal slip of this liquid concealer, plus it covers well and sets to a matte finish. This absolutely cannot be blended once it sets, so you have to get it right the first time. That can be accomplished with practice, but it doesn't take away the bigger issue, which is with the shades. Maybelline really regressed here and for whatever reason created five shades that go on much more pink, rose, or peach than you'd expect.

MAYBELLINE NEW YORK POWDERS

✓☺ BEST **Dream Matte Face Powder** *($8.23)* has a silky-smooth yet dry texture, allowing it to make good on its claim of providing an air-soft matte finish. It is a very good pressed powder for normal to very oily skin. Application is sheer, and applying more doesn't lend a thick, powdery look (though it can make skin look dull, so do use some restraint). Only four shades are available, but they're all beautiful; unfortunately this limited selection only includes options for light to medium skin tones.

✓☺ BEST **Fit Me! Pressed Powder** *($7.99)* is more sheer than most, but leaves a soft matte finish with a subtle, healthy glow. The velvety texture, and the fact that it doesn't look at all powder-like on skin, makes this a great option for all skin types. The 18 shades provide plenty of options for fair to medium skin tones, and this powder's blendability makes finding a suitable match for your skin refreshingly easy. The shades are coded to match exactly the Fit Me! Foundation shades, and while we found that the shades do work together well, these powders fare better than their foundation counterpart, mainly because they lack the orange and yellow undertones some of the Fit Me! Foundation shades have.

✓☺ BEST **Instant Age Rewind Protector Finishing Powder SPF 25** *($9.25)*. This talc-based pressed powder goes on exceptionally smooth and blends perfectly, imparting a soft matte finish best for normal to oily skin due to its super-absorbent ingredients. (It's worth noting that while the finish is a soft matte, it does contain tiny shimmer particles that are noticeable in the daylight.) It controls shine without looking chalky or dry and provides medium coverage in flattering shades suitable for fair to medium-dark skin tones. All that plus a great price and broad-spectrum sun protection from pure titanium dioxide! Although we don't advocate relying solely on a pressed powder for sun protection because most people don't apply powder liberally enough, which is essential when applying sunscreen, when paired with a foundation with sunscreen rated SPF 15 or greater, this is a brilliant option. The anti-aging claim is tied to the goji berry extract that's present. Listed by its Latin name *Lychium barbarum*, there is no proof that goji berry will rewind anyone's age, not to mention that the antioxidants won't remain stable in a product like this. This powder's real anti-aging superstar is the sunscreen!

☺ GOOD **Mineral Power Finishing Veil Pressed Powder** *($7.49)* is a mica-based powder that comes in three very good shades. It leaves a touch of shine on skin, but the effect is more radiant glow than glittery. It has a silky, sheer texture that is best for making normal to dry skin look polished. Those using powder to control shine (oil) will want something more absorbent.

MAYBELLINE NEW YORK BLUSHES & BRONZERS

☺ GOOD **Fit Me! Blush** *($5.51)* has five color categories (Nude, Pink, Coral, Mauve, and Rose) and three skin-tone categories (Light, Medium and Deep). This extensive collection of powder blush is among the widest and most organized you'll find at the drugstore. Aside from a somewhat dry texture that's not easily picked up by a brush, once applied, this sheer blush creates lasting natural-looking color that can be built up to create a more dramatic look. Maybelline has organized the display for their Fit Me! Blush into the three skin-tone groups: Light, Medium, and Deep. When selecting blush, it's very helpful to follow their guideline. Softer blush shades work better on lighter skin tones and more pigmented shades work better on medium and deep color skin tones. Most shades have a somewhat noticeable satin sheen, but the nude tones contain a subtle shine. None of these blush colors flake, something that can't be said about some of the more expensive shiny blushes from high-end lines at the department store. Those looking for blush shades that go on with more noticeable color than Fit Me! Blush offers may want to consider L'Oreal's True Match Blush, which also has an ample selection of shades divided by color intensity.

☺ GOOD **Mineral Power Bronzer Shimmer Loose Powder** *($9.35)* is a loose-powder bronzer that's silky and easy to apply. It imparts a beautiful light bronze color with a radiant, non-sparkling shine. It works great to enliven cheeks, and can be used with any powder blush for more color or heightened dimension. Although pressed bronzing powders are even easier to work with, this is worth an audition if the loose format doesn't bother you. The mini brush packaged with this is quite good, but you'll want a full-size powder or blush brush for best results.

☺ AVERAGE **Dream Bouncy Blush** *($7.99)*. The big deal about this cream-to-powder blush is its unique spongy texture. While that may be interesting, it really is just a gimmick and has little to do with how it applies or performs. As a replacement for Maybelline's excellent (and discontinued) Dream Mousse Blush, this is, sadly, inferior by comparison. The consistency in pigmentation is spotty—that is, some shades go on very sheer and others apply very bright. Hot Tamale, Plum Wine, and Pink Frosting go on bright, while Rose Petal, Peach Satin, and Pink Plum are too sheer if the goal is to add color to your cheeks. The shade selection is a generous mix of peach, pinks, and plums—each leaving a somewhat luminous finish on skin. The biggest problem with Bouncy Blush is the amount of blending required. It is difficult to blend without over-rubbing to the point that it smears the foundation underneath. Using this on bare skin yields better results, but only if you have smooth skin; any dryness or large pores will just look splotchy, plus most shades still require a good amount of layering to get the color to pop. This is an OK option for a soft, natural flush on bare skin, but that's about it.

☹ POOR **Fit Me! Bronzer** *($5.50)* is truly a disappointment. The color is very good, but it has an unpleasantly dry texture that doesn't pick up easily onto a brush, and it has a shiny finish too far from being natural and soft. Another drawback is the small pan size, which means you can't easily use a professional-size brush applicator to get it on evenly. (The smaller the brush, the more likely the powder bronzer will go on in streaks.) In the end, this bronzer just isn't a good fit.

MAYBELLINE NEW YORK EYESHADOWS & PRIMERS

☺ GOOD **Color Tattoo by Eyestudio 24hr Eyeshadow** *($6.99)*. This long-wearing cream-to-powder eyeshadow seems tenacious enough to live up to its 24-hour claim, but we don't recommend keeping any cosmetic around your eyes for that long; after all, at some point you need to sleep, and sleeping in makeup is always a bad idea! Housed in a screw-top jar, application is easy with fingertips or a synthetic brush, with plenty of time to blend. Once the formula sets, it resists creasing, flaking, and smearing until removed. The problem is that once this shadow dries, it tends to exaggerate wrinkly lids. Another use for this is as an eyeshadow primer, which seemed to help (but not completely eliminate) the wrinkly lid issue. We found that layering powder shadow on top of Color Tattoo produced amazingly rich results, but only if you pair your shadow with a complementary shade. Only a handful of these shades will work for daytime wear (Bad to the Bronze and Tough as Taupe are best bets), but if you are looking to amp up your evening look, these could be a fun way to enhance your depth of color while ensuring your eye design will last all night.

☺ GOOD **Eyestudio by Maybelline Color Pearls Marbleized Eyeshadow** *($6.99)* has a texture that's wonderfully silky and not the least bit flyaway, which is what you want from a powder eyeshadow. Application is smooth and even, with a color payoff that's noticeably stronger than what Maybelline's other eyeshadows provide. If only the colors were better! As is, you're left to choose from a preponderance of pink, purple, green, and blue tones. There are some that step outside this Technicolor brightness (consider Bronze Blowout, Khaki Craze, and Mocha Mirage), but it's a shame there aren't more workable options. Depending on how you apply this and because of the marbleized swirl of colors, it can function as a single eyeshadow, a duo, or even a trio (you'd use the darker parts of the marbleized side for intense shading). Every shade has a strong shimmer with sparkling particles, and the particles have a slight tendency to flake, even when applied sheer.

☺ GOOD **Eyestudio by Maybelline Color Plush Silk Eyeshadow** *($9.99)*. This quad eyeshadow set from Maybelline comes in what may be the cheapest, flimsiest plastic packaging around. Given the professional angle Maybelline is going for with their Eyestudio collection, it's really surprising they went so cheap on the packaging. It's almost like what you'd see in a kid's play makeup set sold at a toy store. The shadow itself is very good, if you don't mind intense shimmer coupled with large flecks of sparkles that tend to flake. Application is smooth and pigmentation impressive, at least for the darker shades. Most of the color combinations are workable, but avoid Sapphire Siren, Spirited Seas, and Irresistibly Ivy—all are too blue or green.

☺ GOOD **Expertwear Eye Shadow** *($3.75–$8.30)* doesn't surpass the top picks in this category. What's missing from these shadows is that lush, almost suede-like smoothness and impeccable blending found in superior options. This does have a nice silkiness, but also has a waxy feel that prevents smooth, even blending. Pigmentation is good, as is this eyeshadow's ability to cling to skin. You won't get as much color payoff as you will with eyeshadows from M.A.C. or Stila, but the sheerness is bound to please those looking for softer eyeshadow shades. There appear to be some matte options among the singles, but closer inspection reveals that even these have some shine, so avoid them if matte is your goal. The almost-matte single shades include Vanilla, Earthy Taupe, Champagne Fizz, and Creme de Cocoa. All the duos have a soft shine, but if that doesn't bother you, the best pairings are Indian Summer, Browntones, and Grey Matters. Two of the three shades in each trio set are shiny, but again, there are some attractive combinations, including Almond Satin, Chocolate Mousse, and Impeccable Greys. Among the quads, most sets have at least one matte shade, and at least one shade is suitable for use as powder eyeliner. Half of the quads are assembled as "Smokes," and each contain a thoughtful combination of shades (along with imprinted guidelines) to create a smokey eye. **Expert Eyes Designer Selections Shadow** provides eight powder eyeshadows in one compact, though you get just a small amount of each. Four of the shades are matte and four are shiny.

☺ AVERAGE **Eyestudio Color Explosion Luminizing Eyeshadow** *($10.99)*. Each of these powder eyeshadow palettes includes five shades, intended to create striking shimmery eye designs, but use with caution because the "Luminizing Topcoat" shade (one included in each palette) makes a mess, spilling sparkles everywhere. Aside from that major issue, the four other shimmery shades in each palette are silky-smooth, richly pigmented, and last without creasing. Among the five palettes, only Caffeine Rush has enough neutral options. If you're interested in using the purple, blue, or bright green shades in each palette, then go for it but realize that doing so isn't going to shape or shade your eyes as much as add overly almost clownish, bright color to them.

☹ POOR **Eyestudio Color Gleam Cream Eyeshadow** *($6.99)*. These three-shade palettes of high-shine cream eyeshadow go on sheer, begin caking as you build color intensity, and then crease within minutes. If you have any amount of oiliness on your eyelids, this formula will slip right off; if you have any dryness, it will be exaggerated by all the shine. Adding insult to injury are the shades, which incorporate green, pink, purple, and blue in nearly every palette, except for the bronze-y Neutral Liaisons. Any way you look at it, this is a disappointing product.

MAYBELLINE NEW YORK EYE & BROW LINERS

✓☺ BEST **Line Stiletto Ultimate Precision Liquid Eyeliner** *($7.25)* has a flexible felt-tip brush meant to create "slender lines," which it absolutely does. Rich color is deposited evenly and the formula dries quickly to a patent-leather shine. The formula has impressive wear time and doesn't flake, though anyone with oily eyelids will likely find that this doesn't go the distance as well as the gel-type eyeliners.

✓☺ BEST **Line Stylist Eyeliner** *($7.25)* is another excellent automatic pencil, though this one isn't retractable, so take care not to overextend or you could break the pencil tip. The tip allows you to draw a thin or thicker line, and application is smooth and even. Once set, this feels powdery and stays in place all day.

✓☺ BEST **Unstoppable Smudge-Proof Waterproof Eyeliner** *($7.23)* is an automatic, retractable pencil that applies swiftly without skipping and really doesn't smudge, even with provocation. It's waterproof, too, yet removes easily. The only drawback is its slightly tacky finish. That's a minor issue for such an outstanding pencil, and with the exception of Jade, the color selection is reliable.

☺ GOOD **Define-A-Line Eye Liner** *($5.82)* is supposed to glide on smoothly, and it does. This automatic, retractable pencil needs no sharpening, but includes a built-in sharpener (housed under the sponge-tip smudger) if you desire a finer point. Because this pencil's finish is quite smudge-prone on its own, it is best for creating a smoky eye effect. The shade range offers several variations on brown along with gray and black.

☺ GOOD **Expertwear Brow and Eyeliner** *($5.59)* is an automatic, retractable pencil that can be sharpened to a finer tip than most (the sharpener is built into the pencil). This pencil has a dry texture, which means less smudging. The sheer application and drier finish is well suited to brows.

☺ GOOD **Ultra Brow Brush-On Brow Color** *($5.98)* is a standard, matte brow powder that comes packaged with the standard hard brush that you should toss away and replace with a good soft professional brush. There are two shades, which is limited, but what's available works if it matches your brow color.

☺ AVERAGE **Lasting Drama by Eyestudio Gel Eyeliner** *($9.99)*. The big deal with this gel eyeliner is Maybelline's claim of 24-hour wear. Let's sidestep the fact that wearing eyeliner for 24 hours isn't the best idea (at some point you have to sleep, and sleeping with your eye makeup can cause puffiness and swelling) and focus on the fact that the claim is designed to make this gel eyeliner seem a cut above the rest, most of which cost more than this option. Like all gel eyeliners based on silicone, this goes the distance and definitely wears longer than most eye pencils or liquid eyeliners. But whether or not Maybelline's contribution lasts 24 hours, you'll notice problems within the first 24 seconds. This tends to apply unevenly, necessitating that you go over the lash line repeatedly to achieve a uniform line. Because it sets quickly, building for intensity and even color deposit can cause the formula to clump, requiring more smoothing. Application is surprisingly sheer, which contradicts the "drama" ads for this eyeliner. Maybelline included a full-size eyeliner brush, and it works decently. If only the formula itself were better, this would be an all-around winner.

☺ AVERAGE **Master Precise Ink Pen Eyeliner** *($7.99)* is a felt pen-style liquid eyeliner with an extra-long tip that delivers rich color, but, unfortunately, tends to skip and drag as you apply. The elongated tip is very fine and draws a thin line, but it is not firm enough to deliver a precise line, which means it's a challenge to get the liner exactly where you want it, though the line the brush draws is very thin. As for the 12-hour wear claim, this does set quickly and will last until exposed to moisture, which will allow it to run and smear easily.

☺ AVERAGE **Master Shape by Eyestudio Brow Pencil** *($7.99)* is a dual-ended brow pencil that applies a smooth line with a soft, semi-transparent finish, which definitely helps to avoid an overly drawn-on look. (Harsh, overdrawn brows can really add years to your face!) However, this is a somewhat wide, creamy pencil that needs sharpening, so it doesn't deliver the most accurate line, and keeping it sharpened to a fine point is a chore. A nice touch, however, is the spoolie brush included on the other end of the pencil, which works well to groom and blend brows. Note that this pencil does come in a flattering Auburn shade—a rare find for redheads among brow pencils!

MAYBELLINE NEW YORK LIP COLOR & LIPLINERS

✓☺ BEST **Color Sensational Lipcolor** *($7.49)* is an excellent cream lipstick. It has a smooth, emollient texture that glides on without being too slick and makes lips feel indulgently moist with a soft cream finish. The 48 shades are divided into color families of Pinks, Plums, Reds, and Naturals (tan to brown tones) and each group has a color-coordinated cap that makes it easy to figure out which group you're looking at. Most of the shades have some degree of shimmer finish. Note that you need several layers of this to build what Maybelline describes as "rich, stunning color." This lipstick is prone to feathering into lines around the mouth, but if that's not an issue for you, it is highly recommended. This line also comes in a "**Pearls**" finish, which includes 10 shades of sheer, shimmery lipstick that leaves a more frosty finish than a pearly one.

✓☺ BEST **Color Sensational Lip Gloss** *($6.49)* rises above much of the competition with its supremely smooth texture, luxurious feel on lips, and attractive colors that go on moderately strong and impart a glossy sheen. The shade range is excellent and this isn't the least bit sticky. It's a great option to wear alone because the color deposit approaches that of many lipsticks, although it wears off faster.

✓☺ BEST **SuperStay 24 Color** *($9.99)*. If you've avoided long-wearing lip color in the past because it was either too dry or too slick, this may be the product you've been waiting for. Not only does the color stay put, but also the base coat feels wonderful going on, and the clear coat is a low-shine balm rather than the typical gloss. Packaged in a dual-ended tube, the base coat's slanted sponge-tip applicator is extra-long for precise application, which is so important with long-wearing color. The base coat's texture is thin and has plenty of slip, making it easy to evenly distribute the richly pigmented color. As the base coat sets (which takes about two minutes), the color remains true. The balm top coat doesn't add too much shine, just comfortable moisture, which you can reapply throughout the day. The 20+ flattering shades are true to the packaging, but we were especially impressed with Reliable Raspberry and Perpetual Plum for their universally flattering results. As for the boast of 24-hour wear, don't count on it—you have to reapply the lip balm throughout the day (and night). In terms of the color, we did get eight full hours of wear (including through meals), and it held up beautifully, with little breakdown or movement to the outer edges of the lips. Even better, a makeup remover makes quick work of this at the end of the day.

☺ GOOD **Color Sensational High Shine Lip Color** *($7.49)* is a variation on Maybelline's original, outstanding Color Sensational Lipstick above. This version has a shinier finish and a lighter feel. Also, the shades are primarily sheer, shimmery plums and pinks, but they deposit more of a stain than you typically get from products (such as lip gloss) with such a high level of shine. The only drawback is how quickly the moist finish wears away. That means lots of reapplying if you want to maintain the shiny effect and comfortable wear.

☺ GOOD **SuperStay 14HR Lipstick** *($8.99)* is tenacious, and will certainly get you through 6 to 8 hours of regular wear before you need a touch-up. (Why companies feel the need to exaggerate their wear claims makes no sense—isn't 6 to 8 hours impressive enough?) Although this has a creamier texture than many long-wearing lipsticks, it's not the most comfortable lipstick. It's slightly tacky and you can feel the tackiness on your lips, but to a certain degree the texture and feel is a matter of preference, along with some trade-offs that come with long-wearing lipsticks. The finish is semi-matte, but the color is rich and long-lasting. It smoothes on easily yet the set time is slightly longer than average. Nearly every shade has some degree of shimmer, whether you can see it in the tube or not; even the most matte-looking (Ravishing Rouge) has flecks of sparkle that you'll see once applied.

☺ GOOD **SuperStay 10HR Stain Gloss** *($8.99)* is a completely unique stain-gloss hybrid that deposits the lightweight yet saturated color you'd expect from a stain with a moisturizing finish like a gloss. The hollow, heart-shaped sponge tip-applicator ensures even application, though you'll want to apply a second coat once the first sets to really allow the glossiness of this product to shine. While we love how distinctive this lip stain is, it's not without a few drawbacks. The primary drawback is that it doesn't come anywhere close to living up to its 10-hour wear claim. On average, we got a solid 2 hours of glossiness, and another 2 hours of residual color from the leftover stain beneath. It also tends to darken in drier areas of the lips, so you need to exfoliate lips to get rid of any dry, flaky skin if you want this product to look its best. Shades apply darker and bolder than the color cap suggests (somewhat typical for lip stains), but the lettering is so teeny-tiny on the bottom of the packaging that we had to double and triple check we were getting the shade we wanted.

☹ AVERAGE **Color Sensational Lipliner** *($6.49)*. Although this lip pencil requires routine sharpening, it's a very good option for those who don't mind the chore. It applies evenly and sets to a slightly powdery finish that resists smudging and doesn't fade (at least for the first few hours it's worn). We wish the shade selection were larger, but what's available is great.

☹ POOR **Shine Sensational Lip Gloss** *($5.99)* Sheer lip glosses with wet-looking finishes are a dime a dozen, so when you consider the irritants in this one—coriander oil and fragrance ingredients—it isn't a gloss worth strong consideration. Maybelline's regular Color Sensational Lip Gloss is much better, as are the gloss options from sister company L'Oreal.

MAYBELLINE NEW YORK MASCARAS

✓☺ BEST **Lash Discovery Waterproof Mascara** *($7.77)* lacks the noticeable thickness of its non-waterproof counterpart, but this is otherwise an extraordinary mascara that lifts, lengthens, and leaves lashes with a soft, fringed curl. It's also waterproof and the tiny brush makes application to the lower lashes a cinch.

✓☺ BEST **The Colossal Volum' Express Waterproof Mascara** *($7.77)* doesn't leave lashes as thick and lush as its non-waterproof counterpart, but the worry-free, easy application still leaves most other waterproof mascaras in the dust. Unless you want ultra-thick lashes, you'll be impressed by the results from this mascara, and it is waterproof as claimed. You will need more than a water-soluble cleanser to remove it.

✓☺ BEST **Full 'n Soft Mascara** *($7.77)* ranks as Maybelline's best mascara for those desiring equal parts impressive length and thickness. The balanced application sweeps on without clumps, separates lashes evenly, and wears all day. Marvelous!

✓☺ BEST **Lash Stiletto Voluptuous Mascara Waterproof** *($8.95)* is excellent. We would describe this as a great all-purpose mascara that does everything right but nothing to the extreme. Impressive results occur quickly, and this wears without a hitch. For those times when a waterproof mascara is called for, you simply must check this out. One caution: The curvy brush is meant to emulate the underside shape of a stiletto-heeled shoe, but it's a gimmick that ends up making this mascara trickier to apply than most others, at least until you get the hang of it.

✓☺ BEST **Lash Discovery Mini Brush Mascara** *($6.99)* has a very small brush that initially made us skeptical. Yet this tiny, short-bristled brush lets you be adept not only at getting to each and every lash, but also at expertly lengthening, separating, and providing appreciable thickness without clumping or smearing.

✓☺ BEST **One by One Volum' Express Waterproof Mascara** ($8.15). Although it takes time for this to reach its full potential, you'll be impressed with how beautifully this mascara lengthens, thickens, and separates your lashes. It absolutely won't clump, and smearing occurs only while you're acclimating yourself to using this mascara's large, football-shaped brush. This isn't the mascara to choose if outrageous thickness is your goal, but for a waterproof formula (which this definitely is), it thickens better than most—and wears without flaking, even when lashes get wet.

✓☺ BEST **The Colossal Volum' Express Mascara** ($7.77). Maybelline's Volum' Express mascaras have a stellar track record for producing big, thick lashes. This mascara follows suit, with a huge rubber-bristled brush that still allows you to be surprisingly nimble as you elongate and thicken every lash. The volumizing results are evident almost immediately, though not without some clumping that needs to be smoothed out. Make no mistake, this mascara is not for the lash-timid. It produces Texas-size lashes that keep getting bigger the more you apply (though layering this tends to worsen the clumps and cause slight flaking). This goes slightly beyond the outstanding results from rival Cover Girl's Lash Blast Mascara (orange tube), but with Lash Blast, clumps and a too-heavy appearance are rarely an issue. Either way, both are excellent mascaras to consider.

✓☺ BEST **Volum' Express Mascara 3X, Curved Brush** ($7.77) isn't the best thickening mascara in Maybelline's lineup anymore, but it still excels at creating long, thick lashes without clumps. Results are noticeable immediately, and layering makes lashes slightly more dramatic. The curved brush version produces even faster results than the traditional brush style and makes lashes look slightly more lifted.

✓☺ BEST **Volum' Express The Falsies Mascara Black Drama** ($7.39) demands careful application to avoid getting excess product above and below your lashline, but it produces big, long lashes with decent thickness. You'll see some slight clumping but it's easily combed out. The results are made more dramatic because the "black drama" color is so inky-dark. Although this doesn't replace the effect false lashes can have, it comes close—and is much easier to apply and remove than falsies!

✓☺ BEST **Volum' Express The Falsies Mascara Waterproof** ($7.39) is one of Maybelline's best waterproof mascaras, and among the best anywhere, at any price. You get beautifully big lashes fast, plus expert lash separation and a soft, fringed look that's defined and impactful. Thickness is minimal but this mascara still gives lashes a dramatic update—and without clumping! The brush's variegated bristles allow you to cover and get in between each and every lash for remarkable results, plus this is waterproof. You will need an oil- or silicone-based makeup remover because this won't budge with cleanser alone.

✓☺ BEST **Volum' Express Turbo Boost Mascara 7X** ($7.77) advertises that users will achieve seven times the volume in one stroke, and guess what? It works! This is certainly one of Maybelline's most impressive thickening mascaras, with an application that's quick and clump-free and a lash look that's only for those who covet long, impossibly thick lashes.

☺ GOOD **Full 'n Soft Waterproof Mascara** ($7.77) is said to build "full, soft thick lashes." It does a decent job of fulfilling that claim, albeit with less thickness than you may be expecting. Still, it bests several other waterproof mascaras that make thicker-lashes claims, and this one won't come off in the pool or inclement weather.

☺ GOOD **Great Lash Clear Mascara** ($6.40) is a multipurpose clear mascara that adds a touch of length and a glossy finish to lashes while also grooming unruly brows. The standard formula is similar to that of most other clear mascaras and brow gels, but it does its job without flaking or feeling sticky. It does take a bit longer than usual to dry, but that's a minor quibble for this versatile, affordable product.

☺ GOOD **Great Lash Lots of Lashes** *($6.40)*. We've never been fans of Maybelline's long-standing Great Lash Mascara, and most of the Great Lash spinoffs have been just as average. This entry is a bit of a game-changer, though it doesn't match the performance of many other mascaras from Maybelline or sister company L'Oreal. The main problem with this mascara is its wildly uneven application. It simply takes more time to apply, as the slightly unusual brush shape deposits noticeably more mascara at lash's outer edges yet barely any from the center of lashes in toward the tear duct area. Several coats and the use of a lash comb help even the results, but again, it's more effort than what the best mascaras require to show their stuff. If you have patience, you'll be rewarded with long, defined, and softly fringed lashes. Thickness is scant, but this wears all day without flaking or smearing—and is easy to remove with a water-soluble cleanser.

☺ GOOD **Lash Stiletto Voluptuous Mascara** *($8.95)*. After an unimpressive start this mascara picks up steam and the result is good length and thickness. Although not among Maybelline's best mascaras, this doesn't clump or flake and is easy to remove with a water-soluble cleanser. The curvy brush is meant to emulate the underside shape of a stiletto-heeled shoe, but it's a gimmick that ends up making this mascara trickier to apply than most others, at least until you get the hang of it.

☺ GOOD **Lash Stiletto Ultimate Length Mascara** *($8.95)* claims to do for your lashes what stiletto heels do for your legs. That could mean any number of things, but what this fairly average mascara will do is lengthen well with minimal clumping. This doesn't build much thickness, but it wears well through the day with no flaking or smearing. The long brush takes some getting used to, but the tapered end makes it easy to reach smaller lashes. It doesn't give your lashes a shiny patent finish as claimed; the color deposit is the same as that of any other good mascara.

☺ GOOD **Volum' Express One by One Mascara** *($8.15)* is an excellent mascara to consider if you want appreciable length and slight thickness with beautifully defined lashes. The rubber-bristled brush is shaped so that each and every lash gets smooth, even coverage and clumping is minimal. The tiny amount of clumping is easily smoothed with a lash brush or with subsequent coats of the mascara. In terms of wear, this resists smudging and flaking yet comes off easily with a water-soluble cleanser. What may be a problem for some are the fragrant plant extracts this mascara contains. They may cause undue sensitivity, which is why this mascara did not earn our top rating, despite its other impressive traits.

☺ GOOD **Volum' Express Waterproof Mascara 3X** *($7.77)* builds quickly and makes lashes moderately longer and noticeably thicker without clumps. It is waterproof.

☺ GOOD **XXL 24HR Bold Mascara** *($9.99)* is a lash primer/mascara duo that involves a two-step process of a volumizing base coat with a standard brush plus a color-rich top coat with a fuller, curvy brush. Unlike Maybelline's other XXL mascaras, the primer (base coat) is also pigmented, which really blurs the line between primer and mascara, making the first step feel even more unnecessary than lash primers usually are! The truth is that the black base coat, contrary to its claims of volumizing, did an adequate job of lengthening lashes all on its own, although the finish is slightly ashen, so the shiny black top coat is mandatory. Once the top

The Reviews M

coat went on, it was product overkill—our lashes quickly stuck together and appeared spidery. Used alone, the top coat worked nicely (providing you apply at least two coats), though it lengthened far better than it thickened. As for its claims of lasting 24 hours, this mascara (with and without the base coat) kept lashes soft and clump- and flake-free up until hour 10 before it began to show the usual signs of wear, but we recommend against anyone going 24 hours before removing their makeup.

☺ GOOD **XXL Volume Mascara** *($9.99)* involves a two-step process of a white "lash-building" base coat plus a color-rich top coat that both feature a standard brush. As is the case with most lash primers, this one does little more than give lashes the same benefit that an extra coat of mascara might, and in this case the base coat and the top coat build far more length than volume, which makes the product's name confusing to say the least! Even though it doesn't actually deliver its promise of 11 times the volume of natural lashes, whether you choose to use the primer or not, this mascara applies easily with hardly any clumps. The formula keeps lashes soft, it doesn't flake, and it comes off easily with a water-soluble cleanser.

☺ GOOD **XXL Pro by Eyestudio Waterproof Extensions Mascara** *($8.99)*. This 2-step mascara includes a white "base coat" (lash primer) followed by a regular black mascara. The base coat is supposed to add bulk to lashes, but it goes on so thin the difference is scant. Following with the mascara provides length with buildable thickness, and leads to impressive results. Clumping is ever-so-slight but easily combed out, and this wears well. It is waterproof as claimed and requires an oil- or silicone-based remover—cleanser alone won't take it off completely. Note: Although the base coat helps a bit, the mascara is quite impressive on its own, too.

☹ AVERAGE **Great Lash Big Mascara** *($6.40)* is only marginally better than the original Great Lash Mascara. You won't get any thickness and its lengthening abilities are average. The best we can say is that this darkens and separates lashes well, but you'll notice slight flaking during wear.

☹ AVERAGE **Lash Stiletto Ultimate Length Waterproof Mascara** *($8.95)* takes several coats to build merely average length. The formula is waterproof and applies without clumping, but it flakes a bit during wear. It's an OK option for occasional use if you don't need much more than modest length.

☹ AVERAGE **The Falsies Volum' Express Mascara** *($7.77)*. Using a curvy, bristled brush shaped like a half moon, this wet mascara goes on thick and fast, requiring a lot of nimble comb-through to separate lashes evenly. Does this mascara create lashes that really look like falsies? Yes, to some extent, with caveats. The results were absolutely long, volumized lashes that were almost too dramatic and obvious, not the best for daytime. The trade-off for this extreme look, however, is in the formula's longevity. Within an hour of normal, daytime wear this mascara began flaking like crazy, which likely is due to the number of coats required to achieve an appreciable "falsie" look. Try Maybelline The Colossal Mascara for equivalent results without flaking.

☹ AVERAGE **Volum' Express Turbo Boost Mascara Waterproof 5X** *($7.77)* is said to make lashes five times thicker in one stroke. Its turbo effect is more akin to a standard 4-cylinder engine because it takes its time to get going, and you will be dealing with clumps and uneven application along the way. It builds reasonable length, but is really more for thickening lashes, an area where it does not perform as well as Maybelline's other Volum' Express mascaras. The best reason to consider this is because it's tenaciously waterproof. It requires a silicone- or oil-based makeup remover—a water-soluble cleanser (even those with some oil) won't do the job.

☹ POOR **Great Lash Mascara** *($6.40)*. Great Lash Mascara (regular or curved brush) builds some length, though it takes a good deal of effort to get anywhere, and pales in comparison to most of Maybelline's other mascaras. Great Lash does not build any thickness and it has a tendency to smear. The curved brush version does little to make an unimpressive mascara any better. It may (shockingly) be the #1-selling mascara, but that doesn't mean it's the best. Clearly Maybelline doesn't think so, either, or why would they sell dozens of other mascaras, many of which out-perform Great Lash?

☹ POOR **Great Lash Waterproof Mascara** *($6.40)* is an utterly boring mascara that takes lots of effort for an "Is that all there is?" result. It stays on in the rain or pool, but so do Maybelline's other waterproof mascaras—all of which are preferred to this.

☹ POOR **Illegal Length Fiber Extensions Mascara** *($8.95)* is said to contain 4mm-long synthetic fibers that adhere to lashes to create "instant extensions." The problem with this concept is that ideally, the synthetic fibers should adhere to the ends of lashes in a lengthwise manner, but in fact they adhere to lashes in all sorts of directions, creating lots of clumps in the process. Occasionally a fiber or two will adhere in place at the end of a lash, creating the intended lengthening effect, but that's merely a matter of luck, not technique. Fibers aside, this mascara's performance leaves much to be desired, as its dry formula is prone to flaking and is stubborn to remove.

☹ POOR **Illegal Length Fiber Extensions Waterproof Mascara** *($8.95)* is the waterproof version of the Illegal Length Fiber Extensions Mascara above, and other than being waterproof, the same review applies.

☹ POOR **The Falsies Volum' Express Flared Mascara** *($7.77)* flakes during wear and clumps as you apply. Neither the thickness nor any other aspect of this formula does anything to create anything resembling false eyelashes. As a result, lashes easily turn spidery, clumpy, and just flat-out unattractive. The plastic-bristled brush is curved, which makes even application difficult, especially with such a thickly textured mascara.

MAYBELLINE NEW YORK BRUSHES

☺ GOOD **Maybelline New York Brushes** *($4.50–$8.98)*. Maybelline's brushes aren't bad for their cost, and are worth a look if you're on a tight budget but want some reliable, functional brushes for improved makeup application. Here's how they break down: **Blush Brush** ($5.50) is extremely soft, but firm, and it works decently well; **Expert Eyes Brush 'n Comb** ($4.50) is a standard, feasible brow and lash comb that's affordably priced; **Eyeshadow Brush** ($4.98) is extremely soft, but firm, and it works decently well given its low cost; and **Retractable Lip Brush** ($7.15) is a standard lip brush that travels well, though it could be firmer.

☺ AVERAGE **Face Brush** *($8.98)* feels soft but is too floppy for controlled application of powder, though some women may prefer a "looser" powder brush.

MD FORMULATIONS (SKIN CARE ONLY)

Strengths: The entire line is fragrance-free; some well-formulated AHA products featuring glycolic acid and ammonium glycolate; a selection of good cleansers; some extraordinary moisturizers and serums; very good toner.

Weaknesses: Some AHA products that include alcohol and other irritants; jar packaging; the at-home peel kit is an irritation waiting to happen; adhering to a routine of several MD Formulations products may expose skin to an excessive amount of exfoliation; incomplete routine(s) for blemish-prone skin.

For more information and reviews of the latest MD Formulations products, visit CosmeticsCop.com.

MD FORMULATIONS CLEANSERS

☺ GOOD **$$$ Facial Cleanser** *($32 for 8.3 fl. oz.)* is a basic, slightly creamy but water-soluble cleanser that contains 12% glycolic acid at a pH of 3.8. That's nice, but it's all for naught because the benefit is rinsed from your skin, when in fact is should be left on (though you wouldn't want to do that with a cleanser). It's an option for normal to oily skin, provided you avoid the eye area.

☺ GOOD **$$$ Facial Cleansing Gel** *($32 for 8.3 fl. oz.)* is a basic, fragrance-free, water-soluble cleanser that works well, but the amount of glycolic acid may prove too irritating for use around the eyes. The glycolic acid won't exfoliate skin due to its brief contact with it, and you don't want to leave a cleanser on your face for longer than is needed to cleanse.

☺ GOOD **$$$ Facial Cleanser, Sensitive Skin Formula** *($32 for 8.3 fl. oz.)* includes the AHA glycolic acid (listed as ammonium glycolate) and some soothing agents. The glycolic acid isn't helpful in a cleanser and is an odd choice in a product meant for sensitive skin. Still, this is a gentle, effective cleansing lotion for normal to dry skin, and it's fragrance-free. Note that the amount of glycolic acid makes this an iffy cleanser to use around your eyes.

MD FORMULATIONS TONERS

✓☺ BEST **Moisture Defense Antioxidant Spray** *($28 for 8.3 fl. oz.)* is pricey, but in this case you're getting a well-done spray-on toner. It supplies skin with very good skin-identical ingredients, antioxidants, and a couple of notable soothing agents, all without any irritants or fragrance. You can find similar superior (but less expensive) toners from Paula's Choice.

MD FORMULATIONS EXFOLIANTS & SCRUBS

✓☺ BEST **$$$ Moisture Defense Antioxidant Lotion** *($50 for 1 fl. oz.)* lists urea as the fourth ingredient, and thus has some exfoliating properties; it is also a very good moisturizing agent for dry skin. A lesser amount of lactic acid (likely 2%) boosts the exfoliation potential, and the pH of 3.8 is within range. Even better, this lotion for normal to dry skin is loaded with antioxidants and ingredients that reinforce skin's healthy functioning. A beautiful formulation that's packaged right, too!

✓☺ BEST **$$$ Vit-A-Plus Illuminating Serum** *($65 for 1 fl. oz.)* combines the benefits of AHAs (15%) at a pH of 4 with retinol and other cell-communicating ingredients, plus a good complement of antioxidants, all in packaging that keeps them stable during use. This is highly recommended for normal to dry skin not prone to breakouts (the plant oil and wax may prove problematic for blemishes). The AHA content is likely to be problematic for those with sensitive skin.

✓☺ BEST **$$$ Vit-A-Plus Night Recovery** *($50 for 1 fl. oz.)* is a combination AHA/BHA product with 8% glycolic compound (consisting of ammonium glycolate and glycolic acid) and 1% salicylic acid. The pH of 4 is borderline for exfoliation, but you should see some results. The lightweight texture and reduced amount of thickening agents is preferred for normal to slightly oily skin, but this can be used by all skin types. The amount of antioxidants and water-binding agents isn't expansive, but the concentrations of each are above average. This exfoliant is fragrance-free, which is yet another plus.

☺ GOOD **$$$ Continuous Renewal Complex** *($35 for 1 fl. oz.)* is a basic, fragrance-free, pH-correct AHA moisturizer for normal to dry skin. It does the job to exfoliate skin and renew its texture, though is lacking a range of beneficial ingredients. Between the glycolic acid and ammonium glycolate, the AHA content is at least 10%.

☺ GOOD **$$$ Continuous Renewal Serum** *($53 for 2 fl. oz.)* has a fluid, serum texture but its formula contains a high amount of AHA ingredients. It claims to deliver the same benefits of glycolic acid without the irritating side effects; however, this doesn't contain anything too different from the other products in this line that contain glycolic acid. Despite the contradictory claim, this is an effective (meaning pH-correct), no-frills AHA product for all skin types. It contains approximately 12% AHA.

☺ AVERAGE **$$$ Continuous Renewal Complex, Sensitive Skin Formula** *($35 for 1 fl. oz.)* contains enough AHAs to exfoliate, but the pH of 4.4 doesn't allow that to occur; AHAs do best at a pH of 3 to 4. So this product really isn't worth considering for any skin type (Source: *Cosmetic Dermatology*, October 2001, pages 15-18).

☺ AVERAGE **$$$ Continuous Renewal Serum, Sensitive Skin Formula** *($53 for 2 fl. oz.)* has a more elegant formula than the Continuous Renewal Serum above, but the pH of 4.4 reduces the potential for the AHAs it contains to exfoliate skin.

☹ POOR **Daily Peel Pads** *($30 for 40 pads)* would be recommended as pH-correct glycolic and salicylic acid pads if the formula did not include several irritants, including alcohol, juniper oil, lavender oil, and witch hazel. See the Appendix to learn why irritation is a problem for everyone's skin.

☹ POOR **Glycare Acne Gel** *($30 for 2.5 fl. oz.)* lists alcohol as the second ingredient, which makes it too drying and irritating for all skin types. Alcohol is a problem for all skin types, but for those with oily, acne-prone skin it can trigger more oil production at the base of pores, quickly making oily skin worse—not to mention alcohol won't reduce redness and inflammation from acne (Sources: *Clinical Dermatology*, September-October 2004, pages 360–366; and *Dermatology*, January 2003, pages 17–23.)

☹ POOR **Vit-A-Plus Clearing Complex** *($39 for 1 fl. oz.)* lists alcohol as the second ingredient. Without it, the blend of AHAs and salicylic acid plus retinol in this product would have been great for battling blemishes. See the Appendix to learn why alcohol is a problem for your skin.

MD FORMULATIONS MOISTURIZERS (DAYTIME & NIGHTTIME), EYE CREAMS, & SERUMS

✓☺ BEST **Moisture Defense Antioxidant Moisturizer SPF 20** *($36 for 1.7 fl. oz.)*. Now this is how to formulate a great daytime moisturizer with sunscreen! UVA protection is assured thanks to zinc oxide, and the silky lotion formula feels great and works beautifully for normal to dry skin. Antioxidants are plentiful, the formula includes some good water-binding agents, and it is fragrance-free. "Moisture and protection without a greasy look and feel" is a fairly accurate way to describe this product. Those with slightly oily skin will find this doesn't hold back shine, but those with normal to dry skin will find it leaves a natural matte finish that is comfortable under makeup.

✓☺ BEST **$$$ Moisture Defense Antioxidant Hydrating Gel** *($45 for 1 fl. oz.)* contains effective state-of-the-art water-binding agents, antioxidants, and cell-communicating ingredients in an ultra-light base. Although suitable for all skin types, it's best for those with oily skin seeking an antioxidant-laden gel. This fragrance-free moisturizer would also be worthwhile for someone with rosacea or sensitive skin, too.

☺ GOOD **$$$ Critical Care Calming Gel** *($39 for 1 fl. oz.)* is designed for sensitive or rosacea-affected skin, but its most recent formula contains reduced levels of the anti-irritants green tea and licorice extracts. That's disappointing because although the numerous fruit extracts that now have greater prominence offer antioxidant benefits, they're not proven soothing agents. This is still a good, lightweight gel moisturizer for normal to oily skin—it's just not the best choice for sensitive skin. Technically, Critical Care Calming Gel is fragrance-free but some of the fruit extracts add a scent.

☺ GOOD $$$ **The TEMPS: Oil Control Pore Refiner** *($28 for 0.5 fl. oz.)* is a good silicone-based serum with retinol for normal to oily skin. The blend of silicones leaves a smooth matte finish and this also contains another form of vitamin A (retinyl palmitate) plus tea tree oil, though not in an amount that would be effective against acne-causing bacteria. This can help control oily shine on skin's surface, but cannot control oil production because that is regulated by hormones. This contains fragrance in the form of farnesol. One more comment: This would work well as a retinol-based primer to wear under makeup.

☺ AVERAGE $$$ **Critical Care Shielding Creme** *($85 for 1 fl. oz.)* has a beautifully silky texture built around silicones, and also includes some well-researched antioxidants and ingredients that reinforce skin's structure. Yet for the money, it ends up being a disappointment because of the jar packaging, which won't allow the antioxidants to stimulate skin's healing process. See the Appendix to learn why jar packaging is a problem.

☺ AVERAGE $$$ **Critical Care Skin Repair Complex** *($100 for 1 fl. oz.)* promises to restore the smooth, beautiful skin you were born with, but it cannot replace what time and years of sun damage take away. It's just a lightweight, silky-textured moisturizer in which the effectiveness of the antioxidants is diminished due to jar packaging. MD Formulations should have taken "care" to get this "critical" aspect right!

☺ AVERAGE $$$ **Moisture Defense Antioxidant Comfort Creme** *($45 for 1 fl. oz.)* is a basic moisturizer for normal to dry skin. The antioxidants will become less effective once this jar-packaged product is opened (see the Appendix for details), so the price for this moisturizer is out of line due to its diminished benefits.

☺ AVERAGE $$$ **Moisture Defense Antioxidant Creme** *($55 for 1.7 fl. oz.)* contains a selection of ingredients capable of reinforcing skin and rebuilding its protective barrier as claimed, and that's excellent. What's not so great is that jar packaging will render the many antioxidants ineffective shortly after you begin using this cream. In better packaging, this would be a slam-dunk recommendation for normal to slightly dry skin.

☺ AVERAGE $$$ **Moisture Defense Antioxidant Eye Creme** *($35 for 0.5 fl. oz.)* contains too few impressive ingredients and earns its stripes primarily via cosmetics trickery. The amount of titanium dioxide and iron oxides create a whitening, slightly pearlescent finish that helps mask the appearance of dark circles. It's not as effective as a concealer, and overall not worth considering over many other eye creams—but ultimately, you don't need an eye cream at all (see the Appendix to find out why).

☺ AVERAGE $$$ **Vit-A-Plus Anti-Aging Eye Complex** *($53 for 0.5 fl. oz.)* contains 10% AHAs, but the pH of 4.4 limits their exfoliating properties, though they will serve as water-binding agents. This lightweight moisturizer is an option for slightly dry skin. Vitamins A and E are the only antioxidants on board, but the packaging will keep them stable during use.

☺ AVERAGE $$$ **Vit-A-Plus Anti-Aging Serum** *($50 for 1 fl. oz.)* is a heavier (but not occlusive) version of the Vit-A-Plus Anti-Aging Eye Complex above, with an improved selection of helpful ingredients for normal to dry skin. The pH is too high for the 10% concentration of AHAs to exfoliate, but the vitamin A (as retinyl palmitate) content is good.

☺ AVERAGE **$$$ Vit-A-Plus Intensive Anti-Aging Serum** *($55 for 1 fl. oz.)* is similar to the Vit-A-Plus Anti-Aging Serum above, except it has a higher concentration (20%) of AHAs. Once again, the pH does not permit optimal exfoliation; however, the amount of retinyl palmitate is good.

☻ POOR **The Temps Brighten & Tighten Eye Serum** *($36 for 0.16 fl. oz.)* comes packaged with a roller-ball applicator that allows this water-based solution to glide onto the under-eye area. Contrary to claims, this product doesn't contain any ingredients that can vanquish dark circles or puffiness. Actually, it's a problem for use around the eye area because it contains arnica extract, which can cause contact dermatitis and be very irritating to mucous membranes (Source: naturaldatabase.com). By the way, this also contains PVP/polycarbamyl polyglycol ester (a hairspray-type ingredient) that can also be a skin irritant. See the Appendix to learn why you don't need a special serum (or cream) for the eye area.

MD FORMULATIONS LIP CARE

☻ POOR **Lip Balm SPF 20** *($12 for 0.33 fl. oz.)* contains an in-part titanium dioxide sunscreen, but it's beside the point considering that this contains extracts and oils known to cause irritation, which will just lead to more chapping.

☻ POOR **The Temps Lip Plumping Treatment** *($28 for 0.27 fl. oz.)* is an emollient lip balm that contains some excellent moisturizing ingredients for dry, chapped lips. Unfortunately, the plumping comes from the irritating, potent menthol derivative menthoxypropanediol. The inflammation this causes will make lips swell a little, but causing such inflammation daily isn't a good idea for the health of your lips.

MD FORMULATIONS SPECIALTY SKIN-CARE PRODUCTS

☺ GOOD **Benzoyl Peroxide 10** *($20 for 2 fl. oz.)* works swiftly to kill acne-causing bacteria with its 10% concentration of benzoyl peroxide. You shouldn't start with such a high concentration, but it may be worth stepping up to if your blemishes don't respond to 2.5% or 5% concentrations.

☺ GOOD **$$$ Moisture Defense Antioxidant Treatment Masque** *($26 for 2.5 fl. oz.)* contains approximately 8% AHAs (listed as ammonium glycolate and glycolic acid), but the pH of 4.4 reduces the potential for effective exfoliation. Still, the AHAs have merit as water-binding agents, so they're not wasted in this product. It's otherwise a thick, creamy mask for dry skin that contains some good antioxidants and soothing agents. These ingredients are best left on skin rather than rinsed off.

☺ AVERAGE **$$$ The Temps Wrinkle Filler & Deep Crease Relaxer** *($36 for 0.06 fl. oz.)* is basically positioned as a "Botox-on-the-go" product that is packaged in a pen-style applicator. This nonaqueous blend of silicones feels great on skin, but the peptides in this product won't relax expression lines, although it is reasonable to expect them to attract moisture to skin and, therefore, make lines look less apparent by virtue of hydration. This is gentle enough to use on wrinkles around the eye area.

☺ AVERAGE **$$$ Vit-A-Plus Clearing Complex Masque** *($30 for 2.5 fl. oz.)* contains lactic acid and sodium lactate at a pH of 3.6, so some exfoliation will occur. This is first and foremost a clay mask for oily skin, and the amount of exfoliation won't be great because you'll want to rinse this off after several minutes. The small amount of rosemary oil may cause irritation; see the Appendix to learn why fragrant oils can be problematic.

☺ AVERAGE $$$ **Vita-A-Plus Firming Treatment Masque** *($36 for 2.5 fl. oz.)* is an expensive mask that mixes glycerin and clay so you get some oil absorption without a dry, tight feeling after you rinse. Although that sounds ideal, the formula also contains a couple of heavier, wax-like ingredients that impede rinsing. Although it contains a form of AHA (ammonium glycolate) plus glycolic and salicylic acids, the product's pH is too high for it to function as an exfoliant. The amount of alcohol is potentially cause for concern, but ultimately this mask isn't worth the expense. If you have oily skin and want an absorbent mask, there are less expensive options, and the exfoliant step can (and should) be done separately.

☹ POOR **Glycare Lotion** *($40 for 2 fl. oz.)* contains too much alcohol and causes further irritation due to eucalyptus oil. This is not the way to control excess oil or reduce the appearance of large pores. See the Appendix to find out why irritation is a problem for oily skin.

☹ POOR **My Personal Peel System** *($85)* consists of five separate products meant to be customized according to your skin's needs; however, all of them contain at least one irritating ingredient. The **Power Peel Pads** contain 20% AHAs, but irritate the skin with alcohol, witch hazel, lavender oil, and juniper oil. The **Firming Anti-Wrinkle Booster** only boosts skin inflammation because it contains the menthol derivative menthoxypropanediol. The **Extra Clear Booster** contains irritating grapefruit oil (which won't promote clear skin, but can cause a phototoxic reaction). The **Brightening Booster** contains menthoxypropanediol and lavender oil. The **Post-Peel Restorer** contains strawberry oil, which can cause contact dermatitis and has no established soothing benefit for skin, particularly if it's irritated, as it will be after proceeding through the steps of this at-home peel. What a poorly formulated, expensive mistake!

MEANINGFUL BEAUTY CINDY CRAWFORD (SKIN CARE ONLY)

Strengths: The company provides complete ingredient lists on their website; good fragrance-free cleanser; excellent lightweight moisturizer; sunscreen now rated SPF 20 and includes zinc oxide; packaging that keeps light- and air-sensitive antioxidants stable during use.

Weaknesses: Expensive; the mask contains irritating eucalyptus oil; no products to manage acne, lighten skin discolorations, or exfoliate; difficult to order products that do not come as part of the Introductory Kit; the melon extract talked up in the infomercials isn't more amazing than lots of other antioxidants from plants.

For more information and reviews of the latest Meaningful Beauty Cindy Crawford products, visit CosmeticsCop.com.

MEANINGFUL BEAUTY CINDY CRAWFORD CLEANSER

☺ GOOD $$$ **Cleanse: Skin Softening Cleanser** *($28 for 5.5 fl. oz.)* is a very standard, but effective, water-soluble cleanser that is suitable for all but very oily skin. The lotion-like texture lathers minimally and ably removes makeup and excess oil without drying. Of course, there are much less expensive (this price is just ludicrous) cleansers, but at least Crawford's team did their homework and left out essential oils (or fragrance of any kind) as well as drying detergent cleansing agents. But there are lots of products like this for one-third the price.

MEANINGFUL BEAUTY CINDY CRAWFORD TONER

☹ POOR **Pore Refining Toner** *($36 for 5.5 fl. oz.)* is a toner to ignore due to its mix of beneficial and problematic ingredients. The formula is bound to leave skin confused as well as irritated because of the numerous fragrance ingredients it contains. In some ways this is little more than perfume for your face, but fragrance isn't skin care. There are superior toners to consider that not only cost less, but also have formulas that can make a genuine improvement in your skin. Those are the kinds of toners to use—not problematic concoctions like this, which undoubtedly leave many women wondering why they bothered. By the way, in case you're tempted due to this toner's name, it cannot refine pores. If anything, the irritation it causes may make enlarged pores worse (see the Appendix for details).

MEANINGFUL BEAUTY CINDY CRAWFORD SCRUB

☺ AVERAGE $$$ **Superfine Exfoliant** *($43 for 1.7 fl. oz.).* This simple scrub attempts to be microdermabrasion at home minus the device that's essential to making a microdermabrasion procedure easier, more effective, and less messy (although in truth microdermabrasion doesn't do much more than make skin feel smoother; it's a pretty low-tech anti-aging procedure). This scrub uses alumina crystals as the abrasive agent, and they're buffered in a base of slip agent and nonfragrant plant oil. The plant oil helps cushion skin as you scrub, but it also makes this scrub difficult to rinse (and you don't want the alumina crystals lingering on your face, feeling gritty and interfering with smooth makeup application). There's not much else to this fragrance-free scrub, other than to say it's overpriced and no match for what a good AHA or BHA exfoliant can do.

MEANINGFUL BEAUTY CINDY CRAWFORD MOISTURIZERS (DAYTIME & NIGHTTIME), EYE CREAMS, & SERUMS

☺ GOOD $$$ **Eyes: Lifting Eye Creme** *($42 for 0.5 fl. oz.)* is an option (though not an "extra-rich" one) for dry skin anywhere on the face, but contains nothing that will make "tired-looking eyes feel tightened and lifted." If anything, the witch hazel water can cause irritation, although the small amount in this product is unlikely to cause problems. The antioxidants are impressive, as is the opaque tube packaging, which will help keep them stable. This would be rated higher if it did not contain witch hazel water and fragrance (putting either too close to the eyes isn't a good idea). Check out the Appendix to learn why, in truth, you don't need an eye cream.

☺ GOOD $$$ **Lifting Eye Crème-Advanced Formula** *($28.95 for 0.5 fl. oz.).* If this is the "advanced formula," then is Meaningful Beauty's other eye cream above not worth considering? As it turns out, they're both worth considering based on their formulas, but the truth is you don't need to bother considering an eye cream at all. A well-formulated facial moisturizer (which is what you should be using, because there are plenty of great ones in all price ranges) can and should be used around the eyes, too. This eye cream contains nothing that isn't seen in facial moisturizers, though it does offer mica for a shiny finish. What this fragrance-free eye cream contains is what you should look for in a facial moisturizer: smoothing ingredients, antioxidants, repairing agents, and intriguing water-binding agents to help skin attract and hold moisture. This cannot lift skin anywhere and it won't do much for dark circles or puffiness, but it will make dry skin anywhere on the face look and feel better.

☺ GOOD $$$ **Protect: Antioxidant Day Creme SPF 20** *($35 for 1 fl. oz.)* gets it right with an in-part avobenzone sunscreen and lightweight cream base suitable for normal to dry skin, although those with oily skin won't appreciate this product's finish. The formula contains antioxidants and skin-identical ingredients, which are essential for anti-aging benefits. What keeps this from earning a Best Product rating is the inclusion of several fragrance ingredients. They pose a slight risk of irritation, but their presence doesn't erase the benefits this daytime moisturizer with sunscreen provides.

☺ AVERAGE **$$$ Decollete: Firming Chest and Neck Creme** *($43 for 1.7 fl. oz.)* doesn't contain anything that makes it specific for use on the neck and chest area. What we have here is not a specialty cream, but a good moisturizer that is suitable for dry skin anywhere on the body. Its gel-cream texture belies an emollient formula that contains enough film-forming agent to make skin feel tighter (albeit temporarily). Also on hand is a nice assortment of antioxidants, water-binding agents, and soothing agents, all given more prominence than what you'll find in most moisturizers, but the antioxidants won't remain potent for long due to the jar packaging (see the Appendix for details). This does contain fragrance.

☺ AVERAGE **$$$ Eye Enhancing Serum** *($34.95 for 0.5 fl. oz.)* has a silky texture courtesy of the multiple silicones it contains. It also contains the melon fruit extract that Meaningful Beauty boasts about and, although this is a very good antioxidant, it's by no means the only one nor is it the best (there isn't a single best antioxidant). Beyond the melon fruit, this contains a couple of other antioxidants and a tiny amount of peptide. That's nice but hardly exciting, not to mention nothing about this formula is "super-hydrating" or unique for skin around the eyes. This is fine for use by all skin types, but in truth you don't need a special product for the eye area. A well-formulated facial serum can and should be applied around the eyes, too! See the Appendix to learn more.

☺ AVERAGE **$$$ Line Diffuser Wrinkle Smoothing Capsules** *($52 for 60 capsules)* contain a blend of silicones with thickener, film-forming agent, and a tiny amount of skin-identical sodium hyaluronate along with two peptides. In all likelihood, the peptides aren't going to penetrate far enough into your skin to stimulate collagen production, but they still have value in the top layers of skin. Although this serum in capsule form is fragrance-free, you're better off going with the far better formulated capsule/serum formulas from Elizabeth Arden's Ceramide line. In reality, however, there is no reason to use this kind of expensive, gimmicky packaging, regardless of the formulation. Overall, there are far better formulated products with an impressive range of ingredients and without the marketing gimmick of capsules.

☺ AVERAGE **$$$ Restore: Anti-Aging Night Creme** *($45 for 1.7 fl. oz.)* contains an overall impressive roster of ingredients to help skin look and act younger. That's why the choice of jar packaging is so unfortunate. The ingredients you're paying extra for won't remain potent for long, and that severely diminishes this moisturizer's anti-aging prowess, or any other benefit, other than just being an ordinary moisturizer, and you certainly don't need to spend this much for ordinary.

☹ POOR **Glowing Serum Skin Revitalizer** *($39 for 0.5 fl. oz.)* is a water-based serum that contains an impressive amount of soy protein, which functions as a water-binding agent and has antioxidant ability. The slip agents help this serum feel quite light, while the amount of film-forming agent helps your skin appear smoother. Several other intriguing ingredients are present, too, but none of them make this a must-have serum that's worth its price. A cause for slight concern is the inclusion of fragrant orange oil, which can be irritating (and irritation causes collagen to break down, which isn't the way to look younger). Adding to this concern is the inclusion of several fragrance ingredients known to cause irritation. Your skin would be better off using a fragrance-free serum that contains anti-aging ingredients proven to work rather than strictly providing a skin-smoothing effect.

MEANINGFUL BEAUTY CINDY CRAWFORD SPECIALTY SKIN-CARE PRODUCTS

☺ AVERAGE **$$$ Rich Moisture Masque** *($52 for 2 fl. oz.)*. What a shame this moisturizing mask is packaged in a jar! That means many of the beneficial ingredients it contains won't remain stable after this is opened, not to mention the hygiene issue of dipping your fingers into a water-based product like this. In better packaging, this would be a slam-dunk for dry to very dry skin, though no question it's overpriced. Because this contains fragrance it isn't the best bet for sensitive skin, and again, the poor choice of jar packaging is a deal-breaker. If you're going to spend this much money on a moisturizing mask, make sure it's in packaging (like an opaque tube) that keeps delicate yet essential ingredients protected from light and air degradation.

☹ POOR **Purify: Deep Cleansing Masque** *($32 for 1.7 fl. oz.)* is a water- and clay-based mask that contains a bewildering combination of absorbent and moisturizing ingredients, which makes it inappropriate for dry and oily skin. Even if you have classic normal skin, the fact that this product contains eucalyptus oil makes it too irritating to consider. Eucalyptus has no established benefit for skin, but its tingling effect convinces many consumers that the product they're using is doing something, thus making it seem worthwhile when it isn't.

MERLE NORMAN (SKIN CARE ONLY)

Strengths: Most Merle Norman boutiques willingly provide free samples so you can try before you buy; excellent cleansing lotion for dry, sensitive skin; effective, pH-correct AHA and BHA products; surprisingly good toners; excellent lip balm/lip line filler; good sunscreen and self-tanner.

Weaknesses: Jar packaging is prevalent; the Changing Skin products do not effectively address skin changes resulting from menopause; most of the Clear Complexion products cause more skin problems than they solve; a few very good products are impossible to recommend because they also include irritants; the Miracol and classic Merle Norman products are severely dated formulas that harken back to the days before computers replaced typewriters.

For more information and reviews of the latest Merle Norman products, visit CosmeticsCop.com.

MERLE NORMAN CLEANSERS

✓☺ BEST **$$$ Delicate Balance Calming Cleanser** *($19 for 4 fl. oz.)* is an outstanding cleansing lotion for those with dry, sensitive skin despite its high price. The fragrance-free formula contains several skin-identical ingredients and its emollients remove makeup easily. Merle Norman claims this is safe for those struggling with rosacea, and it is. One wonders why all their other cleansers aren't fragrance- and colorant-free like this one, but without question, this is one of the better Merle Norman cleansers if you have dry skin! Creamy cleansers like this work best when used with a damp washcloth. Not only does this help remove makeup more thoroughly, but also it minimizes the residue cleansers like this can leave if not rinsed thoroughly.

☺ GOOD **$$$ Daily Moisture Milky Cleanser** *($22 for 4 fl. oz.)* is a very good cleansing lotion for normal to dry skin not prone to breakouts, but it's not anything special and it's far more expensive than many other well-formulated cleansers. It has a lightly creamy, silky texture and ably removes all types of makeup. The amount of nonfragrant plant oils is a nice touch for dry skin, but their presence slightly hinders this cleanser's ability to rinse completely. For best results, use this with a damp washcloth, taking special care around your eyes.

☺ AVERAGE **Cleansing Lotion** *($22 for 14 fl. oz.)* is a more fluid version of Merle Norman's Cleansing Cream reviewed below. It is easier to apply and a bit easier to rinse, but still amounts to little more than old-fashioned cold cream. It's an OK option for extremely dry skin not prone to acne, but definitely not preferred over a gentle, water-soluble cleanser, and Merle Norman has some good ones.

☺ AVERAGE **$$$ Foaming Cleanser Normal/Dry** *($21 for 4 fl. oz.)* Is a pricey, water-soluble cleanser that produces copious foam, but the foaming action isn't what's getting your skin clean. That job is done by the detergent cleansing agents in this product, and sadly, most of them are too drying for all skin types, especially for those with dry skin. This removes makeup and rinses without a residue, but if you're going to consider this at all, it's really best only for oily skin.

☺ AVERAGE **$$$ Foaming Cleanser Normal/Oily** *($21 for 4 fl. oz.)* is very similar to Merle Norman's Foaming Cleanser Normal/Dry above. As such, the same review applies.

☹ POOR **Brilliant-C Cleanser** *($21 for 4 fl. oz.)* contains soap-like ingredients that leave a residue you can feel. The amount of potassium hydroxide is high enough to be a drying, irritating experience for all skin types, which is far from brilliant! This cleanser is little more than expensive liquid soap. Vitamin C is useless in a cleanser because its benefit is rinsed down the drain before it can help your skin.

☹ POOR **Cleansing Cream** *($15 for 7.5 fl. oz.)* is a very thick, greasy cleanser that's essentially a classic cold cream. It removes makeup easily, but is very difficult to rinse without a washcloth. Pulling and wiping at the skin to remove cold cream stretches skin and encourages sagging. This definitely is not preferred to a gentle, water-soluble cleanser, and Merle Norman has some good ones.

☹ POOR **Clear Complexion Gel Cleanser** *($21 for 4 fl. oz.)* is a thin-textured gel cleanser medicated with 2% salicylic acid. Regrettably, this active ingredient has little, if any, anti-acne effect due to its brief contact with the skin. If that weren't disappointing enough, the price is definitely too high and the formula contains way too many fragrant plants that can irritate skin, which potentially can trigger more oil production at the base of your pores.

☹ POOR **Skin Refining Cleanser** *($22 for 4 fl. oz.)* is a standard, basic, fragrance-free cleansing lotion that is not recommended due to the amount of potassium hydroxide (that's lye) it contains. Potassium hydroxide can be particularly problematic when used around the eyes, which anyone using this cleanser would be inclined to do.

MERLE NORMAN EYE-MAKEUP REMOVERS

☺ AVERAGE **Very Gentle Eye Makeup Remover** *($14 for 2 fl. oz.)* is a basic, fragrance-free, fairly greasy eye-makeup remover. The oil–based formula easily breaks down even waterproof formulas, but because it leaves a greasy residue, it's best to use it before washing your face, or just forgo using it at all given the far better formulated eye-makeup removers from other lines.

☺ AVERAGE **$$$ Dual Action Eye Makeup Remover** *($18 for 4 fl. oz.)* is a standard dual-phase eye-makeup remover. Its combination of silicone and mild cleansing agents makes quick work of all types of eye makeup. The only drawback is the fragrance, which has no business being included in a product meant for use around the eyes. Paula's Choice Gentle Touch Makeup Remover or Clinique's Take the Day Off Makeup Remover both have better formulas that omit the fragrance.

MERLE NORMAN TONERS

✓☺ BEST **Daily Moisture Toner** *($18 for 6 fl. oz.)* is an impressive, truly moisturizing toner for those with normal to dry skin. It contains helpful emollients, skin-identical glycerin,

---

🖾 Buying skin-care products packaged in jars? See the Appendix to learn why that's a bad idea.

and silicones for a silky finish. Also on hand are a few antioxidants and soothing agents. This contains a tiny amount of fragrance, but given the dearth of well-formulated toners, this is still worth strong consideration if you want to add this step to your skin-care routine.

☺ GOOD **Brilliant-C Toner** *($20 for 6 fl. oz.)* is actually quite impressive, considering that most toner formulas are average to terrible. It contains some very good ingredients for normal to dry skin, including several antioxidants and soothing licorice extract. Some of the plant extracts in this toner have in vitro research attesting to their skin-lightening ability, but on balance you're not going to see much reduction in pigmentation issues—at least not in comparison to what you'll see using products with hydroquinone or higher levels of vitamin C.

☺ GOOD **Delicate Balance Soothing Toner** *($19 for 6 fl. oz.)* is not quite as impressive as Merle Norman's Daily Moisture Toner above, but this alcohol- and fragrance-free option is worth considering for its blend of lightweight hydrating ingredients and soothing agents. True to claim, this would indeed be a beneficial toner for sensitive skin. One wonders why Merle Norman didn't go the fragrance- and colorant-free route for all their products!

☹ POOR **AHA Toner, for Normal/Dry** *($18 for 6 fl. oz.)* misrepresents its AHA (glycolic acid) by trying to convince you that various fruit extracts have the same effect as glycolic and lactic acids—they don't. Plus, this toner's mix of helpful and problematic ingredients is bound to leave any skin type confused (meaning irritated). As such, it is not recommended.

☹ POOR **AHA Toner Normal/Oily** *($18 for 6 fl. oz.)* lists alcohol as the second ingredient, making it too drying and irritating for all skin types (see the Appendix for more details). It also contains witch hazel and menthol, which add to the irritation. Meanwhile, the amount of genuine AHA (lactic acid) in this toner is too low for it to be effective.

☹ POOR **Clear Complexion Toner** *($17 for 6 fl. oz.)* contains irritants rather than ingredients that encourage acne-healing and healthier skin, like so many other anti-acne products. Alcohol, citrus extracts, witch hazel, and cinnamon are not the way to go, whether acne is a concern or not. All these irritate the skin, make acne more inflamed and red, and can trigger oil production at the base of your pores—this product is loaded with mostly the bad stuff.

☹ POOR **Refining Lotion** *($21 for 14 fl. oz.)* contains some good ingredients for all skin types, but is ultimately a lackluster, dated formula that contains enough witch hazel to cause irritation. See the Appendix to learn how irritation hurts everyone's skin.

MERLE NORMAN EXFOLIANTS & SCRUBS

☺ GOOD **$$$ AHA Intensive Complex** *($46 for 1 fl. oz.)* contains fruit extracts and it's a good thing the fruit extracts aren't front and center in this AHA gel. First of all, they don't work like AHAs, and, second, they can be needlessly irritating. As it turns out, this contains an efficacious amount of time-tested AHA lactic acid, and the pH of 3.6 allows it to exfoliate. The texture is beautifully silky and it sets to a smooth matte finish, making this ideal under makeup or for pairing with a moisturizer. Although it's pricey, it is a well-formulated AHA product and one of the better options from Merle Norman. Of course, this is easily replaced by less expensive versions that leave out the irritating plant extracts. An example would be Paula's Choice Skin Perfecting 8% AHA Gel, which provides three times as much product for half the price.

☺ GOOD **$$$ Gentle Polish** *($26 for 4 fl. oz.)* is a gentle, silky, and emollient facial scrub that's best for dry skin. The emollients and mineral oil make this somewhat difficult to rinse without the aid of a washcloth, and, of course, you can skip a scrub altogether and just use a washcloth with your favorite facial cleanser. However, for those with dry skin who prefer scrubs, this is a good option.

☺ AVERAGE $$$ **Micro-Refiner** *($48 for 2.5 fl. oz.)*. This very expensive, fairly abrasive scrub claims to be a great at-home alternative to microdermabrasion treatments. Those treatments aren't as impressive as once thought, and in many cosmetic dermatology practices they've been replaced by laser and other light-emitting treatments. Despite the statistics quoted in the claims, this ends up being a tricky scrub to use because the amount of silicones impedes rinsing. Silicones are difficult to rinse with water and you don't want to leave the scrub particles on your skin. All told, this scrub is easily replaced by a washcloth or any of the facial scrubs we recommend that are sold at the drugstore.

☹ AVERAGE $$$ **Polished Perfection Facial Scrub** *($21 for 4 fl. oz.)* is a fragranced scrub that attempts to polish skin with ground apricot and jojoba seeds. The gel formula lathers slightly, but the abrasive agents aren't buffered enough to ensure gentleness and effectiveness. This rinses easily, but you're better off using a less expensive scrub whose abrasive agent is rounded polyethylene beads so that it is less damaging to skin.

☻ POOR **Derma-Peel System** *($58 for 3 fl. oz.)* is a two-step system that consists of an AHA peel followed by a neutralizer to stop the action of the peel. The **Glycolic Peel Treatment** contains approximately 10% glycolic acid, but the base formula is mostly alcohol, which makes it too drying and irritating for all skin types. In addition, the alcohol causes free-radical damage that weakens collagen. The **Neutralizer** contains mostly water, slip agents, and preservative. You don't need a product like this to stop the action of an AHA peel—rinsing with plain tap water does the same thing, and, as mentioned, water is the main ingredient in this superfluous product.

MERLE NORMAN MOISTURIZERS (DAYTIME & NIGHTTIME), EYE CREAMS, & SERUMS

☺ GOOD $$$ **Brilliant-C Brightening Serum** *($48 for 1 fl. oz.)* is a fairly standard, but good, silicone-based serum. It contains an impressive amount of vitamin C (listed as ascorbyl glucoside), but there is little research pertaining to this ingredient's ability to lighten skin. In contrast, other forms of vitamin C (such as magnesium ascorbyl phosphate or L-ascorbic acid) have a considerable amount of research in this regard (Sources: *Journal of Cutaneous Medicine and Surgery*, March-April 2009, pages 74–81; *Phytotherapy Research*, November 2006, pages 921–934; and *International Journal of Dermatology*, August 2004, pages 604–607). Still, like all forms of vitamin C, ascorbyl glucoside functions as an antioxidant, and Merle Norman included a smattering of other antioxidants, too. The amount of cell-communicating peptides and skin-identical ingredients are on the low side but still worthwhile, making this a good serum for all skin types except sensitive. It contains fragrance and cosmetic pigments that lend a shiny finish to skin.

☺ GOOD $$$ **Fine Line Minimizer** *($46 for 1 fl. oz.)* is a slightly thick, silicone-based serum that can serve as a type of soft spackle for superficial lines and wrinkles. It has the requisite silky texture and the formula includes some proven antioxidants and a skin-identical ceramide. Overall, this is a fairly impressive product, although you can find even more impressive serums for less money from brands such as Olay, Good Skin, and Paula's Choice.

☹ AVERAGE $$$ **Anti-Redness Cream** *($46 for 2 fl. oz.)*. There are so many things about this moisturizer to extol it is hard to know where to begin. Primarily, its strengths are a truly remarkable array of antioxidants, anti-irritants, and skin-repairing ingredients, and a particularly impressive blend of ceramides. It also has a beautiful emollient base that would work wonderfully for someone with dry, sensitive skin. So what went wrong? Unfortunately, all this potential and praise is wasted because Merle Norman, like numerous cosmetics companies, can't give up their reliance on jar packaging despite the abundant research showing how problematic it is for any skin-care product. Jar packaging won't keep the wonderful, beneficial ingredients in this formulation stable once it is opened (see the Appendix for details). Another drawback is the amount of preservative in this formula because it is higher up on the ingredient list than the good stuff. It really should be the other way around. So close, yet still so far.

☺ AVERAGE $$$ **Daily Moisture Cream** *($46 for 2 fl. oz.)*. Given sunscreen is the single most important product you need to use during the day, this product's lack of sunscreen means it should only be a consideration for nighttime use. You could use it during the day if you added a sunscreen or foundation with sunscreen over it but then the question becomes, is it worth it to use two products when you only really need one? On many levels, this would be more than worth it if you have dry skin but, even better, you could use it at night. It is a beautiful formulation with numerous skin-repairing ingredients, water-binding agents, antioxidants, and cell-communicating ingredients. Unfortunately this level of excellence is wasted because of jar packaging (see the Appendix for details).

☹ AVERAGE **Day Creme with HC-12** *($28 for 2 fl. oz.)* isn't the best for daytime use due to its lack of sunscreen. It contains the sunscreen ingredient octyl methoxycinnamate, but because it's not listed as active and because this product does not have an SPF rating, you should not rely on it for daytime use. Otherwise, this is a fairly mundane formula that contains enough wax and plant oils to clog pores. It also contains some plant extracts that can be irritating, making it one of Merle Norman's less desirable moisturizers. The HC-12 in the name refers to the blend of hydrating ingredients—it isn't a special blend that makes it any better than any other moisturizer, including the dozens of others Merle Norman sells and those with far better formulations from other lines.

☹ AVERAGE **Delicate Balance Moisturizer for Sensitive Skin** *($42 for 2 fl. oz.)* is an OK creamy moisturizer for normal to dry skin. The fragrance-free formula contains anti-irritants that can benefit sensitive skin, but lots of other moisturizers offer similar benefit. What's disappointing is many of the skin-identical ingredients that all skin types need are listed after the preservative, which means you're not getting all that much of the good stuff.

☹ AVERAGE $$$ **Intensive Moisturizer** *($38 for 1 fl. oz.)*. The only thing intensive about this moisturizer is its name. This mineral oil–based cream is an antiquated mix of lanolin, waxes, and perfume in a completely ordinary formula that would be suitable for dehydrated skin but your skin deserves so much more than suitability. Using this to take care of your skin would be like using a rotary telephone instead of a cell phone to make a call. We would typically warn you about any skin-care product packaged in a jar container being a problem (see Appendix for details), but because this formula doesn't contain anything even resembling state-of-the-art ingredients, you don't need to worry about that issue. Given this product's extreme shortcomings, including too much fragrance, this is really overpriced for what you get.

☹ AVERAGE **Moisture Emulsion** *($18 for 3 fl. oz.)* is a very dated moisturizer for dry skin that contains mostly mineral oil and lanolin. That's not saying much, and those with dry skin should know they can do a lot better than this product!

☹ AVERAGE **Moisture Lotion** *($13 for 3 fl. oz.)* is a lighter version of Merle Norman's Moisture Emulsion above, and the same review applies.

☹ AVERAGE **Preventage Firming Defense Creme Normal/Dry SPF 15** *($45 for 2 fl. oz.)* is a relatively rich moisturizer with sunscreen that includes titanium dioxide for reliable UVA protection. It has merit for dry skin, but what a shame the jar packaging won't keep the numerous antioxidants and soothing plant extracts stable during use (see the Appendix for details). In better packaging, this fragrance-free moisturizer with sunscreen would earn a Best Product rating.

☺ AVERAGE **Preventage Firming Defense Creme Normal/Oily SPF 15** *($45 for 2 fl. oz.)* is a fragrance-free daytime moisturizer with an in-part titanium dioxide sunscreen that has a soft, silky texture best for normal to slightly dry or slightly oily skin. Regrettably, there are some formula issues, plus the fact that the numerous antioxidants will degrade during use thanks to the jar packaging. The amount of witch hazel distillate is cause for concern because of its alcohol content. It's less of an issue because of the emollients that precede it on the list, but it doesn't help earn this product a better rating, for those who want to mitigate the signs of aging and reduce irritation.

☺ AVERAGE $$$ **Age-Defying Serum** *($55 for 1 fl. oz.)* is a water-based serum that contains some notable antioxidants and cell-communicating ingredients; however, its texture isn't nearly as elegant as that of many other serums available from other lines. The combination of gum-based thickener and slightly tacky slip agents doesn't measure up to the supreme silkiness of today's best serums. Ultimately, this is a tough serum to recommend because it contains potentially problematic comfrey root extract (listed by its Latin name *Symphytum officinale*) and the sensitizing preservative methylisothiazolinone. The preservative is fine for use in rinse-off products, but generally is not recommended for leave-on products such as this serum.

☺ AVERAGE $$$ **Brilliant-C Neck and Chest Cream** *($46 for 2 fl. oz.)* contains far more fragrance than state-of-the-art ingredients, and what little of those are included will degrade due to the jar packaging (see the Appendix for details). Also, the neck and chest don't need specialized products or ingredients that skin elsewhere on the body doesn't also need, so a product like this is superfluous.

☺ AVERAGE $$$ **Changing Skin Eye Complex** *($29 for 0.5 fl. oz.)* contains soy, clover and wild yam, which are not the antidotes to the changes that menopause has on a woman's skin. In fact, there is no research showing that wild yam has a noticeable effect when applied topically on skin. If anything, the research demonstrates topical application of wild yam has little to no effect on menopausal symptoms (Source: *Climacteric*, June 2001, pages 144–150). More recent studies are scarce because the conclusions reached in earlier research were solid. The research concerning soy's potential benefit pre- and post-menopause examined oral consumption, not topical application (Source: naturaldatabase.com). Even if these plants or any other ingredients in this eye cream were effective at treating skin changes resulting from menopause, their effectiveness would begin diminishing as soon as you opened this jar packaging; the air-sensitive ingredients would begin breaking down and wouldn't remain effective. In better packaging, this would be a very good moisturizer for dry skin anywhere on the face. The amount of zinc oxide in this eye cream has a subtle cosmetic whitening effect around the eyes, but nothing in this eye cream is capable of lifting skin as claimed. See the Appendix to find out why products claiming to lift sagging skin cannot work.

☺ AVERAGE $$$ **Changing Skin Night Creme** *($46 for 2 fl. oz.)* has a silkier, lighter texture than Merle Norman's Changing Skin Eye Complex above. Otherwise, the two products are quite similar, so the same basic comments apply. This contains fragrance in the form of ethylene brassylate, so it is not safe for sensitive skin, despite the company's claims.

☺ AVERAGE $$$ **Energizing Concentrate** *($44 for 1 fl. oz.)* is a water-based serum that isn't all that exciting, unless you believe ginseng is an energizing must-have for skin. For the record, ginseng is an intriguing ingredient when taken orally, but it isn't particularly wonderful used topically. Obviously, even Merle Norman doesn't think it's that great an ingredient; otherwise, they'd include it in their other products as well. This serum contains some good skin-identical ingredients and soy for an antioxidant boost, but the overall mix of ingredients isn't the best formula for minimizing signs of aging; it takes a broader cocktail of ingredients (and daily application of sunscreen) to assemble a smart anti-aging skin-care routine.

☺ AVERAGE **$$$ Nighttime Recovery Creme** *($46 for 2 fl. oz.)* comes in jar packaging, which is the Achilles' heel of this otherwise beautifully formulated moisturizer for dry to very dry skin. The emollient-rich formula is loaded with beneficial ingredients for skin, but almost all of them won't retain their potency with repeated exposure to light and air, plus there's the hygiene issue of routinely sticking your fingers into a jar. In better packaging, this moisturizer would unquestionably rate a Best Product, but, as is, you're not getting your money's worth.

☺ AVERAGE **$$$ Wrinkle Smoother** *($48 for 2.25 fl. oz.)* is positioned as one of Merle Norman's best-selling products, which means lots of their customers are walking away with a poorly formulated, badly packaged product. This fragrance-free moisturizer has a lovely silky texture for normal to dry skin and, like most moisturizers of its kind, can make wrinkles appear smoother. The effect is temporary, which is why you need to keep using moisturizer, but it's really disappointing that the most helpful ingredients are squandered due to the jar packaging, which won't keep the best ingredients in here stable after opening (see the Appendix for details). In addition, there is no substantiated research that the peptide in this moisturizer inhibits muscles that lead to expression lines, so this is not a viable alternative to Botox when it comes to reducing wrinkles. Actually, when you think about it, if the muscle-relaxing peptide worked as claimed, it would affect muscles anywhere you applied it. The result, when applied all over the face, would be sagging, droopy skin and the inability to do things like talk and chew food.

☺ AVERAGE **$$$ Wrinkle Smoother Eye** *($30 for 0.5 fl. oz.)* is very similar to Merle Norman's Wrinkle Smoother above, other than containing less silicone. See the Appendix to find out why, in truth, you don't need an eye cream.

☺ AVERAGE **$$$ Wrinkle Smoother Lift & Firm Serum** *($55 for 1 fl. oz.)* is a water-based serum that gets its tightening effect from a high amount of tapioca starch. The starch and lightweight texture of this serum provide a cosmetic tightening effect, but it absolutely cannot lift sagging skin (refer to the Appendix for an explanation) and it can be drying in the long run. As for its alleged Botox-like effects (it's said to reduce the appearance of deep lines caused by facial movement, which is what Botox addresses beautifully), don't count on it. The peptides can be helpful ingredients for all skin types, but they cannot affect muscles beneath the skin that lead to expression lines. If they could, wouldn't your fingers be affected, too? After all, you're using them to apply this serum, right? Although this product does contain some very good ingredients, it contains far more preservative than anything else, which doesn't bode well for your skin.

☹ POOR **Brilliant-C Eye Cream** *($30 for 5 fl. oz.)* is a very disappointing eye cream because the bulk of the formula is water, thickener, and alcohol. The alcohol causes irritation and free-radical damage, which isn't the way to reduce wrinkles anywhere on the face or on the body. What a shame, because this eye cream also contains a broad range of truly beneficial ingredients. Regrettably, the amount of alcohol negates their effectiveness, but more important, you don't need an eye cream (see the Appendix to find out why).

☹ POOR **Brilliant-C Moisturizer** *($46 for 2 fl. oz.)* is very similar to the Brilliant-C Eye Cream above, and the same review applies. The brightening effect you get with this moisturizer comes from mineral pigments that add a subtle sheen and white cast to your skin.

☹ POOR **Matte Oil-Free Moisturizer** *($35 for 2 fl. oz.)* isn't really oil-free as claimed due to the isohexadecane it contains. Despite the way this product is described on the container, it is at best minimally hydrating, and we mean really, really minimally. Along with the silicones in here, which provide a great deal of slip and a silky texture, are absorbent ingredients including nylon-12 and aluminum starch octenylsuccinate, each of that contributes to this product's matte finish. What this blend of silicones and absorbent powders impart is a layer of oil-absorbing ingredients that work more like a basic primer that can be used under foundation if you have oily skin. How long the oil-absorbing properties last on your skin depends on how oily your skin is and the type of other products you are using with it. The claim that this contains optical diffusers that can minimize the appearance of pores is a fancy way to say it leaves an opaque layer over the skin that has some coverage. There are no special diffusing ingredients in here. There are a couple of ingredient concerns: This contains an extract of cinnamon that does have antioxidant properties, but it can also be a skin irritant; it is far better for skin to have a great topical antioxidant that doesn't impart any irritation. This also contains the preservative methylisothiazolinone, which is not the best in a leave-on product. Although this could be an option as an oil-absorbing primer, because it lacks any other beneficial ingredients for skin such as antioxidants or skin-repairing ingredients, it isn't really worth your time or money.

☹ POOR **Revitalizing Eye Gel** *($22 for 0.5 fl. oz.)* is a fragrance-free offering containing astringent witch hazel for its refreshing properties. Unfortunately, this amount of witch hazel is capable of causing irritation due to its tannin and alcohol content. The film-forming agent (think hairspray) and fast-drying formula will make your skin look and feel temporarily smoother and tighter, but overall that benefit isn't worth the risk of daily irritation. This also contains a couple of plant extracts that are a problem for all skin types, which is a shame because lots of helpful ingredients are also part of the formula, although none of them are proven to reduce puffy eyes or under-eye bags. Such problems almost always must be corrected with cosmetic surgery, not with skin-care products.

MERLE NORMAN SUN CARE

☺ GOOD **$$$ SunSense Tinted Self-Tanner** *($22 for 4.2 fl. oz.)* is a very good, silky self-tanning lotion suitable for all skin types except sensitive. (The fragrance this contains isn't the best for those with sensitive skin.) True to claim, this dries quickly without feeling tacky, and the formula is oil-free. It is tinted with melanin and iron oxides so you can see where you've applied it and enjoy an instant sun-kissed appearance as you wait for your "tan" to develop.

☹ POOR **Dual Spectrum SPF 30** *($22 for 4.2 fl. oz.)* is a good in-part avobenzone sunscreen that supplies broad-spectrum protection. The claim of this being gentle enough for "even the most sensitive skin" is completely off base, however, because all the active ingredients have sensitizing potential. That doesn't make them bad ingredients, but they're definitely not what someone with sensitive skin should be applying; instead, they should be applying a sunscreen whose sole actives are titanium dioxide and/or zinc oxide. Despite the broad-spectrum sun protection and the inclusion of several antioxidants, this sunscreen is not recommended because it contains a sensitizing preservative (methylisothiazolinone), which is not recommended for use in leave-on products—just one more reason why this sunscreen is inappropriate for anyone with sensitive skin.

MERLE NORMAN LIP & SMILE CARE

✓☺ BEST **$$$ Lip Revive** *($20 for 0.5 fl. oz.)* is a very good, unusually silky lip balm that does double duty by smoothing and helping to fill in lines on lips and around the mouth. As one of Merle Norman's most intriguing products, it deserves strong consideration by those looking to prime their lips for better results from lipliner and/or lipstick. Emollient, moisturizing ingredients aren't front and center in this lip balm, but there are enough on board that you should be fine unless your lips are markedly chapped, in which case you can apply a more emollient lip balm at night. Lip Revive is fragrance-free, too!

MERLE NORMAN SPECIALTY SKIN-CARE PRODUCTS

☺ GOOD $$$ **Clarifying Clay Mask** *($22 for 3.4 fl. oz.)* is a good, basic clay mask for normal to oily skin. The relatively high amount of titanium dioxide is a bit of a concern because this ingredient tends to be occlusive on blemish-prone skin and it doesn't rinse easily. Still, this deserves credit for omitting needless irritants, such as menthol, and for adding some helpful anti-irritants and antioxidants.

☺ GOOD $$$ **Wrinkle Smoother Lips** *($28 for 0.30 oz.)* is designed for use on lips and around the mouth, with the objective being to soften lines and prevent lipstick from traveling into them. Does it succeed? Partially. The spackle-like, thick yet silky texture temporarily smoothes and fills in superficial lines on the lips and around the mouth—but how long the effect lasts depends on what you've applied beforehand and how often you move your mouth. Most will see some benefit from this product, and its fragrance-free formula contains a smattering of beneficial ingredients. The peptide referred to in the claims cannot prevent the appearance of expression lines. It is often said to work like Botox (Merle Norman isn't stating this, but other companies have) by stopping the impulses that causes muscles beneath skin to contract, which over time leads to fewer expression lines. However, if this peptide could do that, you wouldn't want to apply it around your mouth. Think about what would happen if it affected muscles around the mouth: you'd have trouble keeping your mouth closed, might not be able to smile, and drooling could become an unattractive daily issue. Wrinkle Smoother Lips is worth trying to see how it works for your lines—and it's great this is fragrance-free.

☺ AVERAGE $$$ **Clear Complexion Moisturizer Acne Treatment Cream** *($28 for 2 fl. oz.)*. With just a few changes, this BHA exfoliant for acne-prone skin would be a winner. In the pro column is a 2% concentration of salicylic acid; an effective pH of 3.5 so the active ingredient will work as claimed; and a lightweight, silky lotion base suitable for all skin types. The cons include some potentially irritating ingredients such as grapefruit and orange extract and various parts of the witch hazel plant. Without the potential irritants, this would have easily earned a better rating. Those looking for a fragrance-free alternative that is more cost effective and free of needless irritants should consider Paula's Choice CLEAR exfoliant with BHA.

☺ AVERAGE $$$ **Renew** *($42 for 1 fl. oz.)*. This pseudo-exfoliant claims to boost skin's natural exfoliation while promoting an even skin tone and reducing the appearance of pores. It does have a skin-smoothing texture, but it lacks a significant amount of ingredients that promote exfoliation. Glucosamine, as acetyl glucosamine, can help this process along, but the hydrochloride form (which this product contains) is a pH adjuster (Sources: cosmeticsinfo.org; and *Journal of Cosmetic Science*, July-August 2009, pages 423–428), so the formulation won't help your skin. The type of urea in this product makes it a good moisturizing ingredient, but it's not anything the skin has to have. In the end, this specialty product works best to improve skin texture for normal to dry skin, but it doesn't contain the broad array of ingredients needed to achieve a beautiful complexion.

☹ POOR **Clear Complexion Spot Treatment** *($20 for 0.5 fl. oz.)* is medicated with 2% salicylic acid, but the base formula contains the potent irritants alcohol and witch hazel, each in amounts that will wreak havoc on acne-prone skin. The irritants also can trigger oil production at the base of your pores, leading to worse breakouts and persistent redness—in other words, the opposite of a clear complexion.

☹ POOR **Moisture Rich Facial Treatment** *($22 for 3 fl. oz.)* is a moisturizing mask that contains a wealth of helpful ingredients, but isn't recommended even for brief use because it contains the irritating menthol derivative menthyl lactate, and irritation is always a problem for skin. How disappointing—talk about one bad apple spoiling the whole barrel! This would definitely be a top pick if it did not contain the menthol derivative.

MURAD

Strengths: A few good water-soluble cleansers; a selection of well-formulated AHA products centered on glycolic acid; most of Murad's top-rated products are fragrance-free; the sunscreens go beyond the basics and include several antioxidants for enhanced protection.

Weaknesses: Expensive; no other dermatologist-designed line has more problem products than Murad; irritating ingredients are peppered throughout the selection of products, keeping several of them from earning a recommendation.

For more information and reviews of the latest Murad products, visit CosmeticsCop.com.

MURAD CLEANSERS

☺ GOOD $$$ **AHA/BHA Exfoliating Cleanser** *($35 for 6.75 fl. oz.)* is a good cleanser/ scrub hybrid that contains rounded jojoba beads. The jojoba beads are what exfoliate skin; the AHAs and BHA will not exfoliate because this cleanser is rinsed from the skin before they can be of much benefit, not to mention there's very little of those ingredients in this cleanser.

☺ GOOD $$$ **Renewing Cleansing Cream** *($35 for 6.75 fl. oz.)* happens to be a very good, though still needlessly expensive, cleanser for those with normal to dry skin. It foams slightly and rinses better than you'd think (it contains oils). This contains fragrance and some fragrance ingredients, but their presence is minor and unlikely to be a problem, though use caution when applying this around the eyes.

☺ GOOD $$$ **Refreshing Cleanser** *($29.50 for 6.75 fl. oz.)* is a very standard, but good, water-soluble cleanser for normal to oily skin. The amount of glycolic acid will not function as an exfoliant. This contains fragrance and fragrant plant extracts along with irritant witch hazel, but the amounts used and the fact that this product is designed to be rinsed from skin poses little risk.

☹ AVERAGE $$$ **Energizing Pomegranate Cleanser** *($26 for 5.1 fl. oz.)* is an OK water-soluble cleanser for normal to slightly dry skin. The formula contains small amounts of several questionable ingredients, including witch hazel water, alcohol, and fragrance ingredients known to cause irritation. The antioxidants and minerals are there for show because in order for these ingredients to benefit your skin, they need to be left on rather than rinsed off. Considering the problems this cleanser poses and its high price, there's little reason to consider it over less expensive, better-formulated cleansers at the drugstore.

☹ POOR **Clarifying Cleanser** *($26 for 6.75 fl. oz.)* contains essential oils that have anti-bacterial properties, but they're also very irritating. In addition to the lemon, orange, and lime oils, this irritation-waiting-to-happen cleanser contains menthol. Steer clear!

☹ POOR **Essential-C Cleanser** *($35 for 6.75 fl. oz.)* states it is designed to soothe environmentally stressed skin, but the orange, basil, and grapefruit peel oils do just the opposite, making this a nonessential cleanser. See the Appendix to learn how irritation hurts everyone's skin.

☹ POOR **Soothing Gel Cleanser** *($25 for 6.75 fl. oz.)* irritates rather than soothes due to the number of volatile fragrant oils, along with the potent menthol derivative menthoxy-propanediol. Murad sells this as their redness-relieving cleanser, which is unbelievable. See the Appendix to learn how irritation hurts everyone's skin.

☹ POOR **Time Release Acne Cleanser** *($30 for 6.75 fl. oz.)* had the makings of a very good cleanser for normal to oily skin. It's a cross between a cleansing gel and a lotion, and is capable of removing makeup along with excess surface oil, just like many other less expensive cleansers. The key anti-acne "selling point" for this cleanser is the claim that it kills bacteria on contact and uses a time-release technology to deliver acne medication to the skin for hours. However, there is no acne medication anywhere on the ingredient list listed as active (which would be required according to FDA regulations) or inactive. There is nothing unique about this product except for the claim. This cleanser's only antibacterial ingredient is zinc gluconate, and there isn't any published research indicating that it kills acne-causing bacteria when applied topically. (It does seem to have some effect when consumed orally, but the dosage must be carefully controlled to avoid toxicity.) Topically, zinc gluconate appears to have an anti-inflammatory effect, which is helpful. Even if this were an antibacterial powerhouse against acne, its benefit would be rinsed down the drain because this is not a leave-on product. In this case, you're asked to take Murad's word for it, but don't, research does not support the claims (Sources: *European Journal of Dermatology*, May-June 2005, pages 152–155; and *Dermatology*, volume 203, 2001, pages 135–140). The rinsing aspect also applies to the retinol in this product. Although without question this vitamin A ingredient can be advantageous for those struggling with acne, in a cleanser it won't stay stable and water breaks it down (think rinsing), so what a waste! What you end up getting for a lot of money is a whole lot of ordinary cleanser with menthol thrown in to add irritation into the mix.

MURAD TONERS

☺ AVERAGE **$$$ Hydrating Toner** *($24 for 6 fl. oz.)* offers skin some helpful water-binding agents, but the amount of witch hazel is potentially problematic and keeps this otherwise well-done toner for normal to dry skin from earning a higher rating.

☹ POOR **Clarifying Toner** *($22 for 6 fl. oz.)* lists witch hazel as the second ingredient and also contains menthol and its derivative, menthoxypropanediol. The citronella oil doesn't help matters, and certainly isn't clarifying. See the Appendix to learn why irritating ingredients are bad for everyone's skin.

☹ POOR **Essential-C Toner** *($26 for 6 fl. oz.)* contains a lot of witch hazel and lesser, but still problematic, amounts of citrus and basil oils. This will not balance stressed skin!

MURAD EXFOLIANTS & SCRUBS

☺ GOOD **$$$ Intensive Wrinkle Reducer for Eyes** *($90 for 0.5 fl. oz.)* is a viable option if you're looking for a pH-correct AHA product with approximately 3%-5% glycolic acid. There isn't anything about this formula that makes it a specialized treatment for eye-area skin; it's suitable for normal to dry skin anywhere on the face (see the Appendix to learn why you don't need an eye cream). What's disappointing, especially for this amount of money, is that other than the glycolic acid (which can be found in dozens of products that cost much less), the other state-of-the-art ingredients are barely present—and there are a lot of them. We suppose the tiny amounts of each antioxidant and cell-communicating ingredient might add up to provide some benefit for skin, but at this price you should expect a lot more. Apparently, this product is supposed to be worth it because it contains Dr. Murad's anti-aging Durian Cell Reform, which they claim reverses signs of aging. Durian is a tropical fruit that research has shown to be a potent antioxidant when consumed orally. It contains high levels of antioxidants such as caffeic acid and quercetin, and likely has topical benefit as well, though this hasn't been proven (Sources: *Food and Chemical Toxicology*, February 2008, pages 581–589; and *Journal of Agricultural and Food Chemistry*, July 2007, pages 5842–5849). However, there isn't a shred of published research (including from Murad himself) that demonstrates durian fruit has a pronounced effect on skin wrinkles or firmness. Plus, there are other products that contain the active ingredients in durian and that would be far more effective in protecting skin.

☺ GOOD $$$ **Intensive Wrinkle Reducer** *($150 for 1 fl. oz.)* may be one of the most expensive AHA products around, though it's definitely an effective one, containing at least 10% glycolic acid in a gel base with a pH of 3.2. The formula also contains several outstanding water-binding agents and plenty of antioxidants along with some good anti-irritants. It's a suitable option for all skin types, but you don't need to spend this much money to enjoy the benefits of AHAs. This product did not rate higher because it contains cinnamon bark extract and fragrant components that can be irritating to skin. Cinnamon has antioxidant ability, but its irritation potential when applied topically doesn't help move this product to the top of the must-have list.

☺ GOOD $$$ **Intensive Resurfacing Peel** *($45 for 4 treatments).* You're not getting much product for your money, but housed in each of these tiny vials is a water-based exfoliant serum whose blend of glycolic and salicylic acids is, according to a representative from Murad, between 3% and 5%. Given the pH of 2.8, it definitely will exfoliate skin. The issue is that the 4% glycolic acid (AHA) and the approximately 1% salicylic acid (BHA) it contains are not "intensive" in the least. A 10% concentration of glycolic acid would have been more "intensive." In addition, a pH of 3.5 would have been adequate (and is within the pH range recommended for AHA products by the FDA), and without the extra irritation that results from a product with a pH of less than 3. Either way, the amount of AHA and BHA Murad used isn't akin to what they use in an in-office AHA peel (where concentrations of glycolic acid typically range from 20% to 40%). The bamboo extract in this product provides mild mechanical exfoliation as you wash this product away, but you could easily get the same mechanical exfoliation using a washcloth. This ends up being an effective AHA option that is needlessly expensive and not a substitute for the peels a doctor can perform.

☺ GOOD $$$ **Rejuvenating Lift for Neck and Décolleté** *($55 for 1.7 fl. oz.).* Even though you absolutely do not need separate skin-care products for your neck and chest (the same products you use on your face, assuming those are well formulated, can be applied to the neck and chest, too), this is an effective AHA moisturizer for normal to oily skin. The pH of 3.5 ensures the AHA glycolic acid (the amount isn't listed by Murad but based on the ingredient list it's probably 10%-12%) will function as an exfoliant, but you don't need to spend this much for an effective AHA exfoliant. Should you decide to purchase this product, it's good to know that Murad includes a helpful range of antioxidants, though the formula would be better without the fragrance ingredients of limonene and linalool, as both are known irritants (though the amounts in this product are minimal). One more comment: Despite the claims, this neck and chest product cannot lift sagging skin. It just isn't possible from skin-care products, though this, like any well-formulated AHA exfoliant, will help firm skin, smooth texture, and improve signs of sun damage.

☹ POOR **Complete Reform** *($67 for 1 fl. oz.)* is an AHA product containing approximately 10% glycolic acid and it's pH is within the range needed for exfoliation to occur. The formula also contains some anti-irritants and several antioxidants, including some that you don't often see in skin-care products. All this is what you want from a well-formulated AHA product, so why the Poor rating? Lavender oil. It's a problem for all skin types, and you can find out why in the Appendix.

☹ POOR **Gaga for Glow Facial Scrub** *($20 for 2.5 fl. oz.)* is more a cleanser than a scrub (it contains a small amount of polyethylene beads). The main cleansing agent, sodium C14-16 olefin sulfonate, is too drying and irritating for all skin types. Those with oily skin should know that drying products like this can trigger excess oil production at the base of the pores, leading to skin that is more oily rather than less.

MURAD MOISTURIZERS (DAYTIME & NIGHTTIME), EYE CREAMS, & SERUMS

✓☺ BEST $$$ **Time Release Retinol Concentrate for Deep Wrinkles** *($65 for 0.5 fl. oz.)* is a very good, fragrance-free moisturizer with retinol. The opaque tube packaging works to keep it stable during use, and the silicone-tip applicator is designed so you can easily target deep wrinkles. Despite this, it must be said that retinol and the other anti-aging ingredients this contains can only do so much for deep wrinkles. For example, using this won't replace or surpass what dermal injections like Botox can do. However, retinol definitely works to improve wrinkles and other signs of aging. It's great that Murad included a range of beneficial ingredients, so this isn't a one-note product. The repairing ingredients and antioxidants help boost collagen production and the formula is suitable for all skin types, including sensitive. This contains mineral pigments (mica and titanium dioxide) that have a subtle brightening effect. You can find less expensive moisturizers and serums with retinol, but if you choose to go with Murad, this is a well formulated option.

☺ GOOD **Down for Defense SPF 15 Moisturizer** *($24 for 1.7 fl. oz.)*. With the exception of the potentially irritating mix of fragrance ingredients, this daytime moisturizer with sunscreen is a good option for those with normal to slightly dry or slightly oily skin. UVA protection is provided by avobenzone and the lightweight lotion texture moisturizes without feeling thick or greasy. Murad included an impressive blend of antioxidants and water-binding agents, too. Those looking for a fragrance-free alternative may want to consider Paula's Choice Skin Balancing Daily Mattifying Lotion with SPF 15 & Antioxidants.

☺ GOOD **Energizing Pomegranate Moisturizer SPF 15** *($33 for 2 fl. oz.)* contains an in-part avobenzone sunscreen in a lightweight lotion formula suitable for normal to slightly oily skin. Pomegranate is a very good antioxidant; it's a shame there isn't more of it in here. Still, this is one of the few Murad products not waylaid by needless irritants, and it contains some effective soothing agents. It does contain fragrance.

☺ GOOD $$$ **Anti-Aging Moisturizer SPF 20/PA++ for Blemish-Prone Skin** *($46 for 1.7 fl. oz.)* is a daytime moisturizer with sunscreen that includes avobenzone for sufficient UVA protection and has a fairly light texture that's suitable for normal to slightly dry or slightly oily skin. The question of whether or not it can control acne is simply answered with a resounding "No!" This product does earn its anti-aging stripes thanks to broad-spectrum sun protection and the inclusion of retinol, vitamin C, and other beneficial ingredients, but nothing in this product has the ability to significantly control acne. Retinol can help to some degree by normalizing healthy cell production, but retinol alone doesn't address the bacterial component of acne. It doesn't exfoliate inside the pore lining and it cannot impact how much oil your skin produces. Also a problem is that this daytime moisturizer's texture is created by thickening agents that, while not bad ingredients, aren't the best for someone with oily, acne-prone skin. That said, this is still worth considering for its sun protection and broad complement of helpful ingredients that can improve signs of aging. If you're looking to spend less for an equally effective formula, consider Paula's Choice Skin Balancing Daily Mattifying Lotion with SPF 15 & Antioxidants.

☺ GOOD **$$$ Essential-C Day Moisture SPF 30/PA+++** *($60 for 1.7 fl. oz.)* is a daytime moisturizer with an in-part titanium dioxide sunscreen that is a very good option for normal to dry skin. Although not as impressive as some less expensive options from department store brands, this sits nicely in the Good rating column thanks to its lightweight lotion formula that contains several antioxidants and some good skin-identical ingredients. It is not rated higher because it contains a small amount of fragrance ingredients known to cause irritation.

☺ GOOD **$$$ Essential-C Eye Cream SPF 15/PA++** *($67 for 0.5 fl. oz.)* includes avo-benzone for reliable UVA protection. Although that's good news, the avobenzone and other synthetic sunscreen actives can be problematic when used near the eyes, which is exactly how this product is supposed to be applied. Of course, not everyone's eye-area skin will react negatively to these sunscreen actives, but if you notice any stinging, burning, or redness, discontinue use and consider a mineral-based moisturizer or concealer with sunscreen (it need not be labeled "eye cream"; see the Appendix to find out why you don't need an eye cream). If your eye-area skin can tolerate the sunscreens in this product, it's a good, lightweight eye cream for slightly dry skin.

☺ GOOD **$$$ Oil-Control Mattifier SPF 15** *($39.50 for 1.7 fl. oz.)*. Were it not for a small amount of potentially irritating cinnamon bark extract, this daytime moisturizer with an in-part zinc oxide sunscreen would rate a Best Product. The sun protection is broad-spectrum and the matte-finish base formula is excellent for oily to very oily skin. What's more, the formula contains several antioxidants, including pomegranate, which is known to boost the efficacy of sunscreen actives. A small amount of cell-communicating niacinamide is included along with some anti-irritants, making this an overall well-rounded product that works beautifully under makeup.

☺ GOOD **$$$ Perfecting Serum** *($62 for 1 fl. oz.)* provides normal to very dry skin types with many of the ingredients needed to ensure a healthy barrier and allow skin to repair itself. It's a shame the clear glass bottle will compromise the effectiveness of the vitamin A and antioxidant-rich plant oils. However, the nonfragrant plant oils and lipids will make dry skin look and feel better. This is only recommended if you're willing to store it in a cool, dark place. Keeping the clear bottle away from light will help preserve the potency of the ingredients your skin needs to look and feel better.

☺ GOOD **$$$ Anti-Aging Moisturizer SPF 20/PA++ for Blemish-Prone Skin** *($46 for 1.7 fl. oz.)*. First, there's nothing special for blemish-prone skin in this daytime moisturizer. It provides broad-spectrum protection that includes avobenzone for reliable UVA screening, but it's lotion-like base formula isn't capable of controlling blemishes as claimed. At the very least, this isn't a one-stop solution for blemishes, nor is it an inherently better choice than other lightweight moisturizers with sunscreen. This contains a couple of ingredients with potential anti-acne benefits, but their efficacy pales when compared to gold standards such as salicylic acid (BHA) and benzoyl peroxide. Still, it's worth nothing that this product contains a formidable array of anti-aging ingredients, including retinol, vitamin C, and several antioxidants plus numerous water-binding agents. It would earn our top rating if it did not contain a tiny amount of fragrance ingredients known to cause irritation.

☹ AVERAGE **$$$ Sensitive Skin Soothing Serum** *($49.50 for 1 fl. oz.)* almost makes it as a Best Product. It contains some very good soothing agents, water-binding agents, and antioxidants. It misses the mark only due to the inclusion of ivy extract, arnica flower, and pellitory. None of these plant extracts are what is needed for sensitive skin or for decreasing irritation. They're not present in large amounts, but including them at all wasn't a wise choice. Although this is a risky proposition for someone with irritated, sensitive skin, its texture is suitable for normal to oily or breakout-prone skin.

☺ AVERAGE **Skin Perfecting Lotion** *($33 for 1.7 fl. oz.)* is a surprisingly affordable moisturizer with an impressive amount of retinol. This also contains plenty of antioxidants and some brilliant anti-irritants, though the arnica extract remains a concern and keeps this moisturizer for normal to dry skin from earning a Good rating. Applied topically to otherwise healthy, unbruised skin (arnica is often recommended for bruised areas), arnica can cause contact dermatitis. Its use in any form is not advised if you are pregnant, either (Source: naturaldatabase.com).

☺ AVERAGE $$$ **Hydro-Dynamic Ultimate Moisture** *($65 for 1.7 fl. oz.)* contains a broad assortment of brilliant ingredients that can help ease dryness while improving signs of aging. Unfortunately, the jar packaging means most of the beneficial ingredients won't remain stable after opening, so dry skin cannot take full advantage of this otherwise well-formulated product. See the Appendix for details on why jar packaging isn't the way to go.

☺ AVERAGE $$$ **Renewing Eye Cream** *($73 for 0.5 fl. oz.)* includes some good moisturizing ingredients for normal to dry skin, though none of them are capable of diminishing dark circles or puffiness. This eye cream contains cosmetic pigments that have a brightening effect on dark, shadowed areas, but that effect is strictly cosmetic—your dark circles will be as dark as ever once this is washed off. The amount of iris and clover extracts is potentially irritating, while the amount of the most intriguing (read: anti-aging) ingredients isn't as impressive as it could have been, especially for what Murad is charging. See the Appendix to learn why, in truth, you don't need an eye cream.

☹ AVERAGE **Active Radiance Serum** *($89 for 1 fl. oz.)*. The claims for this product are as disingenuous and as obnoxious as it gets. It is supposed to "Undo sun damage and erase a lifetime of summers," which it absolutely cannot do in any way, shape, or form. Ignoring the exaggeration and facade, this is merely a serum with a helpful amount of glycolic acid. Although research on that ingredient has shown it can help improve sun-damaged skin, it's hardly a panacea for a lifetime's worth of sun damage, anymore than eating broccoli is a cure for a lifetime's worth of smoking. As it turns out, the pH of this product is too high for the glycolic acid to exfoliate, which means you're pinning your hopes on Murad's vitamin C technology, said to deliver "50 times the free radical neutralizing power of prior generations." What prior generations is he referring to? Could it be his own products that contain vitamin C, which means they are no longer worthwhile for skin and he should stop selling them? Either way, there is no substantiated data proving the claims are true and, in fact, there isn't much vitamin C in this serum anyway, so it is an empty message for your skin. Where this serum really comes up short is in including two forms of menthol along with fragrance ingredients known to cause irritation, and that is skin-damaging, not healing (see the Appendix for details).

☹ POOR **Age-Diffusing Serum** *($72 for 1 fl. oz.)* has a lot going for it when you consider this water-based AHA serum's level of silicones, range of antioxidants, and several water-binding agents. Yet, like so many Murad products, too many irritating ingredients with no benefit for skin corrupt its good start. Clove flower and iris extracts are the prime offenders, and further down on the ingredient list, orange, lime, tangerine, and rosewood oils are joined by buchu leaf oil, which contains camphor as a major constituent. See the Appendix to learn why fragrant irritants are a big problem for everyone's skin.

☞ Did you know you don't need an eye cream? It's true! See the Appendix to find out why.

☹ POOR **Age-Balancing Night Cream** *($75 for 1.7 fl. oz.)*. Age Balancing? At what age does age become imbalanced? And, more to the point, can a moisturizer do anything to balance one's age? Of course not. This is another moisturizer with wild yam extract, directed toward those with peri-menopausal and menopausal skin. You might as well use the wild yams for your Thanksgiving feast because they have not been demonstrated to have any effectiveness when used on skin. Soy has estrogenic benefits when eaten, but not from topical application (though it is a very good antioxidant). It's a good thing this is advised for nighttime use—applied during daylight hours, the lime oil in here can cause a phototoxic reaction when skin is exposed to sunlight.

☹ POOR **Begging for Balance Moisturizer** *($22 for 1.7 fl. oz.)* is a standard lightweight moisturizer with a soft matte finish that feels slightly moist. It cannot "shut down shine" as claimed because that would mean your oil glands would stop producing oil, a physiologic activity that cannot be controlled by skin-care products. At best, this can help keep excess shine at bay for a short period of time; how long it lasts depends on how much oil your skin produces. Ideally, those with oily skin who wish to use a moisturizer to get the beneficial ingredients that all skin types need should consider getting those ingredients from a gel or liquid product rather than from a lotion because the ingredients that create a lotion don't work for very oily skin. What about the salicylic acid this product contains? Although it may be present at around a 1% concentration, the pH of the moisturizer prevents it from working as an exfoliant Ultimately, the mix of fragrance ingredients and the sensitizing preservative methylisothiazolinone prevent us from recommending this.

☹ POOR **Correcting Moisturizer SPF 15** *($37 for 1.7 fl. oz.)* provides broad-spectrum sun protection via its in-part zinc oxide sunscreen. The base formula isn't too exciting, and this is a poor option for all skin types because of the peppermint extract and lemon peel oil. See the Appendix to find out how irritation hurts everyone's skin.

☹ POOR **Essential-C Daily Renewal Complex** *($92 for 1 fl. oz.)* contains several light- and air-sensitive ingredients (including retinol), yet it's packaged in a jar. The orange, grapefruit peel, basil, and galbanum oils included here may smell nice, but they also may cause skin irritation. See the Appendix to learn how fragrant irritants damage skin—even if you cannot see or feel the damage taking place.

☹ POOR **Essential-C Night Moisture** *($60 for 1.7 fl. oz.)* contains several fragrant oils, including lavender, thyme, and grapefruit. The extract forms of these ingredients would be preferred, especially thyme, as certain portions of this plant have potent antioxidant activity. None of these irritants are essential for skin at night or at any time of day!

☹ POOR **Perfecting Day Cream SPF 30** *($47 for 1.7 fl. oz.)* contains hydrogen peroxide and lavender oil, two ingredients capable of causing skin-cell death and free-radical damage. There are plenty of well-formulated sunscreens with avobenzone that omit problematic ingredients, so choosing this option would just be an expensive mistake. See the Appendix to learn more about the problems lavender oil causes.

☹ POOR **Recovery Treatment Gel** *($52 for 1.7 fl. oz.)* is supposed to fortify delicate, sensitive skin and make it feel comfortable, but that's not going to happen when you add peppermint, lemon peel oil, and hydrogen peroxide to the mix. See the Appendix to learn why irritation is a big problem for everyone's skin.

☹ POOR **Sleep Reform Serum** *($97 for 1 fl. oz.)*. Because skin cannot tell what time it is and because skin's daily repair is occurring all the time, how is this product supposed to enhance skin's sleep cycle? Is it going to send a signal to cell receptors that the person is asleep now, so let's put the little skin-saving elves to work before the alarm clock buzzes? No, that's not going to happen. In fact, about the only things that will occur from using this serum is that your skin will feel smoother and perhaps a bit tighter (due to the amount of film-forming agent—similar to putting hairspray on the skin). But the downside is the potential for irritation because this serum contains lavender oil, which can cause skin-cell death and serves as a pro-oxidant (Sources: *Contact Dermatitis*, September 2008, pages 143–150; and *Cell Proliferation*, June 2004, pages 221–229) along with other irritating fragrant ingredients. It also contains synthetic coloring agents, which is sad to see in a product supposedly from a dermatologist, and the hormone ingredient melatonin. The only research pertaining to melatonin's effect on skin (as opposed to oral consumption) demonstrates it has a protective effect when skin is exposed to sunlight (Source: naturaldatabase.com). Given that this product is meant for nighttime use, including melatonin seems to be a marketing maneuver, not a skin-care essential. Another ingredient worth explaining is human oligopeptide-1. This is a type of epidermal growth factor whose benefits, if any, and the risk of long-term use on healthy intact skin are unknown. We do know that such growth factors play a role in wound-healing and reducing inflammation, but wrinkles are not wounds and there are many anti-inflammatory ingredients that have stronger safety profiles than epidermal growth factors. One negative of topical application of growth factors is the potential to cause cells to over-proliferate. That's not what aging skin needs, and the possible side effects include cellular changes that could prove unhealthy or cosmetically undesirable (e.g., psoriasis is a skin disorder that involves over-proliferation of skin cells). In short, topical application of growth factors isn't worth the potential risks to your skin, especially given that growth factors do not have any firmly established benefit as an anti-aging wonder.

☹ POOR **T-Zone Pore Refining Gel** *($40 for 2 fl. oz.)* lists alcohol as the second ingredient, which makes this gel too drying and irritating for all skin types. How disappointing, because this otherwise contains the makings of a very good AHA/BHA product for oily skin. See the Appendix to learn more about alcohol in skin care and how irritation makes oily skin worse.

MURAD SUN CARE

☺ GOOD **Oil-Free Sunblock SPF 30** *($31 for 1.7 fl. oz.)* offers an in-part avobenzone for reliable UVA protection and comes in an emollient base that's best for normal to dry skin. This sunscreen is oil-free, but does not provide a matte finish as claimed. There are proportionately fewer absorbent ingredients compared to the number of emollient, creamy ingredients, so this won't make someone with oily skin happy. Murad includes some great antioxidants and even a skin-identical ingredient, which is always welcome.

☹ POOR **Oil-Free Sunblock SPF 15 Sheer Tint** *($26 for 1.7 fl. oz.)* has so much going for it, including a pure titanium dioxide sunscreen, soft tint, and copious antioxidants to keep skin protected from inflammation, so it doesn't make a shred of sense that several irritating ingredients were included, too. Grapefruit, lavender, thyme, and orange oils all have their share of problems for skin, and make this sunscreen impossible to recommend. See the Appendix to learn why fragrant irritants are a problem for everyone's skin.

☹ POOR **Waterproof Sunblock SPF 30 for Face and Body** *($30 for 4.3 fl. oz.)* provides broad-spectrum sun protection that includes avobenzone for reliable UVA screening. The lightweight lotion texture is water-resistant but this sunscreen is impossible to recommend because it contains several fragrant plant oils known to cause irritation. The sunscreen actives can be sensitizing on their own, so adding fragrant oils won't help your skin. See the Appendix to learn how fragrant oils hurt, not help, your skin.

MURAD LIP CARE

☹ POOR **Energizing Pomegranate Lip Protector SPF 15** *($17 for 0.5 fl. oz.)* lacks the UVA-protecting ingredients of titanium dioxide, zinc oxide, avobenzone, Tinosorb, or Mexoryl SX (ecamsule), and is not recommended.

☹ POOR **Soothing Skin Lip & Cuticle Care** *($16 for 0.5 fl. oz.)* is an emollient, Vaseline-based lip balm that contains benzyl cinnamate, the chief fragrant component of balsam peru. It can be very irritating to skin and lips and is solely responsible for the Poor rating this product received.

MURAD SPECIALTY SKIN-CARE PRODUCTS

☹ POOR **Acne Spot Treatment** *($18 for 0.5 fl. oz.)* lists 3% sulfur as the active ingredient, which makes this spot treatment an irritating, drying experience for skin (though sulfur can kill acne-causing bacteria). This has merit as a pH-correct AHA product, but it isn't worth considering over other AHA products that don't contain additional irritants. By the way, although Murad calls out salicylic acid in the claims, the amount of it in this product likely isn't enough to improve acne.

☹ POOR **Acne & Wrinkle Reducer** *($58 for 2 fl. oz.)*. Acne and wrinkles are no fun separately, but are completely exasperating when you're struggling with both at the same time. You can't help feeling you were supposed to stop breaking out once wrinkles started showing up. The myth about acne being all about the teen years just won't die. Nonetheless, you can treat both acne and wrinkles at the same time, but not with this product. Murad's attempt to combine salicylic acid (BHA) with other ingredients typically included in antiwrinkle moisturizers is interesting, but not well executed in this product. First, the amount of salicylic acid is too low for it to have much benefit and the formula's pH is too high for this exfoliant to work as it should if your goal is less acne and a smoother skin texture. A film-forming agent is a major ingredient in this product, and it can provide a smoothing and temporary tightening (not lifting) effect on skin, but that cosmetic effect is not unique and such an ingredient shouldn't be in an anti-acne product. Beyond the initial disappointment over the salicylic acid is the fact that there are as many bad ingredients as good ones in this formula. The offending ingredients include sulfur, silver citrate, and several fragrance ingredients known to cause irritation. Although sulfur is a potent disinfectant that can help ease acne, it is also exceptionally drying and irritating and definitely a problem for fighting wrinkles. The silver citrate, like all forms of silver, can cause a bluish discoloration of the skin, especially in a product meant for daily application, and there is no research showing it has benefit for wrinkles or acne (Sources: http://ec.europa.eu/health/ph_risk/committees/04_sccp/docs/sccp_o_165.pdf; and naturaldatabase.com). Although the amount of silver citrate in Murad's product is probably too low for it to have any effect on skin, we don't think it's worth the risk given that there are brilliant anti-acne and antiwrinkle products available that don't have any potentially problematic ingredients.

☹ POOR **Clarifying Mask** *($37 for 2.65 fl. oz.)* lists 4% sulfur as the active ingredient, which makes this an incredibly drying, irritating mask for acne-prone skin, or for any skin. Sulfur is joined by camphor and lavender oil, which are as appropriate for blemishes as using bacon grease to absorb excess facial oil. See the Appendix to find out how irritating ingredients make oily, acne-prone skin worse.

☹ POOR **Crazy for Clear Spot Treatment** *($16 for 0.5 fl. oz.)* contains a potentially helpful amount of glycolic and salicylic acids formulated at a pH that allows them to work as exfoliants. That's great, but we couldn't overlook the fact that it contains a high amount of sulfur.

Although sulfur is a potent disinfectant, it is also needlessly irritating and drying, which won't make acne-prone skin look better and can hurt skin's healing process. Several anti-irritants are included, too, but their energy will be partially spent defending your skin from the sulfur rather than reducing redness.

☹ POOR **Exfoliating Acne Treatment Gel** *($54 for 3.4 fl. oz.)* features 1% salicylic acid as the active ingredient, but it's in a base that's mostly water and alcohol. The hydrogen peroxide this contains will help kill acne-causing bacteria, but it's such an unstable ingredient that it also triggers intense free-radical damage, yet another reason to run, not walk, away from this anti-acne product. See the Appendix to find out how irritating ingredients make oily, acne-prone skin worse.

☹ POOR **Gentle Acne Treatment Gel** *($44 for 2.65 fl. oz.)* contains a less-than-desirable amount of salicylic acid, as well as a pH that's too high for exfoliation to occur. But the biggest offense is the inclusion of skin cell–damaging lavender oil, which may smell soothing but is far from gentle (see the Appendix for details).

☹ POOR **Post-Acne Spot Lightening Gel** *($60 for 1 fl. oz.)* could have been an effective option for treating hyperpigmentation because it contains 2% hydroquinone along with a good amount of glycolic acid. However, the amount of alcohol makes this too irritating for all skin types (see the Appendix for details). You'll find brilliant options for dark spots in our Best Products chapter at the end of this book.

☹ POOR **Rapid Age Spot and Pigment Lightening Serum** *($60 for 1 fl. oz.)* is a very expensive skin-lightening product that contains 2% hydroquinone. The problem is the alcohol base, which makes this gel too irritating for all skin types (see the Appendix for details). Paula's Choice RESIST Triple-Action Dark Spot Eraser, 2%BHA Gel contains the same amount of active ingredient along with salicylic acid to help exfoliate, and no needlessly irritating ingredients, all for one-third the cost of this skin-lightening product. Knowing this, why spend more than you need to and risk irritation that hurts skin?

MURAD FACE & EYE PRIMERS

☺ GOOD **$$$ Hybrids Skin Perfecting Primer Dewy Finish** *($35 for 1 fl. oz.)* is a good option for those with normal to slightly dry skin. It isn't all that hydrating (those with dry skin will want to apply a moisturizer first), but has a smooth, slightly creamy texture that blends on silky-smooth and sets to a soft dewy finish. Although the finish appears dewy, it doesn't feel moist. Actually, this is an almost weightless product that works very well under foundation. This primer has a sheer tint that goes on almost transparent; only those with porcelain to fair skin tones will find the tint tricky to work with. The only questionable ingredient is cinnamon bark extract, but the amount is likely too low to be a problem.

☺ GOOD **$$$ Hybrids Skin Perfecting Primer Matte Finish** *($35 for 1 fl. oz.)*. This sheer, tinted foundation primer has a fluid lotion texture with a good amount of slip to make blending a pleasure. The pump dispenser tends to spurt product forcefully rather than dispense it smoothly, so be careful! It sets to a soft matte finish that makes skin look refined rather than dry and flat. As mentioned, this is tinted but goes on so sheer that it works for most skin tones. Those with porcelain to fair skin will find the color too dark. Formula-wise, the only cause for concern is the cinnamon bark extract. The amount this product contains is small enough to be of minimal concern, but the formula would be better without it. Because of this primer's finish, it can minimize the appearance of pores, just like a matte finish foundation or powder does. It is best for normal to oily skin.

☺ AVERAGE **$$$ Hybrids Eye Lift Perfector** *($35 for 0.06 fl. oz.)* is a bit difficult to classify. Essentially, it's a sheer, creamy liquid concealer designed for use on the eyelids. The claim is that doing so will increase eyelid firmness by 50% in just 15 minutes. This won't lift sagging or drooping eyelids, but it does contain a potentially irritating film-forming agent (sodium polystyrene sulfonate) that can make eyelid skin feel temporarily tighter. Just because skin feels tighter doesn't mean it is tighter, and nothing is being lifted. If it was, where would the excess skin go? It would simply be lifted up and look strange. This sheer concealer (which is best for creating a subtle brightening effect) is easy to blend and not prone to creasing. It also contains some intriguing anti-aging ingredients, including peptides and antioxidants. However, the amount of film-forming agent is cause for concern and doesn't make this a slam-dunk eyelid concealer/primer worth strong consideration. As for covering dark circles (another claim Murad makes) this is way too sheer to provide meaningful camouflage.

☺ AVERAGE **$$$ Hybrids Eye Lift Illuminator** *($35 for 0.06 fl. oz.)* is similar to the Hybrids Eye Lift Perfector above, only with different claims and the addition of shine. Otherwise, the same comments apply.

N.Y.C. (NEW YORK COLOR) (MAKEUP ONLY)

Strengths: Inexpensive; good finds for powders, eyeshadows, and lip glosses; several outstanding best buys, including lipstick, mascara, pressed powder, and brow pencil; most products are packaged so you can easily see the color.

Weaknesses: Some really inferior products; the makeup brushes really disappoint; the lip-plumping gloss is filled to the brim with potent irritants; limited options for foundation and concealer; several average pencils.

For more information and reviews of the latest N.Y.C. (New York Color) products, visit CosmeticsCop.com.

N.Y.C. (NEW YORK COLOR) EYE-MAKEUP REMOVER

☹ POOR **In A New York Color Minute Eye Makeup Remover** *($3.99 for 2.3 ounces)* begins well, but suffers a bit due to the inclusion of too many detergent cleansing agents (including the drying, irritating sodium lauryl sulfate) that do not make it preferred to other eye-makeup removers, including those from other drugstore brands. It's fragrance-free, and that's always a plus, but not enough to warrant a purchase. We're also slightly concerned about some of the preservatives this contains, as a couple of them aren't the best for use near the eyes.

N.Y.C. (NEW YORK COLOR) FOUNDATIONS & PRIMER

☺ AVERAGE **Smooth Skin Liquid Makeup** *($2.99)*. This basic liquid makeup applies smoothly and provides medium coverage with a soft matte finish. The slightly opaque, flat finish can work for someone with normal to oily skin, but it has a tacky finish that isn't the best. The only really attractive part of this foundation is the price, and if you're on a tight budget it's worth a try. Among the five shades (the range is only for light to medium skin tones), use caution with the slightly peach True Beige, and avoid Natural Tan due to its orange overtone.

☺ AVERAGE **Smooth Skin Perfecting Primer** *($3.99)*. This inexpensive primer has a fluid, lotion-like texture that's not as silky or smooth as many other primers due to the amount of oil it contains. Best for normal to dry skin, this primer hydrates while mica adds a subtle sheen to skin (which may or may not be to your liking; it can look a bit whitish). This would be rated higher if it contained some beneficial ingredients for skin, but it merely contains a tiny amount of vitamin E (tocopheryl acetate). Although this contains fragrance, the scent is nearly undetectable. In the end, a well-formulated moisturizer or serum would work just as well and provide your skin with a range of beneficial ingredients, too.

☹ POOR **Skin Matching Foundation** *($3.99)*. Here's another liquid foundation claiming to intuitively adjust to skin's color and texture. Don't believe it, because it simply isn't possible. The formula for this foundation is actually quite dated—we haven't seen something like this since the 1980s were giving up the "me decade" ghost to the emerging trend of grunge music and flannel clothing! The fragranced formula has a fluid yet creamy texture with almost too much slip, so blending takes longer than it should. Coverage is sheer to medium but can look spotty and choppy even if you blend carefully. Add to that a somewhat tacky finish that feels moist but looks chalky matte and this is a foundation to leave on the shelf! The colors (which are only for light to medium skin tones) look more neutral in the tube than they do on skin.

N.Y.C. (NEW YORK COLOR) CONCEALER

☺ AVERAGE **Cover Stick** *($1.99)* is a standard, lipstick-style concealer with a smooth, surprisingly non-greasy texture that blends well. It provides medium coverage with a soft powder finish (talc is the second ingredient). It has a slight tendency to crease into lines under the eye, but if you prefer a creamy concealer, this works well to cover minor redness or slight discolorations. Among the five shades, the only ones worth using are Light, Medium, and Natural (a beautiful neutral if there ever was one). Avoid the color-correcting Yellow and Green shades; those are shades that never have and never will improve anyone's skin tone.

N.Y.C. (NEW YORK COLOR) POWDERS

✓☺ BEST **Smooth Skin Pressed Face Powder** *($2.99)*. This talc-based powder comes in excellent shades and has a beautifully silky texture and sheer application. Best for normal to dry skin (the finish won't keep excess oil in check for long), this is definitely a pressed powder to try. In fact, we cannot think of another inexpensive powder as unexpectedly good as this one.

☺ GOOD **Smooth Skin Loose Face Powder** *($2.99)* is a good, basic loose powder for all skin types. It provides a bit more coverage than others in this category, has a texture that's thicker than many, but still blends on well. Both shades of this talc-based powder are acceptable, and you get a generous amount considering how inexpensive this product is!

☺ AVERAGE **Color Wheel Mosaic Face Powder** *($4.99)* is eye-catching thanks to its familiar mosaic pattern, yet the texture, while soft, applies a bit thick and tends to look powdery on skin unless applied sheer. Among the six shades, most are best for use as blush or bronzer rather than for dusting all over your face. Both Pink Cheek Glow and Rose Glow come off as peachy on skin, despite names to the contrary. Translucent Highlighter Glow is the most versatile; all the shades have a soft matte finish.

N.Y.C. (NEW YORK COLOR) BLUSH & BRONZER

☺ GOOD **Sun 2 Sun Bronzing Powder** *($4.99)*. This split-pan pressed bronzing powder provides a medium and light bronze tone, both of which are more pigmented than you might expect and as such are best applied in sheer layers until you get the desired intensity. The smooth, dry texture isn't on par with the best bronzing powders available, but is nevertheless impressive for the money. Each duo has sparkling shine, but its effect on skin tends to be subtle.

☺ AVERAGE **Cheek Glow Single Pan Blush** *($2.99)* isn't that great for a powder blush. It's very sheer, but also tends to look more powdery than blush-like on skin. The shade range is attractive and suitable for fair to medium skin tones, but that's only if you want to apply a blush that doesn't look like you've done anything to enliven your cheeks unless you really pile it on.

N.Y.C. (NEW YORK COLOR) EYESHADOWS

☺ GOOD **Metro Quartet Eye Shadow** *($3.99)*. Housed in one slim compact are four shades of powder eyeshadow, each with a plastic overlay embossed with the area the shades are supposed to be applied (a helpful touch). The enclosed, dual-sided sponge tip applicator is impractically small and should not be used in favor of regular-size eyeshadow brushes. As for the texture, it's smooth and sheer, but also dry enough to impede a seamless application and make it tricky to blend shades into a harmonious design. Although the medium to deep shades look dark in the compact, every shade goes on surprisingly soft, so you'll need to do a lot of layering to build a more dramatic or smoky eye design. Although not the best powder shadows, they're acceptable for the price. The best sets include Union Square, Lexington Luxury, and South Street Seaport. All have a slight to moderate amount of shimmer.

☺ GOOD **Individual Eyes Custom Compact** *($4.99)*. This six-product eye palette contains a nude eyelid primer, white pearlescent brow bone highlighter, and four shades of powder eyeshadow whose finishes range from matte to frost. For the price, this is a veritable steal because most of this kit performs very well. The shadows' color deposit is impressive, and the shades—meant to coordinate with eye color, which is advice best ignored—work well together to create a variety of eye-makeup designs. The sleeper hit here is the eyelid primer, which comes in a generously sized pan. It really does enhance and enrich the shadows, as well as extend their staying power. The only miss is the garish highlighter, which is too iridescent to create a sophisticated highlighting effect.

☺ AVERAGE **City Duet Eye Shadow** *($2.99)*. Housed in one slim compact are two shades of powder eyeshadow, each with a plastic overlay embossed with the area the shades are supposed to be applied (a helpful touch). The enclosed, dual-sided sponge tip applicator is impractically small and should not be used in favor of regular-size eyeshadow brushes. As for the texture, it's smooth and a bit waxy, yet also dry enough to impede a seamless application and make it tricky to blend shades into a harmonious design. Although the shades look color-saturated in the compact, each goes on surprisingly soft, so you'll need to do a lot of layering to build a more dramatic or visible eye design. Although not the best powder shadows, they're acceptable for the price—if you can get past the mostly strange, difficult to use pairings. The only workable duo is NYC Times (soft black and white). The others are only for those whose eye design mantra is "bright, bold, and a bit clownish."

☺ AVERAGE **Color Wheel Mosaic Eye Powder** *($3.99)* presents several complementary shades pressed in a mosaic pattern. It seems appealing because you can use whichever shades you prefer or sweep a brush over the entire powder cake and get one shade. The problem with sweeping the brush over all the colors and swirling them together is that you can't go back to using the colors singly—everything gets blended together. But using the shades individually isn't practical either because of the mosaic pattern and no dividers between shades. The smooth, finely milled texture applies well without flaking, and imparts a shiny finish that borders on metallic. The overall effect is more sheer than many powder eyeshadows, which can be frustrating if you're looking for some definition. Among the available blends, avoid Purple Rain and the beyond-too-blue Beyond the Sea.

☹ POOR **Sparkle Eye Dust** *($3.99)*. This loose-powder eyeshadow comes in a cute container designed to minimize mess, a nice touch. The inner portion features a wand with an attached brush, and the brush is actually good. The problem is that this sheer, shiny powder clings poorly, the shine doesn't stay put for long, and the color fades shortly thereafter.

N.Y.C. (NEW YORK COLOR) EYE & BROW LINERS

☺ GOOD **Browser Brush-On Brow Powder with Grooming Wax & Tweezers** *($3.99)* is a rather practical brow kit. Included are a matte powder brow color along with a brow wax (for grooming), a synthetic mini brow brush, and mini tweezers. The brow color is sheer, but builds well, although the included brush is too stiff for soft, feathered application. The metal tweezers won't make you toss out your full-size pair, but they certainly work in a pinch (pun intended). As for the brow wax, this can be mixed with the brow powder for a stronger color or used after the powder has been applied to "set" and groom the brows. There are two shades available (one per kit), and both are great.

☺ AVERAGE **Automatic Eyeliner** *($2.99)* doesn't need sharpening and maintains a pointed tip, which is always a plus. The smooth, no-tug application is how a pencil should be. From that description you might expect a better rating, but this pencil's rich colors remain slightly creamy after application, which encourages smearing, creasing, and fading. They work better if set with a coordinating shade of powder eyeshadow—but then why not just use the powder to line your eyes in the first place?

☺ AVERAGE **Classic Brow & Liner Pencils** *($0.99)* are among the least expensive anywhere, but how do they perform? Well, they do need routine sharpening, which isn't convenient, and application isn't the best either. Whether used for eyelining or filling in brows (the brown-toned shades are best for brows), these pencils require more pressure than usual to apply. With some effort, the result is smooth color that lasts longer than what you get from creamier pencils. Weigh the pros and cons and decide for yourself if the trade-offs are worth the savings.

☺ AVERAGE **Liquid Eyeliner** *($2.99)* doesn't cost a lot, but its performance isn't on par with several other drugstore liquid liners that don't cost much more, such as those from Almay and L'Oreal. The long, thin brush applies color surprisingly well, but the formula remains wet too long, which encourages smearing.

☺ AVERAGE **Waterproof Eyeliner Pencil** *($3.99)*. This standard, needs-sharpening pencil glides on effortlessly and imparts moderately rich color that sets almost instantly to a budge-proof finish. The formula remains tacky once it sets, but that is what contributes to it being waterproof. Just for the record, most eye pencils are waterproof by virtue of their wax- or silicone-based formulas.

☹ POOR **Brow & Liner Pencil Twin Pack** *($1.99)* is not recommended because its creamy, oil-based formula smudges almost instantly after application. It also tends to apply too thick, especially for use on brows.

N.Y.C. (NEW YORK COLOR) LIP COLOR & LIPLINERS

✓☺ BEST **Smooch Proof LIPStain 16H** *($4.99)* is an outstanding lipstain that goes on moist without grabbing unevenly or immediately bleeding into lines around the mouth. Other drugstore lip stains don't come close to the performance, color selection, or feel of N.Y.C.'s Smooch Proof, and the price is almost unbelievable given the product's superior performance

✓☺ BEST **Ultra Moist Lip Wear** *($0.99)*. For less than one dollar, you're getting an emollient cream lipstick that provides rich color and a glossy, slick finish. This isn't for anyone prone to lipstick feathering into lines around the mouth; however, for others it's definitely worth an audition and the shade range, though small, is good.

☺ GOOD **Automatic Lipliner** *($2.99)* applies easily, stays in place, and offers a softer alternative to fully pigmented lip pencils. If one of the two nude pink shades appeals to you, give it a try (it doesn't need routine sharpening).

☺ GOOD **Liquid Lipshine** *($2.49)* proves to be a very good, non-sticky lip gloss with a thin texture and a shiny finish. You can count on about 2 hours of wear, but you'll need to use a lipliner because this does bleed into lines around the mouth.

☺ GOOD **Ultra Last Lip Wear** *($1.99)* is a very standard cream lipstick that isn't too slippery or greasy. It provides a soft gloss finish and the shades apply more sheer than they look. In fact, some of the colors are surprisingly sheer. In terms of staying power, this lipstick's longevity doesn't go beyond that of most other cream lipsticks.

☹ AVERAGE **Kiss Gloss** *($2.99)* comes in a tube and dispenses thick and gooey. Luckily, it doesn't feel gooey on your lips, but it is thick and tends to slide around, which can make kissing rather messy and slippery. All the flavored shades are sheer, but each provides a glossy wet finish that many are bound to love.

☹ POOR **Lippin' Large Lip Plumper** *($3.99)*. Talk about a burning sensation! This sheer, shimmering lip gloss irritates on contact due to its potent blend of cinnamon, ginger, and peppermint oils. If that weren't enough, N.Y.C. also added an irritating menthol derivative to this painful product. Your lips will get inflamed and will swell for a few minutes, but that is neither healthy nor attractive. This also tastes terrible.

N.Y.C. (NEW YORK COLOR) MASCARAS

✓☺ BEST **City Curls Curling Mascara** *($2.99)* really works to curl lashes into an attractive, upswept fringe. Even better, with successive strokes you'll get impossibly long lashes without a clump in sight. Removing this is as simple as using a water-soluble cleanser, and it wears flawlessly. What's not to like, unless you want thicker lashes?

✓☺ BEST **High Definition Separating Mascara** *($4.99)* applies evenly without a clump or flake. The rubber-bristled brush has a tapered end perfect for getting to small lashes or the outer corner of the eye, allowing for lots of definition and separation, and you'll also see thickness and volume. The best part? It lasts, but then washes off completely with a water-soluble cleanser.

✓☺ BEST **Sky Rise Lengthening Mascara** *($1.99)*. If longer, defined lashes are what you're after, this is a bargain of a mascara! The brush makes lashes longer quickly without a single clump, and it removes easily with a water-soluble cleanser.

✓☺ BEST **Big Bold Ultra Volumizing Mascara** *($2.99)* is an excellent mascara, though not for building volume (thickness). Although this adds some thickness, it's better at lengthening and beautifully defining lashes without clumps. Lashes are left fringed, soft, and flutter-worthy, all for under $3! The only drawback to consider is the size of the brush. It's quite large and the chunky design can be awkward to navigate around small eyes or very dense lashes. Still, with practice, this works great and it doesn't take long for lashes to go from "blah" to "wow"!

☺ GOOD **Show Time Volumizing Mascara** *($3.99)* is a good, inexpensive mascara that is better at lengthening and softly defining lashes than adding lots of volume. Lashes simply don't bulk up easily with this mascara, even with multiple coats. It doesn't clump and wears beautifully, but is best for producing long, fluttering lashes rather than dramatic thickness.

☹ AVERAGE **High Definition Volume Volumizing Mascara** *($4.99)* misses the mark with a dry formula and a rubber brush that spells disaster. The unusual alignment of the bristles (one row is extra-spiky and far longer than the others) makes application difficult, and creating definition nearly impossible, especially on short lashes. The formula does thicken, but it also tends to flake by the end of the day. It's easy to remove with a gentle cleanser, but that convenience doesn't compensate for this mascara's other drawbacks.

☺ AVERAGE **Show Time Waterproof Volumizing Mascara** *($3.99)* is seriously under-whelming. Even with lots of effort, the best this does is make lashes slightly longer and a tad thicker. That's far from the "makes lashes 5X thicker" claim on the packaging, although this is waterproof and holds up well all day (no flaking, smearing, or smudging).

N.Y.C. (NEW YORK COLOR) BRUSHES

☺ GOOD **Cosmetic Sponges** *($1.99)*. These basic synthetic makeup sponges come three to a pack, and each has a different shape. This can be helpful for identifying which sponge you want to use for a specific purpose. For example, you shouldn't use the same sponge to apply foundation that you use to blend the edges of blush or contour. With these sponges, you can "assign" duties to each based on its unique (but still functional) shape. Convenient!

☹ POOR **Shadow Applicators** *($0.99)*. These sponge-tipped sticks are not what you should be using to apply eyeshadow. Brushes are always preferred. Even if you were thinking of using these to soften an eye design or smudge a line, the sponges tend to drag over skin, producing uneven, splotchy color.

☹ POOR **Brush Kit** *($1.99)* is laughable. The tiny, doll-size brushes can't come close to a professional application, and aren't even as nice as the throwaway brushes packaged with most blushes and eyeshadows.

NARS (MAKEUP ONLY)

Strengths: Great range of foundation shades; the powder blush; lipsticks; some of the makeup brushes are excellent; tinted lip balm with broad-spectrum sun protection.

Weaknesses: Expensive; average to poor pencils; the mascaras are not impressive given their cost.

For more information and reviews of the latest NARS products (including NARS skin care), visit CosmeticsCop.com.

NARS FOUNDATIONS

✓☺ BEST **$$$ Sheer Glow Foundation** *($42)* has one of the best, most extensive range of shades we've seen in a long time! Whether your skin is porcelain, ebony, or somewhere in between, you're likely to find a good match from this silky liquid foundation. Its silicone-enhanced base has a good amount of slip for precise, controlled blending and it sets to a soft matte finish that looks quite natural. Despite the name, this is neither sheer nor all that glow-y on skin. Coverage is in the light to medium range, and getting to medium coverage doesn't require much foundation. Sheer Glow Foundation is best for normal to oily skin, including breakout-prone skin. The formula contains a tiny amount of antioxidants, but they're not going to impart much benefit to skin. Overall, well done, NARS!

✓☺ BEST **$$$ Sheer Matte Foundation** *($42)* comes in a staggering array of absolutely beautiful, real skin colors. Those with fair and dark skin will be equally impressed, and the fair shades don't make porcelain skin tones look pink or washed out. This has a silky, fluid texture that feels thin but provides light to medium coverage. Blending must be quick because it doesn't take long for this to set to a true matte finish. It is an ideal foundation for oily skin, and contains absorbents that help keep excess shine in check. There are some "off" shades here, so it is wise to shade test in-store before you buy. Be cautious of anything too peachy or ashy. One more comment: The pump for this foundation clogs easily so keep it scrupulously clean between uses.

☺ GOOD **$$$ Powder Foundation SPF 12** *($45)* has a silky texture and seamless application that make it a very good powder foundation choice. Even better, the formula provides broad-spectrum sun protection, though SPF 15 is preferred for minimum daytime protection and anti-aging benefit. Although the SPF rating is disappointing, this deserves a good rating for those seeking a pressed-powder foundation to wear over a regular sunscreen or over a foundation with sunscreen. It provides sheer to light coverage and leaves a soft matte finish with a hint of shine. There are several, gorgeous shades to choose from, suitable for a wide range of skin tones. Some of the tan to dark shades could also work beautifully as bronzing powders for light to medium skin tones.

☹ AVERAGE **$$$ Pro-Prime Multi-Protect Primer SPF 30 Sunscreen** *($32 for 1 fl. oz.)* loses points because its active ingredients do not provide sufficient UVA protection (see the Appendix for details on what actives you should look for). This primer has a thick but smooth texture that softens to a lightweight cream and leaves skin feeling slightly moist with a soft, whitish glow. The formula is best for normal to dry skin, but again, this isn't a time-saving product because the sun protection isn't up to par. Note: The amount of antioxidants in this primer (mentioned in the claims) is disappointingly low.

NARS CONCEALERS

☺ GOOD **$$$ Duo Concealer** *($30)* has a smooth, slightly creamy texture with minimal slip, which makes blending easy and precise. Each compact houses two shades, allowing for customization if you need to mix shades for the best match. This sets to a soft, satin matte finish that covers well with only minor creasing into lines (even less if you blend carefully and set with a dusting of powder).

☹ AVERAGE **$$$ Concealer** *($22)* is a lipstick-style concealer that provides creamy, opaque coverage that can look heavy, as though it's just sitting on skin rather than melding with it. NARS claims this is crease-resistant, but it can indeed slip into the lines around the eyes. Although the shades offer a good variety of neutral colors, this still isn't your best concealer option.

NARS POWDERS

☺ GOOD **$$$ Loose Powder** *($35)* remains one of the messier loose powders to use due to its awkward, over-sized packaging and lack of a sifter. This is otherwise a gorgeous talc- and cornstarch-based powder that looks beautifully natural on the skin, with only a trace of shine. The shades are exemplary for very fair skin to dark skin.

☺ GOOD **$$$ Pressed Powder** *($32)* shares most of the attributes of the Loose Powder above, including a sheer finish that looks natural rather than powdered. The texture is drier than the Loose Powder, too, but that doesn't affect how nice this looks on skin. The shade range offers superb, neutral colors for light to deep tan skin tones.

NARS BLUSHES & BRONZERS

✓☺ BEST **$$$ Blush** *($27)* is definitely the star attraction of this line and it's easy to see why. These have a splendid texture and apply beautifully with a sheer initial application that builds to any depth of color you want. The shade range is extensive, and most of the colors have strong pigment (a plus for women with dark skin). There are several beautiful shades to choose from, some of which are on the shiny side which doesn't always work for daytime makeup, but can look great for a sultry evening look. And yes, the Orgasm shade (the brand's most popular) is gorgeous.

✓☺ BEST **$$$ Multiple Bronzer** *($38)* is a fantastic bronzing option, especially if you prefer a twist-up bronzer with a smooth cream texture that isn't the least bit greasy. Simply dot this over the cheekbone area and blend with fingertips, a brush, or sponge to create a soft bronze effect with a smooth matte finish imbued with subtle sparkles. One caution: Blending must be instant because this sets quickly, and then it lasts. All the shades are beautiful, and produce a natural-looking tan, even for those with fair skin.

☺ GOOD **$$$ Bronzing Powder** *($33)* is pressed and offers natural-looking bronze colors for fair to tan skin tones. It imparts a moderate amount of shine. Although a real tan doesn't sparkle, at least the shine in this bronzer adheres well to skin.

☺ GOOD **$$$ Cream Blush** *($28)* is definitely creamy but not too thick or greasy. It glides over skin, delivering sheer color and a radiant finish. Although the colors look way too intense in their compacts, each goes on translucent and layers well if you want a bit more color. You will find that this works best on dry to very dry skin.

☺ GOOD **$$$ Highlighting Blush** *($27)* is meant to add shine, and it does it well! The silky smooth texture goes on sheer and even, imparting a subtle wash of color and varying degrees of shine depending on which shade you choose.

NARS EYESHADOWS

✓☺ BEST **$$$ Smudge Proof Eyeshadow Base** *($24)* does an impressive job of helping your eyeshadow stay put while minimizing creasing throughout the day, especially for those with oily eyelids. The polymer and talc blend sets to a matte finish, but you must give it a minute to dry. Once set, you can expect a durable canvas for your eye color. The only downside is that the product can leave a faint white cast where it has been applied, but because you'll likely be covering it up with eyeshadow, no need to worry.

☺ GOOD **$$$ Cream Eyeshadow** *($23)* is quite shiny but has a smooth texture and just enough slip to make application and blending easy. However, because the finish stays moist, it won't stay in place and it will fade and crease slightly. The same comments apply to the **Duo Cream Eyeshadow** ($33).

☺ GOOD **$$$ Duo Eyeshadow** *($33)* has a silky-smooth pressed-powder texture, and comes in several shades, all of which have some shine. Among the overwhelming number of shades, it's worth noting that the majority of them feature pairings that are too contrasting or just too colorful for everyday makeup. However, with so many sets to choose from you're bound to find one that works for you.

☺ GOOD **$$$ Eyeshadow** *($24)*. There are a wealth of beautiful shades and finishes to consider with this pressed-powder eyeshadow. The shades with obvious glitter cling poorly and as such, don't come highly recommended, but the matte and shimmer shades perform well. The texture is velvety-smooth and layers well if you want more intensity.

NARS EYE & BROW LINERS

☺ AVERAGE **$$$ Eyebrow Pencil** *($21)* needs sharpening, but if you're OK with that, all these have a suitably dry texture and smooth powder finish that stays in place. The three shades present options for blondes and brunettes, but nothing for redheads or those with raven brows.

☹ POOR **Eyeliner Pencil** *($21)* has an overly creamy texture that is prone to fading and smearing. The shade range contains more trendy colors than it does classics. All in all, this eyeliner pencil just isn't worth it, especially considering you can find superior, retractable options (as opposed to this one that needs routine sharpening) at the drugstore.

☹ POOR **Glitter Pencil** *($24)* is a fairly creamy, thick pencil infused with flecks of glitter. The glitter tends to separate from the pencil's base formula and chip off onto your face, which really isn't the point.

NARS LIP COLOR & LIPLINERS

✓☺ BEST **$$$ Larger Than Life Lip Gloss** *($26)* coats your lips with a smooth, thick, moisturizing layer that is minimally sticky. The flexible brush applicator is unique, with short, thin bristles allowing for control on even the thinnest lips. The high shine finish comes in a variety of attractive shades; some colors go on sheer and shimmery, others have more of a semi-opaque intensity. Either way, this delivers a gorgeous pop of color!

✓☺ BEST **$$$ Pure Matte Lipstick** *($25)* is a superior option for those who like a true matte finish! It has a silky, lightweight texture that feels comfortable (though not overly moist or creamy) and provides rich, lasting color. All the shades have impressive staying power, and while the selection isn't plentiful, what's available is excellent. The finish is soft matte and it won't make lips feel super dry or look "dulled down." If you want to enjoy some of this lipstick's longer wear but have it be more comfortable, consider topping it with your favorite lip gloss.

✓☺ BEST **$$$ Semi Matte Lipstick** *($24)* has an opaque, slightly creamy finish and a good stain. Creamy lipsticks don't get much better than this, and this formula is available in a wide range of colors, including some of the best reds available.

☺ GOOD **$$$ Lip Lacquer** *($24)* isn't the easiest to use due to its glass jar packaging, but its thick, lanolin oil–based texture leaves lips heavily moisturized and beaming, although with a slightly sticky finish that won't be to everyone's liking. The large color palette includes both sheer and strongly pigmented colors, making this one to test before purchasing. This is best applied with a lip brush because the product is difficult to wipe off your finger.

☺ GOOD **$$$ Satin Lipstick** *($24)* has a creamy, bordering on greasy, texture. The shades are fairly opaque yet have a soft gloss finish. There are several shades to choose from, with flattering colors for all skin tones.

☺ GOOD **$$$ Sheer Lipstick** *($24)* has a glossy finish, isn't too slick, and offers coverage that is light rather than genuinely sheer. The colors are great, and extensive!

☹ AVERAGE **$$$ Lip Gloss** *($24)* features several bold colors in a sticky, thick formula whose price is unwarranted for what you get, which is just a gloss, and a rather tacky-feeling one at that.

☹ AVERAGE **$$$ Lip Liner Pencil** *($21)* claims it won't bleed or feather, and although that won't hold true for everyone, this does have a drier finish that should keep those problems in check at least for a few hours. The color selection coordinates well with the many lipsticks (and glosses) this line offers. This would rate a Best Product if it didn't require routine sharpening.

☹ AVERAGE **$$$ Velvet Matte Lip Pencil** *($24)* has a beautifully smooth texture that goes on silky and feels light, and has enough creaminess to look soft yet still wear comfortably. It isn't a true matte, but velvet matte is a fairly accurate description of this pencil's finish. The shade selection is nicely varied. This pencil's creaminess is enough to pose a slight problem for those prone to lipstick bleeding into lines around the mouth, and the routine sharpening this requires is annoying, hence the average rating.

NARS MASCARAS

☺ AVERAGE **$$$ Larger Than Life Lengthening Mascara** *($25)* takes considerable effort to get results that never begin to approach making lashes "larger than life." The rubber-bristled brush feels quite scratchy as it touches the base of lashes, but it manages to produce clean length with impressive lash separation. Not much for thickness, this mascara does a good job of making lashes long and fringed—it just takes more effort than it should to get there.

☹ POOR **Larger Than Life Volumizing Mascara** *($25)* lives up to its name only in respect to the "Larger Than Life" mess it creates during application and wear. We're used to mascaras with big, barrel-type brushes, but this one takes the cake for somehow making it very easy to get more mascara on the skin around your eyes than on your lashes! From start to finish, this is a mess that requires constant touching up. The icing on a the bad cake is this doesn't volumize lashes. It goes on wet and uneven and it's next to impossible to build thickness.

NARS FACE & BODY ILLUMINATORS

☺ GOOD **$$$ Illuminator** *($29)* is a thin-textured, liquid highlighter packaged in a squeeze tube, which makes application using a sponge or fingers incredibly easy. The shades include hues of pink, bronze, and peach, each of which delivers a decent wash of shimmer and luminosity. This isn't the most blendable product because it sets fast, but once it does there's no flaking or fading to speak of. This highlighter is good option for a night on the town, but too shimmery for everyday wear.

☺ AVERAGE **$$$ The Multiple** *($39)* is a chunky, wind-up stick with a creamy yet lightweight texture and soft, sheer colors that would work for cheeks, eyes, and, in some cases, lips. Although all the colors have varying degrees of shine (and go on softer than they appear in the stick), these are an option for a fun evening look, though the price is extraordinary for what amounts to a soft wash of glow-y color.

NARS BRUSHES

✓☺ BEST **$$$ NARS Brushes** *($21–$75)* almost all have a lovely, soft feel and are appropriately shaped for a variety of application techniques. Rated a notch below best is the **Smudge Brush** *($26)*, which has a unique cut and shape that works for smudging or other eyeshadow detail work. It's worth testing if you're in the mood for something different. Steer clear of the **Retractable Lip Brush** *($26)*, which is really too small for most women's lips.

NEUTROGENA

Strengths: Inexpensive; some superior water-soluble cleansers; good topical scrubs; effective AHA and BHA products; several retinol options, all in stable packaging; vast selection of sunscreens, most of which offer excellent UVA protection; good variety of self-tanning products; several fragrance-free options; most Healthy Skin products are state-of-the-art; almost all the foundations with sunscreen provide sufficient UVA protection; the Moistureshine Gloss.

Weaknesses: An overabundance of overlapping anti-aging products that is perennially confusing for consumers; bar soap; most of the toners are irritating or boring; a handful of bland moisturizers and eye creams; some sunscreens lack sufficient UVA protection or contain too much alcohol or problematic preservatives; most of the Deep Clean products are terrible; no effective skin-lightening products; jar packaging; mostly disappointing concealers and eyeshadows; most of the lip balms with sunscreen provide inadequate UVA protection; mostly poor mascaras.

For more information and reviews of the latest Neutrogena products, visit CosmeticsCop.com.

The Reviews N

NEUTROGENA CLEANSERS

✓☺ BEST **Extra Gentle Cleanser** *($6.49 for 6.7 fl. oz.)* is an excellent option for normal to dry or sensitive skin, including those with eczema or rosacea. The fragrance-free, lotion-textured formula contains mild cleansing agents and some good anti-irritants, but these aren't as effective in a cleanser as they are when they are left on the skin.

✓☺ BEST **Fresh Foaming Cleanser** *($6.49 for 6.7 fl. oz.)* is a superb water-soluble cleanser for normal to oily or combination skin. It removes makeup easily and rinses without a trace. This does contain fragrance, though it's not an intense amount.

✓☺ BEST **Neutrogena Naturals Fresh Cleansing + Makeup Remover** *($7.49 for 6 fl. oz.)* is an inexpensive cleanser not "bionutrient rich," which is the term Neutrogena uses to describe the plant extracts. It is, however, a very good water-soluble cleanser for all skin types except sensitive, because the formula includes fragrance. True to its name, this removes makeup, too.

✓☺ BEST **Neutrogena Naturals Purifying Facial Cleanser** *($7.49 for 6 fl. oz.)* is a very good, gentle water-soluble cleanser that's suitable for all skin types except sensitive because it contains fragrance; without fragrance it would have been perfect for sensitive skin as well.

✓☺ BEST **Oil-Free Makeup Removing Cleanser for Acne Prone Skin** *($5.99 for 5.2 fl. oz.)* is a well-formulated cleanser that is suitable for normal to oily skin. It is also fine for acne-prone skin, as are most water-soluble cleansers. The claim that this rinses without a residue is true, but that applies to any well-formulated water-soluble cleanser. This option removes makeup and refreshes skin without the needless irritants (such as menthol and peppermint) that other Neutrogena cleansers contain. Although this does contain fragrance, the amount is minimal, and as such this cleanser deserves our top rating.

✓☺ BEST **One Step Gentle Cleanser** *($6.49 for 5.2 fl. oz.)* removes makeup and leaves skin feeling clean and smooth, all in one gentle step. Its silky texture feels great on skin, lathers slightly, and rinses easily. It also contains milder cleansing agents than many other cleansers. It is highly recommended for all but very dry skin types. It does contain fragrance.

☺ GOOD **Ageless Essentials Continuous Hydration Cream Cleanser** *($7.49 for 5.1 fl. oz.)* is a good, water-soluble cleansing lotion for normal to dry skin not prone to blemishes. It removes makeup easily and rinses surprisingly well without the need for a washcloth. The amount of feverfew extract is not likely cause for concern. One more point: Although this cleanser doesn't strip skin or leave it feeling dry, it isn't capable of providing continuous hydration. You will notice almost immediately that this cleanser doesn't replace the need for a good toner or moisturizer if your skin is dry.

☺ GOOD **Ageless Restoratives Energy Renewal Cleanser** *($7.99 for 5.1 fl. oz.)* is a standard water-soluble foaming cleanser that contains a small amount of polyethylene beads for a mild scrub action. It doesn't energize or renew skin better than any other cleanser used with a washcloth, but this is a good option for normal to oily skin. It removes makeup and rinses easily, but the scrub particles aren't the best way to remove makeup; so, this is best used as your morning cleanser.

☺ GOOD **Healthy Skin Anti-Wrinkle Anti-Blemish Cleanser** *($6.49 for 5.1 fl. oz.)* contains 0.5% salicylic acid, which is too low a percentage to have much of an effect on blemishes, especially when included in a cleanser that is rinsed off shortly after it's applied. This also contains glycolic acid, but the pH of 4.5 is too high for effective exfoliation, and again, it will be rinsed off before it has a chance to work. What's best about this softly fragranced cleanser is the gentle cleansing agents it contains, which are effective for makeup removal and excellent for all but the driest skin types.

☺ GOOD **Oil-Free Acne Stress Control Power-Foam Wash** *($7.49 for 6 fl. oz.)* contains 0.5% salicylic acid, but it's a useless ingredient in a cleanser because it is rinsed down the drain before it has a chance to work. This is otherwise a standard, water-soluble cleanser that's suitable for normal to oily skin. It removes makeup easily and does contain fragrance.

☺ GOOD **Oil-Free Acne Wash Foam Cleanser** *($6.99 for 5.1 fl. oz.)* contains 2% salicylic acid, but that won't help acne in a cleanser because it is rinsed down the drain before it can go to work. This is still a good water-soluble cleanser for normal to oily skin.

☺ GOOD **$$$ Healthy Skin Visibly Even Foaming Cleanser** *($6.49 for 5.1 fl. oz.)* is a cleanser/scrub hybrid, but first and foremost a cleanser and its foaming formula is somewhat drying. It's an OK option for oily skin, but it takes more than a tiny amount of exfoliating beads (listed as polyethylene) to create an even complexion. For example, an uneven skin tone from sun damage cannot simply be scrubbed away. An AHA or BHA exfoliant does a better job, but you also have to be diligent about daily sun protection. This cleanser works well to remove makeup, but overall its appeal is limited compared to many other cleansers, including others from Neutrogena.

☺ AVERAGE **Oil-Free Acne Wash Cleansing Cloths** *($6.99 for 30 cloths)* are a good option for normal to oily skin, but don't forget to rinse the solution from your skin.

☺ AVERAGE **Visibly Bright Daily Facial Cleanser** *($7.49-$7.49 for 6.7 fl. oz.)* is said to transform dull, tired skin into bright and refreshed skin after only four uses. Sounds tempting, but really, any gentle cleanser will make dull skin look fresher and brighter, and it can do that after just one use! This cleanser is a decent option for normal to dry or combination skin, but it's nothing special and doesn't contain anything that makes skin look brighter (though the cleanser itself is infused with shiny pigments for a pretty appearance, that doesn't translate to brighter, shiny skin). The main concern with this cleanser is the amount of fragrance it contains. Fragrance isn't skin care and research has shown fragrance-free is the best way for all skin types to go. If you prefer some fragrance in your cleanser, it's best to look for those whose scent is minimal, as this minimizes the risk of irritation. Bottom line: Although this cleanses well and removes most types of makeup, Neutrogena offers more effective, less fragranced cleansers.

☹ POOR **Deep Clean Facial Cleanser, for Normal to Oily Skin** *($5.99 for 6.7 fl. oz.)* leaves out the menthol found in many other Neutrogena cleansers, but is based around the drying detergent cleansing agent sodium C14-16 olefin sulfonate, so is not recommended.

☹ POOR **Deep Clean Long-Last Shine Control Cleanser/Mask** *($7.49 for 6 fl. oz.)* can be used as a cleanser or a mask, but is not recommended because it contains menthol, which causes irritation that stimulates oil production at the base of the pore. Plus, this cleanser/mask contains several thickening agents, which someone with oily, acne-prone skin doesn't need. What was Neutrogena thinking? The company maintains that their rice protein technology acts like a sponge to absorb excess oil so you get a long-lasting matte finish, but this technology (which doesn't have published research to support the claim) is rinsed down the drain before it has a chance to have any effect. Those looking for shine control without irritation should consider the mattifying products from brands such as Smashbox (Anti-Shine), Clinique (Pore Minimizer), OC Eight, and Paula's Choice (Shine Stopper).

☹ POOR **Neutrogena Naturals Face & Body Bar** *($3.99 for 3.5 fl. oz.)* contains several natural ingredients; however, this is nothing more than a standard bar soap. That means it is too drying and irritating for all skin types. To some extent, the plant oils it contains help offset the dryness, but the other cleansers from Neutrogena Naturals are strongly preferred.

☹ POOR **Oil-Free Acne Stress Control Night Cleansing Pads** *($6.99 for 60 pads)* will stress your skin because of the amount of alcohol. Alcohol not only causes dryness and irritation, but also can trigger oil production in the pore because the irritation triggers the release of androgens, the hormone responsible for causing oily skin. What a shame, because without the alcohol this would've been an effective cleanser with salicylic acid, and the fact that you don't rinse skin afterward means that the salicylic acid would have a chance to get into the pore and work.

☹ POOR **Oil-Free Acne Stress Control Power-Cream Wash** *($7.49 for 6 fl. oz.)* contains a combination of 2% salicylic acid along with approximately the same amount of glycolic acid and a creamy base, all of which may make you think this is an ideal cleanser for normal to dry skin that's blemish-prone. Alas, it isn't, because the AHA and BHA ingredients aren't in contact with skin long enough for them to function effectively as exfoliants, and leaving this on skin for any longer than what's necessary to clean the face will only increase the irritation from the menthol and cleansing agents. Neutrogena knows menthol is a problem for skin, but they consistently use it in most of their anti-acne products because so many consumers love that "refreshing tingle." If the tingle was somehow conveying an anti-acne benefit, we could concede to the sensation, but that's not the case.

☹ POOR **Oil-Free Acne Stress Control Power Gel Cleanser** *($7.49-$7.49 for 4 fl. oz.)* is not recommended because its main cleansing agent (sodium C14-16 olefin sulfonate) is too drying and irritating for all skin types. A cleanser alone cannot "control breakouts," not even if it is medicated with 2% salicylic acid, as this one is. Salicylic acid in a cleanser is essentially useless because it's rinsed down the drain before it can benefit your breakouts. This cleanser is also highly fragranced, and fragrance isn't skin care and definitely not helpful for acne-prone skin. The combined irritation from the cleansing agent and high amount of fragrance may make oily skin worse because irritation triggers excess oil production in the pore lining.

☹ POOR **Oil-Free Acne Wash** *($5.49 for 6 fl. oz.)* purports to be the #1 cleanser recommended by dermatologists for their patients with acne. If that's true, then lots of dermatologists are swayed by advertising and not up to speed on skin-care formulas. A dermatologist should know better than to endorse a cleanser that contains the drying, irritating detergent cleansing agent sodium C14-16 olefin sulfonate as a major ingredient, not to mention the fact that salicylic acid is wasted in a cleanser because it is just rinsed down the drain before it can be effective.

☹ POOR **Oil-Free Acne Wash Cream Cleanser** *($5.99 for 6.7 fl. oz.)* has a slightly creamy texture and contains gentle cleansing agents, but the inclusion of menthol still makes this cleanser too irritating for all skin types. Menthol's refreshing tingle is your skin telling you it's being irritated—see the Appendix for details. Although this cleanser is medicated with 2% salicylic acid and also contains the AHA ingredient glycolic acid, their contact with skin will be too brief for either to have an exfoliating action, so they're essentially wasted.

☹ POOR **Oil-Free Acne Wash Pink Grapefruit Cream Cleanser** *($7.49 for 6 fl. oz)* contains the key ingredient of BHA (chiefly the active ingredient 2% salicylic acid, which is great for blemish-prone skin), but it is rinsed from your face before it has a chance to work. This cleanser produces a creamy lather as claimed, but the grapefruit fragrance can cause needless irritation, as can the menthol. See the Appendix to find out why irritation is a problem for everyone's skin.

☹ POOR **Oil-Free Acne Wash Pink Grapefruit Facial Cleanser** *($7.49 for 6 fl. oz.)* is nearly identical to Neutrogena's original Oil-Free Acne Wash except this version contains grapefruit extract and a grapefruit fragrance. Otherwise, the same comments apply.

☹ POOR **Oil-Free Acne Wash, Redness Soothing Cream Cleanser** *($7.49 for 6 fl. oz.)* contains 2% salicylic acid as its active ingredient and also contains a fair amount of glycolic acid, which could have been helpful, but in a cleanser these ingredients are rinsed down the drain before they have a chance to do much good. Labeling this cleanser "soothing" is a mistake because Neutrogena included menthol, which is one of the least soothing ingredients around, not to mention that it has zero benefit for acne.

☹ POOR **Oil-Free Acne Wash, Redness Soothing Facial Cleanser** *($7.49 for 6 fl. oz.)* contains mild cleansing agents and is water-soluble; it also contains anti-irritants capable of reducing redness, but in a cleanser they are rinsed off the skin too quickly to impart that benefit. The same issue applies to this cleanser's active ingredient of 2% salicylic acid; you need to leave this on the skin to get maximum benefit, but leaving a cleanser on skin is too irritating and damaging for any skin type. That's doubly true for this cleanser because it contains the irritating menthol derivative menthyl lactate. See the Appendix for more details on why irritation is a problem you shouldn't overlook.

☹ POOR **Oil-Free Cleansing Wipes-Pink Grapefruit** *($7.49 for 25 towelettes)* are hugely irritating and drying for all skin types. Forget the pink grapefruit scent because fragrance isn't skin care any more than ice cream is health food. With alcohol as the second ingredient, a high amount of fragrance, the inclusion of potent skin-irritant menthol, and almost nothing of redeeming value for skin, these wipes should be left on the shelf. They are a problem for all skin types, especially if used around the eyes.

☹ POOR **Rapid Clear Oil-Control Foaming Cleanser** *($6.99 for 6 fl. oz.)* is a simply formulated cleanser that contains the strongly alkaline ingredient potassium stearate as the main cleansing agent. That means this cleanser is about as drying to skin as most bar soaps, and as a result is not recommended.

☹ POOR **Skin Clearing Face Wash** *($5.99 for 5.1 fl. oz.)* contains 1.5% salicylic acid, and you'd expect this to have a reasonable chance of promoting clear skin. Unfortunately, it won't do much to minimize blemishes because the active ingredient doesn't remains in contact with your skin long enough; it's just rinsed down the drain. This has good cleansing ability, but it is not recommended because it contains irritating menthol. See the Appendix to find out how irritation damages skin, even when you cannot see or feel it taking place.

☹ POOR **The Transparent Facial Bar, Acne-Prone Skin Formula** *($2.49 for 3.5 ounce bar)* is a variation on the same standard bar soap based on the drying, irritating cleansing agent TEA-stearate and traditional soap ingredients (such as tallow that can clog pores). This bar cleanser is not recommended for any skin type. The same comments apply to Neutrogena's **The Transparent Facial Bar, Original Formula** ($2.49 for 3.5 ounce bar), and **The Transparent Facial Bar, Original Formula, Fragrance-Free** ($2.99 for 3.5 ounce bar).

☹ POOR **Wave Sonic 2-Speed Spinning Power Cleanser** *($16.99 for 14 pads)* is Neutrogena's contribution to the crop of battery-powered cleansing devices. It isn't as elegant as Olay's Pro-X Advanced Cleansing System, but it costs only half as much, so you may be wondering if it's worth it: It isn't. The cleansing pads sold with the Wave Sonic contain the potent irritant menthol, so there is no reason to consider this system over Olay's option, which you can use with their cleanser or the cleanser of your choice, such as a well-formulated water-soluble cleanser.

NEUTROGENA EYE-MAKEUP REMOVERS

✓☺ BEST **Eye Makeup Remover Lotion-Hydrating** *($6.99 for 3 fl. oz.)* is a standard, but effective, fragrance-free eye-makeup remover. If you prefer a makeup remover with a lotion texture rather than a liquid texture, this is absolutely worth considering. It is suitable for all skin types (including sensitive) and deserves our top rating due to its mildness and the good range of skin-conditioning ingredients (some of which also help remove makeup). This product is suitable for taking off waterproof or long-wearing makeup, too.

✓☺ BEST **Oil-Free Eye Makeup Remover** *($6.99 for 5.5 fl. oz.)* is a gentle, fragrance-free, silicone-based dual-phase remover that works well to dissolve eye makeup, including waterproof formulas. Removers such as this may be used before or after cleansing.

☺ GOOD **Extra Gentle Eye Makeup Remover Pads** *($6.49 for 30 pads)* is akin to a silicone-based makeup remover steeped in plush, slightly textured pads. Although pricier than using a liquid makeup remover on a separate cotton pad, there's no denying that the formula works quickly to dissolve makeup, including waterproof formulas. These pads do contain fragrance.

☺ GOOD **Make-Up Remover Cleansing Towelettes** *($6.99 for 25 towelettes)* are cleansing cloths whose specialty is makeup removal, and they do an excellent job of breaking up and dissolving foundation, lipstick, and mascara (including waterproof types). These soft-textured cloths do not contain any needlessly irritating ingredients (such as menthol or arnica), making them safe for use around the eyes.

☺ GOOD **Makeup Remover Cleansing Towelettes-Hydrating** *($6.99 for 25 towelettes)* are a good option if you prefer to remove your makeup with pre-soaked cleansing cloths, although fragrance-free makeup removers are preferred. The soft cloths contain a lotion-like solution that quickly and easily removes all types of makeup with fairly minimal effort. It's not a good idea to use these cloths around your eyes due to the fragrance, but otherwise they work well.

☺ GOOD **Makeup Remover Cleansing Towelettes, Night Calming** *($7.99 for 25 towelettes)* are nearly identical to Neutrogena's regular Makeup Remover Cleansing Towelettes above. The only difference is the fragrance, which the company maintains is relaxing enough to set the user up for a good night's sleep. Given the brief contact this product has with skin, the scent isn't going to do much to induce relaxation. You're better off lighting a scented candle or spraying an air freshener whose aroma makes you feel relaxed.

☺ GOOD **Ultra-Soft Eye Makeup Remover Pads** *($5.99 for 30 pads)* aren't any softer than lots of others, but the price isn't terrible and they work quickly to remove all types of makeup. Suitable for all skin types except sensitive (due to the fragrance, which is always iffy in a product meant for use around the eyes), these are best used before cleansing because the pads leave a bit of a residue.

☹ POOR **Deep Clean Oil-Free Makeup Remover Cleansing Wipes** *($7.99 for 25 wipes)* list alcohol as the second ingredient, which doesn't deep-clean skin as much as it causes dryness, irritation, and free-radical damage. Menthol is also on hand for a second wave of irritation, and the duo makes these wipes a must to avoid, at least if you're concerned about keeping your skin healthy and youthful.

NEUTROGENA TONERS

☹ AVERAGE **Alcohol-Free Toner** *($6.99 for 8.5 fl. oz.)* is an average toner at best because it lacks significant water-binding agents or ingredients that support skin's structure. The formula is OK for normal to slightly dry or slightly oily skin.

☹ POOR **Clear Pore Oil-Eliminating Astringent** *($5.99 for 8 fl. oz.)* contains 45% alcohol followed by witch hazel (which just adds more alcohol), and together these make this astringent too irritating to consider, not to mention the alcohol stimulates oil production in the pore (see the Appendix for details). The pH of this product prevents the 2% salicylic acid from functioning effectively as an exfoliant.

☹ POOR **Oil-Free Acne Stress Control Triple-Action Toner** *($7.49 for 8 fl. oz.)* causes stress (and stimulates oil production) thanks to its irritating, drying alcohol content. The pH of this product is just low enough to allow the 2% salicylic acid to function as an exfoliant, but that comes at the cost of subjecting your skin to the free-radical damage of the alcohol. Not good, and not recommended considering that there are BHA exfoliants available that work against acne and that soothe and even skin without also causing undue irritation. You'll find those in the Best Products chapter at the end of this book.

☹ POOR **Pore Refining Toner** *($6.49 for 8.5 fl. oz.)* lists alcohol as the second ingredient, and also contains witch hazel. It is even more irritating than usual because it also contains peppermint and eucalyptus. The alcohol will stimulate oil production at the base of your pores, which isn't the least bit refining. See the Appendix to learn more about the problems irritation causes.

☹ POOR **Rapid Clear 2-in-1 Fight & Fade Toner** *($6.99 for 8 fl. oz.)* contains 2% salicylic acid as its active ingredient and has a pH that's within range for exfoliation to occur. A well-formulated BHA (salicylic acid) product is a cornerstone of smart skin care when blemishes are a concern, and ongoing exfoliation will help fade marks left by past blemishes. However, the amount of alcohol in this toner is too great to ignore, and it is not recommended. See the Appendix to learn why alcohol is such a problem, and check out the Best Products section to find anti-acne products that are effective yet gentle.

NEUTROGENA EXFOLIANTS & SCRUBS

✔☺ BEST **Oil-Free Acne Stress Control 3-In-1 Hydrating Acne Treatment** *($6.99 for 2 fl. oz.)* gets Neutrogena back into the BHA game, and it's about time! Most of their previous BHA products either contained irritating ingredients (particularly alcohol and menthol) or had a pH that was too high for effective exfoliation to take place. This version contains 2% salicylic acid at a pH of 3.4, and comes in a nearly weightless silicone base that includes anti-oxidants and anti-irritants. Although the inclusion of fragrance and coloring agents is a slight disappointment, it's a relief that Neutrogena omitted menthol or its derivatives, making this an all-around ideal BHA lotion for skin of any type battling blemishes. The only other company that consistently offers well-formulated BHA exfoliants is Paula's Choice.

☺ GOOD **Deep Clean Gentle Scrub** *($5.99 for 4.2 fl. oz.)* is indeed gentle, and makes a very good cleanser/scrub hybrid product for normal to oily skin. The salicylic acid isn't doing the exfoliating; the polyethylene (plastic) beads do that when massaged over the skin.

☺ GOOD **Fresh Foaming Scrub** *($5.99 for 4.2 fl. oz.)* is a good option. It contains cleansing agents, too, and is best for normal to oily skin. Rounded polyethylene (plastic) beads are the scrub agent, and their smooth shape makes them preferred to scrubs that use nut shells or other irregular particles that can abrade the skin, causing more problems than they solve. This scrub rinses easily and, unlike some others from Neutrogena, does not contain irritants like menthol or menthyl lactate. It does contain fragrance.

☺ GOOD **Healthy Skin Anti-Wrinkle Anti-Blemish Scrub** *($7.99 for 4 fl. oz.)* contains 0.5% salicylic acid as an active ingredient and also includes 2% glycolic acid. Neither will exfoliate, however, given their brief contact with the skin before being rinsed down the drain. However, this is worth considering as a cleansing scrub for all skin types except very dry. It is more abrasive than several other scrubs that also contain polyethylene beads, but if used gently can be a helpful addition to your routine.

☺ GOOD **Neutrogena Naturals Purifying Pore Scrub** *($7.49 for 4 fl. oz.)*. Scrubs don't purify pores or lead to clear skin, no matter how well formulated they are (and this is a good, gentle scrub formula). Breakouts cannot be scrubbed away, and, in fact, it's a bad idea to use scrubs over acne lesions because they can hurt the healing process and make already-red skin lesions redder. If acne isn't your concern, this is a workable scrub that helps make all skin types smoother. For breakouts, the best exfoliant is a leave-on product with salicylic acid (BHA).

☺ GOOD **Rapid Clear Acne Defense Face Lotion** *($6.99 for 1.7 fl. oz.)* is an effective BHA product option in the battle against blemishes. With 2% salicylic acid and a pH of 3.6, this can indeed exfoliate skin and help dislodge blackheads. The product features a lightweight moisturizing base that is best for normal to slightly dry skin dealing with blemishes. The only issue is the irritating fragrant extracts it contains (cinnamon and cedar), though they are present in amounts that are likely too low to cause irritation. Still, they are unnecessary additives and prevent this BHA product from earning a Best Product rating.

☹ AVERAGE **All-in-1 Acne Control Facial Treatment** *($7.49 for 1 fl. oz.)* is medicated with 1% salicylic acid and comes in a lightweight yet hydrating base suitable for normal to dry skin. The pH of this product is above 5, which means the salicylic acid cannot function as an exfoliant, yet that's the goal. We would rate the formula higher if the pH were within range for efficacy and if it were fragrance-free (the fragrance really lingers), and also contained a range of soothing anti-irritants or a higher amount of antioxidants for further benefits. This contains a tiny amount of retinol, likely too low to offer much help to acne-prone skin. By the way, this isn't an "all in one" option for acne. Treating acne requires other products, too, such as a gentle cleanser and a topical disinfectant medicated with benzoyl peroxide. Salicylic acid alone is not enough to get most cases of acne under control, and with this product you'll have little hope of seeing fewer breakouts.

☹ AVERAGE **Oil-Free Acne Wash Pink Grapefruit Foaming Scrub** *($7.49 for 4.2 fl. oz.)* is an OK option if you have normal to oily skin and it isn't nearly as harsh on your skin as Neutrogena's Oil-Free Acne Wash Pink Grapefruit Facial Cleanser, but the fact remains that the 2% salicylic acid is wasted due to this scrub's brief contact with skin. Besides, the pH of this scrub is too high for the salicylic acid to function as intended anyway.

☻ POOR **All-in-1 Acne Control Daily Scrub** *($7.49-$7.49 for 4 fl. oz.)* contains menthyl lactate, which is a form of menthol that causes irritation. As such, this scrub is not recommended. See the Appendix to learn why irritation is a problem for everyone's skin, and remember, acne cannot be scrubbed away!

☻ POOR **Blackhead Eliminating Daily Scrub** *($6.99 for 4.2 fl. oz.)* contains menthol and is not recommended. Using a topical scrub over blackheads removes only the top portion of them. That means that the "root" of the blackhead is still inside the pore, so the effect from the scrub is minimal at best, and for that benefit a washcloth would prove just as effective (without the irritation from the menthol).

☻ POOR **Body Clear Body Spray** *($8.49 for 4 fl. oz.)* is medicated with 0.5% salicylic acid, an amount that's OK, but not as effective as 1%–2%, especially if you have stubborn breakouts or blackheads, which is typical for breakouts on the chest, neck, or back. More important, the pH of this product is too high for the salicylic acid to work as an exfoliant. The other concern is the alcohol, which not only causes dryness, promotes free-radical damage, and impairs healing, but also stimulates oil production at the base of the pore.

☻ POOR **Clear Pore Daily Scrub** *($6.99 for 4.2 fl. oz.)* has good intentions, but poor execution. It's medicated with the anti-acne ingredient benzoyl peroxide, but in a scrub this ingredient is rinsed from your skin before it has much chance to work. Speaking of rinsing, the clay in this scrub makes it difficult to rinse and also makes it tricky to spread evenly over your face. Contrary to claim, this scrub is not "gentle enough for daily use." First, clogged pores and breakouts cannot be scrubbed away; the best way to go is a well-formulated, leave-on product with benzoyl peroxide, used with a BHA product whose active ingredient is salicylic acid (and the BHA is applied first). Second, because this scrub contains the irritant menthol, all claims of gentleness should be dismissed. Menthol causes irritation that can trigger more oil production, potentially making breakouts and clogged pores worse, not better.

☹ POOR **Deep Clean Invigorating Foaming Scrub** *($7.99 for 4.2 fl. oz.)* is a below-standard scrub that irritates all skin types with menthol. Menthol is a problematic ingredient and its invigorating feeling is just your skin telling you it is being irritated.

☹ POOR **Deep Clean Long-Last Shine Control Daily Scrub** *($7.49 for 4.2 fl. oz.)* contains the irritant menthol, like most of Neutrogena's scrubs. This product is not recommended; see the Appendix to learn why irritation is a problem for all skin types.

☹ POOR **Oil-Free Acne Stress Control Power-Clear Scrub** *($7.49 for 4.2 fl. oz.)* contains menthol, which makes it too irritating for all skin types. The 2% salicylic acid isn't going to benefit blemish-prone skin when used in a topical scrub because it is basically rinsed down the drain right after it's applied.

☹ POOR **Oil-Free Acne Wash Daily Scrub** *($5.99 for 4.2 fl. oz.)* is nearly identical to the Oil-Free Acne Stress Control Power-Clear Scrub above, and the same review applies.

☹ POOR **Oil-Free Acne Wash, Redness Soothing Gentle Scrub** *($7.49 for 4.2 fl. oz.)* is nearly identical to the Oil-Free Acne Stress Control Power-Clear Scrub above, and the same review applies.

☹ POOR **Rapid Clear Foaming Scrub** *($7.99 for 4.2 fl. oz.)* is nearly identical to the Oil-Free Acne Stress Control Power-Clear Scrub above, and the same review applies.

NEUTROGENA MOISTURIZERS (DAYTIME, NIGHTTIME), EYE CREAMS, & SERUMS

✓☺ BEST **Ageless Intensives Tone Correcting Moisture SPF 30** *($18.99 for 1 fl. oz.)* is a fragranced daytime moisturizer with sunscreen, but doesn't contain a significant amount of ingredients known to lighten skin discolorations (other than what every sunscreen offers skin in that regard). Still, this is a very good option for those with normal to oily skin. The silky formula includes avobenzone for sufficient UVA protection and also includes several antioxidants, cell-communicating ingredients (including retinol), and a tiny amount of anti-irritants. The consistency of this moisturizer with sunscreen allows it to work well under makeup, too. This contains a small amount of the mineral pigment mica, which lends a bit of a shiny finish.

✓☺ BEST **Healthy Skin Anti-Wrinkle Cream, Night** *($12.99 for 1.4 fl. oz.)* is a good, fragrance-free moisturizer with retinol for normal to dry skin. The retinol is packaged to keep it stable, the amount of green tea is impressive, and the formula contains tiny amounts of two forms of Vitamin E. It is definitely one of the better retinol products at the drugstore. Special Note: This line of products is creating a lot of confusion for readers, so we wanted to clarify the information that we have confirmed through Neutrogena regarding these products. Healthy Skin Anti-Wrinkle Cream, Night used to be called Healthy Skin Anti-Wrinkle Cream Original Formula. What is now called Healthy Skin Anti-Wrinkle Cream Original Formula is a different product that has an added SPF 15.

☺ GOOD **Ageless Intensives Deep Wrinkle Anti-Wrinkle Moisture SPF 20** *($18.99 for 1.4 fl. oz.)* provides a convenient, elegant way for you to experience an in-part avobenzone sunscreen in a lightly moisturizing base with retinol and a tiny amount of water-binding agents. This isn't at the same level of formulary excellence as Neutrogena's tinted Healthy Skin Enhancer

SPF 20, but it's worth a try if you have normal to slightly oily skin. This product will not fill in the look of deep wrinkles within two weeks. That's wishful thinking! Neutrogena should have settled for what works and left the other claim to less reputable cosmetics companies.

☺ GOOD **Healthy Defense Daily Moisturizer SPF 50 with Purescreen for Sensitive Skin** *($13.99 for 1.7 fl. oz.)* has a gentle, fragrance-free blend of mineral sunscreens (titanium dioxide and zinc oxide). The lightweight creamy lotion spreads easily, sets quickly, and leaves a satin matte finish on skin. Yes, this feels slightly tacky, but it's also quite tenacious. You can be assured of long-lasting protection, but don't forget to reapply as needed. The only disappointing part of this sunscreen is its lack of antioxidants and skin-identical ingredients, something the face always needs. A teeny-tiny amount of anti-irritant bisabolol is present, but it's clearly an afterthought and unlikely to benefit your skin. Neutrogena did a great job with the aesthetics (this doesn't leave a strong white cast on skin) and those with sensitive skin can pair it with an antioxidant-rich serum such as Paula's Choice RESIST Super Antioxidant Concentrate Serum.

☺ GOOD **Healthy Defense Liquid Moisturizer SPF 50** *($13.99 for 1.4 fl. oz.)* is a fluid, silky daytime moisturizer with sunscreen bound to appeal to those with oily skin or anyone who normally shies away from high-SPF sunscreens due to their thick texture or tacky finish. Beyond the aesthetics, the formula includes stabilized avobenzone for reliable UVA protection, but the amount of antioxidants (which help boost a sunscreen's efficacy and your skin's defenses) is paltry. This deserves a Good rating for its texture (it works great under makeup) and broad-spectrum protection, but antioxidants should've been a more central part of the formula given the claims Neutrogena makes.

☺ GOOD **Healthy Skin Anti-Wrinkle Anti-Blemish Clear Skin Cream** *($13.99 for 1 fl. oz.)* sounds like a treat for consumers battling wrinkles and breakouts, an all-too-common frustration. However, the 2% salicylic acid cannot exfoliate very effectively because the pH is too high. This is worth considering as an antioxidant-rich moisturizer that also contains retinol. It is suitable for normal to dry skin and does contain fragrance. The addition of a few skin-repairing ingredients would've propelled this to our top rating, but it's still a good, affordable option.

☺ GOOD **Neutrogena Naturals Multi-Vitamin Nourishing Moisturizer** *($13.99 for 3 fl. oz.)* is a fragranced moisturizer that contains a mix of natural and synthetic ingredients (which is fine), but the bulk of the ingredients are natural or at least naturally sourced. The formula is best for normal to dry skin and contains an interesting, rarely used Peruvian plant oil known as *Plukenetia volubilis*. This nonfragrant oil is a rich source of essential fatty acids and antioxidants, including vitamin E (Source: *The Journal of Agriculture and Food Chemistry*, December 2011, pages 13043–13049). It's great that Neutrogena included it in an impressive amount because the only other antioxidant (tocopherol) is in short supply. On balance, this isn't a brilliant formula but it's better than what Neutrogena typically offers in the facial moisturizers without sunscreen category. You may also want to check out Paula's Choice Earth Sourced Antioxidant-Enriched Natural Moisturizer ($20.95 for 2 fl. oz.).

☺ GOOD **Rapid Wrinkle Repair Serum** *($20.99 for 1 fl. oz.)* definitely makes skin feel smoother thanks to the silky silicone ingredients it contains. Because of the absorbent aluminum starch ingredient, this leaves a slightly dry finish that won't hydrate, at least not enough for dry areas to improve. As an anti-aging powerhouse, it's a bit on the weak side but not terribly so. Yes, this contains retinol and retinol is an excellent ingredient to fight multiple signs of aging (though it's not the absolute best or the only ingredient to look for). What this could use more of are antioxidants and repairing ingredients to rebuild skin's surface, fight inflammation, and enhance healthy collagen production. This contains the salt form of hyaluronic acid (an ingredient known as sodium hyaluronate), but so do lots of other serums. The mica in here adds shine to skin and that can help boost radiance, but it's a cosmetic effect, not a skin-care miracle.

☺ GOOD **Ultra Sheer Liquid Daily Sunblock SPF 55** *($11.99 for 1.4 fl. oz.)* is for those of you who detest the thick, occlusive feeling of many high-SPF sunscreens. Neutrogena has crafted an exceptionally light, fluid lotion that provides broad-spectrum protection. Stabilized avobenzone provides reliable UVA protection and, true to claim, this works beautifully under makeup. Worn alone, it has a smooth matte finish that won't make normal to oily skin look greasy. The anti-irritant and antioxidants are a nice touch, but their overall low amounts keep this fragranced daytime moisturizer with sunscreen from earning our top rating. Still, the nearly weightless texture and smooth application are something to experience—and you can always pair this with an antioxidant-rich serum, such as those from Paula's Choice.

☺ GOOD **Visibly Even Daily Moisturizer SPF 30** *($13.49 for 1.7 fl. oz.)* isn't a daytime moisturizer with a bounty of antioxidants to help defend skin, but it does provide sufficient UVA protection with stabilized avobenzone. The somewhat creamy lotion texture is suitable for normal to dry skin and includes soybean seed extract as the main antioxidant. All the other beneficial ingredients (of which there are few) are present in amounts likely too small to benefit skin. This is still worth considering as a daytime moisturizer with sunscreen, but it falls short of joining the top brass in this category.

☻ AVERAGE **Ageless Essentials Continuous Hydration Time Released Moisturizer, Night** *($14.49 for 1.7 fl. oz.)* is a basic, lightly emollient moisturizer for normal to slightly dry skin. There is nothing particularly exciting about the formula, so calling it "Ageless Essentials" is a bit like serving a plain baloney sandwich and calling it fine dining. We're concerned about the amount of *Chrysanthemum parthenium* (feverfew) extract in this product. However, it appears that Neutrogena's owner Johnson & Johnson is aware of the irritants in this plant, and so has developed and is using a form of feverfew that does not contain the suspect chemicals (Sources: *Inflammopharmacology*, February 2009, pages 42–49; and *Archives of Dermatological Research*, February 2008, pages 69–80). What's uncertain is whether they're using the irritant-free form of this ingredient in their products (research is one thing, but it's meaningless if it's not carried through to the formulary stage). Either way, it isn't a miracle ingredient and there is more alcohol in this product than any interesting ingredients anyway.

☻ AVERAGE **Ageless Intensives Deep Wrinkle Anti-Wrinkle Eye Cream** *($18.99 for 0.5 fl. oz.)* is a decent lightweight moisturizing cream for use around the eyes or anywhere your skin is experiencing mild dryness (you really don't need a special product labeled "eye cream"; see the Apependix to find out why). It contains a standard array of thickeners and emollients along with silicones, glycerin, several antioxidants (which is good, because none of them are present in any significant amount), an anti-irritant, retinol, film-forming agent, and preservatives. It is fragrance-free and packaged so the retinol will remain stable during use. This eye cream won't reduce the appearance of dark circles or fill in deep wrinkles. The only reason to consider this product is if you want to try an eye-area moisturizer with retinol.

☻ AVERAGE **Ageless Intensives Deep Wrinkle Anti-Wrinkle Moisture, Night** *($18.99 for 1.4 fl. oz.)* has a decent formula with some antioxidants and a skin-identical ingredient with stable packaging, but for the money, Neutrogena offers more impressive moisturizer formulas, as does their competitor Olay.

The Reviews N

❧ Highly fragranced products smell good, but won't help your skin! See the Appendix for details.

☺ AVERAGE **Ageless Intensives Deep Wrinkle Anti-Wrinkle Serum** *($18.99 for 1 fl. oz.)* has a silky, gel-cream texture unlike that of a true serum, and includes a blend of silicones, film-forming agents, anti-irritants, and retinol. A variety of antioxidants is absent here, making this more of a one-note product, with retinol as the star ingredient. However, retinol is without question an anti-aging superstar. The decision about whether to use this retinol serum or one from another brand comes down to formula, and Neutrogena's isn't among the best. That's partly because the amount of film-forming agents in here is potentially problematic. Nonetheless, it is fragrance-free and comes in packaging that will definitely keep the retinol stable. The formula is suitable for all skin types except sensitive.

☺ AVERAGE **Ageless Restoratives Instant Eye Reviver** *($15.99 for 0.5 fl. oz.)* is an average, extremely ordinary lightweight eye cream that is not specially formulated for the eye area, but rather is suitable for slightly dry skin anywhere on the face. It is fragrance-free and contains a smattering of minerals, though none of these or any other ingredient in this product can noticeably diminish puffy eyes or dark circles.

☺ AVERAGE **Anti-Aging Booster Serum** *($20.99 for 0.5 fl. oz.)*. If you believe the claims, this serum is supposed to combine with your anti-aging moisturizer to "activate" and improve every sign of aging you can think of. It doesn't do anything but make your skin feel smoother and softer. Anti-Aging Booster Serum contains copper and zinc; there is research pertaining to copper and its dual role in skin: wound-healing and altering the matrix metalloproteinases (MMP) that contribute to collagen depletion. Applying ingredients that work against this damage is helpful, but this is not the only way to improve aging skin. Zinc is believed to play a co-factor role with copper when it comes to repairing damaged elastin in skin. However, it's not the only game in town, it can't provide anything that other skin-care products can't provide and doesn't substitute for what a cosmetic dermatologist can do to improve skin. (Sources: *Connective Tissue Research*, January 2010, Epublication; *Experimental Dermatology*, March 2009, pages 205–211; and *Veterinary Dermatology*, December 2006, pages 417–423). There is no solid research proving that topical zinc or copper can stop or reverse sagging skin that results from elastin damage.

☺ AVERAGE **Healthy Defense Daily Moisturizer SPF 50 with Helioplex** *($13.99 for 1.7 fl. oz.)* has a lightweight texture that makes it preferred for normal to oily skin. A smattering of antioxidants is included to help bolster skin's environmental defenses. The only drawback is the inclusion of methylisothiazolinone, a preservative that is contraindicated for use in leave-on products owing to its sensitizing potential.

☺ AVERAGE **Healthy Defense SPF 30 Daily Moisturizer, Light Tint** *($13.99 for 1.7 fl. oz.)* is an average daytime moisturizer with sunscreen for normal to slightly dry skin. The in part zinc oxide sunscreen is great, but the sheer-tinted base formula doesn't go the distance.

☺ AVERAGE **Healthy Defense SPF 30 Daily Moisturizer with Helioplex** *($13.99 for 1.7 fl. oz.)* is an average daytime moisturizer with sunscreen for normal to slightly dry skin. The in-part zinc oxide sunscreen is great, but the lightweight base formula doesn't go the distance.

☺ AVERAGE **Healthy Skin Eye Cream** *($11.99 for 0.5 fl. oz.)* lists glycolic acid, but is unable to exfoliate skin due to this product's pH being too high. It is an OK moisturizer for dry skin anywhere on the face, assuming you don't mind adding shine (the mica is what's working as an "optical light diffuser"). In terms of soothing agents reducing puffiness, this product contains a small amount of them, but they will only reduce your puffy eyes if the swelling is caused by external irritants (think allergens), not aging. Healthy Skin Eye Cream is fragrance-free. See the Appendix to learn why, in truth, you don't need an eye cream.

☺ AVERAGE **Healthy Skin Firming Cream SPF 15** *($12.99 for 2.5 fl. oz.)* is similar to many others from Neutrogena, including "regular" sunscreens you'd apply from the neck down. Critical UVA (think anti-aging) protection is supplied by stabilized avobenzone, and this has a lightweight lotion texture best for normal to slightly dry or combination skin. Antioxidants, which can stimulate collagen production for firmer skin, are in short supply, but at least the formula has a few of them.

☺ AVERAGE **Healthy Skin Radiance Cream Boost Radiance SPF 15** *($12.99 for 2.5 fl. oz.)* is a relatively unimpressive daytime moisturizer with sunscreen despite its great name. It's good that critical UVA protection is supplied by avobenzone, but the fragranced formula is mostly ho-hum, and your skin deserves a daily dose of state-of-the-art ingredients. Beyond the sunscreen, the only impressive ingredient in this product is soybean seed extract, but skin needs more than one ingredient to be healthy and fight wrinkles.

☺ AVERAGE **Light Night Cream** *($11.99 for 2.25 fl. oz.)* remains in the Neutrogena lineup, and is still a basic, emollient moisturizer for normal to dry skin. It contains a tiny amount of soy fatty acid, but is otherwise devoid of state-of-the-art ingredients.

☺ AVERAGE **Neutrogena Naturals Multi-Vitamin Nourishing Night Cream** *($13.99 for 1.7 fl. oz.)* contains a mix of natural and synthetic ingredients (which is fine), but the bulk of the ingredients are natural or at least naturally sourced. The formula is best for normal to dry skin and contains an interesting, rarely used Peruvian plant oil known as *Plukenetia volubilis*. This nonfragrant oil is a rich source of essential fatty acids and antioxidants, including vitamin E (Source: *The Journal of Agriculture and Food Chemistry*, December 2011, pages 13043–13049). It's great that Neutrogena included it in an impressive amount because the only other antioxidants are in short supply. Most disappointing is that the antioxidants and plant oil in this moisturizer won't remain stable once opened due to the fact that it's packaged in a jar. That alone makes this hard to recommend, especially given that competing brands at the drugstore offer better moisturizer formulas in packaging that will keep light- and air-sensitive ingredients stable during use. Note: This moisturizer does not contain vitamins B and C as claimed. The plant *Ilex paraguariensis* (also known as yerba mate) contains trace amounts of vitamin C and the B vitamins riboflavin and thiamine, but that's not the same as using pure vitamin B or C.

☺ AVERAGE **Oil-Free Moisture, for Combination Skin** *($9.99 for 4 fl. oz.)* provides lightweight, skin-silkening moisture for its intended skin type, and doesn't contain fragrance. However, your skin deserves more than this basic formula provides.

☺ AVERAGE **Oil-Free Moisture, for Sensitive Skin** *($9.99 for 4 fl. oz.)* is suitable for dry, sensitive skin (and for those with rosacea) because it contains some good emollients and a small amount of water-binding agents. This is also fragrance-free, but that's where the excitement starts and stops. Still, the other attributes make it a worthy for sensitive skin, but there are better options to consider.

☺ AVERAGE **Oil-Free Moisture SPF 35** *($9.99 for 4 fl. oz.)* includes stabilized avobenzone for critical UVA (think anti-aging) protection; however, the base formula doesn't have the type of ingredients all skin types need to look and act healthier. Neutrogena could have made this far better had they included antioxidants, skin-repairing ingredients, and perhaps a cell-communicating ingredient or two. As is, you're getting an ordinary product, when your skin deserves a daily dose of wow! This moisturizer with sunscreen contains the problematic preservative methylisothiazolinone, which generally is not recommended for use in leave-on products due to its sensitizing potential.

The Reviews N

☺ AVERAGE **Rapid Wrinkle Repair Eye Cream** *($20.99 for 0.5 fl. oz.)* differs little from the ingredient list seen on most of Neutrogena's eye creams. Despite an enticing name, this one doesn't distinguish itself, and it certainly isn't the one you should pick because its formula is boring. Besides, you really don't need an eye cream—see the Appendix to find out why!

☺ AVERAGE **Rapid Wrinkle Repair Moisturizer Night** *($20.99 for 1 fl. oz.)*. Despite claims of fast efficacy on wrinkles, this moisturizer with retinol isn't all that impressive. It has a nice, silky texture and leaves normal to dry skin feeling smooth, but the amount of state-of-the-art ingredients (including retinol) is nothing to write home about. Given the priority retinol gets in this product's ads, it's surprising that the formula contains more preservatives and fragrance than this superstar anti-aging ingredient. The same is true for the hyaluronic acid (listed as sodium hyaluronate) and as for the "glucose complex," we're not sure what Neutrogena means by this because none of the ingredients match this description. The ads for this product state that 100% of women had noticeable results in "just one week," but the company doesn't state what those results were. For all we know, 100% of women who tested this product may have reported their skin looked and felt smoother. That's something any moisturizer can do, whether it contains retinol or not. As it turns out, the claim sounds impressive but is most likely no big deal.

☺ AVERAGE **Rapid Wrinkle Repair Moisturizer SPF 30** *($20.99 for 1 fl. oz.)*. This daytime moisturizer with sunscreen includes avobenzone for reliable UVA (anti-aging) protection, so it's off to a good start. The silky lotion formula is suitable for normal to oily or combination skin, but the anti-aging ingredients touted in the product's claims are in short supply, and this ends up being a rather ordinary, boring formulation. Although claimed to produce remarkable results in one week, given the formula, it just isn't going to happen. At best, this provides lightweight hydration and broad-spectrum sun protection, which is important, but hardly unique to this product.

☹ AVERAGE **Ultra Gentle Soothing Cream** *($15.99 for 1.5 fl. oz.)* is a fairly basic emollient moisturizer that's an OK option for dry skin, although it isn't all that gentle or soothing. It is short on soothing ingredients and contains more fragrance than it does the types of ingredients those with sensitive skin need to see improvement. Really, choosing to include fragrance in a product for sensitive skin is just rude. It is hardly a secret that when it comes to sensitive skin, fragrance is a huge no-no. Neutrogena advertises that the fragrance they use was "uniquely developed for sensitive skin," but given they only list the word "fragrance" on their ingredient list, there is no way to check out what they claim! Nonetheless, because sensitive skin can react to all manner of fragrances, it is best for those with reactive skin to stay away from products with any kind of fragrance. Perhaps most disappointing is that the soothing plant extracts this moisturizer does contain won't remain effective after opening because of the jar packaging. See the Appendix for details on the issues jar packaging presents.

☺ AVERAGE **Ultra Gentle Soothing Lotion SPF 15** *($15.99 for 4 fl. oz.)* isn't ultra gentle and it's only minimally soothing. The active ingredients provide broad-spectrum sun protection, but they are not preferred for sensitive skin. When sensitive skin is your chief concern, the best sunscreen ingredients are the mineral actives titanium dioxide and zinc oxide, which pose no risk of irritation; all other sunscreen actives, including those in this product, run the risk of making sensitive skin worse. Ultimately, this is a well-intentioned product with a misguided formula. It is not recommended for sensitive skin, but is an OK option for normal to dry skin.

☹ POOR **Healthy Skin Anti-Wrinkle Cream, Original Formula SPF 15** *($12.99 for 1.4 fl. oz.)* is not actually "Original Formula." Neutrogena repackaged and renamed the real original formula (now sold as Healthy Skin Anti-Wrinkle Cream Night) and slapped "Original Formula" on this version with SPF 15. The results are disappointing because it lacks the UVA-protecting ingredients of titanium dioxide, zinc oxide, avobenzone, Mexoryl SX (ecamsule), or Tinosorb and is not recommended. If this supplied better UVA protection, it would be a good way to combine daily sun protection with antioxidants and the anti-aging ingredient retinol.

☹ POOR **Healthy Skin Face Lotion SPF 15** *($10.99 for 2.5 fl. oz.)* leaves skin vulnerable to UVA damage because it lacks sunscreen agents capable of shielding skin from the entire spectrum of UVA light (see the Appendix for details). What a shame, because the 8% glycolic acid and pH of 3.3 allow exfoliation to occur, which would have made this a convenient, dual-purpose product.

☹ POOR **Oil-Free Anti-Acne Moisturizer** *($5.99 for 1.7 fl. oz.)* contains the irritating menthol derivative menthyl lactate, and is not recommended. The amount of salicylic acid is good for helping acne and blackheads but the pH is borderline for efficacy. Regardless of how effective the salicylic acid may be, the previously mentioned irritant makes this a deal-breaker. Needless irritation can stimulate oil production at the base of the pores, making acne and oily skin worse, not better.

☹ POOR **Oil-Free Moisture SPF 15** *($9.99 for 4 fl. oz.)* doesn't contain oil, but also doesn't provide sufficient UVA-protecting ingredients (see the Appendix to learn which ingredients are critical for this need). Given Neutrogena's sun-savvy marketing campaigns and its roster of impressive broad-spectrum sunscreens, this product should be discontinued—it's not doing anyone's skin any favors, that's for sure.

NEUTROGENA SUN CARE

✓☺ BEST **Sensitive Skin Sunblock SPF 30** *($8.99 for 4 fl. oz.)* remains a good choice for those with sensitive skin, including those struggling with rosacea. The sole active ingredient is titanium dioxide, formulated in a creamy base that is easy to spread. It's disappointing that antioxidants and soothing agents are in short supply, but they're potentially helpful, so this deserves a Best Product rating due to its value for sensitive skin. Note that the amount of titanium dioxide can leave a white cast that's difficult to soften. This sunscreen is an option for use on facial skin, too.

✓☺ BEST **Ultra Sheer Dry-Touch Sunblock SPF 30** *($9.49 for 3 fl. oz.)* really does have a dry finish, and is an outstanding in-part avobenzone sunscreen that begins creamy but quickly dries down to a weightless matte (in feel) finish. The high levels of active ingredients required to net an SPF 30 do leave a very slight sheen on the skin, but it's hardly worth complaining about, especially if you are dealing with oily to very oily skin and have been unable to find a stand-alone sunscreen that doesn't feel heavy or greasy. Those with normal to dry skin will likely find this sunscreen too drying, but it's a winning option for oily and/or breakout-prone skin, and it does contain vitamin-based antioxidants.

✓☺ BEST **Ultra Sheer Dry-Touch Sunblock SPF 45** *($9.49 for 3 fl. oz.)* is very similar to Neutrogena's Ultra Sheer Dry-Touch Sunblock SPF 30, but the SPF 45 version contains a higher amount of active ingredients necessary to reach its higher SPF rating. Otherwise, the same comments apply.

☺ GOOD **Build-A-Tan Gradual Sunless Tanning** *($9.99 for 6.7 fl. oz.)* is a very standard, but good, self-tanning lotion for normal to oily skin. It tans skin with dihydroxyacetone, the same ingredient found in most self-tanners.

☺ GOOD **Pure & Free Baby Faces Ultra Gentle Sunblock SPF 45+** *($11.49 for 2.5 fl. oz.)* is a surprisingly light sunscreen lotion that provides broad-spectrum protection via the mineral actives titanium dioxide and zinc oxide. These sunscreen agents are excellent for sensitive skin, including those struggling with rosacea. If the formula contained a range of skin-repairing and soothing agents, it would be a slam-dunk for sensitive skin. As is, although the formula is fragrance-free, it definitely leaves your skin wanting (and, if it's sensitive, needing) more. Still, on balance, this deserves a Good rating for the sun protection and the pleasant texture. Those with normal to slightly dry skin that's also sensitive will do best with this sunscreen, and it is suitable for use on babies and children. By the way, this isn't free of chemical sunscreens as claimed.

☺ GOOD **Pure & Free Baby Sunblock Stick SPF 60+ with PureScreen** *($9.99 for 0.47 fl. oz.)* has value for those with sensitive, reactive skin. The gentle actives consist of titanium dioxide and zinc oxide, while the base formula is fragrance-free and works well over dry areas due to the protective qualities of the waxes that keep this product in stick form. It is ideal for use on children or adults but the waxy texture can feel heavy and sticky. Note that this sunscreen stick is not recommended for use on breakout-prone areas.

☺ GOOD **Pure & Free Liquid Daily Sunblock SPF 50** *($12.49 for 1.4 fl. oz.)* is a surprisingly light, thin-textured sunscreen that provides broad-spectrum protection via the mineral actives titanium dioxide and zinc oxide. These sunscreen agents are excellent for sensitive skin, including those struggling with rosacea. If the formula contained a range of skin-repairing and soothing agents, it would be a slam-dunk for sensitive skin. As is, although the formula is fragrance-free, it definitely leaves your skin wanting (and, if it's sensitive, needing) more. Still, on balance, this deserves a Good rating for the sun protection and the pleasant texture. Those with normal to slightly dry skin that's also sensitive will do best with this sunscreen.

☺ GOOD **Ultimate Sport Sunblock Lotion SPF 30** *($9.49 for 4 fl. oz.)* isn't formulated with sensitizing preservatives, unlike most of Neutrogena's other Ultimate Sport sunscreens. That's a plus because the active ingredients in this sunscreen (which includes stabilized avobenzone for critical UVA protection) can be sensitizing on their own, especially if they get in your eyes via sweat. This sunscreen has a lightweight, silky texture that makes it easy to apply, and it is best for normal to oily or breakout-prone skin. Contrary to claims, it doesn't resist sweating, water, or being rubbed off—at least not for more than an hour or two. Although this contains film-forming agents that allow the active ingredients to adhere to skin better, they're not completely impervious to being rinsed or rubbed off over time. That means reapplication is necessary, especially during long days outdoors when you'll be active and perspiring (or swimming).

☺ GOOD **Ultra Sheer Dry-Touch Sunblock SPF 55** *($9.49 for 3 fl. oz.)* is definitely sheer, and a great choice for those who find high-SPF products feel thick, greasy, or occlusive. This has a tenacious formula, but should still be reapplied at regular intervals during long days outside or after swimming or perspiring. It offers broad-spectrum sun protection with stabilized avobenzone for sufficient UVA screening. This would be rated higher if it contained some antioxidants to boost skin's environmental defenses. It does contain fragrance.

☺ GOOD **Ultra Sheer Liquid Daily Sunblock, SPF 70** *($12.49 for 1.4 fl. oz.)* has an SPF of 70, which is borderline overkill for most people (the amount of active ingredients needed to reach SPF 70 increases the chance of a sensitized reaction, plus there just isn't that much daylight anywhere in the world—remember, the SPF number is a time factor, not a quality factor). This fluid, silky sunscreen is bound to appeal to those with oily skin or anyone who normally shies away from high-SPF sunscreens due to their thick texture or tacky finish. Beyond the aesthetics, the formula includes stabilized avobenzone for reliable UVA protection, but the amount of antioxidants (which help boost a sunscreen's efficacy and your skin's defenses) is paltry. This deserves a Good rating for its texture (it works great under makeup) and broad-spectrum protection, but antioxidants should've been a more central part of the formula given the price and claims.

☺ GOOD **Wet Skin Kids Beach & Pool Sunblock Lotion SPF 45** *($10.49 for 3 fl. oz.)* can be applied to wet skin, no need to towel-dry first—the chief selling point of this sunscreen lotion. The technology Neutrogena uses supposedly allows the sunscreen ingredients to cling to wet skin without dripping off, meaning even when you're soaked you'll get reliable sun protection. This can be advantageous for active kids even though the formula itself isn't uniquely suited to children's skin (and definitely not for use on babies). Most likely the Wet Skin technology involves a mix of film-forming agents (which are present in the formula) that are fused with the sunscreen actives, allowing them to bond to the skin. Think of it like applying hairspray to damp hair. Even though your hair is wet, the hairspray's film-forming (holding) ingredients cling to your hair, allowing you to style it. Regardless of how they did it, this is an intriguing way to apply sunscreen when you're active and perspiring or swimming. The active ingredients provide broad-spectrum sun protection (and include stabilized avobenzone for critical UVA protection), but what a shame Neutrogena didn't enhance this formula further with beneficial antioxidants (even young skin needs those great ingredients). Despite that disappointment, if you're at the beach or pool and your skin is damp, and you need to reapply sunscreen to yourself or active kids, this can be a great way to go—and it works great to repel water, so the sunscreen stays on skin. One caution: Although this clings well and repels water, you will still need to reapply this at regular intervals to maintain the stated level of protection.

☺ GOOD **Wet Skin Kids Beach & Pool Sunblock Spray SPF 70** *($11.49 for 5 fl. oz.)* is similar to the Wet Skin Sunblock Spray SPF 30 below, save for it containing a higher level of actives needed to reach SPF 70. Otherwise, the same review applies.

☺ GOOD **Wet Skin Sunblock Lotion SPF 45** *($10.49-$10.49 for 3 fl. oz.)* is nearly identical to Neutrogena's Wet Skin Kids Beach & Pool Sunblock Lotion SPF 45 above. The main difference is the marketing angle, with one angled toward kids and this one being aimed at adults. Both work equally well on kids and adults, and so the same review applies.

☺ GOOD **Wet Skin Sunblock Spray SPF 30** *($9.49 for 5 fl. oz.)* can be applied to wet skin, no need to towel-dry first-- the chief selling point of this spray-on sunscreen. The technology Neutrogena uses supposedly allows the sunscreen ingredients to cling to wet skin without dripping off, meaning even when you're soaked you'll get reliable sun protection. Most likely this technology involves a mix of film-forming agents (which are present in the formula) that are fused with the sunscreen actives, allowing them to bond to the skin. Think of it like applying hairspray to damp hair. Even though your hair is wet, the hairspray's film-forming (holding) ingredients cling to your hair, allowing you to style it. Regardless of how they did it, this is an intriguing way to apply sunscreen when you're active and perspiring or swimming. The problem? Like many spray-on sunscreens, the formula contains a high amount of alcohol. The active ingredients provide broad-spectrum sun protection (and include stabilized avobenzone for critical UVA protection), but the alcohol puts your skin at risk of dryness and irritation that hurts healthy collagen production. Ideally, water-resistant sunscreens that omit the alcohol and are rated SPF 15 or greater are the best way to go. These may not have the same coolness factor of Neutrogena's wet-skin application technology, but they're better for your skin, especially if signs of aging are a concern. But, if you're at the beach or pool and your skin is damp, and you need to reapply sunscreen, this can be a great way to go!

☺ GOOD **Wet Skin Sunblock Spray, SPF 50** *($10.99 for 5 fl. oz.)* is nearly identical to the Wet Skin Sunblock Spray SPF 30 above, save for a greater amount of active ingredients needed to reach SPF 50. Otherwise, the same review applies.

☺ GOOD **Wet Skin Sunblock Spray SPF 85+** *($11.49 for 5 fl. oz.)* is nearly identical to the Wet Skin Sunblock Spray SPF 30 above, save for a greater amount of active ingredients needed to reach SPF 50. Otherwise, the same review applies plus one more comment: SPF 85 is overkill for anyone's skin. There simply isn't enough daylight anywhere in the world to warrant such a high level of protection, unless you know you're really going to skimp on application.

☺ AVERAGE **Oil-Free Sunblock Lotion SPF 45** *($8.99 for 4 fl. oz.)* is a good basic sunscreen for normal to oily skin, and includes avobenzone for UVA protection. However, we're concerned that the amount of methylpropanediol (a penetration enhancer) may make this more irritating to skin than other sunscreens. After all, 26.5% active ingredients is a lot for anyone's skin to handle. This is worth trying, but is recommended with caution.

☺ AVERAGE **Sport Face Sunblock Lotion SPF 70+ with Helioplex** *($10.99 for 2.5 fl. oz.)* has an SPF factor of 70, which is overkill for most people because there simply isn't enough daylight to warrant the extended protection, not to mention that the amount of active ingredients needed to establish an SPF this high increases the chance of a sensitized skin reaction. However, this is a good, lightweight sunscreen that contains stabilized avobenzone for sufficient UVA protection. If you don't think you'll apply sunscreen liberally enough to get the amount of protection stated on the label, this may be worth considering (for example, under-applying a sunscreen rated SPF 70 is likely to net you SPF 30). Note that this sunscreen contains a small amount of the preservative methylisothiazolinone. It can be sensitizing when used in leave-on products, though the amount here is likely not cause for concern because it is blended with parabens. Still, its inclusion makes this sunscreen less desirable.

☺ AVERAGE **Ultra Sheer Dry Touch Sunblock SPF 100+** *($11.49 for 3 fl. oz.)* has an ultra-high SPF rating, however, the extra synthetic sunscreen ingredients (which include avobenzone for reliable UVA protection) don't net much added benefit. You will still need to reapply this if you perspire or swim for more than 80 minutes. SPF 100 is well past the boundaries of how much sun protection anyone needs. For example, even if your skin turns pink in the sun after 10 minutes (typical of those with very white, fair skin), you'd be protected for 1,000 minutes or nearly 16 hours. There isn't enough daylight to warrant such protection. The only reason very high SPF ratings have merit is for those who tend to skimp on application. If you're not one to apply sunscreen liberally, you may well be getting SPF 50 instead of the SPF 100 rating, so there is that consideration. However, this sunscreen is difficult to recommend for two reasons: The amount of active ingredients (39% of the formula) increases the risk of a sensitized skin reaction and it contains a preservative (methylisothiazolinone) that is not recommended for use in leave-on products.

☹ POOR **Age Shield Face Sunblock Lotion SPF 70** *($10.99 for 3 fl. oz.)* has a combination of active ingredients that includes avobenzone for UVA protection, but adds up to a sunscreen with a strong potential to irritate skin. This irritation is compounded by the inclusion of the sensitizing preservative methylisothiazolinone, which is not recommended for use in leave-on products.

☹ POOR **Age Shield Face Sunblock Lotion, SPF 110** *($12.49 for 3 fl. oz.)* is nearly identical to the Age Shield Face Sunblock SPF 90 above, only with an even higher SPF rating. Otherwise, the same review applies.

☹ POOR **Clear Face Break-Out Free Liquid Lotion Sunblock SPF 30** *($10.49 for 3 fl. oz.)* is for those of us whose acne breakouts worsen when using sunblock. Wouldn't it be great to find a sunscreen that didn't do this? Although some formulas (those with liquid or very thin textures and liquid foundations with sunscreen) have an edge in this regard, the truth is there's no way to say with 100% certainty that a sunscreen won't make breakouts worse. This sunscreen has a lot going for it in terms of its water-light, silky texture and near-weightless finish. Both of these traits make it preferred for breakout-prone skin. It also provides broad-spectrum sun protection that includes stabilized avobenzone for reliable UVA screening. That's why it's such a shame to report than the company added two fragrant plant extracts (cinnamon and cedar bark) that are known irritants (Source: naturaldatabase.com). Also disappointing is the lack of proven antioxidants and repairing ingredients, both of which are essential for better skin and stronger environmental defense. In essence, this product does some things right but not enough to make this worth trying—there are better liquid sunscreens from Neutrogena as well as other brands, including SkinCeuticals and Paula's Choice.

☹ POOR **Clear Face Break-Out Free Liquid-Lotion Sunblock SPF 55** *($10.49 for 3 fl. oz.)* is nearly identical to the Clear Face Break-Out Free Liquid Lotion Sunblock SPF 30 above, and the same review applies.

☹ POOR **Fresh Cooling Body Mist Sunblock SPF 45** *($8.99 for 5 fl. oz.)* has an in-part avobenzone sunscreen and near-weightless feel but the negatives (too much alcohol and needless inclusion of a menthol derivative) combine to create a product that's effective yet too problematic to recommend. See the Appendix for details on alcohol and irritating ingredients.

☹ POOR **Fresh Cooling Body Mist Sunblock SPF 70** *($10.99 for 5 fl. oz.)* is similar to the Fresh Cooling Body Mist SPF 45, except for a higher amount of active ingredients needed to reach SPF 70. Mist-and-go sunscreens are great, but you don't have to settle for one that exposes skin to alcohol and other irritants. Paula's Choice, Banana Boat, and other lines sell spray-on sunscreens that do not contain needless irritants.

☹ POOR **MicroMist Airbrush Sunless Tan** *($10.99 for 5.3 fl. oz.)* contains the same ingredient (dihydroxyacetone) found in almost all self-tanners, so it's misting action is the only unique feature, and even that isn't that special (lots of companies offer self-tanning sprays). Although this works just fine to turn skin tan in a short period of time, we don't recommend it because it contains a high amount of skin-irritant witch hazel. Given the number of self-tanners that give the same result, why choose one that also irritates your skin? As for the "no-rub" application, unless you can somehow apply this perfectly even from head to toe, you will absolutely have to rub (blend) it into skin.

☹ POOR **MicroMist Tanning Sunless Spray, Deep** *($10.99 for 5.3 fl. oz.)* has the same irritancy potential as the MicroMist Tanning Sunless Spray, Medium below, and the same review applies.

☹ POOR **MicroMist Tanning Sunless Spray, Medium** *($10.99 for 5.3 fl. oz.)* contains too much witch hazel to make it a good choice, especially given the huge number of self-tanning products that work without irritating skin.

☹ POOR **Pure & Free Baby Sunblock Lotion SPF 60+ with PureScreen** *($10.99 for 3 fl. oz.)* has a lot going for it, especially for babies or those with sensitive skin. It's fragrance-free, contains anti irritants, and its active ingredients (titanium dioxide and zinc oxide) are as gentle as it gets in the world of sunscreens. Neutrogena even includes some antioxidants, though it's difficult to ascertain their concentration because the inactive ingredients are listed in alphabetical order rather than in descending order of content, which in this case is permissible because sunscreens are over-the-counter drug products. Unfortunately, Neutrogena chose methylisothiazolinone, a preservative that is contraindicated for use in leave-on products due to its sensitizing potential (Sources: *Actas Dermo-Sifiliograficas*, January-February 2009, pages 53–60; *Archives of Dermatological Research*, February 2007, pages 427–437; and *Contact Dermatitis*, October 2005, pages 226–233). For that reason alone, we cannot recommend this otherwise beautifully formulated sunscreen.

☹ POOR **Sensitive Skin Sunblock Lotion SPF 60+ with PureScreen** (*$10.49 for 3 fl. oz.*) is identical to Neutrogena's Pure & Free Baby Sunblock Lotion SPF 60+ with PureScreen above, and the same review applies.

☹ POOR **Spectrum+ Advanced Sunblock Lotion, SPF 100+** (*$13.49 for 3 fl. oz.*) is yet another Neutrogena sunscreen option. The claims make the Spectrum line seem more "advanced," but the only thing Neutrogena is really getting at is that antioxidants help boost a sunscreen's effectiveness, which researchers have known for quite some time. This sunscreen contains antioxidants, but in amounts so low that they aren't likely to provide any added benefit. How maddening, especially when we know that Neutrogena sells other sunscreens with a much more impressive amount of antioxidants. Beyond the claims, which sound more exciting than they are, you're left with a sunscreen capable of providing protection for more hours than there are hours of daylight. Moreover, the amount of active ingredients needed to reach SPF 100 increases the chance a person will have a sensitized reaction, which is never the goal of sun protection. Add to this the inclusion of the sensitizing preservative methylisothiazolinone and this becomes a questionably advanced sunscreen to avoid.

☹ POOR **Spectrum+ Advanced Sunblock Spray SPF 100+** (*$13.49 for 5 fl. oz.*) has more cons than pros. The chief concern is the SPF rating, which is overkill at best—there isn't enough daylight in most parts of the world to merit even an SPF 50, and certainly not an SPF 100. Also, because of the high amount of active ingredients needed to reach this astronomical SPF rating, it poses a fairly good risk of causing irritation or a sensitizing skin reaction. This risk is compounded by alcohol, which is a main ingredient. Alcohol can cause dryness, free-radical damage, and collagen breakdown, and this sunscreen doesn't contain enough antioxidants to counteract the damage.

☹ POOR **Spectrum+ Face Advanced Sunblock Lotion, SPF 100+** (*$13.49 for 2.5 fl. oz.*) is nearly identical to the Spectrum+ Advanced Sunblock Lotion SPF 100+ above, and the same review applies.

☹ POOR **Ultimate Sport Sunblock Lotion SPF 70+** (*$10.99 for 4 fl. oz.*) claims to replenish electrolytes to "nourish and restore skin balance," but the electrolytes you lose through your skin from perspiration (such as occurs with sports) are best replenished with fluids you drink. You can't replenish them topically and especially not from your sunscreen, which is designed to stay on top of your skin to protect it. Although this sunscreen applies smoothly and is tenacious when it comes to staying put, we cannot recommend it because it contains the preservative methylisothiazolinone, which is contraindicated for use in leave-on products due to its sensitizing potential (Sources: *Actas Dermo-Sifiliograficas*, January-February 2009, pages 53–60; *Archives of Dermatological Research*, February 2007, pages 427–437; and *Contact*

Dermatitis, October 2005, pages 226–233). The active ingredients in this sunscreen can be sensitizing on their own, so you don't want anything else in the formula adding to that potential.

☹ POOR **Ultimate Sport Sunblock Spray, SPF 100+** *($10.99 for 5 fl. oz.)* is similar to the Ultimate Sport Sunblock Lotion SPF 70+ above, save for it containing a higher amount of active ingredients needed to reach the overkill SPF of 100. Otherwise, the same review applies.

☹ POOR **Ultra Sheer Body Mist Sunblock SPF 30** *($9.49 for 5 fl. oz.)* features 3% avobenzone for sufficient UVA protection, but the base formula is mostly alcohol, and that makes it too drying and irritating for all skin types. Oddly, this product still leaves a fairly greasy, slick finish.

☹ POOR **Ultra Sheer Body Mist Sunblock SPF 45** *($9.49 for 5 fl. oz.)* is nearly identical to the Ultra Sheer Body Mist Sunblock SPF 30, except it contains a higher percentage of active ingredients to achieve its higher SPF rating. Otherwise, the same comments apply.

☹ POOR **Ultra Sheer Body Mist Sunblock SPF 70** *($10.99 for 5 fl. oz.)* provides sufficient UVA protection with stabilized avobenzone, but the base formula is almost 70% alcohol. The alcohol means that it dries quickly, but the large amount also means that it causes extreme irritation, free-radical damage, cell death, and irritation, in turn causing collagen breakdown. The trade-off isn't worth it. Add to that the sensitizing potential of the high amount of active ingredients needed to achieve SPF 70 (a sunscreen rating that's borderline overkill for most people) and this is a sunscreen to leave at the store.

☹ POOR **Ultra Sheer Body Mist Sunblock, SPF 100+** *($11.49 for 5 fl. oz.)* is similar to the Ultra Sheer Body Mist Sunblock SPF 70 above, except this version contains less alcohol and a higher amount of active ingredients needed to reach SPF 100+.

☹ POOR **Ultra Sheer Dry-Touch Sunblock SPF 70** *($10.99 for 3 fl. oz.)* achieves its ultra-high SPF number because it contains over 25% active ingredients, including avobenzone for UVA protection. The lotion texture has a smooth feel and a dry, almost weightless finish. However, this product lacks antioxidants and it contains the preservative methylisothiazolinone, which is not recommended for use in leave-on products due to its sensitizing potential (Source: *Archives of Dermatological Research*, February 2007, pages 427–437). Also, SPF 70 means there are an awful lot of sunscreen ingredients for skin to handle. Considering that an SPF 70 product provides about 24 hours of daylight protection (assuming you don't perspire or wash your hands), there just isn't enough daylight to warrant this kind of formulation.

NEUTROGENA LIP & SMILE CARE

✓☺ BEST **Neutrogena Naturals Lip Balm** *($2.99 for 0.15 fl. oz.)* is an affordable lip balm that's about as close to natural as it gets for treating dry, chapped lips. The wax-based formula contains some great emollients and antioxidant-rich plant oils that leave lips smooth, soft, and protected. Because this doesn't contain sunscreen, it is recommended for use only at night.

☺ AVERAGE **Revitalizing Lip Balm SPF 20** *($8.99)* definitely delivers plenty of moisture with a subtle pop of color. Unfortunately, the sunscreen actives do not provide adequate UVA protection, which is essential for anti-aging benefit (see the Appendix for details), making this otherwise very good lip balm difficult to recommend.

☹ POOR **Norwegian Formula Lip Moisturizer SPF 15** *($2.99 for 0.15 fl. oz.)* is advertised as being PABA-free, which is nice (PABA is a sunscreen active that's rarely used because it tends to be irritating), but Neutrogena forgot to include sufficient UVA protection, so this isn't a lip balm with sunscreen that anyone should rely on. It's also unusually greasy and not a good choice to use under lipstick.

NEUTROGENA SPECIALTY SKIN-CARE PRODUCTS

☺ AVERAGE **Ageless Intensives Anti-Wrinkle Deep Wrinkle Filler** *($18.99 for 1 fl. oz.)* achieves a short-lived "filling" effect by virtue of its thick, spackle-like texture. Although texture matters, what's missing are impressive amounts of state-of-the-art ingredients that not only improve the appearance of wrinkles, but also stimulate healthy collagen production and reduce inflammation. You're not getting much of the good stuff here, and your skin deserves more. Although this is an OK option for all skin types, you would do better applying a serum and/or moisturizer that's loaded with proven anti-aging ingredients. Neutrogena went too far with the claims: There is no way that even your deepest wrinkles will be filled out within eight weeks. Even if you pile this on, deep wrinkles will still be apparent because the minor "filling" effect is only temporary. Cosmetic dermatologists certainly aren't going to see a decrease in the number of Botox or dermal filler procedures because of products like this.

☺ AVERAGE **Microdermabrasion System** *($19.99 for 1 kit)* includes a handheld, battery-powered device to which you affix a textured scrub pad. You're directed to wet the pad before use, then turn the device on and massage over your face for a minute or two. Once that's done you rinse and then discard the pad. Sounds easy enough, right? Well it is easy but this system is also not an ideal way to exfoliate your face. It's easy to be too aggressive with devices like this, and the pads aren't all that gentle. Each pad is filled with a cleanser mix that activates with water, but it's the textured pad itself, not the cleansing ingredients, that has the abrasive action. Contrary to claim, this device is in no way comparable to a professional microdermabrasion treatment—but even those treatments don't do much for skin other than make it feel smoother. Ultimately, you'll get better (and gentler) anti-aging results using a well-formulated AHA or BHA exfoliant rather than a glorified scrub. If you decide to try this anyway, it is only recommended for normal to oily skin. Avoid if you have dry or extra-sensitive skin.

☺ AVERAGE **On-the-Spot Acne Treatment** *($5.99 for 0.75 fl. oz.)* contains 2.5% benzoyl peroxide as the active ingredient, which is helpful for blemish-prone skin. The formula's clay and wax base is a confusing mix for skin; the clay can exacerbate the drying effect of benzoyl peroxide, while the wax may make blemishes worse. Still, we suppose this is an OK option for spot-treating a blemish (which you should do only if you rarely break out—regular breakouts require treating the entire face).

☺ AVERAGE **Shine-Control Blotting Sheets** *($6.99 for 60 sheets)* are thin polypropylene plastic sheets. They absorb excess oil and perspiration, but the addition of mineral oil won't keep skin as shine-free as other options.

☹ POOR **Blackhead Eliminating Cleanser Mask** *($7.49)* cannot work as claimed. First, it contains some fairly thick ingredients whose emollient nature can make blackheads worse. Second, although it's medicated with 2% salicylic acid and the pH is within range for exfoliation to occur, this mask won't be left on skin long enough to have much benefit (a leave-on BHA exfoliant is better). Last, the inclusion of the irritating menthol derivative menthyl lactate makes this mask a problem for all skin types. Menthyl lactate can cause irritation that incites more oil production in the pore lining, leading to, you guessed it, more blackheads. Rather than blackhead-eliminating, this mask ends up being more likely to encourage blackheads!

☹ POOR **Clear Pore Cleanser/Mask** *($6.99 for 4.2 fl. oz.)* can disinfect skin because it contains 3.5% benzoyl peroxide, but the clay base makes this too potentially drying, and the menthol only causes irritation. A well-formulated leave-on benzoyl peroxide product would be far better for treating blemishes.

☹ POOR **Rapid Clear 2-in-1 Fight & Fade Gel** *($9.99 for 0.5 fl. oz.)* could have been a great option for skin if it didn't contain alcohol (which is drying, irritating, and causes free-radical damage) and witch hazel water (which is mostly alcohol). Neither of these ingredients is effective at helping to fade marks from acne faster. If anything, the irritation and damage it can cause can disturb the skin's healing process and immune response, which means the marks you're trying to fade may actually last longer.

☹ POOR **Rapid Clear Acne Eliminating Spot Gel** *($7.99 for 0.5 fl. oz.)* is another product that means well by the inclusion of the proven blemish-fighter salicylic acid (in a 2% concentration), but it falters with the pointless inclusion of almost 40% alcohol along with witch hazel extract, cedarwood, and cinnamon. Even without the irritants, the pH of this product is too high for optimal exfoliation to occur. See the Appendix to learn why irritation is a problem for oily skin.

☹ POOR **Rapid Clear On-the-Go Acne Treatment Pen** *($9.99 for 0.7 fl. oz.)* is a cleverly packaged product and is a convenient way to treat a blemish as soon as you feel or see it forming. The problem is the formula, which contains several irritants that will make your acne worse by increasing oil production and hurting your skin's ability to heal, not to mention making red marks worse. The active ingredient is 2% salicylic acid, which is great for acne, but not when it is accompanied by a high amount of alcohol and irritating plant extracts such as cedar and cinnamon. Add to that the fact that the pH of the base product is not low enough for the salicylic acid to exfoliate your skin, and this ends up being another anti-acne product to leave on the shelf.

☹ POOR **Rapid Clear Treatment Pads** *($7.99 for 60 pads)* will rapidly irritate due to the amount of alcohol, an ingredient that also stimulates oil production at the base of your pores. The 2% salicylic acid is nice and potentially effective, but this is not an anti-acne shining star for Neutrogena. All it does is rapidly cause irritation.

☹ POOR **Wave Power-Cleanser and Deep Clean Foaming Pads** *($10.99)* is a battery-powered hand-held device to which you attach dry cleansing pads, wet the pads, and then massage over skin. This is Neutrogena's attempt to compete with pricey facial cleansing devices such as the Clarisonic. Although the device is just fine for those who want a more thorough cleansing (with the pad attached and the device switched on, this is sort of like a powered washcloth for your face), the pads themselves are a problem. The **Deep Clean Foaming Pads** are a bit abrasive and the cleansing solution the pads are steeped in contains menthol, so you'll feel the tingle long after you're done using this as instructed. That tingle is your skin telling you it's been irritated, and irritation damages skin and can trigger excess oil production.

NEUTROGENA FOUNDATIONS

✓☺ BEST **Healthy Skin Enhancer SPF 20** *($10.49)* combines an in-part titanium dioxide sunscreen with retinol and a hint of color, all of which enhance skin due to their respective qualities. Moreover, there is more than just a dusting of retinol in this product, which makes it unique! It has a light, creamy texture and a satin finish appropriate for those with normal to dry skin. If an oily T-zone is an issue, this product should be set with powder to reduce the sheen it leaves on skin. The six sheer shades are great and include options for fair (but not very fair) to tan skin tones. In addition—and this is again unusual for a foundation—plenty of antioxidants are included. Due to this product's translucent bottle packaging, it is necessary to make sure you protect it from excess light exposure. For best results, store in an opaque makeup bag or drawer/cabinet.

✓☺ BEST **Healthy Skin Glow Sheers SPF 30** *($10.99)* is a very sheer, tinted moisturizer that's ideal for normal to slightly oily skin. It has a feather-light texture that glides over skin and sets to a soft matte (in feel) finish. Left behind is almost translucent color and a soft, natural-looking glow. Of course, the glow makes oily areas appear oilier, but if that's not a cause for concern (or if you have slightly dry skin) this will be perfect. The base has several antioxidants to help the in-part titanium dioxide sunscreen keep skin protected. One caution: The Bronze Glow shade does not contain any UVA-protecting ingredients (meaning titanium dioxide, zinc oxide, or avobenzone) and should be avoided. The other shades are all recommended. Due to this product's partially clear tube packaging, it is necessary to make sure you protect it from excess light exposure. For best results, store in an opaque makeup bag or drawer/cabinet.

✓☺ BEST **Mineral Sheers Powder Foundation SPF 20** *($11.99)* provides light to medium coverage, a soft matte finish, and impressive sun protection (from the mineral titanium dioxide) in one sleek mirrored compact. This pressed powder foundation has a smooth, elegant texture that also looks more natural on skin (though it still looks like makeup). Coverage, even when you apply it with a sponge, is more sheer than what you get with a standard pressed-powder foundation. However, this is an excellent way to boost the protection of your foundation or daytime moisturizer with sunscreen. Among the eight mostly excellent shades are options for fair to tan skin tones. Honey Beige 70 is best avoided due to its overt orange tone. This powder foundation with sunscreen is recommended for all skin types.

☺ GOOD **Healthy Skin Compact Makeup SPF 55** *($12.99)* is a very good cream-to-powder foundation that provides great broad-spectrum sun protection and medium to full coverage. Between the luminous finish and moist feel, this is best for normal to dry skin.

☺ GOOD **Healthy Skin Liquid Makeup SPF 20** *($12.49)* has a silky texture, even application, and natural-looking, soft matte finish. Sun protection remains strong with an all titanium dioxide sunscreen, which lends to the finish and opacity of this foundation. The range of shades is impressive, which is good news for those with normal to slightly dry and oily skin, for whom this foundation is ideal. Among the shades, only Soft Beige stands out as being slightly peach on medium skin tones. As for Neutrogena's touted antioxidant blend, antioxidants are barely present and the clear-glass bottle packaging won't keep them protected from light anyway. One caution: Although it is only one of several preservatives in this foundation, consumers should know that Neutrogena added methylisothiazolinone, which has a history of causing sensitized reactions and is not recommended for use in leave-on products. We suspect the amount present won't be an issue, but it's enough to keep this from earning a Best Product rating.

☺ GOOD **Mineral Sheers Loose Powder Foundation with PureScreen SPF 20** *($11.99)* comes housed in a screw-top jar with a sifter and offers sheer coverage with a shiny finish. Those with dry skin take note because this loose powder doesn't accentuate dry spots or lines. Also promising is the built-in broad-spectrum sunscreen of titanium dioxide, something that Neutrogena is calling "non-chemical PureScreen," but that also is found in countless other loose powders and foundations. The eight shades include acceptable options for fair to light skin tones, but anything deeper than #60 Natural Beige has an ashy cast, likely due to the amount of titanium dioxide.

☺ GOOD **SkinClearing Oil-Free Makeup Microclear Technology** *($11.99)* contains 0.5% salicylic acid as the active ingredient but the salicylic acid won't exfoliate skin because the product's pH is well above 4. It may have a slight antibacterial action, but it would be more effective in that respect if the amount were increased to at least 1%. Outside of the active ingredient letdown, this is a very good, lightweight liquid makeup. It smoothes easily over skin, provides light to medium coverage, and sets to a soft matte finish that looks natural. The shade range appears questionable at first glance—many appear too orange or too peach in the bottle—but these overtones are neutralized once blended on skin. Still, consider Buff, Warm Beige, and Soft Beige carefully. This is best for normal to oily skin; the wax content makes it questionable for acne-prone skin, unless your blemishes are mild and not an issue over your entire face.

NEUTROGENA CONCEALERS

☺ AVERAGE **3-in-1 Concealer for Eyes SPF 20** *($8.99)* is positioned as another multi-purpose product, this time combining concealer, eye cream, and sunscreen in one convenient package. As a concealer, this provides smooth, even coverage that looks natural and has a satin finish slightly prone to creasing. The sunscreen is almost 10% titanium dioxide, which also helps enhance coverage. Where it falls short is the eye-cream claim. This product isn't too creamy (not with talc as the third ingredient) and the amount of fragrance is disappointing. There are better concealers with sunscreen from Revlon, but this is still an option.

☺ AVERAGE **Healthy Skin Brightening Eye Perfector SPF 25** *($11.99)* lacks the opacity and the pigmentation to be an effective concealer and lacks the luminosity to be an effective highlighter. As such, it doesn't accomplish its dual purpose especially well. Available in four fair-to-medium shades, only two are convincing: Light is too peach and Medium is too ash. The one thing this concealer does get right is the built-in titanium dioxide sunscreen, which is gentle enough for use around the eyes. However, this product is better suited for minor dark circles below the eyes because its matte finish exaggerates, to a startling degree, the fine lines around lower lids.

☺ AVERAGE **Healthy Skin Smoothing Stick Treatment Concealer** *($6.99)* wins points for providing nearly opaque coverage with one swipe, but this lipstick-style concealer also looks heavy and creases into lines around the eye. It's an OK option for camouflaging small areas of redness, and three of the four shades are decent (Medium is too peach), but the concealers from L'Oreal and Revlon have much more to offer.

☺ AVERAGE **SkinClearing Blemish Concealer** *($8.99)* comes with a click-style applicator with a slanted sponge tip and boasts "skin-clearing" salicylic acid. We are not recommending this for use under the eye because applying salicylic acid so close to the eyes is too risky for getting it into the eyes. However, it can be a concealer for on-the-spot coverage, although it's very dry, difficult to blend, and won't provide adequate coverage over a sizable blemish. Adding to the problem is that between the small amount of salicylic acid (0.5%) and the product's high pH, any benefit for treating blemishes is unlikely.

NEUTROGENA POWDERS

✓☺ BEST **Healthy Skin Pressed Powder SPF 20** *($11.99)* has a formula that's talc-based, with a soft, silky finish and its sunscreen is pure titanium dioxide. The colors are attractive and workable for fair to medium skin tones. Its sunscreen element is a great add-on for extra sun protection over your moisturizer or foundation with sunscreen. As with any pressed powder with sunscreen, we don't recommend relying on this as your sole source of sun protection because liberal application (necessary to reach the SPF on the label) would result in a heavy, "made up" look.

⊗ POOR **SkinClearing Mineral Powder** *($11.99)* is a fragrance-free pressed powder that contains salicylic acid to fight blemishes, but it won't be all that effective because you cannot establish a pH in a nonaqueous product and because it's present only at a 0.5% concentration. Texture-wise, this is unpleasantly waxy and very difficult to pick up with a powder brush or sponge. It's transfer resistant, but that also makes it hard to blend. Further, when you apply it to skin you get no coverage, an uneven finish, and overall disappointing results.

NEUTROGENA BLUSHES & BRONZERS

✓☺ BEST **Healthy Skin Custom Glow Blush & Bronzer** *($11.49)* looks gorgeous on skin. Neutrogena offers six duos, all beautifully coordinated and best for fair to medium skin tones. The blush portion has a satin shine, while the bronzing powder has a sparkling shine, but it's not glaring or garish (and the shine stays in place). Used alone or together (and they're best mixed together with one large blush brush), this offers a smooth texture and even smoother application. This an inexpensive way to give cheeks a healthy glow any time of year!

☺ GOOD **Healthy Skin Blends Sheer Highlighting Blush** *($11.49)* is a pressed powder blush that presents pale to medium pink squares in one compact. The result is akin to a soft pink blush with a hint of shine, and it's best for fair to light skin.

☺ GOOD **Healthy Skin Custom Glow Bronzer** *($12.99)* is a pressed powder that comes in a gradation of bronze-toned shades ranging from light to medium-dark. This lets you customize your level of bronze and adjust for different areas of the face, but it can be tricky to control the color. It goes on very sheer, but can be layered to achieve a deeper tan color. The "glow" part of the name comes from the light sparkle finish, which isn't necessarily what you want if you're going for a natural tan look (a real tan doesn't sparkle), but it is done in a subtle way that bests many other shiny bronzers. One more comment: Because the colors in the compact do not have dividers between them, if you want to use only one shade for a key area, you must be careful how you place your brush. Alternatively, you can swirl your blush or bronzer brush over the whole powder cake and apply like a regular bronzing powder.

NEUTROGENA EYESHADOW

☺ GOOD **Nourishing Eye Quad SPF 15** *($8.99)* is one of the few eyeshadows with built-in sun protection. In this case, the active ingredient is 5% titanium dioxide, which definitely supports this product's SPF rating. How are the eyeshadows themselves? You get one large base shade, with a matte finish, which is the only one of the four that has sunscreen. The three other shades are labeled as highlighter, crease, and accent colors, and each has a soft to moderate shimmer. For the most part, the designations make sense as you survey the available quads. Other than the base shade, which tends to go on more opaque, the other shades in each quad, while silky and easy to apply, impart no more than sheer color with shine. You'll have to layer this extensively to get adequate shaping and shading, but if a softer, diffused look is what you're after, these work great and the shine doesn't flake.

NEUTROGENA EYELINER

☺ GOOD **Nourishing Eyeliner** *($7.49)* is a silicone-based automatic, retractable eye pencil. The tiny amount of vitamins this contains isn't going to nourish the skin along your lash line or stay stable, so forget the "nourishing" claim. This pencil has a smooth application and soft cream finish that won't smudge once set (though it still feels creamy, which is surprising). The other end of this great eye pencil includes a precision sponge tip for softening the line and a built-in sharpener that you can use to refine the pencil's tip. The shades are mostly classic options, but be careful with Twilight Blue, a deep navy hue that is attractive but not for everyone (it looks best with dark-colored eyes).

NEUTROGENA LIP COLOR

✓☺ BEST **MoistureShine Gloss** *($7.99)* has all the best attributes of a lip gloss: it comes with a hygienic wand applicator, has a smooth, non-sticky texture that feels moisturizing but not goopy, and leaves lips looking evenly glossed rather than overly wet. The selection of shades (most are shimmer-enriched) is beautiful and each goes on more sheer than it appears.

☹ POOR **MoistureShine Lip Soother Cooling Hydragel SPF 20** *($6.49)* has a unique balm/lip gloss texture and each of the sheer, juicy colors leaves lips very shiny, but the sunscreen element lacks sufficient UVA-protecting ingredients and the menthol in this product won't do your lips any favors. See the Appendix to find out which UVA-protecting ingredients to look for and to learn why irritants like menthol are a problem.

NEUTROGENA MASCARAS

☺ GOOD **Healthy Lengths Mascara** *($7.49)* delivers impressive results from the first stroke, going on easily and evenly, with nary a clump in sight. The rubber-bristled brush separates lashes beautifully, with enough width to deliver ample volume at the lash line, and the pointed tip provides definition to smaller inner corner lashes. It thickens and lengthens in equal measure for an effect that's not quite high glamour, but definitely glam by most standards. But after this praise comes a major caveat: You might think that simply applying more coats would yield more dramatic results, but, as it turns out, two's the limit. Applying a third coat, you'll find that the mascara begins to clump and the lashes stick together. When used with restraint, this mascara keeps lashes soft during the day, with no smearing or flaking to speak of. This removes easily with a water-soluble cleanser.

☺ GOOD **Healthy Volume Mascara** *($7.49)* includes a large mascara brush that takes practice and patience to achieve the best results. Once accustomed to it, you'll find this builds impressive length and decent thickness quite fast. Clumping is minimal, and what occurs is easy to neaten without a separate brush. This also keeps lashes very soft, yet doesn't flake or smear, and it removes easily with a water-soluble cleanser. The only drawbacks are the claims, because this standard mascara formula doesn't contain ingredients that plump lashes from the inside. If it did, you could forgo mascara after a week or so because your lashes wouldn't need any more plumping from the mascara, and that just doesn't happen!

☺ AVERAGE **Healthy Lengths Waterproof Mascara** *($7.49)* boasts the same rubber-bristled brush with a pointed tip as the regular Healthy Lengths Mascara above, which is a good mascara to consider, but this waterproof formula fails to deliver the same fantastic results. This applies unevenly and causes the lashes to stick together. Successive coats can comb out the minor clumping, but doing so only intensifies the spidery look. While it does lengthen and is waterproof, it's at the expense of your lashes not appearing lush or separated.

☺ AVERAGE **Healthy Volume Waterproof Mascara** *($7.49)* is supposed to build lashes from the inside out thanks to olive oil. There's no research to support that claim and, thankfully, there's only a minute amount of olive oil present, because oil in mascara can make for short-lived, smear-prone, flaky results. Application-wise, this mascara's large brush is an impediment to getting fast, clean results. If you're careful and take it slow, you can build decent length and thickness with minimal clumping and a soft curl. The formula is waterproof and requires an oil- or silicone-based remover when you're ready for it to come off.

NIVEA (SKIN CARE ONLY)

Strengths: Inexpensive; great makeup removers; good facial cleanser for normal to oily skin.

Weaknesses: Several boring formulas; no products to treat breakouts or lighten skin discolorations; anti-cellulite products are a joke; jar packaging

For more information and reviews of the latest Nivea products (including their body-care products), visit CosmeticsCop.com.

NIVEA CLEANSERS

☺ AVERAGE **Visage Pure & Natural Cleansing Lotion** *($8.10 for 6.8 fl. oz.)* is a basic cleansing lotion that's an OK option for normal to dry skin. It's nothing special, but the ingredients it contains help dissolve makeup, allowing it to be rinsed away. In terms of rinsing, you may need to use this with a washcloth to ensure you're not leaving a residue.

☺ AVERAGE **Gentle Cleansing Cream, Dry to Sensitive Skin** *($7.99 for 5 fl. oz.)* is a basic, but good, cleansing cream that is suitable for dry skin, but the inclusion of fragrance doesn't earn it a recommendation for sensitive skin. This cleansing cream removes makeup easily, but ideally should be used with a washcloth to avoid leaving a greasy residue.

☺ AVERAGE **Refreshing Cleansing Gel, Normal to Combination Skin** *($7.99 for 5 fl. oz.)* is an exceptionally standard gel cleanser that is suitable for its intended skin types. The basic, fragranced formula removes makeup and rinses cleanly. There isn't much else to say, other than the formula would be better if it were fragrance- and colorant-free.

NIVEA EYE-MAKEUP REMOVERS

✓☺ BEST **Eye Make-Up Remover, All Skin Types** *($7.99 for 4 fl. oz.)* is an excellent, soothing, fragrance-free eye-makeup remover suitable for all skin types, including sensitive or rosacea-affected skin. The amount of mineral oil leaves a slight residue, but you can get around that by cleansing after you remove your eye makeup. This is one of the better, inexpensive makeup removers at the drugstore.

☺ GOOD **Aqua Sensation Eye Make-Up Remover Pads, All Skin Types** *($7.99 for 24 pads)* contain silicone and the solvent isohexadecane to remove the most stubborn makeup. The plant extracts don't add much to the formula, but they're called out in the claims because of the siren song natural ingredients have for most consumers. Just know that it's neither the cucumber nor the ginseng that is removing your makeup, not to mention that neither will provide much benefit for skin because the pads are packaged in a jar. Price-wise, you'll get more uses from a silicone-enhanced liquid makeup remover, such as those from Almay, Neutrogena, or Paula's Choice. Still, this is a decent option for all skin types except sensitive.

☺ GOOD **Gentle Eye Make-Up Remover, All Skin Types** *($7.99 for 4 fl. oz.)* is not as gentle as Nivea's Eye Make-Up Remover, All Skin Types because it contains fragrance; it is still an effective, relatively mild makeup remover. The amount of oil in the formula means that it's best to use it before washing your face, because you'll want to remove the slight residue this can leave behind.

NIVEA TONERS

☺ AVERAGE **Gentle Toner, Dry to Sensitive Skin** *($6.49 for 6.8 fl. oz.)* is an OK option for normal to dry skin. The inclusion of fragrance negates its use by those with sensitive skin. The price tag is the only attractive thing about this toner, but in comparison with hundreds of other toners in the world of skin care, at least this one doesn't contain alcohol or irritating plant extracts.

☹ POOR **Refreshing Toner, Normal to Combination Skin** *($6.49 for 6.8 fl. oz.)* lists alcohol as the second ingredient, making it too drying and irritating for all skin types (see the Appendix for details). The flower extract this contains offers no benefit to skin, but does add a lot of fragrance, but fragrance is not skin care, it's eau de cologne.

☹ POOR **Visage Pure & Natural Purifying Toner** *($12.10 for 6.8 fl. oz.)* lists alcohol as its second ingredient, making it too drying and irritating for all skin types (see the Appendix for details). The formula also contains a problematic preservative (methylisothiazolinone) that is known to be sensitizing and is generally not recommended for use in leave-on products. Even without these troublesome ingredients, there's practically nothing of value for skin in this toner.

NIVEA SCRUB

✓☺ BEST **Skin Refining Scrub, Normal to Combination Skin** *($5.99 for 2.5 fl. oz.)* is a very good scrub for its intended skin types. Polyethylene beads are the abrasive agent, and they're buffered in a silky, lightweight gel that rinses easily and offers gentle cleansing with minimal fragrance. Well done, and the price isn't bad, either.

NIVEA MOISTURIZERS (DAYTIME & NIGHTTIME) & EYE CREAMS

☺ AVERAGE **Aqua Sensation Eye Cream, Normal to Combination Skin** *($10.99 for 0.5 fl. oz.)* is a basic, rather boring, fragrance-free eye cream formula whose most intriguing ingredients (of which there are barely any) will deteriorate thanks to the jar packaging, not to mention the hygiene issue of dipping your fingers into a jar every day. This will provide light, skin-smoothing moisture, but you don't need a special eye-area product to get that benefit (see the Appendix for details), and this particular option, despite being affordable, shortchanges your skin.

☺ AVERAGE **Light Regenerating Night Care, Normal to Combination Skin** *($7.99 for 1.7 fl. oz.)* is only slightly better than Nivea's classic moisturizer. This product is packaged in a jar and features a ho-hum emollient formula that's merely OK for dry skin. Those with combination skin will find this too heavy. See the Appendix to learn why jar packaging is a problem.

☺ AVERAGE **Rich Regenerating Night Care, Dry to Sensitive Skin** *($7.99 for 1.7 fl. oz.)* is an emollient, oil-rich moisturizer that's an OK but unexciting option for dry skin. The inclusion of fragrance and a fragrant plant make this unsuitable for sensitive skin, despite the claim on the label. Nivea included a token amount of antioxidants, but their activity will deteriorate once this jar-packaged product is opened because those ingredients break down in the presence of air.

☹ POOR **Nivea Crème** *($7.49 for 6.8 fl. oz.)* remains one of the star products for this line, and Nivea describes it as "the mother of all modern creams." First made available in 1911, the jar-packaged formula with its familiar scent is an exceptionally basic blend of mineral oil, Vaseline, glycerin, and wax. All these standbys can make dry skin look and feel better, but there are many more ingredients that have significant benefit for skin—ingredients that weren't even close to being options when Nivea Creme launched. Far from "unmatched," there are dozens upon dozens of moisturizers that offer skin more than this cream does, and without the inclusion of sensitizing preservatives methylisothiazolinone and methylchloroisothiazolinone.

☹ POOR **Visage Pure & Natural Moisturizing Day Care** *($12.50 for 1.7 fl. oz.)* is an exceptionally basic moisturizer that lists alcohol as the third ingredient, putting skin at risk for irritation that hurts its healing process and damages healthy collagen production, not to mention alcohol isn't hydrating. The jar packaging won't keep the tiny amount of antioxidants present stable during use, which is another strike against this product. It contains some natural ingredients, but so do many other moisturizers whose formulas and packaging are superior to this.

☹ POOR **Visage Pure & Natural Soothing Day Care** *($12.50 for 1.7 fl. oz.)* isn't a suitable moisturizer for daytime use because it does not contain sunscreen (which is the only element that separates a daytime moisturizer from one you'd apply at night). Yes, you could apply this in the morning and follow with a foundation rated SPF 15 or greater, but this moisturizer's formula isn't anything to get excited about so that workaround isn't one we'd advise here. The tiny amount of antioxidants this contains will not remain stable because this moisturizer is packaged in a jar (see the Appendix for details). The chief reason this isn't recommended is due to the inclusion of the preservative methylisothiazolinone. It is known to be sensitizing and is generally not recommended for use in leave-on products.

NIVEA LIP CARE

☺ GOOD **A Kiss of Protection Sun Protection Lip Care SPF 30** *($2.99 for 0.17 fl. oz.)* is a standard wax-based lip balm that also contains an in-part titanium dioxide sunscreen. As such, it's an excellent (and affordable) daytime option to keep lips smooth and protected from environmental damage. With SPF 30, you're getting more than a kiss of protection, and that's good!

☺ GOOD **A Kiss of Flavor Cherry Tinted Lip Care** *($2.49 for 0.17 fl. oz.)* is a basic, wax-based tinted lip balm that does a good job of taking care of dry lips. It's housed in a convenient Chapstick-style container. Interestingly, this contains a couple of sunscreen agents, including avobenzone (listed by its chemical name butyl methoxydibenzoylmethane). However, because these are not listed as active, they shouldn't be relied on for sun protection. The ingredient neohesperidin dihydrochalcone is an artificial sweetener that contributes to this lip balm's flavor.

☺ GOOD **A Kiss of Moisture Essential Lip Care** *($2.99 for 0.17 fl. oz.)* is a basic, wax-based lip balm that does a good job of taking care of dry lips. It's housed in a convenient Chapstick-style container. It is irritant-free and a reliable, inexpensive option.

☺ GOOD **A Kiss of Shine Natural Glossy Lip Care** *($3.29 for 0.35 fl. oz.)*. This glossy lip balm with a very sheer tint is a good option for preventing chapped lips while adding an alluring shine without stickiness. Interestingly, this contains a couple of sunscreen agents, including avobenzone (listed by its chemical name butyl methoxydibenzoylmethane). However, because these are not listed as active, they shouldn't be relied on for sun protection.

☺ GOOD **A Kiss of Shine Pink Glossy Lip Care** *($3.29 for 0.35 fl. oz.)*. Except for its sheer pink tint, this glossy lip balm is identical to Nivea's A Kiss of Shine Natural Glossy Lip Care above, so the same review applies.

☺ GOOD **A Kiss of Shine Red Glossy Lip Care** *($3.29 for 0.35 fl. oz.)*. Except for its sheer red tint, this glossy lip balm is identical to Nivea's A Kiss of Shine Natural Glossy Lip Care, so the same review applies.

☺ AVERAGE **A Kiss of Rejuvenation Q10+ Anti-Aging Lip Care SPF 4** *($3.29 for 0.35 fl. oz.)*. Nivea added coenzyme Q10 to this lip balm with sunscreen, but don't expect it to have much antiwrinkle benefit because it has an embarrassingly low SPF rating. Avobenzone is on hand for UVA protection, but SPF 4 is cheating sun-exposed lips for no good reason. A cosmetics company offering this pathetic level of sun protection should be strung up by their claims. This lip balm with a shimmer finish is not recommended for daytime use, but is an OK option once the sun sets.

☺ AVERAGE **A Kiss of Shimmer Pearly Shimmer Lip Care** *($2.49 for 0.17 fl. oz.)*. This standard waxy lip balm contains a lot of mica to add shimmer to the lips, just like you'd get from numerous lip glosses, many of which feel better on lips. Interestingly, this contains a couple of sunscreen agents, including avobenzone (listed by its chemical name butyl methoxydibenzoylmethane). However, because these are not listed as active, they shouldn't be relied on for sun protection.

NU SKIN (SKIN CARE ONLY)

Strengths: Workable AHA and BHA products; some state-of-the-art moisturizers and serums; several products are fragrance-free; almost all sunscreens include sufficient UVA protection, and most have impressive levels of antioxidants; some excellent sunscreens for the body.

Weaknesses: Expensive; drying cleansers; irritating toners; Tri-Phasic White products do not noticeably improve skin discolorations; unimpressive masks and "spa-at-home" products; claims are too far from reality; the AgeLOC products.

For more information and reviews of the latest Nu Skin products, visit CosmeticsCop.com.

NU SKIN CLEANSERS

✓☺ BEST **Creamy Cleansing Lotion, for Normal to Dry Skin** *($16.60 for 5 fl. oz.)* is an outstanding cleanser for its intended skin type. Emollients and plant oils combine with a gentle detergent cleansing agent to remove impurities and makeup without leaving a greasy film. Fans of cleansing lotions, take note!

☺ GOOD $$$ **Clear Action Acne Medication Foaming Cleanser** *($22.30 for 3.4 fl. oz.)* is a medicated liquid-to-foam cleanser that contains 0.5% salicylic acid, which in a cleanser isn't on your skin long enough to exert a benefit. Although this is a good cleanser for normal to dry skin, its oil content is not the best for anyone battling blemishes, and makes it somewhat difficult to rinse completely.

☺ GOOD $$$ **Tri-Phasic White Cleanser** *($28 for 3.4 fl. oz.)* costs a lot for what amounts to a standard water-soluble foaming cleanser for normal to oily skin. Not a single ingredient in this pricey cleanser can "inhibit the expression of discoloration on the surface of skin." Even if it contained effective skin-lightening agents, they'd be of no use because they'd be rinsed down the drain before they had a chance to work.

☹ AVERAGE **Pure Cleansing Gel, for Combination to Oily Skin** *($14.10 for 5 fl. oz.)* is a standard, detergent-based, water-soluble cleanser for its intended skin type, but one that's not highly recommended because of the amount of fragrant plant extracts it contains. See the Appendix to learn why daily use of highly fragrant products is a problem.

☹ AVERAGE $$$ **180º Face Wash** *($34.40 for 4.2 fl. oz.)* is an overpriced, standard, detergent-based cleanser that contains sodium C14-16 olefin sulfate as the cleansing agent, making it potentially too drying and irritating for skin. There are plant oils in it that can cushion some of the dryness, but why use any irritants whatsoever? The vitamin C it contains will be washed away before it has a chance to have any benefit for skin.

☹ AVERAGE $$$ **AgeLoc Gentle Cleanse & Tone** *($47.20 for 2 fl. oz.)* is so expensive that we had to double-check the price for this cleanser to make sure we weren't seeing things! For a huge amount of money you're getting an exceptionally standard water-soluble cleanser that's best for normal to oily skin. It works great to cleanse and remove makeup without a trace of residue, but the price is completely out of line.

☹ POOR **Epoch Polishing Bar** *($10.50 for 3.4 ounce bar)* is a detergent-based bar cleanser that is similar to Dove's original Beauty Bar. Although more gentle than true soap, it is still drying for all skin types and the ingredients that keep it in bar form can clog pores.

NU SKIN TONERS

☺ GOOD **NaPCA Moisture Mist** *($10.30 for 8.4 fl. oz.)* is an above-average fragrance-free, spray-on toner for all skin types. The alcohol-free formula contains several skin-identical ingredients and the cell-communicating ingredient niacinamide. What's missing is a good range of antioxidants; however, this remains one of the few worthwhile toners to consider using. Note: This contains the sunscreen ingredient octyl methoxycinnamate, which some may find sensitizing. Sunscreen ingredients aren't needed in products like this, but they can help prevent the toner from discoloring if stored in a place where the contents are exposed to daylight.

☺ GOOD $$$ **Clear Action Acne Medication Toner** *($19.70 for 5 fl. oz.)* is a fragrance-free, pH-correct BHA toner; however, the 0.5% concentration of salicylic acid is too low to significantly impact blemishes and blackheads. This toner is fragrance-free and contains soothing agents.

☺ AVERAGE $$$ **180° Skin Mist** *($29.30 for 3.4 fl. oz.)* is a good but fairly basic toner in mist form for normal to dry skin. It is fragrance-free.

☹ POOR **pH Balance Mattefying Toner, for Combination to Oily Skin** *($12.80 for 5 fl. oz.)* lists witch hazel as the second ingredient and also contains some problematic plant extracts, making this toner (which doesn't set to a matte finish) too irritating for all skin types. See the Appendix to learn the many ways irritation hurts skin.

☹ POOR **pH Balance Toner, for Normal to Dry Skin** *($13.30 for 5 fl. oz.)* contains witch hazel and camphor, making this a problem toner for any skin type, and it won't restore skin's optimal pH level (our skin is quite adept at doing so on its own), but the irritation this can cause will make dry skin worse. This is far from "hydration and nourishment" for skin!

☹ POOR **Tri-Phasic White Toner** *($33.10 for 4.2 fl. oz.)* lists witch hazel as the second ingredient, making this too irritating for all skin types. This cannot exfoliate away dark spots, as claimed. See the Appendix to learn how irritation hurts everyone's skin.

☹ POOR **Tru Face Priming Solution** *($33.10 for 4.2 fl. oz.)* contains some helpful, amino acid–based water-binding agents for skin, but the amount of witch hazel makes this toner too irritating for all skin types.

NU SKIN EXFOLIANTS & SCRUBS

☺ GOOD **Exfoliant Scrub Extra Gentle** *($13.40 for 3.4 fl. oz.)* contains mostly water, aloe, thickener, seashells (as an abrasive), and vitamins. The seashells can be rough on the skin, so calling this product gentle is a stretch, but it is a good exfoliant for most skin types, even though a washcloth would work as well if not better.

☺ GOOD **Facial Scrub** *($13.40 for 3.4 fl. oz.)* is gentler than the Exfoliant Scrub Extra Gentle above, despite the name difference. This one contains finely milled walnut-shell powder and husk, which work as a scrub, and it can be good for someone with normal to dry skin (but use this gently).

☺ GOOD $$$ **180° AHA Facial Peel** *($53.50)* is an expensive but effective way to exfoliate skin. The first part of this two-step kit is the **AHA Facial Peel**. This provides 18 pads, each steeped in a water-based solution of 10% lactic acid. The pH of 3.5 ensures exfoliation, and no needless irritants are included. You swipe the pad over your skin and let it sit for at least 10 minutes, at which point you use the **AHA Facial Peel Neutralizer**, which consists of pads soaked with a water-based toner that contains some very good soothing agents. The pH of the Neutralizer stops the peel action, but so would rinsing your skin with plain tap water. At least Nu Skin made these pads better than most companies that sell at-home peel kits. Although this kit will exfoliate skin, you're better off spending less money and using leave-on AHA products that contain between 8% and 10% glycolic or lactic acids, which you leave on your skin, and there are plenty of these products available. Both products in this set are fragrance-free.

☺ GOOD **$$$ 180º Cell Renewal Fluid** *($72.60 for 1 fl. oz.)* exfoliates skin with the polyhydroxy acid (PHA) gluconolactone at a 15% concentration and at a pH of 3.2. This is a good alternative to AHA or BHA products, but research has not shown gluconolactone to be a preferred or a gentler option (at least not in a significant way), and a 15% concentration is high and can be irritating for some skin types. This fluid also contains salicylic acid, but the amount is likely too low to boost exfoliation from the gluconolactone. By the way, if you're curious to try a product with gluconolactone, those from NeoStrata (reviewed on CosmeticsCop.com) are just as effective for a lot less money.

☹ AVERAGE **$$$ Polishing Peel Skin Refinisher** *($25.50 for 1.7 fl. oz.)* is a clay- and cornstarch-based scrub that isn't as elegant or as easy to rinse as the two Nu Skin scrubs above. The pumpkin enzymes are too unstable to provide extra exfoliation. This is not similar to a microdermabrasion procedure any more than a mansion is similar to a studio apartment.

NU SKIN MOISTURIZERS (DAYTIME & NIGHTTIME), EYE CREAMS, & SERUMS

✓☺ BEST **$$$ 180º Night Complex** *($62.50 for 1 fl. oz.)* is a brilliant serum for normal to dry skin because it combines ingredients that restore a healthy look and feel to skin while supporting its structural integrity and supplying it with plenty of antioxidants and cell communicating ingredients. Well done, though why couldn't this be fragrance-free like the other 180º products?

✓☺ BEST **$$$ Celltrex CoQ10 Complete** *($45.90 for 0.5 fl. oz.)* supplies skin with a healthy dose of several antioxidants, including ubiquinone (coenzyme Q10). It also contains a cell-communicating ingredient, water-binding agents, and anti-irritants. In short, this fragrance-free, water-based serum is highly recommended for all skin types.

✓☺ BEST **$$$ Clear Action Acne Medication Night Treatment** *($35.50 for 1 fl. oz.)* is worth considering as an antioxidant serum but not as an anti-acne treatment. That's because the amount of salicylic acid is too low (0.5%) and the pH too high for exfoliation to occur. This also contains cell-communicating ingredients (including retinol) and anti-irritants.

✓☺ BEST **$$$ Tru Face IdealEyes Eye Refining Cream** *($43.70 for 0.5 fl. oz.)* was designed to send under-eye bags packing, but this fragrance-free eye cream cannot accomplish what genetics, time, sun damage, and an aging face create. What it can do is moisturize and smooth, while supplying skin with a good amount of stabilized vitamin C and lesser, but still potentially effective, amounts of other antioxidants and cell-communicating ingredients. Despite those abilities, the truth is you don't need an eye cream—even one we rated highly. See the Appendix for details.

☺ GOOD **Moisture Restore Day Protective Lotion SPF 15, for Normal to Dry Skin** *($30.60 for 1.7 fl. oz.)* would rate a Best Product if not for the needless inclusion of St. John's Wort, which can cause a skin reaction in the presence of sunlight. The fact that this product contains sunscreen (in-part zinc oxide) helps offset this, but not enough to make it a slam-dunk recommendation for normal to dry skin.

☺ GOOD **Tri-Phasic White Day Milk Lotion SPF 15** *($45.90 for 2.5 fl. oz.)* includes avobenzone for UVA protection and wraps it in a silky lotion base for normal to slightly oily or slightly dry skin. A greater array of antioxidants and a cell-communicating ingredient would have netted this daytime moisturizer a higher rating.

☺ GOOD $$$ **180° UV Block Hydrator SPF 18** *($52.20 for 1 fl. oz.)* is a great in-part zinc oxide sunscreen for normal to dry skin not prone to blemishes. For the money, this should be brimming with state-of-the-art ingredients, which it's not, but at least broad-spectrum sun protection is assured and fragrance is excluded.

☺ GOOD $$$ **Tru Face Essence Ultra** *($172.10 for 60 capsules)* is a serum for normal to dry skin that includes mostly silicone, thickeners, plant oils, and antioxidants packaged in tiny capsules meant for single use. The packaging is a good way to keep the antioxidants stable, though some may find they need more than one capsule to cover their face, neck, and chest. For the money, the Ceramide capsules from Elizabeth Arden are worth considering first: They cost half as much for the same amount of product and contain equally good ingredients.

☺ GOOD $$$ **Tru Face Line Corrector** *($43.30 for 1 fl. oz.)* is a lightweight, fragrance-free, silicone-based moisturizer that contains palmitoyl-pentapeptide-3 and other peptides. In theory, peptides are cell-communicating ingredients that also function as water-binding agents. The antiwrinkle claims come from studies that were funded by the companies that sell these peptides to the cosmetics industry, so they're hardly impartial, but peptides can reasonably be considered as helpful anti-aging ingredients. This moisturizer is best for normal to slightly oily or slightly dry skin. It is also recommended for sensitive skin.

☺ GOOD $$$ **Tru Face Skin Perfecting Gel** *($48.40 for 1 fl. oz.)* is a water-based serum that contains a blend of skin-identical ingredients and a small amount of antioxidants. Don't believe the claims that this can stave off the first signs of aging and restructure your skin's collagen, because it absolutely can't do that; do believe, however, that it's a good serum for normal to oily skin, and will work well under makeup.

☹ AVERAGE **Enhancer Skin Conditioning Gel** *($12.80 for 3.4 fl. oz.)* is an OK basic ultra-light, gel-based moisturizer for oily skin. It lacks antioxidants but contains several water-binding agents.

☹ AVERAGE **Moisture Restore Intense Moisturizer** *($29.30 for 2.5 fl. oz.)* offers those with dry to very dry skin some helpful ingredients to restore moisture and radiance, but the jar packaging means the antioxidants (of which there's very little) won't remain stable during use (see the Appendix for details).

☹ AVERAGE **NaPCA Moisturizer** *($24.20 for 2.5 fl. oz.)* is an option for normal to dry skin, but what a shame the many antioxidants are subject to breaking down once this jar-packaged product is opened. See the Appendix to learn more about the issues jar packaging presents.

☹ AVERAGE $$$ **AgeLoc Future Serum** *($210.40 for 1 fl. oz.)* is a water-based serum and it is nothing short of amazing (and sad, too) that NuSkin sees fit to charge so much money for this product. You'd think that a serum in this price range would be jam-packed with ingredients that improve aging skin, but this one simply isn't. How this serum is supposed to transform anyone's skin "for unsurpassed anti-aging results" is beyond any research that exists, not to mention that if this is the "ultimate" answer for skin, why doesn't NuSkin stop selling all its other anti-aging, antiwrinkle products? The formula doesn't contain anything exceptional, and, of course, NuSkin doesn't provide substantiated research to support their grandiose claims. They believe the ultimate source of aging is our genes, but that's not entirely true. Genetics plays a role in aging and longevity, yes, but there are numerous other factors that contribute to what we perceive as aged skin and an "older" appearance. Sun damage outdoes genetic inheritance by miles, and unhealthy lifestyle habits (e.g., poor diet and smoking), gravity, physiological processes (such as the fact that we lose bone mass with age yet our skin keeps growing, leading to advanced signs of sagging), and many more factors, both within and beyond our control, all play pivotal roles. To think that aging comes down to genes is foolishness, or at least turning a blind eye to all the other contributing factors mentioned above. Most important for you to know is that NuSkin hasn't unlocked the secret to preventing or reversing aging—doing so is far more complex than what any cosmetic product could ever provide. AgeLoc Future Serum has a silky texture (like countless other serums) and contains some intriguing ingredients, including acetyl glucosamine and a handful of antioxidants, none of which are unique to AgeLoc. The only ingredient worth further explanation is equol. This was a new one for us, and we were surprised to find out it's a substance produced in the intestines as a by-product of digesting soybeans and soy-based foods. According to MedicineNet.com, equol "is a non-steroidal estrogen that acts as an anti-androgen by blocking the hormone dihydrotestosterone." The site goes on to explain that "Equol is chemically unique among the isoflavones (a family of phytoestrogens, plant estrogens). It is the major metabolite of the phytoestrogen daidzein, an isoflavone abundant in soybeans and soy foods." As a class of ingredients, isoflavones from soy have antioxidant ability, but their hormone-disrupting properties make them controversial ingredients to consume due to their potential link to stimulating breast cancer, although this research is mixed and inconclusive (Source: naturaldatabase.com). What about topical application of equol as a by product of soy? There is no research demonstrating it has any benefit beyond offering some protection to skin cells exposed to UVB radiation in a controlled lab setting. Even so, what research exists concludes that more studies are needed to determine the risks and benefits of equol in skin-care products and for oral consumption (Sources: *The Journal of Nutrition*, July 2010, pages 1369S–1372S and 1390S–1400S; *International Journal of Dermatology*, March 2010, pages 276–282; *Immunology and Cell Biology*, March 9, 2010, Epublication; and *Journal of Investigative Dermatology*, January 2006, pages 198–204). As more research is carried out on equol and other isoflavones, we may discover further advantages of these ingredients. But in terms of equol being one-stop shopping for genetic aging, that's not likely to become reality, any more than eating only pomegranates or drinking noni juice can ensure perfect health. If you decide to invest in this serum (a move we advise against), it is suitable for all skin types except sensitive due to the fragrance it contains. OK, one last comment: NuSkin states that based on daily usage, this serum should last for 30 days. That means you'd be spending $2,832 per year, an amount that would be better spent on any of several cosmetic corrective procedure options that will improve your appearance in a way this serum cannot.

☺ AVERAGE $$$ **AgeLoc Radiant Day SPF 22** *($63.80 for 0.85 fl. oz.)* has a price tag that is hard to stomach. What's especially distressing is that you're getting a tiny amount of an expensive product that must be applied liberally to provide the sun protection you expect. Given the cost, you have to consider how liberally you'll apply this product. Used as directed, this would be gone in less than a month, which adds up to an offensive amount of money for an otherwise ordinary sunscreen! It's great that this contains stabilized avobenzone for reliable UVA protection; on the other hand, the base formula, while lightweight and silky, isn't anything special. For what this costs, the formula should be brimming with state-of-the-art ingredients proven to boost skin's environmental defenses and increase healthy collagen production. Such noteworthy ingredients are barely present, which is really disappointing. Still, on balance, this is an effective sunscreen that's suitable for normal to slightly dry or slightly oily skin. Contrary

The Reviews N

☀ Sunscreens must provide reliable UVA (anti-aging) protection. See the Appendix for details.

to claims, this daytime moisturizer doesn't do much to increase skin-cell turnover. It contains a tiny amount of acetyl glucosamine, but likely not enough to encourage exfoliation (Source: *Journal of Cosmetic Science*, July-August 2009, pages 423–428). Considering the anti-aging angle AgeLoc strives for, you'd think they would have used an established, well researched exfoliant such as glycolic acid to support this claim.

☺ AVERAGE $$$ **AgeLoc Transforming Night** *($73.90 for 1 fl. oz.)* is a very standard, shockingly overpriced moisturizer that is packaged in a jar. That means the beneficial ingredients won't remain stable once it is opened (see the Appendix for details). Surprisingly, NuSkin didn't include a significant amount of those ingredients anyway, but that is just adding insult to injury. Adding everything up, this is a near complete waste of money. It has a silky texture and contains some helpful ingredients to prevent dryness and smooth the appearance of wrinkles, but so do countless other moisturizers, many with better formulas and much lower prices.

☹ AVERAGE $$$ **Tri-Phasic White Night Cream** *($45.90 for 1 fl. oz.)* is a lightweight, jar-packaged moisturizer formulated with the ingredient diacetyl boldine, which Nu Skin claims works to disrupt the activation phase of skin pigmentation, when melanin (skin pigment cells) is created. Diacetyl boldine appears to have antioxidant ability, but there is no independent, peer-reviewed research supporting the claim of being able to suppress melanin production. Therefore, we wouldn't count on this otherwise OK moisturizer for slightly dry skin to do anything other than make skin feel softer and smoother.

☹ AVERAGE $$$ **Tru Face Instant Line Corrector** *($63.80 for 0.5 fl. oz.)* is Nu Skin's "works like Botox" product, claiming to relax forehead wrinkles and expression lines. The company's literature for this product mentions the "heavy risks" associated with Botox injections, but the only convincing "risk" they could come up with was the ongoing expense (admittedly, Botox isn't a value-driven procedure). Formula-wise, this silicone-enriched moisturizer contains aminobutyric acid, also known as GABA. However, GABA does not inhibit muscle contractions that lead to expression lines. For a detailed explanation of this ingredient, please refer to the Cosmetic Ingredient Dictionary at CosmeticsCop.com. This product can make skin feel silky-smooth and, to a small temporary extent, fill in superficial lines on the face. It actually could have been a lot more impressive than it is if a broader range of state-of-the-art ingredients had been included.

☹ AVERAGE $$$ **Tru Face Revealing Gel** *($42.10 for 1 fl. oz.)* is an OK lightweight gel moisturizer for oily skin, but isn't likely to have a noticeable impact on pores—at least not to the extent that dry-finish silicone serums can.

☹ POOR **Celltrex Ultra Recovery Fluid** *($34.40 for 0.5 fl. oz.)* has a lot going for it, but ends up being a problem for all skin types because it contains orange and lavender oils. Lavender oil doesn't help skin cells recover; it causes cell death (see the Appendix for details).

☹ POOR **Face Lift, Original Formula** *($32.90)* includes the **Face Lift Powder** and the **Face Lift Activator**. These two formulas are meant to be mixed together and then applied to your skin. The Lift Powder contains egg white, cornstarch, and some water-binding agents. The Activator contains water, aloe, some water-binding agents, and preservatives. This won't lift skin anywhere, and the egg white and cornstarch combined can be skin irritants. This is a gimmicky, ultimately disappointing product.

☹ POOR **Face Lift, Sensitive Formula** *($32.90)* is similar to the Face Lift, Original Formula above, except the egg white is replaced by a gum-based thickener and the **Activator** portion is just a water- and aloe-based toner. This isn't preferred for sensitive skin because the cornstarch can be a problem, and none of this will lift skin one bit.

NU SKIN SUN CARE

✓☺ BEST **Sunright Body Block SPF 15** *($16 for 3.4 fl. oz.)* is an excellent, in-part avoben-zone water-resistant sunscreen for normal to dry skin. It not only provides broad-spectrum sun protection, but also boosts the skin's defenses with antioxidants and soothing agents. Another bonus: The price isn't so high that it's going to discourage liberal application.

✓☺ BEST **Sunright Body Block SPF 30** *($14.40 for 3.4 fl. oz.)* is nearly identical to Sunright Body Block SPF 15 above, and the same review applies.

NU SKIN SPECIALTY SKIN-CARE PRODUCTS

☺ GOOD **Clay Pack** *($13.40 for 3.4 fl. oz.)* is a standard clay mask with small amounts of water-binding agents and antioxidants. It's a good option for normal to oily skin.

☺ GOOD $$$ **Clear Action Acne Medication Day Treatment** *($35.50 for 1 fl. oz.)* contains 0.5% salicylic acid at a pH of 3.5, and although that allows for exfoliation to occur, it would be better if there were more salicylic acid. Still, this contains some lesser-used AHA ingredients (such as mandelic acid) and polyhydroxy acids (PHAs) that likely provide additional exfoliation, and the formula contains anti-irritant green tea and omits fragrance, which is always a plus. This product is suitable for all skin types.

☺ GOOD $$$ **Epoch Glacial Marine Mud** *($23.30 for 7 fl. oz.)* is a mud mask whose mud is said to be mineral-rich, but minerals aren't a cure for skin problems in the least, nor are they nurturing (especially when delivered in dirt—imagine adding that to your diet). Still, this can be a good absorbent mask for normal to oily skin, and it's fragrance-free.

☺ GOOD $$$ **Tri-Phasic White Radiance Mask** *($64.30 for 8 masks)* provides a collection of individually packaged, fragrance-free, pre-moistened masks that contain a good blend of water-binding agents and antioxidants. None of the ingredients in these masks has substantiated research supporting Nu Skin's claims of inhibiting any phase of hyperpigmentation, but they can make skin look and feel better.

☹ POOR **Creamy Hydrating Masque** *($17.90 for 3.4 fl. oz.)* ends up being more irritating than indulgent for skin because it contains lavender and sage oils along with pinecone extract. None of these help protect dry skin from harsh environmental conditions. See the Appendix to learn how fragrant irritants damage skin.

☹ POOR **Epoch Blemish Treatment** *($11.40 for 0.5 fl. oz.)* contains 2% salicylic acid as an active ingredient, but the pH of 4.1 prevents it from functioning optimally as an exfoliant. This is an ineffective option for blemishes, and is irritating for all skin types due to the fragrant oils.

☹ POOR **Galvanic Spa** *($36.10 for 4 treatments)* is a gimmicky "treatment" system consisting of **Galvanic Spa Pre-Treatment Gel**, which is mostly water, slip agent, film-forming agent, and several plant extracts, and **Galvanic Spa Treatment Gel**, which has a similar formula but also contains an ingredient that has a warming effect on skin, along with fragrant plant extracts that can be irritating. The warming effect can stimulate circulation and cause reddened skin, but this effect is more detrimental than helpful due to the manner in which it is caused, via irritation. It would be much more beneficial to stimulate circulation by exercising rather than wasting time and money on this mostly do-nothing duo.

☹ POOR **Sunright Lip Balm SPF 15** *($6.60 for 0.15 fl. oz.)* lacks the UVA-protecting ingredients of titanium dioxide, zinc oxide, avobenzone, Mexoryl SX (ecamsule), or Tinosorb and is not recommended.

☹ POOR **Tri-Phasic White Essence** *($56 for 1 fl. oz.)* contains a good deal of lemon peel extract, whose volatile components can cause irritation. This isn't helped by the lesser amount of peppermint extract, and to top it off, not a single ingredient in this misguided product can have even a slight impact on skin discolorations. Animal testing has shown that lemon peel can cause a phototoxic reaction on skin in as little as three minutes, even when sunscreen is worn (Source: *Photodermatology, Photoimmunology, and Photomedicine*, December 2005, pages 318–321), and it is known to cause contact dermatitis in people, making it something to avoid.

NYX COSMETICS (MAKEUP ONLY)

Strengths: Provides complete ingredient lists on its website; inexpensive for such quality makeup (much of which rivals department store brands); superior blush and eyeshadows; most of the mascaras are terrific!

Weaknesses: Many products are available only from the company's website, which means you can't see or test the colors in person (and the company doesn't offer samples).

For more information and reviews of the latest NYX Cosmetics products, visit CosmeticsCop.com.

NYX COSMETICS EYE-MAKEUP REMOVER

☺ AVERAGE **Eye & Lip Makeup Remover** (*$8 for 2.8 fl. oz.*) is a very standard but good liquid makeup remover that contains silicone and solvents. It quickly removes even the most stubborn or waterproof makeup. This would be rated higher if it didn't contain fragrance and fragrant orange extract, two ingredients you should be wary of using so close to the eyes.

NYX FOUNDATIONS & PRIMERS

☺ AVERAGE **HD Studio Photogenic Foundation** (*$15*) has a creamy, fluid texture that blends to a finish that's satin in appearance yet it feels matte. You'll get medium to almost full coverage and the pigment technology behind this makeup, like many of today's best foundations, allows the coverage to blur imperfections and improve skin tone without feeling or looking like a mask. On balance, the liquid formula is best for normal to dry skin. The shade range covers light to medium-tan skin tones, but beware that some of the shades have a slight unflattering orange-y undertone. A bigger issue (and the reason for this foundation's rating) is the inclusion of strong fragrance which is not only noticeably annoying to the olfactory system, but also irritating to skin (see the Appendix for details).

☹ POOR **Studio Perfect Photo-Loving Primer** (*$12*). This silicone-based foundation primer has a velvety-smooth texture that blends to a powdery-soft, weightless finish. This temporarily creates a nice canvas for makeup, but once the product has had time to set completely, the finish looks chalky. If that wasn't enough disappointment, some of the colors (green and lavender) are odd and this lacks beneficial ingredients to improve skin. In the end, all you're getting is a fairly standard primer that makes your skin feel smooth but look chalky.

NYX COSMETICS CONCEALER

☺ AVERAGE **HD Photogenic Concealer** (*$5.50*) is a concentrated, fragrance-free liquid concealer that provides moderate coverage and doesn't budge. The minimal slip, matte finish formula must be blended quickly before it sets. The dry finish works best for normal to oily skin types to camouflage breakouts or minor redness, but will magnify fine lines and wrinkles so we don't recommend it for the eye area. The shade range covers fair to medium tan skin tones, but watch out for any shades with unflattering pink undertones. Caution: The lightest shades can look a bit chalky, but as you move up the color scale, the lingering chalkiness isn't a problem.

NYX COSMETICS POWDERS

☺ GOOD **Mosaic Powder** *($8)* presents a square mosaic of five shades in one flip-top compact. The color combinations can work as an all-over powder, blush, bronzer, or even as contour, depending on the set you choose. This has a silky-smooth texture and soft, even application. At least one shade in each set has some amount of shine, but the overall finish of each tends to be a muted soft matte. Since color deposit isn't strong, those with medium to dark skin tones well need to layer to get these to show up on their skin.

☺ GOOD **Xtreme Lip Cream** *($6)* gets its name from the "extreme pigmentation with a silky and glossy finish." This is indeed a richly pigmented lip color that has a shiny finish initially, but eventually it wears off and you are left with more of a matte finish (which isn't a bad thing). The creamy, fluid texture goes on smoothly with a wand applicator, and once on lips, it maintains a slightly slick feel that keeps lips comfortable. The staying power is decent, though you will have to reapply it as the day wears on to maintain the rich, shiny finish. The shade selection is hit or miss, but there are enough choices that most women will find a suitable color. The formula is lightly scented, but not enough so to be a cause for concern in terms of irritation.

☺ AVERAGE **Twin Cake Powder SPF 10** *($15)*. This finely milled pressed powder has an almost creamy texture that blends on super smooth. It picks up easily with a brush and offers medium coverage with a semi-matte finish. The color range is impressive with shades for fair to tan skin tones. Formula-wise, this is workable for normal to slightly dry skin. The low SPF rating is the major disappointment here because it is too low to be counted on for sufficient sun protection. SPF 15 is considered the minimum by most medical boards around the world, and while the formula does contain titanium dioxide for UVA protection, it isn't listed as active which is a must to be considered reliable.

NYX COSMETICS BLUSHES

✓☺ BEST **Blush** *($6)* is a standout from NYX Cosmetics. The mica- and talc-based powder blush has a smooth, non-flaky texture and soft, sheer application that builds well for darker skin tones (or simply those who want more color). As for the shades, there are some beautiful options that have a matte or soft shimmer finish. Some of the colors are very shiny, but those are easily avoided or embraced, depending on your preferences and the look you're going for. This fragrance-free powder blush is recommended for all skin types.

✓☺ BEST **Stick Blush** *($6)*. Despite its creamy texture, this blush in twist-up, stick form doesn't feel greasy or slick once blended on bare skin or over foundation. The attractive range of shades can go on with a rich pop of color or more sheer depending on how you apply them, and each adds a radiant glow. For the most part, this cream blush holds up well, though you may experience a bit of fading as the day wears on. The ingredients that keep this product in stick form can be a problem for oily or breakout-prone skin, but otherwise this is worth a try if you're curious about cream blush.

☺ GOOD **Rouge Cream Blush** *($6.75)* has a glossy cream texture that results in a sheer, dewy-shine finish. It blends on incredibly smooth, and while you might think the slick texture would easily rub off, it actually holds up decently throughout the day, though there will be a small amount of fading due to the emollient nature of cream blush. For someone with oily skin, this can look greasy, but otherwise it offers a nice, radiant glow. There is a shade for everyone with colors ranging from nude to pink, coral, red and bronze, some of which contain shimmer. Most of the colors go on sheer but the pigmentation can vary between shades, so start by applying a sheer layer and build from there if needed.

NYX Cosmetics Eyeshadows & Eyeshadow Primer

✓☺ BEST **Eyeshadow** *($5)* is marvelous and definitely a must-see. It has a velvety smooth texture that applies and blends superbly (no flaking), even though most of the colors don't skimp on pigment. The company sells an overwhelming collection of over 100 shades, of which Ulta stores (the primary retail source for NYX in the United States) stock a couple dozen. There are plenty of matte shades in classic neutral to brown tones, and these work beautifully as powder eyeliner or for defining and filling in eyebrows. You'll also find shades with a metallic, shimmer, sheer glow, and glitter finish, with the glitter finish being the least desirable. Given the vast number of shades, there are plenty to avoid, including several pink, red, green, vivid blue, bright yellow, and orange hues, none of which work to create sexy, sophisticated eye shaping and shading. Note that the darker shades tend to grab a bit and require more skill to blend, but they certainly hold up well.

☺ GOOD **HD Eye Shadow Base** *($7)*. This liquid eyeshadow base sets to a powder-like, matte finish that enhances shadow and liner application. The absorbent formula helps keep oily lids at bay and prevents creasing throughout the day. It applies smoothly and evenly with a sponge-tip wand. This comes in a universal, light peach shade that is so sheer it hardly shows, so this is more about the powdery finish than adding color. It's definitely worth considering if you find that using concealer or foundation as an eyeshadow base doesn't do the trick for you.

☺ GOOD **Trio EyeShadow** *($7)* has a very smooth, slightly dry texture that's not quite as elegant as NYX's single eyeshadows above, but is still worth strong consideration. Application is even and color payoff is strong, so a little goes a long way unless you want a dramatic effect. There are several good color sets with neutral options, but unless you want a deliberately colorful eye design that doesn't shape or shade the eye, avoid the many "trendy" trios with difficult-to-work-with combinations of blue, green, bright pink, orange, and turquoise.

☹ AVERAGE **Jumbo Eye Pencil** *($4.50)* is a chunky pencil that requires routine sharpening. It has a soft tip that breaks down if you apply more than light pressure, which doesn't make it any more appealing. Otherwise, this has a creamy texture and smooth application that imparts rich colors, most of which have a shimmer finish that borders on metallic.

NYX Cosmetics Eye & Brow Liners

☺ GOOD **Felt Tip Liner** *($8)* is an excellent liquid eyeliner whose felt-tip pen applicator enables you to create a line that's as thin or thick as you wish. It smoothes on beautifully and deposits color evenly. Dry time is quick and once set this doesn't budge, though you may notice slight fading before the end of the day. This would be rated higher if it did not contain fragrant rosemary extract, a plant that may cause irritation along the lash line.

☺ GOOD **Super Skinny Eye Marker** *($9)* is a very thin felt-tip pen-style marker for eye lining and it does a very good job of giving you control over your eye design. The formula lasts through an average day, although it's not waterproof, and sets to a soft matte finish. The fine tip is perfect for creating a very thin line right next to the lash line, but more dramatic looks are difficult to achieve with such a fine point.

☹ AVERAGE **Auto Eyebrow Pencil** *($4.50)*. This retractable brow pencil earns praise for its easy-to-use design and included brow brush, but in terms of the pencil itself, it's really basic. The pencil has a semi-stiff texture with a matte finish that stays put, and it comes in a range of colors from taupe to black. The rectangular-shaped tip may be wider than some prefer, but it gets the job done.

☺ AVERAGE **Eyebrow Marker** *($9.75)* is a fine-tip felt-style marker with a long enough tip to get between individual hairs, which is great if you want to create brows that don't look "drawn on." However, the water-based formula tends to bleed easily, which defeats the purpose of a precise fine-tip pen. All the shades go on muted and soft, but they have a warm, red undertone that likely won't look natural on fair to light skin.

☺ AVERAGE **Eye/Eyebrow Pencil** *($2.99)* is a very standard, slightly creamy eye pencil that is also workable for filling in brows. It glides on and sets to a slightly moist finish that won't make brow hairs look greasy or matted. This pencil needs routine sharpening, but if that doesn't bother you, the price is right and classic (plus some not-so-classic) shades are available.

☺ AVERAGE **Push-up Bra for Your Eyebrow** *($10)* is a dual-sided brow product that includes a creamy pale pink pencil intended for the brow bone area just under the eyebrow. Once blended, this creates a subtle lifting effect for the brow, but it doesn't do anything that a light-colored matte eyeshadow couldn't. The other end of the pencil is a dry-textured medium brown/taupe brow pencil that needs a lot of sharpening to remain fine-tipped enough to fill in brows convincingly, although the shade should work for a range of blonde to brown brow colors. While this dual-ended eyebrow pencil is a handy product for a touch-up on the go, it is not the best for creating an eyebrow design.

☹ POOR **Eyebrow Cake Powder** *($6)* is a brow-enhancing palette that includes two shades of powder and a setting wax. If you're considering a brow powder, you're better off using a well-chosen matte eyeshadow rather than this product because, oddly enough, the setting wax tends to leak all over the powders. The mess is not surprising considering that this wax is extremely greasy and difficult to work with.

NYX COSMETICS LIP COLOR & LIPLINERS

✓☺ BEST **Matte Lipstick** *($6)* is a phenomenal matte lipstick that goes on surprisingly creamy and then sets to a long-wearing, non-slip finish. Because this can feel a bit dry on the lips, you may be tempted to apply a gloss over it, but that will deter its longevity and ability to stay-in-place. Still, if you don't overdo the gloss, you may find the trade-off for slightly reduced wear is worth it. The shade range has beautiful, full coverage options including hues of berry, red, nude, pink, mauve and more. For those who are used to creamy or glossy lipsticks, a matte lipstick like this one takes getting used to, but you will be amazed by how well it stays put!

✓☺ BEST **Mega Shine Lip Gloss** *($5.50)*. This very good lip gloss includes a longer sponge-tip applicator that comes to a rounded point. It takes some getting used to, but this type of applicator makes it easier to apply gloss precisely. The very smooth texture feels emollient, isn't the least bit sticky, and has a glossy shine. The shade range is enormous, offering a colorless shade and everything beyond that, from hot pink to rich reds and dark browns. Several of the shades have a much stronger color deposit than standard gloss, so this isn't a gloss to consider if your operative word is "sheer."

✓☺ BEST **Soft Matte Lip Cream** *($6)* is a unique matte lipstick! Although its finish is very matte, the texture is slightly creamy and easy to apply with a wand applicator. Once on lips, it maintains a slightly slick feel that keeps lips comfortable. This is a real find because dryness is often the biggest strike against matte lipsticks. The stain is impressive, meaning that you can count on hours of wear. The shades of this lightly scented lip color are exceptional, ranging from soft pinks to deep plums. Caution: Do not over-apply this product because it will lose its beautiful soft finish and become flaky.

☺ GOOD **Black Label Lipstick** *($7.50)* is a fragranced cream lipstick with a smooth, light-weight yet hydrating texture that glides on. It is not for anyone with lines around the mouth, as it tends to make a beeline for those. However, if that's not a concern, then it's a formidable lipstick to consider! It imparts rich, riveting, full coverage color and leaves a comfortable creamy finish. Generally speaking, the color "dot" on the bottle of the lipstick component is a good indicator of how the color looks when applied.

☺ GOOD **Lip Smacking Fun Colors** *($4)* is a standard, but good, cream lipstick that's available in a dizzying array of over 100 shades! Honestly, if you can't find a color you like from this selection, you probably shouldn't be wearing lipstick! Ulta stores (where NYX Cosmetics is primarily sold in the United States) stock perhaps 10% of what's available online. Note: This product is listed on the NYX Cosmetics website as Round Lipstick.

☹ AVERAGE **Jumbo Lip Pencil** *($4.50)* is a chunky, needs-sharpening pencil whose high wax content is inelegant and makes it feel slightly greasy even after it's applied. It quickly creeps into lines around the mouth and the shade selection (at least what Ulta stores stock) is unusually dark (think Goth colors). You can find a broader shade range on the NYX Cosmetics website, but we wouldn't encourage you to try this unless you prefer lipstick in pencil form and don't have lines around the mouth.

☹ AVERAGE **Lip Liner Pencil** *($3.50)* is unremarkable in every respect except for the shades, which include many unusual options. This is worth a look if you can't find a lip pencil to match an atypical shade of lipstick. Note: This is listed on the company's website as Slim Lip Pencil. This pencil requires routine sharpening.

NYX COSMETICS MASCARAS

✓☺ BEST **Doll Eye Mascara Longlash** *($9)* sells itself as a lengthening option, but it actually builds equal parts length and thickness. If really long lashes are what you want, NYX's Doll Eye Mascara Volume is the one to choose. It wears without a hitch and is easy to remove with a water-soluble cleanser.

✓☺ BEST **Doll Eye Mascara Volume** *($9)* excels at quickly creating long lashes you'll want to go out and flutter. The name is apropos because with a few coats you'll have beautifully long lashes resembling those on a doll. This builds slight thickness and doesn't clump, smear, or flake.

✓☺ BEST **Provocateur 1 Brush, 2 Styles** *($6)*. This mascara has clever packaging that allows the single brush to produce either defined and lengthened or bold and voluminous lashes. The mascara wand goes through a wide or narrow wiper, depending on which part of the cap you unwind, and that wiper controls how much mascara is deposited. If you like to change up your mascara from softly defined to bold depending on what you are wearing or where you're going, this mascara might become your new best friend. The wider wiper opening deposits more mascara for more dramatic, voluminous impact. You will experience some amount of clumping, but nothing that can't be smoothed out with a mascara comb, and besides, that's partially how this delivers its bold results. The narrower wiper portion allows for clump-free length and lash separation. Your lashes will look longer, but not much thickness is added. NYX recommends using this option on the bottom lashes and we agree: It works well to enhance lower lashes without overloading them. Whichever version you choose, you'll get flake-free, smudge-proof lashes.

☺ GOOD **La Amourex Boudoir Individual Curl Mascara** *($5.99)* won't curl your lashes on its own; however, if your lashes are already curled, this mascara, like many others, will help them hold their shape. It provides a deep black color for definition and the brush allows good separation with no flaking or clumping as you apply. The curved brush is easy to use, and doesn't pick up any more product than necessary from the tube.

☺ GOOD **Pin-Up Tease Boudoir Individual Curl Mascara** *($5.99)* is definitely not a tease—this mascara follows through on its curling claim and has a brush that provides great separation. The brush is rounded to follow the curve of the lashline and encourage curl, however the angle of the brush does make it difficult to apply mascara to lower and inner corner lashes. Although this leaves lashes with a slight curl on its own, you'll want use a lash curler either before applying this mascara for even more defined curl.

☺ AVERAGE **Doll Eye Mascara Waterproof** *($9)* isn't the least bit waterproof! What a shame! It dissolves (actually, it begins running right down your cheeks) with a mere splash of water. Application-wise, this produces impressive length and slight thickness, but it can go on a bit unevenly.

☹ POOR **Faux Lashes Mascara** *($6)*. This mascara offers softly-fringed, defined lashes but doesn't approach a false eyelash look. It contains tiny fibers that are supposed to adhere to lashes to elongate them. The problem? In order to work, they would have to attach to the ends of lashes in a lengthwise manner, but in reality they stay wherever they land as you apply this. Worse yet, the fibers flake off throughout the day and they can fall into your eye. Ouch!

☹ POOR **Le Chick Flick Boudoir Mascara** *($5.99)* is a blink-and-mess it up mascara. The mess it makes from smudging and flaking as you apply it is laughable (in an ironic sense), and the flaking continues throughout the day. Furthermore, the standard round brush certainly doesn't reach each and every lash as claimed. Once this mascara dries, the formula is tenaciously waterproof; still, it isn't worth considering given the frustrations you'll endure during application and once it sets.

☹ POOR **Le Frou Frou Volume + Length Mascara** *($6)* has a tendency to clump as you apply it and smudges as the day wears on. It does make lashes look longer, but you can forget about the "volume" part of the name because it only adds minimal thickness. We were unimpressed!

☹ POOR **Za Za Zu Luscious Volume Mascara** *($6)* contains tiny fibers that are intended to adhere to lashes to elongate them. The problem is that in order to work, they would have to attach to the ends of lashes in a lengthwise manner, but in reality they go on in all sorts of directions, creating messy-looking lashes in the process. The other issue is that they tend to flake off throughout the day and worse yet, they can flake off into your eye. Ouch, not to mention the mess involved from watering eyes due to mascara fibers causing irritation.

NYX COSMETICS SPECIALTY MAKEUP PRODUCTS

✓☺ BEST **Pore Filler** *($13)* does a nice job of smoothing over pores, and it contains several dry-finish silicones that leave a lasting matte finish to keep excess oil in check. Pores are not hidden entirely (you would need a heavier, more spackle-like product for that), but rather its thick, silky-smooth texture makes them less noticeable. The fragrance-free formula feels surprisingly weightless on the skin and has a peachy-cream tint that sheers to an imperceptible finish, even on darker skin. This is worth an audition, but for best results, be sure to follow with a matte finish foundation or powder.

☹ POOR **Grow Brow Serum** *($25)* is sold as a prescription-free way to grow thicker, fuller brows. We're assuming the prescription product they're trying to compete with is Latisse from Allergan, a product whose active ingredient is approved for lash growth, although many have found that it also works when applied to sparse brows. As with many other lash- and brow-growth products, NYX wants you to believe the peptide and numerous natural ingredients this contains are superior to the drug ingredients that have been proven to work (and proven safe, when used as directed). The ingredients in here have no research proving they stimulate hair growth, and some of the plant extracts are known irritants, and that doesn't help anything. Interestingly, several of the plant extracts in this product have research pertaining to their value as antitumor, anti-inflammatory, antiviral, and even insecticidal benefits, but nothing—and we mean nothing—relates to hair growth, be it brows, lashes, or the hair on your head. As for the peptide ingredient, as mentioned, it shows up in lots of lash-growth products, but there's no proof it works beyond being a good conditioning agent, and conditioning lashes doesn't affect hair growth one bit.

☹ POOR **Shine Killer** *($13)*. Shine Killer? More like "Money-Waster"! Though the silicone-rich, fragrance-free formula blends on velvety-smooth, it does nothing to absorb oil or control oily shine. Don't waste your time or money on this one. Oil-absorbing products from Paula's Choice or Smashbox are strongly preferred, even though they cost a bit more (you may as well spend your money on something that works right?).

OBAGI (SKIN CARE ONLY)

Strengths: Selection of good water-soluble cleansers; prescription-only products with 4% hydroquinone and tretinoin; almost all sunscreens provide sufficient UVA protection.

Weaknesses: Expensive; some products available only via prescription, which can be inconvenient; poor anti-acne products; one skin-lightening product with sunscreen does not provide adequate UVA protection; moisturizers should contain more state-of-the-art ingredients.

For more information and reviews of the latest Obagi products, visit CosmeticsCop.com.

OBAGI CLEANSERS

☺ GOOD **$$$ C-Cleansing Gel** *($32.76 for 6 fl. oz.)* is a very good, though pricey, water-soluble cleanser for normal to slightly dry or slightly oily skin. The amount of vitamin C is impressive, but its benefit is quickly rinsed down the drain. This does contain fragrance.

☺ GOOD **$$$ CLENZIderm M.D. Daily Care Cream Cleanser** *($30.60 for 6.5 fl. oz.)* is a rather uniquely formulated water-soluble, fairly gentle cleansing lotion that is a respectable, though pricey, option for normal to dry skin. Its only letdowns are a couple of problematic fragrant plant extracts, though their negative impact on skin is likely countered by the soothing plant extracts included and the fact they are rinsed off of skin. This cleanser does a thorough job of removing all types of makeup except waterproof formulas.

☺ GOOD **$$$ Nu-Derm Foaming Gel** *($33.70 for 6.7 fl. oz.)* is nearly identical to the C-Cleansing Gel, minus the vitamin C and with the inclusion of some nonirritating plant extracts. Otherwise, the same review applies.

☺ GOOD **$$$ Nu-Derm Gentle Cleanser** *($33.70 for 6.7 fl. oz.)* is similar to the Nu-Derm Foaming Gel cleanser, except this option includes a plant oil that makes it more suitable for its intended skin type. This would be gentler without the fragrance.

☺ GOOD **$$$ Rosaclear Gentle Cleanser** *($32.40 for 6.7 fl. oz.)* is an absurdly overpriced, standard water-soluble cleanser for most skin types. Ironically, the coloring agents and the fragrance make it a problem for extremely sensitive skin or for those with rosacea.

☹ POOR **CLENZIderm M.D. Daily Care Foaming Cleanser** *($30.60 for 4 fl. oz.)* would have been a good gentle water-soluble cleansing lotion if it did not contain menthol and menthyl lactate, both of which make this too irritating for all skin types. See the Appendix to learn how irritation affects everyone's skin for the worse.

OBAGI TONERS

☹ POOR **C-Balancing Toner for Normal to Oily Skin** *($32.40 for 6.7 fl. oz.)* is a basic, problematic toner that isn't worth consideration by any skin type. Witch hazel water is the second ingredient, and this plant's astringent properties, coupled with its alcohol content, are not the way to regulate sebum (oil) production. See the Appendix to learn how irritating ingredients make oily skin worse.

☹ POOR **CLENZIderm M.D. Pore Therapy** *($30.60 for 4 fl. oz.)* is a terrible alcohol-based toner that also contains menthol and two menthol derivatives, making for potent irritation. Note that the inactive ingredient list for this product is in alphabetical (rather than descending) order, which is permissible because this is classified as an over-the-counter drug.

☹ POOR **Nu-Derm Toner** *($33.70 for 6.7 fl. oz.)* contains potassium alum, a potent absorbent and topical disinfectant that can be a skin irritant, and the witch hazel distillate is mostly alcohol, which also can be irritating and drying for skin. Moreover, this product does not return skin to a good pH because the potassium alum has a very high pH, something that is not helpful for skin. Using this product is a big mistake, even if you're committed to using Obagi's Nu-Derm system.

OBAGI EXFOLIANT

☺ AVERAGE **$$$ Nu-Derm Exfoderm Forte** *($58.03 for 2 fl. oz.)* is a good, though very basic, AHA lotion whose glycolic acid content and pH level allow it to exfoliate skin. The amount of wax makes it inappropriate for normal to oily skin; it is best for normal to dry skin not prone to blemishes. There are far better AHA products for a lot less money, which is why this is only rated average despite it being an effective AHA product.

OBAGI MOISTURIZERS (DAYTIME & NIGHTTIME), EYE CREAMS, & SERUMS

✓☺ BEST **Nu-Derm Physical UV Block SPF 32** *($39.31 for 2 fl. oz.)* is an excellent sunscreen for normal to dry or sensitive skin, and for those with rosacea. The fragrance-free formula lists only zinc oxide as the active ingredient, and the silky texture provides skin with the anti-irritant benefit of willow herb extract.

☺ GOOD **$$$ C-Clarifying Serum** *($109 for 1 fl. oz.)* is a prescription-only product that lists 4% hydroquinone as the active ingredient. It is formulated in a simple gel base that contains L-ascorbic acid, a form of vitamin C that has antioxidant benefits. The pH of this serum allows the vitamin C to be efficacious, but also potentially irritating. This is a definite option for lightening skin discolorations related to sun damage or hormones, but would have been even better if Obagi had included a roster of anti-irritants.

☺ GOOD **$$$ Rosaclear Skin Balancing Sun Protection SPF 30** *($44.10 for 3 fl. oz.)* is a wisely formulated sunscreen for those with rosacea; it contains only the gentle mineral active ingredients of titanium dioxide and zinc oxide. The base formula is a bit harder to judge because the inactive ingredients are listed alphabetically rather than quantitatively, but that is allowed for over-the-counter drug products, which is the U.S. regulatory category where sunscreens fall. The fragrance-free formula is creamy and best for normal to dry skin but mostly void of state-of-the-art ingredients, which is really disappointing considering the price. Paula's Choice and Neutrogena have far less expensive mineral-based sunscreens to consider with better formulations. Considering the amount of active sunscreen ingredients, it's good that this is tinted to offset the white cast that such high amounts of these minerals can cause.

☺ AVERAGE **Nu-Derm Action** *($39.31 for 2 fl. oz.)* lightly moisturizes normal to dry skin, but that's the only exciting action this overall bland but fragrance-free product has.

The Reviews 0

☺ AVERAGE $$$ CLENZIderm M.D. Therapeutic Moisturizer *($30.60 for 1.7 fl. oz.)* is a fairly ordinary moisturizer for dry to very dry or eczema-prone skin, but it also has a bit of flare since it contains 20% glycerin. Without this weighty amount of glycerin the review would have simply said that this is an overpriced, simplistic moisturizer easily replaced by any of several standard moisturizers at the drugstore. If Obagi had included anti-irritants, skin-identical ingredients, or antioxidants (which are fundamental components for the skin's barrier repair and healing), it may have been worth the price tag, but as is, it is not an improvement for skin. However, the 20% glycerin content deserves further discussion. Glycerin is an interesting ingredient (glycerin, glycerine, and glycerol are terms used interchangeably in the cosmetics industry). Glycerin is a humectant and extremely hydroscopic, meaning it readily absorbs water from other sources. So, in part, glycerin works because of its ability to attract water from the environment and from the lower layers of skin (dermis) increasing the amount of water in the surface layers of skin. Another aspect of glycerin's benefit is that it is a skin-identical ingredient, meaning it is a substance found naturally in skin. In that respect it is one of the many substances in skin that help maintain the outer barrier and prevent dryness or scaling. Humectants such as glycerin have always raised the question as to whether or not they take too much water from skin. Pure glycerin (100% concentration) on skin is not helpful and can actually be drying, causing blisters if left on too long. So a major drawback of any humectant including glycerin is that they can increase water loss by attracting water from the lower layers of skin (dermis) into the surface layers of skin (epidermis) where the water can easily be lost to the environment. That doesn't help dry skin or any skin type for that matter. For this reason, glycerin (and humectants in general) is always combined with other ingredients so it will soften skin and becomes a fundamental cornerstone of most moisturizers (Source: *Skin Therapy Letter*, February 2005, pages 1–8). Using glycerin is not unique to Obagi but at 20% it is unusual; however, is it an improvement over other products? The research shows a combination of ingredients including glycerin, dimethicone, petrolatum, antioxidants, fatty acids, lecithin, among many others, are excellent for helping skin heal, reduce associated dermatitis, and restore normal barrier function if used on an ongoing basis (Sources *Clinical Experiments in Dermatology*, January 2007, pages 88–90; *American Journal of Clinical Dermatology*, April 2003, pages 771–788; *Journal of Molecular Medicine*, February 2008, pages 221–231; *British Journal of Dermatology*, July 2008, pages 23–34; and *Skin Pharmacology and Physiology*, January 2008, pages 39–45).

☺ AVERAGE $$$ Elastiderm Decolletage Chest and Neck Wrinkle Reducing Lotion *($110 for 1.6 fl. oz.)* is a relatively ordinary, somewhat poorly formulated moisturizer for normal to slightly dry skin, which doesn't contain a single ingredient that's different from what you'll see in numerous facial moisturizers that are equally as boring. There is no research showing skin on the neck or chest requires anything different from skin on the face. More to the point, the "Elasticity Complex" Obagi speaks of will not add to or help rebuild damaged elastin in your skin, anywhere on your body. A reputable doctor with a good conscience would know better than to sell a product with such a foolish claim (and would at least provide a formula that's more impressive than this one).

☺ AVERAGE $$$ Elastiderm Eye Gel *($88.92 for 0.5 fl. oz.)* is said to fill in the missing pieces of the anti-aging puzzle by improving elasticity, but if that's true, then the same claim can be tagged onto almost any other gel-type moisturizer. This contains mostly water, slip agent,

---

⊘ Think "hypoallergenic" means safe for sensitive skin? See the Appendix to find out the truth.

solvents, glycerin, thickener, film-forming agent, emollient, more thickeners, antioxidants, pH adjuster, talc, preservatives, and mineral pigments. One of the antioxidants is a synthetic ingredient, malonic acid, which is a strong skin irritant when used in pure form. Dr. Obagi claims it is part of a mineral complex clinically proven to stimulate elastic production, but there is no research (not even his own) to confirm this. See the Appendix to learn why, in truth, you don't need a special product for the eye area.

☺ AVERAGE $$$ **Elastiderm Eye Treatment Cream** *($88.92 for 0.5 fl. oz.)* is mostly thickeners and film-forming agent. Although it can address the basic needs of dry skin any-where on the face, its antioxidant content is subject to deterioration due to jar packaging (see the Appendix for details). The mineral pigments can have a slight cosmetic brightening effect, but this is an expensive way to achieve such a result.

☺ AVERAGE $$$ **Nu-Derm Exfoderm** *($58.03 for 2 fl. oz.)* is just a standard moisturizer that lists phytic acid as the third ingredient. Phytic acid is a good antioxidant, but not the only one or the best one. Other than that, this is mostly water and thickeners, which makes it a rather mediocre moisturizer for normal to dry skin.

☺ AVERAGE $$$ **Nu-Derm Eye Cream** *($48.68 for 0.5 fl. oz.)* includes some good emol-lients in a simple base of water and aloe gel. Water-binding agents and antioxidants are barely present, making this expensive eye-area moisturizer a less enticing consideration compared to, say, superior options from Lauder or Clinique—but ultimately, you don't need an eye cream, which we elaborate on in the Appendix.

☺ AVERAGE $$$ **Professional-C Serum 5%, for Eyes** *($44.93 for 0.5 fl. oz.)* contains 5% L-ascorbic acid in a liquid base whose main ingredient (propylene glycol) enhances the penetration of the vitamin C. However, the pH above 4 isn't likely to keep the vitamin C stable during use, so the in-usage efficacy of this serum is questionable.

☺ AVERAGE $$$ **Professional-C Serum 10%** *($60.84 for 1 fl. oz.)* contains vitamin C (ascorbic acid) in a glycol base with water, solvent, and fragrance. Just like the 5% version for eyes above, the pH of this means that the vitamin C isn't likely to remain stable during use.

☺ AVERAGE $$$ **Professional-C Serum 20%** *($92.66 for 1 fl. oz.)* has a lot of vitamin C and a less irritating pH than the Professional-C Serum 15% reviewed below, though the amount of sodium lauryl sulfate is still cause for concern and doesn't make this potent option worth choosing over better formulations from SkinCeuticals or Cellex-C.

☹ POOR **C-Exfoliating Day Lotion With Vitamin C SPF 12** *($54.28 for 2 fl. oz.)*. SPF 12 is below the minimum sun protection recommended by almost every medical and dermato-logic organization throughout the world. In fact, most recommend far higher SPFs, especially in sunny environs. Add to that the fact that Obagi is a line created by a physician and the SPF rating is just downright embarrassing. An even greater problem than the rating is the fact that the active ingredients fail to supply sufficient UVA protection, leaving your skin vulnerable to wrinkles. Any sunscreen should contain titanium dioxide, zinc oxide, avobenzone, Tinosorb, Mexoryl SX, or ecamsule. Given that you must apply all sunscreens liberally to get the full benefit of the SPF rating on the label, this product price isn't going to encourage most people to do that. Considering the formulary problems and the price, this isn't a daytime moisturizer with sunscreen that's worth your time or money.

☹ POOR **Professional-C Serum 15%** *($73.94 for 1 fl. oz.)* contains 15% vitamin C as L-ascorbic acid. The main ingredient (propylene glycol) is a penetration enhancer, which means that the vitamin C is going to get further into your skin than it would if this were strictly a water base. However, this much and this type of vitamin C can be irritating, especially when combined with alcohol and fragrance, as is the case here. With any "active" ingredient, be it vitamin C, retinol, or glycolic acid, you don't want to tip the scales in favor of irritation over benefits. There are better ways for skin to enjoy the benefits of vitamin C than this, and in fact this serum ends up being a one-note product. Just like our bodies need more than one nutrient to remain healthy and vital, our skin needs a range of beneficial ingredients. One key ingredient, even when used in a seemingly impressive amount, just doesn't cut it.

☹ POOR **Rosaclear Hydrating Complexion Corrector** *($53.10 for 3 fl. oz.)* is a thick, slightly tinted moisturizer, not recommended for anyone with rosacea or for anyone else because it contains irritating plant extracts, including lavender, cypress, and arnica extracts. These problematic plants are joined by some great anti-irritants, but why use a product whose ingredients are at war with each other instead of an irritant-free formula packed with soothing agents that devote their energy to calming your skin? See the Appendix to learn how fragrant irritants damage skin—even if you cannot see the damage taking place.

OBAGI SUN CARE

☺ AVERAGE **Nu-Derm Healthy Skin Protection SPF 35** *($41.18 for 3 fl. oz.)* is an incredibly bland, boring sunscreen formula whose only saving grace is that it provides broad-spectrum sun protection from its in-part zinc oxide sunscreen. Otherwise, this is drastically overpriced for a formula that does nothing beyond shield skin from sun damage.

☺ AVERAGE **Nu-Derm Sun Shield SPF 50** *($46 for 3 fl. oz.)* is generously sized (well, for Obagi) and contains an in-part zinc oxide sunscreen to ensure broad-spectrum protection. The base formula is lightweight, silky, and easy to apply (which is good because the easier a sunscreen is to apply, the more likely you'll be to use it daily). The main drawback, especially given this product's price, is the low amount of antioxidants. Those helpful ingredients should be present in greater amounts, and it would also be nice to see some repairing and cell-communicating ingredients. One more caution is the preservative methylisothiazolinone. Although it's not present in a high amount, it is known to be sensitizing and generally not recommended for use in leave-on products (Source: *Contact Dermatitis*, October 2006, pages 227–229). Between the problematic preservative, paltry amount of antioxidants, and the price, this is difficult to recommend with enthusiasm.

OBAGI SPECIALTY SKIN-CARE PRODUCTS

☺ GOOD **$$$ C-Therapy Night Cream** *($94 for 2 fl. oz.)* is a prescription-only product because it contains 4% hydroquinone as the active ingredient. The water- and glycerin-based lotion includes a couple of vitamin antioxidants, and it's a good option for normal to dry skin with pigment irregularities that has not responded well to over-the-counter levels of hydroquinone.

☺ GOOD **$$$ CLENZIderm M.D. Therapeutic Lotion** *($63 for 1.6 fl. oz.)* is a very good topical antibacterial for acne-prone skin. The active ingredient, benzoyl peroxide, is the gold standard for killing the bacteria that cause acne, though the price for this product is almost enough to make anyone break out! The formula deserves its rating for its efficacy and lack of needless irritants, but you need to know you don't have to spend anywhere near this much to get an effective benzoyl peroxide product.

☺ GOOD **$$$ Nu-Derm Blender** *($91 for 2 fl. oz.)* is nearly identical to the C-Therapy Night Cream above, and the same review applies.

☺ GOOD **$$$ Rosaclear Metronidazole Topical Gel** *($58 for 1.6 fl. oz.)* is available by prescription only. Its active ingredient is 0.75% metronidazole, the same topical antibiotic used in the brand name prescription product MetroLotion (and Gel and Cream). This fragrance-free formula is closest to that of MetroGel and there's every reason to consider it if you're dealing with rosacea. As for whether or not this is the more cost-effective prescription option, well, that depends on your health insurance coverage.

☺ AVERAGE **$$$ Nu-Derm Clear** *($95 for 2 fl. oz.)* is a prescription-only skin-lightening product formulated with 4% hydroquinone. Although the amount of hydroquinone can be very effective for stubborn discolorations and conditions such as melasma, this isn't nearly as elegant as other prescription-only skin lighteners with hydroquinone (those that come in a creamy base). The amount of sodium lauryl sulfate in Nu-Derm Clear has the potential to cause irritation, and the tiny amount of vitamin-based antioxidants Obagi included doesn't justify this product's price or greatly enhance its efficacy.

☹ POOR **Nu-Derm Sunfader SPF 15** *($74 for 2 fl. oz.)* is a 4% hydroquinone product that also contains a sunscreen with an SPF 15. That is an intriguing concept: mixing a prescription-strength skin-lightening agent with sunscreen. However, this sunscreen doesn't contain the UVA-protecting ingredients of titanium dioxide, zinc oxide, avobenzone, Mexoryl SX (ecamsule), or Tinosorb and, therefore, provides inadequate UVA protection.

☺ AVERAGE **$$$ Elastilash Eyelash Solution** *($60 for 1 tube)* is in the lash-growth game too, trying to compete with the impressive results possible from lash-enhancement products like Latisse. The claims are strictly cosmetic ("the appearance of thicker, fuller lashes" doesn't actually state that your lashes will grow or become longer or thicker), which is good because this does not contain any ingredients known to influence how lashes grow or how long they stick around before shedding. The only ingredient of interest is the type of peptide being used, but this is only interesting because many other products claiming to grow lashes add this peptide, too. We have searched far and wide and have yet to find any research proving this peptide changes lash length, color, or thickness in any meaningful way. For what this costs, you'd be better off using a product we know works, which basically means go for Latisse. Yes, Latisse costs more, but at least you're much more likely to see the results you're hoping for!

☺ AVERAGE **$$$ Nu-Derm Tolereen** *($48.68 for 2 fl. oz.)* costs a lot for what amounts to a very basic hydrocortisone product. Obagi's contains only 0.5%, while most of those at the drugstore (retailing for a fraction of this price) contain 1%. Hydrocortisone is a very good topical aid for minor redness, itching, and inflammation. Keep in mind that hydrocortisone is for sporadic, infrequent use only, because repeated long-term application will break down the skin's collagen and elastin. This product also contains sodium lauryl sulfate, a significant skin irritant, which is an ironic ingredient to put in a product meant to reduce skin irritation.

OLAY (SKIN CARE ONLY)

Strengths: Inexpensive (mostly); several outstanding water-soluble cleansers and scrubs; boon for any consumer in love with cleansing cloths; good AHA exfoliant; all sunscreens include UVA-protecting ingredients; bountiful selection of state-of-the-art serums and some excellent moisturizers; some of the best products come in fragrance-free versions.

Weaknesses: Bar cleansers; no topical disinfectant for blemishes; random products contain menthol; more than a handful of dated moisturizers; jar packaging; several moisturizers with sunscreen don't offer skin much beyond basic sun protection; repetitive formulas within and between the sub-brands make this line confusing and tricky to shop.

For more information and the latest reviews on Olay, visit CosmeticsCop.com

OLAY CLEANSERS

✔☺ BEST **2-in-1 Daily Facial Cloths, Sensitive** *($5.99 for 33 cloths)* are wonderfully soothing and a good, disposable cleansing option for someone with dry, sensitive skin. One side is smooth for cleansing; the other is softly textured for mild, scrub-like exfoliation. The fragrance-free, Vaseline-based (petrolatum) formula is exceptionally gentle, yet thoroughly removes makeup. Keep in mind that because these cloths contain detergent cleaning agents, you still need to rinse your skin after using them because leaving these ingredients on sensitive skin can lead to dryness and irritation. The petrolatum base demands thorough rinsing.

✔☺ BEST **Foaming Face Wash, for Sensitive Skin** *($7.99 for 7 fl. oz.)* is one of the best cleanser values at the drugstore, and is ideal for all skin types, including sensitive or rosacea-affected skin. It is an excellent water-soluble cleanser that removes makeup without leaving your skin feeling dry or tight.

✔☺ BEST **$$$ Pro-X Restorative Cream Cleanser** *($19.99 for 5 fl. oz.)* is a good option for all skin types, but formula-wise it differs little from similar cleansers in Olay's main line. The only difference is the cost, which comes down to marketing rather than a preferential formula distinction. This fragrance-free cleanser is nearly identical to Olay's Foaming Face Wash, for Sensitive Skin above, which costs approximately one-fourth what this Pro-X cleanser does.

☺ GOOD **2-in-1 Daily Facial Cloths, Normal** *($5.99 for 33 cloths)* are nearly identical to the 2-in-1 Daily Facial Cloths, Sensitive above, except this version contains fragrance and isn't quite as gentle.

☺ GOOD **Age Defying Classic Cleanser** *($5.49 for 6.78 fl. oz.)* is a good cleansing lotion/scrub for normal to dry skin, though the beta hydroxy complex will not exfoliate skin due to its brief contact and the too-high pH. What will exfoliate mildly are the polyethylene beads this cleanser contains.

☺ GOOD **Complete Ageless Rejuvenating Lathering Cleanser** *($8.99 for 6.5 fl. oz.)* is a standard water-soluble cleanser that contains gentle scrubbing beads for enhanced cleansing. It doesn't guarantee ageless skin in the least and the antioxidants it contains are rinsed down the drain before they can impact skin, but it's suitable for all skin types.

☺ GOOD **Foaming Face Wash, for Normal Skin** *($6.49 for 7 fl. oz.)* is a standard water-soluble cleanser that's a good option for normal to oily or combination skin. It cleanses without drying and rinses without leaving a residue. The vitamin E this contains isn't all that helpful in a cleanser (it's best used in leave-on products) and in no way does it help skin retain its natural moisture balance. Other less exciting ingredients in this cleanser are responsible for that benefit.

☺ GOOD **Pore Minimizing Cleanser + Scrub** *($7.99 for 5 fl. oz.)*. Although "deep cleansing ribbons" may sound innovative, this is just another cleanser/scrub combination from Olay. They sell plenty of these, and this one isn't any better at minimizing pores than the others, which is to say this won't minimize pores any more than a regular cleanser. This is best used as a scrub by those with normal to oily skin; however, scrubs don't necessarily minimize pores, especially if you overdo it and cause irritation. In addition, scrubs are not as effective at improving the shape of a pore as are well-formulated products that contain BHA, also known as salicylic acid.

☺ GOOD **Pro-X Exfoliating Renewal Cleanser** *($19 for 6 fl. oz.)* is a good option for all skin types, but formula-wise it differs little from similar cleanser/scrubs in Olay's main line. The only difference is the cost, which comes down to marketing rather than a formulary distinction. This fragrance-free cleanser is gentle and leaves skin feeling very smooth—you just don't need to spend this much money for equally good results.

☺ GOOD **Total Effects Lathering Cleansing Cloths** (*$7.99 for 30 cloths*). These emollient, fragranced cleansing cloths produce a mild lather, which many will appreciate despite the fact that lather isn't what's getting your skin clean. The anti-aging benefits said to be built into each cloth are Olay's standard assortment of state-of-the-art ingredients, including niacinamide and green tea. Although the formula steeped onto these cleansing cloths is designed to be left on skin, you're better off rinsing to complete the cleansing process, so the anti-aging ingredients don't count for much. Even if you left the residue on your face, there are far more elegant ways to treat skin to beneficial ingredients. These cleansing cloths are best for normal to dry skin. The tiny amount of salicylic acid is incapable of exfoliating, while the small amount of witch hazel extract isn't cause for concern.

☺ GOOD **Total Effects Nourishing Cream Cleanser** (*$7.99 for 6.5 fl. oz.*) is a standard emollient cleansing cream for dry to very dry skin. It requires a washcloth to avoid leaving a greasy film on skin. This fragranced cleansing cream removes makeup easily.

☺ GOOD **Total Effects Revitalizing Foaming Cleanser** (*$7.99 for 6.5 fl. oz.*) is a great water-soluble cleanser for normal to oily skin. You'll find it builds a soft lather and is capable of removing makeup and rinsing cleanly. It contains fragrance and isn't more revitalizing than similar products, but it certainly cleanses thoroughly.

☺ GOOD **Regenerist Micro-Purifying Foaming Cleanser** (*$8.99 for 6.7 fl. oz.*) is a very good water-soluble cleanser sold with some grand claims. Best for normal to oily skin, the formula isn't capable of cleaning any deeper than other cleansers, and stating that it cleans "to the pore" is a bit strange—pores are part of the skin's surface, so essentially Olay is stating the obvious. Of course a cleanser will "clean to the pore" and remove micro-particles, which we assume means minute pieces of dirt and skin cells. That's what almost any cleanser does.

☺ GOOD **Regenerist Regenerating Cream Cleanser** (*$9.99 for 5 fl. oz.*) is a cleanser/scrub hybrid, and the lotion base allows the polyethylene beads to exfoliate without being too abrasive. It's an OK cleansing scrub for normal to dry skin, but it doesn't detoxify anything.

☺ GOOD **Wet Cleansing Cloths, Normal** (*$5.99 for 30 cloths*). Cleansing cloths seem to be a popular product category for Olay because they sell more than any other company, except for companies that sell baby wipes. This formula is one you can use without rinsing because it doesn't contain detergent cleansing agents, as the others from Olay do. (You should never leave detergent cleansing agents on your skin because they are potentially irritating and can break down skin if left on.) This one is fine for normal to dry skin if you aren't wearing heavy makeup.

☺ GOOD **Wet Cleansing Cloths, Sensitive** (*$5.99 for 30 cloths*) are the fragrance-free version of the Wet Cleansing Cloths, Normal above, and the same review applies. These cloths are suitable for sensitive skin.

☺ AVERAGE **Acne Control Face Wash** (*$5.99 for 6.7 fl. oz.*) is a good water-soluble cleanser for normal to oily skin, but it is unable to control acne. Not only does acne control require far more than gentle cleansing (you also need to exfoliate and kill acne-causing bacteria), but also the active ingredient in this cleanser (2% salicylic acid) is rinsed down the drain before it can provide much benefit in the fight against acne.

☺ AVERAGE **Age-Defying Anti-Wrinkle Wet Cleansing Cloths** (*$14.99*). The antiwrinkle complex referred to for these relatively gentle cleansing cloths is mostly niacinamide, Olay's B-vitamin star ingredient. Although niacinamide is a multi-faceted ingredient for all skin types, it isn't the only antiwrinkle option, not to mention that, regardless of age, no single skin-care ingredient can address all skin needs. The tiny amount of other vitamins present aren't going to be of much help and these cloths don't do a great job of removing long-wearing makeup, but they're an OK option for use in the morning, especially while traveling.

☺ AVERAGE **Foaming Face Wash, Combination/Oily** *($7.99 for 6 fl. oz.)* does foam, but it is a problem for all skin types, including combination/oily skin. It contains two drying cleansing agents, one of which is potassium hydroxide (that's lye), and that causes irritation, which is bad for skin. This cleanser can "de-grease" oily skin and help remove makeup, but you can get that from many other cleansers without the irritation.

☺ AVERAGE **Regenerist Micro-Exfoliating Wet Cleansing Cloths** *($7.99 for 30 cloths)* do not contain cleansing agents or anything capable of exfoliating skin, although the mechanical action of massaging these cloths over skin (similar to using a washcloth) will remove some dead skin cells. The glycol and silicone can help dislodge makeup, but we wouldn't choose these cloths to remove waterproof mascara (Olay claims they do this, but that's debatable). These are an OK option for normal to dry skin if you wear minimal to no makeup.

☺ AVERAGE **Total Effects 7-in-1 Blemish Control Salicylic Acid Acne Cleanser** *($7.99 for 5 fl. oz.)* contains 2% salicylic acid in a base with a pH below 4, but these positive traits are wasted in a cleanser because it is rinsed from the skin before the BHA has a chance to work, not to mention that salicylic acid should not be used near the eyes or mucous membranes. This is an OK option as a scrub cleanser (a small amount of polyethylene beads is included for manual exfoliation) for oily skin.

☹ POOR **2-in-1 Daily Facial Cloths, Combination/Oily** *($5.99 for 33 cloths)* contains the potent irritant menthol along with witch hazel, which make these cloths a problem for all skin types. Irritation of this kind is always a problem for skin. In fact, exposing oily skin to irritants can trigger excess oil production at the base of the pore. In addition, the petrolatum base of these cleansing cloths isn't what oily skin needs because it will add to the greasiness.

☹ POOR **Shine Control Lathering Cleanser** *($7.99 for 6 fl. oz.)* can clean skin and, therefore, temporarily reduce shine (excess oil), just like any cleanser. However, this one also contains cleansing agents (including potassium hydroxide—lye), which is too drying and irritating for any skin type.

☹ POOR **Ultra Moisture Bar** *($6.99 for 6 bars)* is a detergent-based bar cleanser that can be drying for all skin types, and the strong paraffin base doesn't rinse well, leading to residue that may clog pores or other problems inherent in bar cleansers.

OLAY TONERS

☹ POOR **Oil-Minimizing Toner** *($7.99 for 7.2 fl. oz.)* is not recommended for anyone's skin because it contains potent irritants such as alcohol, witch hazel, and menthol. Alcohol causes free radical damage and dryness, while witch hazel and menthol cause irritation. All of that is a problem for skin. This is a prime example of a toner that stands little chance of helping your skin. Unfortunately, this type of toner formula is found far too often in the world of skin care.

OLAY EXFOLIANTS & SCRUBS

✓☺ BEST $$$ **Regenerist Night Resurfacing Elixir** *($31.99 for 1.7 fl. oz.)*. Although Olay positions this as a light glycolic peel (which, in essence, it is), they are also quick to accurately point out that the results from this product are not comparable to a professional AHA peel. We appreciate this honesty, and commend Olay for creating an outstanding AHA exfoliant that's suitable for all skin types. This has a light, silky, serum-like texture that provides slight hydration and a smooth finish. The fragrance-free formula contains between 8%-10% glycolic acid (Olay wouldn't reveal the exact percentage when we asked) and is formulated within the correct pH range for efficacy. More good news: Olay includes some cell-communicating ingredients along with antioxidants and the skin-repairing ingredient glycerin. The company also added shine to the formula, but its effect on skin isn't akin to layering shimmer on your face. Note that the translucent pump bottle packaging should be stored away from light to preserve the efficacy of the antioxidants. Also, although Olay positions this product as a moisturizer, it is first and foremost an AHA exfoliant. Those with dry skin will absolutely need to apply a moisturizer over this.

☺ GOOD **Blackhead Clearing Scrub** *($7.99 for 6 fl. oz.)*. If blackheads are your concern, you need to know that you cannot scrub them away. A scrub can remove the top portion of the blackhead, but it does nothing to address their formation, which occurs deep inside the pore lining, past the skin's surface. This scrub is medicated with the anti-acne ingredient salicylic acid, but its benefit is rinsed down the drain; to help, it must be left on your skin. To reduce blackheads, it is best to use a well-formulated, leave-on product with at least 1% salicylic acid. Otherwise, this fragranced product is more of a cleanser than a scrub, and an OK option for normal to oily skin whether blemishes are present or not.

☺ GOOD **Regenerist Detoxifying Pore Scrub** *($9.99 for 6.5 fl. oz.)*. Forget the pore detoxifying talk surrounding this scrub because there aren't any toxins lurking in pores that need to be scrubbed away. This is a standard cleanser/scrub hybrid whose benefit is more as a cleanser than as a scrub due to the large amount of detergent cleansing agents relative to the amount of polyethylene beads (that's what has the scrub effect). The salicylic acid has no effect on skin because it is rinsed away before it has a chance to work. This rinses cleanly, removes makeup, and is an acceptable option for normal to oily skin.

☹ AVERAGE **Age Defying Classic Daily Renewal Cream** *($10.99 for 2 fl. oz.)* is an option as a BHA product due to its salicylic acid content (approximately 2%), but the pH of 2.3 is unusually low and may prove too irritating for daily use, so proceed with caution. The base formula is best for normal to slightly dry or slightly oily skin.

☹ AVERAGE **Age Defying Classic Night Cream** *($10.39 for 2 fl. oz.)* is similar to the Age Defying Daily Renewal Cream above, and the same review applies.

☹ AVERAGE **Skin Smoothing Cream Scrub** *($7.99 for 6 fl. oz.)* is an OK scrub for normal to dry skin. The amount of sodium lauryl sulfate is potentially a concern because of its drying nature. Although the exfoliant ingredient salicylic acid is included, in a scrub its benefit is rinsed down the drain.

☹ AVERAGE **Regenerist Daily Thermal Mini-Peel** *($24.99 for 6 fl. oz.)* is a topical, nonaqueous scrub that lists magnesium sulfate (commonly known as Epsom salt) as the second ingredient. Massaging it over wet skin (as directed) causes an exothermic (heat-releasing) reaction. While you will feel an intense warming sensation that gets stronger as you continue to massage the product over your skin, the heat doesn't benefit your skin in any way. If anything, heat can be a problem for skin causing capillaries to break and surface, creating red veining on your face. The polyethylene beads will exfoliate skin, but the glycolic acid is useless because the magnesium sulfate keeps this product too alkaline, and AHAs need an acidic pH to exfoliate, though in a cleanser they would just be rinsed away, so all around the AHA is wasted here.

☹ AVERAGE $$$ **Regenerist Microdermabrasion & Peel System** *($31.99)* is a two-part system that includes a **Microdermabrasion Treatment** and **Peel Activator Serum**. The Microdermabrasion Treatment does not contain the usual aluminum oxide crystals. Instead, this bright orange, gel-based scrub contains baking soda (sodium bicarbonate) and silica to polish your skin. You're instructed to apply the exfoliating gel to dry skin and massage for a minute or so. Next, you apply the Peel Activator Serum to fingertips and massage a thick layer over the exfoliating gel. Since the baking soda in the exfoliant gel is alkaline and the serum is acidic, two things happen: a mild, fizzy, foaming action occurs and there's a slight warming sensation. This happens whenever alkaline and acidic products are mixed together. As the skin's pH acclimates to this change, the warming sensation subsides. After another minute of massaging the mixture over skin, you rinse it off. The abrasiveness of the baking soda makes your skin quite smooth, which is where the bulk of this duo's benefit lies. Although the Peel Activator Serum contains the AHA lactic acid and has a pH of 3.8, it is not left on the skin long enough to cause a peeling effect. All this amounts to a somewhat convoluted way to exfoliate skin with a fairly good risk of irritation given the "salt" scrub followed so closely by the AHA peel. We wouldn't suggest using this scrub, but rather just a washcloth with a gentle cleanser that you rinse off—and then apply an AHA or BHA product that you leave on the skin.

☹ POOR **Total Effects 7-in-1 Anti-Aging Cleanser Refreshing Citrus Scrub** (*$7.99 for 6.5 fl. oz.*) contains gentle polyethylene beads to polish your skin, but the formula also contains menthol, which causes irritation, and that's bad for skin (see the Appendix for details). The salicylic acid isn't helpful because you rinse this product from your skin before it has a chance to have any effect, on your skin or in your pores. If you prefer scrubs, this isn't the one to choose.

OLAY MOISTURIZERS (DAYTIME & NIGHTTIME), EYE CREAMS, & SERUMS

✓☺ BEST **Complete Ageless Skin Renewing UV Lotion SPF 20** (*$22.99 for 2.5 fl. oz.*) is an excellent daytime moisturizer for normal to slightly dry or slightly oily skin. UVA protection is assured from avobenzone, and this has a beautifully silky texture that feels great and works well under makeup. Best of all, it treats your skin to a bevy of helpful ingredients, including niacinamide and efficacious levels of antioxidants. The amount of vitamin C is too small to matter and this contains fragrance, but that's not enough to keep it from earning our highest recommendation.

✓☺ BEST **$$$ Regenerist Eye Lifting Serum** (*$24.99 for 0.5 fl. oz.*) is every bit as state-of-the-art as Olay's other Regenerist products. In fact, Eye Lifting Serum differs little from Olay's Regenerist Daily Regenerating Serum Fragrance Free reviewed below, which provides three times as much product for the same price. Both products contain silicones, glycerin, niacinamide (which can increase skin's ceramide and free fatty acid content, among other benefits), several antioxidants, and some anti-irritants. You really can't go wrong with most of the Regenerist serums or moisturizers as long as you keep your expectations realistic. In other words, Olay's claim that these products are able to provide "dramatically younger-looking skin without surgery" is stretching the truth—plastic surgeons have not seen a decrease in new patients since the Regenerist line came on the beauty scene. But the fact remains that this fragrance-free moisturizer is an excellent option for use around the eyes or anywhere on the face. In contrast to Olay's Regenerist Daily Regenerating Serum Fragrance Free, this product contains mineral pigments (including mica) that impart a soft, reflective shimmer to skin. To a slight degree, this can help make dark circles under the eye look less obvious, but the effect is strictly cosmetic. See the Appendix to learn why, in truth, you don't need a special product for the eye area.

✓☺ BEST **Regenerist Touch of Concealer Eye Regenerating Cream** (*$24.99 for 0.5 fl. oz.*) is a very good moisturizer that Olay is positioning as a tinted eye cream. Its concealing ability comes from titanium dioxide (it provides soft coverage) and from standard cosmetic pigments. The base formula is lightweight and very silky, and it treats skin anywhere on the face to exceptional ingredients. Niacinamide, peptides, antioxidants, and skin-conditioning agents combine to make this tinted eye cream a top consideration, though the single shade won't work for everyone's skin tone; it's best for light to medium skin tones. This is a rare makeup product in that it's a concealer that really does offer some skin-care benefit.

✓☺ BEST **Regenerist DNA Superstructure UV Cream SPF 30** *($31.99 for 1.7 fl. oz.)*. This daytime moisturizer with sunscreen's claim of blocking DNA damage sounds impressive, but in fact that's what any well-formulated sunscreen does, and this certainly qualifies. Daily use of an effective sunscreen rated SPF 15 or greater not only protects skin from the pernicious, cumulative DNA damage that results from sun exposure, but also protects against collagen breakdown and other cellular damage that leads to unsightly changes in skin. So, although it's good, this moisturizer with sunscreen isn't the only game in town, nor do you need to spend this much to get an effective sunscreen. That said, there's no denying that, once again, Olay has crafted a sophisticated formula that is suitable for all skin types except sensitive (because of the non-mineral sunscreen actives) and oily. The formula contains stabilized avobenzone for critical UVA protection. The intriguing ingredients are mostly the same ones that show up in other Regenerist moisturizers (and serums), so Olay isn't breaking any new ground here. But, taken together, these ingredients do their part to protect and enhance skin so it is better able to repair itself and, as a result, become healthier, and yes, able to look and act younger.

✓☺ BEST **Regenerist Micro-Sculpting Serum** *($26.99 for 1.7 fl. oz.)*. This water- and silicone-based serum doesn't have any sculpting ability, either on a micro or macro scale. Hydrating and plumping skin that is showing signs of sagging isn't going to make it look lifted—it's not as though this serum is a mini face-lift in a bottle. Skin sags for various reasons, mostly due to sun damage that hinders its support structure, the cumulative effects of gravity, and bone loss. Simply plumping skin with moisture isn't going to lift it and erase signs of sagging, though it will make skin smoother. The reason this is rated so highly is because with each use your skin is treated to a helpful amount of cell-communicating ingredient niacinamide, skin-identical glycerin, and a cadre of other anti-aging ingredients, including peptides, antioxidants, and more cell-communicating ingredients. This serum contains mineral pigments that leave a shiny finish, which is how this manages to make your skin look brighter and more radiant. The shine factor is the most significant difference between this and the other (less expensive) Olay Regenerist serums. This does contain fragrance.

✓☺ BEST **Regenerist Regenerating Serum** *($24.99 for 1.7 fl. oz.)* is a silky, silicone-based serum that contains a fairly broad complement of beneficial ingredients for all skin types. It contains approximately 2% to 3% niacinamide, and, in this amount, it can increase the skin's ceramide and fatty acid content as well as have anti-inflammatory effect to reduce hyperpigmentation (Sources: *The New Ideal in Skin Health: Separating Fact From Fiction*, Thornfeldt Carl MD, Allured Books, 2010, pages 160–161; and *Journal of Cosmetic Dermatology*, April 2004, pages 88–93). Olay claims the peptide this contains can regenerate and intensely hydrate skin. Peptides are cell-communicating ingredients that can help improve skin's appearance and enhance its healthy functioning, but they are not miracle-workers for skin, nor are they all that hydrating on their own. The various types of silicones really give this product its elegant texture and make skin feel unbelievably silky. Regenerist Daily Regenerating Serum won't give aging skin a new lease on life, but its texture and finish make it a very good serum with antioxidants for normal to slightly oily skin. It also runs circles around most products sold as foundation primers, so be sure to consider this if you're of the mindset that a primer is essential to seamless makeup application. This does contain fragrance.

The Reviews O

✓☺ BEST **Regenerist Regenerating Serum Fragrance-Free** *($24.99 for 1.7 fl. oz.)* is, except for the omission of fragrance (which is better for your skin), identical to Olay's original Regenerist Regenerating Serum above, so the same review applies. Because fragrance-free is better for everyone's skin, this version (if you can find it) is preferred.

✓☺ BEST **Regenerist UV Defense Regenerating Lotion SPF 15** *($31 for 2.5 fl. oz.)* has a lightweight base that is suitable for normal to slightly dry or slightly oily skin, while stabilized avobenzone is on hand for UVA (think anti-aging) protection. The formula is loaded with beneficial extras for skin, including a peptide complex, antioxidants, and soothing agents. For the money, this is a drugstore best buy and it wears well under makeup. This contains a small amount of fragrance, likely not enough to be cause for concern.

✓☺ BEST **Regenerist UV Defense Regenerating Lotion SPF 50** *($31 for 1.7 fl. oz.)*. This in-part avobenzone sunscreen feels wonderfully light yet makes skin feel smooth, moisturized, and protected. Yes, there are lighter products out there that carry lower SPF ratings, and many of those are excellent, too. However, those with normal to oily or combination skin who desire or need a high SPF rating should check this product out. It contains an impressive blend of cell-communicating ingredients and antioxidants and works beautifully under makeup. It really does set quickly and won't leave skin feeling greasy. It does contain fragrance.

✓☺ BEST **Regenerist Wrinkle Revolution Complex** *($31.99 for 1.7 fl. oz.)*. Each new Regenerist moisturizer (despite the "Wrinkle Revolution Complex" name, this is absolutely just a moisturizer) essentially repeats the same formula: water, silicone, glycerin, niacinamide, and a blend of the same antioxidants and cell-communicating ingredients. All those ingredients are great; what's bothersome (and confusing for consumers) is seeing them in product after product after product. We wonder why Olay doesn't offer three or four Regenerist moisturizers for different skin types, rather than almost a dozen with the same ingredients, but with different names, claims, and packaging. Slight rant aside, this is a remarkably good formula whose silky texture and lightweight hydrating ingredients are best for normal to slightly dry or slightly oily skin. The anti-aging ingredients Olay includes have some solid research behind them and, over time, they can reduce the appearance of wrinkles (to the extent of skin-care products) and help strengthen skin's surface against moisture loss. The opaque bottle with built-in pump keeps key ingredients stable during use, and the slightly spackle-like texture helps (temporarily) "fill in" superficial lines and wrinkles. As a bonus, this works beautifully under makeup and can easily replace your foundation primer.

✓☺ BEST **$$$ Pro-X Deep Wrinkle Treatment** *($47 for 1 fl. oz.)*. You might think that this product is another of the spackle-type moisturizers that have been showing up at cosmetics counters with a thicker texture meant to temporarily fill in lines and minor wrinkles. It isn't. Instead, this is akin to a lightweight moisturizer, which is being marketed as a specialty treatment by Olay. This doesn't contain a single ingredient that distinguishes it in any meaningful way from other Olay products, but it's worth considering for its blend of cell-communicating ingredients and antioxidants, all in a silky, thin lotion texture that pairs well with other products. Olay's packaging helps keep the vitamin A stable, which is a very good thing. The form of vitamin A included is retinyl propionate, which also appears in Olay's Age Defying line, though jar packaging prevails for most of that line, which makes the vitamin A in those products useless. All told, Pro-X Deep Wrinkle Treatment has the better formula compared with Olay's other products with retinol, but its price should give you pause. If retinol is what you're after, keep in mind that RoC, Neutrogena, and Paula's Choice have compelling options in that category for less money.

✓☺ BEST **$$$ Pro-X Eye Restoration Complex** *($47 for 0.5 fl. oz.).* We disagree with Olay's marketing claims that this is a specialized treatment for the eye area because the ingredients also show up in their facial moisturizers (one more reason you don't need an eye cream; see the Appendix to learn more). However, it cannot be denied that this fragrance-free formula is outstanding in many respects. It feels lightweight yet substantial, makes skin feel incredibly smooth, and treats it to several cell-communicating ingredients as well as a respectable amount of antioxidants, but the caffeine it contains won't brighten or wake up your eyes. As with most eye creams, the claims of diminishing dark circles and puffiness are dubious at best. By the way, this product is very similar to Olay's Regenerist Eye Lifting Serum, which sells for less than $20 for the same amount of product.

✓☺ BEST **Total Effects 7-in-1 Anti-Aging Moisturizer, Mature Skin Therapy** *($22.99 for 1.7 fl. oz.)* is Olay's answer to the needs of women whose skin is suffering from the changes it endures during and after menopause. The seven benefits in one product claim to intensely moisturize skin, reduce wrinkles, enhance skin tone and color, minimize pores, provide free-radical defense, and lift skin. Wow, all this for under $25? Sarcasm aside, this moisturizer for normal to dry skin contains several state-of-the-art ingredients that can improve the appearance and healthy functioning of skin at any age, but without a sunscreen, a major necessary benefit is missing! Antioxidant-wise, this bests all of the other Total Effects products, propelling this to the top of the list. Much of the skin appearance enhancement has to do with visual trickery—the mineral pigments add a subtle soft-focus, brightening effect to dull skin, while niacinamide encourages ceramide production for a smoother surface, which reflects light better. This isn't one-stop shopping for menopausal skin because most of the claims are at best farfetched, but it definitely has many strong points.

☺ GOOD **Age Defying Anti-Wrinkle Daily SPF 15 Lotion** *($14.99 for 3.4 fl. oz.)* is a lightweight, water- and glycerin-based daytime moisturizer that includes an in-part avobenzone sunscreen. Olay draws attention to this product's pro-retinol and BHA content, but the formula contains neither. What it does contain is a small amount of retinyl propionate. Similar to the more commonly used retinyl palmitate, retinyl propionate is a retinoid ester that must be converted to a more active form by enzymes in the skin. Retinyl propionate is apparently more stable and less irritating than retinol, yet offers a similar benefit to skin. However, research on this retinol alternative is scant. And with the most current information coming from dermatologist Zoe Diana Draelos, who is a consultant to Procter & Gamble (Olay's parent company), it's not exactly impartial. Assuming that retinyl propionate is more stable than retinol (and that's only an assumption because there is no substantiated proof) doesn't fully explain why Olay chose to package this moisturizer in a translucent bottle, which doesn't help keep ingredients stable. Still, it's a good option for someone with normal to slightly oily skin. And, as with most of Olay's latest moisturizers, it includes plenty of skin-beneficial niacinamide.

☺ GOOD **Complete All Day UV Moisturizer SPF 15, for Combination/Oily Skin** *($10.99 for 4 fl. oz.)* features an in-part avobenzone sunscreen and the avobenzone is stabilized with octocrylene. The base formula contains an impressive amount of beneficial ingredients such as niacinamide and antioxidant vitamin E, but is best for normal to dry skin. Those with combination or oily skin will likely find this too emollient. The texture of this product makes it workable under makeup, so it's a good choice if your foundation lacks reliable sun protection (or you're not willing to apply your foundation with sunscreen liberally).

☺ GOOD **Complete All Day UV Moisturizer SPF 15, for Normal Skin** *($10.99 for 4 fl. oz.)* is nearly identical to the Complete All Day UV Moisture Lotion SPF 15, for Combination/Oily Skin above, and the same comments apply.

☺ GOOD **Complete Defense Daily UV Moisturizer SPF 30, for Sensitive Skin** *($10.99 for 2.5 fl. oz.)* includes 6% zinc oxide. Although zinc oxide provides excellent broad-spectrum protection, it can also leave a whitish cast on the skin when used in this amount. Because Olay included other synthetic sunscreen active ingredients, this is not a slam-dunk choice for sensitive skin (zinc oxide or titanium dioxide are the most gentle choices for this skin type). This fragrance-free daily sunscreen would be best for normal to slightly dry skin not prone to blemishes.

☺ GOOD **Total Effects 7-In-1 Anti-Aging UV Moisturizer Plus SPF 15, Fragrance-Free** *($21.99 for 1.7 fl. oz.)* contains avobenzone for reliable UVA protection. Typical for Olay moisturizers is the inclusion of the cell-communicating ingredient niacinamide, present in this product at what is most certainly an efficacious amount. Other than a silky texture and fragrance-free formula, that's where the excitement stops. All the other antioxidants and intriguing ingredients are listed after the pH-adjuster (triethanolamine), so they don't amount to much. Still, this is a good daytime moisturizer for normal to oily skin that is prone to blemishes.

☺ GOOD **Pro-X Age Repair Lotion with SPF 30** *($46 for 2.5 fl. oz.)* has a lotion-like texture that slips easily over skin and sets to a lightweight hydrating finish suitable for normal to slightly dry or slightly oily skin. UVA protection is provided by avobenzone, just as it is for almost every daytime moisturizer with sunscreen that Olay offers. The rest of the formula contains cell-communicating niacinamide along with peptides, vitamin E, and glycerin. Glycerin is a good moisturizing agent that's present in hundreds, if not thousands, of moisturizers. Pro-X Repair Lotion with SPF 30 isn't any more reparative than other well-formulated sunscreens, and would've been even better if Olay had included some potent antioxidants (there isn't that much vitamin E in here, and many dermatologists feel a cocktail of antioxidants is best for skin) for extra environmental defense. Still, this is recommended and its cosmetically elegant texture works beautifully under makeup. As with all Pro-X products, this is fragrance-free. Note: This is not rated with a $$$ because size-wise, Olay provides more product than many competing brands (the standard size is 1.7 ounces).

☺ GOOD **Regenerist Eye Derma-Pod** *($24.99 for 24 pods)* is supposed to resurface, fill in lines, and decongest puffiness around the eyes. Each pod is a tiny packet filled with a silicone-based lotion. Squeezing the pod dispenses the product onto the built-in sponge pad, and you're directed to gently dab the product all around the eye, then use the sponge to massage the area in a circular motion for one minute. The sponge and massage action provides a very mild exfoliation for eye-area skin, while the silicone feels smooth and silky. Olay maintains that the massage action is what helps "remove excess under-eye fluids," but the effect is minimal at best, not to mention that puffiness from fluid buildup is usually temporary and related to diet (high in sodium), allergies, or sinus issues, and the latter two are easily remedied by over-the-counter antihistamines or decongestants. Plus you could just massage the area without the little pads and get the exact same results. The solution dispensed onto the sponge differs little from the other serums in Olay's Regenerist line. It contains a significant amount of niacinamide and lesser amounts of peptides along with a couple of antioxidants. These pods aren't a necessary add-on to your skin-care routine, but if you're curious to try them the formula itself is definitely beneficial for skin, either around the eyes or elsewhere, and the massage action is best done carefully because massaging too vigorously can pull delicate skin. Ultimately, though, you don't need a special product for the eye area (see the Appendix to find out why).

☺ GOOD **Regenerist Filling + Sealing Wrinkle Treatment** *($24.99 for 1 fl. oz.)* comes in a medicinal-looking tube and is meant, as the name states, to fill wrinkles and seal in moisture.

The silicone and the plastic-based thickening agent that comprise the bulk of this product will function as minor fillers for wrinkles, but the best results will be seen for superficial lines, not deep, etched wrinkles, and the effect is best described as temporary. However, someone in their late 20s or 30s with the first signs of lines around the eyes or mouth may find this works beautifully (if temporarily) to reduce these signs of aging. Olay omits the niacinamide and instead includes an impressive amount of a cell-communicating peptide and antioxidant vitamin E. This line-filling serum is fragrance-free and includes a mineral pigment to help reflect light away from the skin, which can further improve the appearance of superficial lines.

☺ GOOD **Regenerist Deep Hydration Regenerating Cream** *($24.99 for 1.7 fl. oz.)* contains ingredients capable of hydrating skin (including glycerin and niacinamide), but has a texture those with dry to very dry skin may find too light. Overall, this is a good formula whose only shortcoming is the somewhat disappointing amount of antioxidants.

☺ GOOD **Regenerist Reversal Treatment Foam** *($31 for 1.7 fl. oz.)*. What this propellant-based foaming moisturizer is supposed to reverse is merely the appearance of lines and wrinkles, a claim that can be made for almost any moisturizer. With the exception of the fact that this pressurized product foams, its formula differs little from all the other Regenerist moisturizers. If the foaming effect had some positive action on skin this would be worth the splurge, but no such luck, it's just a novel way to dispense a moisturizer. This is a respectable moisturizer for normal to slightly dry or slightly oily skin (it's heads and tails above anything L'Oreal or Nivea offer)—it just wasn't a necessary or revolutionary addition to Olay's burgeoning Regenerist lineup. The tin oxide and mica cast a subtle shine on skin that has nothing to do with it being regenerated layer-by-layer; it is merely a cosmetic sheen. This product is supposed to be based on Olay's Aquacurrent science, which is their interpretation of the science behind aquaporins. Aquaporins are membrane water channels present in bacteria, plants, and animals (including humans) that help to maintain the water content of cells, including skin cells (Source: ks.uiuc. edu/Research/aquaporins/). As fancy as that sounds, it doesn't take much to facilitate that system—research shows that ingredients as simple as glycerin handle this quite nicely.

☺ GOOD **Total Effects 7-in-1 Anti-Aging Moisturizer Daily Moisturizer** *($22.99 for 1.7 fl. oz.)* is a lightweight moisturizer that contains a good amount of niacinamide and silicones for a silky finish. The formula also contains a couple of good antioxidants. While overall not as state-of-the-art as similar products from Olay's Regenerist collection, this is still a good option for normal to oily skin.

☺ GOOD **Total Effects 7-in-1 Anti-Aging Moisturizer Daily Moisturizer Fragrance-Free** *($22.99 for 1.7 fl. oz.)* is identical to Olay's Total Effects 7-in-1 Anti-Aging Moisturizer Daily Moisturizer, except this version omits the fragrance, which is to your skin's benefit.

☺ GOOD **Total Effects 7-in-1 Anti-Aging UV Moisturizer Plus Touch of Foundation SPF 15** *($22.99 for 1.7 fl. oz.)*. Is this a brilliant way to combine sunscreen, a touch of color, and lots of beneficial ingredients for skin in one apply-and-get-out-the-door product? The answer is a confusing yes and no. The in-part avobenzone sunscreen is a plus, as is the silky texture laced with an efficacious amount of the cell-communicating ingredient niacinamide. It also applies smoothly, blends well, and sets to a soft matte finish. The problem is that the single shade available won't work for all skin tones (it's best for those with light to medium skin tones that are not overtly pink), and although it's sheer, if the color isn't right for you, the difference will be

The Reviews O

Y Did you know alcohol in skin-care products is a big problem? See the Appendix to learn more.

obvious. Olay would have been better off launching this in three or four shades for various skin tones (and they clearly know how to do that given the impressive improvements seen in Cover Girl's foundations; remember, both Cover Girl and Olay are owned by Procter & Gamble). As it turns out, this is a brilliant option only if the single shade matches your skin well enough to look convincing. If that's the case, the formula, which is good but could've ramped up the antioxidants a bit, is best for normal to slightly oily or slightly dry skin. Neutrogena's Healthy Skin Tone Enhancer SPF 20 is a comparable product with a better formula and several shades.

☺ GOOD **Total Effects Touch Of Sun, Daily Anti-Aging Moisturizer** (*$22.99 for 1.7 fl. oz.*) tries to combine two steps—self-tanning and exfoliation—in one product. While the concept is nice and it sounds like a time saver, it is probably far better for your skin to apply them separately. The self-tanning process is enhanced when you exfoliate before you apply the self-tanner, not during. Applying them at the same time can be counterproductive. Besides, the pH of this lotion doesn't permit the salicylic acid to exfoliate, so it's best used as a bland moisturizer with the self-tanning ingredient dihydroxyacetone. You'll get noticeable color from this, but it's a shame that the formula lacks the roster of state-of-the-art ingredients found in Olay's other Total Effects moisturizers.

☺ GOOD $$$ **Pro-X Skin Tightening Serum** (*$46.99 for 1 fl. oz.*). This water-based, thin-textured, fragrance-free serum contains a high amount of the cell-communicating ingredient niacinamide, just as most Olay serums do. Peptides and some antioxidants also are included, along with a film-forming agent that can make skin feel temporarily tighter, which is strictly a cosmetic effect. The formula includes dill extract, and there's one study indicating that at least on human skin samples and on "dermal equivalents" (which is not the same as intact human skin), dill extract has a strong promotional effect on elastogenesis. Elastogenesis is a fancy way of saying elastin synthesis. Healthy elastin is one of the chief components of youthful skin, responsible for its tightness and its ability to bounce back when manipulated. The study demonstrated that dill stimulates key enzymes in skin that trigger elastin production, although no mention was made of dill being able to repair damaged elastin. All we know is that dill seems to have this effect on isolated skin cells responsible for elastin production (Sources: naturaldatabase.com; and *Experimental Dermatology*, August 2006, pages 574–581). In that sense, it's entirely possible that it won't work to provide the results consumers with sagging skin are hoping for (not to mention that elastin damage is only one part of why skin sags as we age). So, dill isn't a slam-dunk anti-aging ingredient, and one in vitro study isn't much to go on, but at least there's a remote reason to include it in the product, which is more than most cosmetics companies can show for the ingredients they often include.

☺ AVERAGE **Active Hydrating Beauty Fluid, Original** (*$10.99 for 4 fl. oz.*) contains mostly water, thickener, glycerin, oil, Vaseline, and more thickeners, plus fragrance and coloring agents to make it smell and look pretty. This is definitely a case where the original isn't the best. Instead, it's uninspiring and minimally helpful for dry skin.

☺ AVERAGE **Active Hydrating Cream, Original** (*$10.99 for 2 fl. oz.*) is active in name only, and is one of Olay's most boring, do-nothing moisturizers. It's an average option for dry skin, nothing more.

☺ AVERAGE **Age Defying Anti-Wrinkle Eye Cream** (*$14.99 for 0.5 fl. oz.*). This light-textured, silky moisturizer for slightly dry skin anywhere on the face contains many commendable ingredients. The problem is that most of the beneficial ingredients will degrade soon after you start using the product because of the jar packaging (something Olay is typically good about avoiding). This product also contains an unusually high number of preservatives, including

DMDM hydantoin, which can be a problem for skin, especially in the sensitive eye area. See the Appendix to find out why, in truth, you don't need to bother with eye creams.

☺ AVERAGE **Age Defying Anti-Wrinkle Night Cream** *($14.99 for 2 fl. oz.)* is similar to the Age Defying Anti-Wrinkle Daily SPF 15 Lotion reviewed above, minus the sunscreen. It is not rated as highly because the jar packaging will not help keep the antioxidant vitamins stable during use. See the Appendix to learn more about why jar packaging is a problem.

☺ AVERAGE **Age Defying Classic Eye Gel** *($10.99 for 0.5 fl. oz.)* has a lightweight, somewhat slippery texture that feels light and refreshing. The amount and type of witch hazel have been changed, and the changes are to your skin's benefit. Still, witch hazel in any form isn't the best for use around the eyes. This eye gel contains some reliable anti-irritants to counteract any potential problems from the witch hazel. However, what you really want is a skin-care product whose ingredients exert all their effort toward helping your skin rather than protecting it from problematic ingredients. All told, this isn't a must-have item. You can get this eye gel's chief benefit by simply applying a cool compress to your eye area (which can be helpful if your puffy eyes are unrelated to aging).

☺ AVERAGE **Age Defying Protective Renewal Lotion SPF 15** *($10.99 for 4 fl. oz.)* contains an in-part zinc oxide sunscreen, but that's the only exciting element in this rather bland moisturizer for normal to slightly dry skin. The moisturizers with sunscreen in Olay's Regenerist and Total Effects lines are more exciting.

☺ AVERAGE **Anti-Wrinkle Mature Skin Night Firming Cream** *($10.99 for 1.9 fl. oz.)*. There is nothing about this product that is unique or special for mature skin or for any age group. Either way, the name is completely obnoxious because it reinforces the erroneous notion that age is a skin type and it isn't. Someone over 50 can have the exact same skin type as someone who is 30, and both would need the exact same type of ingredients. In this case you're getting a fairly ordinary moisturizer with a few beneficial ingredients, but the light- and air-sensitive ingredients (most of which are barely present) will degrade thanks to the jar packaging (see the Appendix for details). Regardless of whether you're 45, 55, or older, this is one of Olay's lesser moisturizers for those with normal to dry skin.

☺ AVERAGE **Anti-Wrinkle Mature Skin Enriching UV Lotion SPF 15** *($13.99 for 4 fl. oz.)*. Although this in-part zinc oxide daytime moisturizer with sunscreen has the basic antiwrinkle action a sunscreen should, it isn't a unique formula for mature skin. Actually, there is nothing about this product that has anything to do with your age—age is not a skin type. There isn't one ingredient in this product that is preferred for older skin, but many of them are too ordinary for words. The sun protection is nice, but other beneficial ingredients are in short supply and the overall formula isn't nearly as good as many others from Olay. Regardless of age, this remains a boring sunscreen that's a passable, but hardly exciting, option for normal to slightly dry skin.

☺ AVERAGE **Complete All Day UV Moisture Cream SPF 15, for Normal Skin** *($10.99 for 2 fl. oz.)* includes avobenzone instead of zinc oxide for UVA protection. The base formula is nothing too exciting, and in fact is one of the more lackluster options in Olay's vast stable of daytime moisturizers with sunscreen. This formula has too many shortcomings to be considered "complete" and the moisture it supplies is not emollient, so it is a good option for those with normal skin, though truly "normal" skin is a rarity. Overall, this just isn't as good as it could be, and as such isn't worth strong consideration.

☺ AVERAGE **Complete All Day UV Moisture Cream SPF 15, for Sensitive Skin** *($10.99 for 2 fl. oz.)* is the lotion version of the Complete All Day UV Moisture Cream SPF 15, for

Normal Skin above. The main difference, besides the lotion texture, is that this version isn't packaged in a jar. Otherwise, the same comments apply.

☺ AVERAGE **Complete All Day UV Moisturizer SPF 15, for Sensitive Skin** *($10.99 for 6 fl. oz.)*. Olay brought back the former version of this daytime moisturizer with sunscreen due to consumer demand. The previous version used avobenzone for reliable UVA protection while the reinstated formula includes zinc oxide, which is preferred for sensitive skin. Although broad-spectrum sun protection is assured, this remains a fairly lackluster formula that, beyond the zinc oxide sunscreen, has no benefit for sensitive skin other than being fragrance-free. One of the actives (octinoxate) isn't the best for sensitive skin, and the base formula is lacking a good mix of soothing anti-irritants.

☺ AVERAGE **Complete Night Fortifying Cream** *($14.99 for 2 fl. oz.)* is a lightweight moisturizer for normal to dry skin, but regrettably the antioxidants it contains will deteriorate due to the jar packaging. Several other Olay products have better formulations in packaging that will keep the air- and light-sensitive ingredients well protected.

☺ AVERAGE **$$$ Total Effects Eye Transforming Cream** *($22.99 for 0.5 fl. oz.)* has a formula similar to Olay's other Total Effects products, meaning you get a blend of such ingredients as glycerin, niacinamide, silicone, emollients, and antioxidants. It features a dry-finish ingredient known as isohexadecane, which prevents it from being too creamy. If you prefer a luxurious-feeling eye cream, this is not the one to choose. Another reason to reconsider before buying this: The formulation is similar to Olay's other Total Effects products, but in this case you're getting less product for your money and it's in translucent jar packaging, which compromises the effectiveness of the antioxidants even before you open it. Last, you don't need an eye cream—we promise. See the Appendix to find out why.

☺ AVERAGE **Pro-X Clear UV Moisturizer SPF 15** *($33 for 1.7 fl. oz.)* doesn't contain anything that makes it special for acne-prone skin. Critical UVA (think anti-aging) protection is provided by avobenzone, but aside from a lighter texture, this isn't a brilliant option for someone with oily, breakout-prone skin also struggling with signs of aging. It lacks the state-of-the-art ingredients skin needs to look and act younger while improving signs of breakouts (such as red marks or uneven skin tone). Without question the sun protection this offers will help prevent further signs of aging due to sun damage, but Olay offers more exciting and less expensive options in their Regenerist line.

☺ AVERAGE **Regenerist Micro-Sculpting Cream** *($31.99 for 1.7 fl. oz.)* purports to be the result of 50 years of Olay research, so you'd expect this to be a breathtakingly unique formula. It's not, and in fact it's very similar to all the other Regenerist moisturizers and serums (we can't imagine what Olay was doing for 50 years because if this is all they came up with, that would not be something to brag about). Increasing hydration can make skin cells plump, but that doesn't restore volume to a face that is sagging due to the complex process of aging. In other words, despite the name, this is not a face-lift in a jar. Actually, the jar packaging does a disservice to the range of antioxidants in this product (it does contain more antioxidants than many Olay products). That leaves you with a decent lightweight moisturizer for normal to slightly dry skin. Note: This moisturizer is available in fragranced and fragrance-free versions. If you decide to try it, go for the fragrance-free version (your skin will thank you)!

☺ AVERAGE **Regenerist Night Recovery Cream** *($24 for 1.7 fl. oz.)* comes in a jar, so the potency of the interesting ingredients such as niacinamide, vitamin E, and green tea is compromised. This also contains lavender and arnica extracts, which won't provide a "mini-lift" to skin, but do have the potential to cause irritation (see the Appendix for details). This has a less impressive formulation than most of Olay's Regenerist products, and if you're already using one or more of those, there is no reason to add this product, especially when there are more state-of-the-art formulas in better packaging available from companies such as Clinique, Neutrogena, and Paula's Choice.

☺ AVERAGE **Total Effects Night Firming Cream** *($22.99 for 1.7 fl. oz.)* doesn't have anything special up its sleeve that makes it ideal for nighttime use. It's a good moisturizer with a silky texture and enough film-forming agent to help make normal to dry skin look smoother. Olay includes some notable anti-aging ingredients, but most of them won't remain stable due to jar packaging. Niacinamide, the star B-vitamin Olay uses throughout their line, is present in an amount that's definitely efficacious. That's great (and niacinamide isn't prone to breaking down in the presence of light or air) but for all niacinamide's benefits, it isn't capable of firming skin to a noticeable degree.

☺ AVERAGE **$$$ Pro-X Hydra Firming Cream** *($47 for 1.7 fl. oz.)*. The cosmeceutical-sounding claims for this moisturizer are tempting, but for the most part, this silky-textured moisturizer for normal to dry skin doesn't distinguish itself from several less expensive Olay moisturizers. It contains some peptides and vitamin E, but all these state-of-the-art ingredients will see their efficacy diminish due to the jar packaging (see the Appendix for details on jar packaging). A similar Olay moisturizer in better packaging (and for a lot less money) is Regenerist Deep Hydration Regenerating Cream.

☺ AVERAGE **$$$ Pro-X Wrinkle Smoothing Cream** *($47 for 1.7 fl. oz.)* has a slightly heavier texture than the Olay Pro-X Hydra Firming Cream above, and because of that, those with dry to very dry skin will likely enjoy this product's performance best, but don't take that to mean this is the antiwrinkle moisturizer you've been waiting for. To Olay's credit, their claims for this moisturizer are accurate: It smoothes the appearance of lines and wrinkles while improving skin's texture. Those benefits are the beginning of any well-formulated moisturizer, and this one certainly qualifies. What holds it back from a better rating is the jar packaging. When you're loading your moisturizer with peptides and also including antioxidants, you should know that consistent exposure to light and air isn't going to keep these fragile ingredients around for long (see the Appendix for details). A less expensive version of this product that comes in better packaging is Olay Regenerist Reversal Treatment Foam.

☺ AVERAGE **$$$ Total Effects 7-in-1 Anti-Aging Eye Cream Line and Dark Circle Minimizing Brush** *($21.99 for 0.2 fl. oz.)* left us wondering why we bothered. Housed inside a pen-style component outfitted with a nylon brush is a tinted eye cream that is meant to improve dark circles. In short, it does very little to make dark circles look better. With product in hand, you depress the button at the end of the component to feed the tinted liquid onto the brush. Once you've dispenses a small amount, you brush it under the eyes, supposedly to even your skin tone and reduce under-eye darkness. The problem is that the tint (which is slightly orange) provides insignificant coverage. A liquid or cream concealer does a much better job at camouflaging dark circles, which is why you'll likely wonder why you bothered! As for the formula, although it contains some good ingredients (niacinamide, vitamin E) none of them can reduce dark circles, improve puffy eyes, or offer special benefits exclusive to the eye area. The brush applicator feels nice, but ultimately this is just a sheer concealer disguised as an eye cream (and it's barely hydrating so those with dry skin won't be happy). You would do much better pairing one of Olay's Regenerist serums with a great concealer!

☺ AVERAGE **$$$ Regenerist 14 Day Skin Intervention** *($26.99 for 0.7 fl. oz.)* promises a skin turnaround in two weeks, all without surgical intervention. You get 14 tiny tubes of product, divided into phases. **Phase 1** is applied nightly for the first week, and is said to "ignite cellular regeneration beneath the skin's surface." It's a water- and silicone-based serum that contains niacinamide, just like all the Regenerist, Total Effects, and Pro-X products Olay sells. However, this also contains lavender (several parts of the plant) along with arnica, and both are troublesome for skin. Other than the gimmick of using this for a week before moving on to the next phase, there is no reason to consider this serum over others from Olay that contain just as much niacinamide and omit the irritants. **Phase 2** is silicone-based and as such has a thicker, spackle-like texture. It won't make your skin look lifted as claimed, but will definitely make it look and feel better, all while supplying your skin with some potent cell-communicating ingredients plus the antioxidants vitamin E and green tea. Phase 2 is also fragrance-free. In summation, Phase 1 is not worth considering over Olay's better serums; Phase 2, on the other hand, is a state-of-the-art serum that stands an excellent chance of strengthening skin's barrier function and allowing it to create healthier new cells. It's up to you to decide if half of this 14-day regimen is worth the expense; we'd recommend you consider one of Olay's Regenerist serums instead.

☺ AVERAGE **$$$ Regenerist Advanced Anti-Aging Eye Roller** *($23.99 for 0.2 fl. oz.)*. The trio of metal ball rollers on this product is designed to be massaged around the eye area to reduce puffiness. Unfortunately, puffiness cannot be massaged away, especially if it is from aging or genetics, when the fat pads beneath the eye weaken and droop beneath the eye area (and also above the eye's crease). Therefore, this pen-style component and its roller-ball applicator mechanism are more gimmicky than useful, though it does a good job of depositing product. The product itself is a water-based serum that isn't nearly as elegant as several other Regenerist formulas, though it does contain a small amount of peptide, and is fragrance-free.

☹ POOR **Total Effects 7-in-1 Anti-Aging Moisturizer Plus Cooling Hydration** *($22.99 for 1.7 fl. oz.)*. Olay definitely didn't need another moisturizer in their Total Effects line, let alone one that adds cooling, and very irritating, peppermint extract to the mix. The formula also contains the menthol derivative menthyl lactate, which is even more irritating than plain old menthol. All this cooling means that your skin is being irritated, not refreshed. See the Appendix to learn why irritation is a problem for everyone's skin.

OLAY LIP CARE

☺ GOOD **$$$ Regenerist Lip Anti-Aging Concentrate** *($24.99 for 0.06 fl. oz.)* is an emollient, shimmery balm that can't change the lines around your mouth. The niacinamide and lecithin are a nice touch and add to the moisturizing effect of this product, but it won't change the age of your lips by even one day. This is packaged in a pen-style component for easy application.

OLAY SPECIALTY SKIN-CARE PRODUCTS

✓☺ BEST **$$$ Pro-X Discoloration Fighting Concentrate** *($47 for 0.4 fl. oz.)*. This lightweight lotion is packaged in a medicinal-looking tube and its pointed applicator speaks to the spot-treatment nature. Spot-treating discolorations can work, but chances are good that you've got more discolorations that haven't become visible yet. In that sense, you're better off treating the entire face with a skin-lightening product—but if you choose to do so with this Pro-X option, you'll be replacing it frequently because this is a very small amount of product.

The pigmentation-fighting ingredients included in this product are niacinamide, acetyl glucosamine, and an Olay-developed skin-lightening agent known as undecylenoyl phenylalanine. Olay's parent company Procter & Gamble has some published research on the latter ingredient, and it is emerging from some other sources, too, indicating there's promise. Research on acetyl glucosamine (a favorite ingredient of Estee Lauder, too) is less compelling but potentially promising when mixed with niacinamide, as is the case here. Speaking of niacinamide, its research is most bankable in terms of melanin-inhibiting effects (Sources: *Journal of Drugs in Dermatology*, July 2008, pages S2–S6; and *The British Journal of Dermatology*, July 2002, pages 20–31).

☺ GOOD $$$ **Pro-X Clear Acne Protocol Kit** *($47)*. With the launch of this kit, Olay is acknowledging what many consumers already know: Acne and wrinkles can and often do occur at the same time, along with other signs of aging. Being out of your teen years or never having had a breakout before doesn't mean you'll reach your 40s or 50s and be blemish-free; quite the contrary, as we hear from many women struggling with these distinct concerns. So what does Olay have to offer? A 3-step kit that includes cleanser, salicylic acid (also known as BHA) treatment, and a moisturizer. Unfortunately, for various reasons, the kit misses the mark for addressing acne and other types of breakouts such as blackheads. **The Acne Pore Clarifying Cleanser** is medicated with salicylic acid, but in a cleanser its benefit is mostly rinsed down the drain. A potential concern is the inclusion of sodium lauryl sulfate, as this can be drying. Most likely it's not a problem because the amount is low, but there are gentler cleansing agents Olay could have included. The cleanser does an OK job of removing makeup, but salicylic acid isn't meant for use around the eyes, so you'll need a different cleanser to take your eye makeup off. Next is the **Acne Skin Clearing Treatment**. This leave-on product contains 1.5% salicylic acid, but the pH is too high for it to function adequately as an exfoliant. This lightweight lotion feels silky, but will do little to improve acne or blackheads. One more comment: The ginger root is a potential irritant, although most likely the amount is too low to be cause for concern—but why include it in the first place? The **Complexion Renewal Lotion** has a fluid, silky texture that those with normal to oily skin will appreciate, and it contains a good amount of the cell-communicating ingredient niacinamide. There is some research indicating niacinamide can help fade red marks from acne, and it offers numerous other benefits to skin, too. If only Olay had included a greater range of this type of ingredient, this product would be worth strong consideration (well, at least if it were sold separately from this kit). As is, it's a decent option, but those looking for anti-aging benefits will do better with one of the moisturizers or serums we recommend in the Best Products chapter. Ultimately, this rather expensive kit doesn't offer much for those struggling with acne and signs of aging. Without a well-formulated BHA exfoliant, breakouts won't improve to a great degree. Also missing is a topical disinfectant with benzoyl peroxide, which is considered the gold standard for fighting acne because it kills the bacteria that cause acne.

☺ AVERAGE $$$ **Pro-X Advanced Cleansing System** *($32)*. Olay made quite a splash in their magazine ads comparing this battery-powered cleansing brush to a competing version that sells for $200. Although the ads didn't name names, there's no missing that they were comparing their inexpensive cleansing brush option to the Clarisonic brush, the "classic" version of these kinds of brushes that sells for, you guessed it, $200. What really surprised us was that Olay was right, up to a point. The performance and ease of use of their 2-speed facial cleansing brush works to an extent like the Clarisonic brush—at a fraction of the cost. Regardless of the speed you choose (low or high), the Olay brush is easy to operate and maneuver around your face. Some may prefer a larger brush head, but most should find this adequate (but use caution around your eyes).Unlike the Clarisonic and similar wannabe devices, Olay's version has a very soft brush head that spins rather than vibrates. As a result, you get gentle yet thorough cleansing that helps ensure all your makeup is removed. You simply need to move the brush around your face, apply light pressure, and let the powered brush go to work. Most people will find this far more gentle than the Clarisonic, and gentle is a good thing. The problem with Olay's brush is that it is flimsy and the brush speed is lackluster (many will find it too slow). The brush head we tested was bent and was used up in about three weeks. That means you'll have to replace the brush head more frequently, an extra unexpected expense. Getting all your makeup off is essential to waking up with better looking skin and avoiding breakouts, and these cleansing brushes can help, but choosing among them isn't easy. We still believe that a soft washcloth with a gentle water-soluble cleanser is a great way to make sure you get all your makeup off at night, but these brushes also are an option, although none of them are quite up to the task when it comes to being gentle and practical. Keep in mind that a cleansing brush works only on the surface of the skin and it doesn't take the place of a well-formulated BHA exfoliant (salicylic acid) or an AHA exfoliant (glycolic or lactic acid), both of which work beyond the surface layers to reach sun damage and clogged pores.

☺ GOOD $$$ **Pro-X Intensive Firming Treatment** *($46.99)* is a two-part product with a rather exorbitant price tag; it's Olay's attempt to create a special identity for their Pro-X products to differentiate them from their Regenerist products. Unfortunately, other than the price, which doesn't help have any impact on your skin, there isn't much reason to spend more for Pro-X. The two new products included in Pro-X Intensive Firming Treatment aren't all that different from other products Olay sells, including those from their ultra-pricey department store brand SK-II. The first part of this routine is the **Intensive Treatment Mask**, which is nothing more than a piece of cloth (you get five in this set) that's designed to fit over the entire face. The cloth is pre-cut so it doesn't cover your eyes, nostrils, or mouth. Steeped into the cloth is a blend of several intriguing ingredients for skin, including niacinamide, caffeine, hyaluronic acid, and a peptide. The formula is similar to, but less expensive (and better) than, any of the SK-II cloth masks. Once you place the mask over your face, you're directed to leave it on for 10 minutes, then remove it and smooth any remaining product into your skin. Although the formula is impressive, the mask delivery system is a silly gimmick, because you could just massage the gel liquid into your skin in the first place. You don't need to steep these ingredients in a mask to obtain their benefit, and ideally they should be left on skin for hours, not minutes. After the mask, you're then supposed to apply the **Skin Tightening Serum** (0.5 ounce). This water-based, thin-textured, fragrance-free serum contains a high amount of the cell-communicating ingredient niacinamide, just as most Olay serums do. Peptides and some antioxidants also are included, along with a film-forming agent that can make skin feel temporarily tighter, which is strictly a cosmetic effect. Overall, these two formulas are good, but you can get similar results from less expensive Olay products or from other well-formulated or better-formulated lightweight moisturizers that are less complicated to apply.

☹ POOR **Pro-X Clear Intensive Refining Sulfur Mask** *($32 for 1.7 fl. oz.)*. Sulfur is a potent disinfectant capable of killing acne-causing bacteria, which is what you want when you're struggling with breakouts. What your skin doesn't need is the dryness and irritation sulfur causes. While it was once widely used for treating acne, sulfur has taken a backseat to gentler and far more effective anti-acne ingredients like benzoyl peroxide and salicylic acid (also known as BHA). Please see the Appendix for details on why irritation is bad for skin.

The amount of sulfur in this absorbent clay mask makes it impossible to recommend. It will help reduce acne-causing bacteria, but the trade-offs aren't worth it, which in the long run can make matters worse. There's also the issue that acne stands a greater chance of improving with the right ingredients when they're applied daily and left on rather than rinsed off skin. Because a mask is designed for brief, occasional use, it is automatically less beneficial than what you do daily to keep your acne or other types of breakouts in check.

ORIGINS

Strengths: Almost none for the skin-care products, save for a couple of average eye-makeup removers; makeup fares better, with several great options, including liquid concealer, powder foundation, loose and pressed powders, liquid blush, bronzing options, brow enhancer, and automatic lip and eye pencils; very good makeup brushes composed of synthetic hair.

Weaknesses: Almost every skin-care product contains potent irritating ingredients that have no established benefit for skin; no products to address needs of those with acne or skin discolorations; no AHA or BHA products; although sunscreens provide the right UVA-protecting ingredients, they also contain irritating ingredients, some of which are phototoxic; the foundations contain irritating ingredients, as do most of the lip color products; average specialty products.

For more information and reviews of the latest Origins products, visit CosmeticsCop.com.

Note: Due to the overwhelming presence of plant-based irritants in Origins skin-care products, please check out the Appendix to learn how irritation damages skin and why daily use of highly fragrant products (whether the fragrance is natural or synthetic) is a problem for all skin types.

ORIGINS CLEANSERS

☹ POOR **A Perfect World Deep Cleanser with White Tea** *($21 for 5 fl. oz.)* contains irritants such as bergamot, spearmint, and lemon peel oils—this is not even close to a perfect world for your skin. All these and many more plant ingredients in this water-soluble cleanser are problematic for skin, and are a must to keep away from the eye area. As for Origins' rarefied silver-tipped white tea, it is barely present. Even if the white tea were a major ingredient in this cleanser, its positive benefit is negated by the litany of irritants present and the fact that it would be rinsed down the drain before it could have a benefit..

☹ POOR **Checks and Balances, Frothy Face Wash** *($19.50 for 5 fl. oz.)* is a very drying, alkaline cleanser that's made even more troublesome because it contains spearmint, lavender, and geranium oils.

☹ POOR **Clean Energy, Gentle Cleansing Oil** *($21 for 6.7 fl. oz.)* begins with several non-volatile, gentle oils suitable for dry to very dry skin, but quickly turns from mild to irritating due to several fragrant oils, including lavender, lemon, patchouli, and cedarwood.

☹ POOR **Mega-Mushroom Skin Relief Face Cleanser** *($27.50 for 5 fl. oz.)* had potential for being a good cleansing lotion for normal to dry skin, but it includes too many irritating essential oils to earn a recommendation. The various mushrooms have antioxidant ability, but even if that translated to topical application, those benefits are just rinsed down the drain.

☹ POOR **Never A Dull Moment, Skin-Brightening Face Cleanser with Fruit Extracts** *($19.50 for 5 fl. oz.)*. The only thing that isn't dull about this cleanser are irritating plant extracts—pine, eucalyptus, grapefruit, and mint oils—which will make your face glow with inflammation.

☹ POOR **Organics Foaming Face Wash** *($25 for 5 fl. oz.)* would have been a great cleanser for normal to dry skin, but the amount of clove, thyme, grapefruit, and patchouli oils makes this an irritating experience for skin, and a distinct problem if it gets near the eyes. The extract form of these plants would be preferred because in most cases, it is a much less concentrated source of irritation.

☹ POOR **Pure Cream, Rinseable Cleanser You Can Also Tissue Off** *($19.50 for 5 fl. oz.)* contains irritating peppermint, tangerine, lime and spruce oils. Regardless of how you decide to remove this cleanser, it's best not to use it in the first place

☹ POOR **Zero Oil Deep Pore Cleanser** *($19.50 for 5 fl. oz.)* claims to leave skin "tingly clean," and that is cause for concern. The tingle you'll feel has nothing to do with cleanliness and everything to do with your skin being irritated. As expected, this water-soluble cleanser for normal to oily skin contains several fragrant oils that cause irritation, which is a distinct problem around the eyes.

ORIGINS EYE-MAKEUP REMOVER

☺ AVERAGE **Well Off, Fast and Gentle Eye Makeup Remover** *($17.50 for 5 fl. oz.)* is a simply formulated, rosewater-based eye-makeup remover (which is more eau de cologne than skin care) that is only slightly less of a problem than all the other Origin products that are loaded with unfriendly skin irritants.

ORIGINS TONERS

☹ POOR **A Perfect World, Age-Defense Treatment Lotion with White Tea** *($21 for 5 fl. oz.)* contains several essential oils (meaning fragrant oils, because essential oils should only be those that are good for your skin) that are extremely irritating to skin, making this product impossible to recommend and far from skin's fountain of youth!

☹ POOR **Organics Purifying Tonic** *($25 for 5 fl. oz.)* lists alcohol as the second ingredient, and also contains vinegar and lavender oil. None of this is helpful for skin, and the calming willow bark extract doesn't stand a chance of soothing skin in the presence of these potent irritants.

☹ POOR **United State Balancing Face Tonic** *($19.50 for 5 fl. oz.)* has an ingredient list that's painful to even look at due to the number of known skin irritants it contains: lavender, alcohol, spearmint, citronella, and witch hazel, along with fragrant plant extracts—this is more eau de cologne than a skin-care product. It certainly won't bring any skin type to a "United State," but it will cause irritation that hurts skin's healing process, damages healthy collagen production, and stimulates more oil production at the base of the pore. That's probably not what you were expecting, which is why this product should be avoided.

☹ POOR **Zero Oil Pore Refining Toner with Saw Palmetto and Mint** *($19.50 for 5 fl. oz.)* is an alcohol based formula (alcohol causes free-radical damage, irritation, and dryness) that also contains a shocking amount of fragrant plant oils and fragrance ingredients known to cause irritation, which can stimulate excess oil production at the base of the pore. The amount of salicylic acid (BHA) is too low and this toner's pH is too high for it to function as an exfoliant. Anyone with oily skin who uses Origins' Zero Oil products will be subjecting their skin to potential irritation that can make oily skin worse.

ORIGINS EXFOLIANTS & SCRUBS

☹ POOR **Brighter by Nature High-Potency Brightening Peel with Fruit Acids** *($37.50 for 40 pads)* is supposed to rival professional peels that contain 30% glycolic acid. Origins attests that they have clinical proof of this, but the details of how they obtained this proof aren't available to the public. That means you have to take their word for it, but this product is so loaded with irritants, you're putting your skin at tremendous risk from a single use. The third ingredient is alcohol and it is closely followed by a litany of fragrant plant oils, all potent irritants. Lime and grapefruit oil can cause a phototoxic reaction when skin is exposed to sunlight, while lavender oil causes skin-cell death (Sources: *Cell Proliferation*, June 2004, pages 221–229; and naturaldatabase.com). The citrus oils contain citric acid, which is one type of AHA; however, citric acid isn't preferred to glycolic acid, an AHA with considerable research behind its efficacy (Sources: *Facial Plastic Surgery*, December 2009, pages 329-336; *Plastic and Reconstructive Surgery*, April 2005, pages 1156–1162; *Cutis*, August 2001, pages 135–142; and *Journal of the European Academy of Dermatology and Venereology*, July 2000, pages 280–284). This peel is in no way, shape, or form preferred to an in-office glycolic acid peel or to daily use of a well-formulated AHA product.

☹ POOR **Modern Friction, Nature's Gentle Dermabrasion** *($37.50 for 4.2 fl. oz.)* is Origins' take on the group of at-home scrub products that purport to mimic the effect of microdermabrasion treatments. Unlike other microdermabrasion scrubs, which contain aluminum oxide crystals, Modern Friction contains rice starch. Rice starch is considerably less abrasive, but before you get too excited, keep in mind that this is an Origins product. That means you can expect irritation, delivered here by a bevy of essential oils: lemon, bergamot, peppermint, and camphor. These oils are not present In meager amounts either, and you will feel a deep-down tingle (irritation) as you massage this scrub over your skin. Without these additives, this would be a great scrub for normal to dry or sensitive skin types. As is, we cannot recommend it.

☹ POOR **Never A Dull Moment, Skin-Brightening Face Polisher With Fruit Extracts** *($26 for 4.4 fl. oz.)* contains eucalyptus, pine, and mint oils, and is absolutely not recommended unless you want to harm rather than help your skin.

ORIGINS MOISTURIZERS (DAYTIME & NIGHTTIME), EYE CREAMS, & SERUMS

☺ AVERAGE **$$$ Plantscription Anti-Aging Eye Treatment** *($42.50 for 0.5 fl. oz.)* has a lightweight texture that is best for normal to slightly dry skin. You may be surprised to find out you don't need an eye cream (see the Appendix to find out why), but if you're intent on using one as part of your skin-care routine, this isn't the greatest option. The chief problem isn't the fragrant irritants typical of Origins skin-care products; rather, it's jar packaging (see the Appendix to learn why jars aren't the way to go). Origins is careful to state that this eye cream doesn't provide surgery-like results on wrinkles, which is absolutely true—it doesn't. It also cannot correct sagging around the eyes, as the numerous factors that cause sagging cannot be addressed by skin-care products, but the product alludes to such claims nonetheless. The plant extract *Anogeissus leiocarpus* bark is supposedly the ingredient that produces antiwrinkle results, but there is no substantiated research proving it can work in any way as Origins claims. Besides, you have to wonder, if this is such an amazing plant, why not include it in all your other antiwrinkle moisturizers and serums? Are those not as good because they lack this supposedly special plant? And, even if this plant extract were remarkable, putting it in jar packaging that routinely exposes it to air and light will quickly render it ineffective.

☺ AVERAGE **$$$ Starting Over Age-Erasing Eye Cream** *($35 for 0.5 fl. oz.)* has a rich texture that those with dry skin will appreciate; however, it contains some problematic plant ingredients that can cause irritation. It also comes in jar packaging so much of the good stuff won't remain potent once you've opened the product. Please see the Appendix to learn why you don't need an eye cream.

The Reviews O

☹ POOR **All Purpose High Elevation Cream Dry Skin Relief** (*$26 for 2.5 fl. oz.*) is claimed to be for those who live in dry, arid climates. Although many of the ingredients in this moisturizer are great for preventing moisture loss and dehydrated skin, the formula contains too many fragrant plant extracts and oils that cause irritation. In short, this isn't an all-purpose solution for combating environmentally dry skin.

☹ POOR **A Perfect World, Antioxidant Moisturizer with White Tea** (*$39.50 for 1.7 fl. oz.*) starts out strong and, at first glance, has all the elements of what other Lauder companies (of which Origins is one) know is necessary to create a great moisturizer to ease dryness and restore skin to a healthier state. What a shame Origins had to include such unnecessary and irritating ingredients as bergamot, lemon, orange, spearmint, and vetiver oils (among others). Among all the Lauder-owned companies, there are plenty of other excellent moisturizers whose best qualities compare favorably to this one from Origins, and those thankfully omit the problematic ingredients that create anything but a perfect world for your complexion.

☹ POOR **A Perfect World For Eyes, Firming Moisture Treatment with White Tea** (*$32.50 for 0.5 fl. oz.*) is the eye-area counterpart to the A Perfect World Antioxidant Moisturizer above. The formulas for both are similar, but the designated eye-area version contains a hefty amount of peppermint, which you will notice causes a tingling sensation as soon as you apply it to your skin. Peppermint is a potent irritant that is not only an unnecessary ingredient but also should never be used around the eyes. This product also contains several fragrant plant and flower oils that will make someone with allergies miserable. See the Appendix to learn why you don't need an eye cream, especially not one like this!

☹ POOR **A Perfect World SPF 25 Age-Defense Moisturizer with White Tea** (*$39.50 for 1.7 fl. oz.*) contains several irritants, including citrus oils such as lemon and bergamot, which can cause a phototoxic reaction when skin is exposed to sun. Yes, this product contains a reliable sunscreen (including avobenzone for critical UVA protection) and has a texture suitable for normal to dry skin, but when you consider how many other SPF-rated products omit the irritating ingredients, there is no reason to select this far-from-perfect one.

☹ POOR **A Perfect World, White Tea Skin Guardian** (*$36.50 for 1 fl. oz.*) is a silicone- and water-based serum that contains some good antioxidants (and in stable packaging), but ultimately just irritates skin due to the bergamot, lemon peel, spearmint, and rosewood oils it contains. Your face will smell great, but that has nothing to do with taking the best possible care of skin. See the Best Products chapter for serums that feel as silky as this, but minus the bad ingredients.

☹ POOR **Balanced Diet Lightweight Moisture Lotion** (*$26 for 1.7 fl. oz.*) is supposed to be the answer for combination skin, but the formula contains several plant based irritants that can make dry patches worse while stimulating excess oil production where skin is shiny. The called-out wheat and soy proteins are barely present and neither of these ingredients "feed" the needs of combination skin. The finish of this moisturizer is not matte enough to help keep oily shine in check, either.

☹ POOR **Brighter By Nature SPF 35 Skin Tone Correcting Moisturizer** (*$43.50 for 1.7 fl. oz.*) contains broad-spectrum sun protection (including avobenzone for reliable UVA protection), but also contains an overwhelming number of fragrant plant extracts and oils. Most of the ingredient list reads like a "who's who" of exceptionally irritating plant extracts. This is

Lavender oil smells great, but fragrance isn't skin care! Find out why in the Appendix.

further proof that just because an ingredient is natural doesn't mean it's a brilliant ingredient for your skin. This product's irritant potential is practically off the charts, and the daily dose of irritation can lead to collagen breakdown and chronic inflammation, even though you may not see the damage. It also is worth mentioning that this product has its share of synthetic ingredients, something the Origins marketing team was hoping you wouldn't notice. The few beneficial ingredients in this product won't remain stable anyway due to the jar packaging. The Paula's Choice Research Team cannot stress strongly enough how much this product is a must to avoid. It is among the most problematic reviewed in this book.

☹ POOR **Eye Doctor, Moisture Care for Skin Around Eyes** *($32.50 for 0.5 fl. oz.)* is not what the doctor ordered! This moisturizer contains wintergreen, mint, and lemon oils, all of which are a problem for skin and increasingly so when used around the eyes. Plus, you don't need an eye cream—see the Appendix to find out why!

☹ POOR **GinZing** *($29.50 for 0.5 fl. oz.)* has a silky texture, but most of the good-for-skin ingredients won't remain stable due to the jar packaging. Unfortunately, Origins' penchant for including irritating, fragrant plants continues with this product, and that is damaging to skin. The main plant is myrtle leaf water, which can cause problems for skin due to its irritating chemical makeup (Source: naturaldatabase.com). As for the other ingredients, the caffeine plus the plant extracts that contain caffeine won't wake up tired eyes or reduce dark circles; caffeine just doesn't have that effect topically. The cosmetic pigments in this eye cream can reflect light away from dark circles, making them appear lighter, but it's strictly a cosmetic effect. See the Appendix to learn why, in truth, you don't need an eye cream.

☹ POOR **Have a Nice Day, Super-Charged Moisture Cream SPF 15** *($38.50 for 1.7 fl. oz.)* contains an in-part titanium dioxide sunscreen, but at only 1%, so we wouldn't bank on it for UVA protection. Beyond that issue, your skin won't have a nice day because this daytime moisturizer irritates with its peppermint base and blend of volatile citrus and mint oils.

☹ POOR **Have a Nice Day, Super-Charged Moisture Lotion SPF 15** *($38.50 for 1.7 fl. oz.)* is the lotion version of the Have a Nice Day, Super-Charged Moisture Cream above, and the same comments apply (though this contains slightly more titanium dioxide).

☹ POOR **High Potency Night-A-Mins Mineral Enriched Oil-Free Renewal Cream** *($39.50 for 1.7 fl. oz.)* delivers a high potency dose of irritation due to the numerous fragrant plant oils it contains. The formula contains some excellent lightweight emollients and smoothing agents for normal to dry skin, but so do many other moisturizers that omit the problematic ingredients. Because this is packaged in a jar, many of the good ingredients won't remain stable during use. Please see the Appendix for further details on the issues jar packaging and fragrant irritants present. The small amount of salicylic acid isn't enough to prompt exfoliation. In short, this is not the way to enrich or renew skin.

☹ POOR **High Potency Night-A-Mins Mineral-Enriched Renewal Cream** *($39.50 for 1.7 fl. oz.)* is just as bad as the High Potency Night-A-Mins Mineral Enriched Oil-Free Renewal Cream above, and the same review applies. Who is green-lighting these products?

☹ POOR **Make A Difference, Skin Rejuvenating Treatment** *($38.50 for 1.7 fl. oz.)* has a silky texture that can translate to smoother skin. The main difference this product makes is the skin irritation caused by the essential oils of citrus, spearmint, and vetiver. The redeeming ingredients can't compete with these irritants, and won't last long due to jar packaging.

☹ POOR **Make a Difference Skin Rejuvenation Treatment Lotion** *($21 for 5 fl. oz.)* will cause irritation, not rejuvenation. Surprisingly short on truly beneficial ingredients, your skin instead is treated to plant irritant after plant irritant, all in the guise of natural ingredients being better for skin. While it's true that many natural ingredients are quite helpful for skin, here's a clear example of several that are not, and skin suffers as a result. How does Origins justify including spearmint and camphor oils (among others) in a product meant to help skin "rebound from dramatic dehydration"? There is no proof anywhere that these irritants serve skin for the better, especially in comparison with plant extracts that do reduce irritation or do have antioxidant properties.

☹ POOR **Make a Difference Ultra-Rich Rejuvenating Cream** *($38.50 for 1.7 fl. oz.)* has a reasonably rich texture, but that's not enough to offset the irritation and resulting cascade of cellular damage from ingredients such as lemon, spearmint, lavender, and bergamot oils. This moisturizer is mostly devoid of helpful ingredients and the few that are present won't last long due to the jar packaging. If you really want to make a difference for your skin, be sure to avoid this product.

☹ POOR **Mega-Bright Skin Tone Correcting Serum** *($55 for 1 fl. oz.)* contains a form of vitamin C (ascorbyl glucoside) with promising research on its ability to lighten discolorations, but it's also fraught with fragrant plant oils and extracts known to cause irritation. Also on board are fragrance ingredients such as eugenol that only add to the irritation. Ingredients like these have no benefit for skin; indeed, the inflammation they cause can mean discolorations last longer and also damage healthy collagen production. What about the plant *Rosa roxburghii* referred to in the claims? As is turns out, there's no research proving this plant improves skin discolorations from acne or sun damage but this plant is a natural source of vitamin C, so it's not too much of a stretch to assume a skin-lightening benefit exists (Source: *Phytotherapy Research*, March 2008, pages 376–383). Although that's exciting, this plant isn't used in an amount that's likely to have much impact on skin. Unfortunately, fragrant irritants take precedence in this silky serum. One ingredient deserves further explanation: dimethoxytolyl propylresorcinol, which is a chemical compound from the *Dianella ensifolia* plant. It is known to inhibit tyrosinase, which is the enzyme in skin that spurs melanin production. There are many ingredients research has shown inhibit the action of tyrosinase, as this is believed to be a fairly efficient way to control hyperpigmentation. Examples of such ingredients are various types of mushrooms, grape seed, 1-propylmercaptan, and arbutin. To date, there is no conclusive research proving that dimethoxytolyl propylresorcinol is the best one, or that its efficacy is comparable to that of hydroquinone. This ingredient is also used in Estee Lauder's Idealist Even Skintone Illuminator, which is a much better product to consider because it doesn't contain the numerous irritants of Mega-Bright Skin Tone Correcting Serum. In terms of brightening, this serum contains small amounts of the mineral pigments titanium dioxide and mica, which helps improve skin tone, but the effect is strictly cosmetic (like makeup), not due to a miraculous plant somehow evening your skin tone. Note that this serum contains salicylic acid (also known as BHA) but the amount is likely too low for it to have an exfoliating effect.

☹ POOR **Mega Mushroom Advanced Skin Relief Face Serum** *($66 for 1.7 fl. oz.)* is NOT calming, soothing, or in any way helpful for sensitive skin. And with the irritants it contains, it is not capable of helping "defend against silent skin-agers as never before." Oh, the irony! On the one hand, as this serum states up front, "Irritation silently simmering within skin's surface may be aging your skin faster than the candles on your birthday cake." And they are right, irritation absolutely can be "silently simmering" beneath skin's surface, causing damage without you actually feeling it, which is why all things irritating must be kept far away from your skin. On the other hand, this product is LOADED with known irritants! All the fragrant oils and many of the plant extracts in this product can cause acute irritation. Despite Dr. Andrew

Weil's name on the product, this is a mega-problem for your skin. It does contain some exotic types of mushrooms that do have antioxidant action, but most of them take second place to the fragrant irritants, such as lavender, orange, grapefruit, patchouli, rosemary, and linalool.

☹ POOR **Mega-Mushroom Skin Relief Eye Serum** *($45 for 0.5 fl. oz.)* lists myrtle leaf water as the second ingredient, which is not recommended for contact with skin due to volatile compounds, including 1,8-cineole, the constituent responsible for this plant's toxicity (Sources: *Journal of Natural Products*, March 2002, pages 334–338; and naturaldatabase.com). Even without the myrtle, this serum contains several fragrant oils that are troublesome for skin, including patchouli, orange, and lavender oils. See the Appendix to learn why you don't need a special product for the eye area—and certainly not an irritating one like this!

☹ POOR **Mega-Mushroom Skin Relief Face Cream** *($61 for 1.7 fl. oz.)* is the cream version of the Mega-Mushroom Skin Relief Face Serum above. It shares many of the same ingredients, but it omits the emollients and thickeners needed to create a cream texture. Between the proven irritating ingredients and problematic jar packaging, this well-intentioned product has too many negatives to make it a calming, age-fighting experience for skin.

☹ POOR **Mega-Mushroom Skin Relief Face Lotion** *($61 for 1.7 fl. oz.)* contains some novel and potentially effective antioxidants, but it's laced with irritants, including a tea of orange and myrtle and fragrant oils of lavender, patchouli, olibanum, and orange.

☹ POOR **Mega-Mushroom Skin Relief Treatment Lotion** *($30 for 6.7 fl. oz.)* contains too many irritating ingredients to make it a smart choice for any skin type, even though several impressive antioxidants are also included. The basil is a problem, as is the lavender, patchouli, orange, geranium, and frankincense oils. If these ingredients are necessary to "address problems that get in the way of skin's healthy appearance," as claimed, how come the other Lauder brands (such as Clinique) don't also contain them?

☹ POOR **Organics Nourishing Face Lotion** *($43.50 for 1 fl. oz.)* contains too many irritating fragrant oils to list, along with several fragrant components. The amount of alcohol is also a potential cause for concern, and one more factor that causes this moisturizer to pale in comparison with several others from the Lauder stable, or from Paula's Choice Earth Sourced Antioxidant-Enriched Natural Moisturizer (which costs less for twice as much product).

☹ POOR **Plantscription Anti-Aging Serum** *($75 for 1.7 fl. oz.)* is a thin-textured, water-based serum that is mostly a prescription for irritation! We agree that the name is brilliant and tempting, but rather than including proven, state-of-the-art anti-aging ingredients, Origins defaulted to using lots of fragrant plant oils that research has shown can damage skin because of the irritation they cause. You may be curious to try this product based on its claims of helping with specific wrinkles, such as furrows between the brows and frown lines around the mouth. Well, the curiosity ends here: There is nothing in this serum that will improve those wrinkles, or wrinkles anywhere else on your face. Etched lines from repetitive facial expressions are not the type of wrinkles that skin-care products can address. We wish that weren't the case, but there is no topical product that works like Botox or dermal fillers. Those cosmetic corrective procedures remain your best non-surgical options for dramatically (and we do mean dramatic) improving expression lines. Origins' claim that your skin will be "more lifted-looking" is telling many consumers what they want to hear, but in reality it's not telling you anything at all. Making skin look more lifted doesn't mean it will actually be lifted. Plus, if skin is sagging and then is lifted, you have to wonder where the excess skin goes? Simply lifting loose skin isn't going to make you look younger, any more than putting Scotch tape on your forehead lines will prevent deeper furrows from forming.

☹ POOR **Starting Over Age-Erasing Moisturizer with Mimosa** *($46 for 1.7 fl. oz.)* is loaded with irritating plant extracts and oils that absolutely don't help aging, don't help wrinkled skin look better because irritation causes collagen to break down, and hinders your skin's ability to heal. If your concern is aging skin, using this moisturizer is a big step in the wrong direction. Origins needs to take a cue from their sister companies, Clinique and Estee Lauder, both of which offer much better anti-aging moisturizers.

☹ POOR **Starting Over Age-Erasing Oil-Free Moisturizer with Mimosa** *($46 for 1.7 fl. oz.)* is a lighter version of the Starting Over Age-Erasing Moisturizer with Mimosa above, and the same review applies.

☹ POOR **VitaZing SPF 15** *($35 for 1.7 fl. oz.)* is a daytime moisturizer with shine that is not recommended because it contains an abundance of irritants. You should be "vitazing-ing" your skin with proven antioxidants, skin-repairing ingredients, and cell-communicating substances, not with fragrant irritants. Like most of the Lauder-owned brands, Origins consistently gets the critical issue of UVA protection right. That's great, and in the case of this product, you're getting an in-part avobenzone sunscreen. The disappointment is that unlike most of the other Lauder-owned brands, Origins fills their products with fragrant plant oils and extracts that potentially cause significant skin irritation. Even if you cannot see or feel the irritation, it is taking place beneath the surface of your skin, causing harm that can lead to collagen breakdown and a host of other problems. Your nose may love the way these unfriendly skin ingredients smell, but fragrance isn't skin care.

☹ POOR **Youthtopia Lift Ultra-Rich Firming Cream** *($52.50 for 1.7 fl. oz.)* contains some excellent rich emollients and smoothing agents for dry to very dry skin, but so do many other creamy moisturizers that omit the problematic ingredients Origins is fond of using. Because this is packaged in a jar, many of the good ingredients won't remain stable during use, which is disappointing given this product's price. Please see the Appendix for further details on the issues jar packaging and fragrant irritants present.

☹ POOR **Zero Oil Oil-Free Moisture Lotion with Saw Palmetto and Mint** *($26 for 1.7 fl. oz.)* is supposed to be a mattifying moisturizer for oily skin, but it doesn't offer a lasting matte finish and certainly won't lead to "zero oil" (though the promise is certainly enticing). Its chief problem is the inclusion of several irritating fragrant plant extracts and oils. For example, this moisturizer contains an unusually high amount of spearmint and citrus oils, the latter of which can cause a phototoxic reaction when skin is exposed to sunlight. In short, this is a really poor formula for any skin type, but especially for oily skin because the fragrant oils can stimulate excess oil production at the base of the pore (see the Appendix for further details).

ORIGINS SUN CARE

☹ POOR **Faux Glow, Radiant Self-Tanner For Face** *($20 for 1.7 fl. oz.)* lists peppermint (ouch!) as the second ingredient, and that makes this otherwise standard self-tanner extremely irritating. And that's before you even get to the orange, spearmint, and rosemary oils—all of them irritants—that are present, too. Instead of this problematic mix, try an irritant-free self-tanner (most of them are, from Coppertone to Neutrogena), and purchase peppermint oil to inhale while waiting for the self-tanner to dry!

☹ POOR **The Great Pretender, Shimmery Self-Tanner for Body** *($19.50 for 5 fl. oz.)* is almost identical to the Faux Glow facial self-tanner above, and the same comments apply.

ORIGINS LIP & SMILE CARE

☺ GOOD **$$$ Organics Soothing Lip Balm** *($15 for 0.15 fl. oz.)* is a very good emollient lip balm that is based around cocoa butter. It is irritant-free (What a pleasant surprise!) and works as claimed to prevent moisture loss and restore softness to dry, chapped lips.

☹ POOR **Conditioning Lip Balm with Turmeric** *($15 for 0.14 fl. oz.)* is a substandard castor oil–based lip balm that leaves lips irritated due to its lime and ginger oils. The lime oil is dangerous to put on your lips if you are going to expose them to sunlight because a phototoxic reaction can occur that can lead to discolorations (Source: naturaldatabase.com).

☹ POOR **Lip Remedy** *($12.50 for 0.5 fl. oz.)* contains a lot of peppermint oil, which is the opposite of being any sort of lip remedy.

ORIGINS SPECIALTY SKIN-CARE PRODUCTS

☹ POOR **Brighter By Nature Skin Tone Correction Serum** *($42 for 1 fl. oz.)* is advertised to be the inexpensive alternative to chemical peels and laser resurfacing. They even use the phrase "no scarring or scorching skin" to make you think that such procedures are disfiguring women left and right, when, in fact, these are extremely rare to nonexistent side effects of peels or lasers. The irony is that this product is supposed to fade sun-induced skin discolorations and prevent their recurrence, yet it contains several fragrant citrus oils that can cause discolorations in the presence of sunlight, a well-documented process referred to as a phototoxic reaction (Sources: naturaldatabase.com; and *Acta Dermato-Venereologica*, April 2007, pages 312–316). As if that weren't bad enough, this contains several other fragrant oils that irritate skin, inciting inflammation that won't help skin discolorations fade. Brighter By Nature is proof that nature doesn't have the best answers for skin discolorations, and is in no way a worthwhile replacement for cosmetic corrective procedures.

☹ POOR **Clear Improvement, Active Charcoal Mask to Clear Pores** *($22 for 3.4 fl. oz.)* is a clay and charcoal mask that would have been a good option for oily to very oily skin if it did not contain so much horsetail extract, which can constrict skin and cause irritation.

☹ POOR **Drink Up, 10 Minute Mask to Quench Skin's Thirst** *($22 for 3.4 fl. oz.)* offers dry skin some relief, but at the expense of causing irritation because this mask contains bitter orange and camphor oils. For a gentler, less expensive alternative, consider Paula's Choice Skin Recovery Hydrating Treatment Mask or the other moisturizing masks recommended in the Best Products chapter.

☹ POOR **Drink Up Intensive Overnight Mask to Quench Skin's Thirst** *($22 for 3.4 fl. oz.)*. This thick-textured, creamy mask contains some great ingredients for dry to very dry skin. Unfortunately, it contains proportionately more bad ingredients, including high amounts of numerous fragrant oils that are potent skin irritants. This may smell intoxicating, but is the aroma worth it if skin has to suffer? This absolutely isn't a mask to wear overnight or even for a few minutes. The irritation it can cause is just too great. Check out the moisturizing masks from Estee Lauder before this because at least Lauder spares your skin pro-aging irritants. What a disaster, and it's so sad people will buy this thinking it's natural and therefore better. There are most certainly some wonderful natural ingredients (think nonfragrant plant oils like jojoba or olive), but fragrant oils aren't among them.

☹ POOR **Mega Mushroom Skin Relief Face Mask** *($35 for 3.4 fl. oz.)* contains various species of mushrooms, just like the other products in the Dr. Andrew Weil for Origins group. Unfortunately, this moisturizing mask for normal to dry skin continues this line's problematic tradition of including several irritating ingredients for skin. The mushrooms are a novel and potentially effective inclusion, and this contains emollient safflower oil and some soothing agents, but that's little consolation when you consider the abundance of fragrant irritants. Both Estee Lauder and Aveda offer nonirritating, wonderfully soothing facial masks packed with ingredients that skin really needs, and without the disingenuous skin-calming claims

☹ POOR **No Puffery, Cooling Mask for Puffy Eyes** *($22 for 1 fl. oz.)* contains several fragrant oils that shouldn't get anywhere near the eyes (puffy or not), and as such this rose water–based product (rose water is mostly fragrance anyway) is not recommended.

☹ POOR **Out of Trouble, 10 Minute Mask to Rescue Problem Skin** *($22 for 3.4 fl. oz.)* gets skin into trouble because it contains camphor. That won't rescue anyone's skin, and those with blemish-prone skin are potentially setting themselves up for more breakouts because of the high amount of zinc oxide in this mask (which also makes it difficult to rinse).

☹ POOR **Spot Remover Acne Treatment Pads Salicylic Acid** *($26.50 for 60 Pads)*. These pads are, like so many others for those battling acne, steeped in a solution that subjects skin to a high amount of damaging alcohol. If the alcohol wasn't bad enough, your reddened, inflamed skin is also bombarded with clove oil, oregano oil, and the fragrance chemical eugenol, all of which are potent irritants despite having antibacterial properties (Sources: naturaldatabase.com; and *Toxicology*, May 2012, Epbulication). So not only are these pads expensive, they're a serious problem for breakout-prone skin because irritation slows healing and stimulates more oil production, potentially leading to more breakouts and blackheads. Last, although the formula is medicated with 1.5% salicylic acid, the pH is well above the range this anti-acne superstar needs to work as an exfoliant. Just bad news all around!

☹ POOR **Super Spot Remover, Acne Treatment Gel** *($13.50 for 0.3 fl. oz.)* is basically a laundry list of irritants, none of which are helpful for making blemishes go away. Alcohol heads the list, but skin is also assaulted with oregano oil, clove oil, and witch hazel. Some of the fragrant oils have disinfecting properties that may work to kill acne-causing bacteria, but there are gentler (and proven) ingredients to use instead. What's sad is that the active ingredient (salicylic acid) is formulated at pH that will allow it to function as an exfoliant. You'll likely see good results against breakouts, but as mentioned above, there are gentler ways to go about battling "spots" and other types of breakouts. Sticking with this will likely lead to dryness and flaking, and the irritation can stimulate more oil production.

☹ POOR **Zero Oil, Instant Matte Finish for Shiny Places** *($13.50 for 0.64 fl. oz.)* lists witch hazel as the second ingredient and also contains camphor oil, making this instantly irritating for all skin types.

ORIGINS FOUNDATIONS

☺ GOOD **Silk Screen Refining Powder Makeup** *($26.50)* is the best and only foundation we recommend from Origins. This talc-based pressed-powder foundation does not contain any of the irritating essential oils that plague their other options. It has an awesome silky texture and smooth, dry finish that provides light coverage. There are 13 shades available, including options for fair to dark skin, and there's not a poor one in the lot. This is recommended for normal to oily skin, though it's not quite on par with similar pressed-powder foundations from Estee Lauder, Lancome, and Laura Mercier.

☹ AVERAGE **$$$ A Perfect World SPF 15 Age-Defense Tinted Moisturizer with White Tea BB** *($35)*. It's interesting for a line that promotes being natural (and that natural is the best way to go), Origins opted to formulate this BB cream with synthetic sunscreen actives. They provide reliable broad-spectrum protection (and include avobenzone for sufficient UVA screening) but to keep with the natural theme, they should've used titanium dioxide and/or zinc oxide. Surprisingly, this contains several effective natural ingredients (alongside synthetic ingredients). Origins' moisturizers typically contain fragrant oils that irritate skin, but they're absent here, leaving you with a lightweight tinted moisturizer-like product best for normal to slightly dry or slightly oily skin. We'd love to rate this higher, but the colors prevented that. Most are far too peach, orange, or copper. Despite the fact that this BB cream goes on sheer, the colors remain obvious and too bright, so they won't work for most skin tones. Sadly, this doesn't end up being a perfect world for skin, though it comes closer than many other moisturizers Origins sells! One more comment: BB creams are typically little more than tinted moisturizers with sunscreen. They're not a must-have product. This option from Origins contains some beneficial extras, but you can find those from other tinted moisturizers whose shades look more realistic.

☹ POOR **Brighter By Nature SPF 30 Skin Tone Correcting Makeup** *($27.50)* is a talc-free pressed-powder foundation with many strong points, including reliable broad-spectrum sun protection. Unfortunately, it contains several fragrant plant oils that are a problem for all skin types.

☹ POOR **Stay Tuned Balancing Face Makeup** *($22)* has a lot in common with sister company Estee Lauder's Equalizer Makeup SPF 10, except the Origins version contains irritating spearmint, geranium, and lavender oils. All these present their share of problems for skin and yet have no balancing effect whatsoever. What a shame, because the shade range is beautiful and this foundation costs less than Lauder's version (but with theirs you're getting an irritant-free product).

ORIGINS CONCEALER

✓☺ BEST **Quick, Hide! Long-Wearing Concealer** *($15)* is a lightweight, water- and silicone-based liquid concealer that provides moderate, buildable coverage without looking thick or heavy. It sets to a satin smooth finish that feels slightly powdery but doesn't look dry or cakey. Once set, this stays in place quite well and holds up throughout the day. There are six shades available, with Light, Light/Medium, and Extra Deep being the best. The Medium shade is too dark for most medium skin tones and is preferred for tan skin. The Deep shade is a bit tricky due to its slight orange tone, but is worth a look by those with dark skin tones. This concealer is suitable for all skin types, and works equally well over dark circles or blemishes.

ORIGINS POWDER

☺ GOOD **$$$ All and Nothing Sheer Pressed Powder** *($25)* is talc-free and available in only one shade. It applies sheer, but will still look too light on tan or darker skin tones. It has a smooth texture and sheer, dry finish that works best for normal to oily skin.

ORIGINS BLUSHES

☺ GOOD **Pinch Your Cheeks** *($12)* is a liquid cheek stain that blends nicely once you get the hang of it (expect to have to practice), and offers a transparent matte finish. This works best on normal, small-pored, even-textured skin. The original shade is now labeled Raspberry, and two additional shades are also available.

☹ AVERAGE **$$$ Brush-On Color** *($21)* is a powder blush with an unusually dry texture yet smooth, even application. Almost all the shades are laden with shine, which makes them a questionable choice for daytime makeup. The least shiny shades include Crimson and Clover, Pink Petal, and Rose Dust. The other Lauder-owned companies have powder blushes that outperform this one, but if you're devoted to Origins, it's not a total disappointment.

ORIGINS EYESHADOWS & EYE PRIMERS

☺ GOOD **Eyeshadow** *($15)* includes 20 shiny selections ranging from subtle to striking. These have a buttery-smooth texture and very nice application that is neither too sheer nor too intense. There are no suitable options for lining the eyes or filling in brows, but at least the shine tends to remain flake-free. Be warned that applying shine over the eyelid can make any amount of wrinkles in that area more noticeable.

☺ GOOD **Underwear for Lids** *($15)* is an eyeshadow primer that also functions as an eyeshadow, assuming you want very soft, pastel-ish and flesh-toned colors imbued with soft sparkles. These twist-up eyeshadow sticks glide on easily and set within seconds to a long-wearing finish that's relatively impervious to creasing. For best results, use Underwear for Lids as a base for eyeshadow. You'll find that, just like a good matte finish concealer, it enhances shadow application, color intensity, and wear, all of which are needed for eye makeup that lasts. Note: Origins also sells Underwear for Lids as "The Smoothing Lid Primer." This product is essentially the same as their regular Underwear for Lids, except the color is a flesh-toned nude with a soft shimmer, not sparkles. It works best for fair to medium skin tones.

ORIGINS EYE & BROW LINERS

✓☺ BEST **Fill in the Blanks Eyebrow Enhancer** *($15)* is a prime pick if you prefer filling in and defining brows with pencil rather than powder. This skinny, automatic, nonretractable pencil applies with ease, isn't the least bit greasy or smear-prone, and has a soft powder finish. The two shades (one for blondes, one for brunettes) are limiting, but everything else about this brow pencil is terrific.

☺ GOOD **Automagically Eye Lining Pencil** *($15)* is an automatic, nonretractable pencil with one of the smoothest applications you're likely to come across. No tugging or dragging here! The pencil's soft texture makes it tricky to draw a thin line, but thicker lines are a cinch. Although you'll notice some fading as the day passes, it stays in place very well.

☺ AVERAGE **Eye Brightening Color Stick** *($15)* is a chubby, stout pencil that comes in one shade—a pale, shimmery silver-blue that is intended to line the inner rims of the eye, a technique that is more theatrical than practical. Also, repeated daily applications put your eyes at risk, as cosmetic coloring agents just don't belong next to the cornea. Yes, it can look striking in photographs, but it's not worth doing on a regular (or even infrequent) basis.

☺ AVERAGE **Just Browsing** *($15)* is a lightweight, softly tinted brow gel with an OK brush that adds natural color and definition to the eyebrow. The number of shades now stands at two (one for blondes, one for brunettes), and overall, we'd recommend Bobbi Brown's Natural Brow Shaper over this because it has a better brush and a wider selection of shades.

ORIGINS LIP COLOR & LIPLINERS

✓☺ BEST **Automagically Lip Lining Pencil** *($15)* deserves consideration if you're looking for an automatic, nonretractable lip pencil whose soft and sheer colors have a drier application but enough stain and silicone-enhanced tenacity to stay on for hours. This is an excellent option for those prone to lipstick bleeding into lines around the mouth. However, just like any anti-feathering lipliner, it won't keep slick glosses or greasy lipsticks from straying past the mouth's border.

☺ AVERAGE **Matte, Sheer,** and **Shimmer Sticks** *($15)* are the original "chubby sticks" that Origins has offered for years, and they're about the only cosmetics company that still does. Why these ever caught on is anyone's guess because they need constant sharpening, and most are too soft to get a controlled lip line. They're all akin to standard, creamy lipsticks in pencil form. The Matte Stick is not matte in the least, and is actually rather greasy. The Sheer Stick is even greasier than the Matte version, but has less pigment. The Shimmer Stick is creamy without being greasy and has a soft metallic finish. This one stands the best chance of lasting beyond your mid-morning break.

☹ POOR **Flower Fusion Hydrating Lip Color** *($16.50)* does contain several plant and flower waxes, and while those are harmless and contribute to this lipstick's creamy but thick texture, the jasmine, tangerine, lavender, and other citrus oils make this way too irritating to use on lips.

☹ POOR **Liquid Lip Color** *($15)* presents lip gloss with a bit more pigment than usual, which means you'll get a semi-opaque, glossy finish. What a shame the mint flavoring is so powerful and irritating, because the selection of colors is enticing.

☹ POOR **Liquid Lip Shimmer** *($15)* contains enough mint to make lips tingle and, depending on how much or how often you apply this, burn. The irritation is not worth it when many other glitter-infused glosses are so widely available.

☹ POOR **Once Upon a Shine Sheer Lip Gloss** *($15)* could just as easily be called "once upon an irritation" because that's what your lips are up against once they come into contact with this peppermint oil–infused gloss. No need to accept an irritating lip gloss when there are so many that don't irritate the lips.

☹ POOR **Rain and Shine Liptint with SPF 10 Sunscreen** *($15)* lacks adequate UVA-protecting ingredients (see the Appendix for details) and loses even more points due to the strong presence of peppermint oil. Plenty of sheer, glossy lipsticks are available that don't run the risk of irritating your lips.

☹ POOR **Smileage Plus Liptint** *($12.50)* is a sheer, glossy tinted lip balm that comes in some enticing, wearable colors and contains several lip-smoothing emollients. What a shame this ends up being irritating for lips due to its essential oils of lime and tangerine. The lime oil is especially problematic for lips exposed to sunlight, as it can cause a phototoxic reaction (Source: *Archives of Dermatological Research*, 1985, volume 278, pages 31–36).

ORIGINS MASCARAS

☺ GOOD **Fringe Benefits Lash-Loving Mascara** *($15)* is a commendable but not extraordinary lengthening mascara that applies without clumps and leaves lashes soft and separated with a slight curl. It's best for those looking for natural rather than dramatic lashes.

☺ AVERAGE **Full Story Lush-Lash Mascara** *($15)* is more like a novella than a full story, at least when it comes to making the most of your lashes. You're in for a letdown if you expect this to perform as claimed because it's one of the most unexciting mascaras around. Repeated coats will provide some length, but no thickness whatsoever. In fact, trying to build anything impressive with this mascara is akin to reading the same chapter in a book over and over while expecting the story to progress.

☺ AVERAGE **Underwear for Lashes** *($15)* is described as a "little lash builder" and is nothing more than a colorless mascara that adds length and bulk to lashes prior to applying a regular mascara. Its formula is nearly identical to that of the Fringe Benefits Lash-Loving Mascara, and two or three coats of that produces the same results as using this before applying the real mascara.

☺ AVERAGE **$$$ Beyond the Fringe** *($18.50)* is a dual-sided lash-enhancing product that includes Origins' **Fringe Benefits Lash-Loving Mascara** and **Underwear for Lashes**, both of which are reviewed above.

ORIGINS FACE & BODY ILLUMINATORS

☺ GOOD $$$ **Sunny Disposition Bronzing Stick for Eyes, Cheeks, and Lips** *($20)* has a smoother-than-silk texture that is easy to apply and imparts a soft, golden bronze color. The single shade is loaded with iridescence so it looks distracting, rather than beguiling, in daylight. However, it is appropriate for evening glamour, and looks particularly attractive when used over self-tanned legs, collarbone, and brow bone. The finish of this product does not feel great on lips, unless you're mixing it with a gloss or balm. For evening use, this is an excellent shimmer product that blends nicely and (best of all) tends to stay put. It is irritant-free.

☹ POOR **Halo Effect Instant Illuminator for Face** *($18 for 0.5 fl. oz.)* has a gorgeous shimmer effect on skin, whether used alone or mixed with foundation. The problem? The liquid formula contains a plethora of irritating essential oils, including peppermint, orange, and lemon. These make Halo Effect impossible to recommend for any skin type.

ORIGINS BRUSHES

✓☺ BEST $$$ **Origins Brushes** *($16.50-$35)* have always been made of synthetic hair, a boon for animal rights activists (or just for animal lovers). The latest incarnations are better than ever—you have to feel these to believe how amazingly soft and luxurious synthetic hair can be. Every brush has a renewed softness and the hairs are cut more precisely to facilitate a professional makeup application. Even the handles have been improved, making the entire collection worth looking at. The **Eye Lining Brush** ($16.50) could stand to be a bit firmer, but some may appreciate its greater flexibility. The **Lip Brush** ($16.50) is standard fare but the price isn't out of line, and it comes with a cap. Check out the **Powder Foundation Brush** ($22.50) which is rated "GOOD" and works well to apply any type of loose or pressed mineral makeup.

☺ GOOD **Brush Cleaner** *($11.50 for 3.4 fl. oz.)* is a spray-on, solvent-based brush cleaner that is scented with plant extracts so it won't leave brushes smelling medicinal. It works well and dries quickly; however, this type of product is best for makeup artists who may be using the same brushes on multiple faces. If you're the only one using your brushes, an occasional cleaning with a basic shampoo or liquid soap will suffice, and in the long run will be less drying on the brush bristles.

PAULA'S CHOICE

Strengths: Fragrance-free products; all products formulated based on extensive published research on how ingredients can benefit skin; uniquely formulated AHA and BHA products; effective skin-lightening options; gentle cleansers; toners that go beyond the norm; all sunscreens provide broad-spectrum protection (including UVA-screening ingredients); proven anti-acne products; antioxidant-rich serums and moisturizers; anti-aging products that work as claimed; gentle yet effective natural products; most foundations provide sun protection and come in a range of neutral colors; unique brow products; on-the-go teeth whitener; lipstick with sunscreen; impressive, reasonably priced makeup brushes; samples are available for most products.

Weaknesses: Only one self-tanning option; limited makeup shades for darker skin tones; does not offer a complete collection of makeup.

Full disclosure: In addition to reviewing thousands of cosmetics products over the past 30 years, Paula also has her own line of products called Paula's Choice. Along with her research team, Paula's goal is to help you find the best products possible for your skin, whether they are from her line or someone else's. Paula's commitment to this is so strong she is the only cosmetics company owner in the world who recommends products other than her own.

Paula and the Paula's Choice Research Team formulate products to meet or exceed the criteria we use to review products from every other brand in this book and on CosmeticsCop.com. We have tried to remain as objective as possible commenting on our products and have, as much as possible, used the same superlatives we use when reviewing other products with great formulas.

For more information about Paula's Choice, including our 100% satisfaction guarantee, call (800) 831-4088 or visit PaulasChoice.com.

PAULA'S CHOICE CLEANSERS

✓☺ BEST **Earth Sourced Perfectly Natural Cleansing Gel** *($16.95 for 6.7 fl. oz.).* This gentle, water-soluble cleansing gel is suitable for all skin types, including sensitive skin. Its silky texture cleanses and removes makeup with naturally derived ingredients, leaving skin feeling smooth and refreshed. Unlike countless other natural cleansers, Earth Sourced Perfectly Natural Cleansing Gel does not expose skin to irritating natural ingredients. Instead, skin is treated to mild yet beneficial natural ingredients proven to help rather than harm skin. Not all natural ingredients are created equal (after all, poison ivy is a natural ingredient!), and now those who prefer skin-care products with as many natural ingredients as possible have an effective alternative.

✓☺ BEST **Hydralight One Step Face Cleanser** *($15.95 for 8 fl. oz.)* is a water-soluble gel cleanser that feels silky and rinses cleanly. Skin is left smooth and refreshed, and this cleanser removes most types of makeup. Best suited for normal to oily/combination skin.

✓☺ BEST **Moisture Boost One Step Face Cleanser** *($15.95 for 8 fl. oz.)* is a water-soluble cleanser with a milky texture and low lather. It works beautifully to remove all types of makeup and rinses without a trace of residue, leaving your skin clean and soft. Best suited for normal to dry skin.

✓☺ BEST **RESIST Optimal Results Hydrating Cleanser** *($16.95 for 6.4 fl. oz.)* is a silky, water-soluble cleansing lotion with an exceptionally gentle formula that works quickly to remove makeup while cleansing normal to dry, sun-damaged skin. Its anti-aging benefit comes from the soothing and moisturizing ingredients it contains. Together, these work to respect and repair skin's barrier function so skin can begin looking and acting younger. For optimal results, follow with Paula's Choice RESIST Advanced Replenishing Toner.

✓☺ BEST **Skin Balancing Oil-Reducing Cleanser** *($15.95 for 8 fl. oz.)* has a cushiony texture that leaves combination to oily skin perfectly cleansed and free of makeup. This is the cleanser to consider if you prefer lots of foam (though the foam itself has no effect on cleansing ability). Your skin is left feeling refreshed and perfectly balanced, never dry or tight.

✓☺ BEST **Skin Recovery Softening Cream Cleanser** *($15.95 for 8 fl. oz.)* feels rich and soothing, and its creamy texture cleanses dry, sensitive skin while leaving it feeling smooth and supple. It does not leave a greasy residue, nor does it require a washcloth for complete removal. However, those using this cleanser to remove heavy makeup may find a washcloth makes the process easier.

PAULA'S CHOICE EYE-MAKEUP REMOVER

✓☺ BEST **Gentle Touch Makeup Remover** *($12.95 for 4.3 fl. oz.)* is a water- and silicone-based, dual-phase liquid that quickly removes all types of makeup, from long-wearing foundations to waterproof mascaras and lip stains. It contains soothing agents and is safe for use around the eyes. Like most fragrance-free makeup removers, it may be used before or after cleansing and is safe for sensitive eyes.

PAULA'S CHOICE TONERS

✓☺ BEST **Earth Sourced Purely Natural Refreshing Toner** *($16.95 for 5 fl. oz.)*. This mild, alcohol-free toner hydrates with 99% plant-based ingredients as it fortifies all skin types with antioxidants. Completely free of irritating plant extracts so prevalent in most other natural skin-care products, this toner only contains natural ingredients proven to benefit skin. This is an excellent option for those with sensitive, reddened skin, as this ultra-soothing toner contains numerous ingredients designed to reduce inflammation while promoting healthy collagen production. As with any well-formulated toner, this also works to remove last traces of makeup around the hairline and jaw and deposits lightweight hydrating ingredients for smoother, healthier-looking skin.

✓☺ BEST **Hydralight Healthy Skin Refreshing Toner** *($15.95 for 6.4 fl. oz.)* contains ingredients that improve skin function while reducing cellular damage, leaving skin feeling refreshed with a nearly imperceptible finish. This also removes the last traces of makeup and works great during summer months as a super-light moisturizer for normal to oily skin with dry patches.

✓☺ BEST **Moisture Boost Essential Hydrating Toner** *($15.95 for 6.4 fl. oz.)* helps optimize normal to dry skin so it functions normally. It contains antioxidants, cell-communicating ingredients, and skin-softening agents that leave a satin-smooth finish while also removing the last traces of makeup. You will see enhanced skin with a radiant finish. Ideal paired with Moisture Boost Hydrating Treatment Cream.

✓☺ BEST **RESIST Advanced Replenishing Toner** *($18.95 for 4 fl. oz.)* is an antioxidant-rich, milky toner that calms your skin from the first application. It contains a unique, concentrated blend of ingredients that restore and rebuild aging skin, allowing it to produce healthy collagen and help reverse signs of sun damage. This toner makes skin feel beautifully soft and look radiantly healthy. It's excellent for those with sensitive skin or rosacea.

✓☺ BEST **Skin Balancing Pore-Reducing Toner** *($15.95 for 6.4 fl. oz.)* is based around the cell-communicating ingredients niacinamide and adenosine triphosphate, both of which improve skin and restore balance while also improving hydration. This toner helps eliminate mild dryness and flaking skin while leaving it feeling smooth. One of our best-selling products, this is a personal favorite of Paula's. It's ideal for normal to oily or combination skin.

✓☺ BEST **Skin Recovery Enriched Calming Toner** *($15.95 for 6.4 fl. oz.)* is truly a moisturizing toner and is ideal for restoring essential elements to dry or very dry, environmentally compromised or sensitized skin. It contains antioxidants, anti-irritants, and essential lipids while being a perfect starting point before applying moisturizer, serum, or sunscreen. It is extremely beneficial for those with rosacea or easily irritated skin.

PAULA'S CHOICE EXFOLIANTS

✓☺ BEST **RESIST Daily Smoothing Treatment 5% AHA** *($25.95 for 1.7 fl. oz.)* is an advanced AHA exfoliant designed to significantly improve the appearance of sun-damaged, wrinkled skin. A pH-correct 5% concentration of glycolic acid (plus 0.5% salicylic acid) exfoliates for improved texture and tone, while a blend of anti-aging ingredients helps the skin look and act younger. The benefits of this daily exfoliant go above and beyond what a traditional AHA product provides. It is suitable for all skin types and provides light hydration that helps enhance skin's radiance.

✓☺ BEST **RESIST Weekly Resurfacing Treatment 10% AHA** *($28.95 for 2 fl. oz.)* is a unique AHA treatment that can reveal younger-looking skin overnight. The 10% glycolic acid is formulated in a liquid base designed to enhance results while infusing skin with calming anti-irritants. The toner-like formula penetrates quickly to exfoliate dry, sun-damaged skin while supplying it with a potent blend of antioxidants. This powerful treatment leads to fewer wrinkles, discolorations, and a significant improvement in skin tone. It may be used once weekly (always in the evening) and left on overnight or rinsed off after 10 minutes. Those with severely sun-damaged skin may find using this treatment 4-5 times per week produces excellent results.

✓☺ BEST **Skin Perfecting 8% AHA Gel** *($19.95 for 3.3 fl. oz.)* pairs an effective amount of glycolic acid in a pH-correct (3.5 to 3.8), silky gel. It exfoliates and smoothes sun-damaged skin and improves signs of unevenness and minor discolorations. Daily use of a well-formulated AHA product such as this helps stimulate healthy collagen production for younger-looking, firmer skin. This is suitable for all skin types.

✓☺ BEST **Skin Perfecting 1% BHA Gel** *($19.95 for 3.3 fl. oz.)* features 1% salicylic acid in a pH-correct formula whose gel texture feels silky-smooth. This is ideal for exfoliating the skin's surface and inside the pore to improve its texture and appearance, while minimizing blemishes and blackheads. The formula contains soothing anti-irritants to reduce redness and inflammation while perfecting skin texture. It is for all skin types but ideal for normal to oily or combination skin.

✓☺ BEST **Skin Perfecting 1% BHA Lotion** *($19.95 for 3.3 fl. oz.)* contains soothing agents and 1% salicylic acid. It exfoliates and improves skin's texture while providing light-weight moisture with a soft matte finish. Formulated for all skin types, but best for normal to combination skin with dry, flaky areas.

✓☺ BEST **Skin Perfecting 2% BHA Gel** *($19.95 for 3.3 fl. oz.)* is similar to Paula's Choice Skin Perfecting 1% BHA Gel above, but has twice the concentration of salicylic acid for those with stubborn blemishes or blackheads. This is suitable for all skin types, but best for combination to oily skin. Potent anti-irritants work to calm redness and reduce inflammation.

✓☺ BEST **Skin Perfecting 2% BHA Liquid** *($19.95 for 4 fl. oz.)* is a one-of-a-kind product that works gently yet effectively to remedy breakouts, dislodge blackheads, smooth the surface of skin while imparting no irritation, and improving skin tone (due to the gentle but functional exfoliation it offers). This product also can calm pre-existing irritation. You can apply this toner-like solution with fingertips or a cotton pad. It works for all skin types struggling with stubborn acne and blackheads, but is best for normal to oily skin.

✓☺ BEST **Skin Perfecting 2% BHA Lotion** *($19.95 for 3.3 fl. oz.)* soothes and softens skin with its combination of water-binding agents and anti-inflammatory ingredients. This is ideal for those with normal to dry skin prone to breakouts. It also contains anti-irritants to calm skin and reduce redness.

PAULA'S CHOICE MOISTURIZERS (DAYTIME & NIGHTTIME) & SERUMS

Please note: Paula's Choice does not offer an eye cream because all the moisturizers can be used around the eye. In fact, it is a waste of money to buy a separate product labeled as an eye cream (or gel or serum) unless it's among those that offer an unusual benefit, such as concealing while supplying skin with anti-aging ingredients. Otherwise, we explain why you don't need an eye cream in the Appendix.

✓☺ BEST **Earth Sourced Antioxidant-Enriched Natural Moisturizer** *($20.95 for 2 fl. oz.)*. Packed with natural ingredients proven to help skin, this silky yet surprisingly rich moisturizer is natural done right! Designed for all skin types, including oily skin struggling with dry, flaky areas, the formula contains 99% plant-based antioxidants, cell-communicating ingredients, and skin-repairing ingredients. This combination works to hydrate and smooth skin plus help it look and act younger. This is one of the few natural skin-care products that doesn't contain any irritating plant extracts or irritating plant-based fragrances. It only contains natural ingredients proven to be gentle yet effective. We honestly don't know why more brands selling natural skin-care products don't take this approach!

✓☺ BEST **Hydralight Moisture-Infusing Lotion** *($19.95 for 2 fl. oz.)* is a lightweight, thin-textured moisturizer for normal to oily/combination skin. It's packed with antioxidants providing a powerhouse of helpful ingredients skin needs to look radiant and healthy. Skin is left feeling fresh and looking matte; this works great under makeup, too. This lotion is ideal for eliminating dry patches without making skin look or feel the least bit greasy.

✓☺ BEST **Moisture Boost Daily Restoring Complex, SPF 30 with Antioxidants** *($20.95 for 2 fl. oz.)* has an innovative lightweight cream texture that provides substantial moisture without a thick, heavy feel. It contains stabilized avobenzone to prevent sun damage and skin discolorations. The formula further boosts skin's defenses with a proven antioxidant complex. Its satin-smooth finish serves as a perfect base for makeup application. This daytime moisturizer with sunscreen is ideal for those with normal to dry skin who want a luxurious moisturizer that protects skin in multiple ways but never feels like a traditional sunscreen.

✓☺ BEST **Moisture Boost Hydrating Treatment Cream** *($19.95 for 2 fl. oz.)* makes skin feel luxuriously soft with its combination of skin-identical ingredients, plant oil, cell-communicating ingredients, and emollients. Its texture works superbly around the eyes, and rivals the best eye creams reviewed in this book. Best suited for normal to dry skin.

✓☺ BEST **RESIST Anti-Aging Clear Skin Hydrator** *($22.95 for 1.7 fl. oz.)*. This specialized moisturizer is formulated for those struggling with oily skin, signs of aging (like fine lines and wrinkles) as well as red marks from acne. It contains a unique blend of proven ingredients that help reduce breakouts without making skin feel dry or flaky. This gentle, fragrance-free formula also treats skin to proven anti-aging ingredients that improve skin tone, texture, and clarity. Its silky, gel-cream texture glides on without feeling slick or greasy, which means it works beautifully under makeup or can be used as the moisturizer step in your nighttime skin-care routine.

✓☺ BEST **RESIST Barrier Repair Moisturizer with Retinol** *($22.95 for 1.7 fl. oz.)* is an advanced moisturizer with retinol that's formulated to provide skin with key ingredients it needs to resist environmental damage that causes wrinkles and other signs of aging. Its restorative blend of emollients, antioxidants, skin-identical substances, and cell-communicating ingredients work to remodel and significantly improve skin, as shown by published research. The state-of-the-art ingredients selected for this moisturizer are proven to generate healthy collagen production, reduce inflammation, and allow skin to repair itself. Suitable for all skin types but its texture and amount of moisture are best suited for normal to slightly dry or combination skin.

✓☺ BEST **RESIST Cellular Defense Daily Moisturizer, SPF 25 with Antioxidants** *($24.95 for 2 fl. oz.)* protects skin from wrinkles and brown spots with a gentle, mineral-based sunscreen. Its elegant lightweight cream texture moisturizes as it treats skin to a range of proven antioxidants. Best for normal to dry skin and designed for use under makeup, this daytime moisturizer won't leave a white cast or feel greasy. It leaves skin smooth and helps brighten a dull complexion. As with any effective sunscreen, daily use ensures skin continues to repair sun damage so it is able to generate healthy collagen to improve wrinkles and other signs of aging. This daytime moisturizer with sunscreen is also a great option for those with sensitive skin, including rosacea.

✓☺ BEST **RESIST Intensive Wrinkle-Repair Retinol Serum** *($29.95 for 1 fl. oz.)* is a silky, fragrance-free serum that utilizes a proprietary blend of highly stabilized retinol, potent antioxidants, and skin-repairing ingredients. Its soothing, silky texture contains proven anti-aging ingredients so all skin types (even breakout-prone skin) will see their skin looking and acting younger. Like all Paula's Choice packaging, this container keeps key ingredients stable during use, and as with all serums, this may be applied under or over your moisturizer. This serum may also be used with other products that contain retinol or with prescription retinoid products such as Retin-A.

✓☺ BEST **RESIST Super Antioxidant Concentrate Serum** *($25.95 for 1 fl. oz.)* works to target the needs of aging skin. This serum supplies skin with an efficacious amount of stabilized vitamin C, a cell-communicating peptide, and other potent, proven antioxidants in a base formula that's silky yet neither matte nor emollient. It is suitable for sensitive skin or those whose skin cannot tolerate retinol. Works beautifully for all skin types as a foundation primer, and may be applied to face, neck, and chest.

✓☺ BEST **Skin Balancing Daily Mattifying Lotion, SPF 15 with Antioxidants** *($20.95 for 2 fl. oz.)*. This daytime moisturizer with sunscreen has a weightless texture someone with oily or blemish-prone skin will love, yet it provides sun protection and supplies skin with potent antioxidants and cell-communicating ingredients, while leaving a matte finish. UVA protection is assured by stabilized avobenzone, which prevents wrinkles and brown spots. The texture and finish of this product are excellent under makeup!

✓☺ BEST **Skin Balancing Invisible Finish Moisture Gel** *($19.95 for 2 fl. oz.)* leaves skin feeling silky while imparting necessary ingredients that maintain and generate healthy skin. It is ideal under makeup, assuming your foundation provides broad-spectrum sun protection. This can easily replace your foundation primer for smooth makeup wear and is also a great moisturizer for men to use after shaving. The texture and finish are best for normal to oily or combination skin.

✓☺ BEST **Skin Balancing Super Antioxidant Concentrate Serum with Retinol** *($25.95 for 1 fl. oz.)* is a weightless combination of beneficial antioxidants, cell-communicating ingredients (including retinol), skin-identical ingredients, and soothing agents. It helps to normalize skin-cell function while its long-lasting matte finish (which also allows this to work as a "primer" under foundation) helps keep oily skin from looking slick. It has a silky, weightless finish that feels elegant and makes skin look smooth.

✓☺ BEST **Skin Recovery Daily Moisturizing Lotion, SPF 15 with Antioxidants** *($20.95 for 2 fl. oz.)* combines titanium dioxide and zinc oxide for gentle daytime sun protection, while pampering normal to very dry skin with a blend of emollients, silicones, lots of antioxidants, and cell-communicating peptides. Surprisingly moisturizing for being so lightweight, it is designed to work well under foundation. It is suitable for sensitive skin including those with rosacea.

✓☺ BEST **Skin Recovery Replenishing Moisturizer** *($19.95 for 2 fl. oz.)* restores vital moisture to dry to very dry skin and has an elegantly creamy texture. Emollients, peptides, antioxidants, and skin-identical ingredients combine to deliver soft, smooth skin with a beautifully healthy glow. This also works beautifully for dry skin around the eyes and is great for those struggling with dry skin and rosacea.

✓☺ BEST **Skin Recovery Super Antioxidant Concentrate Serum with Retinol** *($25.95 for 1 fl. oz.)* revitalizes normal to very dry skin with copious antioxidants, cell-communicating ingredients (including retinol), and efficacious plant oils. This is a great way to improve the appearance and healthy functioning of sun-damaged skin, including wrinkles and loss of firmness.

PAULA'S CHOICE ACNE PRODUCTS

✓☺ BEST **CLEAR Pore Normalizing Cleanser** (*$10.95 for 6 fl. oz.*) is a water-soluble gel cleanser that feels refreshing and offers thorough yet gentle cleansing for blemish-prone skin, whether oily, combination, or dry. It is formulated with an antibacterial agent designed to begin the process of killing acne-causing bacteria. This cleanser removes makeup, doesn't leave a trace of residue, and won't dry out skin.

✓☺ BEST **CLEAR Anti-Redness Exfoliating Solution, Extra Strength** (*$19.95 for 4 fl. oz.*) is similar to our regular CLEAR Anti-Redness Exfoliating Solution, Regular Strength below, except this contains an ingredient that enhances the penetration of 2% salicylic acid into the pores. It is recommended for those with stubborn acne and blackheads. It reduces breakouts and redness while significantly improving skin tone and texture.

✓☺ BEST **CLEAR Anti-Redness Exfoliating Solution, Regular Strength** (*$19.95 for 4 fl. oz.*) is an anti-acne toner whose active ingredient is 2% salicylic acid. It exfoliates skin's surface as well as inside the pore lining to dislodge blackheads, prevent acne from recurring, and reduce redness and inflammation. This light-as-water toner provides a measurable improvement in skin tone, redness, and clarity while leaving skin feeling smoothed and refreshed.

✓☺ BEST **CLEAR Daily Skin Clearing Treatment, Regular Strength** (*$16.95 for 2.25 fl. oz.*) contains 2.5% benzoyl peroxide as its active ingredient, considered the gold standard when it comes to over-the-counter ingredients for acne-prone skin. It has a lightweight lotion base that sets to a soft matte finish. It contains soothing anti-irritants so it remains effective against acne-causing bacteria while being gentle on skin. Regular use will result in a significant improvement of acne.

✓☺ BEST **CLEAR Daily Skin Clearing Treatment, Extra Strength** (*$17.95 for 2.25 fl. oz.*) is nearly identical to the CLEAR Daily Skin Clearing Treatment, Regular Strength, except this version contains double the amount of benzoyl peroxide. It is recommended for all skin types with stubborn acne, and the formulary attributes remain the same as those for the regular strength version: a gentle, soothing lotion designed to quickly kill acne-causing bacteria while leaving a non-greasy, non-drying finish.

PAULA'S CHOICE SUN CARE

✓☺ BEST **Almost the Real Thing Self-Tanning Gel, Face & Body** (*$12.95 for 5 fl. oz.*) is a water-based self-tanner that contains dihydroxyacetone to turn skin a natural tan color. The formula is tinted so you can instantly see where it has been applied, and it dries quickly. It is suitable for all skin colors, which is why we don't offer separate formulas for fair to light and medium to dark skin. The result is a believable golden tan that lasts for 2-3 days before reapplication is needed. Ideal for all skin types and designed for use on the face and from the neck down.

✓☺ BEST **Extra Care Non-Greasy Sunscreen SPF 45, Face & Body** (*$14.95 for 5 fl. oz.*) has a lightweight lotion texture that smoothes easily over skin and provides a soft matte finish. It has a much more elegant feel than many other high-SPF products, and provides sufficient UVA protection thanks to stabilized avobenzone. The formula contains antioxidants to boost skin's environmental defenses and is very water-resistant. Ideal for active people or anyone spending several hours outdoors (be sure to reapply as needed). This sunscreen is ideal for normal to oily or blemish-prone skin but can be enjoyed by all skin types.

✓☺ BEST **Weightless Finish Sunscreen Spray SPF 30, Face & Body** (*$15.95 for 4 fl. oz.*) is a nonaqueous spray that includes avobenzone for sufficient UVA protection and potent antioxidants to help boost skin's environmental defenses. This protects skin beautifully yet feels like you're wearing nothing at all. It is ideal for the whole family, and great for active outdoor enthusiasts. As with any sunscreen, this should be reapplied after swimming, sweating, or toweling off.

PAULA'S CHOICE LIP & SMILE CARE

✓☺ BEST **Brighten Up 2-Minute Teeth Whitener** *($14.95 for 2.5 grams)* comes in a unique portable, twist-up stick, making it an easy way to whiten your teeth anytime, anywhere. It works fast to remove common stains (such as from red wine and coffee) and has none of the mess or fuss of conventional teeth-whitening products. This product safely whitens your teeth with encapsulated hydrogen peroxide. Once you try it, you'll wonder how you ever did without it!

✓☺ BEST **Lip Perfecting Gentle Scrub with Micro-Beads** *($7.95 for 0.5 fl. oz.)* has a gentle formula that works quickly to remove dead, dry, chapped skin without irritating your lips. Excellent used before applying Paula's Choice Lip & Body Treatment Balm or whatever lip balm you prefer. Also ideal before lipstick because it leaves lips flake-free and perfectly smooth.

✓☺ BEST **Lip & Body Treatment Balm** *($10.95 for 0.5 fl. oz.)* is a multi-benefit emollient balm containing protective oils and emollients that prevent moisture loss and restore dry, chapped skin to a normal state. Applying this twice a day can guarantee you never have chapped lips again. It also can be used on elbows and heels to eliminate dry cracked skin in those areas, too.

PAULA'S CHOICE SPECIALTY PRODUCTS

✓☺ BEST **Oil-Blotting Papers** *($6.95 for 100 sheets)* are thin tissue paper–style sheets that quickly soak up excess oil and perspiration without leaving a powdery residue or disturbing makeup. Ideal for use before touching up your makeup with powder, and great for use in humid climates to help keep skin from looking greasy.

✓☺ BEST **Redness Relief Treatment, for All Skin Types** *($15.95 for 4 fl. oz.)* is a unique toner-like product that contains stabilized aspirin and vitamin C to soothe skin and calm irritation. This is ideal as an after-shave product for men or women and is great for use before and after spa or dermatologist procedures.

✓☺ BEST **RESIST Pure Radiance Skin Brightening Treatment** *($26.95 for 1 fl. oz.)* is a targeted treatment for all skin types, including those prone to blemishes. It's specially formulated for anyone struggling with brown spots, uneven skin tone, and a dull complexion. Its lightweight, silky-soft texture instantly provides a more luminous complexion, while an exclusive blend of skin-repairing and antioxidant ingredients target multiple signs of aging. Continued use, coupled with daily application of sunscreen, will prevent discolorations from coming back and keep new discolorations from appearing. A perfect alternative for those who cannot use products that contain hydroquinone.

✓☺ BEST **RESIST Remarkable Skin Lightening Gel, 2% BHA** *($18.95 for 2 fl. oz.)* is an unparalleled treatment for those struggling with discolorations and breakouts. It contains 2% hydroquinone to lighten sun-damaged areas while 2% salicylic acid exfoliates to reduce blemishes and renew surface skin cells. This anti-aging lightener restores an even skin tone by fading skin discolorations caused by the sun or hormones. The silky, breathable gel texture is ideal for normal to oily or blemish-prone skin. Note: In 2013 this product's name will change to *RESIST Triple-Action Dark Spot Eraser, 2% BHA Gel.*

✔☺ BEST **RESIST Remarkable Skin Lightening Lotion, 7% AHA** *($18.95 for 2 fl. oz.)* lightens sun- or hormone-induced skin discolorations with its blend of 2% hydroquinone and 7.4% glycolic acid to help fade brown spots and renew skin's surface. This smooth-textured lotion may be used alone or layered with other products as needed. Ideal for those struggling with wrinkles and an uneven skin tone. Note: In 2013 this product name will change to *RESIST Triple-Action Dark Spot Eraser, 7% AHA Lotion.*

✔☺ BEST **Shine Stopper Instant Matte Finish with Microsponge Technology** *($21.95 for 1 fl. oz.)* is an innovative oil-absorbing product that provides an instant matte finish. The matte finish lasts at least 6 hours and helps reduce the appearance of large pores. Works best when smoothed on under makeup or dabbed on over makeup. You'll notice this product also enhances makeup application and wear—much more than standard foundation primers designed for oily skin!

✔☺ BEST **Skin Balancing Oil-Absorbing Mask** *($15.95 for 4 fl. oz.)* absorbs excess oil with a mix of clay and other absorbent agents. This rinses easily, and the drawing action of the mask also helps to dislodge blackheads. Ideal used with any of the Paula's Choice CLEAR or Skin Balancing products, this mask can be applied as often as needed.

✔☺ BEST **Skin Recovery Hydrating Treatment Mask** *($15.95 for 4 fl. oz.)* prevents dry skin with moisturizing ingredients that help to restore a healthy barrier function and reduce inflammation. Skin is left feeling soft and looking radiant; you can leave this mask on as long as necessary. Those with very dry, dehydrated skin should leave this mask on overnight. It is suitable for use around the eyes, too.

PAULA'S CHOICE HAND & BODY CARE

✔☺ BEST **All Over Hair & Body Shampoo, for All Skin & Hair Types** *($14.95 for 14.5 fl. oz.)* functions as a shampoo for all hair types (including chemically treated) and as a body wash. The lathering formula rinses cleanly and does not contain any ingredients that may be irritating to skin or scalp. It is excellent for use on babies and children, too. It is one of the few truly fragrance-free shampoos available anywhere.

✔☺ BEST **Cuticle & Nail Treatment** *($10.95 for 0.06 fl. oz.)* is an emollient blend of oils and conditioning agents dispensed from a pen-style applicator with a built-in synthetic brush tip. The applicator makes it easy for targeted use to keep nails and the skin around them looking great. May be used on fingernails and toenails and is designed for men or women.

✔☺ BEST **RESIST Skin Revealing Body Lotion, 10% AHA with Antioxidants** *($22.95 for 7 fl. oz.)* contains 10% glycolic acid in a pH-correct, emollient base formula that supplies skin with an array of ingredients it needs to look and feel its best. This is ideal for rough, dry, sun damaged skin. It's an anti-aging body lotion that, with ongoing use, can restore a firmer, smoother, even-toned look to your skin.

✔☺ BEST **RESIST Ultimate Anti-Aging Hand Cream, SPF 30 with Antioxidants** *($15.95 for 1.7 fl. oz.)* blends silky emollient ingredients along with broad-spectrum mineral sunscreens for reliable protection against sun damage. Keeping hands protected from sun exposure helps prevent brown spots and thin, crepey skin that makes hands look older. The formula also contains antioxidants for an additional level of protection and repair, plus ingredients to help improve skin tone. The convenient tube is sized for use on-the-go so you're never without great sun protection for your hands.

✔☺ BEST **RESIST Weightless Body Treatment, 2% BHA with Antioxidants** *($22.95 for 7 fl. oz.)* is an exfoliating body lotion designed to significantly improve skin's texture while supplying lightweight moisture. Excellent for acne on the body or for treating raised red bumps (keratosis pilaris, also known as "chicken skin"), this silky, lightweight lotion reduces roughness, inflammation, and helps skin heal. Daily use will make your skin remarkably smooth, soft, and even-toned, all without a greasy or slippery feel.

✓☺ BEST **Smooth Finish Conditioner, for All Hair Types** *($14.95 for 14.5 fl. oz.)* moisturizes, detangles, and adds shine to hair, all without making it look or feel limp or greasy. This is one of the only fragrance-free conditioners available. It works for all hair types; simply adjust the amount you use to achieve the desired results of smooth, silky, detangled hair. This conditioner is well-suited to the needs of chemically treated hair, too, and may also be used as a leave-in conditioner for protection during heat-styling. This is excellent for anyone struggling with a dry, itchy scalp.

PAULA'S CHOICE FOUNDATIONS

✓☺ BEST **All Bases Covered Foundation SPF 15** *($14.95 for 1 fl. oz.)* has a light, creamy-smooth texture and is ideal for normal to dry or sensitive skin. Its soft matte finish offers light to medium coverage with excellent blendability in five neutral shades for fair (but not very fair) to medium/tan skin tones. It protects skin from sun damage with a pure titanium dioxide SPF 15 sunscreen.

✓☺ BEST **Barely There Sheer Matte Tint SPF 20** *($14.95 for 1 fl. oz.)* is a tinted moisturizer with sunscreen that has a creamy but light texture that slips flawlessly over skin and provides a smooth, satin-matte finish. Its sheer-coverage formula provides a hint of color to even out your complexion while still allowing your natural skin tone to show through. The broad-spectrum titanium dioxide and zinc oxide sunscreen included will help shield your skin from harmful UV rays, making this an ideal all-in-one option for broad-spectrum sun protection and light moisturizing, plus soft color that enhances your skin. It comes in four neutral shades for fair (but not very fair) to medium/tan skin tones. It is suitable for all skin types and also recommended for those with rosacea.

✓☺ BEST **Best Face Forward Foundation SPF 15** *($14.95 for 1 fl. oz.)* is designed especially for normal to very oily, combination, or blemish-prone skin. It has a fluid, ultra-light texture that blends beautifully and sets to a long-wearing matte finish that doesn't look thick or feel heavy. An in-part titanium dioxide sunscreen provides broad-spectrum protection from the sun, eliminating the need for a separate facial sunscreen (provided you apply the foundation evenly over your entire face). Available in four neutral shades for fair (but not very fair) to medium/tan skin, this foundation offers sheer to medium buildable coverage.

PAULA'S CHOICE CONCEALER

✓☺ BEST **Soft Cream Concealer** *($9.95)* features everything a good cream concealer should: It has a smooth texture that blends easily, it covers well without looking thick or cakey, and has a natural satin finish that resembles skin rather than makeup. When lightly set with loose or pressed powder, it remains creaseless for hours. There are two neutral shades to complement fair to medium skin tones, whether used alone or with foundation and powder.

PAULA'S CHOICE POWDER

✓☺ BEST **Healthy Finish Pressed Powder SPF 15** *($14.95)* offers shine control and additional sun protection, with a titanium dioxide- and zinc oxide–based sunscreen. This has a velvety feel and goes on evenly and smoothly without looking chalky or dry. Please keep in mind that we don't recommend relying on any SPF-rated pressed powder as your sole source of sun protection because it is unlikely anyone will layer it thickly enough to achieve optimal sun protection. It is best to use an SPF powder in conjunction with a moisturizer or foundation rated SPF 15 or greater that contains sufficient UVA-protecting ingredients. Three neutral shades are available plus Healthy Tan, which has a soft bronze tone.

PAULA'S CHOICE EYE & BROW LINERS

✓☺ BEST **Brow/Hair Tint** *($9.95)* defines eyebrows and holds them in place with natural-looking color. The brush-on formula is lightweight and flake-proof, and the three shades can also be used to touch up gray hair at the roots between colorings.

✓☺ BEST **Browlistic Long-Wearing Precision Brow Color** *($9.95)* is a cross between a brow pencil and brow tint, with a built-in, felt tip pen–style applicator that allows you to precisely fill in your brows for natural-looking results. Best of all, this really stays put: no running, smearing, or flaking all day, guaranteed! It's available in two shades that are best for those with light to medium brown brows. This type of brow makeup may take some getting used to, but once you get the hang of it you'll likely find it indispensible for lasting, defined brows.

PAULA'S CHOICE LIP COLOR & LIPLINER

✓☺ BEST **Long-Lasting Anti-Feather Lipliner, Clear** *($7.95)* is an automatic, retractable colorless lipliner. It has a smooth application but isn't greasy, and can help prevent feathering (just like most pencils that have this kind of texture). It works beautifully to keep lipstick from bleeding into lines around the mouth. The colorless formula works with any lipstick shade. For best results, do not use with lip gloss (gloss has too much movement and no pencil can keep it from slipping into lines around the mouth).

PAULA'S CHOICE MASCARAS

✓☺ BEST **Great Big Lashes Mascara** *($9.95)* has a flexible brush whose dense bristles provide instant thickening and considerable length with just a few strokes. The flake-free formula goes on smoothly, defining each lash for maximum impact. It also keeps lashes soft and is easy to remove with a water-soluble cleanser or your favorite makeup remover. Several customers have told us they prefer this mascara to best-sellers from Lancome and department store brands.

✓☺ BEST **Illicit Lash Maximum Impact Mascara** *($10.95)* allows you to lengthen and separate your lashes with ease, all while leaving lashes softly curled. The specially-designed rubber-bristled brush ensures you'll reach each lash effortlessly and the formula, which goes on a bit wet, doesn't clump, flake, or smear. Lashes are left soft and dramatically defined, with a touch of thickness.

PAULA'S CHOICE BRUSHES & ACCESSORIES

Paula's Choice offers brushes that correspond with the select makeup products available. The **Powder Brush** ($20.95) has a density and softness that works perfectly to apply Healthy Finish Pressed Powder SPF 15 (or any powder you prefer), while the **Concealer Brush** ($12.95) has expertly tapered synthetic bristles ideal for applying Soft Cream Concealer or the concealer of your choice.

✓☺ BEST **Makeup Application Sponges** *($5.95 for 10 sponges)* are latex-free. They work well for applying foundation and for blending the edges of makeup—an essential step that's all too often overlooked. The sponges may be washed as needed and only need to be replaced when they begin showing signs of wear that hinder a smooth application.

✓☺ BEST **Mini Brush Set** *($38.95)* includes small yet perfectly functional brushes for applying powder, blush, eyeshadow, eyeliner, and brow color. The brushes are tucked inside a nylon pouch with a Velcro closure. It's great as a secondary brush set for office or travel.

PERRICONE MD COSMECEUTICALS (SKIN CARE ONLY)

Strengths: Good cleansers; handful of very good moisturizers for eye area; outstanding tinted moisturizer with sunscreen; well-formulated topical disinfectant; some fragrance-free products.

Weaknesses: Expensive; long on claims not supported by evidence-based science; shortage of products with sunscreen for normal to oily skin; no BHA products; no products to successfully lighten skin discolorations; most Super products aren't at all super.

For more information and reviews of the latest Perricone MD Cosmeceuticals products, visit CosmeticsCop.com.

Special Note: Most of Perricone's anti-aging products contain the ingredient dimethyl MEA. Also known as DMAE, this ingredient is controversial because research has shown conflicting results. It seems to offer an initial benefit that improves skin but these results are short-lived and eventually give way to destruction of substances in skin that help build healthy collagen (Sources: *Aesthetic Plastic Surgery*, November-December 2007, pages 711–718; and *American Journal of Clinical Dermatology*, Volume 6, 2005, pages 39–47).

Interestingly, there is a formulation challenge when using DMAE in skin-care products. In order to maintain efficacy and stability, the product's pH level needs to be at least 10. A pH of 10 is highly alkaline, which isn't good news for skin. A high pH like this can increase bacteria content in the pore plus cause dryness and irritation. Moreover, since almost all moisturizers (including serums and eye creams) are formulated with a pH that closely matches that of human skin (generally 5.5-6.5, which is on the acidic side of the scale), in all likelihood the DMAE used in such skin-care products cannot have any prolonged functionality (Source: *Journal of Drugs in Dermatology*, Supplement 72, 2008, pages S17–S22).

PERRICONE MD COSMECEUTICALS CLEANSERS

☺ GOOD $$$ **Citrus Facial Wash** *($39 for 6 fl. oz.)* is a very standard but good water-soluble cleanser for normal to oily skin. The tiny amount of vitamin C cannot correct a reddened or blotchy complexion, and in a cleanser it is just rinsed away before it can have any benefit as an antioxidant. Besides, sensitized skin would do better with a fragrance-free cleanser, and this one doesn't fill the bill.

☺ GOOD $$$ **Gentle Cleanser** *($35 for 6 fl. oz.)* is a standard detergent-based cleanser is indeed gentle. It is suitable for all skin types except very dry or sensitive; the precaution for sensitive skin is because this cleanser contains more than the typical amount of fragrance. The amount of plant oil is unlikely to be a problem for those with oily skin. Gentle Cleanser removes makeup and rinses cleanly.

☺ GOOD $$$ **Hypoallergenic Gentle Cleanser** *($39 for 8 fl. oz.)* is a fragrance-free cleanser with a lot to like; the main dislike is its price. Without question, you don't need to spend this much for a gentle cleanser that can remove makeup, and there are plenty of brilliant, inexpensive options listed in the Best Products chapter.

☺ GOOD $$$ **Nutritive Cleanser** *($52 for 8 fl. oz.)* is a very standard but good water-soluble cleanser for normal to oily skin. Its only issue is the price, which is way out of line for a standard cleanser.

☹ POOR **Cleansing Treatment Bar** (*$38 for 1 bar*) is a very expensive version of Dove's classic Beauty Bar, except Perricone added glycolic acid, although the pH of this bar cleanser prevents the glycolic acid from exfoliating. Plus, including glycolic acid in a bar cleanser is relatively pointless for skin because it is rinsed from the skin before it can be effective. More problematic for the skin is that the cleansing agents are too drying and potentially irritating for all skin types, and the ingredients that keep this in bar form can clog pores. If you're stuck on bar cleansers, at least try Dove's inexpensive version before paying way too much for this "treatment" bar, which really doesn't treat anything, and may make matters worse for your skin.

PERRICONE MD COSMECEUTICALS TONERS

☺ AVERAGE $$$ **Super Coconut Quench Coconut Water MCT** (*$38 for 4 fl. oz.*) is a fairly basic, not-so-super toner whose best attributes are the inclusion of two skin-repairing ingredients. That's about all there is to extol, and your skin deserves more than what this pro-vides (especially given what this costs). Fans of a coconut aroma, take note: This toner smells of the tropical fruit, even though the added fragrance isn't great for your skin. If you decide to try this toner, it is best for normal to dry skin. This contains a small amount of coconut oil, which is a source of medium chain triglycerides (that's what the MCT in the name means), but there isn't a special benefit to using this type of triglyceride versus other types that show up in skin-care products—they're all beneficial.

☹ POOR **Firming Facial Toner** (*$39 for 6 fl. oz.*) irritates, not firms, the skin because it lists alcohol as the second ingredient (see the Appendix for details). Without it and the tiny amount of eucalyptus, this would have been an interesting toner for normal to dry skin.

☹ POOR **Intensive Pore Minimizer** (*$55 for 4 fl. oz.*) contains approximately 1% salicylic acid, but the product's pH of 6 makes it ineffective for exfoliation or reducing enlarged pores. When pores become clogged with dead skin cells, oil, and cellular debris, they become enlarged. A well-formulated salicylic acid (BHA) product can produce great results, but, despite the name, that's not what Intensive Pore Minimizer does. One more word of warning—the amount of alcohol in this toner is cause for concern. Alcohol causes free-radical damage, cell death, and breaks down collagen, none which is helpful for skin, but it is intensive!

☹ POOR **Super Detox Elixir Watercress Sulphoraphane** (*$30 for 4 fl. oz.*) claims that it "contains the ingredient sulforaphane, abundant in watercress, [which] aids detoxification while helping skin achieve a purified, glowing complexion." Sulphoraphane is a chemical compound found in cruciferous vegetables, such as broccoli and watercress. It has anti-inflammatory, anti-cancer, and antioxidant benefits. Although there is much research about the health benefits of sulphoraphane when eaten (pile on those veggies!), there is little research concerning its value when applied topically to skin, although in vitro research on skin cells has shown it to have antioxidant benefits and potential cell-communicating activity (Sources: *Molecular Biology of the Cell*, December 2010, pages 4068–4075; *Archives of Pharmacal Research*, November 2010, pages 1867–1876; and *Plant Medica*, October 2008, pages 1548–1559). That's a positive thing, but there is not a single ingredient in this toner that is a source of sulphoraphanes. What a strange twist: A complete split between the claims and the content. Perricone maintains that this toner detoxifies your skin, but it doesn't do that. Skin doesn't have toxins that can be pulled out by any ingredient and no one at Perricone's company could identify a single toxin lurking in our skin that the body cannot handle on its own. Aside from the marketing nonsense, what this product will do is cause irritation because it contains various forms of witch hazel, which is a source of alcohol. Alcohol is always a potential cause for concern, but in all likelihood, there is too little in here to cause trouble. Still, there's little that's super about this toner, and the price is needlessly high.

PERRICONE MD COSMECEUTICALS EXFOLIANTS

☺ GOOD $$$ **Advanced Face Firming Activator** *($120 for 2 fl. oz.)* contains AHA (roughly 10% glycolic acid) at a pH that allows exfoliation to occur. It also contains alpha lipoic acid along with some other interesting antioxidants, though some are present in mere window-dressing amounts. Consider this a good AHA lotion for normal to slightly dry skin, though not one that's superior to many other well-formulated (and much less expensive) AHA products. The firming claim has some basis in truth because of the manner in which glycolic acid works when it's correctly formulated. Ongoing use stimulates collagen production, which will result in smoother, firmer skin. We're not talking firm as in you'll think you're in your twenties again—instead, think incremental minor improvements.

☺ GOOD $$$ **Super Brightening Activator Melon Carotenoids** *($38 for 4 fl. oz.)* is a good, though pricey, AHA toner for all skin types. Exfoliation comes from the blend of glycolic and lactic acids this contains along with this product's pH being in range for these ingredients to work as exfoliants. Because of the water-light texture, this must be applied with a cotton pad; it treats skin to benefits beyond exfoliation thanks to the antioxidants and soothing agents it contains. This would earn our top rating if it did not contain fragrance and a fragrance ingredient (limonene) known to cause irritation. The amounts of both are likely too low to be a problem, but no question the formula would be better for your skin without them.

☺ GOOD **Super Firming Activator Red Algae Astaxanthin** *($38 for 4 fl. oz.)* is a very good AHA toner for all skin types. It contains approximately 10% of the AHA glycolic acid, but missed being rated a Best Product because its beneficial extras (such as antioxidants) are a minor part of the formula. Kudos to Perricone for adding them at all, but we'd love to have seen greater amounts being used, and the fragrance being left out (fragrance isn't skin care). This also contains a couple of fragrance ingredients that pose a risk of irritation, though on balance it's a nicely done AHA product in toner form.

☹ AVERAGE $$$ **Concentrated Restorative Treatment** *($52.50 for 1 fl. oz.)*. This moisturizer's star ingredient is a form of vitamin C along with the amino acid L-tyrosine. Although there are mounds of research supporting the topical use of various forms of vitamin C, such research is scant when it comes to L-tyrosine. It is believed this amino acid may affect wrinkles due to its ability to modulate chemicals depleted by stress. Because stress causes the depletion of certain beneficial chemicals in the body, it stands to reason that stress also may take a toll on a person's appearance. However, the benefits of L-tyrosine appear to be much greater when it is consumed orally rather than slathered on the skin (Source: naturaldatabase.com). The other concern about this moisturizer is the jar packaging. After opening the jar, the vitamin C and other antioxidants in this formula lose their effectiveness because they are exposed to air, leaving you with an overpriced moisturizer whose antiwrinkle benefits have been squandered. Although representatives we contacted at Perricone wouldn't divulge the percentage of glycolic acid in this product, it most likely is too low for it to function as an exfoliant.

☹ AVERAGE $$$ **Super Crinkle Eraser Red Algae Astaxanthin** *($48 for 1 fl. oz.)* is a fragranced antiwrinkle product that is actually an AHA exfoliant because one of its main ingredients is glycolic acid. Unfortunately, the pH of this product is above what's necessary for the glycolic acid to work as an exfoliant. This contains some intriguing anti-aging ingredients including alpha lipoic (thioctic) acid and green tea, but one of the main ingredients, dimethyl

MEA, is controversial (see the special note at the beginning of the Perricone line review). Ultimately, this isn't preferred to other AHA products in moisturizing bases, or to other anti-aging "anti-crinkle" moisturizers.

PERRICONE MD COSMECEUTICALS MOISTURIZERS (DAYTIME & NIGHTTIME), EYE CREAMS, & SERUMS

✓☺ BEST $$$ **Advanced Eye Area Therapy** *($98 for 0.5 fl. oz.)* launched with the announcement that it is the evolution of eye-area care, designed to address ALL concerns one might have for aging skin in this delicate place. Although you won't see that claim fulfilled, there is no denying that this is one of Perricone's best formulations. The second ingredient (stabilized vitamin C, an antioxidant), is present in a significant amount, and other antioxidants are plentiful, including alpha lipoic acid, tocotrienols, and borage seed oil. Perricone also included cell-communicating ingredients and some good water-binding agents, making this an all-around fantastic (though pricey) lightweight moisturizer for all skin types. It's fragrance-free, too. Other than the overinflated claims of remedying every eye-area concern, the only other issue we have is that Perricone states this contains "unique ingredients rarely found in one product." None of the ingredients in this product are unique or exclusive to Perricone's formulas, and there is no reason several of his other products couldn't have the same blend of state-of-the-art ingredients. The real question is: Why don't they?

☺ GOOD $$$ **Super First Blush Brightening Serum Melon Carotenoids** *($48 for 1 fl. oz.)* is a good serum in terms of its vitamin C content (Perricone uses a stabilized form of vitamin C known as tetrahexyldecyl ascorbate) and skin-repairing ingredients. Also on hand is the antioxidant ferulic acid, which is known to help protect skin against sun damage. Cause for concern comes from the amount of benzyl alcohol this serum contains and possibly from the amount of rosemary leaf extract. The amount of benzyl alcohol holds this back from our top rating, as does the inclusion of the fragrance ingredient limonene, which can cause irritation on its own, though the amount of it in this serum is likely too low to be problematic. This serum is best for normal to dry skin.

☺ GOOD $$$ **Vitamin C Ester Eye Serum** *($55 for 0.5 fl. oz.)* is a silicone-based moisturizer that contains an impressive amount of stabilized vitamin C and three forms of antioxidant vitamin E. It is worth considering if you're curious to try a modern product with vitamin C that goes beyond being a one-note option. This would be better for the eye area if it didn't contain fragrance. Before investing in this, check out the Appendix to find out why, in truth, you don't need an eye cream (or serum).

☺ AVERAGE $$$ **Acyl-Glutathione** *($175 for 1 fl. oz.)* has a creamy texture suitable for dry skin, but all the good stuff you're paying extra (a lot extra) for simply won't last long and cannot benefit your skin the way it could in better (airtight) packaging. Dr. Perricone sells so many anti-aging moisturizers making the same claims, we wonder how consumers know which one to use? If any of these hyper-expensive products worked to the extent claimed, who'd have wrinkled, sagging skin? It's not that anti-aging ingredients don't help—it's the problem of so many products that over-promise yet under-deliver. The name of this fragranced moisturizer has to do with glutathione, an antioxidant that is synthesized in the human body and responsible for a variety of repair processes. It's a great antioxidant to see in skin-care products, but far from the only or the best one. What's most upsetting about this needlessly expensive moisturizer is that the glutathione, other antioxidants, and peptides won't remain potent for long due to jar packaging. Please see the Appendix for details on why jar packaging is a problem.

☹ AVERAGE **$$$ Acyl-Glutathione Eye Lid Serum** *($115 for 0.5 fl. oz.)* Although this eyelid serum (can you believe now Perricone maintains the eyelid area needs its own product, too?) contains some great ingredients, none of them offer special benefit to loose or wrinkled eyelid skin. What's especially problematic is that the formula contains fragrance ingredients (linalool and citronellol) that are known irritants and ideally should be kept far away from the eyes. What was Perricone thinking? In terms of this serum providing "dramatic tightness" for drooping eyelids, don't bet on it. This isn't an eye-lift in a bottle. The anti-irritants and vitamin-based antioxidants this contains are beneficial for skin anywhere on the face. As for glutathione, it's a great antioxidant and there's an impressive amount of it in this serum, but there's no research proving it tightens skin or is capable of dramatically improving signs of aging. As for the peptides this contains, they're theoretical cell-communicating ingredients but the amount used is paltry, especially considering how expensive this product is.

☹ AVERAGE **$$$ Cold Plasma** *($155 for 1 fl. oz.)* supposedly represents Dr. Perricone's "most comprehensive and efficacious work to date." He should go on record and admit that, oops, all the other anti-aging, antiwrinkle, and neuropeptide products bearing his name cost way too much and don't work as well as Cold Plasma. Of course, that won't happen, and Perricone will continue to sell numerous anti-aging products, each with beguiling claims, misleading hype about miraculous results, and offensive price tags. All the various products in this line are reminiscent of snake oil. Supposedly, Cold Plasma is the result of five years of scientific research. Never mind that Perricone didn't publish any of this research and certainly doesn't make it available in any form to the public. As for the "cold plasma" portion of the name, it refers to an ionized gas that has low energy. What that has to do with skin care is anyone's guess; most likely, Perricone chose the name because it sounds novel and new. Perricone proclaims this product can take care of the 10 signs of aging. Whether your concern is wrinkles, large pores, redness, discolorations, loss of firmness, and on and on, Cold Plasma is alleged to be the cure, promising "extraordinary results." On the other hand, it doesn't even contain a sunscreen, so that's one contributor to signs of aging that it can't address. But there are lots of other issues this product can't address, including acne and loss of firmness. The results that Perricone claims this product can provide are due to what he calls an "ionic-suspension carrier." That does sound impressive and scientific until you realize that ions (an atom or group of atoms that has lost or gained one or more electrons, making it positively or negatively charged) are suspended in lots of products, from skin and hair care to medicines. Using ions in a suspension isn't a guarantee of a superior or groundbreaking anti-aging product; it's just a way to make any moisturizer sound more special than it is, and an attempt to justify the product's cost. Perhaps the most laughable claim made for Cold Plasma is that its technology is said to "understand" your skin. You're asked to believe that this product "determines the nutrients" your skin needs to stay healthy and youthful, which is physiologically impossible. The claim, of course, is absurd, but your skin does need a complex, wide range of ingredients to reach a healthy, youthful state. Unfortunately, Perricone included only a handful of beneficial ingredients in this product, so even if this product could tell what your skin needs, it wouldn't be able to provide it because it isn't in here. What's more, the jar packaging won't keep any of the anti-aging ingredients that are in here stable once it is opened. What a bad joke for the consumer. Is there some sort of consolation prize for a product that purports to give skin everything it needs yet is incapable of doing that? Using this product in lieu of other, less expensive options in better packaging and with even better ingredients is surrendering to the undeserved hype that doctor-designed lines tend to have—and Perricone often leads the pack. And spending this much money on any single skin-care product is foolish, plain and simple.

☺ AVERAGE **$$$ Cold Plasma Eye** *($98 for 0.5 fl. oz.)* is Cold Plasma's eye-area counterpart. Other than the inclusion of an emollient thickening agent suitable for dry skin, the ingredient list and incredibly tempting claims for Cold Plasma Eye is remarkably similar to the original Cold Plasma, which of course begs the question of why a separate version for the eye area was needed, though it does help sell more products. Both versions suffer from outrageous prices and packaging that won't keep key ingredients stable during use. Specific to Cold Plasma Eye, for almost $100, you're getting an eye cream with fragrance ingredients such as farnesol and linalool. These ingredients are bad news for all skin types because the irritation they cause can diminish healthy collagen production—and that's not the way to look younger. Curiously, the original Cold Plasma product is fragrance-free (so the eye area gets fragrance but the rest of the face doesn't?). Without question there are some intriguing ingredients in Cold Plasma Eye; it's just not the breakthrough product it's made out to be and Perricone hasn't published any research to support his claims. Lastly, consider this: If Cold Plasma Eye is such a miracle, why is Perricone still selling numerous other eye-area products, all with similar amazing claims? Wouldn't it be best to admit that those don't work as well and that Cold Plasma Eye is the one to buy? Of course, that won't happen and none of this nonsense will stop many women from buying (literally and figuratively) into the too-good-to-be-true claims.

☺ AVERAGE **$$$ Cold Plasma Sub-D** *($135 for 2 fl. oz.)* is another product from Perricone's Cold Plasma range, despite the original Cold Plasma product being touted as a does-it-all wonder. Clearly Perricone didn't believe his own claims are he would've stopped with the one, so-called revolutionary Cold Plasma moisturizer! The key selling point of this pricey moisturizer is that it reduces sagging and signs of a double chin. However, this does nothing of the sort and is in no way a reliable replacement for a surgical (or even a non-surgical, light-based) cosmetic corrective procedure. As for using this on the neck, it holds no special benefit for skin in this area, and in fact you don't need a separate moisturizer for your neck (a well-formulated facial moisturizer and/or serum can and should be used on the neck, too). Cold Plasma Sub-D contains many of the same ingredients Perricone uses in his other products, including DMAE, which has its share of controversies (see the special note at the beginning of the Perricone line review) and the second ingredient is glycolic acid (the pH of this product keeps it from functioning as an exfoliant). Since the dimethyl MEA (also known as DMAE) is also pH-dependent, it doesn't work with AHAs like glycolic acid. The former requires an alkaline pH for efficacy while the latter requires an acidic pH to work—you simply can't have it both ways. Perhaps most disappointing is that the jar packaging won't keep several key anti-aging ingredients this contains stable once you've opened it. That's a shame but especially so for a moisturizer that costs this much. In the end, Cold Plasma Sub-D isn't worth your time or money. If you're tempted by Perricone's claims, remember his classic quote as seen in a November 18, 2001, *New York Times* article: "If you promise them an unlined face, you can sell them anything!" Note: Many women who've tried this product have commented on its scent, often comparing it to rotten fish. If you decide to try this (and we urge you to reconsider), be sure you're OK with its aroma.

📖 Buying skin-care products packaged in jars? See the Appendix to learn why that's a bad idea.

☺ AVERAGE **$$$ Deep Moisture Therapy** *($85 for 2 fl. oz.)* is a rich-textured moisturizer for very dry skin that contains numerous nonfragrant plant oils whose fatty acid profiles and mix of antioxidants can go a long way toward improving the look and feel of uncomfortably dry, sensitive skin. Unfortunately, all those good ingredients will suffer due to jar packaging. See the Appendix to find how jar packaging undermines the effectiveness of products like this.

☺ AVERAGE **$$$ Face Finishing Moisturizer** *($69 for 2 fl. oz.)* has an emollient texture that's suitable for normal to dry skin. It includes some beneficial antioxidants, but the amounts are disappointingly low. Even if these state-of-the-art ingredients were present in greater amounts, the jar packaging won't allow them to remain stable during use (refer to the Appendix for details). This contains several fragrance ingredients proven to irritate skin, which makes this one of Perricone's weaker moisturizers (the rose scent is potent and lingers).

☺ AVERAGE **$$$ Firming Neck Therapy** *($95 for 2 fl. oz.)* contains many helpful ingredients for dry skin anywhere on the body. Some potent antioxidants are included, but their collective effect doesn't mean much for skin given that they're all listed after the preservative. Even more discouraging is that Perricone switched from airless jar packaging to a traditional jar, so what little potency the antioxidants have will be squandered (see the Appendix for details). The second ingredient in this product is taurine, and it deserves some explanation. A major ingredient in the product is the amino acid taurine. The most abundant source of taurine is human breast milk, but it also occurs in many foods, including meat and fish. Taurine can also be synthesized in the body from hypotaurine and cysteine, and works in the body to promote healthy brain, eye, and heart functions, among other duties. What does any of this have to do with wrinkles or lax skin? Taurine is considered a good antioxidant, but that in and of itself is no reason to seek products containing it. There is research showing that adequate levels of taurine in the body work to protect skin from UVB-induced changes, but it's no substitute for sunscreen and many other ingredients (most of them antioxidants such as green tea or ferulic acid) offer photoprotection as well. Research has also shown (albeit in vitro) that topical application of taurine can reduce epidermal water loss and inflammation in the presence of topical irritants. It also appears to stimulate barrier repair substances such as cholesterol and ceramides, which can help skin repair itself. Moreover, animal research has shown that taurine plays a role in mitigating collagen destruction related to consumption of high-fructose corn syrup, though this research was more concerned with preventing collagen-induced skin changes in diabetics than examining its effect, if any, on wrinkles. In short, taurine is indeed a beneficial ingredient for skin, but there is no published research proving it can lift skin or significantly improve wrinkles or is better than other ingredients that help skin in this manner (Sources: naturaldatabase.com; *Journal of Immunology*, September 2007, pages 3604–3612; *Journal of Cosmetic Science*, January/February 2006, pages 1–10; and *Journal of Diabetes and its Complications*, September/October 2005, pages 305–311). Another ingredient of interest in this product is phosphatidylcholine. (Please refer to the Cosmetic Ingredient Dictionary at CosmeticsCop. com for detailed information about this ingredient.) There is nothing in this product that will improve sagging skin, but hope springs eternal in the world of cosmeceutical skin care.

☺ AVERAGE **$$$ High Potency Amine Complex Face Lift** *($98 for 2 fl. oz.)* does not contain anything that has been proven to lift, tighten, or redefine skin. The second ingredient, L-tyrosine, is a nonessential amino acid that has limited research proving its benefit for skin. Oral consumption is a different story, but topically it isn't a must-have by any means (Source: naturaldatabase.com). This moisturizer contains appreciable amounts of two forms of vitamin C, which is very good for skin. Other antioxidants are present in small amounts, but none of them add up to a face-lift in a bottle. At best, this is a decent lightweight moisturizer for normal to slightly dry skin. The glycolic acid functions as a water-binding agent, not as an exfoliant.

☺ AVERAGE $$$ **High Potency Evening Repair** *($98 for 2 fl. oz.)* is supposed to recharge skin with high amounts of the antioxidant alpha lipoic acid and the controversial ingredient DMAE. Both ingredients are present at impressive levels, but given DMAE's controversial status (see the special note at the beginning of the Perricone line review), it isn't exactly an anti-aging ingredient you can use with confidence (and Perricone has published no research to the contrary). The alpha lipoic acid in here is a very good antioxidant, but you're better off getting this ingredient from a product that doesn't contain questionable ingredients. The amount of retinol and other antioxidants in this moisturizer is too low for them to offer much benefit for skin, which is disappointing given this product's steep price.

☺ AVERAGE $$$ **High Potency Eye Lift** *($98 for 0.5 fl. oz.)* is a lightweight lotion that contains an impressive amount of vitamin C (tetrahexyldyl ascorbate) along with other ingredients that Perricone likes to tout, including DMAE and phosphatidylcholine. Neither works as claimed to reduce any amount of skin aging. DMAE remains a controversial ingredient due to its effect on skin cells; at first it helps protect cells, but within hours it begins to prevent cell growth, which can lead to trouble because new cells aren't there to replace the old ones, which are pre-programmed to die after a certain length of time (see the special note at the beginning of the Perricone line review for more info). Although this product contains some questionable ingredients, it also contains several very good antioxidants, and it's packaged to keep them stable during use. But ultimately, you don't need an eye cream (see the Appendix to find out why) and definitely not one that costs nearly $100!

☺ AVERAGE $$$ **Hypoallergenic Firming Eye Cream** *($65 for 0.5 fl. oz.)* contains great ingredients for dry skin anywhere on the face, but it doesn't distinguish itself in any striking way from most emollient facial moisturizers, further proof that you don't need a product labeled as eye cream for use around the eye area (see the Appendix to find out why). As for the hypoallergenic portion of the name, it's meaningless (we explain why in the Appendix). This is a gentle, fragrance-free formula with some good soothing agents, but that still doesn't tell you whether or not you will have an allergic reaction. The real shortcoming of this product is that most of the beneficial anti-irritants and other anti-aging ingredients won't remain stable due to the jar packaging. Please see the Appendix to find out why jar packaging is a problem. Given the price, the jar packaging, and the fact that you don't need an eye cream, there are few reasons to consider this product.

☺ AVERAGE $$$ **Hypoallergenic Nourishing Moisturizer** *($75 for 2 fl. oz.)* is a fragrance-free moisturizer for dry skin that contains some good emollients along with a nice mix of soothing ingredients and skin-repairing substances to help rebuild the skin's surface. What's disappointing is that many of the key ingredients won't remain stable because this moisturizer is packaged in a jar (see the Appendix to find out why jar packaging is a problem). There's also the issue that many of the intriguing ingredients are listed after the preservative, something you don't want to see, especially in a product that costs this much! Sadly, while this is a good moisturizer with mostly helpful ingredients for sensitive skin, the amount of benzyl alcohol is potential cause for concern, making this less enticing if sensitive skin is your chief concern.

☺ AVERAGE $$$ **Hypoallergenic Peptide Complex** *($98 for 1 fl. oz.)* contains nothing that makes it "dermatologist-grade" because there is no such "grade" available for ingredients or formulations anywhere in the world. It isn't a superior formula, nor do dermatologists have access to any cosmetic ingredients that are not available to "regular" brands. If anything, this serum ends up being a serious disappointment because it contains a potentially irritating amount of benzyl alcohol. What's also disappointing is that most of the soothing, anti-aging ingredients are present only in tiny amounts. At almost $100 per bottle, these good-for-skin ingredients should be a prominent part of the formula, but instead you get mostly standard slip agents, with the only anti-aging ingredient of note being a form of vitamin C (tetrahexyldecyl ascorbate). Even the olive oil–based ingredients are barely present. This isn't money well spent! See the Appendix to learn why the hypoallergenic name and claim is meaningless.

☺ AVERAGE $$$ **Intensive Moisture Therapy** *($125 for 2 fl. oz.)* is an emollient moisturizer for dry skin that is rich in phosphatidylcholine, an ingredient whose major constituent, lecithin, is a phospholipid that occurs naturally in the skin and is believed to have cell-communicating ability. Phospholipids help ensure the integrity of the skin-cell membrane and are effective in protecting and restoring skin's barrier function (Sources: *The Journal of Biological Chemistry*, May 2008, Epublication; *International Journal of Pharmaceutics*, March 2008, pages 263–272; and *Experimental Dermatology*, July 2006, pages 493–500). The price might have been worth it if phospholipids were exclusive to this moisturizer, but that's not the case. The other emollients in this moisturizer are commonplace, and the inclusion of vitamin E, vitamin C, and soy could've provided a good antioxidant boost had Perricone not reverted back to standard jar packaging (see the Appendix to learn why you should avoid anti-aging products packaged in jars). Other antioxidants and some skin-identical ingredients are present as well, but they are listed after the preservative and as such don't amount to much (at least as far as providing any noticeable benefit to skin).

☺ AVERAGE $$$ **Neuropeptide Deep Wrinkle Serum** *($185 for 1 fl. oz.)* is more of a lightweight moisturizer than a serum, and is yet another absurdly overpriced product from Dr. Perricone. With all the neuropeptide products he sells, you'd think he would have a solid backdrop of research to support his claims. You would, however, be wrong: No such research exists, at least not from Dr. Perricone. This allegedly fast-acting "treatment" is supposed to make deep wrinkles a distant memory, but the ingredients it contains cannot do that. Doctors aren't seeing less Botox and dermal filler work due to Perricone's products, and by the time you read this, he'll likely have more antiwrinkle products ready to capture your attention. It's a huge embarrassment that this serum contains mostly water, slip agent, a glycol-based penetration enhancer, plant-based thickener, and preservative. For the cost, it should be brimming with proven ingredients to improve aging skin, but that's not the case. This contains the controversial ingredients DMAE. For more information about this ingredient, please refer to the special note at the beginning of the Perricone line review. The selection of peptides in this product have theoretical cell-communicating ability for skin, but there is no research showing they improve sagging skin or are capable of erasing deep wrinkles in any way. This is fragranced with rose oil, and its fragrant components can cause irritation, though the amount this contains isn't likely to be a problem.

☺ AVERAGE $$$ **Neuropeptide Eye Contour** *($195 for 0.5 fl. oz.)* contains a low amount of neuropeptides but perhaps even more disappointing is that there is no research proving that topical application of neuropeptides has any benefit for skin. As noted cosmetic surgeon Dr. Arthur Perry stated, "The molecular size of these peptides is likely too large for them to penetrate skin and reach their target cells"—and that's assuming these peptides can somehow avoid being broken down by naturally occurring enzymes in the skin. The association between neuropeptides and skin care doesn't have much logic behind it. Neuropeptides are composed of short-chain amino acids and are perhaps best known as being key components of the human brain (think endorphins, the feel-good chemicals our brains release after exercise or other pleasurable activities). How these neuropeptides go about firming skin and reducing sagging isn't explained, nor is there any proof that they reduce dark circles or puffy eyes; but that didn't stop Perricone from claiming otherwise and hoping that consumers will take a (very expensive) leap of faith. Beyond the neuropeptide discussion, this is a basic lightweight moisturizer suitable for normal to slightly dry skin anywhere on the face. It contains some great antioxidants, although half of them are present in amounts too low to be of much benefit for your skin. As with most of Perricone's anti-aging products, this eye cream contains DMAE. See the special note at the beginning of the Perricone review for details on this ingredient.

☺ AVERAGE $$$ **Neuropeptide Facial Conformer** *($495 for 2 fl. oz.)* claims that it "activates surface renewal of the dermis." The dermis is not part of the skin's surface, and there's likely not anything in this hugely expensive moisturizer that affects the dermis layer of skin, at least not to the extent that any permanent change will occur. In many ways, this formula is an embarrassment for the company and a pathetic waste of money for you. There is nothing in this overpriced concoction that is going to whisk away your wrinkles, sagging skin, and other signs of aging. The only thing that is going to "dramatically diminish" is your cosmetics budget. The low amount of neuropeptides in this product is disappointing, but that really doesn't matter because even more disappointing is that there is no research proving that topical application of neuropeptides has any benefit for skin. See the review for Neuropeptide Eye Contour above for more details on how neuropeptides work. Last, for what this costs, it is downright depressing that several of the most beneficial ingredients are listed after the preservative, meaning they are barely present and, therefore, barely effective.

☺ AVERAGE $$$ **Neuropeptide Firming Moisturizer** *($280 for 2 fl. oz.)* is said to have been a secret Perricone kept hidden in his anti-aging vault (perhaps hidden along with all the research he claims to have done but has never published or had peer-reviewed or shown to anyone). The good doctor is said to have developed this formula for his personal use (why wasn't he using his other products all along is a question no one at his company has the answer to), and now he's making it available publicly. So if you have deep pockets and are dealing with wrinkles and sagging facial contours, should you consider this product? Well, at its core, this is just an emollient, jar-packaged moisturizer for normal to dry skin not prone to breakouts. A major ingredient in the product is the amino acid taurine. This ingredient is discussed in detail in the review for Perricone's Firming Neck Therapy above. L-tyrosine is also present in this product. It's a nonessential amino acid, and there is research indicating its benefit for skin, but it's effect in terms of anti-aging prowess is questionable, and it's certainly not capable of making sagging skin a thing of the past (Source: naturaldatabase.com.) To sum up, none of the other scientific or pseudo-scientific ingredients in this outrageously expensive moisturizer can make aging skin look young again. Most of them have potential benefit, just not in a way that jibes with Perricone's claims.

☺ AVERAGE $$$ **Super Bright Eyed Melon Carotenoids** *($50 for 0.5 fl. oz.)* contains some intriguing ingredients with the potential to help skin anywhere on the face look and act younger. The problem? Jar packaging. The fact that it's packaged in a jar means the beneficial ingredients won't remain stable once it is opened. Another point: Although we know it's hard to believe, the truth is you don't need an eye cream. See the Appendix to learn more about the problems jar packaging presents and find out why you don't need to bother with eye creams.

☺ AVERAGE $$$ **Super Daylight Savings SPF 25 Moisturizer** *($38 for 1 fl. oz.)* is a daytime moisturizer with sunscreen that has a slightly thick, lotion-like texture with a noticeably strong fragrance. The fragrance doesn't linger, but regrettably the formula contains the kind of fragrance ingredients (such as limonene) that cause needless irritation. That's a shame because otherwise this provides gentle broad-spectrum sun protection with zinc oxide as its sole active ingredient. Despite the high amount of zinc oxide, this moisturizer goes on almost translucent, leaving no visible white cast once set. The amount of zinc oxide also lends this product a finish that feels a bit dry, yet it still moisturizes. We know, that doesn't make a lot of sense but nevertheless it's how the product feels. The translucent bottle packaging isn't the best, as it compromises the effectiveness of the antioxidants (if you keep the product on your counter and it is exposed to daylight). If you decide to try this, make sure you store it in a dark place. The base formula contains some very good antioxidants, though the amounts are low. We're a bit concerned about the amount of coconut alcohol in this product; combined with the fragrance ingredients it makes this moisturizer with sunscreen a problem for anyone with sensitive skin. On balance, although the formula has its drawbacks (including its price, which may discourage liberal application), it is an OK option for normal to dry skin not prone to breakouts.

☺ AVERAGE $$$ **Super Hyper Hydrator Coconut Water MCT** *($40 for 1 fl. oz.)* contains some intriguing ingredients to help replenish and restore dry skin. What a shame that many of the beneficial extras won't hold up due to the jar packaging (see the Appendix for details). What about the MCT ingredient Perricone touts? MCT refers to medium-chain triglycerides, the primary source of fat in coconuts. There is no research proving this type of triglyceride is better for dry skin than countless other triglycerides, derivatives, or numerous emollients and oils. It's a helpful ingredient for dry skin, but it's neither the best nor the only option. Like many products in Perricone's main line, this contains the controversial ingredient DMAE. Refer to the special note at the beginning of the Perricone line review for details on this ingredient.

☺ AVERAGE $$$ **Super Night Recharge Red Algae Astaxanthin** *($50 for 1 fl. oz.)* is packaged in a clear bottle and that's a problem for the antioxidants this contains. Although a clear bottle is better than a jar in terms of keeping these air-sensitive ingredients stable once you've opened the package, it still demands careful storage away from light because light also causes delicate ingredients to break down before they can benefit your skin, and that includes the retinol in this moisturizer. As for the formula, it has a great silky cream texture that is suitable for normal to slightly dry skin. It contains some impressive antioxidants, although several of them are present in small amounts that don't justify this product's steep price. In essence, you're shortchanging your skin of the antioxidants it needs and, for what Perricone is charging, should be present in abundance. This contains the fragrant plant oil *Litsea cubeba*, a plant whose chemical constituents can cause irritation, although that's unlikely given the small amount (Source: *Food and Chemical Toxicology*, May 2006, pages 739–746).

☹ POOR **Chia Serum** *($75 for 1 fl. oz.)* is an oil–based serum that is capitalizing on the current nutrition craze for chia seeds. If you're not familiar with chia seeds, they're a rich plant source of omega-3 fatty acids, specifically, alpha-linolenic acid. Like all fatty acids, this has benefit for skin, especially dry skin. Also, like most plant oils, chia oil is a good source of antioxidants. It isn't a miracle or must-have ingredient for skin; rather, it's just another good, nonfragrant plant oil to consider. Clearly Perricone would agree chia oil isn't the best, as he sells several other serums and moisturizers that contain other plant oils. This serum contains a few other plant oils as well as antioxidant vitamins (A, C, and E) and fragrance. Despite an impressive roster of ingredients for dry skin, the second oil on the list, *Aleurites moluccana*, is problematic. Also known as tung seed, candlenut, or kukui oil, it is known to cause "acute contact dermatitis" when applied to skin (Source: naturaldatabase.com). Of course, not everyone will respond this way, but this oil has other precautions, too: It can induce sweating and the plant is a natural source of the poison hydrogen cyanide, which is why the seeds are considered toxic if consumed in their raw, unprocessed state. None of this is good news for your skin, and it makes Chia Serum an iffy product to consider, despite an overall good assortment of ingredients.

PERRICONE MD COSMECEUTICALS LIP & SMILE CARE

☺ AVERAGE $$$ **Lip Plumper** *($35 for 0.48 fl. oz.)* is a creamy lip moisturizer that contains some good antioxidants, but those won't create fuller lips. The amount of urea may prove sensitizing to lips, which will temporarily make them look plump, but that's by virtue of irritation. Still, urea is a better choice than mint or spice irritants. As with most of Perricone's anti-aging products, this product contains DMAE. See the special note at the beginning of the Perricone line review for details on this ingredient.

☺ AVERAGE $$$ **Super Lush Lips Coconut Oil Tocotrienols** *($20 for 0.5 fl. oz.)* is a buttery lip balm that contains excellent ingredients to protect lips from moisture loss and chapping. Almost every ingredient is a source of antioxidants, and that's always helpful, but the jar packaging is a real disappointment, making this product a no-go at any price. Because this antioxidant-rich lip balm is packaged in a jar, none of the antioxidants will remain stable once it is opened. What a shame; in better packaging, this lip balm, though pricey, would've earned our highest rating.

PERRICONE MD COSMECEUTICALS SPECIALTY SKIN-CARE PRODUCTS

☺ AVERAGE $$$ **Super 3-Minute Facial Ginger Gingerols** *($50 for 2 fl. oz.)* claims to deliver "intense, tingling hydration," so we were concerned that this product would contain irritating ingredients because "tingling" often means irritation. As it turns out, however, the only problematic ingredient in this product is ginger root extract, and there's not much of it present. So, this turns out to be little more than a moisturizing mask for dry skin. The fact that it's packaged in a jar is the real problem because none of the beneficial ingredients (of which there are surprisingly small amounts, given what this product costs) will remain stable once it is opened (see the Appendix for details).

☺ AVERAGE $$$ **Vitamin C Ester 15** *($120 for 4 tubes)*. If you're curious to try a product with a high amount of stabilized vitamin C, this is an intriguing option. But before we discuss this product in more detail, you need to know that skin care isn't as simple as one superstar ingredient. For all of vitamin C's benefits (which include stimulating collagen production and lightening brown spots), the truth is your skin needs more than one great ingredient to look and act younger. Although it may seem impressive that the four 0.34 fl. oz. tubes of product that comprise Vitamin C Ester 15 contain 15% vitamin C (listed as ascorbyl palmitate), the vitamin C is really the only point of interest. The other ingredients are mundane and definitely don't justify this product's price. We're also not thrilled to see fragrance and a couple of fragrance ingredients known to be irritating. High amounts of vitamin C can pose an irritation risk on its own, so adding fragrance ingredients to the mix isn't the best move. The tiny amount of antioxidant vitamin E and skin-repairing sodium hyaluronate are mere window dressing and can be ignored. Ultimately, your skin deserves more than what this can provide, but if you're willing to settle for a one-note product with a high concentration of a proven anti-aging ingredient (and your budget extends to what this costs) then this is worth a look.

PERRICONE MD COSMECEUTICALS FOUNDATION

☺ GOOD $$$ **No Concealer Concealer SPF 35** *($45 for 0.3 fl. oz.).* The name for this fragrance-free product is strange because essentially, it is a concealer. It provides light coverage and offers the benefit of gentle sun protection with its mineral-based active ingredients. The formula dispenses somewhat thick but softens to a light cream that's easy to blend, though you'll notice some opacity right away due to the amount of mineral active ingredients. Combined with the soft peach tint (only one shade is offered and it's best for light to medium skin tones) and soft matte finish, you absolutely get some coverage, negating the "no concealer" name. In addition to coverage and broad-spectrum sun protection, this concealer is also laced with several anti-aging ingredients, including peptides, repairing ingredients, and antioxidant vitamins. Because this product provides sun protection, the inactive ingredients are listed in alphabetical rather than descending order (which is permissible per FDA regulations because SPF-rated products are regulated as over-the-counter drugs). Unfortunately, the alphabetical listing makes it difficult to tell how much of the anti-aging ingredients you're getting—and given this product's cost, you want to know if they're present in a meaningful amount or just window dressing. As for the neuropeptides, they have theoretical cell-communicating ability for skin, but there is no research showing they improve sagging skin around the eyes or are capable of erasing wrinkles in any way. Not even Perricone has published research on what these peptides can do; instead, he just makes the claims and most likely assumes women will trust him because he's a doctor. This contains the controversial ingredients DMAE (listed as dimethyl MEA). For more information about this ingredient, please refer to the special note at the beginning of the Perricone line review. The inclusion of DMAE keeps this concealer from earning a higher rating, though its strong points make this worth a look, as there are few good concealers with sunscreen.

☹ POOR **No Foundation Foundation SPF 30** *($55 for 1 fl. oz.)* is available in one shade, and we couldn't help but think the tint was simply to offset the white cast from the high concentrations of mineral active ingredients it contains. The sunscreen is great and this feels surprisingly light and practically blends itself. The formula even contains an impressive amount of stabilized vitamin C. Perricone added several other intriguing ingredients, too, but they're listed after the preservative and don't count for much. What keeps this foundation from earning a higher rating is the inclusion of several fragrant oils. They're not present in large amounts, but they certainly aren't something to put in the "pro" column for this pricey foundation. Two more comments: There is too little glycolic acid for it to function effectively as an exfoliant and the product's pH is too high for exfoliation to occur. Perricone includes a drug ingredient (Teprenone) off-label in this product. Teprenone is the brand name for a drug known as geranylgeranylacetone, which is used to treat gastric ulcers and is being researched as an option for slowing age-related hearing loss (Sources: *Brain Research*, May 2008, pages 9–17; and *Digestion*, October 2007, pages 215–224). What do hearing loss and ulcers have to do with aging skin? One of the key ways geranylgeranylacetone works is by influencing heat shock proteins. These proteins help other proteins interact as they should at the cellular level, which affects many systems in the body. Heat shock proteins are most active during times of stress, such as exposure to cigarette smoke and exposure to sunlight. When heat shock proteins are reduced (which ultimately is what you want because that means reducing inflammation), cells appear to live longer. Perhaps Perricone theorized that geranylgeranylacetone (as Teprenone) may also have a helpful effect when applied topically. After all, the skin is a source of heat shock proteins, and it is certainly exposed to enough stressful situations that an ingredient that can help these proteins function more efficiently would be a benefit. However, there's no research proving that topically applied geranylgeranylacetone has any effect on heat shock proteins within skin. Moreover, as previously mentioned, Perricone is using a drug ingredient in a cosmetic product, which means the consumer is the guinea pig. We'd consider this with caution, if at all.

PETER THOMAS ROTH

Strengths: Provides complete ingredient lists on website; most products are fragrance-free; very good AHA products; good selection of water-soluble cleansers and scrubs; some excellent sunscreens, benzoyl peroxide products, and many antioxidant-rich formulas.

Weaknesses: Expensive; mostly lackluster toners; mostly boring to potentially irritating masks; no BHA products that do not include at least one needless irritant; jar packaging; several products that purport to work like cosmetic corrective procedures when they don't even come close to comparing.

For more information and the latest Peter Thomas Roth reviews, visit CosmeticsCop.com.

PETER THOMAS ROTH CLEANSERS

✓☺ BEST **$$$ Gentle Foaming Cleanser** *($32 for 6.7 fl. oz.)* is indeed gentle, has a mild foaming action many consumers will appreciate, and works beautifully to remove makeup. Best for normal to oily skin, this fragrance-free cleanser is highly recommended, although you don't need to spend this much money for a good fragrance-free cleanser.

☺ GOOD **$$$ Chamomile Cleansing Lotion with Natural Herbal Extract for All Skin Types** *($32 for 8.5 fl. oz.)* would be a great water-soluble cleanser for any skin type, but because it contains fragrance those with rosacea or sensitive skin should consider it carefully. This will remove makeup well and contains soothing plant extracts.

☹ AVERAGE **$$$ Anti-Aging Cleansing Gel** *($35 for 8.5 fl. oz.)*. This may be Peter Thomas Roth's best-selling cleanser, but what that mostly means is that lots of his customers are spending way more than is necessary for a good water-soluble cleanser. The salicylic acid and glycolic acid absolutely have anti-aging benefits for all skin types, but not when they're used in a product that's quickly rinsed from skin. This cleanser contains citrus extracts that can be a problem when used around the eyes. For a lot less money and a gentler yet just-as-effective cleanser, consider the options from CeraVe, Boots, and Paula's Choice.

☹ AVERAGE **$$$ Beta Hydroxy Acid 2% Acne Wash** *($35 for 8.5 fl. oz.)* lists 2% salicylic acid as an active ingredient, but this is rinsed from the skin before it can work the way it should. This is otherwise a very simple fragrance-free cleanser for all skin types except very dry.

☹ AVERAGE **$$$ Glycolic Acid 3% Facial Wash** *($32 for 8.5 fl. oz.)* may contain 3% glycolic acid, but without the right pH and given this cleanser's brief contact time with skin, it doesn't matter. It is otherwise a very standard, fragrance-free, water-soluble cleanser for normal to oily skin.

☹ AVERAGE **$$$ Un-Wrinkle Creme Cleanser** *($38 for 6.7 fl. oz.)*. This fragrant, creamy cleanser for dry skin is a bit greasy, but it does remove makeup and leave your skin feeling smooth. Most will find that you need to use a washcloth for complete removal, and it's best not to leave residue from this cleanser behind because the fragrant base can cause irritation. What would make this cleanser even better (aside from easier rinsing, no fragrance, and a more realistic price tag) would be if it contained an array of barrier-restoring ingredients to help skin begin the process of repairing itself.

PETER THOMAS ROTH TONERS

☺ AVERAGE **$$$ Aloe Tonic Mist** *($32 for 8.5 fl. oz.)* is a very basic, alcohol-free spray-on toner that contains mostly water, aloe (which is primarily water), soothing agents, and a dusting of antioxidants. It is fragrance-free and suitable for all skin types.

☺ AVERAGE **$$$ Conditioning Tonic** *($32 for 8.5 fl. oz.)* is an exceptionally basic toner whose salicylic acid content is far too low to be effective, regardless of pH. Countless other less expensive toners offer your skin more than this. If you want the exfoliating benefits of BHA in toner form, consider the options from the Paula's Choice CLEAR collection.

☺ AVERAGE **$$$ Glycolic Acid Clarifying Tonic** *($32 for 8.5 fl. oz.)* is a substandard toner that contains a frustrating mix of helpful and irritating ingredients, plus the pH is too high for the glycolic acid to function as an exfoliant.

PETER THOMAS ROTH EXFOLIANTS & SCRUBS

✓☺ BEST **$$$ Glycolic Acid 10% Moisturizer** *($45 for 2.2 fl. oz.)* is an ideal AHA moisturizer for normal to dry skin. Glycolic acid at a pH of 3.8 ensures exfoliation, while emollients and antioxidants help dry skin look and feel better, all without added fragrance. Well done, though there are less expensive, equally elegant AHA exfoliants listed in the Best Products chapter.

☺ GOOD **$$$ Botanical Buffing Beads** *($36 for 8.5 fl. oz.)* is a scrub that contains jojoba beads as the abrasive agent. They're quite gentle and a good option for normal to dry skin. However, they cannot open clogged pores and emulsify sebum (oil) as claimed. In contrast, because jojoba oil's molecular structure is so similar to our skin's oil, it is much more likely to contribute to rather than remedy clogged pores.

☺ GOOD **$$$ Glycolic Acid 10% Hydrating Gel** *($48 for 2 fl. oz.)* is an excellent fragrance-free AHA product for all skin types, and the pH of 3.6 ensures efficacy. The amount of antioxidants and other beneficial extras isn't enough to earn our highest rating, but it's still good.

☺ AVERAGE **$$$ Un-Wrinkle Peel Pads, for All Skin Types** *($36 for 60 pads)* are alcohol-free pads that contain 20% glycolic acid, a level that is close to peel strength, but before you get too excited, know that the pH of the solution is almost a 6, which is well beyond the level needed for the acid to exfoliate skin. There is no reason to consider these pricey pads (though they're certainly not a problem for skin); the many antioxidants and retinol will not remain stable due to jar packaging.

☹ POOR **Gentle Complexion Correction Pads** *($36 for 60 pads)* contain an unimpressive amount of salicylic acid, but would have merit as an AHA product if the base did not contain so much alcohol. See the Appendix to learn why alcohol is the opposite of gentle!

☹ POOR **Max Complexion Correction Pads** *($36 for 60 pads)* share the core problems of many anti-acne pads: an alcohol-based solution and a pH too high for salicylic acid to exfoliate, which won't help blemished skin in the least. The amount of alcohol in these pads will stimulate oil production at the base of your pores and won't help reduce the redness that goes hand-in-hand with acne. When it comes to anti-aging benefits, alcohol isn't what you want either, because it breaks down collagen.

☺ AVERAGE **$$$ Anti-Aging Buffing Beads** *($36 for 8.5 fl. oz.)* is made to sound like an advanced scrub capable of polishing away wrinkles, but the company uses the term "fine lines," which aren't true wrinkles but the lines that occur from dryness. Using a scrub over dry skin and following with a moisturizer can eliminate fine lines, but won't help wrinkles. What's iffy about this jojoba bead scrub (an abrasive agent that is quite gentle) is the inclusion of the drying detergent cleansing agent sodium C14-16 olefin sulfonate as a main ingredient. The glycolic and salicylic acids are present in amounts too small to exfoliate skin. This is an OK, needlessly pricey scrub for normal to oily skin.

☹ AVERAGE **$$$ Blemish Buffing Beads** *($36 for 8.5 fl. oz.)*. The fact that jojoba oil is the second ingredient in this body scrub makes it unsuitable for blemish-prone skin. However, the oil keeps the detergent cleansing agent sodium C14-16 olefin sulfonate from being as drying as it typically is. This is otherwise a very basic scrub whose cinnamon bark content isn't going to do your skin any favors. Overall, it is a problematic formula that fights against itself, putting your skin in the boxing ring as well. The inclusion of 1% salicylic acid may seem helpful, but this anti-acne superstar is of little use in a rinse-off product because its contact with skin is too brief for it to be effective. For best results, treat acne from the neck down with a leave-on products that contains salicylic acid, such as Paula's Choice RESIST Weightless Body Treatment with 2% BHA.

☹ AVERAGE **$$$ Clinical Peel & Reveal Dermal Resurfacer** *($58 for 3.4 fl. oz.)*. This tube-packaged product aims to provide manual exfoliation from aluminum oxide crystals and "chemical" exfoliation from pumpkin enzymes and the AHA ingredient lactic acid. As it turns out, this is more a scrub for oily skin than anything else—it's not a peel per se because the amount of lactic acid is likely too low to exfoliate, and the pumpkin enzymes are, at best, an unreliable way to exfoliate. They're unreliable because enzymes are extremely unstable in cosmetic formulations and unlikely to be of much benefit in a product like this, which is meant to be rinsed from the skin after only a few minutes. Also, there's no research proving pumpkin enzymes are effective for exfoliation. There isn't much else to say about this product, other than that as a scrub (which is really the only exfoliating ingredient in this ridiculously expensive product), it will leave skin feeling softer and smoother, assuming you use it gently and rinse thoroughly.

☹ POOR **Laser-Free Retexturizer Exfoliating Scrub** *($38 for 2 fl. oz.)*. Before we discuss this artificially colored scrub's formula, we need to state that the name is just silly. "Laser-free" is supposed to imply laser treatments a dermatologist performs, but really it means that this product is free of lasers. Well, duh! Come on, Peter Thomas Roth, have a little more respect for consumers. Anything that's *not* a laser is, by definition, laser-free! This scrub claims to do just about everything under the sun to improve skin texture and tone, and it's said to be incredible for all skin types, even acne-prone. It isn't. In fact, this scrub is a problem for all skin types, especially acne-prone skin (if you have acne, a scrub isn't the way to go; acne cannot be scrubbed away). The abrasive agent (polyethylene) is quite gentle, but the cleansing agent employed is needlessly drying and this contains a high amount of skin-irritant cinnamon bark. The glycolic acid (an AHA) is useless in a scrub because its benefit is rinsed down the drain before it can help your skin. If you want the benefits of AHA (and without question an AHA exfoliant is preferred to a scrub), Peter Thomas Roth and other brands offer excellent options. This glorified scrub ends up being overpriced and not capable of making good on its claims of "dramatically younger looking" skin.

PETER THOMAS ROTH MOISTURIZERS (DAYTIME & NIGHTTIME), EYE CREAMS, & SERUMS

✓☺ BEST **$$$ Clini-Matte All Day Oil-Control SPF 20** *($48 for 1.7 fl. oz.)*. Aside from the all-day oil control claim being misleading (those with oily skin will see shine in a matter of hours; you won't be matte all day), this is an impressive daytime moisturizer with sunscreen for those with oily skin. Avobenzone is on hand for critical UVA protection; it has a silky, weightless texture that treats skin to mattifying ingredients and beneficial antioxidants; and it has skin-identical ingredients. It's also fragrance-free and an excellent option for use under makeup, easily replacing any foundation primer you may be using. Again, this cannot "regulate oil levels" (that's a function controlled by hormones, not skin-care products), but it can help absorb surface shine while providing a matte finish, albeit not one that's going to last from morning 'til night.

✓☺ BEST **$$$ Retinol Fusion PM** *($65 for 1 fl. oz.)* is a very good nonaqueous, silicone-based serum with retinol. It also includes antioxidant vitamins C and E along with a cell-communicating ingredient and anti-irritant. The fragrance-free formula is best for normal to dry skin. The amount of alcohol is so small as to not be cause for concern; likely it's present to make an ingredient in this serum more soluble. As for the amount of retinol, the company claims it is present at 1.5%. Based on the ingredient list, there's no reason to dispute this; however, be aware that this amount of retinol increases the risk of side effects such as redness and flaking. Despite the packaging, which is capable of letting in some air, the company maintains the retinol is encapsulated, which should protect it from the minor amount of air exposure that occurs with each use.

✓☺ BEST **$$$ Sheer Liquid SPF 50 Anti-Aging Sunscreen** *($52 for 1.7 fl. oz.)* is a very good, though overpriced, daytime moisturizer with sunscreen. Best for normal to oily or combination skin, the thin, lightweight lotion texture is fragrance-free and provides reliable UVA (think anti-aging) protection with avobenzone. The formula contains some proven antioxidants and its semi-matte finish works well under makeup (and really does feel sheer). In many ways, this is similar to Paula's Choice Extra Care Non-Greasy Sunscreen SPF 45. That product is sold for use from the neck down but absolutely can be used on the face, too (not to mention it costs a fraction of what Roth is charging and comes in a larger size). Whether you go with Roth's option, Paula's Choice, or another sunscreen we recommend, what counts is you're getting environmental protection with antioxidants to boost skin's defenses.

☺ GOOD **$$$ FIRMx Growth Factor Extreme Neuropeptide Serum** *($150 for 1 fl. oz.)*. This water-based serum (amazing that a product that costs this much is based on the least expensive cosmetic ingredient around) is supposed to activate youth, which it can't, but who knows what "youth activating" really means. It could mean almost anything. Aside from marketing nonsense, it turns out this is a very intriguing serum, though not for the reasons Roth wants you to believe. The company claims it contains 52% growth factor, but the bulk of the formula is standard cosmetic ingredients, so 52% isn't possible from an actual content point of view, and you wouldn't want it to be because real growth factors can turn on skin cancer cells just as easily as they can turn on healthy skin cells. Moreover, none of the ingredients in this product qualify as growth factors, at least not directly. Some peptides function as growth factors, and peptides play a role in the formation and activity of various growth factors, but there is no research proving that any of the peptides in this serum influence growth factors that contribute to youthfulness. The only research on the peptides in this product was performed by the companies that sell them for use in skin-care products (and again, what about all the other peptides Roth includes in his anti-aging products?). Despite that information, it's possible that the peptides in this product function as cell-communicating ingredients. They definitely have potential value, but the reality is the research just isn't there yet. However, when peptides are combined with the antioxidants and other intriguing ingredients in this serum, you get a truly beneficial product. It is an understatement to say that you don't have to spend this much to get a great product for your skin.

The Reviews P

☺ GOOD **$$$ Max All Day Moisture Defense Cream with SPF 30** *($42 for 1.7 fl. oz.)* is a good daytime moisturizer for normal to dry skin. The in-part titanium dioxide sunscreen provides sufficient UVA protection, and the formula includes antioxidants (though they should have been given more prominence).

☺ GOOD **$$$ Oil-Free Moisturizer** *($42 for 1.7 fl. oz.)* supplies skin with a good, though not incredibly impressive, blend of beneficial ingredients. Antioxidants join retinol, anti-irritant allantoin, and a tiny amount of skin-identical mucopolysaccharides to create a lightweight moisturizer for normal to slightly dry skin. The thickening agents this contains may be problematic for acne-prone skin, but you'd have to experiment with this to see how your skin responds.

☺ GOOD **$$$ Un-Wrinkle, for All Skin Types** *($120 for 1 fl. oz.)* is a rose-scented serum loaded with peptides in a proportion that the company claims tops out at 23%, thereby enabling this product to make dramatic antiwrinkle claims that might have you canceling that appointment for Botox or dermal fillers. Yet there is no research showing that higher concentrations of peptides can have an effect that matches (or even comes reasonably close to) what's possible from these in-office procedures. Here are details about the key peptides in this product: SYNr-AKE comes from Pentapharm, whose website describes it as a "peptide with an Age Killing Effect. Mimics the neuromuscular blocking properties of Waglerin 1, a polypeptide found in the venom of the snake *Tropidolaemus wagleri.*" This snake is a type of viper, and Waglerin-1 is a peptide (composed of 22 amino acids) that is derived and purified from the venom. There is information on how this peptide performs on neurons in the brain and on its relation to GABA (gamma amino butyric acid), a common ingredient in products claiming to work like Botox. However, information on how this ingredient works when blended into cosmetic products is lacking. Waglerin-1 is said to be another blocker of the neurotransmitter acetylcholine, which triggers muscle contractions. But if it worked as claimed, when applied topically it would relax muscles in your fingers, too, and what would happen if you used too much at once or accidentally got it too near the area around your eyes or mouth? (Sources: *Journal of Pharmacology and Experimental Therapeutics*, July 1997, pages 74–80; and *Brain Research*, August 1999, pages 29–37). The SNAP-8 peptide is said to target the "wrinkle formation mechanism" in the same manner as Botox injections. Although there is no substantiated research to support that claim, keep in mind that not even Botox works like Botox when it's applied topically. Fear the needle or not, if you want Botox to work it must be injected into, not dabbed on, your skin. SNAP-8 (technically, acetyl octapeptide-3) is the trade name for an ingredient manufactured by Centerchem. Of course, the only efficacy studies performed for this peptide were conducted by the manufacturer, and done in vitro rather than on human skin (Source: centerchem.com/PDFs/SNAP-8%20Tech%20Lit%20Aug05.pdf). What you need to keep in mind is to not get lost looking for high doses of peptides claiming to work like wrinkle-erasing or plumping procedures a dermatologist can provide. They do not and physiologically cannot work the same, or even come close. Peptides are exciting anti-aging ingredients, just not capable of replacing in-office procedures regardless of the percentage a brand may tout. The best reason to consider using this serum is not for its litany of peptides or antiwrinkle prowess (which it is most certainly lacking), but for its antioxidants and water-binding agents, all in stable packaging. This is a costly way to get those ingredients, but they nevertheless are the most substantiated, useful ingredients in this product.

☺ GOOD **$$$ Ultimate Creme in a Tube** *($48 for 1.7 fl. oz.)*. This very emollient, heavy-duty facial moisturizer is only for dry to very dry skin. Its blend of rich ingredients works well to make dry skin feel smooth and comfortable, and it contains a good blend of skin-repairing ingredients and antioxidants. The only drawback is the inclusion of grapefruit peel extract, but it's likely present in an amount too low to be cause for concern. Although this is pricey, it's worth considering if you've struggled to find a facial moisturizer that makes your dry skin feel better for more than a couple of hours. Kudos to Peter Thomas Roth for not packaging this in a jar, which would have negated the effectiveness of the antioxidants the formula contains.

☺ GOOD $$$ **Un-Wrinkle Eye** (*$100 for 0.5 fl. oz.*) makes the same "look years younger" claim as the other Un-Wrinkle products, but doesn't have nearly as interesting a formula, at least not if you're looking for a peptide-rich product (there's no pressing need to do that, but peptides do get a lot of buzz). This has purpose as a lightweight moisturizer for slightly dry skin anywhere on the face, and it contains some good antioxidants in packaging that will keep them stable during use. However, this will not lead to lineless eyes, and in truth you don't need an eye cream at all (see the Appendix to find out why).

☺ AVERAGE $$$ **Anti-Aging Cellular Eye Repair Gel** (*$42 for 0.76 fl. oz.*) is sold as a revolutionary eye treatment whose benefits for wrinkles go beyond retinol. The company's Firme-CELL-4 technology is allegedly responsible for this feat. It combines four peptides (including the works-like-Botox argireline, also known as acetyl hexapeptide-3) said to have a synergistic effect on reducing deep lines and wrinkles. Before you get too excited, there is no substantiated research to support this claim. Peptides have theoretical cell-communicating ability and likely play a role in encouraging healthy skin functioning, but whether or not they can affect deep wrinkles is unknown; they probably can't. In contrast, retinol has mounds of research pertaining to its ability to improve skin's appearance and stimulate collagen production. Besides, beyond the peptides, this gel is mostly slip agent, thickener, and preservatives, which is hardly worth opening up your pocketbook for.

☺ AVERAGE $$$ **FIRMx Neck & Decollete Creme** (*$135 for 1.5 fl. oz.*) is said to contain ingredients that stimulate natural cell activity that somehow works only for the skin on the neck and chest. We wish we could say they've succeeded in creating a remarkable product to remedy signs of aging on the neck and chest, but they haven't, although they certainly found a price tag that makes it seem that way. In reality, this is just a moisturizer with a smattering of unusual ingredients, but our analysis of these ingredients (some of which are tongue twisters on a grand scale) did not reveal any special properties or benefits for aging skin, below the jawline or elsewhere. This product does contain a peptide blend for which there is one study (not published in a peer-reviewed or scientific dermatology journal, so its results are suspect) involving 41 women between the ages of 56 and 65. Half of the women applied a cream with the peptide blend; the others applied a placebo cream. After twice daily use for 8 weeks, the results revealed a 9% increase in skin tightening and 8% increase in firmness compared with the placebo product. Not only is the sample size too small for these results to be reliable, but also the concentration of the peptide blend used in the study was 2.5%, well below what this Roth product contains. Also of interest: The study did not involve application to the neck or chest, which is how this product is marketed, but instead to the forearms and face (Source: personalcaremagazine.com/Print.aspx?Story=6594). The study also did not compare the results to those from other well-formulated skin-care products that include a sunscreen to see how that would measure up. This contains some good anti-aging ingredients for skin anywhere on the

👁 Did you know you don't need an eye cream? It's true! See the Appendix to find out why.

The Reviews P

face or body, but most of them (including the peptide blend mentioned above) will not remain effective because this product is packaged in a jar, and jars don't keep beneficial ingredients stable. Please see the Appendix for details on the problems jar packaging presents. More to the point, there isn't one iota of research or any physiological information showing that skin on the neck or chest needs an ingredient different from the skin on the face. The whole notion is ludicrous.

☺ AVERAGE $$$ **Laser-Free Resurfacer** *($75 for 1 fl. oz.)*. Stating that this is a "laser-free serum" is a bit odd and not the least bit distinctive because serums aren't lasers. As it turns out, this water-based serum cannot come close to approximating what a laser procedure can do for signs of aging. The formula isn't terrible, but you'll still need to keep that appointment with your cosmetic dermatologist! Besides, Laser-Free Resurfacer has its share of controversial ingredients: ethyl perfluoroisobutyl ether and ethyl perfluorobutyl ether. These ingredients are said to generate oxygen, which isn't helpful for aging skin (antioxidants are all about protecting skin from oxidative damage), and are sources of fluorocarbons (chemically inert compounds), which increase the oxygen content in liquids. As an aside, fluorocarbons also are responsible for much of the ozone depletion that occurs in the atmosphere. In all likelihood, these ingredients won't remain stable in cosmetics and as such cannot generate oxygen on your skin.

☺ AVERAGE $$$ **Laser-Free Regenerator Moisturizing Gel-Cream** *($68 for 1 fl. oz.)*. Before we discuss this red-tinted moisturizer's formula, we need to explain why skin-care products cannot work like a laser to improve signs of aging: lasers use specific colors and calibrated wavelengths of light which, when properly administered (by a trained medical professional) target and break up pigment cells and/or broken blood vessels (capillaries) in the lower layers of your skin. When these specific colors are targeted, the results work from the lower layers of your skin (beyond where cosmetics can reach) to the surface, so you'll see signs of redness and brown discolorations go away (or at least noticeably fade). Because laser treatments essentially wound skin in a carefully controlled manner, they stimulate cells in skin that manufacture healthy collagen, which helps improve wrinkles and enhance firmness. Lots of skin-care ingredients can stimulate healthy collagen production (and when skin isn't being damaged by sunlight and other aggressors, it loves making healthy collagen on its own), but the type of collagen stimulation you get from laser treatments is beyond where skin-care ingredients can target. The best solution is to combine a state-of-the-art skin-care routine (which includes daily sun protection) with the appropriate cosmetic corrective procedures, be they laser or dermal fillers. What about the red resin dragon's blood that's said to be a "centuries old native secret" (though clearly the secret is out)? It's extracted from a fruit that is part of the history of Chinese medicine. It has long been used as a coloring agent for pottery and ceramics. Are you sensing that none of this has to do with anti-aging or wrinkles? You're right, it doesn't! In fact, we couldn't come up with a single viable study or other piece of information proving dragon's blood resin has any benefit for skin, aging or not. It seems to be a gimmicky, novel ingredient but that's about it. And of course, there's no association between dragon's blood and laser treatments! Beyond the dragon's blood being a whole lot of nothing, this moisturizer contains a very good blend of ingredients for all skin types. Silky silicones are joined by cell-communicating ingredient niacinamide and a range of antioxidant plant extracts, some of which are fragrant (which isn't skin care). Unfortunately, most of those ingredients plus the peptides won't remain stable because this moisturizer is packaged in a jar. See the Appendix to find out more about the problems jar packaging presents.

☺ AVERAGE $$$ **Max Anti-Shine Mattifying Gel** *($35 for 1 fl. oz.)* is merely a blend of silicones and a dry-finish solvent. It produces a matte finish, although without ingredients that offer more absorbency, don't expect shine-free longevity. Also, for the money, the company could have included at least one antioxidant and a single skin-identical ingredient.

☺ AVERAGE $$$ **Mega Rich Intensive Anti-Aging Cellular Creme** *($85 for 1.7 fl. oz.).* None of the peptides in this moisturizer have research that proves they can affect deep wrinkles or expression lines. At best, this moisturizer will make normal to dry skin feel better, but the many antioxidants are subject to deterioration because of jar packaging, making this a mega waste of money. Some of the plant extracts in this moisturizer are known irritants, yet another reason to skip this pricey product.

☺ AVERAGE $$$ **Mega Rich Intensive Anti-Aging Cellular Eye Creme** *($65 for 0.76 fl. oz.)* is mainly problematic because of the jar packaging. Not only is jar packaging unsanitary for a water-based product like this, but also it causes many of the anti-aging ingredients to break down upon repeated exposure to light and air. It's such a shame, as this product is loaded with the type of ingredients skin needs to look and act younger. Despite an impressive formula yet poor packaging, the truth is you don't need an eye cream (see the Appendix to find out why).

☺ AVERAGE $$$ **Retinol Fusion AM Moisturizer SPF 30** *($78 for 1.6 fl. oz.).* This thick-textured, fragrance-free, slightly creamy daytime moisturizer with sunscreen provides reliable UVA protection from zinc oxide. The zinc oxide is joined by a standard synthetic sunscreen active, and isn't present in an amount that leaves a white cast on your skin. Although the formula contains retinol and is packaged to keep it stable, that's about the only exciting aspect. This is mostly standard thickeners and preservative, so the price is completely out of line for what you get. Peter Thomas Roth includes a handful of other antioxidants, too, but none of them are present in an amount that justifies the price or makes this a must-have product.

☺ AVERAGE $$$ **Ultra-Lite Anti-Aging Cellular Repair** *($52 for 1.5 fl. oz.)* makes the same antiwrinkle, our-peptides-pack-a-punch claims as several other Peter Thomas Roth products. Peptides are present in this product, but there is no proof they can affect collagen and elastin production or improve the appearance of wrinkles and expression lines. The smattering of antioxidants is not helped by jar packaging (see the Appendix for details). Lastly, this contains a skin-confusing blend of helpful and irritating plant extracts, making it a poor contender for anti-aging and cellular repair

☺ AVERAGE $$$ **Un-Wrinkle Creme** *($110 for 1 fl. oz.).* What a great, simple name for an anti-aging moisturizer! And what a shame it's packaged in a jar, which means several of the important ingredients will break down shortly after it's opened (see the Appendix for details). This has a rich, creamy texture and includes several emollients to make dry skin look and feel better. It also contains several peptides, and those are among the ingredients Roth is referring to in the company's mention of "Un-Wrinkle technology" that relaxes wrinkles. Supposedly, these and other anti-aging ingredients are combined at a seemingly impressive 29% concentration, but the poor choice of packaging wouldn't keep these delicate ingredients stable even if it were a 100% concentration, so the claim looks good on paper only. Even considering the number of anti-aging ingredients in this moisturizer, the 29% boast is still quite a ways off from what's typically included in facial moisturizers (unless Roth is counting standard cosmetic ingredients like glyceryl stearate and cetyl alcohol). Regardless of the percentages and how the company did the math, the bottom line is that this moisturizer would've earned an enthusiastic recommendation were it not for its problematic packaging. Yes, it's needlessly expensive, too, but in better packaging this kind of formula is one where over-spending wouldn't be a waste.

The Reviews P

☺ AVERAGE $$$ **Un-Wrinkle Illuminator Instant Brightening Moisturizer** *($68 for 1.7 fl. oz.)* marries the concept of anti-aging ingredients with multi-colored shiny pigments meant to add a radiant glow to skin. The glow from these "optical diffusers" is supposed to blur deep wrinkles and expression lines, but it really doesn't work that way. Unless it's really subtle, shine tends to magnify wrinkles and fine lines. The sheer but noticeable shine this moisturizer provides isn't going to fool anyone into thinking you look younger, though the pigment blend helps enliven a dull or sallow complexion. It terms of this product's merit as a moisturizer, it is only for those with normal to combination or minimally dry skin. Those with dry skin or markedly dry areas will find this lacks the moisture their skin needs. Anti-aging ingredients include peptides, vitamin C, niacinamide, and a bounty of antioxidant plant extracts. All in all, there are quite a few beneficial ingredients, which makes it all the more disappointing that Roth included irritants such as eucalyptus and arnica. Also disappointing is that there is more alcohol in this moisturizer than state-of-the-art anti-aging ingredients. Ultimately, the problematic ingredients make it not worth strong consideration.

☺ AVERAGE $$$ **Un-Wrinkle Night** *($110 for 1 fl. oz.)* is like a science project in a jar! It contains several peptides and claims to firm skin, improve its tone, minimize pores, reduce wrinkles, repair damage, and prompt collagen production. All of a sudden the price seems not so bad, until you realize that there isn't any research proving that the multiple peptides in this moisturizer can reach any of the goals mentioned in the claims. Another disappointment is that the jar packaging won't keep the retinol and antioxidants stable during use. And the "mega dose" of glycolic acid amounts to a mere dusting, not to mention that this product's pH won't permit exfoliation. As a moisturizer, this is suitable for normal to dry skin and it doesn't contain fragrance. Otherwise, this is really pricey for what you get, and a letdown when you consider the jar packaging. By the way, the manner in which most of the peptides in this product are said to work is by interrupting the chemical pathways that occur beneath the skin and that allow us to make facial expressions—this isn't possible. However, assuming these "100% active" peptides could do that, the results would be potentially frightening (as in you wouldn't be able to smile, chew, or keep your eyes completely open).

☹ POOR **Instant FIRMx Eye** *($38 for 1 fl. oz.)* contains a high amount of irritating, drying ingredients, notably sodium silicate. Combined, these can constrict skin and make it feel temporarily tighter, but the daily irritation can damage healthy collagen production, eventually making wrinkles and sagging around the eyes look worse. If that weren't bad enough, this also contains problematic plant extracts that cause further trouble for skin anywhere on the face. Please see the Appendix to learn why you don't need a special product for the eye area.

☹ POOR **Instant FirmX Temporary Face Tightener** *($35 for 1.7 fl. oz.)*. The October 2010 issue of *Good Housekeeping* magazine proclaimed this product to be among the best firming options for women concerned with sagging skin. A recommendation from this well-respected magazine means a lot, so we regret that in this instance, we disagree with their assessment. This does make your skin feel firmer and tighter, but this sensation is not equivalent to skin actually being firmer or tighter. Rather, the feeling comes from the high concentrations of alkaline, drying ingredients that have a constricting effect on skin. In particular, sodium silicate is highly alkaline (Source: *American Journal of Contact Dermatitis*, September 2002, pages 133–139). Application-wise, you're supposed to apply this to clean skin, wait five minutes, and then remove it with warm water. Any white residue that remains (and you will see some) is supposed to be tapped into the skin. This method of application is supposed to be a quick fix that removes the cosmetically undesirable film this leaves behind while allowing the key ingredients to remain.

The problem? Whatever the "key ingredients" are, they're removed with the rinsing. Nothing in this formula can hold up to removal by water, so, essentially, you're waiting for this to start feeling uncomfortably tight and then removing it before the sensation becomes intolerable.

☹ POOR **Laser-Free Resurfacing Eye Serum** *($58 for 0.5 fl. oz.)* is a very light eye cream that is minimally hydrating, but can be an OK option for slightly dry skin. On balance, though, it's a perfect example of why you don't need a special product for the eye area. Not only are most of the good ingredients this contains also used in Roth's facial moisturizers, but this contains plenty of fragrant and other ingredients that should not be used around the eyes due to the risk of irritation (irritation that can make wrinkles, puffiness, and dark circles worse, not better). Some who have tried this commented on how it improved their dark circles a bit, and it will—but only because it contains mica, a shiny mineral pigment that helps reflect light away from shadowed, darker areas. Mica shows up in thousands of products; you don't need to buy an eye serum like this to gain its benefit (although shine itself isn't skin care, it's a cosmetic effect). Ultimately, despite some beneficial ingredients, this eye serum is a mixed bag. Many of the plant extracts (one is a type of bacteria) are little more than fragrance with no established benefit for skin, and the amount of alcohol is also cause for concern due to the free-radical damage and dryness it causes. This serum also contains a large range of preservatives, including some that are known to be sensitizing. What are those doing in a product meant to be applied so close to the eye? As for the dragon's blood, please refer to the review above for Roth's Laser Free Regenerator Moisturizing Gel-Cream above. As for the name, anything that's not a laser is, by definition, laser-free! This eye product does not work like a laser.

☹ POOR **Power K Eye Rescue** *($100 for 0.5 fl. oz.)* includes several antioxidants front and center, but none of them will do much good for your skin because of the jar packaging (see the Appendix for details). In addition, vitamin K cannot affect dark circles or brighten skin when applied topically, and although arnica has a history of being used for bruising, it is ill-suited for use around the eye, not to mention that very few cases of dark circles are from actual bruises.

☹ POOR **Radiance Oxygenating Serum** *($65 for 1 fl. oz.)* is a classic example of cosmetics double-talk because it claims to provide oxygen to skin, while also supplying antioxidants. Given that these two actions are diametrically opposed, how can anyone's skin possibly benefit? The answer is it can't, and it may actually make matters worse. Although this water-based serum doesn't contain pure oxygen, it contains fluorocarbons (chemically inert compounds), which increase the oxygen content in liquids. Peter Thomas Roth's theory and claim is that by increasing the oxygen content of this serum users will be giving skin a potent dose of oxygen with each application. If that's their claim, then one must surmise that no one at the company has taken note of any of the research indicating that oxygen isn't going to help your skin resist wrinkles or look younger. Exposing skin to more oxygen than it is already will simply generate more free-radical damage (Sources: *International Journal of Cosmetic Science*, October 2008, pages 313–322; and *Human and Experimental Toxicology*, February 2002, pages 61–62). In contrast, applying antioxidants to skin (and consuming them as part of a healthy diet) is supposed to reduce the very damage oxygen exposure causes. See what we mean about opposite actions? Even if increasing the oxygen that is delivered to skin was somehow beneficial, this serum would not be recommended because it contains the irritating menthol derivative menthyl lactate along with peppermint extract. Without question, neither of those ingredients are helpful for skin, regardless of age or concern. See the Appendix to learn how irritation hurts everyone's skin.

☹ POOR **Un-Wrinkle Turbo Face Serum** *($150).* You may be drawn to this serum due to its claims of zoning in on the most stubborn wrinkles, such as the vertical lines between the brows, forehead lines, and marionette lines at the sides of the mouth. But before you spend what Roth is asking, know that this serum is not the solution—and it's certainly not a replacement for cosmetic corrective procedures such as Botox or dermal fillers. It looks impressive that this serum contains several different peptides, but regardless of the number, what matters is that none of them have substantiated research proving they offer your skin a miraculous (or even somewhat impressive) antiwrinkle benefit. Theoretically, all of them are good cell-communicating ingredients, and that's important, but peptides are not the end-all, be-all of anti-aging skin care. Even if you wanted to try a serum with multiple peptides, this isn't the one to go for. Not only is the price outrageous, but two of the main ingredients are irritants. Fragrant rose water and alcohol in the amounts this serum contains will cause irritation that hurts your skin's ability to look and act younger. Assuming the peptides work to stimulate collagen production, what good is that when the amount of alcohol causes collagen breakdown? Talk about opposing forces! This artificially colored serum contains other beneficial ingredients including some good antioxidants, but the core ingredients are a problem that cannot be overlooked.

PETER THOMAS ROTH SUN CARE

✓☺ BEST **Uber-Dry Sunscreen SPF 30** *($26 for 4.2 fl. oz.)*. This in-part avobenzone sunscreen has a name that fits, because the base formula feels nearly weightless and provides a silky-matte finish that's sure to please those who dislike the often thick, tacky texture of many high-SPF sunscreens. This earns its stripes not only for providing broad-spectrum sun protection, but also for being fragrance-free and treating skin to antioxidant vitamins and phospholipids. It is an excellent sunscreen option for all skin types, particularly normal to oily skin (and there is no reason this cannot be used on facial skin).

✓☺ BEST $$$ **Ultra-Lite Oil-Free Sunblock SPF 30** *($26 for 4.2 fl. oz.)* is a very good in-part avobenzone sunscreen whose antioxidant-rich formula is suitable for normal to slightly dry skin. This is also fragrance-free and while it does not contain any oil, some of the thickening agents may be problematic for blemish-prone skin.

☺ GOOD $$$ **Anti-Aging Instant Mineral SPF 45** *($32)* is a loose powder foundation with sunscreen that's best for oily, sensitive skin. It contains high amounts of the sunscreen actives titanium dioxide and zinc oxide (this likely provides more protection than SPF 45, but as with any powder, you'd really have to apply a lot to get the stated amount of protection). The base formula has a light, smooth, and dry texture without obvious shine. This sheer powder is dispensed from a cylindrical component onto a built-in powder brush. The brush isn't the softest, but works to apply this loose powder evenly while minimizing mess. The powder goes on sheer and translucent, and does a good job of keeping oily shine at bay. It's a good way to add to your daily sun protection, even if you're just touching up to tone down shine. As for the peptides and antioxidants this contains, they're a nice touch but it's questionable as to how stable they'll be in a powder base. They're not bad additions and in fact they may offer anti-aging benefits (the sunscreen does that for sure), but just how much is up for debate.

☺ GOOD $$$ **Instant Mineral SPF 30** *($30 for 0.17 fl. oz.)* is very similar to the Anti-Aging Instant Mineral SPF 45 loose powder with sunscreen above, and the same review applies.

☺ GOOD $$$ **Oily Problem Skin Instant Mineral SPF 30** *($30)*. The mineral sunscreens in this tinted loose powder are a great way to get broad-spectrum protection, plus they have the secondary benefit of providing coverage to help even out the complexion. The downside is that the amount of titanium dioxide and zinc oxide is likely to contribute to, rather than help, clogged pores, but that's always a risk with these two ingredients. This loose powder is housed in a cylindrical applicator with a built-in brush. It has a dry texture and absorbent finish that's ideal for oily skin, but again, if blemishes are a concern the amount of mineral actives may prove problematic. This contains a potentially effective amount of salicylic acid, but the pH is not within range for exfoliation to occur. Although the company positions this product as being perfect for acne-prone skin, it is preferred for oily skin not struggling with blemishes (or dealing with occasional breakouts). By the way, the main ingredient in the base formula is a mineral known as illite, which has a clay-like texture and a luminosity similar to that of mica. Despite that, the mineral actives in this powder keep it from being noticeably shiny. This would be a worthwhile sunscreen addition for someone with oily skin and rosacea.

PETER THOMAS ROTH LIP CARE

☺ AVERAGE **$$$ Un-Wrinkle Lip** *($30 for 0.34 fl. oz.)*. Talk about high tech! This water-based lip moisturizer contains several peptides the company refers to as "100% active," while the Maxilip complex is made to sound like a topical way to reproduce the results of collagen lip injections. Don't count on either class of ingredient coming close to what's possible with lip injections. Assuming that the peptides remain stable (active) as they penetrate the lips and surrounding skin, there's no proof that any peptide blend stimulates collagen production to the extent that lips will be noticeably fuller or less lined. The silicones and waxes in this product can help to temporarily fill in superficial lip lines and lines around the mouth, but nothing magical is taking place, it's just fleeting cosmetics trickery, which is helpful, but doesn't change anything. Peptides aren't throwaway ingredients for skin (they have water-binding properties and theoretically cell-communicating ability), but to think they can restore what time, smoking, and sun damage depletes (or what was never there in the first place, as in taking thin lips to a full-on pout) is fantasy. The peppermint extract in this product poses a slight risk of irritation, and the resulting inflammation may make lips ever-so-slightly larger for a small amount of time.

☹ POOR **Lips to Die For Pink Bombshell Lip Balm** *($20 for 0.4 fl. oz.)*. This sheer, pale pink lip balm contains the menthol derivative menthone glycerin acetal. You'll feel the cool tingling sensation almost instantly, and it intensifies the longer this balm is on lips, all of which means your lips are being acutely irritated.

☹ POOR **Un-Wrinkle Volumizing Lip Treatment** *($28 for 0.15 fl. oz.)* is a sheer-tinted lip plumper that contains several peptides, but none of them have been proven by published research to make thinning lips fuller. This product will not provide results even remotely close to what's possible from lip injections with filler such as collagen; in fact, ongoing use of this lip plumper can damage healthy collagen production. That's because it contains the potent menthol derivative menthone glycerin acetal, which is what makes your lips tingle. Unfortunately, that tingle is your lips telling you they're being irritated, not volumized, and the minimal plumping you may see from this "treatment" isn't worth the risk irritation presents.

PETER THOMAS ROTH SPECIALTY SKIN-CARE PRODUCTS

✓☺ BEST **Lashes to Die For Platinum** *($125 for 0.16 fl. oz.)*. This lash growth product, which is exclusive to Sephora, is a more potent version of Peter Thomas Roth's original Lashes to Die For product, which is no longer available. In theory, this should work better and faster than the original because it contains more of the active ingredient. That active ingredient is 17-phenyl trinor prostaglandin E2 serinol amide, the same type of ingredient used in the drug product Latisse, which you've seen female celebrities advertise as growing their lashes. Prostaglandins are believed to work by prolonging the growth cycle of eyelashes (and, it stands to reason, other hair, such as eyebrows). There isn't any substantiated proof that the prostaglandin analogue Roth chose works as claimed, but women are seeing results from this product and, as mentioned, it should work better, at least in theory, and faster than the original Lashes to Die For. Most should see impressive results after 8 weeks of daily use. If you're curious to try a lash growth product that stands a good chance of working, this is a viable, fragrance-free option. Just be aware that the same potential side effects of other prostaglandin analogues (such as bimatoprost) apply here, too. That means skin along the lash line (where this is applied) could turn blue, the color of your eye (the iris) could change to brown, and you could experience irritation, redness, and extreme tearing. Also, if you're using medicated eye drops to manage glaucoma, make sure you talk with your ophthalmologist before considering this or any other lash growth product.

☺ GOOD $$$ **Aloe-Cort Cream** *($30 for 2.2 fl. oz.)* is a very standard lotion that contains 1% hydrocortisone as the active ingredient. It's an option for occasional use on minor skin irritations and itching, but for the money you'll get just as much efficacy from less expensive hydrocortisone creams at the drugstore.

☺ AVERAGE $$$ **Cucumber Gel Masque** *($45 for 5.3 fl. oz.)* is an overpriced water-based mask that contains a mixture of irritating and nonirritating plant extracts. It should not be considered calming or capable of reducing under-eye puffiness, at least not any better than using a cold compress to relieve swelling.

☺ AVERAGE $$$ **De-Spot Skin Brightening Corrector** *($75 for 1 fl. oz.)* contains only a small amount of ingredients with limited research pertaining to their ability to lighten dark spots and improve an uneven skin tone. The two skin-lightening ingredients are azelaic acid and the mineral ingredient zeolite. Research on azelaic acid is intriguing, but the concentration must be 15% or greater for it to have an effect on skin discolorations, which is far from the case with this product. You'll find such concentrations of azelaic acid only in prescription products such as Azelex or Finacea (Sources: *Cochrane Database of Systematic Reviews*, volume 7, July 2010; and *Journal of the American Academy of Dermatology*, December 2006, pages 1048–1065). As for the zeolite, a single in vitro (petri dish) study indicates it has the potential to suppress excess melanin (skin pigment) production. However, at this time, it's a novel approach without published research supporting its efficacy on human skin (Source: *Biological and Pharmaceutical Bulletin*, January 2010, pages 72–76). So, although this zeolite may have benefit, it would be far better to seek out skin-lightening products with proven ingredients, such as hydroquinone (still the gold standard), forms of vitamin C, niacinamide, arbutin, or kojic acid. All these have considerably more research than the zeolite, which makes it less compelling. On balance, this serum-like skin lightener contains some intriguing ingredients, but most of them are present in tiny amounts that belie this product's high price. Although this appears to be fragrance-free, it contains a small amount of fragrant plant extracts. The formula is suitable for normal to dry or oily skin, but its benefits for brown spots or uneven skin tone are questionable at best.

☹ POOR **Acne Spot And Area Treatment** *($32 for 1 fl. oz.)* lists 5% sulfur as its active ingredient. Although sulfur is a potent disinfectant, it is very drying and irritating on skin. For that reason, it is not preferred to benzoyl peroxide or even tea tree oil. The pH of 3.1 serves only to make the sulfur more irritating, but it does allow the blend of glycolic and salicylic acids to exfoliate.

☹ POOR **AHA/BHA Acne Clearing Gel** *($45 for 2 fl. oz.)* contains 2% salicylic acid in the correct pH range for exfoliation to occur, but the amount of alcohol makes this too potentially drying and irritating for acne-prone skin. See the Appendix to learn more about the problems alcohol presents.

☹ POOR **Radiance Oxygenating Masque** *($50 for 3.4 fl. oz.)* doesn't contain pure oxygen; its water-based formula contains fluorocarbons (chemically inert compounds) that increase the oxygen content in liquids and also contribute to ozone depletion in the atmosphere. It is certainly possible that this mask will incite free-radical damage in your skin, and even if it didn't, the formula still contains several plant extracts known to irritate skin. The "brighteners" in this mask are nothing more than cosmetic pigments—and there are plenty of products that give skin a soft glow without risking oxidative damage and irritation.

☹ POOR **Sulfur Cooling Masque** *($40 for 5 fl. oz.)* severely irritates skin due to its 10% concentration of sulfur along with eucalyptus oil. This mask is not recommended.

PETER THOMAS ROTH FOUNDATION & PRIMER

☺ AVERAGE **$$$ Un-Wrinkle Foundation SPF 20** *($45)*. The name for this liquid foundation is not credible because the active ingredients do not supply sufficient UVA protection. This isn't a treatment makeup for wrinkles any more than eating a pan of brownies is a treatment for weight loss! The formula contains some peptides that typically are reserved for anti-aging serums and moisturizers, but there's no substantiated proof that any of them work to make skin look younger. Even if they did, the insufficient sun protection leaves skin vulnerable to more damage and wrinkles. This has a slightly creamy texture that blends smoothly, providing medium coverage and a satin finish that's somewhat glow-y. If the sun protection were better, this would be a suitable option for normal to dry skin. As is, you should think twice before considering any of the mostly neutral shades this foundation offers. The Deep shade is slightly peach.

☺ AVERAGE **$$$ Un-Wrinkle Primer** *($38 for 0.8 fl. oz.)* has an unbelievably silky texture that sets to a soft matte finish. The silicone base helps create an even canvas for your face so your makeup applies smoothly. With all the anti-aging ingredients and claims they make at stake, Peter Thomas Roth made a good decision to put this in air-tight packaging, but they missed the boat by housing it in a clear bottle and not fully protecting it from sunlight, which quickly breaks down several of the key ingredients. When you think about the fact that you are paying $38, the packaging should ensure that your skin benefits as much as possible from the anti-aging ingredients!

PETER THOMAS ROTH CONCEALER

☺ GOOD **$$$ Un-Wrinkle Concealer & Brightener** *($35)* isn't a bad option for a 2-in-1 concealer and highlighter. One end supplies a liquid concealer that offers full coverage and sets to a matte finish. The other end is a shimmering, white liquid "brightener" that blends into skin for a soft, glistening highlight on the inner corners of the eyes, brow bones, or cheekbones. The only downfall is that the concealer is offered in only two shades (Light-Medium and Medium-Deep), so its appeal is limited. If you're curious about the antiwrinkle claims for this concealer/brightener duo, the concealer portion contains some intriguing ingredients that are helpful and that, potentially, exert some anti-aging action, but not to the extent that your eye area will become unwrinkled!

PETER THOMAS ROTH MASCARA

✓☺ BEST **$$$ Lashes to Die For The Mascara** *($22)* is meant to serve as the partner product for Peter Thomas Roth's lash growth product, Lashes to Die For Platinum. That product should work about as well as Allergan's Latisse (available by prescription-only) because it contains the type of ingredients (known as prostaglandin analogues) that stimulate lash growth.

Cost-wise, they're about the same. Roth's Lashes to Die For The Mascara doesn't contain any ingredients that stimulate lash growth. It's just an expensive mascara, albeit a very good one, hence the rating. You'll get an impressive amount of length, moderate thickness, and a clean, clump-free application that wears beautifully. The rubber-bristled brush combines stubby and elongated bristles in a pattern than produces drama at the base of lashes and a soft, fringed effect at lash tips. It removes easily with a water-soluble cleanser. It's overpriced, but you aren't likely to be disappointed by its performance.

PHILOSOPHY (SKIN CARE ONLY)

Strengths: Relatively inexpensive; some of the best products are fragrance-free; very good retinol products; selection of state-of-the-art moisturizers; innovative skin-lightening product.

Weaknesses: Irritating and/or drying cleansers; average to problematic scrubs; at-home peel kits far more gimmicky than helpful; some products contain lavender oil; several products include irritating essential oils.

For more information and reviews of the latest philosophy products, visit CosmeticsCop.com.

PHILOSOPHY CLEANSERS

☹ POOR **clear days ahead oil-free salicylic acid acne treatment cleanser** (*$20 for 8 fl. oz.*) is medicated with anti-acne salicylic acid, but in a cleanser this ingredient is rinsed down the drain before it can benefit your skin (not to mention the pH of this cleanser is above the range salicylic acid needs to exfoliate). You're directed to massage this over your skin for 60 seconds, but doing so is ill-advised because the formula contains a couple of problematic ingredients. Chief among them is the main cleansing agent, sodium C14-16 olefin sulfonate. It can be quite drying, even for those with oily skin, and massaging this over your face for a minute only makes the potential dryness worse. Of lesser concern but still worth mention is the orange extract that lends this cleanser its citrus scent and the tiny amount of hydrogen peroxide, which can kill acne-causing bacteria, but also causes acute free-radical damage because it's so unstable. All told, there are gentler, less expensive cleansers those with acne-prone skin can consider. Paula's Choice CLEAR Normalizing Cleanser is one; you'll find others from Neutrogena as well as Clean & Clear (but choose carefully because both of those brands sell problematic cleansers, too).

☹ POOR **purity made simple mineral oil-free facial cleansing oil** (*$25 for 5.8 fl. oz.*) may be free of mineral oil, but it is loaded with fragrant oils known to cause irritation. The irony is that despite its bad reputation, mineral oil is among the gentlest, safest cosmetic ingredients in use, and the fragrant plant oils are among the worst, at least if your goal is healthy, younger-looking skin. Like most cleansing oils, this contains oil-like emollients and ingredients that, when mixed with water, form a milky emulsion that moves easily over the skin and removes all types of makeup, all without leaving a greasy residue. If not for the problematic fragrant oils, this would be worth a try, assuming you have normal to dry skin not prone to breakouts. As is, this is simply way too irritating to get even a provisional recommendation.

☹ POOR **purity made simple one-step cleansing bar for face and body** (*$20 for 7 fl. oz.*) is a problem for all skin types because of its form (bar cleansers tend to be drying and difficult to rinse), but also it is loaded with drying, soap ingredients and numerous irritating fragrant oils. This cleanser would be a mistake to use anywhere near the eyes because it contains black pepper oil, which is a potent irritant; in fact, according to the Environmental Protection Agency, it is used as a repellant for animals.

☹ POOR **purity made simple, one-step facial cleanser** *($20 for 8 fl. oz.)* is overloaded with irritating ingredients. The fact that it is listed as "Best of Sephora" merely means that lots of Sephora customers are using a cleanser that is hurting their skin. Fragrant oils are abundant in this cleanser, and all of them contain volatile components that are irritating to skin. Philosophy also included black pepper extract, just in case the fragrant oils weren't irritating enough. Those of you who use this cleanser may not see the irritation it causes because most of the irritation is taking place under the skin, where collagen is being damaged and free-radical damage is being generated, but it is happening nonetheless. For the health of your skin and your beauty budget, please consider switching to a truly gentle water-soluble cleanser.

☹ POOR **purity made simple one-step facial cleansing cloths** *($20 for 45 cloths)* are incredibly fragrant and an exercise in disaster for your skin. Although capable of cleansing and removing most types of makeup (waterproof and long-wearing formulas don't budge all that much), each cloth is steeped in potent plant-based irritants. Fragrant oils of sandalwood, sage, and amyris may smell great but what's good for your nose is a surefire way to cause skin irritation—even if you cannot see it happening. Repeated irritation from fragrant irritants like the ones in these cloths can cause collagen breakdown and hurt skin's healing process—two ways to stop looking younger and potentially stir up problems you'll be looking to correct with other products!

PHILOSOPHY EYE-MAKEUP REMOVER

✓☺ BEST **just release me dual-phase, extremely gentle, oil-free eye makeup remover** *($18 for 6 fl. oz.)* is a very good silicone-enhanced makeup remover that works beautifully to remove all types of makeup, including waterproof. It is fragrance-free and contains a good mix of soothing agents. You don't have to spend this much for a good makeup remover, but for those who choose to do so, this works great for all skin types.

PHILOSOPHY TONER

☹ POOR **hope springs eternal** *($20 for 5 fl. oz.)* is a spray-on toner—and misguided attempt to try to convince users that seawater is a rich source of nutrients for skin. There are nutrients in seawater, but there also are a lot of pollutants from animals, industry, and actual sewage, not to mention that the salt in seawater is drying and irritating. Our seas are not the pristine sources of life they're made out to be, and spraying seawater on your face isn't going to "feed" skin and give it a healthy glow. Beyond the seawater, you're getting a lot of fragrance and very small amounts of beneficial ingredients, making this a toner to avoid, though you can "hope" that philosophy eventually will offer a toner worth purchasing. One more comment: This toner contains the sensitizing preservative methylisothiazolinone, which is generally not recommended for use in leave-on products. Between this preservative and the high amount of fragrance, you've got a toner that puts skin at high risk for damaging irritation.

PHILOSOPHY EXFOLIANTS & SCRUBS

☺ GOOD $$$ **the microdelivery purifying peel, one-minute purifying enzyme peel** *($40 for 3 fl. oz.)* contains an effective amount (likely 8%-10%) of the AHA lactic acid along with enzymes, natural AHA-sound-alikes, and the BHA salicylic acid. Among those, only the lactic and salicylic acids are reliable exfoliants. The fruit extracts don't have exfoliating ability and the enzymes are notoriously unstable (not to mention that they can cause needless irritation and have nothing to do with purifying skin). The selling point of this AHA peel is that your skin is renewed and all-around better looking in one minute. That sounds great, right?

Not so fast: For AHAs and BHA at this concentration to really benefit your skin, they must be left on the skin, preferably for several hours. So, if used as philosophy directs (i.e., rinse within one minute), the exfoliants barely have time to begin working before they're rinsed off. Because the pH of this product allows exfoliation to occur, you should leave it on for five to ten minutes before rinsing. Don't want to spend this much? Not a problem: The benefits this product provides are attainable from other AHA or BHA products whose textures are more elegant and that are supposed to be left on your face for enhanced results. Please see the Best Products chapter for a list of brilliant AHA and BHA exfoliants.

☺ AVERAGE $$$ **the great mystery one-minute daily facial** *($25 for 5 fl. oz.)* is basically glycerin, water, sea salt, and thickeners, along with some token marine plant extracts and a tiny amount of lavender oil. Salt can be a problem for the skin due to its high pH and irritation potential, though it does work as a scrub, but for that purpose a simple washcloth will work even better. The only mystery is why more people don't do that instead of bothering with all these scrub particles scraping and abrading their faces.

☺ AVERAGE $$$ **the microdelivery exfoliating wash** *($25 for 8 fl. oz.)* contains a gentle detergent cleansing agent, but the clay it contains can be a bit drying for all but oily skin. The apple amino acids may sound farm fresh, but they have no ability to exfoliate skin, especially not in a product that is quickly rinsed away.

☺ AVERAGE $$$ **the microdelivery peel** *($68)* is a two-step at-home peel kit that ends up being more trouble than it's worth. Step 1 involves the **Vitamin C/Peptide Resurfacing Crystals**. This is essentially a baking soda scrub that contains silica for additional exfoliation and antioxidant vitamins, none of which will remain stable once this jar-packaged scrub is opened. You massage the Resurfacing Crystals over your skin for up to one minute, then apply Step 2, the **Lactic/Salicylic Acid Reactivating Gel**. This gel contains mostly water and lactic acid, and its pH of 2 interacts with the alkaline pH of the baking soda in the Resurfacing Crystals, which is what provides the immediate sensation of warmth. The warm feel doesn't mean the vitamin C and peptides are suddenly active, as philosophy claims; it's merely a chemical reaction. Not surprisingly, it leaves your skin very smooth after rinsing, just as it would be if you used a standard scrub with a washcloth. The lactic acid functions as an AHA product (with a pH that's definitely irritating), but its contact with skin is too brief to do much, so this is essentially a very expensive, potentially irritating baking soda scrub.

☹ POOR **the microdelivery mini peel pads** *($35 for 60 pads)* contain eucalyptus, tangerine, lemon, lavender, and orange oils, which make these AHA pads (lactic acid is on hand for exfoliation) too irritating for all skin types. If you want an effective AHA product that is free of needless irritants, consider the less expensive options from Alpha Hydrox, Neutrogena, or Paula's Choice.

☹ POOR **the microdelivery triple-acid brightening peel** *($68 for 12 pads)*. This fragrance-free at-home peel includes 12 individual applications, each with a pre-soaked pad that's packaged in its own pouch. You're supposed to use one peel per week, so this should last up to three months. Although that makes the price seem reasonable, the formula is a problem. Not only is the amount of alcohol cause for concern (see the Appendix for details), this contains barely any exfoliating ingredients (really the only contender is mandelic acid) and the pH is not within range for it to exfoliate. The azelaic acid is a good "brightening" ingredient due to its impact

♦ Irritating ingredients are a problem for all skin types. Find out why in the Appendix.

on melanin (skin pigment) production, but it needs to be used in a much greater amount than what this peel offers. All told, this ends up being a waste of time and money, and of course there's "zero downtime" because this doesn't work remotely like a doctor-administered facial peel.

☹ POOR **the oxygen peel kit** *($55)* is a two-step kit that contains oxygen foam and catalase enzyme capsules. The foam portion contains a good deal of hydrogen peroxide, which is not recommended for anyone, while the capsules contain the enzyme catalase, which is responsible for the elimination of peroxide. Taken together, this is a do-nothing duo that is not akin to any type of in-office professional peel.

PHILOSOPHY MOISTURIZERS (DAYTIME & NIGHTTIME), EYE CREAMS, & SERUMS

✓☺ BEST **$$$ miracle worker miraculous anti-aging neck cream** *($45 for 2 fl. oz.)* deserves its rating but before we begin complimenting this fragrance-free product's formula, it must be stated up front that you do not need a separate moisturizer for your neck. If you're using a well-formulated facial moisturizer (and you should be) you don't need a separate, special product for the neck. This product illustrates this beautifully because, despite being sold as a neck cream, the ingredients it contains are found in facial moisturizers, too. That doesn't mean this neck cream isn't worth considering; it is, provided you apply it to your face, too (no reason not to do this). The emollient formula is best for dry skin and contains a great blend of cell-communicating ingredients, antioxidants galore, and some helpful repairing and soothing ingredients. We restate that none of these ingredients are unique to skin on the neck, but without question they will help the neck (and, as mentioned, the face) look smoother, feel softer, and be better able to repair signs of aging. What this neck cream will not do is lift sagging skin or prevent a "corded" look that occurs with age as the platsyma muscle shifts. Those concerns can only be addressed via cosmetic surgery, not skin care, so please do not waste your money on neck creams if those are your concerns.

✓☺ BEST **$$$ miracle worker spf55 miraculous anti-aging fluid** *($57 for 1.7 fl. oz.)* isn't a miracle worker—that is, it doesn't significantly differ from the other daytime moisturizers with sunscreen we recommend—it is an outstanding option due to its combination of broad-spectrum sun protection and anti-aging ingredients. The light, fluid texture is ideal for normal to oily skin prone to breakouts. Critical UVA (think anti-aging) protection is supplied by stabilized avobenzone, and skin is treated to an impressive mix of antioxidants, a cell-communicating peptide, and beneficial plant extracts. As a skin-caring bonus, the formula is fragrance-free. One concern: Given this product's cost, you may not apply it as liberally as you should. Liberal application is essential to get the amount of sun protection stated on the label, so be sure you're OK with needing to repurchase this product every couple of months (that's about how often you're likely to go through it with daily application to your face and neck). As well-formulated as this moisturizer with sunscreen is, there are less expensive options from other brands.

☺ GOOD **$$$ eye hope advanced anti-aging eye cream** *($49 for 0.5 fl. oz.)* is one of philosophy's better moisturizers. It is suitable for dry skin anywhere on the face, but ironically isn't the best for use in the eye area because it contains fragrant sandalwood extract. That's really the only strike against this otherwise well-formulated product. It contains mineral pigments that add shine to skin to improve the appearance of dark circles, but it does not contain any ingredients that have a permanent effect on lightening dark circles. The same is true for the eye puffiness–reducing claims, although that doesn't change the fact that this is overall a very good moisturizer in packaging that keeps the light- and air-sensitive ingredients stable during use. See the Appendix to learn why, in truth, you really don't need an eye cream.

☺ GOOD **$$$ hope in a tube** *($33 for 0.5 fl. oz.)* is a thick, emollient-rich, fragrance-free cream that will take excellent care of dry, dehydrated skin anywhere on the body, but it won't firm skin one iota. Of course, given the small amount of product, this is best reserved for use on the face, and would work well around the eyes if that area is dry. Classic moisturizing standbys such as glycerin, petrolatum, and mineral oil comprise the bulk of the formula, and philosophy included a few antioxidants, too.

☺ GOOD **$$$ miracle worker miraculous anti-aging eye cream** *($60 for 0.45 fl. oz.)* is a good though not miraculous eye cream for normal to slightly dry skin around the eyes or anywhere on the face. The formula blends classic and state-of-the-art ingredients, though some of the classics (like wax) are dated and don't give this product the most elegant or silky texture. If you want to experience an efficacious amount of retinol along with some good cell-communicating ingredients and smaller amounts of antioxidants, this is worth considering. It's packaged to keep the light- and air-sensitive ingredients stable during use, which is critical to maintaining efficacy during use. Despite our enthusiasm for this product's anti-aging benefits, please know that you don't need an eye cream! There is not a single ingredient in this eye cream that doesn't show up in facial moisturizers, too, including those with retinol. Note that the tiny amount of alcohol in this eye cream is unlikely to be problematic.

☺ GOOD **$$$ when hope is not enough facial firming and lifting serum** *($40 for 1 fl. oz.)* contains mostly water, film-forming agent, slip agents, glycerin, water-binding agents, anti-oxidants, anti-irritant, pH adjuster, fragrance, and preservatives. It is a worthwhile, serum-type moisturizer for normal to slightly oily skin because it supplies hydrating agents, antioxidants, and cell-communicating ingredients without thickeners, oils, or oil-like ingredients. This product won't lift skin (see the Appendix for details), and it won't help minimize facial hair growth as claimed because it contains no ingredients with proven ability to do that.

☹ AVERAGE **$$$ eyes wide open instant refreshing eye gel** *($45 for 0.85 fl. oz.)* is an OK, lightweight moisturizer for slightly dry skin anywhere on the face. The fragrance-free formula is suitable for use around the eyes, but you don't need a special eye-area product (see the Appendix to find out why). This cannot de-puff eyes or make them look more awake, at least not anymore than using a cold compress or splashing the face with cold water will make one look more alert. The amount of film-forming agent (think hairspray) this eye gel contains may make skin feel temporarily tighter, but that's not the same as actually tightening loose skin, and it has no impact on puffiness—though it does pose a risk of irritation.

☹ AVERAGE **$$$ help me retinol night treatment** *($38 for 0.75 fl. oz.)* is a moisturizer with retinol that works best for normal to very dry skin not prone to blemishes (the amount of wax can aggravate breakouts). Content-wise, retinol isn't given more prominence here than it is in several drugstore lines. Although this is stably packaged and fragrance-free, the overall formula isn't as exciting as the options on our Best Retinol Products list at the end of this book. Note that contrary to claim, this product cannot "clear congested pores." Not only is the texture quite thick, but also retinol is not an exfoliant. Retinol can change how skin cells are created (making damaged cells healthier), but it does not exfoliate like an AHA or BHA product.

☹ AVERAGE **$$$ hope in a jar, original formula** *($39 for 2 fl. oz.)* is sold as philosophy's world-famous therapeutic moisturizer, but it's a rather ordinary formula that does not contain lactic acid as claimed. Instead, this has lauryl lactate, which is the ester of lauric and lactic acids. Although the product has a pH of 3.2, lauryl lactate does not have exfoliating abilities; rather it functions as an emulsifier and enhances the spreadability of creams. Jar packaging won't keep the antioxidants in this product stable, and it's really not deserving of its alleged worldwide fame.

☺ AVERAGE **$$$ hope oil-free moisturizer SPF 30** *($39 for 2 fl. oz.)* is an OK, though needlessly pricey daytime moisturizer with sunscreen for normal to slightly dry or slightly oily skin. The promised matte finish isn't all that matte and it won't keep oily areas shine-free for long. Although this provides very good broad-spectrum sun protection (zinc oxide is among the active ingredients), for the money it lacks a sufficient amount of antioxidants and anti-irritants. This ends up being too ordinary for the face when better formulated sunscreens abound in the world of skin care. As for the oil-free claim, take note: Although the formula doesn't contain oils, it does include some ingredients that feel like oils, so this isn't as light as philosophy would have you believe.

☺ AVERAGE **$$$ miracle worker miraculous anti-aging moisturizer** *($57 for 2 fl. oz.)* is a beautifully silky moisturizer for normal to dry skin, so it is a huge shame that it's packaged in a jar. The formula contains several beneficial antioxidants (including an impressive amount of a vitamin C derivative) and nonfragrant plant oils, but all of them will become less potent with each use given the daily exposure to light and air. This is a gentle fragrance-free formula, so again, it's a shame that the ingredients you're paying extra for won't hold up for long because of the packaging. See the Appendix for further details and research supporting why jar packaging is a problem you shouldn't overlook.

☹ AVERAGE **$$$ miracle worker miraculous anti-aging retinoid pads and solution** *($72 for 60 applications)* is ridiculously packaged. You get 60 pads along with a 2-ounce bottle of solution. The directions tell you to pour the entire contents of the solution into the jar of pads, steeping all of them at once. Why philosophy didn't just do that ahead of time is a good question, but it may be because they wanted to keep the air-sensitive ingredients in the solution stable. The thing is, once you've soaked the pads and toss the bottle, you're exposing the delicate ingredients to air and light with each use. The solution is a form of silicone with solvents that aid penetration; these solvents have an oxygenating effect when mixed with water, so it's a good thing this is a nonaqueous product. Then again, we don't know what happens when these solvents contact skin and mix with its water content, but, theoretically, it could prompt oxygenation that leads to free-radical damage. philosophy includes a type of retinol they refer to as HPR, an acronym for hydroxypinacolone retinoate. The company maintains that this form of retinol boosts surface cell turnover rate without irritation. The lack of irritation is the big sell here; lots of consumers concerned with mitigating signs of aging know that a prescription retinoid (such as Renova) is a better option than a cosmetic, but that tolerance is an issue for many, and for some it means that retinoids are best avoided. Does philosophy have the answer for those whose skin cannot tolerate traditional retinoids? Possibly, but you'll have to take their word for it because there is no substantiated research proving that hydroxypinacolone retinoate is a viable option for treating wrinkled, sun-damaged skin. However, there is research demonstrating that other forms of retinoate, such as retinyl retinoate and retinyl gallate 6, improve wrinkles and enhance healthy collagen production without notable irritation (Sources: *The British Journal of Dermatology*, August 2009, Epublication; and *Bioorganic and Medicinal Chemistry*, June 2008, pages 6387–6393). Of course, there are volumes of research attesting to retinol's ability to improve aging skin in numerous ways, but we suppose simply touting "plain" retinol in this product wouldn't make it seem like such a miracle worker. Getting back to the ingredient hydroxypinacolone retinoate; the only information pertaining to its efficacy comes from Grant Industries, the company that sells this ingredient to cosmetics brands. Their sole study on the effectiveness and claims for this retinoid involved five people, which is not nearly a large enough sample to declare that this retinoid is the one to beat (Source:http://grantinc.

The Reviews P

com/cosmetics/active_series/granactive_rd 101.php). It's a leap of faith (a lo-o-o-ong leap) that the retinoid in miracle worker is going to work as claimed. There are antioxidants in the formula to support the company's anti-aging claims, but if you follow directions and pour the solution over the pads, you're rendering both the retinoid and the antioxidants less effective with each use—and without those ingredients, this product won't be of much use to anyone.

☺ AVERAGE $$$ **when hope is not enough replenishing cream** *($48 for 2 fl. oz.)* is an emollient moisturizer whose best, price-justifying ingredients will break down once this jar-packaged product is opened. This will help dry skin look and feel better, but so will many less expensive moisturizers.

☺ AVERAGE **when hope is not enough smoothing vitamin c/e/peptide cream for neck and decollete** *($35 for 2 fl. oz.)* is a creamy, emollient-rich moisturizer that covers the basics for those with dry skin thanks to its blend of restorative ingredients, but it isn't as state-of-the-art as many other moisturizers and does not contain anything special for skin on your neck or chest (decollete). Given the product's name, the vitamins and peptides should be higher up on the list than they are. However, the overall blend is good and the formula contains some proven antioxidants. What's missing is a more impressive blend of skin-repairing ingredients and some anti-irritants to help skin recover from previous damage.

☹ POOR **27 wishes multi-purpose skin nurturing balm** *($18 for 1 fl. oz.)* contains irritating fragrant oils, none of which help solve "multiple skin concerns." If anything, using this product can potentially create more problems than you started with, and that's the wrong way to go about solving a problem! This balm-like moisturizer starts out well, with skin-repairing glycerin as the first ingredient and some very good, nonfragrant emollient plant oils. It also includes two forms of vitamin E for an antioxidant boost, but the numerous irritating oils that follow spell trouble for all skin types. Please see the Appendix to learn why irritation from fragrant ingredients is bad.

☹ POOR **divine illumination** *($85 for 1.6 fl. oz.)* is a very fragrant moisturizer that softly illuminates skin with the mineral pigments titanium dioxide and mica. This cosmetic effect can be pretty, but you can get it from countless other products that don't subject your skin to the irritating fragrant oils that are present in divine illumination. Moreover, the antioxidants in this moisturizer won't remain potent for long due to the jar packaging. The amount of niacinamide means it can have a positive effect on skin discolorations, but this ingredient is available in other products (such as those from Olay or Paula's Choice) that not only cost less but also spare your skin the irritation and skin damage that will result from the alcohol in this product (the fourth ingredient). See the Appendix to learn why alcohol in skin care is a problem.

☹ POOR **hope in a bottle** *($39 for 2 fl. oz.)* contains an unspecified amount of salicylic acid, but regardless of the amount, the pH of this moisturizer is too high for preferred levels of exfoliation to occur. It is not recommended because it contains lavender oil (see the Appendix for details) and lacks any significant amounts of beneficial ingredients.

☹ POOR **hope in a jar, extra-rich moisturizer for normal to dry skin** *($39 for 2 fl. oz.)* is completely inappropriate for any skin type because it contains lavender and sage oils, both of which have components that are irritating to skin and destructive to cells (see the Appendix for details).

☹ POOR **hope in a jar oil-free moisturizer for normal to oily skin** *($39 for 2 fl. oz.)* is misnamed because it's actually packaged in a tube, which is preferred to a jar anytime a formula contains light- and air-sensitive ingredients as this product does. While technically oil-free, a main ingredient in this somewhat thick lotion is a plant wax blend that acts similarly to oil, except it's heavier. Those with oily, shiny skin won't find this moisturizer reduces either issue, and in fact it may make skin oilier. Why? Because like many philosophy moisturizers, this contains lavender oil, a fragrant irritant with no established benefit for skin. Lavender oil, even when used in small amounts, can cause skin-cell death and enhance oxidative damage. Meanwhile, the irritation it prompts can stimulate more oil production at the base of the pores, making matters worse. Without the lavender oil (and this product smells strongly of it), this would be a good moisturizer for normal to dry skin. See the Appendix for further info on lavender and how irritation hurts oily skin.

☹ POOR **hope in a jar SPF 20 extra-rich moisturizer for normal to dry skin** *($39 for 2 fl. oz.)* provides hope for protecting your skin from the sun thanks to this daytime moisturizer's in-part avobenzone sunscreen. It also contains small amounts of several beneficial ingredients for skin, such as antioxidants and cell-communicating peptides. The texture of this product makes it best for its intended skin types, but the formula has one major weakness that makes it impossible to recommend: lavender oil. This fragrant oil won't do the same favor for your skin as it might for your nose. See the Appendix to find out why avoiding lavender oil is a skin care must!

☹ POOR **hope in a jar SPF 25 daily moisturizer for all skin types** *($39 for 2 fl. oz.)* is similar to philosophy's hope in a jar oil-free moisturizer for normal to oily skin above, except this is a bit thicker and contains an in-part avobenzone sunscreen. Otherwise, the same comments apply.

☹ POOR **keep the peace super soothing moisturizer for redness and sensitivity** *($38 for 2 fl. oz.)* is marketed to those with sensitive, dry skin, and does contain some excellent ingredients to help reinforce skin's surface and reduce inflammation. That's why it's so disappointing to report that it also contains a high amount of lavender oil. Although this fragrant plant oil has a soothing aroma, fragrance isn't skin care. In fact, lavender oil can cause skin-cell death and enhance oxidative damage. This is also packaged in a jar, which won't keep key ingredients stable during use. See the Appendix to learn more about the problems associated with lavender oil and jar packaging.

☹ POOR **keep the peace super soothing serum for redness and sensitivity** *($38 for 0.9 fl. oz.)* is supposed to calm redness and irritation, and improve sensitive skin. Although the formula (which is best for dry skin) contains some excellent restorative and soothing ingredients, it is a problem for sensitive skin due to the inclusion of lavender oil. Regrettably, that single ingredient means this serum is a poor choice for sensitive skin. And remember, even if you cannot see or feel the damage, it's still happening and keeping your skin from improving to a greater degree. Refer to the Appendix for details and research on why lavender oil is bad for skin.

☹ POOR **miracle worker miraculous anti-aging concentrate** *($62 for 0.95 fl. oz.)* has a name that's a bad joke and a formula that's even less funny. The "breakthrough" technology in here is like saying a skateboard is the latest in transportation. Although this serum does contain some very good antioxidants along with peptides, which, in theory, have cell-communicating ability that may result in younger-looking, healthier skin, there is nothing in here unique to philosophy. What keeps this serum from earning a recommendation is the inclusion of the preservative methylisothiazolinone, which is contraindicated for use in leave-on products due to its sensitizing potential (Sources: *Chemical Research in Toxicology*, February 2005, pages 324–329; *Contact Dermatitis*, November 2001, pages 257–264; and *European Journal of Dermatology*, March 1999, pages 144–160). Interestingly, when we perused online consumer reviews of this product, we noticed several women wrote that they experienced red, stinging skin, which isn't surprising given the inclusion of methylisothiazolinone. Ironically, philosophy

The Reviews P

likely included this preservative to replace parabens, and parabens have a pretty stellar track record for not causing skin reactions. Despite the claims to the contrary, parabens are not the evil, harmful group of preservatives many brands make them out to be. Perhaps the real miracle is how philosophy can convince women that this product is the anti-aging serum to buy! We would be far more convinced if philosophy's formula were supported by published research, but that's not the way most cosmetics brands operate.

☹ POOR **shelter, untinted SPF 30** *($25 for 4 fl. oz.)* would rate a Best Product for sun protection if it did not contain lavender oil (see the Appendix for details). The in-part titanium dioxide sunscreen and silky lotion base with plentiful antioxidants could have been a great option for those with normal to dry skin.

☹ POOR **the oxygen boost daily energizing oxygen elixir** *($50 for 1 fl. oz.)* is a serum-like product that's a classic example of cosmetics double-talk because its claims lead you to believe it provides oxygen to skin, while also supplying antioxidants to fight signs of aging. Given that these two actions are diametrically opposed, how can anyone's skin possibly benefit? The answer is it can't, and it may actually make matters worse. Although this water-based serum doesn't contain pure oxygen, it contains a fluorocarbon (chemically inert compound), which increases the oxygen content in liquids. Research has made it abundantly clear that oxygen, despite the fact that we need it to stay alive, is also a source of free-radical damage throughout the entire body (Sources: *Phytotherapy Research*, November 2010, Epublication; *Current Drug Metabolism*, June 2010, pages 409–424; and *Human and Experimental Toxicology*, February 2002, pages 61–62). Giving your skin more oxygen than what occurs naturally is anti-aging in the wrong direction: pro-aging! This product also lists alcohol as its second ingredient. Alcohol causes dryness, free-radical damage, and hinders healthy collagen production (see the Appendix for details). The formula also contains some plant extracts known to cause irritation, which will only make matters worse. The mineral and metal pigments this contains cast a subtle glow to skin, but that's a makeup effect, not a boost of radiance from skin getting more oxygen. Please don't fall for this product's appearance on skin because you can achieve this effect from many other products that don't put your skin at such risk of damage.

PHILOSOPHY SUN CARE

✓☺ BEST $$$ **here comes the sun age-defense water-resistant SPF 30 UVA/UVB broad-spectrum sunscreen** *($26 for 4 fl. oz.)* is a very good, fragrance-free, water-resistant sunscreen that includes avobenzone for sufficient UVA (think anti-aging) protection. It has a silky, somewhat thick lotion texture that's best for normal to dry skin. As for the "age defense," you're getting that in spades with any well-formulated sunscreen because unprotected sun exposure is a major cause of most signs of aging. But philosophy went further by including several antioxidants and repairing ingredients to boost skin's defenses in and out of the sun. If you're going to spend in this range for a sunscreen for use from the neck down, this is the kind of formula you want to use, because it goes beyond just protecting skin from sunburn.

✓☺ BEST $$$ **here comes the sun age-defense water-resistant SPF 40 UVA/UVB broad-spectrum sunscreen for face** *($30 for 2 fl. oz.)* is strikingly similar to the here comes the sun age-defense water-resistant SPF 30 product above, and the same review applies. Both of these sunscreens may be applied to the face, and you're getting a better deal with the SPF 30 version.

☺ GOOD $$$ **here comes the sun gradual glow self-tanner for body** *($28 for 4 fl. oz.)* is a standard, but good, self-tanner. Although the name says "body," which implies from the neck down, this can also be applied to the face. It's actually a better formula than the version philosophy offers for the face, though like their facial self-tanner, this body version contains fragrance ingredients that pose a risk of irritation. The amounts are low, which is good, but if self-tanner is something you apply often, consider a fragrance-free formula to spare your skin from irritation. In addition to dihydroxyacetone (DHA), the ingredient in most self-tanners that bronzes skin, this also contains the slower-acting self-tanning ingredient erythrulose, so you get color in a few hours that deepens within a day or so. That's nice, but not unique to this product. The amount of DHA in this self-tanner makes it suitable for fair to medium skin. Ultimately, this would earn our top rating if not for the concern over the fragrance ingredients. Unlike many self-tanners, this contains some notable antioxidants and repairing ingredients. As such, it goes beyond merely turning skin tan.

☺ AVERAGE **$$$ here comes the sun age-defense gradual glow self-tanner for face** *($26 for 2 fl. oz.)* is a standard, but good, self-tanner that is marketed for use on facial skin but it may be applied anywhere on the body. Whether or not you want to do that comes down to price (there are countless self-tanners that produce great results yet cost much less than this) and whether you want to expose your skin to the fragrance ingredients this self-tanner contains.

☺ AVERAGE **$$$ here comes the sun age-defense very water-resistant SPF 30 UVA/ UVB broad-spectrum spray sunscreen for the body** *($26 for 4 fl. oz.)* has so much going for it, including reliable broad-spectrum protection and antioxidants aplenty. Unfortunately, the base formula contains enough alcohol to be potentially irritating for all skin types. Not only is alcohol an irritant on its own, but also when joined with the active ingredients in this sunscreen, it increases the chance that your skin will suffer a sensitized reaction. Without the alcohol, this would be a good, though pricey, spray-on sunscreen for all skin types. philosophy's range of antioxidants is truly impressive; what a shame the base of the formula doesn't reach the same feat.

PHILOSOPHY LIP & SMILE CARE

☺ AVERAGE **$$$ kiss me tonight** *($20 for 0.3 fl. oz.)* has an exceptionally emollient base that takes very good care of dry, chapped lips, although the formula would be better without fragrance, and it is very fragrant! Caution is warranted because this contains a small amount of neem leaf extract. This plant is known to be problematic with long-term use when ingested, and given that we ingest a certain amount of lip balm each time we apply, this may end up being an issue. Ingestion of neem leaf can lead to liver and kidney problems, but the dosage must be higher than it is in this product. Neem is not recommended for ingestion by pregnant women (Source: naturaldatabase.com).

☹ POOR **kiss me very emollient lip balm** *($10 for 0.5 fl. oz.)* is emollient like the name states, but it also contains a high amount of peppermint oil, which makes it too irritating for regular use. The tingle from the peppermint may feel refreshing, but it's your lips telling you they're being irritated—and this irritation can lead to collagen breakdown and worsen chronically dry, chapped lips.

☹ POOR **kiss me very emollient SPF 20 lip balm clear** *($12 for 0.5 fl. oz.)* has a sunscreen whose actives do not provide sufficient UVA protection plus it contains irritating peppermint oil. This is a step in the wrong direction, philosophy! The same review applies to **kiss me very emollient SPF 20 lip balm red** ($12 for 0.5 fl. oz.).

☹ POOR **kiss me exfoliating lip scrub and facial** *($15 for 0.5 fl. oz.)* is an emollient sugar-based scrub for lips that works to remove dry, flaky skin and leave it smooth. The problem? Peppermint oil, which only causes irritation, which will make dry, flaky lips worse in the long run.

☹ POOR **kiss of hope SPF 15** *($16 for 0.12 fl. oz.)* has two major flaws that make it not worth considering: The sunscreen fails to provide sufficient UVA protection (see the Appendix for details) and the base formula contains an unusually high amount of fragrance. Whether on your lips or face, fragrance isn't skin care. Your lips may feel kissable with "kiss of hope" on them, but they'll still be vulnerable to sun damage.

PHILOSOPHY SPECIALTY SKIN-CARE PRODUCTS

✓☺ BEST **$$$ clear days ahead oil-free salicylic acid acne treatment & moisturizer** *($39 for 2 fl. oz.)* is a very good BHA (salicylic acid) exfoliant for acne-prone skin. It's medicated with 1% salicylic acid and its pH of 3.6 ensures it will function as an exfoliant. Surprisingly, the formula doesn't contain irritants such as fragrant oils or alcohol—a rarity in anti-acne products—and it's fragrance-free! The silky, slightly hydrating lotion texture treats skin to a beneficial blend of fatty acids (which may help reduce inflammation from acne) as well as cell-communicating ingredients and antioxidant vitamin E (listed as tocopheryl acetate). Really, the only drawback is the price; you can spend half as much yet get nearly twice the amount of product with the BHA exfoliants from Paula's Choice. But if you're sold on philosophy, this is definitely one of their better products to consider.

✓☺ BEST **$$$ miracle worker dark spot corrector** *($62 for 1 fl. oz.)* claims to treat brown spots and other discolorations from sun damage and is a great contender with ingredients backed by published research! The lightweight, fragrance-free hydrating lotion texture contains several ingredients capable of interrupting the process that causes brown spots to form and stick around. Chief among them is niacinamide, but others include two forms of stabilized vitamin C, some great antioxidants, and a novel ingredient known as undecylenoyl phenylalanine. This white powder is composed of amino acids and appears to work by interfering with the pathways in skin that cause excess melanin production (melanin is what these spots are made of). Concentrations of at least 2% are needed for noticeable results, and that appears to be in line with what philosophy used in this product. Other research has shown that this ingredient works even better when combined with niacinamide, which is the case here (Sources: *Journal of Cosmetic Dermatology*, September 2011, pages 189–196 and December 2009, pages 260–266; and *Clinical Experiments in Dermatology*, July 2010, pages 473–476). In addition to the skin-lightening and brightening ingredients, this contains several repairing ingredients to bring about further improvements in skin tone and texture. And it is packaged to ensure the ingredients remain stable during use, which is precisely what you want (and especially at this price). Suitable for all skin types except very oily, miracle worker dark spot corrector ranks among philosophy's best products. It deserves strong consideration if your skin is unable to tolerate the gold standard lightening active hydroquinone (whether over-the-counter or prescription). Keep in mind that as with any skin-lightening product, daily use of a well-formulated sunscreen rated SPF 15 or greater (and greater is better) is essential (really, really essential) to prevent existing brown spots from becoming worse and to stop new brown spots from appearing. Don't bother with any skin-lightening product if you're unwilling to commit to daily sun protection, rain, clouds, or shine.

☺ GOOD **$$$ clear days ahead fast-acting salicylic acid acne spot treatment** *($18 for 0.5 fl. oz.)*. We struggled with how to rate this BHA exfoliant for acne-prone skin. On the one hand, it's medicated with 2% BHA (salicylic acid) and its pH of 3.5 ensures it will work as an exfoliant. The silky, fragrance-free lotion formula also contains some anti-irritants and cell-communicating ingredients that are helpful for (and indeed the formula is suitable for) all skin types. On the other hand, this is pricey for such a tiny amount of product (though, cutting philosophy some slack, they do sell this as a spot treatment) and the amount of alcohol is potential cause for concern. We could smell the alcohol emanating from this BHA exfoliant, though based on the formula the amount is likely less than 3%. Ultimately, we decided to rate this as "GOOD" due to its efficacy and potential to help breakout-prone skin—but we're adding the caveat that there are other, less expensive BHA exfoliants you may want to consider, including those from Paula's Choice, that do not contain alcohol.

☹ POOR **clear days ahead overnight repair salicylic acid acne treatment pads** *($39 for 60 pads)*. Like countless anti-acne products that came before it, these clear days ahead pads contain a high amount of skin-damaging alcohol. See the Appendix to learn why alcohol is a problem for all skin types, and learn how irritating ingredients make oily, acne-prone skin worse. The pads are steeped in a solution that contains 0.5% salicylic acid as well as the AHA ingredients glycolic and mandelic acids. The combined amount of these ingredients plus the formula's pH of 3.6 ensures exfoliation occurs, but the alcohol is too big a risk to ignore—there are other exfoliants that work without causing undue irritation.

☹ POOR **keep the peace super soothing instant relief mask for redness and sensitive skin** *($40 for 4 fl. oz.)* features a blend of absorbent clay and moisturizing ingredients. That's a strange mix because the absorbent clay keeps the moisturizing ingredients from hydrating as well as they otherwise would and the moisturizing ingredients work against the absorbent action of the clay. This could be overlooked and we could recommend this mask as an OK option for normal to slightly oily skin, but the formula is problematic for its intended audience of those with sensitive skin. Although philosophy includes some good soothing agents and antioxidants, they added skin-damaging lavender oil. See the Appendix to learn why this fragrant plant oil is bad for everyone's skin.

☹ POOR **lasting hope instant refreshing moisture mask** *($25 for 2 fl. oz.)* is a nicely formulated mask for dry skin. Although this contains some reparative, hydrating ingredients, the lavender oil is a strong skin irritant, even in low amounts, which makes this mask impossible to recommend. See the Appendix for further details on lavender oil.

PHYSICIANS FORMULA

Strengths: Inexpensive; almost all products fragrance-free; outstanding cleansers; pressed powders with broad-spectrum sunscreen; several bronzing powder options (primarily for fair to light skin tones); one of the only lines at the drugstore selling matte finish eyeshadows; the loose powder; most of the blushes; good liquid liner; excellent automatic brow pencil.

Weaknesses: Dated moisturizer formulas; several sunscreens lack sufficient UVA protection; jar packaging; several of the makeup products epitomize wasteful packaging; the shade selection for almost all the foundations and concealers is awful; tons of gimmicky products that don't perform as well as you'd think but are eye-catching in their compacts; the lip color and lip plumper; mostly average to disappointing mascaras; Organic Wear products either have undesirable textures or contain irritating ingredients.

For more information and reviews of the latest Physicians Formula products, visit CosmeticsCop.com.

PHYSICIANS FORMULA CLEANSERS

✓☺ BEST **Gentle Cleansing Lotion, for Normal to Dry Skin** *($7.25 for 8 fl. oz.)* is a very standard, but also very good, fragrance-free cleansing lotion for its intended skin type.

It is also recommended for those with sensitive skin who cannot tolerate detergent cleansing agents. You will need a washcloth for complete removal.

✓☺ BEST **Hydrating & Balancing Cleanser** *($11.95 for 5 fl. oz.)* is a very good water-soluble cleanser for all skin types except very dry. The fragrance-free formula produces a mild lather and works well to remove most types of makeup without leaving skin dry or tight. It rinses without a residue and doesn't contain potentially irritating ingredients, which is exactly how a well-formulated cleanser should be.

☺ GOOD **Redness Relief Cleanser, Formula RX 301** *($11.95 for 5 fl. oz.)* is an emollient, creamy cleansing lotion that is indeed an option for dry, sensitive skin. It contains gentle ingredients to cleanse and remove makeup, but because this doesn't rinse easily on its own, you'll want to use it with a washcloth to avoid leaving a noticeable residue. As for redness relief, this contains some proven soothing plant extracts and the formula is fragrance-free, always an important consideration for those struggling with sensitive, reddened skin. The soothing ingredients are a nice touch, but keep in mind that these types of ingredients provide the most benefit when included in leave-on products. This missed our top rating due to the rinsability issue mentioned above and also because it contains artificial coloring agents, which really don't belong in a product marketed to sensitive skin.

☹ AVERAGE **Wrinkle Corrector & Firming Cleanser, Formula RX 101** *($11.95 for 5 fl. oz.)* contains nothing "correcting" or firming; it's just an extremely standard, mineral oil–based cleanser. However, because of the amount of mineral oil it contains, it can soften skin and, to a minor extent, soften the appearance of wrinkles as you cleanse. That's nice, but it doesn't change the fact that this cleansing lotion is difficult to rinse without the aid of a washcloth, and any gentle cleansing lotion can help soften the appearance of wrinkles, especially if your skin is dry. This removes makeup easily and its formula makes it best for dry skin. Although fragrance isn't listed, this contains the ingredient ethylene brassylate, whose sole function in skin-care products is … fragrance. The amount isn't high, and this is a rinse-off product so the fragrance is less cause for concern, but for best results, stick with cleansers that are truly fragrance-free.

PHYSICIANS FORMULA EYE-MAKEUP REMOVERS

✓☺ BEST **Eye Makeup Remover Lotion, for Normal to Dry Skin** *($4.75 for 2 fl. oz.)* has a formula that's remarkably similar to the Gentle Cleansing Lotion, for Normal to Dry Skin above, except this version is marketed as a makeup remover. It works in that capacity, even removing waterproof mascara, but if you're already using or considering the Gentle Cleansing Lotion, you don't need this too.

☹ POOR **Organic Wear 100% Natural Origin Eye Makeup Remover Liquid** *($6.95 for 4 fl. oz.)* contains plant extracts that may be organic, but that doesn't inherently make them better for your skin. The orange fruit water base, coupled with radish root extract and lavender oil, are not what you want to apply because they are irritating and problematic for skin anywhere on the face, especially around the eyes. Ouch!

☹ POOR **Organic Wear 100% Natural Origin Eye Makeup Remover Pads** *($6.95 for 60 pads)* contain fragrant orange fruit water as a main ingredient and also contain the potent irritants lemon peel and lavender oils. These are a mistake to use anywhere near the eyes or on the face for that matter, and, organic or not, lavender causes skin-cell death and increases oxidative damage (see the Appendix for details).

☹ POOR **Organic Wear 100% Natural Origin Facial Makeup Remover Lotion** *($6.95 for 5 fl. oz.)* would be a good option if not for the amount of orange fruit water and the inclusion of lavender oil. You'd be better off removing your makeup with pure jojoba, safflower, or olive oil—all of which are natural and have none of the cell-damaging effects.

☹ POOR **Organic Wear 100% Natural Origin Makeup Remover Towelettes** *($6.95 for 25 towelettes)* contain far too many "natural" irritants to make them a wise choice for makeup removal. Using an organic, nonfragrant plant oil would be a much better solution.

PHYSICIANS FORMULA TONERS

☺ AVERAGE **Instant Skin Calming Spray, Formula RX 321** *($19.95 for 4 fl. oz.)* is one of the better toners available at drugstores, although considering how most toners are average to poor formulas, that's not really saying much. This deserves credit for being alcohol- and fragrance-free and for including a good group of soothing plant extracts and standard but effective water-binding agents. It's a good option for normal to dry or sensitive skin, but there are better toners outside the drugstore environment. For example, Paula's Choice Skin Recovery Toner contains soothing plant extracts like this toner, but also contains a range of proven skin-repairing and cell-communicating ingredients, plus other beneficial substances. Had this Physician's Formula toner included a broader range of ingredients, it would've earned our highest rating.

☹ POOR **Pore Refining Skin Freshener, for Normal to Dry Skin** *($6.95 for 8 fl. oz.)* is mostly water and alcohol, and as such is an undesirable option, especially for dry skin. See the Appendix to learn why alcohol is bad news in skin care products.

PHYSICIANS FORMULA MOISTURIZERS (DAYTIME & NIGHTTIME), EYE CREAMS, & SERUMS

☺ AVERAGE **Deep Wrinkle Corrector Day & Night Cream, Formula RX 121** *($19.95 for 1.7 fl. oz.)* is sold as a day and night cream, but we don't advise using it during the daytime unless you're willing to pair it with a separate product rated SPF 15 or greater. This contains the AHA ingredient lactic acid, and the company states it is a 3% concentration, which, combined with this product's pH, means the lactic acid will provide some exfoliating benefits. Although 3% lactic acid isn't much (for AHAs, a range of 5%-10% is considered best), you should see some benefit. Although this product has merit, it also has two considerable drawbacks: Jar packaging won't keep several key ingredients stable once the product has been opened (see the Appendix for further details), and the formula falls short on offering a good array of proven anti-aging ingredients. It does contain some antioxidants, including a teeny-tiny amount of antioxidant vitamins, but their benefit is lost due to the poor choice of jar packaging. Although fragrance isn't listed, this contains the ingredient ethylene brassylate, whose sole function in skin-care products is fragrance.

☺ AVERAGE **Hydrating & Balancing Moisturizer SPF 15 Formula Rx211** *($19.95 for 1.7 fl. oz.)* is a very basic, overpriced daytime moisturizer with sunscreen. Although it may seem inexpensive compared to similar options from drugstore brands such as Olay or Neutrogena, the formula here just isn't exciting enough to justify the cost. This provides broad-spectrum sun protection and includes stabilized avobenzone for critical UVA protection, but so do lots of other daytime moisturizers that treat skin to beneficial ingredients such as antioxidants and repairing substances. This lightweight formula is merely an OK option for normal to slightly dry skin. It cannot balance anything. Interestingly, one of the plant extracts (*Tremella fuciformis*) is a species of tree fungus that produces a flowering fruit. This plant extract has no known benefit for skin.

☺ AVERAGE **Hydrating Eye Cream, Formula RX 222** *($19.95 for 0.5 fl. oz.)* is a light-weight eye lotion (it doesn't have a true cream texture) that feels silky and contains some very good hydrating ingredients. However, in many ways, its formula is so similar to a lightweight facial moisturizer that it's further proof of why you don't need an eye cream (see the Appendix to find out why). One concern is the plant extract *Fraxinus excelsior* bark. As stated on the Natural Medicines Comprehensive Database website: "Avoid use due to lack of safety and effectiveness information … there is very little scientific information about this product." We concur because this is a plant whose benefits and risk are not established, so why chance it? What's frustrating is that this fragrance-free eye cream also contains ingredients proven to help signs of aging, yet on balance it's ultimately an unexciting formulary.

☺ AVERAGE **Intensive Wrinkle Corrector Eye Cream, Formula RX 122** *($19.95 for 0.5 fl. oz.)* has one major problem, other than being incapable of truly improving dark circles, puffiness, or wrinkles—the amount of magnesium silicate it contains. This ingredient is used to make creams opaque and to boost thickness, but it tends to have a dry, somewhat absorbent finish that can magnify, not reduce, the appearance of wrinkles. Because it's the third ingredient listed, it's not surprising that this eye cream isn't as moisturizing as it claims to be. Beyond the magnesium silicate issue, another concern is the plant extract *Fraxinus excelsior* bark, discussed in the review above. What's frustrating is that this eye cream also contains some ingredients that are proven to help signs of aging, yet on balance, the formula has more against it than for it, including an over reliance on waxy ingredients that are the hallmark of a dated formula. Last, the truth is you don't need an eye cream (see the Appendix to find out why).

☺ AVERAGE **Redness Correcting Moisturizer, Formula RX 312** *($19.95 for 1.7 fl. oz.)* has a green tint. The company maintains that the green tint instantly neutralizes redness, but all it really does is replace more obvious redness with another color that you'll then have to conceal with makeup (unless you want to go about your day looking seasick). In short, green helps a bit to cancel red, but essentially you're replacing one discoloration problem with another—and how is that helpful? Although this moisturizer contains some good ingredients to improve dryness and reduce redness from sensitive skin, it's disappointing that it also contains the fragrance ingredient ethylene brassylate. Although not labeled "fragrance," this ingredient's sole function is just that: fragrance. A lesser concern, but still worth mentioning, is the inclusion of artificial coloring agents. Ideally, a moisturizer for sensitive, reddened skin should be fragrance- and colorant-free and loaded with repairing and soothing ingredients. This contains some great soothing ingredients, but loses points in other areas where it counts, hence, its neutral rating.

☺ AVERAGE **Redness Relief Moisturizer, Formula RX 311** *($19.95 for 1.7 fl. oz.)* is, except the omission of the green tint, nearly identical to the Redness Correcting Moisturizer, Formula RX 312, above, and the same basic comments apply.

☺ AVERAGE **Ultra-Hydrating Day & Night Cream, Formula RX 221** *($19.95 for 1.7 fl. oz.)* isn't "ultra hydrating" because its core ingredients are lightweight, not emollient, and one of them (isododecane) is known for its silky, dry (not moisturizing) finish. So the name is misleading, but is there a reason to consider this anyway? Not really. In many ways, this is a boring formula whose price is on the embarrassing side given the number of moisturizers in the same price range that have better formulas. It's great that this is fragrance-free, but where are the antioxidants and cell-communicating ingredients all skin types need to look and act younger? Even if they were present they wouldn't remain effective for long because this moisturizer is packaged in a jar. It ends up being an average option for normal to combination skin, but your skin deserves better than average!

☺ AVERAGE **Wrinkle Corrector & Firming Moisturizer SPF 15, Formula RX 111** *($19.95 for 1.7 fl. oz.)* provides broad-spectrum protection and includes stabilized avobenzone for reliable UVA (think anti-aging) protection. That means we're off to a good start in terms of keeping skin protected from wrinkles—if only the rest of the formula kept pace with the benefits sun protection provides. As is, this is an OK option for normal to dry skin. The formula has a small amount of water-binding agents and a plant-based antioxidant, but that's about it in terms of extra anti-aging ingredients. The lactic acid in this formula functions as a water-binding agent, not as an exfoliant, owing to the amount included and because the pH of the product is too high for exfoliant efficacy. Although fragrance isn't listed, this contains the ingredient ethylene brassylate, whose sole function in skin-care products is fragrance.

☹ POOR **Firming & Lifting Booster, Formula RX 124** *($21.95 for 1 fl. oz.)* is supposed to firm and lift skin while adding "cushion" to thinning skin, but mostly what it does is feel tacky thanks to its underwhelming formula that treats skin to precious few proven anti-aging ingredients. Instead, you get a blend of water with a somewhat sticky slip agent and a film-forming agent that may make your skin feel a bit tighter, but that's not the same as actually tightening and firming (or lifting) skin (see the Appendix for details). This contains the AHA lactic acid in a potentially helpful amount to exfoliate skin (definitely an anti-aging benefit), but the pH of this serum prevents this AHA from exfoliating. Actually, the amount of trietha-nolamine (a common pH-adjusting ingredient typically used in much lower amounts) may make this product feel constricting due to its basic (alkaline) nature. It's considered safe for use in low amounts, but it's listed third in this product, which means it's very likely to put your skin at risk of irritation

PHYSICIANS FORMULA SUN CARE

✓☺ BEST **Sun Shield For Faces Extra Sensitive Skin SPF 25** *($8.95 for 4 fl. oz.)* is a good, gentle sunscreen for someone with sensitive skin that is normal to dry, including rosacea-affected skin. The Best Product rating pertains to this sunscreen's value for sensitive skin. Other skin types should consider a sunscreen that is loaded with antioxidants, which this formula is lacking. Clinique Super City Block Sheer contains SPF 25, mineral sunscreens, and antioxidants so that would give someone with sensitive skin an even better product than this (but ounce for ounce, Physician's Formula's option costs a lot less).

☺ AVERAGE **Bronze Booster Self-Tanning Bronzing Veil** *($14.95)* is a butterscotch-scented product liquid bronzer with shimmer that also has self-tanning action, courtesy of dihydroxyacetone and erythrulose. Combined, you get instant color and shimmer from the cosmetic pigments plus a sunless tan that develops in a few hours and continues to darken over the next couple of days. It sounds wonderfully convenient, but unless you apply this all over the face and neck, the results once the self-tanner develops will look blotchy and uneven. Rather than combining these products, Physician's Formula should recommend using a self-tanner first (perhaps in the evening) and, once it has developed, augmenting the tan with a liquid bronzer with soft shine. As is, this Bronzing Veil is tricky to get right and the built-in brush applicator doesn't do a thing to promote even, streak-free application. If you decide to try this anyway, it's available in two shades suitable for fair to medium skin tones.

The Reviews P

⚘ Highly fragranced products smell good, but won't help your skin! See the Appendix for details.

☹ POOR **Sun Shield Sunless Tanning Lotion SPF 20** *($9.95 for 6 fl. oz.)* lacks the UVA protecting ingredients of titanium dioxide, zinc oxide, avobenzone, Tinosorb, or Mexoryl SX (ecamsule), and is not recommended.

PHYSICIANS FORMULA LIP CARE

☹ POOR **Plump Potion Needle-Free Lip Plumping Cocktail** *($9.75)* is packaged to resemble a syringe (so much for allaying fear of the needle!) and only provides lips with a cocktail of irritants, including menthol and menthyl nicotinate. These ingredients cause inflammation and increase blood flow to the lips, resulting in a slight increase in fullness—but such irritation is not the key to younger-looking, smoother lips

PHYSICIANS FORMULA SPECIALTY SKIN-CARE PRODUCTS

☹ POOR **Dark Spot Corrector & Skin Brightener, Formula RX 123** *($21.95 for 1 fl. oz.)* contains an extract from daisy as its chief lightening (or, truer to the product name "brightening") effects. Also known as tansy, this plant extract has only anecdotal evidence of skin-lightening ability, and, despite being a good antioxidant, it can cause severe contact dermatitis (Source: naturaldatabase.com). The amount in this product makes it a cause for concern because the irritation potential is high, and that's never the goal (see the Appendix for details on the problems irritation causes). This also contains the AHA lactic acid, but the amount is too low and this product's pH is too high for it to function as an exfoliant, so you won't get that benefit. You may love the silkiness of this serum, and it does contain cosmetic pigments for an instant brightening effect, but if your concern is dark spots or uneven skin tone, this doesn't have what it takes to improve matters—and the irritation from the daisy extract may make things worse.

PHYSICIANS FORMULA FOUNDATIONS & PRIMERS

✓☺ BEST **Healthy Wear SPF 50 Powder Foundation** *($14.95)* is a fragrance-free pressed-powder foundation that delivers results as impressive as its SPF rating. Its creamy smooth texture translates into easy application with the included sponge and it leaves a soft matte finish that's flattering for all skin types. The powder has a noticeable opacity, which makes it a contender for those looking for medium to full coverage from their powder foundation. Like other Healthy Wear products, the neutral shades are limited, and the four options offer nothing for dark skin tones. Its water-resistant claims are mostly true, although exposure to any moisture beyond a moderate mist will require a touch-up. By the way, although this powder foundation contains antioxidants, they aren't likely to remain stable because this product is packaged in a compact.

☺ GOOD **Mineral Wear Talc-Free Correcting Primer** *($10.95)* has a mineral-based broad-spectrum sunscreen, making it somewhat unique for a primer. The packaging is a twist-up tube with a flat brush dispenser. Although the brush feels soft, its synthetic bristles gunk up easily, a fact that poses hygiene issues because the brush is nearly impossible to clean without compromising the product inside. If you apply this with your fingertips, it does go on smoothly, feels lightweight, and dries to a subtle, yet luminous finish (with the exception of the Green shade). In fact, for a primer with a satisfactory SPF, the texture and finish is impressive, and it looks beautiful underneath foundation or powder. Unfortunately, aside from the sunscreen, there are no beneficial ingredients for skin. Also, given that you must apply sunscreen liberally to get the protection rated on the label, it's doubtful that anyone will use the amount they should. Consider this a nice boost to your foundation or moisturizer's sun protection, but not your only means of defense.

☺ GOOD **Mineral Wear Talc-Free Mineral Tinted Moisturizer SPF 15** *($12.95)* contains a mineral sunscreen (titanium dioxide) as the sole active ingredient. Its initially fluid texture blends well and sets to a moist finish suitable for normal to dry skin. Worth noting is that this tinted moisturizer feels heavier than many others. All four shades are worthwhile and all go on sheer, and there are options for light to tan skin tones. The very small amount of lavender oil is unlikely a cause for concern.

☺ GOOD **Youthful Wear Cosmeceutical Youth-Boosting Foundation & Brush SPF 15** *($14.95)*. This fragrance-free cream foundation with a zinc oxide sunscreen claims to make your skin look 10 years younger plus restore firmness and elasticity to sagging skin. Although the formula contains some anti-aging ingredients (and, of course, the sunscreen counts as anti-aging), this foundation is far from a face-lift in a tube! What it has going for it is a smooth, ultra-silky texture that dispenses thick (like spackle), but quickly softens into a sheer-coverage makeup that improves skin tone and texture without looking or feeling heavy or mask-like. You get a soft matte finish that won't emphasize wrinkles, but it won't make them disappear or look lifted, either. In essence, if you keep your expectations realistic and have normal to oily skin, you're likely to enjoy this foundation. The included mini foundation brush with synthetic bristles feels smooth and soft, though it's not quite as elegant as most full-size foundation brushes. Whether you use the brush, a sponge, or your fingers, the result is seamless sheer to light coverage. Only three shades are available, which is limiting, but all are workable for fair (but not porcelain) to medium skin tones. Our only concern is that as the sole active ingredient, the percentage of zinc oxide is a bit on the low side. We'd like to see at least 2% zinc oxide, with 5% being even better to ensure reliable protection.

☹ AVERAGE **Healthy Wear SPF 50 Tinted Moisturizer** *($14.95)* goes on greasy and retains a noticeable sheen even after it sets to a finish that practically stains skin. The amount of film-forming agents contributes to the long wear and supports the water-resistant claim, and this does hold up through moderate perspiration or humidity. For a tinted moisturizer, this is surprisingly pigment-rich, which means that you'll have to get the color just right if you want it to look convincing. Unfortunately, finding the right shade is easier said than done, because the four available shades just don't vary that much: The lightest shade is too dark for fair to light skin tones and the deepest shade is too light for dark skin tones. Add to that issue the inclusion of drying alcohol (although there's not a lot of it), and this is a product that you're better off skipping. What a shame, because the in-part zinc oxide and titanium dioxide sunscreen provides excellent sun protection.

☹ AVERAGE **Mineral Wear Talc-Free Mineral Liquid Foundation** *($11.95)* has an odd name not only because most liquid foundations are talc-free, but also because talc is a mineral! This water- and silicone-based foundation is dispensed from its tube onto an attached sponge. The sponge is a bit small for application to the entire face, but it smoothes the product well. Despite an initially attractive texture, this sets to a strong matte finish that appears chalky and tends to just sit on the skin rather than mesh with it, which is not good. Out of the available shades, the only real-skin shades are Classic Ivory and Natural Beige. Although not a total loss, this is only worth considering by those with very oily skin who desire medium coverage.

☹ POOR **Beauty Spiral Brightening Compact Foundation** *($9.95)* is a cream-to-powder makeup that "spirals" two colors together. It's eye-catching, but that's all this substandard foundation has going for it. The thick texture offers sheer coverage and a dry, powdery finish that just doesn't feel or look great on the skin. The three colors are passable, but there are far more elegant cream-to-powder foundations from Cover Girl or Revlon, and their options include sun protection.

☹ POOR **Beauty Spiral Skin Brightening Liquid Foundation** *($9.95)* is a sheer, light-textured foundation that has an uneven, slightly pasty-looking finish due to the high amount of titanium dioxide. The two shades are passable, but nothing this chalky can have any sort of brightening effect.

☹ POOR **CoverToxTen50 Wrinkle Therapy Foundation** *($12.95)* is one of a few foundations claiming to work like Botox, without painful injections. One of the main ingredients is GABA (gamma amino butyric acid). Please refer to the Cosmetic Ingredient Dictionary at CosmeticsCop.com for an in-depth discussion of this ingredient. Suffice it to say, GABA does not work to smooth wrinkles; not even Botox works for this purpose if it is applied topically rather than injected. Another anti-aging ingredient touted on the package is vitamin C (as tetrahexyldecyl ascorbate), but there is so little present in this foundation, your skin won't even notice it. Although it is clever and convenient that this initially creamy liquid foundation is dispensed onto a built-in brush, it does little to enhance application. It also doesn't change the fact that no matter how much blending you do, this foundation always looks heavy and somewhat opaque with a flat, slightly chalky finish. It is not the answer to camouflaging wrinkles; in fact, its finish tends to emphasize them and most of the colors go on too peach or pink to recommend.

☹ POOR **Le Velvet Film Makeup SPF 15** *($5.25)* is an old-fashioned cream-to-powder foundation that goes on surprisingly moist and creamy and can be blended out fairly sheer. The SPF is part titanium dioxide, which is great, but the finish is somewhat chalky and none of the colors resemble real skin tones, making this one to avoid.

☹ POOR **Organic Wear 100% Natural Origin Tinted Moisturizer SPF 15** *($11.95)* has all manner of organic certification and contains lots of organically sourced ingredients, something that will appeal to many consumers. It even has a titanium dioxide sunscreen, which is great. The problem is that, organic or not, the overall formula is terrible. Alcohol is the second ingredient (which causes free-radical damage, dryness, and irritation), and that is followed by lavender oil (which causes cell death), adding up to a natural disaster for all skin types. Despite the claims, this contains a few synthetic ingredients, so don't be fooled. However, as stated, there is no way we would recommend anyone try this product. The texture isn't pleasant to deal with, it is very fragrant (even though Physicians Formula labels it fragrance-free—if lavender oil isn't fragrance, we don't know what is), and most of the four shades are too pink or rose to look convincing.

☹ POOR **Organic Wear Liquid Foundation SPF 15** *($13.95)* is a fragrant foundation that may be certified organic, but that doesn't mean it's not without considerable problems. The titanium dioxide sunscreen is fine, but the base formula feels and looks heavy on skin. This foundation's texture and finish make skin look worse instead of better. Even more distressing, it contains the potent irritants lemon and lavender oils as well as colloidal silver, which can cause a permanent bluish discoloration on skin. This is absolutely not recommended, nor is it the least bit comfortable or natural-looking on skin.

PHYSICIANS FORMULA CONCEALERS

☺ AVERAGE **Blemish Rx Blemish-Healing Concealer** *($8.95)* plays the medicinal angle of this liquid concealer to the hilt by packaging it in a component that resembles a syringe, right down to the dosage markers on the side and a needle-like tip. It is "medicated" with

1.7% salicylic acid, but the pH is not low enough to permit exfoliation, a major way salicylic acid helps banish blemishes. This must be shaken before use (the formula tends to separate) and it then dispenses as a thin liquid that supplies modest coverage and a soft matte finish. Although nothing in this formula is likely to aggravate blemishes (there's a tiny amount of cinnamon bark extract, likely not enough to be a problem), most people will want more coverage than this provides. It is an OK option for those with oily skin whose blemishes don't need serious camouflage.

☹ AVERAGE **Gentle Cover Concealer Stick** *($6)* is a thick, lipstick-style concealer that provides moderate coverage with a heavy-looking, crease-prone finish. This is only recommended for those who refuse to consider the many superior concealers at the drugstore.

☹ AVERAGE **Mineral Wear Talc-Free Mineral Concealer Stick SPF 15** *($7.65)* has 26% titanium dioxide, so sun protection is assured—but we were also anticipating an opaque, dry texture and chalky finish and sadly, those suspicions were confirmed. Overall, this looks too obvious and heavy on skin, especially if you need extra coverage on trouble spots. The shade range only compounds the less-than-desirable finish this concealer has.

☹ AVERAGE **Mineral Wear Talc-Free Mineral Correcting Concealer** *($8.95)* comes as a trio: a corrector (in either Yellow or Green), concealer (Light only), and highlighter (Pink only). Each product is packaged in their own rectangular tube that interlocks with the others (sort of like Legos) so that you can keep the set together. Physicians Formula calls this "ultra convenient," but there's nothing convenient about using three products when one would suffice! Unfortunately, the packaging is the most interesting thing about this product. Using a corrector means that you almost always trade one discoloration problem for another that also must be covered. Shouldn't a good concealer alone be able to do the job on its own? This soft matte finish concealer is decent, but not exceptional, especially because it comes in only one shade that's suitable for light skin tones. All three product tubes are equipped with a wand applicator, which is a great way to apply the nicely textured liquid highlighter. It's a shame that it's a shimmery iridescent pink, which we absolutely do not recommend for anyone trying to combat redness on their face.

☺ AVERAGE **Youthful Wear Cosmeceutical Youth-Boosting Concealer** *($12.95)* isn't cosmeceutical or youthful, at least not if you interpret that to mean the formula is chock-full of anti-aging ingredients. The name is more for marketing purposes than it is about a superior, youth-giving formula. You get two concealers plus a circular, roller-ball blending tip that's built into the cap. Removing the purple top (which includes a clear cap to cover the roller-ball blending tool) reveals a twist-up stick concealer. The bottom portion of the component houses a yellow-tinted liquid concealer that can be used alone or blended with the stick concealer. Among the two concealers, the stick formula is preferred for its lightweight yet creamy texture and smooth, even blending. It provides fairly good coverage and creases minimally if set with powder. The liquid concealer sets quickly, so blending must be fast, and many will find it too yellow to work on anything but notably dark, purplish circles. Even then, this is a tricky product to use on dark circles because the yellow is bright enough that the result can look sickly rather than seamless. One limitation is that this is available only in one shade set, which is best for light skin tones. The blending tool works well at first, but once you get excess product on it, the roller ball becomes stuck and difficult to roll under the eyes. A concealer brush and/or a sponge are much better tools, or you can use a clean fingertip to dab and blend.

☹ POOR **Circle Rx Circle Control Concealer** *($8.95)* is only "just what the doctor ordered" if your doctor is in favor of runny concealers that dispense too heavily and look opaque and chalky on skin. Yes, this conceals dark circles, but so do many other concealers whose finish doesn't call attention to itself (and also comes in much better colors).

☹ POOR **Concealer 101 Perfecting Concealer Duo** *($7.25)* doesn't make the grade as an introduction to concealers, at least not if one of your prerequisites is shades that resemble skin. The texture, coverage, and finish of this concealer are quite nice, but that doesn't mean a thing when the unnatural skin colors scream "obvious" over whatever you're trying to hide.

☹ POOR **Conceal Rx Physicians Strength Concealer** *($8.95)* has a ridiculous name because there is no such thing as a physician's strength concealer. The company claims this liquid concealer is the prescription for "any and all imperfections" due to its coverage capability. This does provide full coverage that can camouflage dark circles, redness, or bruising, but the result is heavy and chalky and none of the colors resemble real skin tones in the least.

☹ POOR **Gentle Cover Cream Concealer SPF 10** *($5.45)* is a mineral oil- and wax-based concealer with a wand applicator and a titanium dioxide sunscreen. This formula will easily crease into any lines around the eye. The Yellow and Green shades are horrid, while Light is barely passable.

☹ POOR **Mineral Wear Talc-Free Mineral Cream Concealer SPF 10** *($7.65)* provides sun protection via 15% titanium dioxide, but that amount also gives this liquid concealer an unusually opaque finish, which doesn't make the four awful shades look any better.

☹ POOR **Powder Finish Concealer Stick SPF 15** *($5.45)* is a creamy stick concealer with titanium dioxide as one of the active ingredients for sun protection. That's great, but the only flesh-toned shade (Light) is too pink to look natural (especially with this concealer's thick texture), and the powder finish is minimal—it tends to stay creamy and creases easily.

PHYSICIANS FORMULA POWDERS

✓☺ BEST **Mineral Wear Talc-Free Mineral Face Powder SPF 16** *($13.95)* is an outstanding pressed powder! This talc-free, mica-based pressed powder protects skin from sun damage with its titanium dioxide and zinc oxide sunscreens, which is great. The texture feels wonderfully creamy for a powder, and becomes almost like a second skin after application. It can get powdery (dusty, if you will) as you swirl the brush over the compact, but we suspect this is because the powder isn't pressed as tightly as others. This fragrance-free powder comes in a neutral range of four shades best for fair to medium skin tones. It is a brilliant way to add to the sun protection you're getting from your daytime moisturizer or foundation with sunscreen, and is highly recommended. Note that the tiny, flat brush this comes with should be tossed in favor of a full-size professional powder brush.

✓☺ BEST **Youthful Wear Cosmeceutical Youth-Boosting Illuminating Face Powder** *($13.95)* There isn't anything particularly youthful or the least bit "cosmeceutical" about this fragrance-free pressed-powder's formula. It's merely a very good pressed powder with enough low-glow shine to double as a highlighter. In fact, this powder with shine is best used as a highlighter rather than dusted all over, unless you want a completely shiny face. The texture is buttery smooth and almost seems to float on your skin, enlivening it with a soft glow without making it look dull or chalky. When strategically applied with a full-size powder brush (not the terrible brush included in the base of the compact), this is an excellent way to add dimension and appeal to your makeup design, especially for evening glamour. Of all the Youthful Wear products, this is the one to buy, assuming you have fair to light skin, because only one shade is available.

☺ GOOD **CoverToxTen50 Wrinkle Formula Face Powder** *($12.95)* is a talc-based pressed powder with GABA, which is said to work like Botox to reduce wrinkles and expression lines. It doesn't work as claimed but this sheer, creamy-feeling powder is a very good option for normal to dry skin. The three shades appear slightly pink in the compact, but go on soft enough so as not to be a concern. There are no shades for medium to dark skin tones. Just to be clear: Although this is recommended, it does not do a better job of reducing the appearance of wrinkles than any other recommended powder (and, generally speaking, powdering isn't the way to make wrinkles less apparent).

☺ GOOD **Magic Mosaic Multi-Colored Custom Pressed Powder** *($13.95)* is a tightly pressed, talc-based powder that features overlapping circles of tone-on-tone colors. Applying this to skin produces a uniform color that is quite sheer and nonintrusive, though it does have a dry texture. The Light Bronzer/Bronzer shade has noticeable shine, while the other options have a very subtle shine that's suitable for daytime.

☺ GOOD **Mineral Wear Talc-Free Mineral Correcting Powder** *($13.95)* is a super-soft mica-based pressed powder that does a good job of evening out skin tone as well as adding some luminosity. Calling this a "corrector," however, is a bit of a stretch—then again, so is calling it "mineral" (not that anything mineral really matters to skin anyway). With pastel pink, green and yellow powders swirled into a light base, it appears undeniably neutral on skin, but it's not enough to combat any significant discoloration. If you like a soft glow, this would work as a setting powder, especially seeing as it doesn't look blotchy or cake easily. The clear plastic compact comes with a small half-moon brush, and its scratchiness aside, it's inadequate for this kind of use. Even though this "mineral" powder is pressed, it's still quite messy to work with.

☺ GOOD **Mineral Wear Talc-Free Mineral Airbrushing Loose Powder SPF 30** *($13.99)*. This fragrance-free loose mineral powder with titanium dioxide and zinc oxide for broad-spectrum protection is housed in an orb-like jar that includes a tiny buffing brush. The brush helps blend this powder, but you can use (and may actually prefer) a full-size powder brush. This powder has a silky, almost creamy texture that can be a bit messy to apply, but it blends well, setting to a soft, satin finish that provides light coverage. The satin glow is due to the mica and boron nitride this powder contains, which helps offset the dry, matte finish from the high amounts of mineral actives. Three shades are available; each goes on a bit darker than it looks in the container. The shades are limited to those with light to light-medium skin tones. Be aware that this foundation's texture and finish absolutely emphasize fine lines and wrinkles, as well as enlarged pores or uneven skin texture. Also, don't rely on this powder as your sole source of sun protection because you're not likely to apply it liberally enough to get the stated level of protection. Powders with sunscreen are best used over a foundation or daytime moisturizer with sunscreen. This mineral foundation is best for normal to slightly dry skin that's sensitive.

☺ GOOD **Mineral Wear Talc-Free Mineral Illuminating Powder Duo SPF 16** *($13.95)* is a very good option for those looking for sheer coverage and luminosity along with a boost of broad-spectrum sunscreen protection! Packaged in a dual-chambered dome with a too-small brush (which you might as well toss out), the two powder sifters each contain a different shade and finish of powder. What's nifty is that the sifters can be opened individually or together depending on the look you are trying to achieve. The highlighting shade lends a subtle glow, while the contouring powder helps shape facial features, although its finish is far from matte. Swirled together, the powders create a beautifully even effect that's neither overly shiny nor too dry. What impressed us most about this powder is how easily it applies and stays put. Like many mineral powders, it does settle into lines around the eyes, but it doesn't cake or streak on skin. This duo is available in three shades that suit fair to medium skin tones only. It is worth considering if you find the dual loose-powder concept appealing, and don't mind a small amount of shine.

☺ GOOD **Organic Wear 100% Natural Origin Pressed Powder** *($13.95)* is a talc-free, mica-based pressed powder whose formula is on the dry side but still feels silky and is easy to apply and blend. The range of nine shades is superb due to the neutral tones of each, and there are options for fair to tan skin tones. This powder is best for normal to oily skin, and provides a touch more coverage than standard pressed powders.

☺ GOOD **Youthful Wear Cosmeceutical Youth-Boosting Mattifying Face Powder** *($13.95)* is a very good, sheer pressed powder whose silky-smooth texture applies easily and leaves a soft matte finish. The formula isn't youth-enhancing or cosmeceutical in the least, so you can ignore those portions of the name. The skin-conditioning ingredients this contains (although only a tiny amount) are a nice touch, but their inclusion doesn't make this powder an age-defying wonder—it's just a good pressed powder for normal to oily skin. Sadly, only one shade is offered, although it's suitable for light (not fair) skin tones. This powder is fragrance-free.

☹ AVERAGE **Bamboo Wear Bamboo Silk Face Powder Refill** *($9.95)* claims that it "remineralizes" skin, which is nothing more than marketing nonsense, as are its "lifting and toning" claims. What you can count on from this finely milled talc-based pressed powder is much more illumination than coverage, making it best as a finishing powder over a moisturizer or foundation with sunscreen. All three shades contain enough shimmer to be unflattering for oilier skin types, with Translucent having a definite pink cast to it. Now, let's address the Bamboo Wear line's claims about sustainability. While we commend Physicians Formula for bringing the environmental issue to the forefront (cosmetics are notorious for wasteful packaging), it's difficult to take their intent seriously given the product's completely unnecessary double-plastic packaging. Even worse, Physicians Formula markets the additional purchase of the Bamboo Wear Compact as a way to "waste less," but that, too, is extraneously packaged! Refillable compacts are indeed a great way to conserve, but in this case rather than "waste less," the message seems to be "spend more."

☹ AVERAGE **Mineral Wear Airbrushing Loose Powder SPF 30** *($13.95)* is a prime example of a promising formula that just doesn't perform well. The powder has a smooth texture that's easy to pick up with a brush, but when applied it looks very dry and flat on skin. The three shades provide sheer coverage, but are all nearly indistinguishable variations of light to medium skin tones. Although the mineral actives titanium dioxide and zinc oxide do provide great broad-spectrum protection, it leaves your skin dry, accentuating fine lines and adding an unnatural chalkiness to skin.

☹ AVERAGE **Mineral Wear Talc-Free Mineral Airbrushing Pressed Powder SPF 30** *($13.99)*. This talc-free pressed mineral powder with sunscreen contains titanium dioxide and zinc oxide for gentle, effective broad-spectrum protection. Although that's great, this powder (and it's odd "wavy" design) has an unusually dry, slightly chalky texture that isn't as smooth or elegant as many other pressed powders with sunscreen, mineral-themed or not. Application and blending can be tricky because this tends to grab and drag over the skin, though it's OK if applied with a big, fluffy powder brush. (The enclosed brush is useless and should be discarded.) The other issue with this powder is that it looks heavy and can become cakey on skin. The three shades (for fair to light skin tones only) are good, but the trade-off is a powder that will be noticeable and will feel heavy on your skin. This is best used sparingly over a liquid foundation or daytime moisturizer with sunscreen—but there are better pressed powders with sunscreen to consider.

☹ AVERAGE **Mineral Wear Talc-Free Matte Finishing Veil** *($12.95)* is a loose powder packaged in a container that is attached to a sifter which feeds the powder onto the built-in brush. The corn- and aluminum starch–based powder feels weightless and has a very dry texture and finish that is only suitable for very oily skin. Further limiting its appeal, the sole shade is only suitable for those with fair skin.

☺ AVERAGE **Mineral Wear Talc-Free Mineral Loose Powder** *($11.95)* contains mica and zinc oxide instead of talc, which adds up to a mineral-based loose powder (but talc is a mineral, so almost all powders meet the criteria). The zinc oxide causes this light-textured powder to feel dry and look somewhat thick and pasty on skin, but that effect is offset to some extent by the mica's shine. The dry finish of this powder is best for oily skin, but you'll have to be OK with the shine it leaves behind, which kind of defeats the purpose of using powder.

☺ AVERAGE **Organic Wear 100% Natural Origin Loose Powder** *($13.95)* has a 100% natural claim that is misleading and what is odd about this mica-based loose powder is that it isn't difficult to create a powder composed of entirely natural ingredients—lots of lines offer this, but Physicians Formula, for all their 100% natural origin posturing, didn't! The powder has an initially grainy, powdery texture that transforms to a silky-smooth feel that applies evenly. Due to the absorbent nature of the minerals and clay, this leaves skin looking a bit too powdered and matte, almost as if it has a grayish cast. Another oddity is that almost all the shades are interchangeable, so there are no options for medium to dark skin tones.

☺ AVERAGE **Pearls of Perfection Multi-Colored Powder Pearls** *($12.95)* are large pots of colored, talc-based powder beads, available in bronze, flesh, and shiny highlighting shades. They're fun in concept, but the execution is messy and not worth the effort. Still, if you're a fan of Guerlain's Meteorites Powder for the Face, this is quite similar and only one-fourth the price.

☹ POOR **Happy Booster Glow & Mood Boosting Powder** *($13.95)* comes imprinted in a heart-shaped design that's lovely to look at, but it's fragrant and the irritating ingredients aren't going to make your skin happy. See the Appendix to learn why daily use of highly fragrant products, including makeup, is a problem for skin.

☹ POOR **Talc-Free Mineral Wear Correcting Pebbles** *($13.95)* creates more problems than it solves. These green, pink, yellow, and nude-colored powder pebbles (which disconcertingly resemble loose teeth) all mix together to create one "balancing" shade with shimmer that is supposed to correct and illuminate; unfortunately, it really doesn't do either. The colors don't combine in a convincing way, and it doesn't cover very well because it goes on too sheer, and the little coverage it does provide is uneven. Another issue is that the compact with the loose-powder pellets is filled past the brim, which makes it difficult to control how much of the crumbly powder ends up on your brush, leading to a potentially spotty, caked-on appearance and a mess in the compact.

PHYSICIANS FORMULA BLUSHES & BRONZERS

☺ GOOD **Baked Bronzer Bronzing & Shimmery Face Powder** *($11.95)* is similar to the Baked Pyramid Matte Bronzer below, except this version is imbued with large flecks of gold shine, whether used wet or dry. The shine clings well either way, and wet application intensifies the color and won't streak, assuming you blend it carefully.

☺ GOOD **Baked Pyramid Matte Bronzer** *($11.95)* is a good pressed-powder bronzer that comes in two semi-matte colors. Dry application produces sheer color and an almost matte finish that can be layered for more intensity. Wet application reveals stronger color and a shimmer finish, though you have to blend carefully to avoid streaking (this isn't a problem once the powder dries).

☺ GOOD **Bronze Booster Glow-Boosting Pressed Bronzer** *($14.95)* is a good, talc- and mica-based pressed bronzing powder. Its texture is smooth and dry, application is decent, and the color payoff is softer than you might expect, yet workable for lighter skin tones. The Fair to Light shade is too flesh-toned to work as bronzer; the other shades are better and impart a subtle shine.

☺ GOOD **Mineral Wear Talc-Free Mineral Blush** *($11.95)* is a mica-based pressed-powder blush that has a beautifully silky texture and smooth application. The color payoff is great, while the radiant (rather than sparkling) finish is attractive. The Nude Glow shade is closer to overall skin color than what you'd want from a blush, but the other shades are soft and well suited for application to cheeks.

☺ GOOD **Shimmer Strips Custom Blush & Highlighter** *($11.95)* is a smooth, dry-textured striped blush that's a good way to get shiny cheeks. The highlighting portion of the product's name is from the shine, but it's intense enough so as to make truly subtle highlighting impossible. As mentioned, you get stripes of color in one compact. When swirled together with a brush, the color reads as one soft shade on skin, with the color impact taking a backseat to the high degree of shine. The gleaming finish wears well without flaking.

☺ GOOD **Solar Powder SPF 20 Face Powder** *($12.95)* is a talc-based, pressed bronzing powder that includes an impressive titanium dioxide–based sunscreen. The two shades go on sheer, and each has three colors, representing a picture of the sun setting over a beach (it sounds odd, but fits the theme). Swirling a powder brush over the entire powder cake results in one uniform color with a tiny amount of shine. Although it would be nice if a greater range of skin-tone shades were available, this pressed bronzing powder with sunscreen is one to consider, especially if you want to pair it with a foundation that contains sunscreen for a touch of bronze color without the sun damage.

☺ AVERAGE **Bamboo Wear Bamboo Silk Face Bronzer Refill** *($9.95)*. What you can count on from this finely milled talc-based pressed-powder bronzer is a very sheer bronzing effect, with little streaking or grab. The powder applies beautifully, but all three shades have enough of a gold cast and iridescent shimmer to make this a bronzer with very limited appeal.

☺ AVERAGE **Bronze Booster Glow-Boosting Season to Season Bronzer** *($14.95)* earns the "season to season" part of its name due to the four varying levels of bronze color it contains (indicated as Winter, Spring, Summer, and Fall). The intention is to allow you to customize the level of bronze throughout the year; however, because there are no dividers between the shades, it's tricky to get anything from your brush without swirling all four shades together. They even include a special brush that is supposed to allow you to use the colors individually or together, but trust us, it's no better than using a regular brush; in fact, it's worse. There are two sets, one for light to medium and the other for medium to dark skin tones. The problem with either set is the overtly glittery finish that looks distracting, instead giving off a faux-tan glow. Otherwise, the pressed-powder texture blends on evenly and offers true tan colors.

☺ AVERAGE **Cashmere Wear Ultra-Smoothing Bronzer** *($13.95)* is yet another bronzer that tries to pass off large flecks of sparkle as a great way to look tan, but be careful with a glittery approach to making your skin look naturally tan. Although the powder is very soft and smooth, the wide stripe of glittery gold powder means that you look artificially sparkling instead of naturally sun-kissed.

☺ AVERAGE **Magic Mosaic Multi-Colored Custom Blush** *($10.95)* looks pretty in its pressed-powder compact, but this blush is so sheer and difficult to pick up on the brush that you'll be left wondering why you bothered unless your goal is the faintest hint of blush. Even the Soft Mocha/Mocha shade (for bronzing) goes on so soft no one will believe you've been kissed by the sun. Still, this does have a matte finish.

☺ AVERAGE **Mineral Wear Talc-Free Bronzing Veil** *($12.95)* has the same formula and packaging as the company's Matte Finishing Veil but comes in a slightly orange/bronze shade that is an OK option for medium skin tones, but not for all-over use.

☺ AVERAGE **Organic Wear 100% Natural Origin Blush** *($11.95)* has plenty of natural ingredients, yet ends up being difficult to apply due to its dry, powdery texture. Moreover, its flat matte finish on skin isn't attractive, even for those shades with a noticeable shimmer. The overall effect is a blush that tends to sit on top of skin rather than mesh with it, which is what the best powder blushes do. The brush that's included in the paper-wrapped compact is not sufficient for a smooth application.

☺ AVERAGE **Organic Wear 100% Natural Origin Bronzer** *($13.95)* looks pretty and will appeal to natural enthusiasts due to its formula and "from the earth" packaging. However, as far as pressed bronzing powders go, this doesn't come close to benchmark status. Smooth and dry, it is difficult to pick up a sufficient amount of powder with a brush, and as such this applies sheer and uneven. With patience you can get satisfactory results and a soft glow finish, but lots of other bronzing powders do this quickly and seamlessly. We wish this were a better product because the shade range is gorgeous, with options for fair to medium skin.

☹ POOR **Bronze Booster Glow-Boosting Loose Bronzing Veil** *($14.95)* is a loose, talc-based bronzing powder that is more trouble than it's worth. A small amount of powder is housed in the center of a cylindrical component with a built-in brush. You open the cap and turn the bottom of the component to the desired number on the center dial. This determines how much powder is dispensed onto the brush. After you've dialed in the amount, simply brush on wherever you want a hint of bronze color. Sounds easy, right? Mostly it is; the problems lie in the dry texture of the powder coupled with its sheerness and the harsh feel of the brush. This is not a comfortable product to apply, and you need to keep brushing it on to see any color, a process that becomes painful. Why someone would choose this over a standard bronzing powder is beyond reason—it isn't worth the gimmick.

☹ POOR **Bronze Booster Glow-Boosting Pressed Shimmer Bronzer** *($14.95).* This bronzer's packaging is novel in concept but failed to impress us during use. It comes with a kabuki-style brush that pops through the lid but is a bit on the scratchy side, so we wouldn't recommend using it unless you were stranded without your regular brushes. In terms of performance as a bronzer, it's equally disappointing. The pressed-powder texture is a bit on the stiff side and takes additional strokes to adhere to the brush. The ultra-shimmery formula is overly shiny and distracting, plus not all the shades look natural (watch out for copper undertones).

☹ POOR **Happy Booster Glow & Mood Boosting Blush** *($11.95)* comes imprinted in an adorable heart-shaped design that's pretty to look at, but its fragrant and irritating formula isn't going to make your skin happy. See the Appendix to learn why daily use of highly fragrant products is bad for skin.

☹ POOR **Healthy Wear SPF 50 Bronzer** *($14.95)* is a bronzer that packs a broad-spectrum sunscreen punch; however, this one misses the mark, providing neither convincing color nor easy application. Each of the four shades includes flecks of shimmer, and it seems like the deeper the shade the more sparkle you get. More of an issue is that this pressed-powder bronzer tends to streak, even if you don't use the scratchy brush included in the compact. Add to that problem the odd cantaloupe-orange cast each shade leaves behind, and this is a bronzer that you can and should do without.

☻ POOR **Organic Wear 2-in-1 Bronzer Blush** *($13.95)* includes a pressed bronzer and blush that can be used independently or swirled together for a sheer glow. The brush is too small for practical use, but the real deal-breaker is the strong odor of the powder itself, likely from the plant oils going rancid due to the packaging.

PHYSICIANS FORMULA EYESHADOWS

✓☺ BEST **Bright Collection Shimmery Quad Eye Shadow** *($6.75)* is identical to the Matte Collection Quad Eye Shadow below, except with these sets all four shades have shine (which tends to stay in place, making these highly recommended if you prefer shiny eyeshadows). Otherwise, the same basic comments apply.

✓☺ BEST **Matte Collection Quad Eye Shadow** *($6.75)* has some of the best neutral color combinations around, with a welcome silky texture and matte finish that applies and blends beautifully. There are only three quads available, but each is excellent, though not every set has a suitable shade for eyelining.

✓☺ BEST **Shimmer Strips Custom Eye Enhancing Shadow & Liner** *($10.95)*. There's only one issue with these strips of powder eyeshadows (each one provides nine shades in arrangements of three sets of tone-on-tone colors) and that is the mistaken notion that blue eyes need blue eyeshadow, green eyes need green eyeshadow, and so on. Matching your eyeshadow to your eye color is not the way to showcase your eyes. All it does is put two similar colors in proximity, drawing attention away from what you're using eyeshadow to emphasize. In every other respect, unless you don't want shine, these eyeshadows have a remarkably smooth texture and an even, flake-free application (unless you overdo it when using them wet). The offerings for Hazel and Brown eyes feature the best color combinations. The Green group is good if you ignore or downplay the green shades, while Blue is the trickiest because blending blues and peaches with gray tends to produce a muddy yet pastel-looking result. Each set includes one shade dark enough to work as powder eyeliner, making these convenient, all-in-one options to shape and shade the eye.

☺ GOOD **Baked Collection Wet-Dry Eye Shadow** *($7.95)* offers three well-coordinated, shiny eyeshadows in one compact. Most of the trios have one darker shade to use as eyeliner, and these have smooth, dry textures that blend nicely and last, plus the shine doesn't flake. True to the name, these may be applied wet or dry (most powder eyeshadows have this feature), with wet application intensifying the color and shiny finish. Watch out for Baked Spices—the orange tones aren't the easiest to work with. Baked Sweets has the same issue with its colors.

☺ GOOD **Organic Wear 100% Natural Origin Eye Shadow Duo** *($7.95)* has wording that says "100% natural origin" instead of "100% natural." That's how Physician's Formula gets around the fact that not every ingredient in this powder eyeshadow is natural. (Have you ever seen glyceryl caprylate at your local farmer's market?) It's a bit deceptive because the average consumer interprets the wording in the name as meaning that this product is 100% natural, but it isn't. That said, although the shade selection is limited, these shadow duos have a smooth but dry texture that applies well. Color intensity is sheer, but these layer well for more intensity, although you won't be able to create a deep smoky eye look. Among the duos, the best are Brown Eyes Organics and Hazel Eyes Organics. The other duos are too blue or green to recommend. Each duo has a soft shine that clings well and is suitable for daytime wear.

✦ Exposing oily skin to irritating ingredients makes it worse! See the Appendix to learn more.

One caution: This product contains a tiny amount of the fragrance chemical cinnamic acid, which may cause allergic contact dermatitis (Source: *American Journal of Contact Dermatitis*, June 2001, pages 93–102).

PHYSICIANS FORMULA EYE & BROW LINERS

✓☺ BEST **Brow Definer Automatic Brow Pencil** *($5.95)* ranks as one of the best brow pencils at any price, and the shade selection includes options for all but red or auburn brows. It applies smoothly and allows you to build color in sheer layers, which makes for natural-looking brows. The slightly thick powder finish lasts without smearing, while the brow comb (built into the cap) finishes things with precision.

✓☺ BEST **Eye Booster 2-in-1 Lash Boosting Eyeliner + Serum** *($10.95)* has no research showing that any ingredient in this product is going to grow even a single eyelash. Aside from the hype, what you do get is an outstanding, pen-style liquid eyeliner with an incredibly precise brush, smart packaging, and impressive staying power. Simply put, this is one of the best liquid eyeliners available anywhere at any price.

✓☺ BEST **Eye Definer Felt-Tip Eye Marker** *($6.95)* looks like a fine-tipped marker and applies like a liquid eyeliner. The felt tip is firm yet comfortable, making it easy to draw a continuous thick or thin line. You'll find this dries almost immediately and wears all day without chipping, smearing, or fading

☺ GOOD **Shimmer Strips Custom Eye Enhancing Eyeliner Trio** *($10.95)* comes with three retractable eyeliner pencils in shades that are meant to bring out your natural eye color. They tell you that the container with the purple, brown, and black shades is supposed to be for someone with brown eyes; purple, green, and black are supposed to be for those with green eyes; hazel eyes get two different shades of purple and one black; and if you have blue eyes the blue, brown, and black set is meant for you. However, follow this guideline at your own peril—selecting a color of shadow or liner based on eye color is an extremely dated way of doing eye makeup. As far as performance goes, these eyeliners go on smooth, are easy to blend, and stay put once they set. The color combinations, on the other hand, don't necessarily bring out the intended eye color. For example, blue eyeliner doesn't enhance blue eyes; rather, it competes with them. Don't be fooled by the name of this product, which implies a shimmery finish; in reality, this has more of a dark metallic finish and some of the shades are actually matte.

☺ GOOD **Shimmer Strips Gel Cream Liner** *($10.95)* is available in "Custom Eye Enhancing" and "Glam" versions. These cleverly packaged gel eyeliner trios are on the shimmery side, which increases the chance of getting glitter in your eye. That said, they nevertheless are smoothly textured and long-lasting, as long as you apply with your own fine-tip eyeliner brush.

☹ AVERAGE **Fineline Brow Pencil** *($4.25)* needs sharpening and comes in three decent shades. It has a standard, dry texture. If you don't mind routine sharpening, this is one of the least expensive reliable brow pencils.

☹ AVERAGE **Mineral Wear Talc-Free Mineral Eye Liner Pencil** *($6.95)* contains a couple of minerals but the very same ones show up in almost every eye pencil being sold (because they help create the color or add texture to the pencil). This is not a unique option; it's just another standard, creamy eye pencil that needs routine sharpening.

☹ AVERAGE **Organic Wear 100% Natural Origin Eyeliner** *($7.95)*. The main ingredients in this pencil show up in many other eye pencils that don't make organic certification claims, so unless you're gung-ho on your makeup being approved by the Ecocert group, there's no need to choose this pencil. It needs routine sharpening and remains creamy enough to smudge and smear. It's OK if you want a smoky eye design or are willing to pair it with a powder eyeshadow, but why not just line your eyes with the longer-lasting powder eyeshadow and skip the pencil?

☹ POOR **Eye Definer Automatic Eye Pencil** ($5.50) is a twist-up, retractable eye pencil that is greasier than most, which means it can smear and smudge easily, and it does.

PHYSICIANS FORMULA LIP COLOR

☹ POOR **Plump Potion Needle-Free Plumping Lipstick** ($9.95) is a creamy, smooth-textured lipstick that plumps lips with three potent irritants: menthol, benzyl nicotinate, and the menthol derivative ethyl menthane carboxamide. It actually hurts to wear this; we'd rather have a needle injection of collagen or another filler substance because at least the injection sites are numbed before such procedures! Without the trio of irritants, this would be a very good cream lipstick with beautiful full coverage colors.

PHYSICIANS FORMULA MASCARAS

☺ GOOD **PlentiFull Thickening Mascara** ($5.20) is a credible mascara to consider if you primarily want a lengthening mascara that, with several coats, builds moderate thickness without clumps or smearing. The tiny amounts of botanicals (aloe and chamomile) has no impact on lashes.

☺ GOOD **Plump Potion Lash Plumping and Stimulating Mascara** ($9.75) makes wallflower lashes the talk of the party in no time thanks to its dense brush that deposits a lot of mascara to quickly thicken lashes. You'll get some minor clumps along the way, but they can be smoothed out without a separate brush. Unless you don't want dramatic lashes in an instant, the only downside of note is that if this gets on your skin (such as the eyelid or lash line), it is very difficult to correct without the help of a makeup remover. Most mascara smudges can be remedied with a cotton swab, but this one won't budge. By the way, none of the ingredients the company uses in an effort to stimulate lashes actually have that effect. Even if they did, the amount of said ingredients in this mascara is insignificant.

☺ GOOD **To Any Lengths Lash Extending Mascara** ($5.20) is excellent for substantial but not excessive length and clean, clump-free definition. Don't expect any thickness from this, but as a lengthening formula this wins high marks, and it wears all day without smearing or flaking.

☺ AVERAGE **AquaWear Waterproof Mascara** ($5.20) will build some length, but no thickness, and is fairly waterproof. Contrary to the claim here, no waterproof mascara can condition lashes, nor do lashes need conditioning. However, this does make lashes feel softer than a typical waterproof mascara.

☺ AVERAGE **Eye Booster 2-in-1 Day & Night Lash Boosting Serum** ($10.95 for 0.16 fl. oz.) is a brush-on lash serum that cannot work to make lashes longer, thicker, or darker. Granted, the company isn't directly claiming that, but that's the underlying implication for just about every "lash boosting" product being sold—or why bother to use them? The simple formula's only intriguing ingredient is a peptide (myristoyl pentapeptide-17) that shows up on several other lash-growth products, including the pricey option from Jan Marini Skin Research (reviewed on CosmeticsCop.com). Regrettably, there's no research proving this peptide does a thing for lashes. In contrast, we know from years of research that prostaglandin analogues (such as the active ingredient in prescription Latisse) DO work to give you longer, thicker lashes. There's no harm in trying this, and the price is realistic—but don't expect results beyond softer lashes.

☺ AVERAGE **Organic Wear 100% Natural Origin Jumbo Lash Mascara** ($9.95) performs adequately, adding more thickness than length to lashes. Its oversized round rubber brush definitely deposits lots of mascara, but it lacks a tapered end to create definition and separation.

☺ AVERAGE **Organic Wear 100% Natural Origin Mascara** *($9.95)* has a thin application but builds decent length without clumps. Thickness is scant and this is prone to minor flaking. It is unusually fragrant due to its orange fruit water base. The natural waxes it contains are found in numerous mascaras, yet they're not used to impressive effect here.

☺ AVERAGE **Shimmer Strips Custom Eye Enhancing Mascara Duo** *($10.95)*. Unfortunately, this dual-ended rubber-brush mascara is yet another product marketed to enhance your eye color. One end houses a black mascara that performs satisfactorily, with little clumping or smearing, but the other end houses a sickly grass green mascara for green eyes, bright royal blue for blue eyes, and so on. While the colored end of the mascara does deliver lots of color to every lash and dries to a vivid hue, it's a look that is simply unnatural and unflattering, no matter what your eye color. This deserves an average rating, but only for the reasonable performance of the black mascara.

☹ POOR **Mineral Wear Talc-Free Mineral Mascara** *($7.95)* makes a strange claim because mascaras are rarely made with talc (and it's not a harmful ingredient for eyelashes anyway). The mineral component comes from the mineral water, which is the main ingredient in this mascara. The product applies heavily from the get-go, and quite wet. It takes several minutes to dry, during which time you run the risk of smearing, making this a poor contender among other mascaras. Another downer is how difficult this is to remove. A water-soluble cleanser and two rounds of a silicone-based eye-makeup remover weren't enough (though the formula does wear well once it finally sets).

PHYSICIANS FORMULA FACE & BODY ILLUMINATORS

☺ GOOD **Summer Eclipse Bronzing and Shimmery Face Powder** *($12.95)* casts an equal amount of shimmer and sun-kissed bronze tint on the skin. The tightly pressed, talc-based powder applies sheer and even, and the shine clings better than you might think. It's best for evening glamour when you want shine without overdoing it.

☺ GOOD **Virtual Face Powder Multi-Reflective Face Powder** *($10.95)* is a talc-based pressed powder that attempts to minimize lines and wrinkles by diffusing light. It doesn't work in that manner, however, because it is so shiny that any flaw or wrinkle it's applied over is magnified. However, this is perfect if you have smooth, unlined skin and want a shiny powder with a dimensional effect that clings well. All four shades are enticing if strong shine is your thing.

☺ AVERAGE **Mineral Wear 100% Mineral FaceBrightener** *($13.95)* is a clay-based pressed powder with shine that has a very dry texture and sheer color deposit. It isn't pleasurable to work with and the shine flakes almost immediately. The colors are suitable only for fair to light skin tones, but it's not really worth the effort or expense.

☹ POOR **Shimmer Strips Custom Bronzer, Blush, & Eye Shadow** *($12.95)* tries to compete with Bobbi Brown's popular Shimmer Brick Compacts, but fails due to its dry, thick texture that applies unevenly. The shimmer tends to sit (and look piled) on the skin no matter how little you use, whereas Brown's option (and Laura Mercier's) mesh with and use shimmer to highlight skin.

PHYSICIANS FORMULA SPECIALTY MAKEUP PRODUCTS

☺ AVERAGE **Shimmer Strips Custom Eyeliner, Eye Shadow & Highligher** *($10.95)* resembles a traditional pencil, but at either end are sponge-tip applicators that twist in and out of small amounts of loose powder. One side has darker powder for lining; the other has a lighter shade for shadow and highlighting. The concept is great because the powder really

The Reviews P

does stick to the applicators, going on smoothly and blending well, although there's very little product for the money. The major drawback is the small number of shadow options, all of which are shiny (hence the "Shimmer" part of the product name), but also continue with the notion that the eye color should be matched with your eyeshadow color: Blue tones for blue eyes, greens for green eyes, and so on. Add to that the suggestion that one should highlight the browbone with these same coordinating colors and you've got a product that should be considered very carefully.

☺ AVERAGE **Organic Wear Face Sculpting Trio 3-in-1 Highlighter, Face Powder, Bronzer** *($13.95)* is housed in an eco-friendly cardboard compact. You get a talc-based pressed powder, powder bronzer, and powder highlighter. There are no dividers between the products and the crescent shape of each makes it difficult to hone in on one unless you're using a small brush, which isn't that practical for applying powder or bronzer. More important, the color payoff of this product is minimal, especially for the bronzer, so forget about sculpting your features. Each product has the same formula, and the texture is best described as overall smooth with an underlying graininess that hinders application. Buying organic is one thing, but whether you do so or not, you shouldn't be left wondering why you bothered.

PROACTIV SOLUTION (SKIN CARE ONLY)

Strengths: Effective, elegant-textured AHA, BHA, and skin-lightening options; all sunscreens provide sufficient UVA protection; good options for controlling excess oil breakthrough.

Weaknesses: Several products contain irritating ingredients that do not help acne-prone skin; some gimmicky products that no dermatologist-created line should be selling (they should know better).

For more information and the latest ProActiv reviews, visit CosmeticsCop.com

PROACTIV SOLUTION CLEANSERS

☺ AVERAGE **$$$ Renewing Cleanser** *($20 for 4 fl. oz.)* is a water-soluble cleansing lotion that uses 2.5% benzoyl peroxide as the active ingredient. A benzoyl peroxide wash may sound convenient, but it's a problem if used around the eyes, plus in a cleanser, it's in contact with the skin only briefly, which makes it not nearly as potent as when it is used in a leave-on product. This contains tiny spherical beads for a scrub action, but should be used with caution over acne lesions. Acne cannot be scrubbed away, and getting too zealous with this cleanser can cause further inflammation that will make acne look worse, not better.

☹ POOR **Deep Cleansing Wash** *($20 for 16 fl. oz.)* cannot help unclog pores as claimed because its 2% salicylic acid is washed down the drain before it can go to work inside the pore lining. More of an issue is that this cleansing scrub contains irritant menthol, which won't help anyone have clearer skin.

☹ POOR **Clear Zone Body Pads** *($22 for 75 pads)* are dual-textured pads medicated with 2% salicylic acid. Although the pH of the solution in which the pads are soaked allows exfoliation to occur, the amount of alcohol and the inclusion of witch hazel do not make these a must-have option for blemished skin. See the Appendix to find out how alcohol and the irritation it causes makes oily, acne-prone skin worse.

☹ POOR **Makeup Removing Cloths** *($15 for 45 towelettes)* are not adept at removing makeup thoroughly because they lack cleansing agents or solvents, and they contain enough lavender to cause problems for skin. The cleansing cloths from Olay are preferred to and less expensive than this.

☹ POOR **Medicated Cleansing Bar** *($18 for 5.25 fl. oz.)*. Despite being medicated with anti-acne superstar salicylic acid, this is still a standard bar cleanser and not recommended for any skin type, acne or not. Bar soaps and bar cleansers share the same issue of being drying (though bar cleansers are generally less drying than true soaps) and leaving a residue on skin that interferes with how other skin-care products work. This particular bar cleanser has a high amount of fragrance, too, and for all skin types that's irritation waiting to happen. Any gentle, water-soluble cleanser is preferred to Medicated Cleansing Bar—and don't forget that with "medicated" cleansers, the active ingredient is rinsed from skin before it has much chance to work!

PROACTIV SOLUTION TONER

☺ GOOD **$$$ Revitalizing Toner** *($20 for 4 fl. oz.)* is a good 6% AHA exfoliant in toner form. However, when it comes to most kinds of breakouts, research indicates that BHA (salicylic acid) rather than AHA is the best way to exfoliate for breakout prevention. Salicylic acid can exfoliate within the pore as well as on the surface of the skin because it is lipid soluble (meaning it can penetrate oil). AHAs exfoliate primarily on the surface of the skin because they are water-soluble and can't work beneath the surface. The amount of witch hazel is unlikely to be irritating, but it keeps this from earning a higher rating. You can find excellent BHA exfoliants for acne from Paula's Choice as well as others in the Best Products chapter, plus a pricier but effective option from ProActiv.

PROACTIV SOLUTION EXFOLIANTS

✓☺ BEST **Clarifying Night Cream** *($27 for 1 fl. oz.)* is a well-formulated BHA lotion that includes 1% salicylic acid at an effective pH of 3.6. As further enticement, the formula also includes retinol and several antioxidants, all in stable packaging. This is highly recommended for normal to dry skin battling blackheads and blemishes. Clarifying Night Cream does contain fragrance.

☹ POOR **Mild Exfoliating Peel** *($20 for 1 fl. oz.)* is mild to the point of being ineffective because the 0.5% salicylic acid won't work efficiently at this product's pH level. Further, with alcohol and witch hazel heading up the ingredient list, this peel is far from "calming"; rather it is irritating and drying (see the Appendix for details).

PROACTIV SOLUTION MOISTURIZERS (DAYTIME & NIGHTTIME), & SERUMS

✓☺ BEST **Replenishing Eye Serum** *($24 for 0.5 fl. oz.)* is a silky, silicone-enhanced serum that can be used anywhere on the face. It doesn't contain anything special for the eye area, but instead is loaded with ingredients that benefit skin regardless of what body part it touches. Replenishing Eye Serum contains some excellent skin-identical ingredients along with proven antioxidants in a fragrance-free formula that is suitable for all skin types, including sensitive skin. See the Appendix to find out why, in truth, you don't need a special product for the eye area.

☺ AVERAGE **Oil Free Moisture with SPF 15** *($25 for 1.7 fl. oz.)* is a basic, fragrance-free sunscreen for normal to oily skin. The in-part zinc oxide sunscreen may be a problem for someone struggling with blemishes, but it does contribute to this product's matte finish and UVA protection. The formula contains methylisothiazolinone, a preservative that is not recommended for use in leave-on products and is known for causing contact dermatitis (Source: *Contact Dermatitis*, August 2007, pages 97–99). As such, this becomes a less desirable option.

☹ POOR **Daily Oil Control** *($19 for 1.7 fl. oz.)* lists alcohol as the second ingredient and although that can de-grease skin, it is also very irritating, causes free-radical damage, and can stimulate oil production at the base of your pores. This is a poorly formulated product that's not something a dermatologist should willingly endorse.

The Reviews P

☹ POOR **Green Tea Moisturizer** *($25 for 1 fl. oz.)* contains a lot of green tea and vitamin A, two antioxidants with considerable value for all skin types. The problem is that the amount of iris root extract (also known as orris root) can cause allergic or sensitizing skin reactions and there is no research showing it to be beneficial for skin (Source: *Botanical Dermatology Database*, http://bodd.cf.ac.uk/BotDermFolder/BotDermC/CACT.html). What a shame, because this is otherwise a great moisturizer for normal to dry skin.

PROACTIV SOLUTION SUN CARE

☺ GOOD **Daily Protection Plus Sunscreen SPF 15** *($19 for 4 fl. oz.)* is a good in-part avobenzone sunscreen for normal to oily skin. It provides a lightweight but short-lived matte finish and contains a tiny amount of vitamin-based antioxidants. The amount of salicylic acid is too low to affect blemish-prone skin, although the pH is within the ideal range.

PROACTIV SOLUTION SPECIALTY SKIN-CARE PRODUCTS

✓☺ BEST $$$ **Advanced Blemish Treatment** *($18 for 0.33 fl. oz.)* is a topical disinfectant for acne. It contains 6% benzoyl peroxide as its active ingredient, and is alcohol-free. This is a very effective, soothing option to help combat acne-causing bacteria. Although it's recommended, you should know that there are less expensive benzoyl peroxide products to consider, including those from Neutrogena, Clearasil, and Paula's Choice.

✓☺ BEST **Dark Spot Corrector** *($22 for 1 fl. oz.)* combines 2% hydroquinone with approximately 4% glycolic acid at an effective pH of 3.3. This is an outstanding option to fade sun- or hormone-induced brown skin discolorations, while also improving skin's texture and reducing inflammation with antioxidants. The opaque packaging ensures the hydroquinone will remain stable during use.

✓☺ BEST **Repairing Treatment** *($29 for 2 fl. oz.)* is a very good topical disinfectant for acne. The active ingredient is 2.5% benzoyl peroxide and it is blended in a silky lotion base that contains an anti-irritant. It's pricey for what you get, but is definitely worth considering as part of a battle plan for blemishes. This does contain fragrance. By the way, ProActiv's claim that Repairing Treatment contains "prescription grade benzoyl peroxide" is meant to make it sound like a superior choice. However, the only difference between prescription-grade and over-the-counter benzoyl peroxide is the amount used and the other drugs it's combined with. It's not about better results.

☺ GOOD $$$ **Oil Blotter Sheets** *($10.95 for 130 sheets)* are standard, powder-free pieces of paper that work quickly to absorb excess oil and perspiration. They're on the pricey side, but at least you get an abundance of papers.

☺ AVERAGE $$$ **Refining Mask** *($20 for 2.5 fl. oz.)* is a standard clay mask that also contains 6% pure sulfur. Sulfur can be a good antibacterial agent, but its irritant properties outweigh its benefit for most people. There are better ways to disinfect skin than this, but this is a potential option for short-term use if your acne hasn't responded to benzoyl peroxide. Our strong suggestion is to use this only on acne-prone areas to minimize the dryness and irritation sulfur can cause. This irritation will be offset to an extent due to the inclusion of linoleic acid, a fatty acid that can reduce inflammation in the pore lining (Source: *Cosmetic Dermatology*, April 2008, pages 211–212)

☹ POOR **Medicated Pore Cleaning System** *($18)* is further proof that the dermatologists behind this line are frustratingly endorsing both helpful and harmful products for those with acne. This two-step system includes **Pore Strips** and a **Pore Cleansing Solution**. The

Pore Strips are like Scotch tape for skin, and include alcohol, peppermint oil, and menthol to further irritate and inflame skin. The Pore Cleansing Solution doesn't fare much better because it contains a lot of alcohol and irritating arnica extract. This is a mistake from any angle. There is nothing medicated about alcohol, menthol, or peppermint.

REVLON (MAKEUP ONLY)

Strengths: Superior foundations with sunscreen and each of them provide sufficient UVA protection (though one has a disappointing SPF 6); several outstanding concealers and powders; one of the best cream blushes around; great cream eyeshadow and liquid eyeliner; a beautiful selection of elegant lipsticks, lip gloss, and lipliner; some worthwhile specialty products.

Weaknesses: Average eye and brow pencils; inaccurate claims surrounding their Botafirm complex; mostly average to disappointing mascaras.

For more information and the latest Revlon reviews, visit CosmeticsCop.com

REVLON FOUNDATIONS

✓☺ BEST **Age Defying Makeup with Botafirm SPF 20** *($13.99)* is slightly more emollient than its designation for normal/combination skin would suggest, but it does have a finish that's almost matte. It provides broad-spectrum sun protection with titanium dioxide and zinc oxide. Texture- and application-wise this provides seamless medium coverage without a heavy feel. This foundation features 12 shades that tend to go on lighter than they appear in the bottle. The best news: With the exception of the too-peach Honey Beige, there's not a bad shade in the bunch, and there are options for light to dark (but not very fair or very dark) skin tones. Do keep your "age defying" expectations for this foundation realistic because this won't firm skin or reduce the look of expression lines.

✓☺ BEST **Age Defying Makeup with Botafirm SPF 15 Dry Skin** *($11.99)*. This liquid foundation earns brownie points right off the bat for its broad-spectrum sun protection, but that's as close to an "age-defying" benefit as you'll get. Despite claims, it won't firm skin or reduce expression lines, and though Revlon did include some good antioxidants, they are in such low concentrations that the added benefit is slim to none. That's not to say this isn't otherwise a good foundation, because it certainly is! It blends on seamlessly to provide sheer to medium coverage. The slightly moisturizing formula works well for dry skin without feeing greasy or heavy. Add that to the fact that the shade range features neutral options for light to medium-deep skin tones, and you've got yourself a winner (well, unless you have fair skin)! Note: This contains fragrance in the form of methyldihydrojasmonate.

✓☺ BEST **ColorStay Makeup with Softflex for Normal to Dry Skin SPF 15** *($12.99)* contains zinc oxide and titanium dioxide for broad-spectrum sun protection, and although it's not emollient enough to please those with dry skin, it has a beautiful satin-matte finish that feels slightly moist and provides medium to nearly full coverage (if layered). Those with dry skin looking for a long-wearing foundation with sunscreen will find that this pairs well with a moisturizer. This isn't nearly as difficult to remove as the original ColorStay Makeup, and it's much easier to blend because it is forgiving of any mistakes rather than setting and refusing to budge. There are several shades, and nearly all are praiseworthy. The only shades to avoid are the too-pink Fresh Beige and the slightly orange Cappuccino.

✓☺ BEST **New Complexion One Step Compact Makeup SPF 15** *($12.99)* ranks as the best cream-to-powder foundation at the drugstore, hands down, and it includes titanium dioxide as the only sunscreen active. It applies superbly; has a light, silky texture; and sets to a

The Reviews R

soft, natural-looking powder finish that is best for normal to slightly oily or slightly dry skin. (Just keep in mind that moisturizer must be applied over any dry spots or this foundation will exaggerate them.) Coverage goes from sheer to medium. The shades are mostly neutral, but avoid Natural Beige and Cool Beige. Tender Peach is fairly true to its name, but may work for some light skin tones. Regrettably, there are no shades for very light or very dark skin tones.

✓☺ BEST **PhotoReady Compact Makeup SPF 20** *($13.99)*. This cream-to-powder foundation comes in packaging where the makeup is covered by a flexible screen that you press to deposit the product onto your sponge. It looks a bit odd, but it makes even application effortless! Once applied, this makeup creates sheer, blendable coverage that you can build up as needed for more coverage. The texture begins quite creamy, but sets to a very lightweight, slightly powdery finish that's flattering for all skin types (but the thickening agents and waxes may cause problems for those with blemish-prone skin). The sole active sunscreen is titanium dioxide, which is great news for those sensitive to "chemical" sunscreens. Plus, this active ingredient provides critical broad-spectrum protection. The shades provide options for fair to medium skin, but be forewarned that the screen on top of the compact makes it very difficult to determine what the makeup actually will look like on your skin. We were surprised at the significant tonal differences between how this looked on skin and how it looked in the package. For example, the somewhat pink-looking Medium Beige had obvious orange undertones on skin. You'll need to experiment with the different shades to get it right, so make sure you're purchasing at a store with a flexible return policy!

☺ GOOD **Age Defying with DNA Advantage Cream Makeup SPF 20** *($12.99)*. This silky, lightweight cream foundation provides light to medium coverage and leaves a satin finish with a slight sheen. Though this is called a "cream makeup," it has more slip and provides less coverage than one would expect from a cream. It does, however, provide a good amount of moisture, making this a very good option for all skin types except oily. We love the texture, coverage, and pump packaging, but the most exciting thing about this foundation is the formula, as it provides sufficient UVA/UVB sun protection and a host of skin-beneficial ingredients, with no added fragrance or irritants. The only notable drawback is the limited shade selection, which is suitable only for light to medium skin.

☺ GOOD **PhotoReady Makeup SPF 20** *($13.99)*. Are you ready for your close-up? Revlon believes you will be after applying this liquid foundation with a mineral (titanium dioxide and zinc oxide) sunscreen. Given the promise of "perfect, airbrushed skin in any light," we're betting this foundation is one many women will be inclined to try. But should they? Yes, but not for the reasons Revlon wants you to believe—this isn't Photoshop in a bottle! This foundation has a beautifully silky texture that's a pleasure to blend, but its smooth matte (in feel) finish isn't the picture of airbrushed perfection. In fact, unless you apply several layers of this foundation, minor discolorations such as broken capillaries or freckles are still visible. Coverage remains in the light to medium range. We mentioned the finish was matte in feel, but because Revlon added prismatic shiny particles to this makeup it doesn't offer a matte look. The shine is relatively subtle but still evident, especially in daylight. Also worth noting is that the amount of mineral sunscreens lends this foundation an absorbent finish that feels uncomfortably dry unless your skin is oily (or prepped with a good emollient moisturizer). As for the shades, they're mostly good, with the emphasis toward those with light to tan skin tones. Avoid orange-toned Cappuccino and consider the peach-tinged Cool Beige carefully.

☺ GOOD **PhotoReady Perfecting Primer** *($11)*. This fragrance-free, sheer-tinted primer has a silky-cream texture that blends on beautifully to even out skin tone and temporarily fill in pores. The satiny-smooth matte finish controls excess shine, but the effect won't last for hours and hours. The formula allows foundation to apply smoothly over it or it can be worn alone. Our only complaint was that Revlon didn't add more antioxidants and other skin-beneficial ingredients, but this primer performs well nonetheless.

☺ AVERAGE **ColorStay Makeup with Softflex for Combination/Oily Skin SPF 6** *($12.99)* is downgraded from the get-go because of its unusually low SPF rating. This is an area where Revlon typically excels, and the SPF 6 rating is frustrating given the minimum to look for is SPF 15. Still more perplexing is the fact that this version of ColorStay Makeup has a higher percentage of active ingredients than the Normal to Dry Skin version (which is rated SPF 15). If you're willing to pair this with an effective sunscreen rated SPF 15 or higher, it has a superb texture that blends effortlessly and allows enough time to do so before setting to a solid, but not flat-looking, matte finish. It's tricky to get less than medium coverage from this, but you can buff away any blending mistakes, it wears beautifully, and it removes with a water-soluble cleanser. If the sunscreen were rated SPF 15 or higher, this would have been a slam-dunk recommendation for normal to very oily skin. Several shades are available for fair to dark skin tones, almost all of which are wonderful. Avoid Natural Beige and Golden Caramel. Note: The Caramel, Toast, Rich Ginger, Cappuccino, Mahogany, and Mocha shades do not offer any sun protection.

☺ AVERAGE **$$$ ColorStay Aqua Mineral Makeup SPF 13** *($13.99)* is a loose powder foundation with sunscreen that has a unique "wet" feel on your skin. The wet sensation is supposed to indicate that the powder is hydrating, but that effect is nothing more than pure gimmick. Topically applied water (even the coconut water in this product) alone cannot hydrate skin—if anything, it only leaves skin drier once the water evaporates.

☹ POOR **PhotoReady Airbrush Mousse Makeup** *($12.99)* is much more like a hair mousse than anything resembling airbrushed makeup. When dispensed (even when you're being careful), it shoots out in a bubbly mound, which quickly begins to dissolve into a puddle of creamy liquid foundation that feels wet and runny as you apply. As you might imagine, it's difficult to get even application with a foundation whose consistency is bubbly, and indeed the biggest problem with this foundation is its tendency to streak and apply unevenly. It does provide light to medium coverage, but its gimmicky delivery system, difficult-to-use texture, and unnaturally shiny finish are major, and ridiculous, drawbacks. If the texture and application aren't enough to dissuade you, this foundation is also loaded with flecks of shimmer that tend to sink into lines and exaggerate wrinkles. All told, this foundation has no redeeming qualities.

REVLON CONCEALERS

☺ GOOD **ColorStay Under Eye Concealer SPF 15** *($9.99)* nets its excellent sun protection from a combination of titanium dioxide and zinc oxide, two gentle active ingredients well suited for use around the eyes. This click-pen concealer has a built-in, angled sponge-tip applicator that dispenses a slightly thick but blendable concealer. It smoothes over skin, provides decent coverage (this isn't the best choice for very dark circles), and has a satin finish. Overall, this is a great option for normal to dry skin. It poses minimal risk of creasing into lines under the eye, and most of the shades are superbly neutral. Avoid Light/Medium, which has a peachy cast that doesn't soften enough to look natural.

☺ AVERAGE **ColorStay Blemish Concealer** *($9.99)* contains 0.5% salicylic acid, which is on the low side for handling blemishes, but the pH of this concealer prevents it from working as an exfoliant anyway. It provides uneven, often insufficient, coverage (especially for blemishes), and it never sets to a true matte finish, so slippage and fading will be issues, not to mention that it looks slightly chalky on skin. The shades are nearly perfect (though Light/Medium is a bit pink), but that's not enough to make this liquid concealer an easy recommendation. Check out L'Oreal's excellent True Match Concealer instead; its formula is fine for blemish-prone skin.

☹ POOR **PhotoReady Concealer SPF 20** *($9.99)* is a disappointing cream stick concealer with sunscreen. It lacks the opacity required to convincingly cover discolorations or blemishes, and it's not recommended for use under the eye because its texture is too creamy, which makes it slip into lines around the eye and make wrinkles more pronounced.

REVLON POWDERS

✓☺ BEST **Age Defying with DNA Advantage Powder** *($13.99)* is an outstanding fragrance-free pressed powder for normal to oily skin. The talc-based texture applies seamlessly and feels weightless. Skin looks refined and polished without appearing dull, dry, or too powdered. The soft matte finish is imbued with a hint of shine, but it's not overtly sparkling and is suitable for daytime wear. All the shades offered are great and best suited for light to medium-tan skin tones. Those with porcelain to fair or dark skin tones are out of luck, at least until Revlon decides to expand the palette. As for anti-aging benefits, the formula contains a peptide and some good repairing ingredients along with a tiny amount of antioxidant from cherries. The peptide and antioxidants won't remain stable in this type of packaging, but the repairing ingredients are a nice touch and likely contribute to this powder's finish (which, by the way, does a good job of not settling into lines and large pores). One caution: This powder contains the sunscreen ingredient ethylhexyl methoxycinnamate. Although not a bad ingredient, caution is warranted if you apply this powder around your eyes. Some will find this ingredient sensitizing for use near the eyes, though most won't find it to be a problem.

☺ GOOD **ColorStay Pressed Powder** *($9.99)* claims to wear for 16 hours over makeup, and, yes, it can stay that long (assuming you keep your hands off your face and you don't perspire or live in a humid climate), but your oily areas will undoubtedly need a touch-up at some point during the day well before 16 hours. This pressed powder lists the shiny mineral pigment mica as the main ingredient. Mica isn't a bad ingredient, but it has an inherent shine those with oily skin won't appreciate, not to mention it only keeps skin looking shine-free for a fraction of the 16-hour claim. It has a silky texture that feels a bit waxy and isn't the easiest to pick up with a brush. Still, this applies smoothly and sheer and doesn't look dry, thick, or powdery. Those with normal to combination skin (without very oily areas) will do best with this powder. The shades are mostly good. Translucent is OK for fair skin but can go on too white, so be careful. The range is best for fair to tan skin; there are no shades for dark skin tones. The darkest shade (Medium Deep) will be too peach for some tan skin tones, so consider this carefully.

☺ AVERAGE **PhotoReady Powder SPF 14** *($12.99)*. It's odd and disappointing that Revlon, a company known for their nearly spotless record of offering makeup with reliable UVA protection, missed the mark with this mica-based pressed powder. Its sole active ingredient is octinoxate, which doesn't quite cut it when it comes to protecting skin from the entire range of UVA radiation. What a shame, because this is otherwise a very good pressed powder, at least if you don't mind its shiny (radiant) finish. Application is sheer and smooth, giving skin a polished look without dulling its natural glow. All the shades are great, but the pickings are slim and it lacks options for very light and dark skin tones. As for the "PhotoReady" part of the name, this powder isn't any more adept at prepping skin for flashing camera lights than any other good powder, including others that provide better sun protection.

☺ AVERAGE **PhotoReady Translucent Finisher** *($12.99)* is a very dry pressed powder that has noticeable flecks of shine and far too much opacity to be labeled translucent. Not only is the finish dry, but the powder is also absorptive, which means more drying throughout the day and an exaggeration of any amount of dry skin. The lone shade can be best described as a luminous alabaster, and will work only on the very fairest skin tones. Like many dry-textured powders, this one is unusually dusty, making it a mess to apply.

REVLON BLUSHES

✓☺ BEST **Cream Blush** *($9.79)* is misnamed because this is really a cream-to-powder blush. However, if you're looking for a smooth alternative to powder blush and have normal to slightly dry or slightly oily skin (that's not oily in the cheek area), this is an outstanding option. The color selection is small but well edited, meaning every shade is a winner, though each shade has a touch of shimmer (but it's light enough so it's not distracting). Note that all the shades go on softer than they appear. This blends so easily that it is easy for the color to go "out of bounds" as you apply it, so you may need to practice before you get it to go just where you want it to be. It is best to apply this as a series of dots along the cheekbone and onto the apple of the cheek, then carefully blend each dot together to form one smooth wash of color. The compact features a cleverly concealed mirror that pops out at the touch of a button. Very sleek, and the mirror is just big enough for quick lipstick touch-ups or to check for mascara smudges.

☺ GOOD **Matte Powder Blush** *($9.79)* is a very good sheer powder blush with a genuine matte finish. Revlon took the matte name literally and delivered a beautiful yet small range of pastel-ish colors best for fair to light skin tones. The texture is silky and you'll need to layer this if you want more than a soft wash of color, but it's worth considering if you've been dismayed by the lack of good matte blushes and want a soft hint of color.

☺ AVERAGE **PhotoReady Sculpting Blush Palette** *($11)*. This pressed-powder blush palette consists of one "contour" shade (a bronze color for most of these palettes), one blush shade, and one highlighter (a lighter, shimmery shade). There are various color combinations available, and for the most part, the shades work well together. Our major complaint is the colors go on with such low intensity that they hardly show up, requiring a lot of layering. Part of that problem is because the pressed powder texture is a bit on the stiff side, making it harder to pick up with the brush. However, if a subtle sculpting effect is what you're going for, you can give this a whirl.

☺ AVERAGE **Powder Blush** *($9.79)* doesn't impart much color, even with successive applications. It has a silky texture with results that are so soft it's almost like wearing no blush at all, though you are left with sparkles. The sparkles aren't readily visible as you're eyeing the shade in the compact, but don't be fooled—they're part of each shade. This blush is only recommended if you want a hint of color and don't mind sparkly cheeks.

REVLON EYESHADOWS & EYE PRIMERS

✓☺ BEST **CustomEyes Shadow & Liner** *($8.99)* includes four powder eyeshadows and a soft matte powder eyeliner in each container, which makes it incredibly convenient to use and an incredible value. The powder eyeshadows have a creamy smooth texture and blend on beautifully. Each shade leaves behind a varying degree of shine. Most of the sets are well assembled with universally flattering modern shades you can use to create a variety of eye designs.

✓☺ BEST **Illuminance Creme Eyeshadow** *($6.50)* offers four shades of cream-to-powder eyeshadow in a sleek, slim, mirrored compact. Most cream eyeshadows tend to crease and can be troublesome to blend with other colors, but these hold up quite well and go on softly. Your choices are limited if you prefer neutral tones, but those who enjoy cream eyeshadows should strongly consider these. Powder eyeshadows may be applied before or after for different effects, and to give the cream shadow greater staying power. Note that this type of eyeshadow is not the best for anyone with oily eyelids.

☺ GOOD **Colorstay 16 HR Eye Shadow** ($7.49). Can a powder eyeshadow really last 16 hours without fading or creasing? It's hard to say for sure, because so much depends on application (how much of the color you actually apply), how oily your eyelids are, whether or not you use moisturizer on your eyelids, and what other makeup products you use, such as matte concealer, foundation, or powder over the eye. Overall, this product is really too sheer to make it for 16 hours. These quads do indeed have the potential to last for a good part of the day, but it takes a lot of effort to layer the sheer shadow to adequately shape and shade the eye. Part of the difficulty is the powder's light texture, which doesn't pick up easily with a brush and can apply unevenly (especially a problem with the shinier shades). Blending isn't effortless, but it can be done with some patience and good makeup brushes. We love the low price and the fact that most of these quads are well coordinated (Decadent and Addictive are especially great), but note that each of these Colorstay quads has some degree of shine.

☹ AVERAGE **PhotoReady Eye Primer + Brightener** ($9.99) has a thin texture and dry finish that tends to exaggerate fine lines and dry areas once it sets. That's not a huge concern if you intend to use it as a shadow primer (which is easily accomplished using your concealer instead of an extra product like this), but for under-eye brightening, as Revlon recommends, you'll need to prep with a moisturizer and blend quickly before this pale pink fluid sets, which ends up being more trouble than it's worth. As a brush-on shadow primer, it helps powder eyeshadow adhere to skin while evening out the skin tone beneath, but it doesn't significantly extend eyeshadow wear-time compared with doing nothing to prep the eyelid. The sole pale pink shade limits its use to those who have fair to light skin.

☹ POOR **Luxurious Color Perle Eye Shadow** ($4.99) is sparkly and the mirror-like shiny particles cling poorly. It suffers from a dry texture and uneven color deposit that makes blending difficult. This is one to skip!

REVLON EYE & BROW LINERS

✓☺ BEST **ColorStay Liquid Liner** ($7.29) has a brush that enables you to paint a thin or thick line with precision and ease. The formula dries in a flash, so get this on correctly right from the start because once it sets it won't budge all day. This is assuredly worth a look for those who prefer liquid eyeliner or who have trouble getting pencil eyeliners to last.

✓☺ BEST **ColorStay Liquid Eye Pen** ($8.99) has a pointed, flexible felt-tip applicator that makes this a breeze to apply, even if you don't have a very steady hand. The formula dispenses evenly and sets quickly to an immovable finish. Smearing, smudging, and fading simply don't happen with this eyeliner. The only drawback is that the color intensity isn't as strong as that of standard liquid eyeliners. That means the initial application is a bit softer, but if you're adept, you can lay down a second coat for additional emphasis. All the shades are recommended.

☺ AVERAGE **Brow Fantasy Pencil & Gel** ($7.39) combines a standard brow pencil with a sheer brow gel in one component. The pencil needs sharpening; you get a very small amount (it's roughly a quarter of the length of a standard brow pencil); and the brow gel, while completely non-sticky, imparts almost zero color and does not contain the type of ingredients that keep unruly hairs in place. This is more a blah product than a fantasy.

☺ AVERAGE **ColorStay Brow Enhancer** *($8.99)* provides a tinted wax and brow bone highlighter in one component. The wax is essentially a twist-up brow pencil housed in a retractable base. It definitely has a waxy texture and unless applied sparingly can make brow hairs look and feel coated. Unlike the best brow pencils, the finish of this one remains slightly tacky. The highlighter is simply a twist-up cream-to-powder eyeshadow that leaves a gleaming finish wherever it is used. It applies smoothly and is minimally crease- and fade-prone. If you opt to give this a whirl, all the shades are workable, including the Blonde tone.

☺ AVERAGE **ColorStay Creme Gel Eyeliner** *($9.99)*. Eyeliner aficionados know that the advantage of cream-gel eyeliners is their longevity and dramatic effect. A good eyeliner will last all day and then some, even if you have oily eyelids. However, the drawback is that this type of eyeliner requires a nimble, thin-tipped brush and a fair amount of skill to apply it. That's largely the problem with Revlon's Colorstay Creme Gel Eyeliner: The included brush is too short and bulky to create a thin or precise line, and the texture of the eyeliner is somewhat goopy and hard to work with. If you opt to use a different brush, you'll find that you can apply this liner evenly, but only if you take care to always blot and smooth the excess liner from the brush first. The texture is dry, which can result in tugging and skipping a bit over the lids; however, patient application will be rewarded with color that's rich and long-lasting. Although this has its strong points, ultimately, its weaker elements add up to a frustrating experience that's not preferred to other long-wearing gel eyeliners.

☺ AVERAGE **ColorStay Eyeliner** *($7.49)* is a twist-up, retractable pencil that has almost too much slip and a tip that's soft enough to flatten and become unusable with moderate pressure. Once this sets in place though, it does stay quite well without feeling tacky. If you're willing to acclimate to this pencil's quirks, it is one to consider.

☺ AVERAGE **Grow Luscious Lash Liner** *($7.69)* is a decent pencil liner. The creamy texture glides on smoothly, allowing ample time to blend, after which it sets to a dry, smudge-proof finish. The shades include black, brown, gray, and emerald green—all of which deposit a bold, smooth line of matte-finish color. We only wish Revlon had made this a retractable pencil instead of one that you have to routinely sharpen. The implications of lash growth are 100% false.

☺ AVERAGE **Luxurious Color Eyeliner** *($9.99)* is a relatively standard eye pencil that needs routine sharpening. The color intensity is strong (Revlon compares it, accurately, to that of a liquid eyeliner), yet the color can be smudged and softened for a smoky effect. It is mildly prone to smearing and some fading, but the rich colors last, making this an option for those who prefer pencils and don't mind sharpening.

REVLON LIP COLOR & LIPLINER

✓☺ BEST **Colorburst Lip Butters** *($5.99)*. With a rich texture somewhere between that of a lip balm and a lipstick, Revlon's Lip Butters are wonderfully moisturizing treats for lips. Packaged like traditional lipsticks, they slick on easily, leaving a soft wash of sheer color with just the right amount of color and a shiny finish. These are sheer enough to be versatile for daytime or casual wear, but vibrant enough to get noticed. A wide array of truly gorgeous shades means there's an option for everyone!

☀ Sunscreens must provide reliable UVA (anti-aging) protection. See the Appendix for details.

The Reviews R

✓☺ BEST **ColorStay Lipliner** *($7.99)* is a retractable, twist-up pencil that really holds up against greasy lipsticks and, true to its name, stays put. The variety of shades do a formidable job of keeping lipstick anchored in place, making this a must-try if you're prone to feathering.

✓☺ BEST **Super Lustrous Lipstick** *($7.99)* is fantastic. Whether you choose a creamy or frost (shimmer) finish, you get a moderately creamy lipstick that feels comfortable without being too slick or greasy and has better-than-average staying power. This is a very good creamy lipstick with a staggering range of shades.

✓☺ BEST **Super Lustrous Matte Lipstick** *($7.99)* is indeed matte and you can wear it with little risk of having it move into lines. It definitely has a matte finish and a slightly dry texture, but if you are tempted to put on a gloss, it will bleed into lines around the mouth. If that issue doesn't apply to you, this is absolutely worth trying.

☺ GOOD **Colorburst Lipgloss** *($7.99)* has enough opacity and stain that it could be considered a liquid lipstick. While it does provide lots of shine, it doesn't appear glossy or overly thick—in fact, the texture is pleasantly thin and it doesn't feel the least bit sticky. Colors range from sheer gold to fiery red, and each is packaged in a tube with an elongated sponge-tip applicator that's easy to use. You'll get a couple of hours of wear from this gloss, which is above average, but the trade-off is a significant amount of bleeding into lines around the mouth (and because the gloss is so pigmented, it's very noticeable). A good lipliner (like Paula's Choice Long-Lasting Anti-Feather Lipliner) will help stave off the creeping color, but that drawback still prevents this from earning a higher rating.

☺ GOOD **Colorburst Lipstick** *($8.99)* is a good, lightweight cream lipstick that offers nearly full coverage and a soft cream finish. This is worth considering, but it lacks the wow factor of today's best lipsticks.

☺ GOOD **Super Lustrous Lipgloss** *($6.99)* is a standard lip gloss with an angled, sponge-tip applicator and smooth application that finishes glossy and feels slightly sticky. The beguiling shade selection offers sheer and dramatic hues that can be worn alone or to add pizzazz to a lipstick. This reasonably priced gloss competes nicely with more costly options from luxury lines such as Chanel and Yves Saint Laurent.

☺ AVERAGE **Moon Drops Lipstick** *($8.99)* has been around for decades, and even the bright green packaging hasn't changed. Although this is a good, traditional cream lipstick, its fragrance is knock-your-socks-off strong and that also affects how this tastes, which is to say not pleasant. The vast array of shades favors bright, bold hues (fans of orange lipstick, take note).

☺ AVERAGE **Just Bitten Lip Stain + Balm** *($8.99)* has a felt-tip marker–style applicator on one end and a colorless stick of lip balm on the other. Once you've applied the stain and its set on your lips, the clear balm top coat is meant to deliver moisture to lips and add a bit of shine. While it does both those things beautifully, the stain itself doesn't perform very well. First, the scented stain has a strange tackiness, and it grabs to dry spots and seeps into lines quickly, so you may want to prep with a liner. Subsequent coats of the stain (required to even out the color) create dark spots and increase the chance of feathering, but an even coat can be done with patience. There are some lovely jewel-toned shades, as well as softer pinks and mauves, but they all are darker and brighter than they appear in packaging. If you are patient and have a very light and even touch, you might see good results, but there are lip stain products that are far less tricky that you can pair with your favorite lip balm.

☺ AVERAGE **ColorStay Mineral Lipglaze** *($8.99)*. Never mind the fact that the only minerals in this gloss are mica and iron oxides, the same cosmetic pigments that show up in thousands of lipsticks and glosses—what about Revlon's claim of 8-hour wear from a lip gloss?

Well, due to the high amount of (very synthetic) film-forming copolymer, that claim is basically true. This wand-applied lip gloss wears and wears (though the top layer will come off on coffee cups or anything else your lips touch). The problem is that the long-wear and lingering color come with the trade-off that your lips constantly feel slightly tacky. This isn't a silky, slick gloss with a wet-looking shine; it's a tenacious gloss with a shimmering finish that doesn't feel as good as it should. This is a tough sell, but if you're willing to tolerate the drawbacks, it may be worth a try (it certainly wears longer than standard lip gloss).

☹ POOR **ColorStay Ultimate Liquid Lipstick** *($10.99)* is supposed to be a lip paint and top coat in one, thus negating the need to use the numerous two-step long-wearing lip products on the market. That's an admirable goal, but Revlon failed miserably. This liquid lipstick applies smoothly and feels like a lightweight gloss, but within minutes after it dries, your lips literally feel like the moisture is being sucked right out of them. We tried applying more product, thinking that because the top coat was built in, it would offer some relief from the parched feeling. That didn't happen. Instead, our lips continued to feel dry. About an hour later, the color began flaking and looking all-around unattractive. Revlon maintains this wears for 12 hours, but we suspect most women won't tolerate the way it feels for longer than 12 minutes, so their long-wearing claim won't be put to the test. What a shame, because the concept is exciting and the shade range is beautiful.

REVLON MASCARAS

✓☺ BEST **Fabulash Mascara** *($6.79)* promises fuller, clump-free lashes, and it delivers—big-time! You'll get a clean application that defines each lash while lengthening and thickening in the right proportions to produce dramatic but not over-the-top lashes. Add to this the fact that lashes stay soft without flaking or smearing, and Fabulash deserves an enthusiastic round of applause!

☺ GOOD **CustomEyes Mascara** *($8.99)* claims it can create either "Length & Drama" or "Length & Definition" by adjusting the applicator setting, which is part of the container, but the difference between the two "bristle alignments" is negligible at best. However, the results on either setting are impressive: lots of thickness, moderate lengthening, and no smudging or flaking throughout the day. The widely spaced bristles on the rubber brush don't do much in the way of separation or individual lash definition.

☺ GOOD **Grow Luscious Plumping Mascara** *($8.99)* has a heavy but workable application from a large, long brush that can be tricky to maneuver if your eye area is small or if your brow bone is very close to the crease of your eye. Those willing to experiment with this mascara will find it builds impressive thickness without clumps and you'll get surprisingly good length, too. Despite the name, this doesn't "plump" lashes or contain anything that will stimulate healthier lash growth. This mascara contains the same standard ingredients found in most mascaras, and the tiny amount of nonfragrant plant oils Revlon added won't enhance the natural growth cycle of your lashes as claimed. The conditioning ingredients do help keep lashes soft, but softness has nothing to do with how lashes grow. If you're willing to test out Revlon's brush, this is recommended and is better than their other Grow Luscious mascaras.

☺ GOOD **Lash Fantasy Total Definition Primer & Mascara** *($8.99)* is worth considering. The Primer step is essentially a colorless mascara that's applied first, followed by a regular mascara. Using the Primer versus not using it makes a subtle difference, but whether you do both steps or just apply the mascara, you'll enjoy substantial length and thickness in nearly equal measure. Lashes are perfectly defined without a clump in sight, and this wears beautifully all day.

☺ GOOD **Lash Fantasy Total Definition Waterproof Primer & Mascara** *($8.99)*. Just as with Revlon's non-waterproof Lash Fantasy Total Definition Primer & Mascara, this two-step product owes its successful results to the lash primer. Sweeping the primer through lashes and immediately following with mascara produces prodigiously long, appreciably thick lashes. You'll need a lash comb handy unless you want a heavier, dramatic look. Clumping is kept to a minimum, but you may notice some minor flaking if application is overzealous. The mascara applied alone is a snooze; all you get is patchy definition and mediocre length without much thickness, even with successive coats. Whether you use the lash primer with or without the mascara, the formulas are waterproof and require more than a water-soluble cleanser for complete removal.

☺ GOOD **PhotoReady 3D Volume Mascara** *($8.99)* has a large but short brush with ultra-fine rubber bristles that coat lashes evenly, creating appreciable thickness and length. Without any clumping, smudging, or flaking, this mascara holds up to all-day wear, but still comes off easily with a makeup remover. However, given the large brush size and short wand length, this isn't a very nimble mascara, especially if you like to get into the inner corners of the eye.

☺ AVERAGE **Grow Luscious by Fabulash Mascara and Lash Enhancer** *($8.99)*. Revlon wants you to use this mascara not only for longer, thicker lashes, but also because they maintain it will "complement the natural growth cycle of your lashes." Just like many cosmetics companies are doing these days, they want you to believe this can work like Latisse, the prescription-only lash-growing product being advertised all over the television and magazines. There are no cosmetic products that work like Latisse or that can affect one eyelash. Just like the hair on your head, eyelashes have a growth cycle. Depending on which phase lashes are in (growth, resting, or shedding), you can expect eyelashes to shed and grow every 30-45 days. Of course, this doesn't happen to every lash at the same time, which is why most people don't notice when old lashes fall out and are replaced by new ones. However, being very careful with its language, Revlon never claims that they can affect the growth of eye lashes; rather, they use clever marketing language so you will think that's what they mean. Revlon states their mascara can "complement the growth" of your lashes. Well, "complement" simply means something that accents what you are using, such as a good red wine complements a steak dinner. All Revlon is really stating is that their mascara goes nicely with the growth cycle of your lashes, which is what any mascara in the world can do. Slick, huh? There are no ingredients in this mascara that affect eyelash growth—this isn't a cheap way to enjoy the benefits of the prescription-only lash-growth product Latisse. Instead, it's just a decent mascara with an awkward, overly large brush that hinders quick application. If you can get the hang of the huge brush, this works OK to make lashes remarkably longer and slightly thicker. The problem is that it applies unevenly and tends to smear along the lash line during wear. That's not good news, and really, there's no need to tolerate that given the number of superior mascaras at the drugstore.

☺ AVERAGE **Grow Luscious by Fabulash Mascara & Lash Enhancer Waterproof** *($8.99)*. Revlon wants you to know that 94% of women who applied this mascara saw longer lashes, which is about as shocking as stating that washing your face is a good way to remove makeup. Really, any mascara can cause a high percentage of women to admit that, yes, their lashes look longer. Big deal! As it turns out, this mascara isn't impressive. You get average length and minimal thickness and the large brush can make application tricky. It is all too easy to get mascara where you don't want it (on the eyelid or under-brow area) and the results you get on your lashes aren't worth the cleanup. Most disappointing (and unusual) is that this actually looks flaky on lashes but doesn't actually flake. The formula is waterproof but there are lots of better waterproof mascaras at the drugstore. As for this making lashes able to grow stronger, no way.

☹ POOR **CustomEyes Waterproof Mascara** *($8.99)*. The main selling point with this waterproof mascara is that you can "dial in" for subtle length and definition or for more drama. The cap of this mascara can be rotated to the number one or two positions. Setting it to number one deposits more mascara on the brush and dialing it to number two deposits less. Regardless of which position you set, both go on too heavy and quickly make your lashes look spiky. This mascara is waterproof, but it is also difficult and time-consuming to remove; you essentially have to chip away at lashes and the formula becomes goopy and runny as you work to take it off.

☹ POOR **Fabulash Mascara Waterproof** *($6.99)* lengthens and provides decent thickness, but also it clumps as it is applied, goes on unevenly, and flakes throughout the day, not to mention it makes your lashes feel dry and crispy.

RIMMEL (MAKEUP ONLY)

Strengths: The pressed bronzing powder; some of the best mascaras at the drugstore; powder eyeshadows; excellent automatic eye pencil; Lasting Finish Lipstick is a must-see.

Weaknesses: Packaging that isn't very user-friendly; average concealers; several lackluster eyeshadow options; none of the Extra Super Lash mascaras earn their impressive-sounding names; potentially problematic eye-makeup remover.

For more information and the latest Rimmel reviews, visit CosmeticsCop.com.

RIMMEL EYE-MAKEUP REMOVER

☺ AVERAGE **Gentle Eye Makeup Remover** *($7.59 for 4.2 fl. oz.)* is a relatively standard, non-silicone–based eye-makeup remover whose formula is hindered a bit by the inclusion of sodium lauryl sulfate, a cleansing agent known for being a potent skin irritant. There isn't a lot of it in the product, but this strong detergent cleansing agent is best kept away from the sensitive eye area, so this isn't worth considering over gentler options found in the Best Products chapter.

RIMMEL FOUNDATIONS & PRIMER

☺ GOOD **Fix & Perfect Foundation Primer** *($7.59)*. A sheer peach tint that dissipates quickly is what you'll get when you apply this silky, lightweight primer. The powdery matte finish it provides helps keep excess oil in check and creates a smooth surface to apply makeup. Best for normal to oily skin, this is a good, inexpensive product to consider if you've been curious about whether a primer would be helpful or whether it would be a needless addition to your makeup routine.

☺ GOOD **Lasting Finish 25 Hour Foundation** *($7.13)*. In terms of a lasting finish, this liquid foundation delivers, thanks to its silicone-enhanced formula and silky matte finish. This has a beautiful texture suitable for normal to oily skin, and does an above-average job of looking more skin-like than flat. This is especially impressive when you consider the amount of coverage it provides. Although it can be blended on sheer, the standard amount provides nearly full coverage, yet it doesn't look heavy. The best shades include Ivory, Soft Beige, and True Ivory. The options for medium skin tones are not worth considering because of their obvious pink or peach tones.

☺ GOOD **Match Perfection Foundation SPF 15** *($5.68)* earns high marks for its built-in broad-spectrum sun protection and beautiful creamy texture, which feels surprisingly lightweight. The liquid formula is ideal for normal to combination skin that's slightly dry. Equally impressive is this foundation's natural-looking coverage, blending ability, and hint-of-dew finish. Where this product falls short is its staying power (you need to use a powder for this to stay put all day, especially on oily areas), and the clear glass screw-top bottle is hard to use. A pump dispenser and an opaque bottle would've been a nice touch.

☺ AVERAGE **Clean Finish Foundation** *($4.99)* is a liquid foundation with a blendable, creamy texture that provides medium coverage—but that's where the positives end. Five minutes into wear, there are signs of trouble. The first and most obvious drawback is that this foundation, regardless of the shade, changes color over time. It begins by turning a pale tone of orange, and then continues darkening. It also feels heavy on skin and the coverage doesn't last. Of the numerous shades, there are plenty of options for light to medium skin tones. The semi-matte finish and formula are best for most skin types, but overall you just can't trust the color, and when it comes to foundation, that's everything.

RIMMEL CONCEALERS

☺ GOOD **Match Perfection Skin Tone Adapting 2-in-1 Concealer & Highlighter** *($5.99)*. This liquid concealer dispenses through a squeeze tube onto a built-in brush for mess-free application. Although the brush works for applying this, you may still want to use your fingers to blend it completely. It offers light to medium coverage for concealing imperfections, but as far as highlighting goes there really isn't anything special about this. Rimmel claims that this concealer's Smart-Tone technology mimics your skin tone, but it's impossible for any makeup to intuitively adjust itself to a wide variety of skin tones. In reality, the limited color range is hit or miss (watch out for shades with peach undertones). This is a good concealer if one of the shades works with your skin tone. The soft matte finish holds up well throughout the day and doesn't creep into fine lines like creamy concealers do.

☺ AVERAGE **Hide the Blemish Concealer** *($5.19)* is a very greasy, lipstick-style concealer that doesn't cover that well, though it does come in three very good colors. An emollient, wax-based concealer like this is the last thing you want to place over blemishes, at least if the goal is to not make them worse! If you prefer this type of concealer, it would be OK over non-blemished areas, but if you're using it under the eye, creasing is inevitable.

RIMMEL POWDER

☺ AVERAGE **Stay Matte Pressed Powder** *($5.79)* has a smooth texture and non-powdery, but dry matte finish laced with a tiny amount of shine. Those with oily skin will find this doesn't stay matte for long, but it doesn't look thick or cakey, either. While not the most elegant-feeling powder, it's a good, inexpensive option for normal to slightly oily or slightly dry skin. There are three shades, with no options for medium to dark skin tones. This contains a small amount of fragrance ingredients known to cause irritation, which is what keeps this from earning a better rating.

RIMMEL BLUSHES & BRONZERS

✓☺ BEST **Natural Bronzer** *($5.79)* is a talc-based pressed-powder bronzer that has a beautifully smooth texture and application. Shine from each of the three shades is so subtle as to be almost nonexistent, making this a fine choice for daytime wear. Speaking of the shades, all have potential, but the orange tinge of Sun Light makes it trickier for fair to light skin tones to pull off, and it's too light for medium skin tones.

☺ GOOD **Lasting Finish Blendable Powder Blush** *($4.99)* has a silky-smooth texture and is picked up easily with a brush, and it contains enough pigment so it really does last on skin. The four shades are all flattering pink and berry hues, and all contain enough shimmer to create a striking, luminous finish, but without noticeable flecks of sparkle. Depending on the size of your blush brush, the small pan size Rimmel uses may be an issue.

☺ GOOD **Lasting Finish Blendable Powder Blush & Highlighter** *($4.99)* has a silky-smooth texture and the colors are pigmented enough to really last on your skin. Each of the trios features a dark, richly pigmented shade, a lighter more luminous shade, and a frosty highlighter shade with larger flecks of sparkle. However, the small pan size makes it difficult to use the three shades separately, which is frustrating, unless you are happy with the shiny shade you get by swirling all three together.

☺ GOOD **Sunshimmer Shimmering Maxi Bronzer** *($8.99)* is a very good (and very large) option for those looking for a pressed-powder bronzer. In the package, the bronzer definitely seems shinier than it actually appears on skin due to a thin layer of golden sparkles on top designed to look like waves on a shore. Once the gold sparkles are brushed away, what lies beneath both shades is a soft, somewhat shimmery bronzer without a trace of orange. The talc-based powder goes on sheer and even, with little streaking, though it does grab on damp or oily spots.

RIMMEL EYESHADOWS

☺ GOOD **Glam'Eyes Mono Eye Shadow** *($3.32)* has a smooth, blendable powder texture that provides more coverage than most shadows. There are no truly matte shades, but some have a flattering, subtle luminosity.

☺ GOOD **Glam'Eyes Quad Eye Shadow** *($5.42)* provides four shades of powder eyeshadow in coordinating colors, so you can create a wide variety of looks. There are no truly matte options, but most quads contain at least two shades with minimal shine—meaning no large flecks of sparkle, just slight luminosity.

☹ AVERAGE **Glam'Eyes Trio Eye Shadow** *($4.92)* provides three shades of powder eyeshadow in coordinating colors, so you can create a variety of looks. There are no truly matte options, but all contain at least one shade with minimal shine.

RIMMEL EYE & BROW LINERS

✓☺ BEST **Exaggerate Waterproof Eye Definer** *($5.67)* gets an A+ for its ease of use and wearability. The texture is soft enough to glide on lids, but not so creamy that it smudges all over the place. The pigment goes on rich and doesn't fade as the day wears on, and, true to name, it's also waterproof. This retractable pencil also comes with a sharpener for sculpting a precise, fine tip, as well as a soft smudging tool for smooth blending. And did you notice the price? We're talking bona-fide beauty bargain here!

☹ AVERAGE **Professional Eyebrow Pencil** *($3.09)* has a drier, stiffer texture than most standard brow pencils, but its finish really lasts and application is soft and even. This includes a brush built into the cap, which can come in handy. It would be rated higher if it didn't need sharpening.

☹ AVERAGE **Soft Kohl Kajal Eye Pencil** *($3.19)* needs sharpening so it isn't as convenient as an automatic/retractable pencil. Although it is creamy and glides on with minimal effort, it has a longer-lasting finish and is less prone to smudging than you'd expect.

☹ POOR **Special Eyes Precision Eye Liner Pencil** *($3.09)* is a poor eye pencil choice, even if the prospect of sharpening thrills you. It's way too creamy and smears with minimal provocation. Even without provocation, you'll notice fading way too soon.

☹ POOR **Glam'Eyes Professional Liquid Eye Liner** *($5.99)* is a standard liquid liner that comes with a long, skinny brush that can be hard to control along the lash line. Although some may prefer this type of brush, the formula takes too long to dry (even when applied lightly) and it smears easily.

The Reviews R

RIMMEL LIP COLOR & LIPLINERS

✓☺ BEST **Lasting Finish Lipstick** *($4.92)* promises 8-hour wear, and almost makes it to that mark. Color intensity is strong, which lends staying power, but this is still a cream lipstick that comes off on coffee cups and other objects (and it certainly won't last through a meal without a touch up). That said, you'll find this to be one of the better (and least expensive) elegant cream lipsticks available at the drugstore. It feels supremely smooth and light, yet leaves lips comfortably moisturized with a soft gloss finish (or shimmer, depending on the shade chosen). We'd put this up against any department store lipstick, that's for sure!

✓☺ BEST **Stay Glossy Long-Lasting Lipgloss** *($4.99)* doesn't live up to its 6-hour wear claim. On average, we got about 2 hours of wear before it was time to reapply, which is still fairly tenacious for a lip gloss, but nowhere near what Rimmel promises. The texture is sumptuously plush, without any residual stickiness or grainy feel. A balm-like texture and an elongated sponge-tip applicator make applying this lip gloss a delight. There are nearly two dozen shades, with options for everyone—from sheer shimmers to bold opaques. Despite Rimmel's exaggerated claims about how long this wears, this moisturizing and affordable lip gloss still deserves our highest rating.

☺ GOOD **Exaggerate Automatic Lip Liner** *($6.49)* is an automatic, retractable lip pencil that is creamy without veering into greasiness. It stays on quite well and the colors are rich with pigment. It doesn't apply as smoothly as others (you have to apply a fair amount of pressure to get the color to show up), but for the money, this is a safe bet.

☹ AVERAGE **1000 Kisses Stay On Lip Liner Pencil** *($3.59)* is a standard, needs-sharpening pencil. It has a smooth and comfortably creamy texture and stays on as well as most other pencils, which is to say, well, but not well enough to withstand even one kiss, much less a thousand!

☹ AVERAGE **Moisture Renew Cream Lipgloss SPF 15** *($6.15)*. Labeling this a cream lip gloss is a stretch because it's simply a thin-textured lip gloss with sunscreen that imparts sheer color and lots of shine. Most of the shades have tiny flecks of shimmer that add to the glossy finish, but it can look odd as the lip color begins to fade. Another problem is that this lip gloss does not include the ingredients needed to shield your lips from the sun's entire range of damaging UVA rays, which is essential for anti-aging benefits (see the Appendix for details).

☹ AVERAGE **Moisture Renew Lipstick SPF 18** *($6.47)* is a very standard cream lipstick that isn't worth strong consideration due to its intense fragrance and unpleasant taste. Though it applies smoothly and the colors have moderate pigmentation with a soft cream finish, the active sunscreens don't provide sufficient UVA protection, which is a huge mark against this lipstick. See the Appendix to find out which UVA-protecting ingredients you need for reliable protection.

RIMMEL MASCARAS

✓☺ BEST **The Max Volume Flash Mascara** *($6.83)* is a grand slam for those who want lush, thick, beautifully separated lashes. The large brush proves surprisingly nimble, and its bristles allow you to coat the lashes sufficiently for dramatic results without clumping. Once set, this won't smear or flake, yet it removes with a basic water-soluble cleanser. The claims of 14 times more volume don't come true, but this produces impressive results fast.

☺ GOOD **Extra Wow Lash Mascara** *($3.99)*. If you want full, thick lashes, this is a good mascara to try. The formula is smudge-free and flake-free, and adds volume with minimal clumping. You also get some lengthening though this works best to add bulk and volume to lashes.

☺ GOOD **Lash Accelerator** *($8.53)*. While this mascara claims to include "Grow-Lash Complex," there just aren't any ingredients in the formula proven to grow even a single lash. However, that doesn't mean this isn't a worthwhile mascara! Those looking for length and subtle thickness will appreciate this mascara's nimble brush and slightly wet formula that deposits evenly over the length of each lash. Lashes stay soft to the touch, with no smearing or flaking. This produces elegantly sweeping lashes without over-the-top drama (although you can get to dramatic if you apply enough coats), which makes this a very good option for daytime wear.

☺ GOOD **Sexy Curves Full Body Mascara** *($5.99)*. This mascara's caterpillar-like spiral brush (they describe it as a "triple plump brush") looks cool and is surprisingly easy to use despite its larger size. You can build length quickly without a hint of clumping and this leaves lashes defined with a soft fringed curl. Is the result "sexy"? Well, we suppose it can be depending on your criteria for sexy lashes. The results don't replicate false eyelashes or build prodigious thickness, but many will still find it impressive, not to mention the price is attractive, too! The one drawback is that this tends to smear along the lashline during application and, to some extent, during wear.

☺ GOOD **Volume Flash Scandaleyes Mascara** *($6.99)* is said to capture and plump every lash. Although this isn't a bad mascara, the name and claims don't come true. Instead, you get decent length that takes quite a bit of effort to achieve anything close to dramatic. You won't get any clumping, likely because despite an extra-large brush, the mascara formula itself is on the thin side. That means thickness is scarce so consider this a lengthening mascara only. If that's what you're after, you won't be disappointed.

☹ AVERAGE **Extra Super Lash Curved Brush Mascara** *($3.59)* performs just as well as the straight brush version below, but is the one to choose if you want a more defined curl.

☹ AVERAGE **Extra Super Lash Mascara** *($3.59)* remains a reliable lengthening mascara that applies clump-free and tends to not flake or chip, but thickness is harder to come by. It isn't all that super, but it does the job.

☹ AVERAGE **Glam'Eyes Day2Night Mascara** *($6.99)* has clever packaging that allows the single brush to produce different results. It works because the mascara container has two different wipers. Inside any mascara tube, the wiper is what cleans the brush and controls how much mascara is deposited when you remove the wand prior to application. With Day2Night Mascara, you can remove the wand in one of two ways, depending on which part of the cap you unwind. Regrettably, neither side is all that impressive. The Length option goes on sparse and thin and provides very little length; you basically just get some lash darkening and subtle definition complete with some smearing (but no clumps). The Volume side promises up to 12x more volume, but it nearly keeps your lashes on mute! Thickness is minimal and this ends up performing similarly to the Length option, albeit with a wetter, gloppier application. This can be smoothed out with several strokes of the brush, but the results just aren't impressive enough to warrant the effort.

☹ AVERAGE **Lycra Lash Extender Mascara** *($7.49)* makes a big deal of the fact that it contains the synthetic, amazingly stretchable fiber Lycra. Used in mascara, it is supposed to increase lash length by 60% and curl by 50%, all while helping lashes hold their shape for 14 hours. It sounds impressive, but isn't value added because, for all its ballyhoo, Lycra Lash Extender Mascara doesn't produce results anyone would consider "instant" or "dramatic." With several coats you can elongate lashes, and it sets to a soft, eye-opening curl. But thickness is scant, some clumping occurs along the way, and the performance plateaus far too soon to make good on the claims.

☺ AVERAGE **Sexy Curves Mascara** *($7.19)* has what Rimmel calls a "Triple Plump Brush," which is likely to entice those with skimpy lashes. The problem is that the excessively curvy brush makes it unnecessarily difficult to get an even application of mascara onto your lashes. If you're willing to put in the work, you'll be rewarded with longer and slightly thicker lashes. You won't get, as Rimmel claims, lashes that are 70% curlier, because Sexy Curves does little to help curl the lashes.

☹ AVERAGE **Sexy Curves Waterproof Mascara** *($7.19)* has a very scratchy brush and getting it too close to the base of your lashes (where you definitely want to deposit mascara) hurts. You need several coats to produce average length, and don't count on thickness. This doesn't clump, but neither do lots of other mascaras that out-perform this one. As for the waterproof claim, it isn't one you can rely on for fail-safe results; at best, this is slightly waterproof.

☹ AVERAGE **The Max Volume Flash Bold Curves Mascara** *($6.83)* is mostly a mess. From its awkward, unnecessarily large curved brush to its application, this isn't one of Rimmel's better mascaras. The biggest obstacle is its heavy and uneven application. Some lashes get sparse coverage, while others get too much, so you're spending extra time separating and combing through lashes with a brush to make this look halfway decent. As for maximum volume, this barely makes it past an audible whisper. With lots of effort and comb-through (plus smearing along the way), you can achieve decent length, but really, why bother?

☹ AVERAGE **The Max Volume Flash Waterproof Mascara** *($6.83)* is a lackluster waterproof mascara that comes with a standard, straight-bristle wand. The best thing about it is that it doesn't clump or flake and is relatively easy to remove. Otherwise, you're left with a basic mascara that doesn't do much to add length or thickness.

☹ AVERAGE **Volume Accelerator Mascara** *($7)*. Rimmel claims this mascara contains an "Exclusive Grow-Lash Complex," but in reality it doesn't include any ingredients proven capable of growing fuller, longer, or darker lashes. It adds length, but does so in a way that leaves lashes looking clumpy at the tips, and the thickening effect comes at the expense of lashes becoming stuck together. To make matters worse, the lackluster formula leaves lashes stiff, tends to flake, and the large brush head is difficult to use without getting mascara on the surrounding skin.

ROC (SKIN CARE ONLY)

Strengths: Some well-packaged products with retinol; all the sunscreens provide sufficient UVA protection; relatively inexpensive for a line that revolves around anti-aging.

Weaknesses: Mediocrity reigns supreme, so few of the formulas are particularly exciting; antiwrinkle claims tend to go too far; jar packaging.

For more information and reviews of the latest RoC products, visit CosmeticsCop.com.

ROC CLEANSER

☺ AVERAGE **Daily Resurfacing Disks** *($9.99 for 28 discs)* consist of a basic, gentle cleanser steeped into discs that are textured on one side to approximate the effect of a scrub or washcloth. It doesn't get more ordinary than this, and we mean really ordinary. The claim is that you can diminish lines and wrinkles after just one week of use, but the reality is that wrinkles cannot be scrubbed away. What's most likely happening is that the abrasiveness of the disc's textured side is causing low-grade inflammation. The inflammation makes your skin swell, and, voila, wrinkles (or, more specifically "fine lines") are less apparent. The problem? This type of inflammation, when experienced daily, can end up making matters worse by leading to collagen breakdown and over-manipulation of your skin. It's easy to overdo it, and when it comes to daily skin care, gentle is always best.

ROC MOISTURIZERS (DAYTIME & NIGHTTIME), EYE CREAMS, & SERUMS

✓☺ BEST **Multi Correxion 4-Zone Daily Moisturizer SPF 30** *($27.99 for 1.7 fl. oz.)*. This daytime moisturizer with an in-part avobenzone sunscreen is said to target four distinct zones of your face. Reading the claims for this product, we couldn't help but wonder why RoC is still selling their other antiwrinkle and anti-sagging products. This one supposedly does it all, so what are the others for? The good news is that the formula contains several anti-aging ingredients, including antioxidants along with retinol. It's difficult to determine how much of these beneficial ingredients are actually in the product because RoC opted to list the inactive ingredients in alphabetical order rather than in descending order of content. That's permissible because, being a sunscreen, this is an over-the-counter drug by U.S. regulations—but that doesn't really help the consumer determine the relative amounts of the different ingredients. We're going to give RoC the benefit of the doubt and assume they included efficacious amounts of these ingredients. Even with that vote of confidence, however, this product will not be able to help with deep forehead wrinkles, sagging skin around the eyes, or a less-than-taut jaw line. You just have to get over believing these illogical, mythical claims that most cosmetics companies taunt you with. The factors that cause sagging and a gradual loss of youthful contours cannot be addressed by skin-care products, regardless of how well they're formulated (see the Appendix for details). Deep forehead lines will look less apparent with any moisturizer. Despite the fact that this doesn't come close to being a face-lift in a bottle, it is a very good daytime option for normal to slightly dry or slightly oily skin. Those with oily skin, take note: This product contains mica and has a slightly shiny finish.

✓☺ BEST **Multi-Correxion Night Treatment** *($27.99 for 1 fl. oz.)*. Although this moisturizer isn't a "comprehensive anti-aging solution" for your skin, it is a light, silky moisturizer that treats your skin to an impressive amount of vitamin C (ascorbic acid) along with the cell-communicating ingredient retinol. The texture of this product makes it best for those with normal to slightly dry skin. If your skin is dry to very dry, you will want to pair this with a separate moisturizer or serum. This definitely deserves consideration if you're curious to see what a well-formulated retinol product will do for your skin. It currently stands as the best retinol product RoC offers, which of course begs the question of why they have so many other products with retinol!

☺ GOOD **Multi-Correxion Eye Treatment** *($24.99 for 0.5 fl. oz.)*. There is much to like about this lightweight, silky-textured eye cream, but its treatment benefits don't extend to diminishing dark circles and puffiness (so much for the multi-correction claim). What this will do is provide a light dose of moisture along with the antioxidant benefit of vitamin C, vitamin E, and soy protein. Also on hand is an impressive amount of the cell-communicating ingredient retinol, and this product's packaging will keep it stable during use. The combination of ingredients can help skin look better, and that includes improving the appearance of wrinkles. This would be rated a Best Product if it did not contain fragrance. We can concede to fragrance in an otherwise well-formulated facial moisturizer, but not in a product meant for use in the eye area (see the Appendix to learn why you don't need an eye cream). This is suitable for normal to slightly dry skin.

☺ GOOD **Multi Correxion Skin Renewing Serum** *($27.99 for 1 fl. oz.)*. RoC has stepped up their game with this well-formulated serum that's best for normal to oily skin, although suitable for all skin types except sensitive. The silky formula contains some very good antioxidants as well as the cell-communicating ingredient retinol (in packaging that ensures prolonged stability).

The addition of a range of skin-identical (aka skin-repairing) ingredients and some anti-irritants would elevate this to Best Product status, but it remains worth considering, especially if you're looking to replace your foundation primer with something that offers a lot more benefits and that works great under makeup. Note that this contains mica, which lends a soft shine finish.

☺ GOOD **Retinol Correxion Deep Wrinkle Daily Moisturizer SPF 30** (*$19.99 for 1 fl oz.*). Those with normal to dry skin looking for a daytime moisturizer with retinol would do well to consider this product. The in-part avobenzone sunscreen (using Neutrogena's Helioplex technology, though RoC doesn't advertise this; both companies are owned by Johnson & Johnson) has a smooth texture and satin finish. The pH is above 4.5, which means the glycolic acid won't function as an exfoliant. But this does contain retinol and comes in packaging that keeps it stable. Although this should have a better blend of antioxidants and cell-communicating ingredients, it deserves praise for the aforementioned positive traits.

☹ AVERAGE **Multi Correxion Lift Anti-Gravity Day Moisturizer SPF 30** (*$27.99 for 1.3 fl. oz.*) is an extremely average daytime moisturizer with sunscreen whose product name and claims promise more than it could possibly deliver. Please see the Appendix for details on why this product's lifting and anti-gravity claims won't come true. In terms of anti-aging, the only benefit you can rely on from this product is broad-spectrum sun protection. Critical UVA (the sun's most aging rays) protection is provided by stabilized avobenzone, and this has a lightweight cream texture that's best for normal to dry skin. We're not sure what RoC's Protient Plus ingredient is, but this product contains merely standard thickeners and silicones, which help dry skin look and feel better, but are not known to provide firmer skin. RoC included a synthetic antioxidant (pentaerythrityl tetra-di-butyl hydroxyhydrocinnamate), but there is no research proving its benefit for skin over and above the benefits you get from any of the other stable antioxidants found in lots of skin-care products.

☹ AVERAGE **Multi Correxion Lift Anti-Gravity Night Cream** (*$27.99 for 1.7 fl. oz.*) is a lightweight moisturizer for normal to slightly dry skin with a tempting name, but it isn't capable of correcting multiple signs of aging, which includes lifting skin or somehow stopping the eventual toll gravity takes. The formula isn't an anti-aging powerhouse; instead, it's a fairly standard moisturizer with grand claims that are not supported by independent published research or based on what we know is and isn't possible when it comes to controlling the effects of gravity. Although this moisturizer contains some good antioxidants, they will not remain stable once this product is opened because it is packaged in a jar. See the Appendix for details on why jar packaging is a problem for any anti-aging moisturizer. RoC claims their Protein Plus firming technology helps to tighten the skin, but they don't explain how this technology works or which ingredients make up this "technology." Most likely it is tied to the ingredient tetrahydroxypropyl ethylenediamine (THPE). RoC's parent company Johnson & Johnson did a double-blind study that examined topical application of a moisturizer containing 2.5% THPE on 41 women. Not surprisingly, the results showed the skin treated with THPE looked firmer, "more lifted," and younger compared with skin that received a placebo moisturizer without this ingredient. This may be due to the effect THPE has on surface skin cells: It is believed to modify the cell surface and increase cell tension. In theory, this would "pull" skin cells tighter and result in skin that gets a lift, but the study results showed that after 8 weeks of use, skin treated with THPE was lifted only by 14%. That's not much of an improvement, and what we don't know is whether or not THPE's effect on skin is more detrimental than helpful. After all, causing skin cells to become tense is what most astringent, drying ingredients do, and it's not the healthiest approach (Source: *Journal of*

Drugs in Dermatology, October 2011, pages 1102–1105). Using products with high amounts of THPE on a daily basis may not be the best idea if the result of making skin cells tense is irritation. Right now, we don't know if that's the case, but we do know that irritation hurts skin's healing process and its ability to look and act younger. Plus, the small sample of only 41 women is not exactly a sweeping assessment of effectiveness. Ultimately, the unknowns associated with THPE, along with the jar packaging and the lack of other state-of-the-art anti-aging ingredients, makes this moisturizer a less desirable option. Note that there is not enough glycolic acid (an AHA) in this moisturizer for it to work as an exfoliant. In low concentrations like this, it functions as a water-binding agent.

☺ AVERAGE **Multi Correxion Lift Anti-Gravity Serum** *($27.99 for 1 fl. oz.)*. This serum's name may make you think you've found a face-lift-in-a-bottle, but that's not what you'll actually get from using this product. This rather lackluster formula's second ingredient is a starch that, when dry, makes skin feel smoother and a bit tighter. Making skin feel tighter is not the same as actually tightening it, which is where the ingredient tetrahydroypropyl ethylenediamine comes into play, as discussed in the review above for RoC's Multi Correxion Lift Anti-Gravity Night Cream. Ultimately, the amount of starch in this serum (which can feel uncomfortable) makes it an iffy option. If you're going to spend this much, your skin will do better with a serum loaded with antioxidants, skin-repairing ingredients, and cell-communicating ingredients proven to help it look and act younger, without potential irritation.

☹ AVERAGE **Retinol Correxion Deep Wrinkle Night Cream** *($22.99 for 1 fl. oz.)* is a fairly standard moisturizer with retinol. Best for normal to dry skin, it has a creamy yet lightweight texture that smoothes on easily and works well under moisturizer (assuming you need more moisture than what this provides; this is fine to use on its own, too). The amount of retinol and stable packaging ensures efficacy, but the amount of glycolic acid is too low to function as an exfoliant (but does have water-binding properties). This would earn a higher rating if it offered a better range of anti-aging ingredients. The tiny amount of vitamin C (ascorbic acid) is little more than an afterthought, and the formula could use a better range of skin-repairing ingredients. Still, it covers the basics for a moisturizer with retinol if that's all you're after.

☺ AVERAGE **Retinol Correxion Deep Wrinkle Serum** *($22.99 for 1 fl. oz.)* has a silky, silicone-enhanced texture that's suitable for all skin types: It contains an impressive amount of vitamin E, but there's still more fragrance in here than there should be. You can find better retinol products from other drugstore lines and those listed in the Best Products chapter.

☺ AVERAGE **Retinol Correxion Eye Cream** *($22.99 for 0.5 fl. oz.)* contains only a tiny amount of retinol (it's listed after the preservatives) and as such this isn't a top choice if retinol is what you're after. This is otherwise a standard lightweight but hydrating eye cream for slightly dry skin. It does not contain fragrance, which is nice, but you still don't need an eye cream (see the Appendix to find out why).

☺ AVERAGE **Retinol Correxion Sensitive Night Cream** *($22.99 for 1 fl. oz.)* is supposedly designed for skin that's sensitive to retinol. That's fine; this does contain a much lower amount of retinol than what RoC typically includes in its products. What puzzled us was the inclusion of a potentially sensitizing sunscreen ingredient (ethylhexyl methoxycinnamate) and fragrance. Neither ingredient is the best for sensitive skin, whether the product contains retinol or not. Therefore, this turns out to be a questionable choice for someone with sensitive skin. Although RoC is up front about this not containing much retinol, they also included only a tiny amount of other anti-aging ingredients. In the end, this is a barely passable option for normal to dry skin that isn't sensitive.

The Reviews R

☺ AVERAGE $$$ **Multi Correxion Lift Anti-Gravity Eye Cream** *($27.99 for 0.5 fl. oz.)* is a decent emollient eye cream that is suitable for use anywhere on the face. You don't need a product labeled as being just for the eye area (see the Appendix to find out why), but if you choose to use one anyway, it shouldn't be packaged in a jar like this one is. Jar packaging exposes key ingredients to degrading light and air, so that with each use these beneficial ingredients become less stable and less able to improve your skin. Despite a tempting name, this fragrance-free eye cream isn't the answer for sagging skin. It cannot fight "multiple signs of aging caused by the downward pull of gravity" because gravity's pull is but one factor that causes the eye area to look older. There are no cosmetic ingredients that overcome what gravity eventually does to the skin, all over the body. We wish that weren't the case, but it's the truth. See the Appendix for further details on what you can do to help aging skin. At best, this eye cream will moisturize dry skin and make wrinkles less apparent (as any moisturizer will), plus it will brighten the eye area because it contains mica for shine and titanium dioxide for a subtle white cast. Both effects are more like makeup than skin care, but it explains RoC's claims that this eye cream makes the eye area look more awake—in the fight against wrinkles, however, this comes up short!

☺ AVERAGE $$$ **Retinol Correxion Sensitive Eye Cream** *($22.99 for 0.5 fl. oz.)* is said to be better for sensitive skin because it contains only a tiny amount of retinol. The idea is that this is an option for women whose skin cannot tolerate "normal" amounts of retinol or for those who are trying a retinol product for the first time. There is a logic to that, but lots of women can tolerate the "regular" amounts of retinol present in skin-care products (typically 0.025% and up) just fine, even if they are using it for the first time. Using products with lower concentrations may eliminate the problems (redness, flaking) that may accompany one's initial use of a retinol product, but you also will be sacrificing some of the benefit. On the other hand, although the antiwrinkle results may not be as dramatic if you use only the tiny amount present in this product, ongoing use can still produce equivalent results, especially if you're diligent about daily sun protection. In the long run, this eye cream ends up being a one-note song because, while retinol is a great ingredient for skin, it is not the only one. Skin does much better with an array of beneficial ingredients. Think about it like your diet: Green tea may be good for you, but if you drink only green tea, you will become malnourished or worse. Although this product's lightweight texture is silky and it provides some hydration, the formula lacks the skin-repairing and antioxidant ingredients that all skin types need to look and act younger. There is nothing special about this product that makes it better for the eye area. Yes, it's fragrance-free, but all your skin, from head to toe, does better when fragrance is omitted; it's not as though only eye-area products shouldn't have fragrance. Fragrance is a source of irritation, so it is best to minimize exposure to it, no matter what skin-care product you use or where you apply it.

ROC SPECIALTY SKIN-CARE PRODUCTS

☺ GOOD **Retinol Correxion Deep Wrinkle Filler** *($21.99 for 1 fl. oz.)*. RoC has lots of products they describe as "breakthrough formulas," but it's simply marketing hype, not real science or fact. The ingredient list doesn't make this a breakthrough any more than reverting to a typewriter would be a step forward in communication! The formula is mostly water, thickeners,

---

⊘ Think "hypoallergenic" means safe for sensitive skin? See the Appendix to find out the truth.

sunscreen agent (there is no SPF rating so you cannot rely on this for sun protection), silicones, emollient, retinol, hyaluronic acid, and preservatives. It's a good option if you're looking for a standard moisturizer with retinol, but it would have been far better if more state-of-the-art ingredients were included because retinol is not the only answer for skin. This is best for normal to slightly dry skin.

☺ AVERAGE **$$$ RoC Brilliance Day Rejuvenating Moisturizer, SPF 20 Protection** ($49.99) is a two-product kit that uses what RoC terms e-pulse technology, but it doesn't bring anything new to the table. If you're considering this kit, here are the basics: It claims to reduce wrinkles and firm skin by increasing elastin production. In addition to a daytime moisturizer with sunscreen, you get a serum (labeled **Day Activating Serum**) meant to be applied beforehand. The minerals in the serum are supposed to generate an electrical charge of some kind owing to the copper and zinc it contains. The serum needs to be paired with the moisturizer to cause an electric charge (or pulse), but there is no independent research showing the micro-current triggering ingredients can have a visible effect on skin or that other ingredients can't function the same or even better. Back to the claims about the combination of products being able to stimulate elastin repair or produce new elastin. Lots of companies make this claim because producing healthy elastin is important for skin. Elastin fibers provide support and give skin its ability to bounce back after being manipulated. As elastin becomes damaged from genetic, environmental (sun damage) aging, gravity, muscle laxity, fat movement, and hormonal loss, changes to skin structure occur. As a result, the fibers become too weak for skin to snap back as it once did. Can RoC's kit rescue your skin from sagging? Of course not. Even assuming the products in this kit could generate more elastin, it's not going to prevent sagging because elastin degradation is only one aspect of what causes skin to sag—there are significant pieces of the puzzle still missing. There is research pertaining to copper and its dual role in skin—wound-healing and altering the matrix metalloproteinases (MMP) that contribute to collagen depletion. Applying ingredients that work against this damage is helpful, but this is not the only way to improve aging skin. Zinc is believed to play a co-factor role with copper when it comes to repairing damaged elastin in skin, but again, it's not the only game in town; it does not replace anything a cosmetic dermatologist can do to improve skin and it doesn't provide anything that other skin-care products can't provide (Sources: *Connective Tissue Research*, January 2010, Epublication; *Experimental Dermatology*, March 2009, pages 205–211; and *Veterinary Dermatology*, December 2006, pages 417–423). There is no solid research proving that topical zinc or copper can stop or reverse sagging skin due to elastin damage. Step 2 in this set is the **Day Rejuvenating Cream with SPF 20**. Not surprisingly, this in-part avobenzone sunscreen is a lightweight moisturizer that provides broad-spectrum sun protection but contains barely a dusting of antioxidants. That's not to say that this is useless, although it's far less exciting than it could've been, especially for what RoC is charging.

☺ AVERAGE **$$$ RoC Brilliance Eye Beautifier** ($49.99). This eye-area duo isn't going to improve sagging skin or get you anywhere close to what RoC describes as "brilliantly beautiful" results. It's not an eye-lift for under $50! Please see the review above for RoC Brilliance Day Rejuvenating Moisture with SPF 20 Protection for key details of the e-pulse and elasticity-triggering claims. This set contains the same serum as the SPF 20 version, but this time it's packaged with an eye cream. A significant ingredient in the **Eye Beautifying Cream** is the chelating agent tetrahydroxypropyl ethylenediamine. Guess what chelating agents do? They deactivate metal ions by making them a part of their complex ring structure. In other words, the presence of a chelating agent in the Eye Beautifying Cream prevents the copper and zinc in the accompanying serum from exerting their ion-based energy, which is supposed to be the crux of how this kit exerts its anti-aging benefits. Unbelievable!

☹ AVERAGE $$$ **RoC Brilliance Night Recharging Moisturizer** (*$49.99*) is, save for the sunscreen being replaced by a regular moisturizer, very similar to the RoC Brilliance Day Rejuvenating Moisture with SPF 20 Protection above. The first step in this kit is **Night Activating Serum**, which is the same serum found in the other RoC Brilliance kits. Step 2 in this set is the **Night Recharging Creme**. This moisturizer is a very basic, slightly emollient formula that contains mica and titanium dioxide for shine and thus provides a brightening effect, which is a cosmetic benefit, not skin care. There is a lot missing in this product, including skin-identical ingredients, antioxidants, or, ironically, proven cell-communicating ingredients. We wish there were something extra to extol about this kit, but there isn't. It's a classic case of marketing hoopla for products that cannot work as claimed. This mineral serum/moisturizer duo isn't going to improve sagging skin or get you anywhere close to what RoC describes as "brilliantly beautiful" results. This isn't a face-lift for under $50! One last, but important, comment: A significant ingredient in the Night Recharging Creme is the chelating agent tetrahydroxypropyl ethylene-diamine. Guess what chelating agents do? They deactivate metal ions by making them a part of their complex ring structure. In other words, the presence of a chelating agent in the Night Recharging Creme prevents the copper and zinc in the accompanying serum from exerting their ion-based energy, which is supposed to be the crux of how this kit works!

ROC SPECIALTY PRODUCTS

☹ AVERAGE **RoC Brilliance Anti-Aging Face Primer** (*$23.99 for 1 fl. oz.*) is a standard silicone-based formula that is nearly identical to the serum packaged with RoC's Brilliance products reviewed above. What's interesting is that in the Brilliance kits, RoC maintains that the serum and accompanying product (such as eye cream) must be used together to generate the "pulse" of electricity, but according to the claims for this primer, the pulse is generated without the need for the second product! It appears that not even RoC believes their own claims, at least not as it relates to needing two products to generate the electric charge to improve skin; we wish they'd make up their minds. This product's value as a primer is mostly due to the silky-smooth finish it leaves behind. The formula contains tiny amounts of vitamin E (tocopheryl acetate) and copper, but you can achieve greater anti-aging benefits, plus prime your skin for makeup, by applying a serum from our Best Products list at the end of this book.

☹ AVERAGE $$$ **RoC Brilliance Eye and Lash Anti-Aging Primer** (*$24.99 for 0.5 fl. oz.*) is nearly identical to RoC's Brilliance Anti-Aging Face Primer above. The only points of difference are that the eye version doesn't make claims about micro-current technology for fewer wrinkles and its formula contains titanium dioxide for a subtle brightening effect. Not a single ingredient in this primer will lift skin or promote fuller-looking lashes. If anything, applying this silicone-heavy formula to lashes may interfere with your regular mascara application and wear, resulting in smearing and your mascara breaking down (when ordinarily this wouldn't happen). Please see the Appendix to learn why products claiming to lift skin cannot actually do this—and find out what works instead. All this primer will do is make skin around the eyes or elsewhere on the face feel softer and smoother.

SEPHORA

Strengths: Inexpensive; some good cleansers and makeup removers; the Blotting Papers; good powder foundation; impressive blush and shiny eyeshadow options; great metallic finish eyeliner; awesome brow kit; bountiful selection of lipsticks and lip glosses; a couple of very good mascaras; several outstanding makeup brushes; testers are available in-store for each product, and sales pressure is practically nonexistent.

Weaknesses: Mostly average to below-average toners, moisturizers, and sunscreens; no reliable options for those dealing with acne or skin discolorations; some SPF-rated products (including foundations) lack sufficient UVA-protecting actives; the lip plumper is too irritating; too many disappointing eye-makeup products, including several disappointing eyeliners and brow pencils; unappealing shimmer powders.

For more information and the latest Sephora reviews, visit CosmeticsCop.com.

SEPHORA CLEANSERS

☺ GOOD **Supreme Cleansing Oil** *($14 for 6.4 fl. oz.)* is a very good though basic cleansing oil for normal to dry skin. The mineral oil–based formula contains an emulsifying ingredient, so when this is mixed with water it forms a milky fluid that becomes easier to rinse than if you were removing makeup with plain mineral oil. The formula contains several plant oils, too, so this is best used before cleansing with a water-soluble cleanser or with a washcloth. Used on its own, it removes all types of makeup but can leave a slightly greasy residue. It does contain fragrance. Note that cleansers like this aren't the best bets for blemish-prone skin.

☺ GOOD **Supreme Cleansing Foam All In One Cleanser** *($15 for 5 fl. oz.)* is a very good though basic water-soluble cleanser for most skin types. It has an impressive blend of detergent cleansing agents known for being gentle and effective. What kept this otherwise well done cleanser from being "supreme" are a few drawbacks you shouldn't ignore. Where it falls down the most is the amount of fragrance, which is a problem if you're going to be using this over the eye area to remove makeup (as is recommended on the label). One of the marketing claims about this product is that it is supposed to contain an ingredient called HydroSenn +. Sephora says this ingredient is more hydrating and longer-lasting than hyaluronic acid. Whether or not that's true is irrelevant given this is a cleanser and the ingredient would be broken down by the cleansing agents it contains and then immediately rinsed down the drain before it could have any benefit. There isn't one ingredient in here with research showing it to be more hydrating than any other ingredient in the cosmetics world including hyaluronic acid. Even if we were to suspend conventional wisdom and believe Sephora's claim about HydroSenn + being better than hyaluronic acid, hyaluronic acid is hardly the best ingredient for skin hydration as there are many, many others. In fact, a blend of hydrating ingredients would be best of all, something this product doesn't contain.

☺ GOOD $$$ **Purifying Cleansing Gel** *($12 for 4.2 fl. oz.)* is a very standard but good water-soluble cleanser for normal to oily or combination skin. Its formula isn't anything special but it removes makeup and rinses cleanly, leaving skin smooth and refreshed. Its only drawback is the rather strong fragrance. Fragrance isn't skin care and there are plenty of gentle, fragrance-free cleansers that would be a better option for your skin.

☺ AVERAGE **Express Cleansing Wipes** *($9 for 25 wipes)* are little more than water, vegetable oil, and preservative. They contain a tiny amount of cleansing agents, so it's the oil that works to remove all types of makeup—but the oil also leaves a somewhat greasy film on skin that you'll most likely want to rinse (so you may as well just use a regular cleanser). Actually, considering the amount of fragrance and fragrance ingredients the formula contains, you should rinse. Those ingredients aren't the best to leave sitting on your skin. Express Cleansing Wipes are suitable for normal to dry skin.

☺ AVERAGE **Triple Action Cleansing Water** *($14 for 5 fl. oz.)* is a fluid, somewhat hydrating cleanser that's best for normal to dry skin. The mix of fatty acids, silicone, and plant oil helps dissolve most types of makeup, and this rinses fairly well. Sephora maintains this contains "cleansing spheres" that capture and remove dirt and makeup, but that's essentially true for almost any cleanser, as the science behind that claim is the basis for how surfactants (cleansing agents) work to remove oil and debris from skin. The only drawback of this cleanser is its high amount of fragrance and inclusion of fragrance ingredients known to be irritating. Because of this, this isn't advised for use around the eyes.

SEPHORA EYE-MAKEUP REMOVERS

☺ GOOD **Waterproof Eye Makeup Remover** *($9.50 for 4.2 fl. oz.)*. Other than the pointless addition of artificial coloring agents, this is a very good, fragrance-free eye-makeup remover for all skin types. The silicone-enhanced formula removes all types of makeup (including waterproof formulas) quickly and smoothly, so you won't need to pull and tug at the delicate eye area.

☺ AVERAGE **Instant Eye Makeup Remover** *($8.50 for 4.2 fl. oz.)* is a very good, fairly gentle, fragrance-free eye-makeup remover. It contains a tiny amount of water-binding agents and soothing plant extracts, but why Sephora felt they needed to add coloring agents and a splash of alcohol is a good question. The coloring agents don't benefit skin and the alcohol, while present in a very low amount, isn't the best ingredient to use near the eye itself. Given the number of makeup removers that are alcohol-free and don't have an artificial tint, this one becomes a less desirable option. Still, it works to remove most types of eye makeup without leaving a residue.

SEPHORA TONER

☹ POOR **Instant Refreshing Toner** *($12 for 6.76 fl. oz.)* has so many problems it is impossible to tell you about them in an instant, but we'll do our best to be brief. Except for glycerin, there is far more fragrance in here than beneficial skin-care ingredients, and fragrance is never skin care. It also contains a small amount of witch hazel, which can be a skin irritant and the extract form can also contain alcohol. See the Appendix for details on why daily use of fragrant or irritating products is bad for all skin types. One of the marketing claims about this product is that it is supposed to contain an ingredient called HydroSenn +. Sephora says this ingredient is more hydrating and lasts longer than hyaluronic acid. It's important to realize this product doesn't list anything called HydroSenn + on the ingredient label, so there is no way to know which ingredient or ingredients Sephora is alluding to. There isn't one ingredient in here with research showing it to be more hydrating than any other ingredient in the cosmetics world, including hyaluronic acid. Even if we were to suspend conventional wisdom and believe Sephora's claim about HydroSenn + being better than hyaluronic acid, hyaluronic acid is hardly the best ingredient for skin hydration; there are many, many others. In fact, a blend of hydrating ingredients would be best of all, something this product doesn't contain.

SEPHORA EXFOLIANTS & SCRUBS

☺ AVERAGE $$$ **Double Duty Exfoliator + Mask** *($18 for 1.69 fl. oz.)* is more a scrub than a mask, so that's how we categorized it. Sephora maintains that the scrub action comes from the jojoba beads, but it doesn't. Instead, the combination of cellulose (the second ingredient) and polyethylene (synthetic) exfoliating granules is what helps smooth and refine skin. The thickening agents this contains make is somewhat difficult to rinse, but we suspect Sephora included them so this could also function as a moisturizing mask. It can do that, but it's not the most elegant formula around. Consider this an OK scrub for normal to dry skin not prone to breakouts, and use it occasionally, if at all, as a mask.

⊗ POOR **Smart Dual Action Exfoliator** *($24 for 4.2 fl. oz.)* is, from almost any perspective, as dumb as dirt. Let's start with the way this truly ordinary, barely passable scrub is packaged to make it look like you're getting something more than what it is. It comes packaged in a single jar with a divider between two formulas, one white and the other green. You're supposed to use the "white" scrub all over your face, including around the eyes, and then follow with the "green" scrub just in the T-zone. The white scrub formula is a mixture of mineral oil and synthetic scrub particles with way too much fragrance and synthetic coloring agents. It is an understatement to say neither synthetic scrub particles nor synthetic coloring agents are good for the eye area. The green scrub is a mix of cleansing agents, relatively abrasive scrub particles of tapioca starch, some alumina, and way too much fragrance. This formula for the T-zone makes a bit more sense but harsh scrubs such as this can tear into skin, causing problems such as dryness, flaking, and irritation. Overall, the ordinary formula leaves much to be desired. (See the Appendix to learn why fragrance is a problem for all skin types.)

SEPHORA MOISTURIZERS (DAYTIME & NIGHTTIME), EYE CREAMS, & SERUMS

☺ AVERAGE $$$ **Age Defy Eye Cream** *($24 for 0.5 fl. oz.)* has a formula that amounts to little more than waxes, glycerin, and mineral oil; labeling this 'age defying' is like calling a skateboard a Mercedes. The lackluster formula is practically void of anti-aging ingredients such as antioxidants, skin-repairing ingredients, or cell-communicating ingredients. For the few beneficial ingredients this does contain, they are so far at the end of the ingredient list they are barely worth mentioning, and your skin won't notice. What certainly defies rational thinking are the claims that this product can tackle dark circles, puffiness, and lines around the eyes. There is nothing in here remotely capable of living up to that hope. Because this doesn't contain sunscreen, it would actually make all those concerns worse if you used it during the day. In fact, as shocking as this sounds, you don't even need a separate product labeled as an eye cream (we explain why in the Appendix). Please refer to the review above for Instant Refreshing Toner for a discussion of the HydroSenn + complex this contains.

☺ AVERAGE **Age Defy Moisture Cream SPF 15** *($30 for 1.69 fl. oz.)*. Although this daytime moisturizer contains titanium dioxide, which is typically a great option to provide much needed UVA protection, the amount in here is 0.5%, which isn't enough to do much of anything protective. Adding to this product's disappointing profile is the mundane formulation of mostly waxes and mineral oil and the lack of proven anti-aging ingredients such as an array of antioxidants, skin-repairing ingredients, and cell-communicating ingredients. Although this contains a small amount of beneficial ingredients, it isn't enough for skin to get what it needs to be younger. There is more preservative in here than the good stuff. But even if it was enough of the good stuff, the jar packaging it comes in wouldn't keep the vitamin E stable (see the Appendix to find out why jar packaging is a problem for any anti-aging skin-care product). Also see the review for Instant Refreshing Toner above for a discussion of the HydroSenn + complex.

☺ AVERAGE **Age Defy Night Moisture Cream Sleeping Beauty** *($30 for 1.69 fl. oz.)* is a standard moisturizer for normal to dry skin. Despite claims of being able to activate collagen synthesis, it contains barely any ingredients known to do that, though it will make dry skin feel soft and smooth. What really sets this back is the jar packaging (see the Appendix for details). This also contains a few of fragrance ingredients known to be irritating, though the amounts are likely too low to matter. Ultimately, this isn't an age-defying formula, especially not the way it's packaged.

☺ AVERAGE **Flawless Moisturizing Lotion SPF 15** *($22 for 1.69 fl. oz.)* has more flaws than positives. This daytime moisturizer contains titanium dioxide for UVA protection, but the amount in here is 0.4%, which isn't enough to do much of anything protective. Ideally, you want to see at least 2% titanium dioxide when it is joined by other sunscreen actives. Another flaw is this product's utterly mundane, albeit emollient formulation of shea butter and waxes. There is far more preservative and fragrance in here than anything beneficial for skin. What this product lacks is an array of antioxidants, skin-repairing ingredients, and cell-communicating ingredients. Although it contains a small amount of beneficial ingredients, they are a mere dusting, certainly not enough for skin to get what it needs to be younger. See the review for Instant Refreshing Toner above for a discussion of the HydroSenn + complex.

☹ POOR **Instant Depuffing Roll-On Gel** *($15 for 1.5 fl. oz.)*. This roller-ball applicator contains a gel that you're supposed to rub over your eye area to reduce puffiness. You can roll this around all day and it won't change the puffiness around your eye one iota, at least not any more than gently massaging a well-formulated moisturizer over the area can do. There are many reasons why the eye area can be puffy; some of it can be genetic or it can be related to allergies or falling asleep in makeup (which causes irritation and swelling). It can also be from sagging skin that occurs when fat pads under the eye shift, which causes "undereye bags." Regardless of the cause, this product isn't going to change any of that. The formula leaves much to be desired. It is a rather simple combination of mostly glycerin and film-former (think hairspray). Although it does contain some ingredients that have antioxidant and anti-irritant properties, it also contains cinnamic acid, a component of cinnamon that can be irritating, especially for the eye area. See the Appendix to find out why you don't need a special product for the eye area.

☹ POOR **Instant Moisturizer** *($20 for 1.69 fl. oz.)* is little more than water, wax, and preservative, making it one of the worst offerings from Sephora, and that's really saying something given how below-average almost all their other skin-care products are. The smattering of antioxidants in this product is barely worth mentioning, especially considering the jar packaging won't keep them stable once it is opened. (See the Appendix to learn why jar packaging is a problem.) The subtle glow this moisturizer imparts is from the mica it contains. Mica is a shiny mineral used in thousands of products to add shimmer to skin. Although it can look nice, it is strictly a cosmetic effect, not skin care. See the review for Instant Refreshing Toner above for a discussion of Sephora's HydroSenn + complex.

☹ POOR **Super Loaded Age Defy Serum** *($32 for 1 fl. oz.)* is about as far from super as you can get. It does have a silky-smooth application with a matte finish but that's where the positives stop. It's otherwise a strange mix of water, silicone, absorbent, and film-forming agent (think hairspray), with far more fragrance and preservative than anything beneficial. Silicone is a great ingredient for skin, but the tiny amount of peptides and vitamin E in here isn't even vaguely enough to give skin what it needs to act and look younger. See the review for Instant Refreshing Toner above for a discussion of Sephora's HydroSenn + complex.

SEPHORA LIP CARE

☺ GOOD **Super Nourishing Lip Balm** *($5 for 0.12 fl. oz.)*. This lipstick-style lip balm contains some good emollient ingredients to help keep lips smooth, soft, and flake-free. It can feel a bit waxy, but the wax component also helps this last longer before needing to be reapplied. If this didn't contain fragrance, it would be a top pick; however, it's still a good option and, owing to its packaging, is great for on-the-go use.

SEPHORA SPECIALTY SKIN-CARE PRODUCTS

☺ GOOD **Matte Blotting Papers** *($8 for 100 sheets)*. Sephora offers different versions of these oil-blotting papers. All of them are dusted with calcium carbonate, an absorbent, powdery ingredient more commonly known as chalk. The tissue paper–thin papers absorb excess oil and perspiration and deposit a sheer layer of powder. Among the options, the ones to consider are **Natural** (which is fragrance-free), **Vitamin C + E**, and **Tea Tree Oil**, though those ingredients have no impact in this kind of delivery method. Avoid the **Lavender**—fragrance can irritate skin, no matter what kind of product it's in, because the volatile oil that provides the fragrance is always irritating for skin.

☺ GOOD **Tricks of the Trade Immediate Wrinkle Filler** *($20 for 0.42 fl. oz.)* is a thick, nonaqueous cream based on silicones and talc. It feels very silky and goes on lighter than you might expect. The silicones have a soft spackle effect on minor lines and wrinkles, temporarily smoothing their appearance. This also reduces the appearance of large pores, though how long that effect lasts depends on what other products you apply and how oily your skin is.

☺ AVERAGE **Matte Blotting Film** *($10 for 50 sheets)* are blotting papers of a synthetic material coated with mineral oil and a polymer blend. They do an average job of absorbing excess oil, but are not as efficient as tissue-paper blotters.

☺ AVERAGE **$$$ Instant Moisture Mask** *($15 for 4 packets)* includes four 0.35-ounce packets of a gel-like mask that you mix with water prior to use. The product comes with a small plastic shaker bottle to mix the contents before application, but really, this mask isn't anything special, unique, or even fun. It's mostly sugar (sorbitol) plus starch, and an amino acid plus a plant extract and fragrance. Its hydrating abilities are minimal, especially for those with dry skin. We suppose this is an OK option for slightly dry skin (when mixed as directed the texture is a goopy gel you can slather on), but if you're taking the time to use a mask (perhaps as part of a spa night at home), there are dozens of better options that don't require mixing prior to use.

SEPHORA FOUNDATIONS & PRIMER

✓☺ BEST **Matifying Compact Foundation** *($20)* is an outstanding talc-based pressed-powder foundation for those with normal to oily skin. It has a silky application and sheer matte finish that looks practically seamless on skin. True to claim, this really does make your complexion "look like sheer perfection," assuming that you don't have any discolorations or blemishes, in which case you should use this foundation with the appropriate concealer. Sephora provides a huge range of shades with options for fair to dark skin tones. Consider the following shades carefully due to slight overtones of rose, copper, peach, or gold: R30, D32, D33, R33, D40, and R55. On the other hand, avoid D34, R40, and R50 because they don't resemble real skin tones. Shade D65 is an impressive non-ashen dark tone.

☺ GOOD **Perfecting Tinted Moisturizer SPF 20** *($21)* has a texture with the perfect amount of slip, allowing it to glide over skin and blend well. While it does contain a decent amount of skin-beneficial ingredients like antioxidants and peptides, the real boon to this formula is the inclusion of the UVA-protecting sunscreen avobenzone, something that few tinted moisturizers can boast! Although the formula will work for all skin types, those with oily skin will appreciate its light feel and matte finish. Like most tinted moisturizers, you can't count on this one for anything more than sheer coverage, though it does leave a significant veil of color behind. In fact, the only thing preventing this from earning our highest rating is that all the shades (except for Nude) revealed peach or orange undertones after they set. These overtones are less obvious because this product is so sheer, but check the result in natural light so you can be sure it looks right on your skin.

☺ GOOD $$$ **Mineral Foundation Compact SPF 10** *($22)* is a good pressed-powder foundation. Application-wise, the powder's slightly creamy texture goes on smoothly and provides sheer to medium coverage with a soft matte finish. It is best for normal to dry or slightly oily skin; those with pronounced oily areas will find this isn't absorbent enough. The SPF 10 rating comes from pure titanium dioxide, which provides broad-spectrum sun protection and, like all broad-spectrum sunscreens, an anti-aging benefit. However, SPF 15 is the recommended minimum rating by medical boards and organizations all over the world, so this shouldn't be used alone for your sun protection unless you wear another sunscreen product of SPF 15 or greater underneath it.

☹ POOR **Tricks of the Trade Anti-Shine Primer** *($18 for 1 fl. oz.)* isn't one you'll want to add to your makeup routine. Generally speaking, a primer isn't essential and certainly not preferred to using an antioxidant-rich serum, many of which have silky, primer-like finishes and as such perform double duty. The trick is on you if you choose this Sephora product, however, because the formula contains enough alcohol to cause irritation and the finish of this gel-textured primer remains tacky. Any of the primers from Smashbox (a brand Sephora sells in many of their stores) are preferred to this.

SEPHORA CONCEALERS

☺ AVERAGE **Lasting and Perfecting Corrector** *($15)*. This dual-ended retractable pencil has two different shades and shapes of cream concealer at either end (one end is broad and rounded, the other is finely tipped). The coordinated shades are intriguing because you can dot and mix them to match your skin tone nicely, and once it sets to a matte finish, it does last longer than most concealers. The formula's thick texture certainly provides full coverage, but with very little slip. The dryness resists blending so concealing anything bigger than a small blemish is tricky, if not impossible. The inclusion of salicylic acid is wasted here because without a base and a pH that enables it to penetrate the pore lining, it's not able to heal blemishes or prevent new ones.

☺ AVERAGE $$$ **Perfecting Cover Concealer** *($16)* has a smooth, ultra-matte finish that is so absorbent even oily skin types may find the formula a bit too drying. If you have any wrinkles, the dry appearance will make them more noticeable, too. On the plus side, the liquid formula stays put once it sets, provides medium to full coverage for concealing blemishes, and its texture won't make breakouts worse. Just be aware that the finish of this concealer will draw more attention to any dry areas of skin that you have.

☺ AVERAGE $$$ **Concealer Palette** *($22)* presents four creamy concealers in a compact, and comes with a brush that's too small to use unless you like a challenge. This applies well and provides nearly opaque coverage, which results in a heavy look. The creaminess means this is prone to creasing, but setting it with powder minimizes this effect. The flesh-toned palette is neutral, but the color-correcting palette is not. All told, this is an OK option only for those seeking full coverage. Note: These palettes are sold as part of the **Buildable Cover Complexion Kit**, available in Light, Medium, and Tan. Twenty-two dollars reflects the price of the kit.

SEPHORA POWDERS

☺ AVERAGE **Highlighting Compact Powder** *($15)* is an average pressed powder with shine. It has a dry texture and sheer application that imparts more shine than is warranted, at least for daytime makeup. The shine clings marginally well, but Sephora sells better versions of this type of product from brands such as Benefit, Stila, and Dior.

☺ AVERAGE **$$$ Sculpting Disk** *($24)*. Housed in one giant compact slightly larger than a CD are three stripes of pressed powder separated by a plastic divider. The center stripe, the largest, is a regular, flesh-toned pressed powder. To the left is a peachy tan bronzing powder; to the right is a pale peach highlighting powder. All three have a decently smooth, dry texture and soft application. Those with light skin tones can use these shades to "sculpt" the face, but doing so is tricky and the color combinations aren't going to work for all light skin tones.

SEPHORA BRONZERS

☺ GOOD **Bronzer** *($15)*. This pressed-powder bronzer has a silky-dry texture that glides on skin without looking cakey or chalky. The shades include varying intensities of bronze with a shimmer finish (Aruba, Maui, and Maldives) or a matte finish (Los Cabos and Bora Bora). Beware that the Maui shade looks more orange than tan, and the Bora Bora shade has slightly peachy undertones; however, the Los Cabos shade is a great option for a natural-looking, matte finish tan (remember, a real tan never sparkles).

☺ GOOD **Sun Disk** *($22)* is a pressed-powder bronzer that is as large as a CD. While it won't fit into most makeup bags, the talc-based formula applies smoothly and imparts sheer, buildable peachy tan color that is best for fair to light skin tones. The shine is toned down, making this a suitable bronzing powder for daytime.

SEPHORA EYESHADOWS & EYE PRIMER

✓☺ BEST **Colorful Mono Eyeshadow** *($12)* offers a huge assortment of shades that come in three finishes: matte, metallic, and glittering. Among them, the mattes (which really are matte!) and metallic (most of which produce a subtle shine that doesn't look metallic at all) are the best. Avoid the glittering shades at all costs; not only is the glitter blatantly obvious and overdone, but also the formula has a dry, grainy texture that clings poorly, so the glitter flakes immediately. The matte and metallic shades have a smooth, non-powdery texture that applies evenly and deposits soft color. You'll need to layer for more than nuanced shading and shaping, but we suspect most women will prefer how softly these apply at first. Those interested in matte powder eyeshadows should not miss this collection.

☺ GOOD **$$$ Colorful Eye Shadow Palette** *($24)* is a collection of powder eyeshadow quads that are talc-based and have a smooth, dry texture. The dryness hinders application a bit, but the shadows are still workable if applied in sheer layers. The most versatile quads are Kiss From ___ (you're supposed to fill in the blank), and Taupe Model.

☺ GOOD **Perfecting Eye Primer** *($14)* promises smooth, lasting eye makeup free from creasing, plus it is said to provide anti-aging benefits. Like most eyeshadow primers, this has a silky texture and (eventually) sets to a powder-like matte finish that enhances makeup application. It goes on slightly greasy and slips a lot as you blend but doesn't feel heavy (nor does it impart any color). The formula isn't anti-aging in the least, though it does have a minor, temporary smoothing effect on less-than-taut eyelids. This will not moisturize eyelid skin and in fact some may find it feels noticeably dry; however, it does work to prevent shadows from creasing. It is an option for those with oily eyelids and the formula is fragrance-free.

☺ AVERAGE **Colorful Duo Eyeshadow** *($16)* includes two eyeshadows in one compact with a divider between the shades. The texture is smooth, but powdery enough to make flaking during application an issue unless you blend in sheer layers. The shade range is hit-or-miss; roughly half are too odd or contrasting to work for an attractive eye design. Duo No. 05 and Duo No. 06 are matte, while Duo No. 07 is the best one if you want a smart pairing of shades with shine. Shades labeled "shimmer" have a more obvious, glitzy shine than those labeled "metallic."

☺ AVERAGE $$$ **Baked Moonshadow Trio** *($17)* comes in various shade combinations with either glitter, iridescent, or shimmer finishes. The colors go on sheer, but can be layered for a more dramatic look, and the shine adheres well to skin without feeling grainy or flaking. The tricky part of this eyeshadow is how to apply one color at a time given that the three shades are housed in a small, circular compact without any dividers between them. Furthermore, some of the color combinations don't complement each other, and the colors are completely unrelated, which makes for a contrasting eye design that can look like a rainbow instead of a nuanced design.

SEPHORA EYE & BROW LINERS

✓☺ BEST **Doe Eyed Felt Eyeliner** *($12)* is an excellent liquid liner that's every bit as good as pricier options from Yves Saint Laurent and Lancome. This has a calligraphy-style felt-tip brush that works beautifully whether you want a thin or thick line. Color deposit is intense and the formula dries quickly, so smearing isn't an issue. Once set, this is difficult to budge, so long-wear is guaranteed (and removal takes more effort than usual). The only drawback is that each shade is bright and has a shiny finish. The Blue shade is a shocking bright teal and Green is an olive-gold tone that's an attractive alternative to basic brown. As long as you don't mind the shiny finish and more obvious colors, this is a liquid liner to audition!

✓☺ BEST **Retractable Brow Pencil "Waterproof** *($12)* gets an A+ for ease of use and performance! It has a soft powder finish that isn't the least bit greasy or prone to smearing, and the twist-up applicator ensures you always have a fine-point tip for precise control. The colors are natural looking, with one blonde shade and three varying shades of brown. All that, and it comes with a small brow comb on the opposite end so you can tame and blend brows! Brilliant, and a fairly good value, too!

✓☺ BEST $$$ **Arch It Brow Kit** *($35)* is just about one of the cutest and most practical brow kits we've ever seen. Packaged in a chic leather case about the size of a change purse is a compact that houses brow powder, brow wax, and two synthetic brushes, a mini clear brow gel, a full-size pair of tweezers, brow stencils, instructions, and a larger (but too scratchy) brow brush. The brow powder is matte, and although the accompanying wax looks too dark to coordinate with the powder, it applies sheer. The instructions indicate how to use the stencils (three shapes are included) to perfect your brows, and although they're brief they're also accurate. If you are new to the practice of brow tweezing and shaping, this kit will get you off to a great start and is highly recommended!

☺ GOOD **Jumbo Liner 12HR Wear Waterproof** *($12)*. This wide-tipped pencil creates a thick, dramatic line that can be blended out to be used as an eyeshadow (assuming you want a stronger color for your eyeshadow design). The richly pigmented, creamy texture goes on easily and evenly and blends well on initial application, but it quickly sets to a dry finish that is surprisingly resistant to creasing and water. There are a variety of bold, metallic colors offered, as well as your typical brown, black, and gray. Overall, this eyeliner is best for those who prefer a thick line along with impressively long wear. However, it isn't any more waterproof than other pencils; pencils just don't wash off all that easily. Although this pencil needs routine sharpening, its pros outweigh that issue, and as such it deserves its rating. However, twist-up pencils that don't require sharpening are more convenient.

☺ GOOD **Lash & Eyebrow Mascara** *($8)* has a dual sided brush that works well and the colorless formula remains non-sticky, though you can find clear brow gels for less money at the drugstore.

☺ GOOD **Waterproof Smoky Cream Liner** *($10)* applies smoothly and resists flaking. The color selection includes both traditional and vibrant shades, and the colors go on somewhat sheer, but can be layered to create a more dramatic line. This type of eyeliner is best applied with a fine-tip brush. Because this formula doesn't set instantly, you have time to blend before it dries, which is great if you're creating a smokey eye design. It is waterproof as claimed, and even holds up well on oily skin.

☺ AVERAGE **Kohl Expert** *($8)* claims to be "deeply pigmented," but the result is much softer than that claim would lead you to believe. Still, this is a very good eyelining option if you prefer a soft or smudged look and a matte finish that will make it through the day. The lone Brun Perfect shade is universally flattering for lining eyes because it's neither too black nor too brown, and its smooth texture means that it won't tug or pull eyelids. The only aspect that keeps this pencil from earning a higher rating is its need for routine sharpening.

☺ AVERAGE **Liner Electro** *($8)*. With an impressive array of colors, this needs-sharpening eyeliner pencil would be an affordable option for those looking to glam up their look for a fun night out or special occasion. The texture is creamy, blends nicely, sets to a very durable finish, and comes off easily with a water-soluble cleanser. Some shades (Black Electro, Mauve Electro) have a matte finish beneath tiny flecks of sparkle, but most shades have a metallic finish with lots of shimmer, with no flaking to speak of. The overall effect is very striking, although its appeal and occasions for use are clearly limited. The low rating is due to the sharpening required, which is a hassle and inefficient when you're in a hurry.

☺ AVERAGE **Nano Eyeliner** *($5)*. This pencil needs routine sharpening and the "nano" in the name refers to how small it is (about half the size of a regular eye pencil); it's got nothing to do with the formula. This has a minimally creamy texture and smooth application, though it goes on a bit thick. Because the finish stays creamy, this is best used when you intend to smudge the line. The colors feature mostly glittery or shimmer finishes.

☺ AVERAGE $$$ **Retractable Waterproof Eyeliner** *($12)*. The trade-off for this automatic, retractable eye pencil's waterproof finish is that it remains tacky to the touch. That's not a big deal because you shouldn't be touching your eyes anyway if you want it to last, but those who draw a thick line may notice the tacky feeling during wear, especially if you have deep-set eyes and small eyelids. This pencil applies easily and most of the shades provide an intense, metallic shine, plus there are some truly odd colors that do little to emphasize the eye. Still, classic black is available and some of the metallic shades can be fun for evening makeup.

☹ POOR **Kohl Pencil** *($8)* is a below-standard pencil that drags and tugs during application, along with a creamy finish that won't stay in place for long.

☹ POOR **Kohl Waterproof Eyeliner** *($9)* lives up to its waterproof claims (in fact, it was a bit tough to remove completely, even with makeup remover). It doesn't deliver the results you would expect from any type of eyeliner. The problems are numerous: It drags across the eyelid, it's difficult to blend (even using the included rounded rubber smudger), and each of the three shades is too sheer to achieve the emphasis eyeliner is intended to provide.

SEPHORA LIP COLOR & LIPLINERS

✓☺ BEST **Retractable Waterproof Lip Liner** *($12)*. Sephora has created a wonderfully smooth lip pencil that never requires sharpening and is retractable. True to its name, this is waterproof, although to be fair, most lip pencils are impervious to water so the designation is irrelevant. The long-wearing formula comes in a small but well-edited range of basic and bright colors.

✓☺ BEST **Rouge Cream Lipstick** *($12)* offers an incredibly impressive and inexpensive collection of cream lipsticks that smooth on easily, without any greasiness or notable bleeding. Though these are not long-wearing lipsticks (you'll have to reapply after a meal), the formula provides a good stain, wears comfortably, and has staying power beyond that of a standard cream lipstick or gloss. The richness of the colors is striking, both on lips and in the tube—even the lighter shades have considerable pigment—and all leave a comfortable semi-matte finish. Of the 20+ shades, there are flattering options for all. Those looking to avoid shimmer or frosted finishes, take note: There's not a single fleck of frost or sparkle in the entire Rouge Cream collection.

☺ GOOD **Glossy Gloss** *($10)*. This squeeze-tube gloss leaves lips feeling smooth and moisturized with a velvety, non-sticky finish. It's available in a vast array of sheer colors, some of which impart a shimmer or iridescent finish, and all of which have a high shine effect. The delectable fragrances each shade has pose a slight risk of irritation, but otherwise, this lip gloss offers a variety of fun and beautiful colors!

☺ GOOD **Lip Attitude Glamour** *($12)* is a good creamy lipstick with a glossy finish and attractive group of sheer to light coverage colors. The longevity of each shade is brief at best, but that tends to be the norm with sheer lipsticks anyway, so it doesn't make this less worthy of consideration.

☺ GOOD **Lip Attitude Star** *($12)* has an elegantly smooth, creamy feel that moisturizes lips without feeling thick. Each shade leaves a soft to moderate shimmer, but has minimal stain, so frequent touch-ups will be necessary. Still, this is a very good, modern cream lipstick with a shade range that's bound to please.

☺ GOOD **Maniac Long-Wearing Lipstick** *($12)* promises "the satiny radiance of a second skin," and although it doesn't feel quite that light, for a creamy lipstick this is not nearly as thick-textured as many. It applies smoothly and imparts nearly opaque color with a satin finish. The shade selection is well rounded, but small by Sephora standards, offering mostly shimmer- or glitter-infused colors. As for the long-wearing claims, this doesn't fade within an hour, but it also doesn't make it past lunch without a touch-up either, making it a decent lipstick.

☺ GOOD **Shimmer Harmony Gloss Palette** *($12)*. Can't decide on a lip gloss shade? You could go with this sleek palette, which contains six shades of soft, creamy lip gloss. The drawback is that the shades deposit almost no color, so you're basically left with a translucent sheen that's not the least bit sticky.

☺ GOOD **Ultra Shine Lip Gloss** *($14)* does leave lips ultra-shiny as well as glittery. This showy gloss isn't for the demure, and its slightly thick application feels a bit sticky, but that contributes to its high-gloss finish. Give this a sniff before purchasing to make sure the fruit scent appeals to you.

☺ GOOD **Ultra Vinyl Lip Pencil** *($12)*. If you're looking for an alternative to traditional lipstick, this is a fantastic option. This jumbo-size lip pencil has a unique creamy wax texture that provides richly pigmented color with intense shine. Despite the slick texture, the color holds up quite well, but it can wear away unevenly, so don't go too long without checking to make sure your lips aren't in need of a touch-up. The color selection ranges from vibrant shades of pink and red to caramel and coral, some of which have a shimmer finish. This lip pencil requires routine sharpening, which is always frustrating, but if you can find your sharpener and not whittle down to nothing trying to get a tip, it's an interesting way to get lipstick on.

☺ AVERAGE **Cream Lip Stain** *($12)* is for those who desire the long staying power of a lip stain with the opacity of traditional lipstick. Once the creamy-liquid texture sets, the stain looks and feels too dry and matte, so for comfortable wear, finish the look with a lip gloss or balm. That said, the color really lasts, even with gloss on top of it. The shade range is just so-so, but you may find a workable option if your preferences match what's available.

☺ AVERAGE **Maniac Mat Long-Wearing Matte Lipstick** *($12)* is a true matte lipstick whose application is smooth and even, imparting pure, rich color with a soft matte finish. The problem is that within minutes this lipstick becomes uncomfortably tacky. Lips feel slightly stuck together, which reminded us of how the old ultra-matte lipsticks felt. This does a good job of not cracking or balling up and it wears longer than a cream lipstick, but it's definitely one to test before purchasing.

☺ AVERAGE **Nano Lip Liner** *($5)*. The name of this standard, needs-sharpening pencil has to do with its tiny size. We imagine it will be used up or barely usable within a month or so. That's especially true because this pencil is too creamy and the colors have minimal stain, so they don't last long on lips. Knowing this, the price isn't such a value!

SEPHORA MASCARAS

✓☺ BEST **Atomic Volume Mascara** *($15)* has a misleading name because it doesn't produce lots of volume (i.e., thickness). What it does do easily and copiously is make lashes wonderfully long and beautifully defined, especially if you want a soft, fringed look without clumps. Some comb-through is needed to avoid a slightly spiked look, but otherwise this works well and wears without a hitch. It leaves lashes noticeably soft and removes easily with a water-soluble cleanser.

✓☺ BEST **Lash Plumper** *($12)* pledges to "fatten your flutter" (meaning lashes) and does so quickly! This is an awesome mascara if your goal is length and volume without clumps. The brush is a bit larger than standard, but once you adapt, it isn't too tricky to reach even the shortest lashes. This wears all day without a hitch and comes off easily with a water-soluble cleanser.

☺ GOOD **Le Waterproof Mascara** *($12)* adds volume to lashes without the clumping or that "crunchy" lash feel you can get with some mascaras. The formula is resistant to water and smudging and does a good job of holding curl throughout the day, but it doesn't add much length. Overall, this mascara isn't ultra-dramatic, but it's just enough to give you an enhanced look that won't appear overdone.

☺ AVERAGE **Lash Stretcher Mascara** *($15)* is supposed to be like false lashes in a tube, but it isn't. The formula adds bulk and drama to lashes with tiny fibers, but for all the good they may do appearance-wise, they end up being a nuisance. That's because they tend to flake as the day wears on, depositing themselves in your eye or on your cheek. As you can imagine, that gets annoying pretty quickly, and doesn't make the enhanced results (which are messier than what you can achieve with false eyelashes) worth it.

☺ AVERAGE **Professional Clear Natural Mascara** *($10)* is a very standard, colorless gel mascara that has minimal impact on lashes beyond slightly darkening them and creating

Did you know alcohol in skin-care products is a big problem? See the Appendix to learn more.

a minimal groomed look. This actually works better as a brow gel, but isn't worth the splurge over similar products from Cover Girl or Maybelline.

☺ AVERAGE **Lash Plumper Waterproof** *($4)* isn't nearly as impressive as its non-waterproof counterpart. The full, plump-bristled brush allows you to build ample length and definition with some thickness. Clumps are absent, but this has the uncommon tendency to dry with tiny balls of product at the very tip of your lashes. It's not a deal-breaker, but it doesn't make for the cleanest look. This is waterproof, and removing it requires something with oil, where you'll find it tends to come off in pieces and flecks rather than just a smear of dissolved color.

☺ AVERAGE **$$$ Outrageous Volume Mascara** *($15)* ends up being a miss. The long, somewhat thick brush is outfitted with spiky rubber bristles of various lengths that grab onto lashes and coat them evenly. That's basically what happens, but coat after coat proves how futile it is to try and build thickness (volume) that gets anywhere near "outrageous." At best, this pricey mascara lengthens and separates lashes without clumping, though on the downside it is unusually prone to smearing before it sets. We ended up with mascara on lashes as well as smudged along the upper and lower lash line—and this was us being very careful while applying! Your experience may differ, and this does wear well, but ultimately it's not an easy product to recommend.

SEPHORA BRUSHES

✓☺ BEST **Sephora Brushes** *($10–$41)*. Sephora's Brushes present some prime choices, especially for applying eyeshadow and powder eyeliner. Over 50 brushes are available, with the best ones being the **Pro Powder Brush #50** ($38), **Pro Natural Domed Powder Brush #59** ($36), **Pro Foundation Brush #47** ($27), **Pro Oval Blending Brush #27** ($20), **Classic Bronzer Brush #44** ($26), **Classic All Over Shadow Brush, Small #22** ($13), **Pro Natural All Over Shadow Brush #12** ($18), **Classic Angled Blush Brush #40** ($28), **Pro Gel Eyeliner Brush #26** ($16), and **Professional Platinum Air Brush #55** ($34). The **Vanity Brush Set** ($48) is practical, beautifully packaged, and absolutely worth a look.

☺ GOOD **Sephora Collection I.T. Brushes** *($14-$40)*. We found that these brushes (the initials stand for "Intelligent Tools") are a well-thought-out set that's designed to be user-friendly. The colored handles are eye catching and are categorized for different uses: Pink for the face area and blue or purple for the eye area. Another handy feature is the cap, which not only protects the bristles, but also makes each brush self-standing when turned upside down. The ergonomically tapered handles add an element of sleekness that sets these brushes apart from the competition. Beyond aesthetics, these brushes also rate highly as a collection in terms of functionality due to bristle flexibility, softness, and density. The **Smudge** ($22), **Crease** ($24), **Medium Shaper** ($20), and **Blending** ($24) brushes are all pretty standard. The **Brow Filler** ($14) and **Slanted Eyeliner** ($18) brushes perform exceptionally well because they are dense enough to function properly, but not so stiff that they become rigid or scratchy. The **Slanted Eyeliner** brush is quite thin so you can achieve a high level of precision and detail. The **Round Powder Brush** ($40) is great for use on the body because it covers a large surface area, although perhaps a little too large for the average person's face. There are a few brushes that you can do without in this collection: **Stippling** ($32), **Face Contour** ($30), and **Highlighting Fan** ($24) are all unnecessary and it is highly unlikely you would use them at all unless you were a makeup artist. The **Concealer Brush** ($28) is a bit wide for precision while the **Angled Synthetic Blush Brush** ($35) and **Angled Natural Blush Brush** ($32) are basically identical, so you would only need to decide whether you wanted synthetic or natural hair. Of the two foundation brushes, the regular **Foundation Brush** ($30) is the stronger option because it has just the right amount of bristle density and flexibility and has a better shape for more controlled use. The **Natural Foundation Brush** ($36) is better designed for powder foundation.

☺ GOOD $$$ **Deluxe Antibacterial Brush Set** *($60)*. This seven-piece brush set is housed in a well-made fabric carrying case with a smart tri-fold design that makes for easy storage. All the brushes are composed of synthetic hair, and they're exceptionally soft yet dense enough to apply their "assigned" product professionally. The **Lip/Eyeliner** brush has a square-cut head, which isn't the best for lips and can be awkward for eyelining, too, although some may find this cut preferable. You may be wondering about the antibacterial claim (we certainly were). Sephora maintains that these brushes repel and destroy bacteria, yet, when questioned, no one at Sephora could explain exactly how they do this. We asked if they were treated with an antibacterial chemical, and no one was sure. The Seattle-area salespeople we dealt with even called Sephora Corporate and they couldn't provide a reliable answer, either. If these brushes are treated with an antibacterial substance, does it hold up to repeated use or repeated washings? Even if it did, the kind of antibacterial properties this could provide would be practical only if you used your brushes on other people; it wouldn't affect acne-causing bacteria that exist deep in the pores. Despite the fact that no one at Sephora seems to know what makes these brushes antibacterial, they are still a good, relatively inexpensive set of brushes.

☹ AVERAGE $$$ **Double-Ended Brushes** *($18–$35)*. Sephora's collection of double-ended brushes offers some practical pairings, but storage is an issue with each one. Adding these to a standard brush case or roll inevitably means that one end of each brush is likely to be squished or forced out of shape. The only solution is to store these on their side, which is how Sephora had most of the testers displayed. If these brushes with their vivid dyed hair appeal to you, the best among them are the **Double-Ended Winged Brush** ($18), which is ideal for versatile eyelining; the **Double-Ended Smokey Eye Brush** ($18), which can be used for lining the eyes, filling in brows, and applying dramatic crease shading; and the **Double-Ended Perfect Complexion Brush** ($35), which works well for those who like to use a brush to apply liquid foundation followed by another to dust on loose powder. Just be aware that in your makeup bag these can end up not looking as pretty or being as functional over time.

SEPHORA SPECIALTY MAKEUP PRODUCTS

☺ GOOD **Flirt-It Lash Duo** *($8)* is a kit with pre-cut strips of false eyelashes and adhesive. It's well priced and a basic kit for beginners interested in experimenting with this type of product. The second version features rhinestones at the lash base for a sparkling effect.

☺ GOOD **Makeup Bags** *($10–$50)*. You will not be disappointed by Sephora's vast selection of **Makeup Bags**. The variety is astounding. The selection tends to vary by store, so if you want to see everything that's available, check out the Sephora website.

☺ GOOD **Tricks of the Trade Eyeshadow Transformer** *($6)*. The purpose of this product is to turn any powder eyeshadow into a liquid liner. You apply the clear fluid (like eyeliner) over your powder eyeshadow, which deepens the color and forms a long-wearing finish that keeps the color from fading or smearing. It's easier to use than liquid liner, and worth checking out if you're curious to see the effect and/or need help getting your powder eyeliner to last.

SERIOUS SKIN CARE

Strengths: Provides complete ingredient lists on website; several good cleansers; some impressive serums (with and without retinol) and primers; one effective BHA (salicylic acid) product; effective AHA (glycolic acid) pads; effective 5% benzoyl peroxide product; the lip line–filling products (though the effect is not akin to dermal fillers as claimed).

Weaknesses: Too many products, which makes determining what to buy incredibly confusing; several good formulas hampered with needless irritants; no effective skin-lightening options; jar packaging for many moisturizers, which allows the important, but unstable, ingredients to degrade; average masks; the at-home peels are terrible; too many gimmicky products; very small assortment of sunscreens, especially considering all the anti-aging products; the Glucosamine and Calstrum sub-brands are mediocre; irritating lip plumper.

For more information and reviews of the latest Serious Skin Care products, visit Cosmetics-Cop.com.

SERIOUS SKIN CARE CLEANSERS

☺ GOOD $$$ **A-Wash, Vitamin A Gel to Foam Cleanser with Triple Peptides** *($49.50 for 16 fl. oz.)* is a water-soluble cleanser that contains peptides and some skin-identical ingredients. In a cleanser, these peptides are rinsed from the skin before they can penetrate (which is what you want peptides to do to obtain results), but the skin-identical ingredients help make this cleanser more conditioning than a standard, detergent-based cleanser. It is a good, though pricey, option for normal to slightly dry to slightly oily skin.

☺ GOOD $$$ **Daily Ritual, Acne Medication Cleanser** *($21 for 4 fl. oz.)* contains 2% salicylic acid, but this anti-acne ingredient isn't going to be effective in a product that is quickly rinsed from skin. This is otherwise a good water-soluble cleanser for normal to dry skin. The tiny amount of jojoba wax beads provides a mild abrasive action. Because of the salicylic acid and the exfoliant beads, you should not use this cleanser in the eye area.

☺ GOOD $$$ **Olive Oil Emulsifying Cleanser** *($49.50 for 12 fl. oz.)* is an oil–based cleanser that contains an emulsifier that turns it into a softly foaming cleanser when mixed with water. It is a good cleanser option for those with dry to very dry skin, but likely will require use of a washcloth for complete removal. The price is over-the-top for what ends up being a fairly ordinary emollient cleanser that removes makeup.

☺ AVERAGE $$$ **C-Clean Vitamin C Cleanser** *($22.50 for 4 fl. oz.)* has nothing unique for mature skin. Age is not a skin type, and whether a woman considers her skin "mature" or not may have more to do with signs of sun damage and aging than issues such as dryness, oiliness, redness, or acne, which can affect women in their 20s as well as their 30s, 40s, 50s, 60s, and beyond. You can ignore the vitamin C and line-reducing claims because any benefit this antioxidant vitamin could have is rinsed down the drain. It's still a decent, overpriced cleanser that is as standard as they come, with over-the-top claims that waste your money. Note that the numerous citrus extracts this contains pose a risk of irritation, especially if you use this cleanser around your eyes.

☺ AVERAGE $$$ **Glycolic Cleanser** *($19.95 for 4 fl. oz.)* contains a hefty amount of glycolic acid and has a pH low enough to allow exfoliation. Sounds great, but you're not going to get that benefit unless you leave this on your skin for several minutes, which poses a serious problem for your skin. You never want to leave detergent cleansing agents on your skin for any longer than you have to, which should be just a few seconds because they can be extremely drying if left on skin longer than necessary. As is, this cleanser is a good option for normal to oily skin, but only if you take care to completely avoid the eye area (due to the low pH and the potential for glycolic acid to get into the eye).

☹ POOR **Clear Wash, Acne Medicated Targeted Cleanser** *($16.50 for 4.2 fl. oz.)* is medicated with 1% salicylic acid, which is an effective anti-acne ingredient but whose contact with skin as a cleanser will be too brief for it to work as intended. Even if you left this on your skin for several minutes, the pH is too high for exfoliation to occur, plus the peppermint oil causes instant irritation (see the Appendix to learn why irritation makes oily skin worse).

☹ POOR **Glucosamine Skin Resurfacing Cleanser** *($21 for 5 fl. oz.)* is supposed to be an acid-free way for those with sensitive skin to exfoliate. That may sound intriguing, but the ingredient that is meant to have exfoliating properties, acetyl glucosamine, doesn't have research supporting that benefit, and definitely would not have that benefit in a cleanser where it is rinsed off before it can work. Moreover, the amount of acetyl glucosamine is tiny, so even if it did work as claimed this wouldn't be the product to test out. This cleansing lotion also is not the best option for sensitive skin because it contains sodium lauryl sulfate, a well-known skin irritant.

SERIOUS SKIN CARE TONERS

☺ AVERAGE **$$$ Glucosamine Hydrating Facial Mist** *($18 for 4 fl. oz.)* isn't the toner to choose if your goal is to dissolve dead skin cells because acetyl glucosamine does not function as an exfoliant. However, it does function as a good water-binding agent, and as such this is a good, though basic, one-note toner for all skin types. Skin needs more than this single ingredient to function optimally.

☹ AVERAGE **$$$ Resveratrol Drench Pre Soaked Pads** *($36.50 for 60 pads)* are just toner soaked into pads in a jar container. The solution is mostly grape water with a slip agent, soy, preservative, fragrance, and coloring agent. The ingredient resveratrol is probably not in here; the ingredients on the label list *Pichia* resveratrol ferment, which isn't the same as pure resveratrol, but only a minute amount of the ferment is present anyway. Even if it were present in a larger amount, *Pichia* resveratrol ferment is neither the only nor the best antioxidant around; it is merely one of many antioxidants to consider. Grape water is also a dubious antioxidant. If it had benefit, you could take grape juice out of your refrigerator and use that instead; we are not recommending that, we're just pointing out the lack of benefit. However, even if this product were better formulated and contained a more state-of-the-art assortment of beneficial ingredients, the jar packaging wouldn't keep any of it stable. Antioxidants break down in the presence of air, and jar packaging allows air in (see the Appendix for details).

☹ POOR **Reverse Mist Firming Facial Mist with Argifirm** *($21 for 2 fl. oz.)* is a spray-on toner that contains gum-based thickener and a protein from milk known as casein. Combined with the film-forming agent sodium polystyrene sulfonate (yes, it's as synthetic as it sounds), this product will constrict skin and make it feel temporarily tighter. Unfortunately, the sodium polystyrene sulfonate is present in an amount that's likely to be more irritating than beneficial for skin—and this irritation is made worse by the numerous fragrant oils in this toner. Geranium, clary sage, lavender, rosemary, and more are on hand to hurt your skin's healing process and delay or diminish healthy collagen production (which is what happens when skin is consistently irritated). Please, for the health and appearance of your skin, do not take this product seriously and certainly don't purchase it, unless you intend to use it as an air freshener, not skin care.

SERIOUS SKIN CARE EXFOLIANTS & SCRUBS

☺ GOOD $$$ **Resveratrol X5 Concentrate Drench** *($34.50 for 1 fl. oz.)* is sold with the premise that it contains resveratrol, an antioxidant from red grapes, which is a premier ingredient for those concerned with aging. Without question, research shows that resveratrol Is a potent antioxidant. However, it isn't the only and certainly not the best option. Searching for one miracle ingredient isn't the answer for beautiful skin. Just like our bodies require a variety of nutritious foods for good health, our skin has the same need for a range of beneficial ingredients. The real reason to consider this is because it's an effective AHA exfoliant. It contains approximately 5% glycolic and lactic acids (5% total, not 5% of each AHA) in a pH that ensures effectiveness. The resveratrol is an antioxidant bonus, as is the tiny amount of stabilized vitamin C. This product is best for normal to dry skin not prone to breakouts.

☺ GOOD $$$ **Serious Firming Facial Pads** *($32.50 for 60 pads)* contain approximately 8%-10% glycolic acid at an effective pH to ensure exfoliation. The inclusion of witch hazel rather high on the ingredient list doesn't make this as gentle as many competing AHA products in gel or lotion form, but the potential irritation from it is likely countered by the soothing agents in the formula. The minuscule amounts of amino acids have no effect on skin.

☺ AVERAGE **Continuously Clear Nano Hydra+ Cream** *($27.50 for 2 fl. oz.)* contains 0.5% salicylic acid as the active ingredient. That amount is as low as you'd want to go to combat blemishes and blackheads, but in this product it cannot exfoliate because the pH is not within the correct range. The base formula contains too many oils and thickeners to make someone with oily, blemish-prone skin happy and the fragrant oils can cause excess irritation. See the Appendix to find out why the jar packaging this comes in is far from optimal.

☺ AVERAGE **Glycolic Cream** *($32.50 for 2 fl. oz.)* contains an effective amount (between 8%-10%) glycolic acid and is formulated within the correct pH range for exfoliation to occur. Its emollient, somewhat greasy texture is best for dry to very dry skin, but this product isn't without some drawbacks. Chief among them are the citrus extracts, which are known irritants. Although the amount in this AHA moisturizer isn't high, it would be better without them (they do not exfoliate). It would also be nice to see a greater amount of antioxidants in this product, but even if that was the case, it's a letdown due to jar packaging (see the Appendix for details). You'll get moisture and skin-smoothing exfoliation from this product, but not much else.

☺ AVERAGE **Repairz-It Nano Hydra+ Youth Formula Oil Free Skin Hydrator** *($26.50 for 2 fl. oz.)* contains 0.5% salicylic acid as the active ingredient. That amount is as low as you'd want to go to combat blemishes and blackheads, but in this product it cannot exfoliate because the pH is not within the correct range. The base formula is creamier than what most people battling blemishes would want, at least if their acne is accompanied by oily skin (as is usually the case). This is an OK moisturizer for normal to dry skin but what a shame it won't exfoliate.

☺ AVERAGE $$$ **Glowbrasion, Micro-Fine Face Polish** *($26.50 for 1.7 fl. oz.)* is a topical scrub that exfoliates skin with a combination of polyethylene beads, sand, and salt. Serious Skin Care claims it won't scratch or abrade skin because they've cushioned these scrub agents in an emollient base, but that's not a guarantee you won't overdo it and hurt your skin. You can easily go overboard with this scrub, so if you decide to try it, scrub gently. This contains a couple of plant extracts that have the potential to cause irritation and the jar packaging is not a sanitary way to use any skin-care product.

☺ AVERAGE $$$ **Glucosamine Phyto-Pumpkin Scrub** *($21 for 2 fl. oz.)* is an oil–based topical scrub for dry to very dry skin. Sucrose (sugar) is the granular abrasive agent, and it is buffered by several oils. The oils help cushion skin, but they impede rinsing, so you may need to follow with a washcloth (which can also be used in place of any scrub, especially in place of this overpriced mixture).

☺ AVERAGE $$$ **Olive Oil Deep Facial Peel** *($26 for 4 fl. oz.)* is an exceedingly odd combination of ingredients that offers little benefit for skin, and if anything, would end up confusing it. The peeling is supposed to come from the enzyme papain, but papain is an unstable ingredient that definitely won't remain active in the jar packaging. The canola oil and cornstarch base is a strange mixture, the oil being greasy and the cornstarch absorbent. Those with dry skin would be better off exfoliating with a well-formulated AHA moisturizer and applying plain olive oil to dry areas afterward.

☹ POOR **Buff Polish, Facial Exfoliation Treatment** *($21 for 4 fl. oz.)* is a cleanser/scrub hybrid that contains several irritating ingredients, including lemon, balm mint, and jasmine oils. It is not recommended, but do check out the Appendix to learn how irritation hurts everyone's skin.

☹ POOR **Glycolic Retexturizing Pads** *($34.50 for 60 pads)* contain glycolic acid in an amount that's likely less than 5%. Despite being the second ingredient, the company confirmed the amount of AHA was below the 5% they use in their Glycolic Cleanser. The pH is within range for exfoliation to occur, but it's also below pH 3, which is needlessly irritating. The witch hazel extract and potassium hydroxide (lye) are cause for concern as both are potent skin irritants when used in high amounts. The pad's solution contains some helpful water-binding agents and antioxidants, but it's almost too little, too late—not to mention the antioxidants won't remain stable due to jar packaging (see the Appendix for details).

☹ POOR **Glycolic Serum Extreme Renewal** *($34.50 for 1 fl. oz.)* contains an effective amount of glycolic acid, but its pH isn't within range for exfoliation to occur. Even if it was within range, this serum contains irritating citrus extracts and lavender oil. See the Appendix for details on why lavender oil is bad for skin. For better results without needless irritants, consider Paula's Choice RESIST Weekly Resurfacing Treatment with 10% Alpha Hydroxy Acid.

SERIOUS SKIN CARE MOISTURIZERS (DAYTIME & NIGHTTIME), EYE CREAMS, & SERUMS

✓☺ BEST **A-Force XR, Retinol Serum** *($37.50 for 1 fl. oz.)*. This water-based serum contains an impressive amount of vitamin A (mostly as retinyl palmitate), along with a smaller but still efficacious amount of retinol. The formula also contains a good anti-irritant as well as antioxidants, including vitamin C and green tea. Although glycolic acid is present, the amount is too low for it to function as an exfoliant; however, it has water-binding properties for skin, and that's helpful. This serum is best for normal to dry skin; the castor oil will be a problem for those with oily or breakout-prone skin. The only slight drawback is that it contains fragrance.

☺ GOOD **A-Eye XR** *($26.50 for 0.5 fl. oz.)* is a lightweight eye-area moisturizer that contains a good amount of retinol and comes in packaging that will keep it stable during use. It is not rated higher because, despite the fact that it contains beneficial ingredients in addition to the retinol, it contains potential irritants such as horsetail, witch hazel, and elderflower, all of which have an astringent or constricting effect on skin. The amounts are small enough that they aren't likely to be a problem, but they're worth calling out because this product is designed to be used near the eye, and retinol as an active ingredient can cause problems by itself on the skin, so staying away from any additional risk is best.

☺ GOOD **InstaGleam, Glowing Facial Moisturizer** *($32.50 for 1.7 fl. oz.)* is a very good sheer-tinted moisturizer that imbues skin with soft bronze color and a soft shine. Best for dry skin, this smoothes on evenly and treats skin to an impressive mix of beneficial ingredients, including retinol. This would be nearly perfect if it contained sunscreen, too. Without the sunscreen, you're missing one of the main conveniences of using a tinted moisturizer as part of your daytime routine.

☺ GOOD **Rulinea-FX Topical Regenerating Eye Cream for Aging Skin** *($21.25 for 0.65 fl. oz.)* is yet another eye cream from a line that already has too many eye-area options. If any of them worked as claimed, why would they keep offering more, all with similar line-diminishing claims? Overall, this is an impressive moisturizer for dry skin anywhere on the face. Some of the plant extracts pose a slight risk of irritation, but the amounts of these potential irritants are likely too small to matter. Despite our enthusiasm, see the Appendix to learn why you don't need an eye cream.

☺ GOOD $$$ **Nanofill Topical Collagen** *($27 for 0.5 fl. oz.)* is supposed to be the answer to getting collagen into skin because Serious Skin Care claims to have made the collagen molecule very small via nanotechnology. OK, so let's assume they're right and that the hydrolyzed collagen molecules in this product really are able to penetrate the skin. Does that mean they'll seek out and attach to your skin's own supply of collagen? No, of course not; but there are lots of consumers who would likely make that association. In contrast, the purified highly concentrated collagen (whether animal sourced or bioengineered) used for injections is a relatively thick gel that is injected just under the wrinkle, filling it out. Over time, this collagen breaks down, and then you must have another injection. So, even if nano-sized collagen was being used in this product (which it isn't), it won't bind to the collagen in your skin; even the collagen fillers don't do that. And keep in mind how small nano-sized particles are—if Serious Skin Care is really using such small particles of collagen, there's not much to stop them from penetrating where you don't want them to go (which is one of the reasons nanotechnology in cosmetics is controversial). By the way, the ingredient *Pseudoalternomonas* ferment extract is a form of bacteria sold by cosmetic ingredient supplier Lipotec. According to the company, this bacteria has an amazing ability to increase skin's collagen production. If that were true, then presumably Serious Skin Care wouldn't need to tout their nano-sized collagen molecules because the bacteria would go to work and super-stimulate skin to produce more collagen to fill lines. Of course, there is no published, peer-reviewed research supporting the claims for *Pseudoalteromonas* ferment, just Lipotec's unduplicated studies (as you might expect, Lipotec's study of its own product shows results that are nothing short of miraculous). In the end, this is a good fragrance-free moisturizer for normal to slightly dry skin not prone to blemishes, and it can be used around the eyes.

☺ GOOD $$$ **Seramins Free Radical Quencher Multi Vitamin Facial Serum** *($39.95 for 1 fl. oz.)* claims to be packed with antioxidants, a claim that, for the most part, is true. Blended into hydrating slip agents and silicones are numerous antioxidants, from soy to vitamin C. Tried-and-true antioxidants (e.g., vitamin E) are joined by the trendier ones (e.g., resveratrol and melon fruit) in a serum that's suitable for all skin types. We're not sure why the company thought coloring agents were needed, but perhaps their intent was to give this serum a more medicinal look, which is also done quite nicely by the amber glass bottle packaging. The only cause for concern is the ingredient dimethylaminoethanol. Also known as DMAE and listed as dimethyl MEA, it's controversial because research has shown that when applied to skin it offers immediate protective benefits to cells, but this is followed by a decrease in cell growth up to and including cellular growth coming to a halt (Sources: *Aesthetic and Plastic Surgery*, November-December 2007, pages 711–718; and *The British Journal of Dermatology*, March 2007, pages 433–439). There isn't much DMAE in here, but the concern over this ingredient isn't something you'll hear from Serious Skin Care when their spokesperson is doing on-air presentations exclaiming how wonderful this serum is supposed to be.

☺ AVERAGE **A-Copper Oil Control Serum with Copper Peptides** *($28.50 for 1 fl. oz.)* is a water-based, somewhat sticky-feeling serum that contains two forms of copper, yet the lack of research attesting to copper's antiwrinkle prowess means this isn't a serum anyone should choose over others that contain proven ingredients, such as a wide range of antioxidants, skin-identical ingredients, exfoliants, sunscreens, and on and on. Moreover, the inclusion of sodium polystyrene sulfonate (an ingredient found in firm-hold hairspray products) may cause irritation and doesn't have a pleasant after-feel on skin.

☺ AVERAGE **C-Cream SPF 30, Vitamin C Ester Protective Daytime Moisturizer** *($26.50 for 2 fl. oz.)* contains numerous citrus fruit extracts that put a damper on an otherwise brilliantly formulated daytime moisturizer for normal to dry skin. Stabilized avobenzone is on hand for sufficient UVA protection and this contains some helpful moisturizing ingredients for normal to dry skin. But the citrus extracts make this sunscreen a potential problem, especially for sensitive skin. Parts of this product's formula are worthy of a higher rating, but taken as a whole, an average rating and a caution are warranted. Despite the name, this product's vitamin C content is on the low side, unless the company is referring to the irritating citrus extracts being a natural source of this vitamin.

☺ AVERAGE **Eye Help, Daily Moisture Eye Cream** *($19.95 for 0.5 fl. oz.)* has a silky-smooth texture yet this ordinary, boring eye cream for normal to slightly dry skin doesn't offer much beyond a nice texture. The effectiveness of the plant extracts and their antioxidant ability will be squandered once this jar-packaged product is in use. None of the ingredients in this eye cream will promote firmer skin. It is fragrance-free, though, but ultimately it's just further proof of why eye creams are unnecessary (see the Appendix to find out why).

☺ AVERAGE **Glucosamine Acid-Free Skin Resurfacing Moisturizer** *($22 for 4 fl. oz.)* is a moisturizer for normal to dry skin that doesn't contain any exfoliating ingredients, so the resurfacing claim is farfetched. This can deliver "immediate hydration," but so can any moisturizer when applied to dry skin, so the urgency behind that claim is not tied to anything unique about this product. Most of the antioxidants are present in amounts too small to matter, though at least it's better than nothing.

☺ AVERAGE **Glucosamine Skin Refining Eye Cream** *($19.50 for 0.5 fl. oz.)* leaves you with little to get excited about. Although suitable for normal to dry skin anywhere on the face, the amount of the mineral pigments mica and titanium dioxide lend a slightly opaque shiny appearance to this cream, hence the "brightening" effect. The intriguing ingredients don't amount to much, so at best this is a below-average fragrance-free moisturizer. See the Appendix to learn why, in truth, you don't need an eye cream.

☺ AVERAGE **Glucosamine Skin Resurfacing Serum** *($26.50 for 1 fl. oz.)* contains acetyl glucosamine as the second ingredient; however, it cannot resurface skin—at least not in the same manner as using a well-formulated AHA or BHA product. Acetyl glucosamine is similar to the skin-identical ingredient glycosaminoglycans, so it functions as a water-binding agent and can help hold moisture in skin. The pore- and redness-reducing claims aren't in acetyl glucosamine's bag of tricks, but the antioxidants can exert an anti-inflammatory benefit. In the end, this isn't as impressive as serums listed in our Best Products chapter.

☺ AVERAGE **NanoSeal Topical Collagen Treatment & Hydration Sealer** *($29.95 for 1.7 fl. oz.)* contains collagen, which absolutely cannot be absorbed into your skin and fuse with the collagen there to fill in lines and wrinkles. There is no research to the contrary, either. Collagen injections cannot be replaced with lotions and potions in any way, shape, or form. Even if collagen (nano-size or not) could fuse with the collagen in your skin, how would your skin know when it was getting too much or where in the skin it was going? What if you used this too often and added so much collagen to your skin that you ended up with a lumpy, distorted face? Or if the collagen spread evenly all over, it would puff up evenly, and the same wrinkles would still be there because the entire face would have equal collagen growth. Of course, there's no chance of that happening because applying collagen of any kind topically can't impact skin in any way, other than it being a moisturizing agent. Beyond the collagen issue, this is an ordinary moisturizer that's a barely passable option for normal to dry skin. Normally we'd comment on the problem jar packaging presents, but there's so little of value in here that the packaging really doesn't matter.

☺ AVERAGE **Olive Oil Moisture Cream for Face and Neck** *($27.50 for 2 fl. oz.)* is packaged in a jar. First-pressed or not, the antioxidant benefits and stability of the olive oil in this moisturizer for dry to very dry skin will be compromised because of the packaging (see the Appendix for details). That's unfortunate, because otherwise this is an exceptionally emollient formula that contains some good antioxidants and a cell-communicating ingredient.

☺ AVERAGE **Olive Oil Moisture Replenishing Eye Balm** *($19.50 for 0.5 fl. oz.)* is a very rich balm that is based on a blend of a nonfragrant plant oil and cornstarch, which helps keep things from getting too greasy and likely enhances spreadability. Rather than use this product (the rosemary oil it contains is an irritant), you can treat areas of very dry skin to plain olive or canola oil from your kitchen cupboard. As is, this product should not be used routinely around the eyes because of the fragrant rosemary oil and because this is just a really boring ordinary group of ingredients that leave skin wanting so much more. See the Appendix to learn why, in truth, you don't need an eye cream.

☺ AVERAGE **Replicate & Renew Plant Stem Cell Eye Cream** *($32.50 for 0.5 fl. oz.)* is a very basic eye cream that contains standard thickeners and a tiny amount of antioxidant plant extracts, despite the name and claims. The fruit cell culture from a type of apple known as *Malus domestica* cannot bring its regenerating power to improve wrinkles and other signs of aging around the eyes. Here's why stem cells in skin-care products do not work as claimed: Stem cells need to be alive in order to function as stem cells. Once these delicate cells are added to skin-care products, they are long dead and therefore useless. It's actually a good thing that stem cells in skin-care products can't work as claimed because one stem cell study has revealed the potential risk of cancer they pose. Plant stem cells such as those derived from apples, melons, or rice cannot stimulate stem cells in human skin, though being from plants these ingredients likely have antioxidant properties. It's a good thing plant stem cells can't work as stem cells in skin-care products; after all you don't want your skin to absorb cells that can grow into apples or watermelons! There are also claims that because a plant's stem cells allow a plant to repair itself or survive in harsh climates, these benefits can be passed to human skin. How a plant functions in nature is unrelated to human skin and these claims are completely without substantiation. This ends up being an OK eye cream for dry skin, but in truth you don't need an eye cream at all if you're already using a well-formulated facial moisturizer and/or serum.

☺ AVERAGE **SuperMel C, An Antioxidant Rich Beauty Cream** *($39.50 for 1.7 fl. oz.)* is packaged in a jar, so can forget about getting much antioxidant benefit from using this product because the packaging will routinely expose it to degrading light and air. The meager amounts of antioxidant included make it all the more disheartening. By the way, just because the antioxidants in this product are encapsulated does not mean they are impervious to light and air. Most ingredient encapsulations use a lipid (fat) membrane, and the lipids are prone to oxidation, too.

☺ AVERAGE **SuperMel C, An Antioxidant Rich Eye Cream** *($24.50 for 0.5 fl. oz.)* is a good, though unexciting, moisturizer for dry skin anywhere on the face. The melon extract, present in an extremely small amount, contains superoxide dismutase as one of its constituents, but in this small amount, so what? See the comments above for SuperMel C, An Antioxidant Rich Beauty Cream, because they apply to the eye cream version, too.

☺ AVERAGE **SuperMel C, An Antioxidant Skin Beauty Cocktail** *($73 for 4 fl. oz.)* is supposed to be an antioxidant powerhouse, but ends up falling a bit flat. The olive and sunflower seed oils have antioxidant ability and the packaging will keep these oils stable during use; however, this product does not contain superoxide dismutase as claimed. Even if it were encapsulated, as the label states, it would still have to be listed on the ingredient statement, and it isn't. Despite this omission, it is worth noting that a constituent of the melon extract in this product is superoxide dismutase (Source: *Journal of Agricultural and Food Chemistry*, May 2008, pages 3694–3698), but the amount of melon extract is next to nothing, which makes its ability to impart the beneficial component to skin at best remote. This is a relatively unexciting overly hyped moisturizer for dry skin.

☺ AVERAGE $$$ **Capominerale Mineral Rich Facial Creme** *($26 for 0.5 fl. oz.)* claims that this is densely packed with minerals, which it isn't because they are barely present. The minerals that it does contain—malachite and hematite—can't penetrate skin and there is no research showing they have any benefit anyway. Aside from the outlandish promise of minerals being the skin-care answer for your wrinkles or other concerns (what a sad joke), this moisturizer doesn't qualify as state-of-the-art, but it's an OK option for normal to dry skin not prone to blemishes.

☺ AVERAGE $$$ **Creamerum Evolve** *($89 for 1 fl. oz.)* is an expensive, lightweight cream for normal to dry skin that contains many intriguing ingredients, but ultimately it's not among the better options, especially at its price. This contains some plant extracts (sugar cane, sugar maple, orange) that are often said to function like AHAs such as glycolic acid. That sounds great and oh-so-natural, but the truth is these ingredients cannot and do not function like AHAs and there's no research proving otherwise. If anything, the orange and lemon extracts this contains pose a risk of irritation. We love that several antioxidants made their way into this formula, but some of the plants are fragrant and the inclusion of gold (yes, as in jewelry) is cause for concern because gold is known to cause contact dermatitis (Source: *Cutis*, May 2000, pages 323–326). There's no research showing gold (or the precious metal platinum also present in Creamerum Evolve) have any benefit for skin. The bulk of this formula is worthwhile, but wouldn't you rather use a less expensive moisturizer that only treated your skin to beneficial ingredients and no potential troublemakers?

☺ AVERAGE $$$ **InstaGleam, Illuminating Facial Serum** *($36.50 for 1 fl. oz.)* is a lightweight serum that contains mineral pigments that add a soft shimmer to skin. Although it contains some intriguing ingredients such as peptides, soy protein, and niacinamide, all of these are listed after the film-forming agent PVP. Most often used in hairstyling products, PVP can make skin feel tacky and may cause irritation when present in the amount here. That drawback keeps this serum from earning a higher rating.

☺ AVERAGE $$$ **NightWorks, Luxurious Night Cream** *($36.50 for 1.7 fl. oz.)* is a very standard emollient moisturizer whose big claim is that its ingredients are time-released throughout the evening. Although that's nice, it is hardly unique to this product, and in fact, makes you wonder why all the other Serious Skin Care products don't use the same technology. Although this has merit for very dry skin, it is not recommended over countless other moisturizers because it contains the plant irritants lavender, orange, and lemon. The citrus ingredients aren't a large part of the formula, but the amount of lavender is cause for concern (see the Appendix to find out why, plus learn why this product's jar packaging is a problem).

☺ AVERAGE $$$ **O3 Mega Omega 3 Restoring Beauty Therapy** *($32.50 for 1 fl. oz.)* is trying to be more than a one-note product. This olive oil–based moisturizer (which isn't in the least therapeutic) also contains glycerin along with a cell-communicating ingredient and some silicones. There are omega fatty acid oils in the product, which is good for skin, but they are hardly unique to this product. When this simple ingredient list is added up, you end up with a decent moisturizer for dry skin, but little else.

☺ AVERAGE $$$ **Replicate & Renew Double Power Concentrate** *($46.50 for 1 fl. oz.)* is the serum version of Serious Skin Care's Replicate & Renew Plant Stem Cell Cream reviewed below. It is said to contain twice the amount of the showcased apple stem-cell ingredient found in the Replicate & Renew Plant Stem Cell Cream, which makes us wonder why anyone would consider that product. After all, if this apple stem-cell ingredient is so amazing, why not go for a higher dose? And who knows how much of it your skin needs? How inane! As it turns out, no surprise here, domestica fruit cell culture isn't the antiwrinkle answer. The only research on its benefit for skin comes from the company that sells the ingredient to cosmetics brands, and the study was done in vitro, not on actual human or animal skin. Even if this ingredient has some protective potential for skin cells, then the same would be true of hundreds of other ingredients, from sunscreens to antioxidants and cell-communicating ingredients such as retinol or niacinamide. Aside from the stem cell issue, this serum has a silky texture and a decent but unexciting assortment of emollient, nonfragrant plant oils, antioxidants, and cell-communicating ingredients, but not enough to set it apart or warrant a better rating.

☺ AVERAGE $$$ **Replicate & Renew Plant Stem Cell Cream** *($44.95 for 1.5 fl. oz.)* is an emollient moisturizer for dry skin that is another antiwrinkle product from a company that already sells a dizzying amount of them. Serious Skin Care claims to be serious about getting rid of wrinkles; they just can't make up their mind about which of their myriad products really works because they sell numerous products making the same claims. Aside from their vast array of other miracle products, this new option is supposed to be an infusion of stem cells into your skin from a certain species of apple. We've discussed this ingredient (*Malus domestica* fruit cell culture) before—the manufacturer and the cosmetics companies that add it to their formulas tout it as being able to restore skin. The Domestica Fruit Cell Culture is based on plant callus cells and claimed to be from a rare Swiss apple tree (of course it has to be rare; the marketing story wouldn't be nearly as interesting if the apple tree were in Detroit or Seattle). Plant callus cells are formed when a plant is wounded. The cells surrounding the wound turn into stem cells; that is, they change and become cells that can produce wound-healing plant tissue. After the wound has healed, these callus cells remain stem cells (they are totipotent) and can continue to make whatever cells the plant needs. The Swiss apple tree in question also has substances

Lavender oil smells great, but fragrance isn't skin care! Find out why in the Appendix.

that give the tree longevity. That's really good news for the plant, but whether or not it is good news for your skin is simply a guessing game, supported only by the in vitro research performed by the ingredient manufacturer, who claims that it shows some protective benefit. Even if this ingredient has some protective potential for skin cells, then the same would be true of hundreds of other ingredients, from sunscreens to antioxidants and cell-communicating ingredients such as retinol or niacinamide. This is not a miracle or a new must-have ingredient for skin, despite its association with stem cells, a technology which in plant or human form has yet to be developed for wrinkles. The potential risks where stem cells are concerned are just ignored by these companies because that side of the story gets in the way of a good sales pitch. Given the unknowns, this ends up being just another moisturizer packaged in a jar, which means the really beneficial ingredients it contains won't be of much help to your skin for long, not even the all-important fruit extract.

☺ AVERAGE **$$$ Reverse Lift, Firming Eye Cream** *($24.50 for 0.5 fl. oz.)* is a really basic, almost embarrassing eye-cream formula that the company claims should be used by women in their 40s and 50s. It contains acetyl hexapeptide-3, a peptide that some companies claim relaxes muscles like Botox does, but it absolutely cannot even remotely have that effect on skin. Even Botox doesn't work like Botox when applied on the surface of the skin. That's about as exciting as this formula gets; it contains a teeny amount of antioxidants and helpful plant extracts and the amount of soybean oil will provide antioxidant benefits. This eye cream won't lift skin in the least or reverse even one second of aging, but it can make skin feel smoother and softer. See the Appendix to learn why, in truth, you don't need an eye cream.

☺ AVERAGE **$$$ Rulinea FX Intensive Plus Wrinkle Serum** *($59.95 for 1.7 fl. oz.)* is a potentially good antioxidant serum for all skin types, though it's not without some concerns. Chief among them is the ingredient dimethyl MEA. Also known as DMAE, it's controversial because research has shown that when applied to skin it offers immediate protective benefits to cells, but this is followed by a decrease in cell growth up to and including cellular growth coming to a halt (Sources: *Aesthetic and Plastic Surgery*, November-December 2007, pages 711–718; and *The British Journal of Dermatology*, March 2007, pages 433-439). There isn't a lot DMAE in here, but the concern over this ingredient isn't something you should take lightly, especially if your skin-care routine includes multiple products with dimethyl MEA. It's disappointing that several of the good-for-skin ingredients are listed after the preservative; for a product at this price point, you want to see as much of the good stuff up front as possible. The skin firmers referred to in the claims are likely the film-forming agent glyceryl pullulan, which is included in many serums and moisturizers for its smoothing ability. Note that the amount of glycolic acid in this serum is too low for it to function as an exfoliant.

☺ AVERAGE **$$$ Skincandescence, Illuminating Skin Serum** *($44.50 for 1 fl. oz.)* is a water- and olive oil–based moisturizer that contains a small amount of arbutin, a plant ingredient whose hydroquinone content has skin-lightening ability, though likely not when present in such a small amount. Another ingredient, diacetyl boldine, is said to disrupt the activation phase of the melanin production process (remember, melanin is the pigment that darkens skin cells). Diacetyl boldine appears to have antioxidant ability, but there is no independent, peer-reviewed research supporting the claim that it can suppress melanin production. Although you shouldn't rely on this serum for lightening skin imperfections, it is an OK option as a moisturizer for dry skin.

☺ AVERAGE **$$$ Super Eye Creamerum** *($44.50 for 0.5 fl. oz.)* is an eye-area moisturizer with a shiny finish. The bismuth oxychloride functions as a thickening and opacifying agent, while also lending a subtle brightening effect to the eye area (the effect is strictly cosmetic). Normal to dry skin will do best with this product, though again, it isn't as impressive or as "super" as it could have been—and you don't need an eye cream, anyway (see the Appendix for details).

☹ POOR **4 Million IU A Cream XR-Time Release Retinol Cream** *($39.50 for 2 fl. oz.)* contains anti-aging vitamin A in a moisturizing base for normal to dry skin. The formula is also littered with fragrant oils that cause irritation. Irritation from fragrant oils is pro-aging, which means this isn't the product to help you "put your best face forward every day." If anything, using this is a big mistake if your goal is younger, healthier-looking skin. Many other companies, from RoC to SkinCeuticals and Paula's Choice, offer expertly formulated retinol products that give your skin all the good and none of the bad.

☹ POOR **C-Eye, Vitamin C Ester Eye Beauty Treatment** *($21.50 for 0.5 fl. oz.)* contains a high amount of irritating citrus extracts too great to ignore, and none of them have any notable benefit for wrinkles or eye-area skin. Without the citrus extracts, this would be an OK lightweight vitamin C moisturizer for normal to slightly dry skin. The amount of film-forming agent (think hairspray) is another potential source of irritation, though some may find it makes skin around the eyes feel a bit tighter (but skin feeling tighter isn't the same as tightening loose, sagging skin). See the Appendix to learn why, in truth, you don't need an eye cream.

☹ POOR **C Morning Magic Overnight Cream** *($31.50 for 2 fl. oz.)* is an AHA moisturizer for dry skin that contains a helpful amount of the AHA glycolic acid and is formulated at a pH to ensure exfoliation occurs. Unfortunately, the formula contains a range of irritating citrus extracts along with a preservative (methylisothiazolinone) that is contraindicated for use in leave-on products due to its sensitizing potential. Given this product's vitamin C-themed name, it's disappointing that it contains so little vitamin C. This had the potential to be an excellent AHA moisturizer but too many missteps were made to make this a safe bridge to cross.

☹ POOR **C-Serum, Vitamin C Ester Skin Conditioner** *($28.50 for 1 fl. oz.)* is a non-conditioning ultra-light moisturizer that contains far too many irritating citrus extracts to make it worthwhile for any skin type. Lots of companies offer much better vitamin C formulations, including N.V. Perricone, MD Skincare by Dr. Dennis Gross, Jan Marini (reviewed on CosmeticsCop.com), and SkinCeuticals. Those brand's products cost more, but at least you're getting the goods without several extraneous irritants taking precedence over the beneficial ingredients. Also concerning is the high amount of film-forming agent (think hairspray) this product contains. As the second ingredient, it can be an irritant though you may initially notice it makes your skin feel tighter.

☹ POOR **COQ10, Around the Clock Antioxidant Beauty Treatment** *($39.50)* is based around the entire concept of providing 24-hour antioxidant protection to skin. However, whether you use the **Daytime** or **Nighttime** version, both expose your skin to a damaging amount of alcohol (listed as ethanol in the nighttime version). Talk about counterproductive! Alcohol generates free-radical damage! How foolish is that? Furthermore, in both products, the only antioxidant of note is ubiquinone (coenzyme Q10). If you assume that round-the-clock antioxidant protection is possible, it would take more than one antioxidant to do the job. Also worth mentioning is the skin cell–damaging lavender oil present in the Nighttime version and the fact that the Daytime version doesn't contain sunscreen. This kit is an anti-aging joke, with ingredients that cause more problems than they help.

☹ POOR **Eyetality Total Eye Evening** *($36.50)* is another one of the over a dozen eye creams, all with the same basic claims from Serious Skincare. And here's another one that's said to be the total solution. So, does the company really think that their other eye creams aren't all that good for your skin? Probably not, because they're still selling those, too. Obviously, none of the other eye creams from Serious Skin Care worked to get rid of wrinkles, dark circles, or puffiness, because now this one is the answer. However, it isn't an answer to any eye issue you're having. This particular option brings nothing new to the table, but there's plenty of reasons to avoid it, chief among them being the jar packaging (see the Appendix for details). Even in better packaging, this eye cream is a problem for all skin types due to the fragrant irritants it contains. Lemon oil, lavender, and arnica are a problem for all skin types, and lemon oil near the eyes?! Seriously?! It's really disappointing that this eye cream also contains some helpful ingredients. Whether you choose to use an eye cream or not (and you absolutely don't need to use one), your skin deserves only the good ingredients and none of the bad.

☹ POOR **Eyetality Total Eye Morning with Wand** *($32.50 for 0.5 fl. oz.)*. Although Serious Skin Care included some beneficial ingredients (none of which are unique for the eye area), they're joined by questionable ingredients (platinum has no established benefit for your skin) and, further down the ingredient list, several potent irritants (including lemon oil). Moreover, the good ingredients will lose their potency due to the jar packaging, which allows antioxidants and other beneficial ingredients to break down when they are exposed to air every time the product is opened. See the Appendix for more details on jar packaging and to find out why you really don't need an eye cream.

☹ POOR **Firma-Face XR All Over Skin Tightener** *($36.50 for 1.5 fl. oz.)* is a water-based serum that contains a high amount of absorbent ingredients that can constrict skin and make it feel temporarily tighter. Of chief concern is the second ingredient, sodium silicate. This is an alkaline ingredient with antiseptic properties, and is a known irritant (Source: *American Journal of Contact Dermatitis*, January 2002, pages 133–139). This serum contains some intriguing ingredients (such as retinol), but none that aren't found in other products (including many from Serious Skin Care) that don't risk irritation. This serum will make skin feel tighter, but it cannot lift skin. Even if it could, where would all the loose skin go? Simply pulling lose skin higher (which is what "lifting" would do) would only look strange, not youthful. See the Appendix to find out the extent skin care can help sagging.

☹ POOR **InstA-Tox Temporary Facial Firming Wrinkle Smoothing Serum** *($28.50 for 0.75 fl. oz.)* is the company's works-like-Botox product (something numerous cosmetics companies have added to their product lines over the past few years). Serious Skin Care does state that the effect of their serum isn't as dramatic as the effect you get from the actual medical procedure, but they also state that the results are still "remarkable." What a joke! It isn't dramatic, remarkable, or anything resembling good skin care. The alkaline pH of this mineral-heavy serum can cause skin irritation, resulting in inflammation that will temporarily reduce the appearance of wrinkles. This product does not provide moisture—on the contrary—it can draw moisture from the skin due to sodium silicate's irritating, astringent quality (Source: *American Journal of Contact Dermatitis*, September 2002, pages 133–139). Just about any serum or moisturizer is preferred over this mistaken concoction.

☹ POOR **Pure-Pep Pure Peptide & Neuropeptide Concentrate** *($59.95 for 1.7 fl. oz.)* is another anti-aging serum. The question begs to be asked, how many anti-aging serums does one brand need? Offering variety for different skin types and preferences is one thing, but Serious Skin Care offers so many serums, most with overlapping claims, that we wonder how their customers figure out which one to buy. This serum is all about peptides, at least if you believe the name. The ingredient list tells a different story because the formula does not come close to containing 30% peptides. But even if it did, so what? For most peptides, we don't know for certain how much is necessary in order for them to be beneficial. And more important, with many peptides, we're not sure if they're reaching their target areas within skin's uppermost layers. That's because our skin has defensive enzymes that break down fragile peptides before they reach their targets, so any benefit they may have isn't all that impactful. Peptide science in terms of skin care is getting better at stabilizing peptides so they remain active longer when applied to skin, but even assuming this serum's peptides could hit an anti-aging bull's eye each time, one ingredient crashes the party and brings everything down: bergamot oil. This citrus oil is known to cause contact dermatitis and can also cause brown spots or other discolorations when applied to skin that's exposed to sunlight without sun protection (Source: naturaldatabase. com). Because of this one (serious) misstep, this gel-like serum is not recommended.

☹ POOR **Resveratrol Drench Age-Defying Facial Cream** *($32.95 for 1.7 fl. oz.)* has a lot of problems that defy reasoning for this moisturizer. First, the jar packaging won't keep the air-sensitive ingredients that this contains stable. There also aren't many other interesting ingredients in here that are helpful for skin, but even more significant, this product does not contain the potent antioxidant resveratrol, even though that ingredient is in the name. According to Serious Skin Care, the resveratrol in this moisturizer comes from *Pichia* ferment extract, a type of yeast, but that doesn't make it resveratrol. According to information from the company that sells this ingredient to cosmetics companies, the usage level must be between 2%-5% for efficacy, yet that's not the amount Serious Skin Care added to this product; in fact, they included only about 0.1%. There is more alcohol here than yeast extract. Even if this yeast extract could provide skin with any amount of antioxidant activity, it won't hold up against repeated exposure to light and air.

☹ POOR **Reverse Lift, Firming Facial Cream with Argifirm** *($29.95 for 2 fl. oz.)* is a jar-packaged moisturizer for normal to dry skin that contains the works-like-Botox ingredient argireline. Please refer to the Cosmetic Ingredient Dictionary at CosmeticsCop.com for details on this ingredient. Suffice it to say, it does not work like Botox or have remarkable wrinkle-reducing ability. This product is not recommended because it contains menthol, which is irritating for skin (see the Appendix to learn how irritation hurts skin).

☹ POOR **Reverse Neck Neck & Decollatage Firming Lotion with Argifirm** *($29.50 for 2 fl. oz.)* is a pathetic mix of mineral oil, lanolin, alcohol, and sodium polystyrene sulfonate; it also contains menthol, thus adding irritation to a mundane formula. This absolutely cannot tighten or streamline sagging skin along the neckline or jawline or anywhere. By the way, this also contains a high amount of acetyl hexapeptide-3, an ingredient that's often said to work like Botox injections "without the needle." It doesn't do that (at least not to the extent of antiwrinkle results possible from Botox injections) but assuming it did, you wouldn't want that all over your neck. If this peptide were able to paralyze muscles in your neck, you wouldn't be able to turn your head, nod, look up, and possibly not even be able to chew and swallow food or drinks. It's a good thing this peptide doesn't come remotely close to working like Botox!

☹ POOR **Reverse Serum, Firming Facial Serum with Argifirm** *($26.50 for 1 fl. oz.)* contains several problematic ingredients incapable of lifting or firming skin. It will cause irritation due to some plant extracts along with camphor, menthol, and the potent menthol derivative menthoxypropanediol. The redeeming ingredients are so few and far between, it's impossible to recommend this serum.

☹ POOR **Rulinea-FX Topical Aging Skin Regenerating Cream** *($32.50 for 2 fl. oz.)* is all about the power of penetrating botanicals that is said to be at the heart of this moisturizer's formula. Although it does contain several helpful plant ingredients with documented evidence of their benefit for skin, the inclusion of peppermint oil (which doesn't have a regenerating effect on skin) is a major strike against it. Without the peppermint oil, this would've been one of Serious Skin Care's better moisturizing formulas. See the Appendix to learn how irritation from peppermint oil damages skin.

☹ POOR **Total Youth Recall, All Over Facial Firmer** *($44.50 for 1.7 fl. oz.)* is primarily a blend of water with acrylate-based film-forming agents (think hairspray) along with drying, irritating, free-radical–generating alcohol. There is no redeeming quality to this product whatsoever.

SERIOUS SKIN CARE SPECIALTY SKIN-CARE PRODUCTS

✓☺ BEST **$$$ Clearz-It Acne Medication** *($17.50 for 2 fl. oz.)* is the only topical disinfectant we know of that combines an effective amount of benzoyl peroxide (in this case, 5%) with a high amount of tea tree oil, also known to have disinfecting properties for skin. The lightweight lotion formula is suitable for all skin types experiencing acne, and it's fragrance-free.

✓☺ BEST **Clearz-It Nano Hydra+ On-the-Spot Treatment Acne Medication** *($18.50 for 2 fl. oz.)* is an exceptional topical disinfectant that contains 5% benzoyl peroxide as its active ingredient. Serious Skin Care's website lists the active ingredient as 0.5% salicylic acid, but that is incorrect based on what's printed on the product itself (we also called the company to confirm). Mistakes aside, as mentioned, topical benzoyl peroxide is the gold standard for over-the-counter products for killing acne causing bacteria, and Serious Skin Care's fragrance-free version comes in a lightweight, antioxidant-rich formula. Antioxidants can reduce inflammation (and acne is an inflammatory disorder), so their inclusion is a plus. The formula also contains a good mix of skin-identical and cell-communicating ingredients (including retinol) that help counteract the potentially drying effect benzoyl peroxide has for some people. Tea tree oil also is included, and it likely contributes (in a small way) to this product's antibacterial action.

☺ GOOD **Clarify, Acne Medication Clarifying Treatment** *($17.50 for 2 fl. oz.)* contains 2% salicylic acid at a pH of 4.1, so some exfoliation will occur. There are more effective, less expensive BHA products available (such as those from Paula's Choice), but this lightweight, simply formulated anti-acne product is an option.

☺ GOOD **Reverse HD, High Definition Diffuser with Argifirm** *($24.50 for 1 fl. oz.)* is a silicone-heavy serum that contains shimmer pigments to add a glow to skin. The effect isn't necessarily soft-focus, but this can be considered a good primer-type product to use pre-makeup.

☺ AVERAGE **Glycolic 3, Cleansing, Exfoliating and Tightening Mask** *($19.50 for 5 fl. oz.)* contains a tiny amount of glycolic acid so this mask isn't going to exfoliate skin, making it at best a standard absorbent product for oily skin. It contains some good plant-based soothing agents, though the witch hazel distillate can make this more drying than other clay masks because this form of witch hazel is mostly alcohol.

☺ AVERAGE **Repairz-It, Youth Formula Oil Free Skin Hydrator Acne Medication** *($26.50 for 2 fl. oz.)* isn't a bad product; however, it is not effective for its intended purpose due to a low amount of salicylic acid and a pH of 4.5, so exfoliation is only minimally able to take place. There isn't any other reason to consider this product; it's an average moisturizer that may contribute to the clogged pores due to the amount of wax it contains.

☺ AVERAGE **Reverse Facial, Five Minute Firming Mask** *($22.50 for 2 fl. oz.)* cannot firm and lift skin, although it would be great if it could. All you can expect is oil absorption and a slight tight feeling after rinsing (but that isn't related to skin being firmed or lifted in any way). The aluminum chlorohydrate (the main ingredient in some deodorants) makes this clay mask extra-drying, and it is advised only for oily to very oily skin.

☺ AVERAGE $$$ **Probiotics Skin Balancing Beauty Treatment Mask** ($34.50 for 1.7 fl. oz.) contains a small amount of probiotics. Probiotics are "friendly" strains of bacteria that have some impressive, documented benefits when consumed orally. When it comes to topical application, there's almost no research to go on, not to mention that in all likelihood probiotics in skin-care products won't remain stable through the manufacturing process. This mask isn't as desirable as many others due to the small, but potentially problematic, amount of irritating plant extracts. Given that there's no valid reason to seek out skin care with probiotics, why not consider a moisturizing mask that treats your skin to the ingredients it needs to improve?

☺ AVERAGE $$$ **C-Extreme Results** ($44.50 for 2 fl. oz.). This two-part product begins with the application of **C-Resurface**, a baking soda-based gel scrub that contains vitamin C and fragrant citrus oil. The vitamin C is wasted in a rinse-off product and the baking soda creates a pH that is too high and not the best for skin. After rinsing, you apply the **C-Potion**, which is a lactic acid–based exfoliant whose pH is too high for exfoliation to occur. This is a very expensive way to scrub skin and treat it to a vitamin C "potion," which isn't nearly as impressive as it should be.

☺ AVERAGE $$$ **Correc-chin Firming Beauty Cream for the Chin, Neck and Jawline** ($36.50 for 2 fl. oz.) is supposed to contain a special ingredient used in French products, so it must be good (right?), because French women have great skin (right?), because….Well, suffice it to say, if you've been to France, you know that is absolutely not true. Second is the claim that it contains an ingredient that has research showing it works against cellulite. There is no independent research showing any ingredient works on cellulite, at least not to the degree that Serious Skin Care claims. Third is the claim that this answer to cellulite is now helpful for the chin, neck, and jawline, too. Aside from the absurdity that any cosmetic formulation can lift skin, there is no research showing any ingredient from France, or anywhere else, has reduced cellulite to a significant degree. Quite frankly, this is cosmetics marketing at its worst. All you're getting from this product is a blend of water, glycerin, algae, a natural starch made from yeast, and several thickening agents. The remainder of the formula is mostly plant oils (one of which is an irritant) and preservatives. None of the ingredients in this product, alone or together, can improve sagging skin anywhere on your body. Physiologically that is impossible from a topical skin-care product. Skin-care products cannot address the complex factors that cause skin to sag and our profiles to lose their contour. We know how tempting it is to search for products and try for a quick fix but, please, save your money and put it toward a procedure that really will make a difference.

☺ AVERAGE $$$ **Unmasked, Acne Medication Sulfur Mask** ($22 for 2.5 fl. oz.) doesn't contain any sulfur, at least not if the company-supplied ingredient list is correct. It would work well to absorb excess oil and rinse cleanly from the skin, but it's a shame the effect of the anti-irritant licorice is canceled out by irritating cinnamon bark extract. The tea tree oil could be helpful as a disinfectant, but the jar packaging wouldn't help keep it or any of the other potentially helpful plant extracts in this mask stable (see the Appendix for details).

☹ POOR **Clear Pads, Acne Medicated Pre-Soaked Wipes** ($19.95 for 45 wipes). The 2% salicylic acid steeped onto these cleansing pads would be much better for skin if it weren't for the base of strong alcohol in this formula. As such, the alcohol is too irritating and drying for all skin types (plus it generates free-radical damage), and the formula's pH is too high for the salicylic acid to function as an exfoliant.

☹ POOR **Continuously Clear, Acne Medication Moisture Replenishing Cream** ($24.50 for 2 fl. oz.) is an anti-acne moisturizer that contains 0.5% salicylic acid and is formulated at an effective pH. The rating is due to the high amount of paraffin, which can contribute to clogged pores, plus the rosemary oil is needlessly irritating.

☹ POOR **Light Fraxion Light Beauty Therapy in a Bottle** *($49.95 for 1.8 fl. oz.)*. We're not sure where to begin with the insane, absurd clams this product asserts. The misleading notions are couched in carefully worded marketing lingo to suggest that this lightweight lotion is somehow related to the light-based treatments performed in a doctor's office. You're supposed to believe that putting this on and then going out into the sun will provide the skin-renewing benefits that doctor-performed procedures like Fraxel can provide, ergo the distorted name Fraxion. It can't do that, not even remotely. Going out in the sun with this on will not convert the sun's energy into red light because the red light is already in the environment and there is no way to get around the damage UV light causes when you're not wearing sunscreen. That claim about how to use this product is reprehensible. Plus, because this contains bergamot oil, going out in the sun with this on is a big problem: Bergamot oil is phototoxic due to a chemical it contains known as bergapten. When you apply bergamot oil to unprotected skin and then expose it to sunlight, it can cause a reaction that leads to brown spots and other problems. This contains the cult favorite noni plant that has a devoted following of believers (and sellers of the juice and supplements) who proclaim this plant is the answer for long life. There is research showing it is a good antioxidant, as well as having other health properties, but it is hardly the only plant extract to have those properties. Noni isn't a must-have for skin.

☹ POOR **Olive Oil Hydration Mask** *($24.50 for 2 fl. oz.)* is a facial mask designed for dry skin that shouldn't contain clay (bentonite) as a main ingredient, followed by another absorbent ingredient, as this product does. If you're thinking that it must be good for oily skin, you'd be fooled again because the thickeners and plant oils in here aren't going to do that skin type any favors either. Ironically, this ends up being ideal for normal skin, but if your skin is truly normal (meaning no discernible oily or dry areas), you don't need a mask!

☹ POOR **ProRemedy Mineral Acne Medication** *($24.50 for 0.9 fl. oz.)* does contain 2% salicylic acid as its active ingredient, which is great for blemish-prone skin, but the pH is too high for it to work well as an exfoliant. Moreover, this product contains the potent irritant sulfur, which can cause dry, flaky skin. This product is far from an intelligent way to remedy acne or blackheads. Added to this mess is jar packaging, and stability is compromised, which in the case of some of these ingredients is a good thing.

☹ POOR **Serious Conceal Acne Treatment Pen** *($19.50 for 0.05 fl. oz.)* contains 10% sulfur, a potent amount of this antibacterial agent. There is definitely research showing sulfur has a positive effect on acne, but not in comparison to benzoyl peroxide. Plus, sulfur can be irritating, especially at this concentration. In addition, research indicates that sulfur works better when paired with salicylic acid (BHA) (Source: *Journal of Drugs in Dermatology*, July-August 2004, pages 427–431). What is most problematic about this formula is the amount of thickeners, titanium dioxide, and zinc oxide it contains, which could potentially clog pores. There are far better options to consider.

☹ POOR **Skincandescence Brightening Pen** *($24.50 for 0.12 fl. oz.)*. Housed in a pen-like package complete with built-in applicator is a silicone-based white, spackle-like product that helps temporarily fill in superficial lines. The amount of titanium dioxide adds a cosmetic brightening effect, but that's about it. This contains bergamot fruit oil, a citrus oil that is notorious for causing a phototoxic reaction when skin is exposed to sunlight, resulting in discolorations. It's counter-intuitive (to say the least) to add this problematic ingredient to any product claiming to help those with an uneven skin tone!

SERIOUS SKIN CARE SPECIALTY MAKEUP PRODUCTS

☹ POOR **HydraPixel Correct Micro Hydrating Corrective Coverage** *($34.95 for 1.7 fl. oz.)* is a cross between a foundation primer and a light coverage foundation. Essentially, it's a slightly thicker version of Serious Skin Care's HydraPixel Micro Hydrating Pixelated Skin Match reviewed below. Other than providing a bit more coverage, the same review applies.

☹ POOR **HydraPixel Micro Hydrating Pixelated Skin Match** *($34.95 for 1.7 fl. oz.)* is a cross between a foundation primer and a sheer coverage foundation. The silicone-heavy formula has a beautifully silky texture that sets to an almost instant matte (in feel) finish that lends a subtle glow to skin. This works really well to add a subtle but helpful "soft focus" effect to skin and is compatible with most foundations. Regrettably, there's one ingredient in this product that's a deal-breaker. Bergamot oil is one of the most irritating citrus oils around and contains a chemical constituent capable of causing skin discolorations upon exposure to sunlight. We had to wipe this off our skin almost immediately due to a burning sensation. The good news is that you're not really missing out because this product's best attributes are found in the top-rated foundations, foundation primers, and serums at the end of this book.

SHISEIDO

Strengths: Most of the sunscreens provide sufficient UVA protection and present a variety of options for all skin types, whether you're looking for titanium dioxide, zinc oxide, or avobenzone; a handful of good (but not great) moisturizers; worthwhile oil-blotting papers; foundations with sunscreen that provide sufficient UVA protection; pressed powder with sunscreen for oily skin; the Perfect Rouge Lipstick is one of the best creamy lipsticks at the department store; mostly good mascaras.

Weaknesses: Expensive; several drying cleansers; boring toners; a few sunscreens offer insufficient UVA protection; no AHA or BHA products; no products to effectively manage acne; no reliable skin-lightening options despite a preponderance of products claiming to do just that; irritating self-tanners; gimmicky masks; jar packaging; uneven assortment of concealers (and some terrible colors); average to disappointing eye and brow shapers; average makeup brushes.

For more information and the latest Shiseido reviews, visit CosmeticsCop.com.

SHISEIDO CLEANSERS

☺ GOOD $$$ **Pureness Refreshing Cleansing Sheets, Oil-Free, Alcohol-Free** *($18 for 30 sheets)* are cleansing wipes suitable for all skin types, but their cleansing ability isn't such that makeup removal is swift. The *Palo azul* wood extract in this product has no documented benefit for skin.

☺ GOOD $$$ **Pureness Refreshing Cleansing Water, Oil-Free, Alcohol-Free** *($22 for 5 fl. oz.)* is suitable for all skin types, but its cleansing ability isn't such that makeup removal is swift. The *Palo azul* wood extract in this product has no documented benefit for skin but the fragrant plant extracts of peony and rosemary are potentially problematic to use around the eyes.

☺ GOOD $$$ **The Skincare Extra Gentle Cleansing Foam** *($30.50 for 4.7 fl. oz.)* is a standard, glycerin-based foaming cleanser that is an option for all skin types except very dry. It removes makeup completely and rinses well.

☺ GOOD $$$ **The Skincare Rinse-Off Cleansing Gel** *($30 for 6.7 fl. oz.)* doesn't rinse completely due to its silicone content, but this is a new twist on standard, water-soluble cleansers and is a consideration for normal to oily skin. The tiny amount of alcohol is not likely to be a problem for skin. This is capable of removing all but the most stubborn types of makeup.

☺ AVERAGE **$$$ Ultimate Cleansing Oil, for Face & Body** *($25 for 5 fl. oz.)* is marketed as a cleanser that will remove long-wearing makeup and water-resistant sunscreens, and although it can do that, the formula is mostly mineral oil, which you can buy for a few dollars at any pharmacy around the world.

☺ AVERAGE **$$$ Benefiance Creamy Cleansing Emulsion** *($35 for 6.7 fl. oz.)* is a very standard, water- and oil–based cleansing cream for dry to very dry skin. This is essentially glorified cold cream and, although it removes makeup in a flash, you'll need a washcloth to avoid the greasy residue it leaves behind.

☺ AVERAGE **$$$ Benefiance Extra Creamy Cleansing Foam** *($35 for 4.4 fl. oz.)* is a foaming, creamy-textured, water-soluble cleanser that contains alkaline cleansing agents capable of causing dryness for most skin types.

☺ AVERAGE **$$$ White Lucent Brightening Cleansing Foam** *($35 for 4.7 fl. oz.)* is a standard, water-soluble foaming cleanser whose detergent cleansing agents can be slightly drying. This is a decent option for oily skin, but it will not whiten skin.

☹ POOR **Future Solution LX Extra Rich Cleansing Foam** *($55 for 4.2 fl. oz.)*. This ludicrously overpriced cleansing foam is not worth considering, either in the present or the future. Its core ingredients are similar to those found in products throughout the Shiseido line, so why this costs so much more is pure marketing, not formulary excellence. As it turns out, this isn't as good as many of Shiseido's less expensive cleansers because it contains too much potassium hydroxide (lye). This foaming cleanser is too drying for all skin types and completely incapable of "retaining skin's essential moisture."

☹ POOR **Pureness Deep Cleansing Foam** *($22 for 3.6 fl. oz.)* contains potentially drying cleansing agents and irritates skin with menthol, making this a cleanser to avoid. See the Appendix to learn how irritation makes oily, acne-prone skin worse.

☹ POOR **Pureness Foaming Cleansing Fluid** *($22 for 5 fl. oz.)* contains potassium myristate as its main cleansing agent. A constituent of soap, it can be drying for most skin types.

☹ POOR **The Skincare Gentle Cleansing Cream** *($30 for 4.3 fl. oz.)*. More slick than creamy, this cleanser does a good job of removing makeup, but the amount of alcohol it contains makes it a problem for all skin types, especially if you intend to use this around your eyes. Far from gentle, this cleanser is not preferred to the numerous silicone-enhanced makeup removers or water-soluble cleansers we recommend in the Best Products chapter.

☹ POOR **The Skincare Purifying Cleansing Foam** *($30.50 for 4.6 fl. oz.)* contains the drying, alkaline cleansing agent potassium myristate, which makes this cleanser/scrub hybrid a problem for all skin types.

SHISEIDO EYE-MAKEUP REMOVERS

☺ AVERAGE **$$$ The Skincare Instant Eye and Lip Makeup Remover** *($26 for 4.2 fl. oz.)* is a water- and silicone-based makeup remover that is below standard due to its alcohol content. Several other companies offer a better version of this type of makeup remover for a lot less money, including Almay, Neutrogena, and Paula's Choice.

SHISEIDO TONERS

☺ AVERAGE **$$$ Pureness Balancing Softener, Alcohol Free** *($24 for 5 fl. oz.)* is an OK toner for normal to oily skin, but it absolutely cannot create stronger skin that resists adult acne, as claimed.

☺ AVERAGE $$$ **The Skincare Hydro-Balancing Softener, Alcohol-Free** *($36 for 5 fl. oz.)* is an OK toner for all skin types. It provides water-binding agents, but that's it, so it's up to you to decide if spending this much for such a basic formula is worthwhile.

☺ AVERAGE $$$ **White Lucent Brightening Balancing Softener Enriched W** *($48 for 5 fl. oz.)* claims to brighten skin, which is merely a cosmetic claim that's not the same as lightening discolorations. Regardless of claims, this is a product to avoid not only for the sake of your pocketbook (the price is just absurd for what you get), but also because the formula is mostly water, slip agents, and alcohol, which is about as softening and enriching as a day in the desert. Alcohol causes free-radical damage, collagen depletion, and hurts the skins ability to heal. The fourth ingredient is xylitol, a sugar that has no benefit for skin, and it doesn't get much better from there.

☹ POOR **Benefiance WrinkleResist24 Balancing Softener** *($44 for 5 fl. oz.)* doesn't have what it takes to help aging skin resist wrinkles. Its formula is so do-nothing that it would be laughable if it weren't so expensive (wasting money on bad skin-care formulas is never funny). Despite the name and the impressive claims, this irritant-heavy toner is not recommended because irritation is always bad for skin (see the Appendix for details).

☹ POOR **Benefiance WrinkleResist24 Balancing Softener Enriched** *($44 for 5 fl. oz.)* doesn't have what it takes to help aging skin resist wrinkles. It contains far too much skin-damaging alcohol along with a lot of fragrance—two ingredients that keep aging skin from really looking younger (see the Appendix for details).

☹ POOR **Future Solution LX Concentrated Balancing Softener** *($90 for 5 fl. oz.)*. The most concentrated parts of this toner are water, slip agent, and, shockingly, alcohol. Unbelievable! The token amounts of intriguing ingredients don't justify this product's price or claims, and the alcohol isn't going to help skin counteract future signs of aging! That's like sending a woman concerned with wrinkles out into the sun with a bottle of mineral oil and lemon juice, and wishing her good luck on looking younger! There aren't words fit for print to state just how bad a formula this is, and the price is a slap in the face to anyone concerned with taking the best possible care of their skin.

☹ POOR **Pureness Anti-Shine Refreshing Lotion** *($24 for 5 fl. oz.)* contains a low amount of salicylic acid and has a pH that prevents it from functioning effectively as an exfoliant. This also contains enough alcohol to cause dryness, yet also stimulate oil production in the pore and cause irritation, all of which won't help treat acne in the least.

☹ POOR **The Skincare Hydro-Nourishing Softener** *($36 for 5 fl. oz.)* amounts to mostly water, slip agent, alcohol, and glycerin. There's enough alcohol to make this a non-softening problem for all skin types, and the peppermint extract only makes matters worse (see the Appendix to learn the many ways irritating ingredients hurt skin).

☹ POOR **White Lucent Brightening Toning Lotion, Cool** *($48 for 5 fl. oz.)* lists alcohol as its second ingredient (refer to the Appendix for details on alcohol) and contains numerous other irritants, too. This toner is a problem for all skin types, and that's a shame because it contains some helpful skin-lightening ingredients.

SHISEIDO EXFOLIANTS & SCRUBS

☺ GOOD $$$ **Pureness Pore Purifying Warming Scrub** *($24 for 1.7 fl. oz.)* doesn't make much sense as a scrub product designed for someone with oily skin and clogged pores because its main ingredient is mineral oil, followed closely by petrolatum (Vaseline). Although neither of these ingredients poses a risk of clogging pores, both have a thick, greasy texture that won't make someone with oily skin happy. This scrub is actually very good for someone with dry skin. The polyethylene beads (standard for most scrubs) are buffered by the mineral oil base, leaving skin with a soft, smooth feel along with some residual moistness. The warming effect is in the name only, because this scrub contains nothing to warm the skin (although the mechanical action of scrubbing can create a slight sense of warmth). This product does contain fragrance.

☺ AVERAGE **$$$ Bio-Performance Super Exfoliating Discs** *($65 for 8 discs)* are said to work like microdermabrasion, and manually exfoliate skin due to their texture and a mixture of talc and rice bran. These discs differ little from those sold in many drugstore lines; save your money and use a damp cotton washcloth instead (or better yet, an AHA or BHA exfoliant).

SHISEIDO MOISTURIZERS (DAYTIME & NIGHTTIME), EYE CREAMS, & SERUMS

✓☺ BEST **$$$ Bio-Performance Super Eye Contour Cream** *($55 for 0.53 fl. oz.)* is an excellent emollient moisturizer suitable for dry to very dry skin anywhere on the face. It is stably packaged, to the benefit of the many vitamin- and plant-based antioxidants it contains. Despite our praise, the fact is you don't need an eye cream (see the Appendix to find out why).

☺ GOOD **Extra Smooth Sun Protection Cream SPF 38 PA+++, for Face** *($32 for 2 fl. oz.)* needs a bit of explanation because of its PA+++ designation. This rating system was developed in Japan (where Shiseido is based) as a means to quantify the level of UVA protection a sunscreen can provide. "PA" stands for Protection-Grade of UVA. A PA+ rating signifies some UVA protection (which would apply to most sunscreens today), while a PA++ means moderate UVA protection, and PA+++ symbolizes high UVA protection. Because this particular sunscreen contains over 9% zinc oxide, it qualifies for its PA+++ rating. (This system is not recognized in the United States, Canada, Australia, or throughout Europe.) The fragranced base formula is suitable for normal to oily skin not prone to blemishes. This would be rated higher if it included greater amounts of antioxidants and did not contain a potentially problematic plant extract. Still, it has an admirably lightweight texture and silky-smooth finish and definitely provides broad-spectrum sun protection.

☺ GOOD **Ultimate Sun Protection Cream SPF 55 PA+++, for Face** *($35 for 2 fl. oz.)* is an in-part zinc oxide sunscreen for normal to combination skin that's not prone to breakouts. It definitely covers the broad-spectrum bases and has a silky texture. It's a shame the amount of antioxidants is so low, because in a sunscreen that costs this much they should be plentiful. See the review for Extra Smooth Sun Protection Cream SPF 38 above for an explanation of the PA+++ portion of the name.

☺ GOOD **White Lucent Brightening Moisturizing Emulsion** *($59.50 for 3.3 fl. oz.)* is an OK lightweight lotion for normal to slightly dry or slightly oily skin, but it cannot lighten discolorations, not even a little. The sleek packaging will keep the antioxidants stable during use, but they would be more potent without the alcohol that precedes them on the list.

☺ AVERAGE **$$$ Benefiance Concentrated Neck Contour Treatment** *($52 for 1.8 fl. oz.)* is primarily a blend of water, silicones, and slip agents along with film-forming agents and some antioxidants, none of which are specific to the neck area. This serum-like product also contains potentially irritating ingredients, although the small amounts mean they are likely inconsequential. This product has no hope of making lines on the neck a thing of the past, and there are products from other lines that are better formulated than this gaffe.

☺ AVERAGE **$$$ Benefiance NutriPerfect Eye Serum** *($76 for 0.5 fl. oz.).* The infusion of nutrients in this serum is claimed to counteract hormonal changes that cause skin to look aged, but they absolutely cannot do that. Hormonal changes that take their toll on skin must be addressed medically, not with cosmetics. It is very disappointing that this product contains not only fragrance, but also several fragrance ingredients known to cause skin irritation, which causes collagen to break down. What are those doing in a product meant to be used around the eyes?! The sole intriguing ingredient in this serum is carnosine, an amino acid that has anti-inflammatory and antioxidants properties, but these potentially positive effects are muted by the inclusion of denatured alcohol. For the money, this serum should've been significantly better, and it definitely won't make good on its claims to restore youthful vitality to aging eye-area skin.

☺ AVERAGE $$$ **Benefiance NutriPerfect Night Cream** (*$94 for 1.7 fl. oz.*) is Shiseido's answer for women dealing with skin changes that occur during and after menopause. With claims talking about restoring skin's density, renewing its vitality, and strengthening skin weakened by hormonal shifts, this is truly a disappointing and vastly overpriced moisturizer. Other than the addition of carnosine, this differs little from the dozens of other emollient moisturizers for normal to dry skin Shiseido sells. Carnosine is composed of amino acids and has benefit as an anti-aging ingredient for skin because of its antiglycation properties, but it is not a superior ingredient to address the many skin changes that occur during and after menopause. For example, it cannot stop skin sagging from loss of estrogen, cannot stimulate collagen production, and cannot correct decreased oil gland functioning that leads to dry skin (Sources: *Pathologie Biologie*, September 2006, pages 396–404; and *Life Sciences*, March 2002, pages 1789–1799). The amount of fragrance, relaxing or not, is greater than the amount of vitamin-based antioxidants, but those won't last long once the product is opened because the jar packaging won't keep them stable (see the Appendix for details).

☺ AVERAGE $$$ **Benefiance Wrinkle Lifting Concentrate** (*$63 for 1 fl. oz.*) is sold with the promise of, what else, lifting wrinkles. But Shiseido goes on to claim that this product allows skin to resist future wrinkles, something that's not possible without an effective sunscreen, which is absent here. The showcased ingredient in this product is chlorella extract. According to Shiseido, this reinforces the presence of a protein in skin that's critical to halting the wrinkling process. But none of that is substantiated, and even if it were, there's so little chlorella that your wrinkles wouldn't even notice. Chlorella is an algae and, like almost all species of algae, can act as a water-binding agent and antioxidant on skin. A good question for Shiseido: If this ingredient is that important for stopping wrinkles, why isn't it in every "antiwrinkle" product this line sells? This product is chiefly a lightweight moisturizer that contains more alcohol than it does beneficial ingredients for skin. At best, this is a substandard moisturizer for slightly dry skin that has no positive effect on wrinkles—either past, present, or future.

☺ AVERAGE $$$ **Bio-Performance Advanced Super Revitalizer (Cream) Whitening Formula N** (*$98 for 1.7 fl. oz.*) contains a selection of plant extracts and vitamin C (as ascorbyl glucoside), which have some research showing them to be effective for skin-lightening. However, due to jar packaging, none of these potentially efficacious ingredients will remain stable during use. See the Appendix to learn why jar packaging is not the way to go.

☺ AVERAGE $$$ **Bio-Performance Advanced Super Revitalizing Cream** (*$75 for 1.7 fl. oz.*) isn't advanced when compared to today's state-of-the-art moisturizers, but it does contain several ingredients (including glycerin, squalane, fatty acids, and silicone) that are helpful for dry skin. The tiny amounts of antioxidants will suffer from the jar packaging (see the Appendix for details). The pigments this contains produce a slight glow on skin, but don't mistake that for skin being revitalized.

☺ AVERAGE $$$ **Bio-Performance Super Corrective Serum** (*$80 for 1 fl. oz.*) is drastically overpriced and its core ingredients don't have a prayer of prompting skin's regenerative powers to fight the effects of time. It's mostly water, silicones, slip agents, talc, film-forming agent, minerals, and the type of alcohol used in most peel-off masks (polyvinyl alcohol), which is not great news for your face. These ingredients can make your skin feel tighter, but the effect is strictly cosmetic. There is considerably more fragrance and preservative in this serum than there are state-of-the-art ingredients capable of helping skin look and behave in a younger manner. In summation, this is a big waste of time and money.

☺ AVERAGE $$$ **Bio-Performance Super Restoring Cream** *($98 for 1.7 fl. oz.)* is sold as an unparalleled age-defying cream, which doesn't explain why Shiseido sells dozens of other moisturizers with this same claim. After all, if this is *the one*, why bother with the rest of them? As it turns out, this is a very good moisturizer for dry skin. Yet it ends up being disappointing because of jar packaging, which hinders the effectiveness of the impressive amount of antioxidants in this product (see the Appendix for details).

☺ AVERAGE $$$ **Future Solution LX Total Regenerating Cream Night** *($260 for 1.7 fl. oz.).* Labeling this a "high performance" moisturizer is intended to convince you that the price is worth it, but in reality it's a bit like going back to a typewriter after using a computer; the formula is marketed as advanced, but the ingredient list is circa 1970. This product is all about marketing rhetoric—it's all fluff with no substance. A couple of the ingredients are mildly interesting, but the jar packaging won't keep them stable (see the Appendix for details). The rest are there as fragrance, as preservative, or as simple emollients meant to make dry skin look and feel better; a $5 moisturizer can do the same thing (really)!

☺ AVERAGE $$$ **Future Solutions LX Ultimate Regenerating Serum** *($225 for 1 fl. oz.)* is just another overpriced serum that contains far more fragrance and preservative than state-of-the-art ingredients to help your skin look and act younger. Because of the silicone this contains, it has a silky, lightweight texture that works well under a moisturizer, but the same is true for many serums regardless of their price. This serum does contain a unique, amino acid-derived ingredient known as piperidinepropionic acid. According to a press release from the company, "Shiseido discovered the protein Serpin b3 is a factor in blocking the barrier function that protects the body from external stresses such as dryness and ultraviolet rays and has independently developed the amino acid derivative 1-piperidine propionic acid. Moreover, on human skin, 1-piperidine-propionic acid suppresses the production of Serpin b3 and results in improvement of the barrier function, moisture retention ability and skin texture and smoothness. These results have proven that application of 1-piperidine-propionic acid leads to improved skin quality." Sounds great and there's nothing wrong with touting a unique discovery, but what isn't mentioned is how many other ingredients offer similar benefits or go beyond what this amino acid derivative can do. Niacinamide has similar benefits and goes above and beyond, as do many other antioxidants and cell-communicating ingredients. It's interesting that research on this ingredient mentions its ability to protect skin from ultraviolet rays (sunlight). Again, many other ingredients do this, too, but none of them replace the need for a well-formulated sunscreen. Because this serum doesn't provide sun protection, it cannot make good on its claim to counteract "all signs of aging." After all, sunlight causes most of what we identify as signs of aging, so without sunscreen as part of your daily routine, even the best anti-aging serums won't be of much help. In the end, despite the novel ingredient, this serum simply isn't worth

🔊 Wondering why that product claiming to lift sagging skin didn't work? See the Appendix!

the cost. It poses a risk of irritation due to the fragrance ingredient it contains, which would be one more issue the amino acid–derived ingredient mentioned above would need to fight against, which isn't helpful for anyone's skin.

☺ AVERAGE $$$ **Future Solution Total Revitalizing Cream** *($230 for 1.8 fl. oz.)* is said to work on every aspect of skin to alleviate all signs of aging, from wrinkles to sagging. But, without a sunscreen, don't bet on this for any future protection against wrinkles, dark spots, and loss of resilience. For the money, this should be brimming with a who's who of today's top ingredients for helping skin function at its best, but it isn't. Even if some of those were included, they'd suffer from the unfortunate choice of (pretty) jar packaging. This ends up having OK potential but it's ultimately a waste of money ($230 for jar packaging? Are they kidding?).

☺ AVERAGE **Pureness Matifying Moisturizer, Oil Free** *($33 for 1.6 fl. oz.)* is a nearly weightless lotion for normal to oily skin, though its alcohol content may cause problems (see the Appendix for details). Still, this is an option for those who need a bit of hydration with a matte finish.

☺ AVERAGE **Pureness Moisturizing Gel-Cream** *($33 for 1.4 fl. oz.)* provides a hint of moisture along with a tiny amount of water-binding agent. It is an average option for normal to oily skin.

☺ AVERAGE $$$ **Revitalizing Cream** *($140 for 1.4 fl. oz.)* is an incredibly basic, shockingly priced moisturizer for dry to very dry skin. Not a single ingredient in this emollient product is justified by the cost, and jar packaging won't keep the two forms of vitamin E stable during use (see the Appendix for details on why jar packaging sells your skin short).

☺ AVERAGE $$$ **Sun Protection Eye Cream SPF 32 PA+++** *($32.50 for 0.6 fl. oz.)* deserves kudos for its in-part zinc oxide sunscreen and silky-cream texture, but it sorely lacks sufficient amounts of state-of-the-art ingredients for skin, and given the price that's an insult. Although the sunscreen is very good, this doesn't compete favorably with similar products from the Lauder-owned lines at the department store (including their relatively inexpensive Good Skin line, which is sold at Kohls). Still, it would work as sunscreen.

☺ AVERAGE **The Skincare Multi-Energizing Cream** *($44 for 1.7 fl. oz.)* is far from an intensive treatment for dull, dehydrated skin, but is an okay jar-packaged moisturizer for normal to dry skin.

☺ AVERAGE $$$ **The Skincare Night Moisture Recharge, Enriched** *($42.50 for 1.8 fl. oz.)* contains more thickening agents than The Skincare Night Moisture Recharge, Regular reviewed below, but is otherwise an equally uninspired moisturizer with a very small amount of the star ingredient, yuzu seed extract.

☺ AVERAGE **The Skincare Night Moisture Recharge, Light** *($42.50 for 2.5 fl. oz.)* contains mostly water, glycerin, silicone, and alcohol. The few intriguing ingredients are listed after the preservative, making this yet another disappointing, boring, fluid moisturizer.

☺ AVERAGE **The Skincare Night Moisture Recharge, Regular** *($42.50 for 2.5 fl. oz.)* is a lightweight moisturizer that's an average option for normal to slightly dry skin. Shiseido maintains that the yuzu seed extract (present in a next-to-nothing amount in this product) is a "breakthrough ingredient" that encourages the skin to produce more hyaluronic acid. There is no research anywhere to support this claim, but yuzu is a popular citrus fruit in Japan and Korea, and the peel does have considerable antioxidants. However, that's all related to eating the fruit and its skin, not putting it on your skin (Source: *The Journal of Agricultural and Food Chemistry*, September 2004, pages 5907–5913).

☺ AVERAGE **Urban Environment Oil-Free UV Protector for Face SPF 42 PA+++** *($30 for 1 fl. oz.)* is a super-light, almost weightless daytime moisturizer with sunscreen. Its silky fluid texture spreads easily and sets (quickly) to a soft matte finish. Those with oily or combination skin will likely find the finish pleasing; if you have any dry areas or if you have normal to dry skin this will likely feel uncomfortable, though you can always prep skin with a separate moisturizer. Broad-spectrum sun protection is assured thanks to the in-part zinc oxide sunscreen. This product's only drawbacks are the amount of alcohol it contains and that it is noticeably fragrant (perhaps to conceal the odor from the alcohol). The amount of alcohol is cause for concern in terms of irritation (refer to the Appendix for details), which is a shame because this has such a great finish for oily skin. The formula contains a tiny amount of antioxidants, most likely too little to offer much benefit to skin and definitely not enough to prevent free-radical production (though in truth no product can stop that process completely). With some minor formulary tweaks, this would be a slam-dunk. As it, it's recommended with reservations. See the review for Extra Smooth Sun Protection Cream SPF 38 above for an explanation of the PA+++ portion of the name.

☺ AVERAGE **Urban Environment UV Protection Cream for Face/Body SPF 35 PA+++** *($30 for 1.7 fl. oz.)* is nearly identical to the Urban Environment UV Protector for Face SPF 42 PA+++ above, except this has a lower SPF rating. Otherwise, bearing in mind this product is misnamed as being a "cream," the same review applies.

☻ AVERAGE **$$$ White Lucent Brightening Moisturizing Cream** *($59.50 for 1.4 fl. oz.)* costs a lot of money for a really basic, jar-packaged moisturizer that cannot lighten discolorations. It has an emollient texture, but the amount of alcohol is potential cause for concern, and this also contains some plant extracts that can be irritating. See the Appendix for details on the problems with jar packaging, alcohol, and irritating ingredients.

☺ AVERAGE **$$$ White Lucent Brightening Serum for Neck & Decolletage** *($76 for 2.6 fl. oz.)*. Without question, a woman's neck and chest area (decolletage) take a beating from sun and environmental exposure. Just as sun protection is a must for your face, you want to extend the same benefit to your neck and chest, too. Doing this doesn't require special products, and this serum is a case in point: It contains nothing unique for skin on the neck or chest, and absolutely cannot prevent discolorations from appearing (you need a well-formulated sunscreen for that). What about lightening existing discolorations? This does contain some plant extracts with limited research pertaining to their ability to work in that manner, and the vitamin C (ascorbic acid) may help, too. The problem is that all these potential skin-lightening ingredients are present in small amounts, so any benefit will be minor—and that's not what you want if you're going to spend this much on a single skin-care product. Shiseido includes more preservative and mica (a mineral pigment that imparts shine) than state-of-the-art ingredients, which is a big disappointment. At best this product will make dry skin anywhere on the body feel softer and smoother. Whether you want to spend this much for those results is up to you.

☹ POOR **Benefiance Energizing Essence** *($56 for 1 fl. oz.)* cannot energize skin, but it contains enough alcohol to cause irritation. Another concern is the inclusion of tranexamic acid. This synthetic ingredient is a drug used to control bleeding during surgical procedures, and it has no purpose or business being in a skin-care product (Sources: drugs.com; and *The Journal of Thoracic and Cardiovascular Surgery*, September 2000, pages 520–527).

☹ POOR **Benefiance NutriPerfect Day Cream SPF 15 Sunscreen** *($90 for 1.7 fl. oz.)* lacks the UVA-protecting ingredients of titanium dioxide, zinc oxide, avobenzone, ecamsule, or Tinosorb and is not recommended. The cell-communicating ingredient carnosine and the few antioxidants in this formula will soon become useless due to the jar packaging (see the Appendix for details), making this product an expensive mistake for its target audience of women age 50 and older (and remember, age isn't a skin type).

☹ POOR **Benefiance WrinkleResist24 Day Emulsion SPF 15** *($52 for 2.5 fl. oz.)* does not include the ingredients needed to shield your skin from the sun's entire range of damaging UVA rays, which is essential for anti-aging benefits. See the Appendix to learn which active ingredients you should be seeking.

☹ POOR **Benefiance WrinkleResist24 Intensive Eye Contour Cream** *($55 for 0.51 fl. oz.)* is a very basic, overpriced eye cream that's little more than water, standard thickener, mineral oil, Vaseline, and wax. It will feel rich and soothing over dry skin, but so will plain Aquaphor Healing Ointment for mere pennies per use. This contains a small amount of skin-repairing ingredient sodium PCA and a tiny amount of vitamin E, but not enough to warrant the expense or make this eye cream the one to buy. Besides, even with greater amounts of vitamin E or other antioxidants, the jar packaging won't keep those ingredients stable during use. What a letdown! By far the worst element of this eye cream is its fragrance and the presence of fragrance ingredients (such as hexyl cinnamal) known to be irritating. Fragrance is not only a problem for all skin types, but also it can be especially problematic in products meant for use so close to the eye. No element of fragrance is "age-defying"; if anything, the irritation it causes is pro-aging! In the end, this product is further proof of why eye creams are not necessary (see the Appendix for details).

☹ POOR **Benefiance WrinkleResist24 Night Emulsion** *($55 for 2.5 fl. oz.)*. Although this moisturizer for dry skin contains some good emollients, the overall formula is stunningly basic and absolutely not worth the price. Many of the intriguing ingredients are listed after the preservative, so they don't count for much. Last, this contains numerous fragrance ingredients known to cause irritation (see the Appendix to find out why daily use of highly fragrant products hurts skin).

☹ POOR **Bio-Performance Super Refining Essence** *($76 for 1.8 fl. oz.)* is a water- and glycerin-based serum that contains some good water-binding agents and small amounts of vitamins E and C. The problem is that it also contains numerous fragrant components, which can cause irritation, and that isn't what should be applied to freshly scrubbed skin.

☹ POOR **Future Solution LX Eye and Lip Contour Regenerating Cream** *($130 for 0.54 fl. oz.)* contains some of the least expensive cosmetic ingredients around, so the price is a joke! Far from a "powerful restoring treatment," all this can really do is make dry skin anywhere on your face feel somewhat smoother and softer, just like thousands of other moisturizers, and only temporarily. This product contains far more fragrance and fragrance ingredients than the brilliant anti-aging ingredients you'd expect at this price point. Plus, the few intriguing ingredients in this product will quickly degrade thanks to the jar packaging, making this very close to an all-around beauty budget burn. See the Appendix for details on jar packaging and to learn why you don't need a special product for your eye area.

☹ POOR **Future Solution LX Protective Day Cream SPF 15** *($240 for 1.7 fl. oz.)* can't fully protect skin because it doesn't contain the right UVA-protecting ingredients, which means it's not a "solution" for anyone's "future"! The base formula is mostly disappointing, too. At this price, it should be loaded with state-of-the-art ingredients proven to repair damage and help skin look and behave in a younger manner. Instead, it's mostly water, silicone, slip agents, thickener, and alcohol. There is only a small amount of alcohol and so it's unlikely a cause for concern, but this product is woefully short on beneficial ingredients, and what little there is will break down thanks to the jar packaging. See the Appendix to find out more about jar packaging and which sunscreen actives are needed for optimal anti-aging benefits.

☹ POOR **The Skincare Day Moisture Protection SPF 15 PA+, Enriched** *($40.50 for 1.8 fl. oz.)* is a slightly more emollient version of The Skincare Day Moisture Protection SPF 15 PA+, Regular below, but other than that the same review applies.

☺ POOR **The Skincare Day Moisture Protection SPF 15 PA+, Regular** *($40.50 for 2.5 fl. oz.)* lacks sufficient UVA-protecting ingredients (see the Appendix for details), which makes this daytime moisturizer—especially with its lackluster base formula—a resounding disappointment. What is extremely detrimental is that the PA+ is supposed to represent Japan's standard for some level of UVA protection. This system applies only to sunscreens manufactured in Japan, and does not imply superiority, as clearly evidenced here.

☹ POOR **The Skincare Eye Moisture Recharge** *($40.50 for 0.54 fl. oz.)* has a substandard formula that subjects skin to more alcohol than state-of-the-art ingredients. It also contains fragrance, which isn't what you want in a product meant for use around the eyes, and peppermint, another problem. Last, almost all the really intriguing ingredients (including the thiotaurine Shiseido spotlights) are listed after the fragrance and preservative. This is a "why bother?" product if ever there was one, and huge proof of why eye creams are superfluous (see the Appendix to find out more).

☹ POOR **White Lucent Anti-Dark Circles Eye Cream** *($55 for 0.53 fl. oz.)*. There are so many things wrong with this eye cream that we don't know where to begin. First, it's fragrant. Really fragrant. Fragrance is not only a problem for all skin types, but also it can be especially problematic in products meant for use so close to the eyes. This also contains several fragrance ingredients known to cause irritation, which won't improve skin anywhere on the face. Next up is the amount of alcohol. There's more alcohol (the skin-damaging, youth-subtracting kind) than there are state-of-the-art ingredients. And the teeny-tiny amount of impressive ingredients won't remain effective for long because this eye cream is packaged in a jar. The formula is supposed to be an intensive treatment with cutting-edge technology, but it ends up being a big step backward, relying on standard cosmetic pigments for a subtle brightening effect that's more makeup than skin care. Nothing in this eye cream can improve dark circles (whether related to sun damage or circulation issues). The only intriguing ingredient this contains is potassium methoxysalicylate. This ingredient's reported function is "skin bleaching agent" so we were curious to see if there was any research to support its use for lightening dark circles from sun damage. Regrettably, there isn't—at least nothing substantiated. The only research pertaining to melanin (the pigment that can be an underlying cause of some cases of dark circles and brown spots from sun damage) and this ingredient was done by Shiseido. Apparently, this ingredient was developed by Shiseido, yet the only research they allude to mentions in vitro, meaning it wasn't done on human skin. Therefore, it's a gamble as to whether or not this will be truly effective. And it won't be effective on dark circles caused by genetics, nor would it have any impact on puffiness. Last, there's no information to let you know if this ingredient is stable with repeated exposure to light and air—which is what will happen with daily use of this eye cream. See the Appendix to learn why jar packaging is a problem, and find out why, in truth, you don't need an eye cream.

☹ POOR **White Lucent Brightening Massage Cream N** *($52 for 2.8 fl. oz.)* is a basic, unimpressive moisturizer that contains more alcohol than ingredients with potential skin-lightening ability (and jar packaging won't keep these ingredients stable anyway, as explained in the Appendix).

☹ POOR **White Lucent Brightening Moisturizing Gel** *($59.50 for 1.4 fl. oz.)* contains enough alcohol to cause dryness and irritation, and there's more salt in here than any potentially helpful skin-lightening agents. We truly feel sorry for the women buying these products!

☹ POOR **White Lucent Brightening Protective Emulsion W SPF 15** *($54.50 for 2.5 fl. oz.)* lacks the UVA-protecting ingredients of titanium dioxide, zinc oxide, avobenzone (also known as butyl methoxydibenzoylmethane), ecamsule, or Tinosorb and is not recommended. Even with the right UVA-protecting ingredient, this would be an embarrassingly bad formula for the money. By the way, this does contain avobenzone (listed by its chemical name of butyl methoxydibenzoylmethane), but because it's not among the active ingredients, it cannot be relied on for sufficient UVA protection.

SHISEIDO SUN CARE

☺ GOOD $$$ **Daily Bronze Moisturizing Emulsion, for Face/Body** *($36 for 5 fl. oz.)* is a self-tanning lotion that works the same way as any self-tanner with dihydroxyacetone. Considering the volatile fragrant components in this product, you're better off trying one of the subtle self-tanners from Jergens (reviewed on CosmeticsCop.com), Dove, or Olay.

☺ AVERAGE $$$ **Extra Smooth Sun Protection Lotion for Face & Body SPF 38 PA+++** *($34 for 3.3 fl. oz.)* includes an in-part zinc oxide sunscreen and does have an extra smooth lotion texture thanks to its silicone-enhanced base formula. Regrettably, there's more alcohol and talc in this sunscreen than there are the beneficial extras (think antioxidants) that skin needs to fight environmental damage. This is an OK option for normal to oily skin, but the price is out of line for what you get.

☺ AVERAGE $$$ **Ultimate Sun Protection Lotion for Face & Body SPF 60 PA+++** *($39 for 3.3 fl. oz.)* is similar to Shiseido's Extra Smooth Sun Protection Lotion for Face & Body SPF 38 PA+++ except it has a higher concentration of zinc oxide, which increases the SPF rating considerably. It has a silky lotion texture and adheres excellently to skin thanks to the amount of zinc oxide and silicones this contains; Shiseido's claim of very water-resistant is valid. It's good that this contains some water-binding agents to help hydrate skin, but antioxidants are in short supply. For the money, this should be a more well-rounded sunscreen; however, without question it will provide excellent broad-spectrum protection without a thick, heavy feel. Note that this amount of zinc oxide can leave a perceptible white cast on skin. See the review above for Shiseido's Extra Smooth Sun Protection Cream SPF 38 for an explanation of the PA+++ portion of the name.

☹ POOR **Brilliant Bronze Tinted Self-Tanning Gel, for Face/Body** *($30 for 5.4 fl. oz.)* is available in a light or medium tan shade, but both versions list alcohol as the third ingredient, making this tinted self-tanning gel an irritation waiting to happen. See the Appendix to learn why alcohol is a problem for all skin types. The same review applies to Shiseido's **Brilliant Bronze Quick Self-Tanning Gel, for Face/Body** ($30 for 5.2 fl. oz.).

☹ POOR **Refreshing Sun Protection Spray SPF 16 PA+, for Body/Hair** *($28 for 5 fl. oz.)* includes avobenzone for UVA protection, but is an alcohol-based product, which makes it a problem for all skin types (see the Appendix for details), as does the orange oil that is present.

SHISEIDO LIP CARE

✓☺ BEST $$$ **Sun Protection Lip Treatment SPF 36 PA++** *($20 for 0.14 fl. oz.)* is a very good lip sunscreen that includes an in-part titanium dioxide sunscreen and emollients to keep lips soft and smooth. The added bonus of an antioxidant and anti-irritant make this even better.

☹ POOR **Benefiance Full Correction Lip Treatment** *($36 for 0.5 fl. oz.)* makes claims similar to Olay's Regenerist Anti-Aging Lip Treatment, but the Shiseido formula is not nearly as interesting, plus it irritates lips with menthol and has only a scant amount of antioxidants. The waxlike thickeners in this product can help temporarily fill in vertical lip lines, but so can Olay's, for less money and with a much better formula.

☹ POOR **The Skincare Protective Lip Conditioner SPF 10** *($22.50 for 0.14 fl. oz.)* lacks the UVA-protecting ingredients of titanium dioxide, zinc oxide, avobenzone, Mexoryl SX (ecamsule), or Tinosorb, and is not recommended.

SHISEIDO SPECIALTY SKIN-CARE PRODUCTS

☺ AVERAGE **The Skincare Moisture Relaxing Mask** *($34 for 1.7 fl. oz.)* contains many of the same ingredients Shiseido uses in all its moisturizers, which means those would be appropriate for masking, too. This version supplies dry skin with an OK selection of emollients and some water-binding agents, but is truly a superfluous product.

☺ AVERAGE $$$ **Benefiance Pure Retinol Instant Treatment Eye Mask** *($62.50 for 12 pairs)* is basically a gimmicky mask that has a very tiny amount of retinol. The bulk of this formula is water, slip agents, silicone and alcohol, making it an average option that costs far more than it should.

☺ AVERAGE $$$ **Benefiance Pure Retinol Intensive Revitalizing Face Mask** *($62.50 for 4 masks)* has a formula very similar to the Benefiance Pure Retinol Instant Treatment Eye Mask, but this option includes pre-cut mask sheets for the upper and lower eye area. It is not intensive if you are looking for a potent dose of retinol, and won't do much beyond providing mild hydration for slightly dry skin.

☺ AVERAGE $$$ **Bio-Performance Intensive Skin Corrective Program** *($300)* has an eyebrow-raising price accompanied by claims that make this combination of products sound like a NASA project for aging skin. Something Shiseido refers to as "Bio-Recharger MC" is said to strengthen skin by "optimizing the calcium-magnesium ion distribution," the result of which is allegedly smoother, firmer skin. Shiseido talks about ion exchange in relation to this product. Briefly, an ion is any atom that has either lost or gained an electron. When an ion loses an electron, it becomes positively charged and is called a cation. When an ion gains an electron, it becomes negatively charged, and is called an anion. Ion exchange is a natural process that occurs in many different substances. Skin can act as an ion exchange medium due to its water content, and cosmetics chemists the world over know that various cosmetic ingredients, used alone or in combination, can make a product positively or negatively charged. Shiseido's idea seems to be that aging skin needs an infusion of calcium and magnesium ions in order to regain its youthful appearance. In reality, these minerals play a minor role (at best) in skin function and appearance; they certainly aren't critical ingredients to look for in the quest for the ultimate antiwrinkle product because they cannot be absorbed into the skin. This kit consists of two products, neither of which is impressive or worth even one-fourth the cost. The **Serum Essence** is the portion that contains the calcium and magnesium, very tiny amounts of both. It is mostly a blend of water and slip agents with alcohol, a humectant, and preservative. Talk about boring, and the alcohol, while not likely to cause irritation, is a letdown. The **Balm** is a nonaqueous blend of silicone with Vaseline, film-forming agents, and wax. It can function as a spackle for wrinkles, but the effect is temporary—plus the amount of fragrant components in this product is likely to cause irritation. All told, this set is an utter disappointment, with a price tag that is over-the-top for what you get by any standard. Consumers looking to spend this much on an antiwrinkle product would do better with the various options from DDF, M.D. Skincare by Dr. Dennis Gross, or even the products from Dr. Perricone. All of them have overinflated claims, too, but at least many of the formulas approach or surpass the current state-of-the-art, which this Shiseido duo absolutely does not.

☺ AVERAGE $$$ **Pureness Matifying Stick, Oil Free** *($25 for 0.14 fl. oz.)* is a silicone-based stick that contains the absorbent ingredient silica, so it does provide a matte finish. However, the waxes that keep this in stick form should not be applied over blemish-prone areas.

☹ AVERAGE $$$ **Pureness Oil-Control Blotting Paper** *($18 for 100 sheets)* consists of blotting papers laced with clay to provide oil absorption and a lasting matte finish. The rosemary extract isn't the best, but without question these work to keep excess shine in check.

☹ AVERAGE $$$ **White Lucent Intensive Brightening Mask** *($68 for 6 masks)* contains a handful of intriguing ingredients, but none of them are present in impressive amounts. The small amount of ascorbic acid (vitamin C) won't fade discolorations or even provide much antioxidant benefit. You're getting mostly water, slip agents, alcohol, and the water-binding sugar xylitol. None of this is brightening or whitening, and some of the plant extracts can be irritating, although it's not likely given the small amounts found in this mask.

☹ POOR **Benefiance Firming Massage Mask** *($48 for 1.9 fl. oz.)* contains tranexamic acid, a synthetic drug that has no proven purpose in a skin-care product. One study that involved applying a 2%-3% concentration of the drug to guinea pig skin indicated severely reduced melanin formation resulting from concentrated UV exposure (Source: *Journal of Photochemistry and Photobiology*, December 1998, pages 136–141). In contrast, another study showed that topical applications of vitamin E (as alpha tocopherol) and ferulic acid (another antioxidant) were more effective at inhibiting melanin production than a higher dose of tranexamic acid, and did so while having an added, potent antioxidant benefit (Source: *Anticancer Research*, September/October 1999, pages 3769–3774). Given the precautions and side effects associated with oral administration of tranexamic acid and the unknowns of topical application, it is an ingredient that is best avoided.

☹ POOR **Pureness Blemish Clearing Gel** *($20 for 0.5 fl. oz.)* contains a barely effective amount of salicylic acid and the pH of this gel is too high for it to function as an exfoliant. Further, the amount of alcohol this contains makes it too irritating and drying for all skin types (see the Appendix for details).

☹ POOR **Pureness Pore Minimizing Cooling Essence** *($28 for 1 fl. oz.)* lists alcohol as the second ingredient, and that, coupled with the menthol in this product, produces its "cooling essence" on skin. These two ingredients cause needless irritation and won't do a thing to benefit blemish-prone skin, nor will they reduce the appearance of pores, as Shiseido claims. Instead, the alcohol will trigger oil production at the base of your pores (see the Appendix for details).

☹ POOR **The Skincare Purifying Mask** *($30 for 3.2 fl. oz.)* has clay to absorb excess oil, but so do many other masks for oily skin, and most of those don't contain irritating eucalyptus oil.

☹ POOR **White Lucent Intensive Spot Targeting Serum** *($125 for 1 fl. oz.)* lists alcohol as its second ingredient. That makes it too drying and irritating for all skin types, not to mention that alcohol causes free-radical damage and causes collagen to break down. This contains a dusting of ingredients with limited research pertaining to their skin-lightening ability, but for this much (or really, any amount of) money your skin deserves what works. For what Shiseido is charging, you'd be better off getting a prescription for 4% hydroquinone, which considerable research has shown is excellent for skin discolorations and for treating melasma (Source: *American Journal of Clinical Dermatology*, volume 7, 2006, pages 223–230).

SHISEIDO FOUNDATIONS & PRIMERS

✓☺ BEST $$$ **Dual Balancing Foundation SPF 17** *($38.50)* is another foundation proclaiming it can balance oily areas while providing moisture to dry spots. It isn't possible. Shiseido's balancing claims are just as out of whack as other foundations with similar claims, but the foundation itself exceeds them by offering superior sun protection (featuring in-part titanium dioxide) and a fluid, silky texture that applies like a second skin. Once blended, this sets to a natural matte finish that gives skin an attractive dimensional (rather than flat) quality. It's well suited for combination skin, but not because it is simultaneously controlling oil and maximizing moisture. You'll net light to medium coverage and the selection of shades is promising. The following shades are noticeably pink or peach and best avoided: B40, B60, and I60.

✓☺ BEST $$$ **Perfect Smoothing Compact Foundation SPF 15** *($31)* is a pressed-powder foundation whose sole active ingredient is titanium dioxide. The powdery texture is exceptionally silky and leaves skin looking beautifully smooth and polished rather than dry. The satin matte finish is laced with subtle sparkles that are not distracting for daytime wear. You can get sheer to light coverage that never looks powdery and the formula blends seamlessly. All but one of the shades is stellar, and each goes on more neutral than it looks (which is good, because some of them appear too peachy-gold in the compact). Only O60 may be too gold for some medium skin tones; the rest are highly recommended for those looking for a powder with reliable sunscreen. This foundation is suitable for all skin types except very oily.

✓☺ BEST $$$ **Sheer Mattifying Compact SPF 22** *($30)*. Wow! This talc-based pressed-powder foundation with an in-part titanium dioxide sunscreen is about as close to perfect as it gets. The texture is unbelievably silky and wonderfully light—you'll notice right away how this seems to float over skin without feeling the least bit like makeup—and provides a silky matte finish. The finish enlivens skin rather than making it look dry or chalky. This isn't the powder foundation for those seeking significant coverage, but it's ideal for those with normal to oily skin seeking sheer to light coverage that looks incredibly skin-like. The shade range favors warm-toned (meaning yellow) shades, and almost all of them are great. Shade O60 is a bit too golden yellow, but that's the only color worth skipping. There are no shades for dark skin tones, but plenty for fair to light skin.

✓☺ BEST $$$ **Stick Foundation SPF 15-18** *($38.50)* has a wonderfully smooth, light texture and a titanium dioxide sunscreen that blends with ease, builds from sheer to almost full coverage, and dries to an absorbent powder finish thanks to the amount of clay it contains. It's best for someone with normal to slightly dry or slightly oily skin, since several waxes in it can be problematic for those with breakouts and/or oily skin. Among the shades, avoid B20, which is quite pink, and the noticeably peach B60 and I60. The I00 shade is a beautiful option for someone with very fair skin.

✓☺ BEST $$$ **Sun Protection Compact Foundation SPF 34 PA+++** *($27)* is a talc-based pressed-powder foundation that includes an in-part titanium dioxide sunscreen for sufficient UVA protection. It has a smooth texture that's drier than normal, but that's to be expected given the amount of titanium dioxide. What counts beyond sun protection is the natural matte finish this powder leaves while providing sheer to light coverage. All the shades apply more neutral than they appear in the compact, so don't reject a particular color without trying it first—you may be surprised.

✓☺ BEST $$$ **Sun Protection Liquid Foundation SPF 42 PA+++** *($35)* deserves much praise not only for offering substantial sun protection via its in-part titanium dioxide sunscreen, but also for having a silky, lightweight texture that blends easily. It offers a sheer matte finish but can provide medium to nearly full coverage if needed, all without feeling thick or looking heavy. The silicone-enhanced fluid is ideal for normal to very oily skin and an excellent option for outdoor wear when you're active because it stays in place and is water-resistant. That doesn't mean you can apply it once and sit by the pool or play volleyball all day, but it is one of the few foundations that provide sufficient sun protection and keep looking fresh even through strenuous activities. Of the shades available, SP40 and SP50 are a bit too peach for most medium skin tones. The other shades are great options for light and dark (but not very dark) skin.

☺ GOOD $$$ **Lifting Foundation SPF 16** ($43.50) claims to provide "full coverage as beautiful as bare skin," but that's taking it too far (even though it's fun to imagine). With almost 10% titanium dioxide as the active ingredient, this creamy, thick foundation doesn't provide its complete coverage without looking like makeup. It spreads and blends well yet is very concentrated—a tiny dab covers half the face, but you'll likely need more than that to ensure sufficient sun protection (unless you're applying this foundation over a regular sunscreen). It has a silky, matte finish that appears somewhat chalky, something that's more apparent with the darker shades. Among the shades, the only poor choices are B60 (very peach) and the slightly peach shades B20 and I40. Lastly, this foundation won't lift the skin—the real reason to consider it is if you need significant coverage and want a foundation with sunscreen.

☺ GOOD $$$ **Smoothing Veil SPF 16** ($33.50) is a silicone-based makeup primer with an in-part titanium dioxide sunscreen. This colorless, solid cream leaves a soft, opalescent finish that feels very silky. It's an extra step whose line- and pore-filling benefit won't be all that noticeable, at least not any more than a foundation can provide. For the most part this is just a great way to get sun protection if your favored foundation does not include sunscreen or lacks effective UVA protection. This is suitable for all skin types.

☺ GOOD $$$ **The Skincare Tinted Moisture Protection SPF 20** ($38 for 2.1 fl. oz.) contains plenty of titanium dioxide for broad-spectrum protection. The amount of titanium dioxide also contributes enough coverage to make this more like a foundation than a tinted moisturizer. It has a slightly creamy, elegantly silky texture that blends superbly and sets to a soft matte (in feel) finish that leaves skin with a subtle, healthy glow. The Medium and Medium Deep shades are borderline peach, but acceptable; there are no shades for fair or dark skin tones. This would earn a Best Product rating if it didn't contain a small amount of peppermint leaf extract, which can cause irritation.

☹ AVERAGE $$$ **Pore Smoothing Corrector** ($30) is a primer with a slightly creamy and notably silky texture that provides a soft, weightless finish. It doesn't have the type of soft spackle texture needed to truly fill in large pores (an effect that is always temporary), but, as with similar primers or serums, this will make your pores appear smoother. If you're using a mattifying serum or similar type of product, you won't need Pore Smoothing Corrector. In addition, the amount of alcohol in this product is potentially concerning due to the risk of irritation it presents (see the Appendix for details). The formula also contains a tiny amount of eucalyptus, another irritant that won't help pores become smaller.

☹ AVERAGE $$$ **Sun Protection Stick Foundation SPF 35 PA++** ($27). This tiny stick foundation (you only get one-third of what liquid foundation typically provides) earns our recommendation for reliable broad-spectrum sun protection, thanks to its in-part titanium dioxide sunscreen. But, given the small amount of product, if you apply it as you should apply a sunscreen (which means liberally), it will be gone in a week or so. That means you cannot and should not rely on it for regular sun protection unless you are willing to buy at least two per month. Aside from the sun protection issue, this stick foundation has a creamy texture and is easy to apply. It imparts sheer color with a smooth finish that's best for dry skin not prone to breakouts. Out of the shades, Beige is slightly pink, Ochre is slightly yellow but workable, and the colorless shade (Translucent) is worth considering.

☹ POOR **Advanced Hydro-Liquid Compact SPF 15** *($40)* has a silky-smooth texture and soft satin matte finish, which together provide light to medium coverage. The sun protection comes from pure titanium dioxide (a lot of it, so this isn't the best choice for breakout-prone skin) so broad-spectrum protection is assured. So why the low rating? For all its attributes, this foundation contains two fragrant plant oils (rosemary and lavender) that serve as potent irritants. They're not present in a great amount (same for the isopropyl alcohol), but even small amounts can be a problem, and both definitely add a noticeable scent to this foundation.

☹ POOR **Perfect Refining Foundation SPF 16** *($38.50)*. This thin-textured liquid foundation has some strong points, especially for oily, blemish-prone skin. It feels weightless and provides impressive coverage and a lasting matte finish. Sadly, the inclusion of alcohol and lavender oil (the scent of both is detectable as you blend) is a problem for skin because they cause irritation (see the Appendix for details). Although this foundation has strong points, there are lots of great foundations available that don't have this one's problems.

☹ POOR **Refining Makeup Primer SPF 21** *($30)* has a lightweight cream texture that glides over skin and leaves a silky finish. It has a soft, pale peach tint that lends a subtle glow that many will find attractive, and it contains broad-spectrum sun protection for added anti-aging benefit. The problem? The formula contains lavender oil, enough that the scent is obvious. Even in small amounts, lavender oil is a problem for skin (see the Appendix for details).

SHISEIDO CONCEALERS

✓☺ BEST **$$$ Natural Finish Cream Concealer** *($25)* is packaged in a squeeze tube and has a liquid-cream consistency that smoothly blends over skin for a flawless finish. The semi-matte finish offers medium to full coverage that camouflages imperfections without settling into fine lines. Colors range from very light to deep in neutral shades, making this an all-around great (though pricey) choice for all skin types.

☹ POOR **Corrector Pencil** *($18)* is a standard, dry-finish pencil that comes in three average but workable colors. This provides good coverage, but application is an issue, and it looks quite obvious on the skin while also being too stiff to soften.

SHISEIDO POWDERS

☺ GOOD **$$$ Pressed Powder** *($32)* comes in colors suitable for fair skin and has a talc-based formula that feels smooth but is more powdery than the best options in this category. It's a good option if you have light skin and want a sheer, basic pressed powder, but that's about it.

☺ GOOD **$$$ Translucent Loose Powder** *($35)* is a mica- and talc-based loose powder with a gossamer texture and nearly invisible finish on skin. Although this powder appears pure white in the jar, it goes on translucent and is suitable for all skin tones except very dark. Brushed on, it makes skin look beautifully polished and won't interfere with the color of your foundation.

☺ GOOD **$$$ Translucent Pressed Powder** *($32)* looks almost white in the compact but it goes on nearly translucent. Those with porcelain to light skin tones will do best with this powder, but it's sheer and translucent enough to work for some medium skin tones, too. Because this doesn't deposit much color, it's best for taming shine and absorbing excess oil thanks to its slightly dry matte finish. The finely milled texture blends well and means this powder won't look, well, too powdery on your skin, assuming you apply it with a brush rather than the enclosed sponge. Translucent Pressed Powder is best for normal to oily skin, and is an option for breakout-prone skin, too.

SHISEIDO BLUSHES & BRONZER

☺ GOOD $$$ **Accentuating Color Stick** *($33)* has a slick, silicone-based texture that is quick to dry out if you don't replace the cap tightly after each use. Think of this as a hybrid cream-to-powder blush that is best applied over moist skin (applying it over powdered skin assures a spotty, streaked look). Each shade goes on almost as bright as it looks, but blending softens the effect and the product sets to a natural matte finish.

☺ GOOD $$$ **Bronzer** *($35)* is an excellent bronzing powder offered in believable tan shades best for fair to medium skin tones. The soft, smooth texture isn't the least bit powdery and applies sheer so you can build to your desired level of bronze. The refined finish has a hint of shine, but it's subtle enough that you can wear this during the day and not look like you have glittering cheeks. Blending can be a bit tricky because this has a slight tendency to grab on skin. For best results, apply over a powdered finish and have a sponge ready to soften any hard edges.

☺ GOOD $$$ **Luminizing Satin Face Color** *($30)* is sold in flattering blush tones of pink and coral and two highlighter shades (white and gold). This high-quality pressed powder offers a slightly iridescent finish and sophisticated glow without being overly shiny. It blends smoothly and quickly builds color with just a couple strokes of the brush. This is an attractive option for those not bothered by the price.

SHISEIDO EYESHADOWS

✓☺ BEST $$$ **Shimmering Cream Eye Color** *($25)* is housed in a glass jar with a screw-on lid. Its texture is silky and each shade is highly pigmented—talk about a shock of color! A little goes a long way and several of the shades work great to add depth or highlight the eye area. Speaking of the shades, each has sparkling shine that's attractive without being overly shiny. The colors themselves are a mixed bag; some are brilliant while others are too bold or difficult to work with (but are fine if you want a colorful eye design). Favorites include BK912, SV810, BR306, and BR709. In terms of longevity, once the formula sets it stays put quite well; no smudging, smearing, or fading was noticed—and these take some effort to remove (have an oil- or silicone-based makeup remover handy). All told, if this type of eyeshadow appeals to you, it's well worth a look. The formula can be applied under or over regular powder eyeshadows, a nice bonus to an already-great eyeshadow.

☺ AVERAGE $$$ **Luminizing Satin Eye Color** *($25)* has a silky, slightly powdery texture that applies evenly with just a slight tendency to flake. Brushed on in sheer layers, this builds dimensional color and comes in some attractive, shades (including pastels) that are a twist on traditional shades. Each has some amount of shine, but it clings well. Watch out for the vivid yellow, violet, and green shades, at least if your goal is to use eyeshadow to shape and shade the eye rather than to add a shock of color.

☺ AVERAGE $$$ **Luminizing Satin Eye Color Trio** *($33)* has a silky, slightly powdery texture that applies evenly with just a slight tendency to flake. Brushed on in sheer layers, this

---

☞ Buying skin-care products packaged in jars? See the Appendix to learn why that's a bad idea.

builds dimensional color with varying degrees of shine (that's the "luminizing" part). If only the color combinations were better! Blues and greens predominate, but there are some workable combos.

SHISEIDO EYE & BROW LINERS

☺ GOOD $$$ **Accentuating Cream Eyeliner** *($26)* is Shiseido's version of the numerous gel eyeliners offered at cosmetics counters. Their version shares the same formula basics and easy-to-apply traits as the others, yet its finish remains slightly tacky, and that can affect weartime. The included synthetic, angled eyeliner brush is a nice touch, but not enough to propel this above the frontrunners in this category.

☺ AVERAGE $$$ **Automatic Fine Eyeliner** *($29)* is another liquid eyeliner with a brush that is only capable of applying a thick line. The color seeps into the brush much like ink in a fountain pen, making it hard to control how much comes out at once, but this can be workable once you adapt to its peculiarities.

☺ AVERAGE $$$ **Eyebrow and Eyeliner Compact** *($30)* presents a brow powder and powder eyeliner (either may be used wet or dry) in one compact. The brow tones are good for those with brown or black hair only, yet each applies smoothly considering the dry texture, and the color builds well. Oddly, each duo has a slight amount of shine, which doesn't add much to the result (eyebrows aren't supposed to shine). As for the included applicator, it is best tossed in favor of full-size brushes.

☺ AVERAGE $$$ **Smoothing Eyeliner Pencil** *($20)* is dual-ended, with a needs-sharpening pencil on one end and a super soft sponge tip on the other. It applies evenly, with just enough creaminess to blend, and then sets quickly. The color goes on somewhat sheer, making this a good, albeit overpriced, pencil option for smudging rather than for creating deep, bold lines. The two color options are black and brown, the latter being more of a muted taupe than a rich brown.

☹ POOR **Natural Eyebrow Pencil** *($20)* is an eyebrow pencil that isn't worth considering unless you enjoy exerting much more pressure than you would need to with almost any other eyebrow pencil to achieve decent results. The brush on the other end of this needs-sharpening pencil is fine, but it cannot soften this pencil's hard, waxy finish.

SHISEIDO LIP COLOR & LIPLINER

✓☺ BEST $$$ **Perfect Rouge Lipstick** *($25)* is truly one of the most elegant lipsticks we have ever reviewed. In stick form this collection of sheer cream lipsticks appears no different from the hundreds of others on the market. But once applied, the silky smooth texture and beautiful subtle shimmer is gorgeous. This is shimmer done right and it includes a touch of glossy shine. The color selection is vast and ranges from light to dark so there is little doubt you'll find more than one to love.

☺ GOOD $$$ **Perfect Rouge Tender Sheer Lip Color** *($25)* is a hybrid between a lipstick and a lip gloss. It comes in a regular lipstick tube, but looks and feels more like a wet shine lip gloss with sheer color. The creamy texture is exceptionally moisturizing, but not sticky like you might experience with a gloss. The shade range is limited, one of which—Natural Wine—you should avoid, because most will find this shade too dark. But, all other factors considered, this is worth a try.

☺ AVERAGE $$$ **Luminizing Lip Gloss** *($22)* is an average lip gloss with a high price tag. The collection comes in a range of translucent shades that offer a shiny finish with a hint of sparkle. The texture is pleasant, offering an ample coating without feeling super sticky, and the brush applicator is standard and easy to use. Just don't fall for the claim that this product offers long-lasting color; as with most lip glosses, this will wear off long before lunch.

☺ AVERAGE **$$$ Shimmering Rouge** *($25)* is a very standard, overpriced cream lipstick whose creamy texture borders on greasy. The glossy finish is imbued with shimmer while the shade range offers some good bright and muted colors that provide moderate coverage. This is said to plump lips but cannot do so, at least not more than any other lipstick with a glossy finish (the light reflected from the gloss finish creates the illusion of fuller lips, but that's not the same as actually making lips plump).

☺ AVERAGE **$$$ Smoothing Lip Pencil** *($20)* has a rounded lip brush at one end and a needs-sharpening pencil at the other. It's an adequate lipliner, but nothing to write home about—especially at this price! It has a somewhat creamy finish, which means there's still potential for feathering, but the finish does allow for even application with very little drag.

☹ POOR **Perfect Rouge Glowing Matte Lip Color** *($25)* is too matte for its own good. The texture is semi-tacky and it can look a bit cakey, especially if your lips are a bit dry or chapped. The color selection is limited and each color is semi-transparent, so you don't get much intensity.

SHISEIDO MASCARAS

☺ GOOD **$$$ Lasting Lift Mascara** *($23)* has a long, thin spiral brush that allows you to reach every lash and extend it for a defined, separated (and, OK, lifted) result. Length is more prominent than thickness, but successive coats add volume.

☺ GOOD **$$$ Perfect Mascara Defining Volume** *($24)* is a very good mascara for those seeking a heavier, more voluminous effect. Although this goes on a bit wet and clumps slightly, a few seconds with a lash comb neatens everything and helps you create lashes that are long (but not outrageously so) and impressively thick. This does not remove easily with a water-soluble cleanser, so be sure you have a silicone- or oil–based makeup remover handy!

☹ POOR **Nourishing Mascara Base** *($24)* is an overpriced, "Why bother?" product that will do nothing to nourish or condition lashes, although it does make them feel soft, if not a little greasy, which is a problem when trying to keep mascara from smearing.

☹ POOR **Perfect Mascara Full Definition** *($24)* defines lashes while adding volume and length without clumping. It leaves lashes flexible, flake-free, and smudge-free. Although all that is nice, the formula contains so much alcohol (specifically, isopropyl alcohol, also known as rubbing alcohol) that you can smell it the instant you open the cap, and throughout the day it can cause itchy, red, irritated eyes. That's what happened to us and we suspect it will happen to you, so heed our warning and leave this one at the cosmetics counter!

SHISEIDO BRUSHES

☺ AVERAGE **$$$ Shiseido Brushes** *($18–$50)*. The straightforward collection of Brushes is supposedly approved by fashion makeup artist Tom Pecheux, and if that's true he must prefer brushes that are mostly too floppy and soft for anything but very sheer application. The **Foundation Brush** ($30) is notably small. The brush head simply isn't practical for daily use on the entire face. It's best for adding foundation or powder to smaller areas, so perhaps this is worth considering if you want a tool to supply extra coverage in key areas without the foundation looking too thick or caked.

SK-II (SKIN CARE ONLY)

Strengths: Some well-formulated moisturizers and serums; all the sunscreens provide sufficient UVA protection.

Weaknesses: Shockingly expensive, especially for the wide assortment of mediocre products; unreliable skin-lightening products; AHA/BHA products that contain an ineffective amount of exfoliant; no products to help manage blemishes; jar packaging.

For more information and reviews of the latest SK-II products, visit CosmeticsCop.com.

Note: Most SK-II products contain an ingredient the company refers to as Pitera. This ingredient is a trade name for *Saccharomycopsis* ferment filtrate (SFF), a form of yeast purportedly unique because of the fermenting and filtering process it goes through before being added to these products. As it turns out, many forms of yeast have anti-inflammatory properties and antioxidant properties, including SFF (Source: *Journal of Dermatologic Science*, June 2006, pages 249–257). Other than that, all the information about Pitera comes from papers presented at medical conferences, not from published studies. Presenting papers at medical conferences is not the same thing as publishing the results of studies. The standards for presenting a paper at a medical conference are different from the requirements for publication of study results in most medical journals. Supposing Pitera is a wonder ingredient (which it isn't), this doesn't explain how it rates when compared with other "wonder" ingredients because there are no comparison studies. Hundreds of ingredients—ranging from green tea to superoxide dismutase, epigallocatechin-3-gallate, eicosapentaenoic acid, beta-carotene, pomegranate, and curcumin to vitamin E, vitamin A, and on and on and on—have stellar reputations, and there's copious documentation to prove it. Bottom line: Pitera isn't special or magical; it just seemingly gives SK-II license to charge way too much money for products that, without the Pitera, are strikingly similar to what you'll find from Olay. Both Olay and SK-II are owned by Procter & Gamble.

SK-II CLEANSERS

☺ AVERAGE **$$$ Facial Treatment Cleanser** *($70 for 4.2 fl. oz.)* is a decent, basic, water-soluble, detergent-based cleanser that is an option for normal to oily skin, if only the cost weren't so ludicrous. It does contain Pitera and a few other interesting extras, but in a cleanser they will hardly be on your face before they are rinsed down the drain.

☺ AVERAGE **$$$ Facial Treatment Cleansing Oil** *($60 for 8.4 fl. oz.)* is mostly mineral oil with a few thickening agents, plant extracts, and, of course, Pitera. This is one of the most expensive containers of mineral oil we've ever seen! The few beneficial extras in here aren't nearly enough to make up for the absurd price and the absence of any unique benefit for skin.

SK-II TONERS

☺ GOOD **$$$ Cellumination Mask-In Lotion** *($75 for 3.4 fl. oz.)* has a confusing name, but despite that, this product (it's not a mask or a moisturizer) ends up being a good toner for all skin types. The formula contains a nice mix of water-binding agents, the cell-communicating ingredient niacinamide, an anti-irritant, and vitamin C (as ascorbyl glucoside). Although there's much to like about this toner, the price isn't likely to put a smile on your face—and without question you don't need to spend this much to get an effective toner. In fact, companies such as Paula's Choice offer more well-rounded, fragrance-free formulas (Cellumination Mask-in Lotion contains fragrance) for considerably less money. If you're sold on SK-II and have a prodigious budget this toner is an option, though it's not the oasis of hydration it's made out to be.

☺ AVERAGE $$$ **Facial Treatment Clear Lotion** *($60 for 5 fl. oz.)* is an exceptionally standard toner that is mostly water and Pitera. There is a tiny, and we mean really tiny, amount of a good water-binding agent, even smaller amounts of salicylic acid, and two AHAs. While the pH is low enough for them to function as exfoliants, the amount of BHA and AHAs is far too low for them to be effective. Spending this much money on what is a basic toner would have to be based only on your faith in Pitera because every other ingredient is easily replaced by better formulations for far less money.

☹ AVERAGE $$$ **Facial Treatment Essence** *($155 for 5 fl. oz.)* is supposed to contain "the most concentrated amount of Pitera of all the SK-II skincare products—around 90% pure SK-II Pitera." Indeed, that is all this contains, other than some slip agents, water, and preservatives. What a waste, and what a strange gimmick to thrust on women the world over. There is no substantiated research proving Pitera is a must-have for skin. Even if it were an amazing ingredient, skin needs more than just one great ingredient to be at its healthy, youthful best.

SK-II EXFOLIANT

☹ AVERAGE $$$ **Skin Refining Treatment** *($150 for 1.7 fl. oz.)* is an ordinary salicylic acid (BHA) cream with a ridiculous price. Other than Pitera—and we have no idea why every SK-II product has to have this ingredient—there is no reason to spend this much of your hard-earned money on what amounts to a decent, though basic BHA product. One word of warning: At 2.3, the pH of this product is unusually low, which means there is a high potential for irritation. Also, the jar packaging isn't the best (see the Appendix for details). But given that this fragrance-free product contains the teensiest amount of an antioxidant and some aloe water, even that can't really make a difference.

SK-II MOISTURIZERS (DAYTIME & NIGHTTIME), EYE CREAMS, & SERUMS

✓☺ BEST $$$ **Cellumination Essence Hydrating Serum** *($220 for 1 fl. oz.)* is far and away one of the most impressive products SK-II offers. Unlike most of their other serums, this one contains a brilliant blend of cell-communicating ingredient niacinamide with silky slip agents and an impressive blend of antioxidants. Its lightweight texture is ideal for normal to oily skin; those with dry skin will find this serum doesn't provide enough moisture. The niaciamide stands a good chance of helping to fade skin discolorations, though you don't have to spend this much to get that ingredient. As for the claims, all they're really stating is that this serum makes skin's surface smoother so it is better able to reflect light. Of course, hundreds of products make skin smoother, so this is hardly the only option out there. It's plain physics that smoother skin reflects light and looks more "illuminated" (or "cell-uminated," if you prefer) than skin with a rough, uneven texture. Although this serum deserves its rating, you should know that Olay's Pro-X and Total Effects lines offer similar serums that cost a lot less. The SK-II line has no shortage of serums, and all of them are expensive.

✓☺ BEST $$$ **Signs Wrinkle Serum** *($175 for 1 fl. oz.)* is an impressive mix of water-binding agents, cell-communicating ingredients, antioxidants, nonfragrant plant oil, and other helpful ingredients that all skin types need. The texture of this serum enables it to serve as a sort of soft spackle for lines, but the effect is fleeting, and, once again, you can get the same effect from many other products that cost less—a lot less—than this. This fragrance-free serum is suitable for all skin types. It is similar to but has a more elegant formula than serums from the Olay Regenerist line. It pains us to rate this serum among the best, because in no way do we believe even half the hype with SK-II's star ingredient Pitera, a strain of yeast. Supposedly, monks who lived in the mountains somewhere used it to make their rice wine and subsequently their skin maintained its youthful appearance. We ask you: Who comes up with this insanity and why do so many women believe it?

☺ GOOD $$$ **Facial Treatment UV Protection SPF 25** *($120 for 1 fl. oz.)* leaves us with one big concern, and that is how likely you'll be to apply it liberally. Liberal application is necessary for sufficient sun protection, yet if you applied this daily to your face and neck (and were applying enough each time) you'd be replacing this each month, which adds up to $1,440 per year! That's especially shocking when you consider this formula (which provides broad-spectrum protection and includes zinc oxide for critical UVA screening) isn't extraordinary and absolutely not indicative of its price. The Pitera ingredient present in every SK-II product has no special benefit for sun-exposed skin and, although this contains some proven repairing and antioxidant ingredients, these show up in many other daytime moisturizers, too. The texture of this product makes it best for normal to oily skin and the fragrance-free formula is suitable for breakout-prone skin. The rating we assigned is warranted due to this product's formula, not for its price.

☺ GOOD $$$ **Whitening Source Brightening Derm Specialist** *($190 for 1.7 fl. oz.)* is supposed to even your skin tone. To that end, it contains niacinamide and a form of vitamin C (ascorbyl glucoside), both ingredients with promising to impressive research behind their abilities to fight brown spots and sun damage that results in, you guessed it, an uneven skin tone. The real problem with this skin-lightening serum is its price! The core lightening ingredients are found (in efficacious amounts) in numerous other products, including some from Olay (whose parent company Procter & Gamble also owns SK-II), Paula's Choice, Clinique, and Estee Lauder. You absolutely do not need to pay anywhere near this amount for a brilliant skin-lightening product. If you decide to indulge, this is best for normal to slightly dry or oily skin. Its silicone content makes skin feel very silky. Thankfully, the DNA ingredient this contains cannot affect the DNA in your skin (doing so could lead to numerous problems).

☻ AVERAGE $$$ **Advanced Eye Treatment Film** *($95 for 0.5 fl. oz.)* is mostly Pitera, and the price is shocking. This is all about Pitera, and banking on that is not a reliable investment. See the note at the beginning of the SK-II review to learn more about Pitera. And check out the Appendix to find out why you don't need a special moisturizer for the eye area.

☻ AVERAGE $$$ **Cellumination Cream** *($150 for 1.7 fl. oz.)* is the moisturizer version of SK-II's Cellumination Essence Hydrating Serum above. Although these two products have much in common, the moisturizer has a thicker, creamier texture and happens to be packaged in a jar, which is why it isn't rated as highly as the Cellumination serum. See the Appendix to learn why jar packaging is a problem. In better packaging, this would be a very good (though still absurdly priced) moisturizer for normal to combination or slightly dry skin.

☻ AVERAGE $$$ **Facial Lift Emulsion** *($125 for 3.3 fl. oz.)* is a decent, though ordinary, fragrance-free, lightweight moisturizer for normal to dry skin that contains too little antioxidants and water-binding agents, especially given its outrageous price. It absolutely cannot lift skin (see the Appendix to find out why).

☻ AVERAGE $$$ **Facial Treatment Repair C** *($160 for 1 fl. oz.)* doesn't contain vitamin C, despite the name. In fact, all it contains is Pitera, water, slip agents, water-binding agent, and preservatives. The one thing you may be gleaning from this product lineup is that whatever effect Pitera has, Procter & Gamble must believe it takes a lot of it to provide a benefit. Otherwise, why not just offer one super-Pitera product and call it good, and have this option be something else that is proven to be beneficial for skin?

☺ AVERAGE **$$$ LXP Ultimate Revival Cream** *($350 for 1.7 fl. oz.)*. There's no reason in the world to spend this much for a moisturizer (which is essentially all this is), especially one that's packaged in a jar. As soon as you open the deluxe, sculptural packaging several light- and air-sensitive ingredients will begin to deteriorate, making this moisturizer less effective for anti-aging with each use (see the Appendix for details). Besides, if this is SK-II's "ultimate treatment for skin" then what are all their other "treatment" products for? Are they not as good because most of them cost less and aren't billed as "ultimate"? And what about the fact that there are far more formulary similarities than differences between all the SK-II moisturizers, despite varying claims and wildly different prices? In the end, this would be a very good (though still absurdly priced) moisturizer for normal to dry skin had the company chosen better packaging. This does contain fragrance.

☺ AVERAGE **$$$ LXP Ultimate Serum** *($265 for 1.7 fl. oz.)* has SK-II's allegedly miraculous Pitera ingredient, no big surprise, so unless you're a firm believer in Pitera, there is no reason in the world to spend this much for a serum. There are plenty of brilliantly formulated serums that cost less than $60 and offer skin a broader range of anti-aging benefits than this one. Besides, if this is SK-II's "ultimate" serum, then what are all their other serums for?

☺ AVERAGE **$$$ Signs Up-Lifter** *($265 for 1.3 fl. oz.)* contains an even more concentrated version of yeast, called Pitera 4. It's there along with many of the same ingredients you find in Olay's Regenerist products, and that means this is a good, fragrance-free moisturizer for normal to dry skin. There are a few extras in Signs Up-Lifter, like *Padina pavonica* extract, from a form of algae that has some antioxidant properties. But as it turns out, a comparison study (our favorite kind) found that a different form of algae had far more potent antioxidant abilities, namely *Caulerpa racemosa* (Source: *Journal of Experimental Marine Biology and Ecology*, July 2005, pages 35–41). This also contains *Crithmum maritimum* extract, another form of algae. There is some research that shows *Crithmum maritimum* has some antioxidant properties, but there is also research showing it can be cytotoxic (toxic to cells) (Source: *Journal of Natural Products*, September 1993, pages 1598–1600). In the greater scheme of things, these extras add up to a whole lot of nothing.

☺ AVERAGE **$$$ Skin Signature Cream** *($205 for 2.8 fl. oz.)* is very similar to other moisturizers from SK-II, including some they sell for almost double the price of this one. What's the difference? Good question! From a formulary standpoint the differences are shockingly minor and definitely not deserving of such wide swings in prices (though even SK-II's most inexpensive moisturizer is easily replaced by a similar product from Olay). It's not a bad formula, but nothing special and absolutely not worth its price. The price becomes even more disappointing when you consider the jar packaging. This type of packaging won't keep key ingredients stable during use, and that includes the antioxidants. The formula has merit for normal to dry skin, but so do lots of others that cost considerably less and come in better packaging.

☺ AVERAGE **$$$ Skin Signature Eye Cream** *($110 for 0.5 fl. oz.)* is not one you should spend your money on, unless you believe that Pitera (the star ingredient that sets Procter & Gamble-owned SK-II apart from the company's Olay brand) is worth the hefty expense, there is no reason to consider this jar-packaged eye cream over any product from Olay Regenerist or Pro-X. Pitera is not even remotely a miraculous or even close to a must-have ingredient for skin, and there's not a shred of published, substantiated research that can refute that statement. Signs Eye Cream contains basic emollient ingredients that moisturize dry skin anywhere on the face, helping to improve barrier function, but the jar packaging is a problem for the stability of the teeny amount of beneficial ingredient it does contain. See the Appendix to find out why you don't need an eye cream, especially not one packaged in a jar.

☺ AVERAGE $$$ **Skin Signature Melting Rich Cream** *($250 for 1.7 fl. oz.)* is a fragrance-free moisturizer similar to SK-II's Skin Signature Cream above. As such, the same basic comments apply.

SK-II SPECIALTY SKIN-CARE PRODUCTS

☺ AVERAGE $$$ **Facial Treatment Mask** *($90 for 6 mask)* is just water, Pitera, slip agents, and preservative. It does contain sodium salicylate, but the pH of the product, combined with the characteristics of this type of salicylate, render it a poor choice for exfoliation.

☺ AVERAGE $$$ **Signs Eye Mask** *($110 for 14 pairs)* comes in at almost $400 for 1 ounce of product, making it the most expensive SK-II item. Oddly, you don't even get the "concentrated" amount of Pitera that's present in several other SK-II products. For the money, even if you were a Pitera adherent, this isn't the way to get the stuff on your skin. It has some interesting ingredients, but again, nothing that would rank it above Olay Regenerist or Pro-X. The few additional plant extracts in here aren't worth the extra expense or time to apply this mask. For example, it contains *Chrysanthellum indicum* extract (from golden chamomile), which has some research showing it reduces irritation and improves the appearance of rosacea. However, the studies didn't compare the extract with other anti-irritant ingredients or protocols, only with a placebo (Source: *Journal of the European Academy of Dermatology & Venereology*, September 2005, page 564).

☺ AVERAGE $$$ **Skin Signature Mask 3-D Redefining Mask** *($145 for 6 masks)* is a two-piece cloth mask set that includes pre-soaked, specially cut pieces designed for the upper and lower portions of your face. You press and mold the damp cloths to your skin, leave on for up to ten minutes, then remove the cloths and massage the product that remains into your skin. None of this is essential, nor does it have anything to do with 3-D effects or any sort of lifting of your skin. The ingredients these cloths are steeped in are very standard and not unique to SK-II. In fact, even the best ingredients this mask contains show up in numerous other products, such as those from Olay Regenerist and Total Effects. This mask contains film-forming agents (think hairspray) that can leave your skin feeling tighter, but skin feeling tighter isn't the same as it actually becoming tighter (or lifted). It's merely cosmetics trickery to make you think the product is doing something effective. Ultimately, masks like this are a waste of time and money (mostly money). Their best ingredients can be obtained from less expensive products (such as serums) that you apply daily and leave on skin. Last, there's no valid, substantiated research proving Pitera does anything close to miraculous for aging skin.

☺ AVERAGE $$$ **Whitening Source Derm Revival Mask** *($160 for 10 masks)* is a two-piece cloth mask set that includes pre-soaked, specially cut pieces designed for the upper and lower portions of your face. You press and mold the damp cloths to your skin, leave on for up to 20 minutes, then remove the cloths and massage the product that remains into your skin. None of this is essential, especially when you consider the whitening ingredients in this mask are found in all the other Whitening Source products from SK-II, as well as several less expensive products from Olay, whose parent company (Procter & Gamble) also owns SK-II. There is no research proving SK-II's Pitera ingredient has any effect on uneven skin tone or brown spots, not to mention that when it comes to skin lightening, what you do daily is far more important than what you do occasionally, which is likely how you'd use this mask (as a "special" treat, perhaps once per week). All told, the formula for this mask is relatively simple and not worth the investment.

☺ AVERAGE **$$$ Whitening Source Skin Brightener** (*$135 for 2.6 fl. oz.*) consists mostly of silicone, yeast (Pitera), slip agent, and niacinamide, so it's absolutely not worth its inflated price. Sadly, this is just one more example of how incredibly out-of-hand this segment of the cosmetics industry has become. If you were hoping this moisturizer would be the answer for your skin discolorations, it might, but you don't have to spend anywhere near this much to see if those ingredients will improve your dark spots. Any of the products with niacinamide from Olay's Regenerist would work at least as well (and possibly better) against skin discolorations and at a fraction of the cost. This product's best attribute is making skin feel silkier; all the plant ingredients and antioxidants will deteriorate quickly once you begin using this jar-packaged moisturizer (see the Appendix for details).

☹ POOR **Whitening Source Clear Lotion** (*$70 for 5 fl. oz.*) is a toner-like, skin-lightening product that doesn't contain anything of significance to banish skin discolorations. If you want to see how niacinamide might work on your discolorations, you can purchase any of the serums or lightening products from Olay's Regenerist or Total Effects lines (Procter & Gamble owns both SK-II and Olay, and Olay has the better products). It's particularly egregious that SK-II included (and brags about) peppermint extract, which serves only to irritate skin and offers no whitening (though consumers may think the product is working because it tingles). Pitera, the star ingredient found throughout the SK-II line, is front-and-center in this product. Please refer to the note at the beginning of the SK-II review for a detailed explanation of Pitera.

SKINCEUTICALS (SKIN CARE ONLY)

Strengths: Great line to shop if you're looking for well-formulated vitamin C and retinol products; some outstanding sunscreens (including for sensitive skin), and every one provides sufficient UVA protection; one effective AHA product; good self-tanner; several fragrance-free products.

Weaknesses: Mostly problematic cleansers and toners; fruit and sugar extracts trying to substitute for AHA products when the real deal is much better; ineffective BHA products; jar packaging; several overpriced products touting one superstar ingredient when skin does best with a cocktail of beneficial ingredients.

For more information and reviews of the latest SkinCeuticals products, visit CosmeticsCop.com.

SKINCEUTICALS CLEANSERS

✓☺ BEST **$$$ Purifying Cleanser** (*$32 for 8 fl. oz.*) is a very good, fragrance-free, mild cleanser for all skin types. Although it's expensive and you can find equally great cleansers for less money, if you choose to spend more than is needed, this won't disappoint. OK, actually it might disappoint, at least if you were hoping the AHA ingredient glycolic acid in this cleanser will exfoliate skin. It cannot do that in a cleanser owing to its brief contact with skin and the fact that in a gentle cleanser like this, the pH is not within the range required for glycolic acid to function as an exfoliant.

☺ AVERAGE **$$$ Clarifying Cleanser** (*$33 for 5 fl. oz.*) contains 2% salicylic acid along with the AHAs glycolic and mandelic acids. Although the pH of this cleansing scrub would allow chemical exfoliation, the acids are not in contact with skin long enough for that to occur. This is a good, water-soluble option for normal to oily skin, but keep it away from the eye area.

☺ AVERAGE **$$$ Gentle Cleanser, for Sensitive Skin** (*$33 for 8 fl. oz.*) is a cleansing gel/lotion hybrid that has surprisingly minimal cleansing ability, and the orange oil it contains isn't something that you should apply to sensitive skin. This is an OK option for normal skin when minimal to no makeup needs to be removed.

☺ AVERAGE **$$$ Simply Clean, for Combination or Oily Skin** *($33 for 8 fl. oz.)* does a good job of cleansing and removing makeup for its intended skin types. However, it doesn't deserve a higher rating due to the problematic plant extracts it includes.

☹ POOR **Foaming Cleanser** *($33 for 5 fl. oz.)* contains several irritating plant extracts, including arnica, ivy, and pellitory, all of which make this otherwise fine water-soluble cleanser not recommended.

☹ POOR **LHA Cleansing Gel** *($36 for 8 fl. oz.)* is a water-soluble cleanser that is fairly standard and definitely overpriced for what you get. It is not recommended because it contains the potent skin-irritant menthol. The cooling sensation from menthol is not a sign it's working; it's a sign your skin is being irritated and that's never the goal with cleansing. This cleanser cannot offer "cell by cell exfoliation" as claimed. It contains the AHA glycolic acid and BHA salicylic acid, but in a cleanser these ingredients exfoliate minimally, if at all, due to their brief contact with skin.

SKINCEUTICALS TONER

☹ POOR **Equalizing Toner, for Combination or Oily Skin** *($30 for 8 fl. oz.)* is mostly water, various plant extracts that don't work like AHAs, and aloe, though the amount of witch hazel is potentially irritating, as are the rosemary and thyme extracts. Last, the orange oil is a fragrant irritant (see the Appendix to find out why fragrance is a problem for skin). Altogether, this toner isn't equalizing—it's bound to make combination skin worse and the irritants can stimulate excess oil production at the base of the pores.

SKINCEUTICALS EXFOLIANTS & SCRUBS

☺ GOOD **$$$ Retexturing Activator Bi-Functional Resurfacing and Replenishing Serum** *($72 for 1 fl. oz.)* sounds like an active, multitasking product, but it isn't. Based on the claims and ingredient list, this is essentially just an AHA-like exfoliant that contains a form of urea instead of conventional glycolic or lactic acids. Other than that, it contains absolutely nothing else that is beneficial for skin. For the money, that is just rude. We have no idea what SkinCeuticals means when they refer to this exfoliant's "paradoxal compound" in their claims, and no one at the company could tell us. "Paradox" refers to a contradiction in terms. What does that have to do with your skin or a product's benefit? No one seems to know. Marketing terminology aside, what this product contains is a high amount of urea. That's good because it can exfoliate and soften your skin, but there is no research demonstrating that the hydroxyethyl urea, which is what this product contains, has the same benefit as plain urea. What urea does is increase skin cell turnover the same way an AHA product does. You'd think SkinCeuticals would publish a study comparing their compound with standard exfoliant ingredients, but no such information exists; you simply need to take their word for it, and spend a lot money in the process. Bottom line: You don't have to spend anywhere close to this amount to get equal or better results from an exfoliant. There certainly isn't any research proving urea in any form is superior to AHAs (e.g., glycolic acid) or BHA (salicylic acid). Although this is an option, and this exfoliant is suitable for all skin types, think twice before trying this instead of less expensive exfoliants whose ingredients have lots of research attesting to their efficacy.

☺ AVERAGE **$$$ C + AHA Exfoliating Antioxidant Treatment** *($133 for 1 fl. oz.)* is a good option if you're looking for a stabilized vitamin C serum that contains a blend of 10%

AHAs along with an effective, though potentially irritating, amount of vitamin C in its pure form (ascorbic acid). Vitamin C is not the sole answer for skin and there are less irritating yet still effective AHA products for far less money, but this is an option.

☺ AVERAGE $$$ **Micro-Exfoliating Scrub** *($28 for 5 fl. oz.)* is a basic scrub that uses diatomaceous earth as the abrasive agent. This ingredient is made from fossilized sea algae. Although that sounds natural and safe, the truth is this scrub agent is a problem for all skin types because the particles have jagged edges that can scratch and tear at skin. If diatomaceous earth is buffered with emollients or oils the risk is reduced, but that's not the case with this scrub. Considering its price and formula, this scrub ends up being a tough recommendation even for those with hardy, oily skin.

☹ POOR **Conditioning Solution** *($30 for 8 fl. oz.)* is a toner-like product that may feel weightless as claimed, but its formula stands an excellent change of irritating your skin, a fact which leads to a host of other problems. Essentially a toner with the AHA glycolic acid and BHA salicylic acid, these ingredients cannot work to exfoliate because the pH of Conditioning Solution is outside the range AHAs and BHA need to work. Moreover, the amount of alcohol and inclusion of fragrant eucalyptus oil make this a deal-breaker for all skin types. See the Appendix to find out the many ways irritation hurts your skin.

☹ POOR **LHA Solution** *($36 for 8 fl. oz.)* would be an intriguing product to consider if its formula didn't contain a potentially irritating amount of alcohol. Listed as the second ingredient, alcohol causes dryness and free-radical damage, and can hinder healthy collagen production. The blend of AHA glycolic acid, BHA salicylic acid, and LHA (lipo hydroxy acid, a type of exfoliant exclusive to L'Oreal, the company that owns SkinCeuticals) is able to exfoliate skin thanks to this product's pH being within range for efficacy, but there are other AHA or BHA products that work just as well without the threat irritation presents—and many of the better options cost less. By the way, there is no substantiated research proving LHA is superior to AHAs or BHA.

SKINCEUTICALS MOISTURIZERS (DAYTIME & NIGHTTIME), EYE CREAMS, & SERUMS

✓☺ BEST $$$ **Retinol 0.5 Refining Night Cream with 0.5% Pure Retinol** *($54 for 1 fl. oz.)* makes many anti-aging claims, and because it contains a significant amount of retinol the chief claims you can bank on are building collagen and stimulating cell regeneration. However, since other ingredients can also do that, or at least assist in the process, it's a bit overly optimistic to hang all your hopes on one specialized ingredient such as retinol. Fortunately, this water- and silicone-based serum contains many other beneficial ingredients for healthy skin, including ceramides, cholesterol, lecithin, antioxidants, and the anti-irritant bisabolol. The opaque bottle with pump applicator helps maintain the stability of the retinol, which is a prerequisite for products with this ingredient. Retinol 0.5 is suitable for all skin types. Getting back to the claims, SkinCeuticals boasts that this serum will also minimize pore size and correct blemishes. The first claim rests on a subjective judgment. The second claim that retinol is able to correct blemishes is at this point more theoretical than proven. In contrast, tretinoin (the active ingredient in Retin-A) has considerable research supporting its use as a prescription acne treatment. While it's definitely possible that using a retinol serum like this will result in fewer blemishes, it's not as much a sure thing as using a tretinoin product. The benefits of retinol versus tretinoin are that retinol has significantly fewer and comparably minor side effects, but the trade-off is reduced efficacy (Source: *Cosmetic Dermatology*, volume 18, issue 1, supplement 1, January 2005, page 19). This product is not recommended for daytime application because it contains photosensitizing St. John's wort.

✓☺ BEST **$$$ Retinol 1.0 Maximum Strength Refining Night Cream with 1.0% Pure Retinol** *($59 for 1 fl. oz.)* is similar to SkinCeutical's Retinol 0.5 product above, except it contains twice as much retinol. Caution is warranted because using retinol at this level (1%) poses a slight risk of side effects that are similar to, but less pronounced than, those caused by topical tretinoin, including redness, flaking/peeling, and possibly stinging. These effects should be short term as the skin acclimates to retinol, but if they do not dissipate or if they worsen with continued use, stop using the product; retinol at this strength may not be right for your skin. Note that this product is not recommended for daytime use because it contains the plant extract St. John's Wort (listed by its Latin name of *Hypericum perforatum*), which has the potential to trigger a negative reaction on sun-exposed skin. As with any retinol or anti-aging product, daily application of a sunscreen rated SPF 15 or greater is a must.

☺ GOOD **$$$ C E Ferulic Combination Antioxidant Treatment** *($146 for 1 fl. oz.)* comes complete with all manner of anti-aging claims, but the only ones you can bank on with this product (based on a significant amount of research) are its abilities to reduce free radicals and to defend skin against oxidative stress. It reportedly contains 15% L-ascorbic acid, a form of vitamin C considered an excellent antioxidant and anti-inflammatory agent (Sources: *Experimental Dermatology*, June 2003, pages 237–244; and *Bioelectrochemistry and Bioenergetics*, May 1999, pages 453–461). Because L-ascorbic acid is stable only in low-pH formulations (Source: *Dermatologic Surgery*, February 2001, pages 137–142), the good news is that this product's pH of 3 is low enough to allow this form of vitamin C to be effective. Also present in this water-based antioxidant serum are vitamin E and ferulic acid. Vitamin E, appearing here as alpha tocopherol, also has a well-established reputation as an effective antioxidant (Sources: *Radiation Research*, July 2005, pages 63–72; *Annals of the New York Academy of Sciences*, December 2004, pages 443–447; and *Journal of Investigative Dermatology*, February 2005, pages 304–307). Ferulic acid provides antioxidant and sun-protective benefits to skin while enhancing the stability of topical applications of vitamin E (Sources: *International Journal of Pharmaceutics*, April 10, 2000, pages 39–47; *Anticancer Research*, September-October 1999, pages 3769–3774; *Nutrition and Cancer*, February 1998, pages 81–85; and *Free Radical Biology and Medicine*, October 1992, pages 435–448). C E Ferulic Combination Antioxidant Treatment is suitable for all skin types. Its brown glass packaging helps keep its high level of antioxidants stable, although an airless pump applicator would have been better than the dropper tip, because that requires you to remove the cover with each use, exposing the oxygen-sensitive antioxidants to air. That and the lack of repairing ingredients like ceramides and cell-communicating ingredients is what keep this product from earning a higher rating. If you opt to use this, take care to replace the dropper tip immediately after each use.

☺ GOOD **$$$ Physical Fusion UV Defense SPF 50** *($32 for 1.7 fl. oz.)* is a great and, for SkinCeuticals, surprisingly affordable daytime moisturizer with sunscreen. Gentle, broad-spectrum sun protection is supplied by the mineral sunscreens titanium dioxide and zinc oxide. This is also fragrance-free, which makes it good for those with sensitive or rosacea-affected skin. The combined amount of mineral sunscreens may be problematic for breakout-prone skin, but the texture is so light it's definitely worth a try (those with breakout-prone skin always need to experiment to find products that work without promoting more breakouts). In a smart move, SkinCeuticals added a soft, flesh-toned tint in an effort to eliminate the white cast most mineral-based sunscreens have. The fluid, sheer texture feels great and provides light hydration and a satin matte finish those with normal to slightly dry skin will find appealing. If you have oily areas this is workable, but you likely will see some shine coming through before midday.

The texture and finish of this product means it works well under makeup, while the sheer tint has only a minimal effect on your foundation color. This can be worn alone without making your skin tone look "off" or dark; that is, unless you have porcelain skin, in which case you'll look a bit tanned. With all this praise, you may be wondering why this isn't a Best Product. One word: antioxidants. SkinCeuticals includes only a teeny-tiny amount of them, yet antioxidants are a great addition to your daytime moisturizer with sunscreen, especially if you're spending this kind of money. If you decide to try this product (and it is worth trying, especially if regular sunscreens tend to cause your skin to sting), we recommend applying it over an antioxidant-rich serum such as Paula's Choice RESIST Super Antioxidant Concentrate Serum.

☺ GOOD $$$ **Serum 10 AOX+** *($86 for 1 fl. oz.)* is a water-based serum that contains 10% L-ascorbic acid along with penetration-enhancing ingredients, stabilizers, and a couple of water-binding agents. SkinCeuticals added the antioxidant ferulic acid to their vitamin C serums because research has shown it helps boost efficacy, although the only research on topical application of these antioxidants was done in part by Dr. Pinnell, founder of SkinCeuticals (Source: *Journal of Investigative Dermatology*, October 2005, pages 826–832), so it's not exactly impartial. Still, there is enough research on ferulic acid's antioxidant effects when taken internally to rationalize (and further research) its use in skin-care products.

☺ GOOD $$$ **Serum 15 AOX+** *($99 for 1 fl. oz.)* is identical to the Serum 10 AOX+ above, except this version provides 15% L-ascorbic acid. Keep in mind that this amount of vitamin C at the pH that's needed for it to be effective may prove more irritating than beneficial for skin (a fact SkinCeuticals mentions on their website and in literature for this product). This is not the type of product you'd want to use nightly with other products such as those with retinol, AHAs, BHA, or topical prescription retinoids because such a combination may send skin into irritation overload, so proceed cautiously to see how your skin reacts. Piling on excess amounts of anti-aging ingredients with a "more is better" mentality can absolutely backfire!

☺ GOOD $$$ **Serum 20 AOX+** *($118 for 1 fl. oz.)* is similar to the Serum 10 AOX+, except this pricier version increases the vitamin C content to 20%. Otherwise, the same comments and precautions made for the other two AOX+ Serums apply here, too. Interestingly, relatively recent research on formulating vitamin C into skin-care products shows that a thickened microemulsion, not a solution as used here, does a better job of keeping the antioxidants stable (Sources: *Drug Delivery*, April 2007, pages 235–245; and *Pharmaceutical Development and Technology*, November 2006, pages 255–261).

☹ AVERAGE $$$ **A.G.E. Interrupter** *($152 for 1.7 fl. oz.)*. The A.G.E. in this product's name refers to advanced glycation end-products (AGE), which are not good for the body or the skin. AGEs are formed by the body's major fuel source, namely glucose. This simple sugar is essential for energy, but it also binds strongly to proteins (the body's fundamental building blocks), forming abnormal structures—AGEs—that progressively damage tissue elasticity. Once generated, AGEs begin a process that prevents many systems from behaving normally by literally causing tissue to cross-link and become hardened (Source: *Proceedings of the National Academy of Sciences*, March 14, 2000, pages 2809–2813). SkinCeuticals' theory is that by breaking these AGE bonds you can undo or stop the damage they cause. AGEs and free-radical damage may be inextricably linked (Sources: *European Journal of Neuroscience*, December 2001, page 1961; and *Neuroscience Letters*, October 2001, pages 29–32), but none of the studies indicate that there are any substances that can be included in skin-care products to affect this process. Specific to this product, the only ingredient it contains that is known to inhibit the formation of AGEs in skin is one that L'Oreal did the research on. Because L'Oreal owns SkinCeuticals, this research can hardly be considered impartial. Surprisingly, the blueberry extract L'Oreal used in this study (and in this product) did not fare as well as aminoguanidine, another ingredient known to inhibit AGEs (Source: *Experimental Gerontology*, June 2008, pages 584–588). Knowing this, why would you want to purchase this SkinCeuticals product when the parent company's own research shows that what they're including to inhibit AGEs is not as effective as another ingredient that they didn't include? If anything, this product is a big step backwards for SkinCeuticals. It's mostly slip agents, silicones, and wax, plus the questionable AGE-inhibiting blueberry extract, although even if this extract could help, it won't remain potent for long thanks to the jar packaging (not to mention that there's hardly any of it in this product). For $150, you have every right to expect a whole lot more than this no-better-than-average product provides. See the Appendix to learn why jar packaging is not the way to go.

☺ AVERAGE $$$ **AOX+ Eye Gel** *($85 for 0.5 fl. oz.)* is an expensive, lightweight eye-area moisturizer that has, as the name states, a gel texture. The ingredients creating this texture help hydrate but, combined as they are, also lend this gel a slightly tacky finish. Although the formula contains some notable antioxidants (including ascorbic acid, better known as vitamin C), it contains more skin-damaging alcohol than these helpful anti-aging ingredients, making this much less desirable. Specific to the eye area, this gel doesn't contain any ingredients that help improve puffiness or dark circles; if anything, the potential irritation from the alcohol can worsen both concerns—and it certainly won't help reduce wrinkles or other signs of aging. For the money, this is one to skip, but do check out the Appendix to learn why you don't need an eye cream (or gel).

☺ AVERAGE $$$ **Eye Balm Rehabilitative Emollient, for Aging Skin** *($81 for 0.5 fl. oz.)* has a lot going for it, including copious antioxidants and a cell-communicating ingredient, all wrapped up in a lightweight lotion texture for all skin types. What a shame the jar packaging won't keep the state-of-the-art ingredients stable during use (see the Appendix for details and to learn why, in truth, you don't need an eye cream).

☺ AVERAGE $$$ **Face Cream Rehabilitating Cream, for Aging Skin** *($140 for 1.67 fl. oz.)* offers normal to dry skin several rehabilitating ingredients, including good antioxidants and plant oils. However, the ylang-ylang and geranium oils are bad news, and keep this moisturizer from being truly state-of-the-art. See the Appendix to learn why fragrant oils are pro-aging.

☺ AVERAGE $$$ **Hydrating B5 Gel Moisture Enhancing Gel** *($70 for 1 fl. oz.)* is a simple hydrating mix of a water-binding agent, vitamin B-5 (also known as panthenol), and a preservative. It is suitable for all skin types but your skin needs more than what this provides.

☺ AVERAGE $$$ **Phyto Corrective Gel Calming Complexion Gel** *($60 for 1 fl. oz.)* is a water-based serum whose water-binding agents can benefit all skin types, while the Uva ursi extract's arbutin content may have a positive impact on skin discolorations. This would be rated higher if not for the amount of thyme extract and the nebulous "herbal fragrance."

☺ AVERAGE $$$ **Renew Overnight Dry Nighttime Skin-Refining Moisturizer, for Normal to Dry Skin** *($59 for 2 fl. oz.)* provides more fruit acids masquerading as AHAs, while jar packaging ruins the effectiveness of the antioxidants in this moisturizer for normal to dry skin. For the money, you're better off investing in a separate AHA product and a stably packaged moisturizer with state-of-the-art ingredients.

👁 Did you know you don't need an eye cream? It's true! See the Appendix to find out why.

☺ AVERAGE **$$$ Renew Overnight Oily Nighttime Skin-Refining Moisturizer, for Normal or Oily Skin** *($59 for 2 fl. oz.)* claims to hydrate skin and exfoliate with "a blend of hydroxy acids." Those acids are not AHAs and BHA, but rather sugar and fruit extracts. Unfortunately, these do not work like AHAs or BHA, and in fact the citrus fruit extracts can cause irritation. This is capable of hydrating normal to oily skin, but some of the emollient ingredients aren't the best for use on blemish-prone skin. The formula also includes orange oil for fragrance, which is another source of irritation. It's possible that the irritating ingredients in this moisturizer will stimulate more oil production at the base of the pores, making this a tough sell for those with oily skin that needs hydration for dry patches.

☹ POOR **A.G.E. Eye Complex** *($86 for 0.5 fl. oz.)* is a classic case of using impressive claims and anti-aging acronyms to make it sound like *the* eye cream for anyone concerned with wrinkles, dark circles, and puffiness. The formula is mostly water, glycerin, silicone, dry-finish solvent (not the best for the eye area), wax, and thickeners. The tiny amounts of vitamins C and E along with plant extracts and peptides are there only for show, not effect—and none of them will last long once this jar-packaged product is opened. None of the ingredients in this eye cream have substantiated research proving they have a remarkable (or even mildly exciting) effect on dark circles or puffiness. The blood vessel-strengthening, lymphatic drainage, and hemoglobin-eliminating claims are pure fiction. What's fact is that the inclusion of the menthol derivative menthoxypropanediol will cause irritation, especially when used around the eye. Please don't misinterpret this to mean the product is working, because it isn't—at least not in the way you may be hoping. See the Appendix to learn more about issues concerning jar packaging and irritating ingredients and to learn why you don't need an eye cream.

☹ POOR **Daily Moisture Lightweight Pore-Minimizing Moisturizer, for Normal or Oily Combination Skin** *($60 for 2 fl. oz.)* begins well with its water-based blend of several species of algae and a light moisturizing agent, but all in all this contains too many potentially problematic plant extracts to make it a slam-dunk for normal to oily skin. Algae extracts cannot make pores smaller, but the cinnamon and ginger may make them appear smaller by virtue of the inflammation they cause—yet that's a negative for the long-term health of your skin.

☹ POOR **Emollience Rich, Restorative Moisturizer, for Normal or Dry Skin** *($60 for 2 fl. oz.)* not only features jar packaging that undermines the efficacy of its many antioxidants (see the Appendix for details), but also this emollient cream is bound to cause irritation due to the volatile essential oils it contains. Ouch!

☹ POOR **Eye Cream Firming Treatment** *($70 for 0.67 fl. oz.)* contains a single ingredient that makes it a deal-breaker for use anywhere on the face. Juniper oil (listed by its Latin name of *Juniperus communis*) is considered a skin irritant due to its many volatile fragrant components (Sources: naturaldatabase.com; and *International Journal of Toxicology*, Volume 20 Supplement, 2001, pages 41–56). What a shame because this is otherwise an extraordinarily well-formulated eye cream despite not being able to help with puffiness, dark circles, or sagging skin. All those concerns are not what the ingredients in this eye cream can fix (especially sagging, which must be corrected via cosmetic surgery, not skin-care products). However, it does contain several state-of-the-art ingredients that help skin resist further signs of aging—but it's all for naught thanks to the juniper oil.

☹ POOR **Phloretin CF** *($152 for 1 fl. oz.)* comes complete with claims on its years of research, patents, and new cosmeceutical buzzwords such as "biodiverse" and "broad-spectrum treatment." Aside from the company's exemplary marketing efforts, the product does deserve some discussion in terms of its single unique ingredient, phloretin (because other than that, this is one boring ordinary, potentially skin-damaging product). Phloretin is a white crystalline flavonoid that results from the decomposition or hydrolysis of phlorizin. Naturally, your next question is: What's phlorizin? It's a bitter substance extracted from the root bark of apple trees and from apples, so phloretin does have a natural origin (though what it takes to get phlorizin out of the apple tree to turn it into phloretin is hardly a natural process; you're not going to use phloretin to flavor pie). As for phloretin's value for skin, in vitro and animal research has shown that it has antioxidant ability, can interrupt melanin synthesis to potentially reduce skin discolorations, inhibits the formation of MMP-1 (which breaks down collagen), and also serves as a penetration enhancer, which, as you'll see below, is not a good thing in the case of this product (Sources: *The FEBS Journal*, August 2008, pages 3804–3814; *Phytochemistry*, April 2007, pages 1189–1199; *Biological and Pharmaceutical Bulletin*, April 2006, pages 740–745; *European Journal of Pharmaceutics and Biopharmaceutics*, March 2004, pages 307–312; and *International Journal of Pharmaceutics*, April 2003, pages 109–116). Although there are compelling reasons to consider phloretin as another potent, beneficial antioxidant to improve skin's appearance and healthy functioning, in the case of this product it is completely wasted. Why? Because the amount of denatured alcohol in this serum negates any antioxidant benefit of the phloretin. The inclusion of alcohol is extremely disappointing because alcohol causes free-radical damage, cell death, and irritation (see the Appendix for details). Phloretin may be the antioxidant du jour, but not in this product. Please keep in mind that despite the published research for phloretin and Skin-Ceuticals's claims, it is not the best antioxidant to "attack damage on every level." There are lots of brilliant antioxidants in skin-care products, but there isn't a miracle or magic bullet out there.

☹ POOR **Phloretin CF Gel** *($152)* is a serum-like gel that is said to contain 10% vitamin C (ascorbic acid), an amount that's impressive but also potentially irritating given that the acid form of vitamin C has a stronger potential for irritation than other forms such as ascorbyl glucoside or magnesium ascorbyl phosphate. More troubling, though, is that if the vitamin C is truly present at 10%, that means there's at least the same amount (or more) of alcohol—the kind that causes dryness and free-radical damage, and hurts healthy collagen production. That's not good news for anyone's skin and ends up being a burn considering what this product costs! See the review above for Phloretin CF to learn more about the ingredient phloretin.

☹ POOR **Skin Firming Cream** *($110 for 1.67 fl. oz.)* lists sandalwood extract as the third ingredient and also contains fragrant juniper oil, which makes this otherwise good but overpriced moisturizer a problem for all skin types. See the Appendix to learn why daily use of highly fragrant products is pro-aging, not the other way around.

SKINCEUTICALS SUN CARE

✓☺ BEST **$$$ Physical UV Defense SPF 30** *($38 for 3 fl. oz.)* is a creamy sunscreen that contains only titanium dioxide and zinc oxide as its active ingredients, making it an excellent choice for sensitive skin, including those with various forms of dermatitis and rosacea. It is fragrance-free. The creamy texture combined with a high amount of mineral actives makes this an iffy choice for those with breakout-prone skin, so if that describes you, look for mineral-based sunscreens with a light, fluid texture, such as SkinCeuticals Physical Fusion UV Defense SPF 50.

✓☺ BEST **$$$ Sport UV Defense SPF 45** *($37 for 3 fl. oz.)* is a very good, in-part zinc oxide sunscreen for normal to very dry skin not prone to blemishes. The fragrance-free formula contains antioxidant vitamins that have proven to be positive additions to sunscreens. It is water-resistant, not waterproof, because no sunscreen is 100% impervious to water (which is why reapplying after sweating or swimming is mandatory).

☺ GOOD $$$ **Daily Sun Defense SPF 20** *($38 for 3 fl. oz.)* has an in-part zinc oxide sunscreen and does not contain fragrance, but for all SkinCeuticals talk about antioxidants (particularly vitamin C), it is disappointing that not a single antioxidant shows up in this sunscreen for normal to dry skin not prone to blemishes.

☺ GOOD **Sheer Physical UV Defense SPF 50** *($32 for 1.7 fl. oz.)* is a lightweight, very fluid sunscreen with only titanium dioxide and zinc oxide as the sole active ingredients. You must shake it before using to disperse the mineral actives. When applied liberally, as sunscreen should be, this is absolutely not transparent on skin, despite the claims, unless you have extremely white skin. The thin texture and soft matte finish make this best for normal to oily skin, but titanium dioxide and zinc oxide can be a problem for blemish prone skin in large amounts, as is the case here. Still, the texture is light, and not everyone with breakout-prone skin will have a problem with higher amounts of these mineral actives, so experimentation is in order. The only unique thing about this product is the SPF rating. Most mineral sunscreens are not rated higher than SPF 30 because the amount of active ingredients needed to surpass SPF 30 leads to a formula that's aesthetically undesirable, although, depending on your skin color, you might find that not to be the case. As for the artemia extract mentioned in the claims, it is indeed a plankton, but more accurately, it's a species of brine shrimp that, as far as skin care is concerned, has no documented benefit. SkinCeuticals must not think too highly of it anyway because the amount of it in this sunscreen is barely a dusting. It is disappointing that antioxidants are practically absent from this formula, but perhaps SkinCeuticals expects their customers to use this with one of their antioxidant scrums.

☺ GOOD $$$ **Ultimate UV Defense SPF 30** *($38 for 3 fl. oz.)* is very similar to the Daily Sun Defense SPF 20 above, except that this one contains the higher percentage of active ingredients necessary to attain an SPF 30 rating. Otherwise, the same comments apply.

SKINCEUTICALS LIP CARE

✓☺ BEST $$$ **Antioxidant Lip Repair Restorative Treatment, for Damaged or Aging Lips** *($38 for 0.3 fl. oz.)* has an interesting texture in an overall emollient (and fragrance-free) formula that provides lips with an impressive selection of antioxidants, water-binding agents, and a peptide, which theoretically has cell-communicating ability. If you're going to spend this much for a lip product, it might as well be loaded with extras like this one is! However, this doesn't contain sunscreen, and so should only be used at night.

SKINCEUTICALS SPECIALTY SKIN-CARE PRODUCTS

☺ GOOD $$$ **Clarifying Clay Masque Deep Pore Cleansing Skin-Refining Masque** *($46 for 2 fl. oz.)* is a standard, but good, clay mask for normal to very oily skin. The fruit and sugar extracts do not exfoliate skin like an AHA product would. This should be thoroughly rinsed because comfrey extract can be irritating if left on skin.

☹ AVERAGE $$$ **Hydrating B5 Masque** *($52 for 2.5 fl. oz.)* is an exceptionally boring mask that is absolutely not worth the money. The claims make it seem like the ultimate moisture oasis for dry, parched skin, but it is primarily water, glycerin, pH-adjusting agent, and gel-based thickener. Big deal!

☹ AVERAGE $$$ **Pigment Regulator Daily High Potency Brightening Treatment** *($85 for 1 fl. oz.)* is said to be proven as effective "as the leading medical standard for treating hyperpigmentation." They must be referring to hydroquinone. Long considered the gold standard for treating sun- or hormone-induced skin discolorations, hydroquinone has a controversial reputation, despite years of safe use when properly formulated and used as directed. Nevertheless, lots of cosmetics lines are offering alternatives to this skin-lightening staple. Is Pigment Regulator a viable option for treating your discolorations? Maybe, but it's a long shot, and for the money you may want to make sure SkinCeuticals has a generous return policy. According to SkinCeuticals (who didn't publish their clinical research), Pigment Regulator is as effective as hydroquinone. It supposedly works due to its combination of 2% kojic acid, 2% emblica, and a 10% blend of exfoliating agents. A quick look at the ingredient list reveals that these percentages don't add up. Think about buying a chocolate cake and the chocolate is way down on the ingredient list. Emblica, also known as Indian gooseberry, has no research supporting its ability to lighten skin discolorations. Like most plants, it has antioxidant ability and also appears to be anti-mutagenic and antimicrobial. We found one study that compared emblica with an extract from cashew leaves. The outcome was that cashew not only reduced melanin (skin pigment) activity in skin, but also had a greater antioxidant capacity than emblica (Sources: *The Medical Journal of Malaysia*, July 2008, pages 100–101; and naturaldatabase. com). Although emblica isn't an ingredient to bank on for skin-lightening, it has antiwrinkle potential because of its ability to inhibit collagen breakdown while promoting healthy collagen production (Source: *Journal of Cosmetic Science*, July-August 2009, pages 395–403), but there are dozens of ingredients that provide this benefit and more. As for kojic acid, there is research showing it has skin-lightening properties (Sources: *International Journal of Molecular Sciences*, May 2009, pages 2440–2775; *Biological and Pharmaceutical Bulletin*, August 2002, pages 1045–1048; *Analytical Biochemistry*, June 2002, pages 260–268; and *Cellular Signaling*, September 2002, pages 779–785). There also is some controversial research that has shown kojic acid to have carcinogenic properties (Sources: *Mutation Research, Genetic Toxicology and Environmental Mutagenesis*, June 2005, pages 133–145; and *Toxicological Sciences*, September 2004, pages 43–49). Also lacking is research showing that kojic acid is superior to hydroquinone. Although we know kojic acid is one of many potential alternatives to hydroquinone, it is neither the best nor any more effective than many others, and it has its own risks. All things considered, this is an expensive way to see if SkinCeuticals' cocktail of ingredients will improve your discolorations. The amount of glycolic acid, while not 10%, is likely enough for exfoliation to occur, and this product's pH of 4 allows that to happen. However, unless you're opposed to using hydroquinone, there are less expensive over-the-counter products to consider. Please see our list of the Best Skin-Lightening Products at the end of this book for our top-rated options with and without hydroquinone.

☹ POOR **Blemish + Age Defense Salicylic Acid Acne Treatment** *($80 for 1 fl. oz.)* is a product that has a goal to target acne along with signs of aging, including discolorations. Lots of people struggle with wrinkles, uneven skin tone, and breakouts, and all of them are wondering "Why me?" We understand your frustration and are thrilled to tell you which products can truly help. Regrettably, this isn't one of them. This does contain the proven acne fighter and anti-aging superstar ingredient salicylic acid, with a decent 1.5% concentration at a pH of 3.4. It also contains a smaller amount of the AHA glycolic acid, which may provide an additional exfoliating boost and help fade discolorations. SkinCeuticals also uses a unique ingredient they label as diocic acid. Listed as octadecenedioic acid, it's a synthetic or naturally derived wax-like fatty acid. According to limited research, octadecenedioic acid has anti-inflammatory properties and works to lighten skin discolorations, but its exact method of action is not fully understood. It seems to function as a cell-communicating ingredient and works to reduce excess melanin production that leads to skin discolorations (Sources: *International Journal of Cosmetic Science*,

August 2006, pages 263–267, and April 2005, pages 123–132). What's not certain is how much of this ingredient is needed to provide benefit. SkinCeuticals maintains they're using 2%, but to date, there's no relevant data to support that amount as being optimal for improving brown skin discolorations. Ultimately, things go downhill due to the inclusion of a large amount of alcohol, which is the main ingredient (and lends this product a potent medicinal scent). See the Appendix to learn of the many problems alcohol causes for all skin types.

☹ POOR **Phyto + Botanical Gel, for Hyperpigmentation** *($78 for 1 fl. oz.)* lists thyme extract as the second ingredient, which makes this arbutin-enhanced, skin-lightening gel a problem for all skin types. Chemical components of thyme have been shown to be irritating for skin (Source: naturaldatabase.com).

SKINMEDICA (SKIN CARE ONLY)

Strengths: Many of the moisturizers and serums are truly state-of-the-art formulas; every sunscreen provides sufficient UVA protection; good cleansers; and several products are fragrance-free.

Weaknesses: Expensive; the acne products are terrible and do not feature a topical disinfectant; no reliable AHA or BHA exfoliants; the unknowns about daily topical use of human growth factors make the TNS subcategory of products a potentially risky endeavor.

For more information and the latest SkinMedica reviews, visit CosmeticsCop.com.

SKINMEDICA CLEANSERS

✓☺ BEST **$$$ Sensitive Skin Cleanser** *($34 for 6 fl. oz.)* is an interesting water- and oil–based cleanser that does not contain detergent cleansing agents. The oil and emollient ingredients help remove makeup, while the plant-based additives are known for their anti-irritant effect. With no fragrance, coloring agents, or known irritants, this is indeed an appropriate cleanser for someone with sensitive skin, assuming it is normal to dry and not prone to breakouts. This is best used with a washcloth to ensure complete removal.

☺ GOOD **$$$ Facial Cleanser** *($34 for 6 fl. oz.)* is a standard, but very good, water-soluble cleanser for normal to slightly dry or oily skin. It's pricey for what you get, but it does remove makeup and it does not contain problematic ingredients. If you choose to spend this much on a facial cleanser, it should be a gentle formula such as this (though it would earn a higher rating if it were fragrance-free).

☹ POOR **Purifying Foaming Wash** *($40 for 5 fl. oz.)* will only make matters worse for those struggling with acne. This liquid-to-foam cleanser contains several irritants, including camphor oil, sage, and menthol. In addition, the main detergent cleansing agent is known to be drying, and the 2% salicylic acid is wasted because you rinse it off before it has a chance to get into the pores and work. See the Appendix to learn how irritating ingredients worsen oily skin.

SKINMEDICA TONERS

☹ AVERAGE **$$$ Rejuvenative Toner** *($34 for 6 fl. oz.)* is said to contain "exfoliating alpha-hydroxy acid," but ingredients such as sugarcane, bilberry, and citrus extracts cannot exfoliate skin the same way as standard AHAs such as lactic and glycolic acids. This toner is an OK mix of water-binding agents and a tiny amount of vitamin-based antioxidants. It would be rated higher if not for the irritation potential from the witch hazel and citrus extracts (plus, ideally, your skin doesn't need the artificial coloring agents this toner contains).

☹ POOR **Purifying Toner** *($34 for 6 fl. oz.)* contains alcohol and menthol, making this another irritating toner for blemish-prone skin. These ingredients hurt skin's healing process, risk making red marks from acne worse, and can stimulate oil production at the base of the pores. A final disappointment: The 2% salicylic acid cannot exfoliate skin because this toner's pH is too high.

SKINMEDICA SCRUB

✓☺ BEST **$$$ Skin Polisher** *($40 for 2 fl. oz.)* is a fragrance-free cleanser/scrub hybrid that contains jojoba beads for gentle exfoliation. Although not a scrub for anyone on a budget or who prefers a more granular feel, it is a suitable option for normal to very dry skin.

SKINMEDICA MOISTURIZERS (DAYTIME & NIGHTTIME), EYE CREAMS, & SERUMS

✓☺ BEST **$$$ Age Defense Tri-Retinol Complex ES** *($75 for 1 fl. oz.)* is an outstanding fragrance-free moisturizer with retinol. Not only are you getting proven anti-aging ingredient retinol in opaque packaging to ensure its stability, it's in an elegant base that also treats normal to dry skin to emollients and antioxidants. The only drawback is the amount of retinol this contains. The company claims to be using a blend of retinoids (retinol, retinyl palmitate, and retinyl acetate) that equal 1.1%. Assuming this claim is honest, it could be too much of a good thing. Retinoids are potent and not everyone's skin tolerates them. With a higher percentage of retinol you're putting skin at risk for sensitivity and flaking, especially if you've never used a product with retinol/retinoids before. However, if you've already acclimated to retinoids and want to try something stronger, this is worth a go. Just keep in mind that (as with prescription retinoids) more is not necessarily better. Pay close attention to how your skin responds and adjust the frequency of usage accordingly.

✓☺ BEST **$$$ Rejuvenative Moisturizer** *($54 for 2 fl. oz.)* is an outstanding moisturizer for normal to dry skin. In many ways this rivals both similarly priced and more expensively priced moisturizers from Estee Lauder. Vitamin E is prominent, but this also contains stabilized vitamin C, tocotrienols, plant-based anti-irritants, and notable emollients. This does contain fragrance and a tiny amount of fragrance ingredients (such as linalool), but that's forgivable considering the tiny amount and the preponderance of good-for-skin ingredients.

☺ GOOD **Ultra Sheer Moisturizer** *($54 for 2 fl. oz.)* has its strong points, but ends up being a less impressive version of SkinMedica's superior Rejuvenative Moisturizer above. The formula is oil-free and has a lighter texture, but the thickening agents it contains aren't the best for someone battling blemishes. This is a good option for normal to dry skin, especially if you want a moisturizer that blends vitamins C and E without an everything-but-the-kitchen-sink approach.

☺ GOOD **$$$ Hydrating Complex** *($80 for 1 fl. oz.)* is a good, lightweight water-based serum that's suitable for all skin types. It contains an impressive amount of skin-identical ingredient hyaluronic acid along with several water-binding agents that won't make oily skin feel greasy. It is also unlikely to exacerbate acne, but that can be said for many serums. Those with dry skin will definitely need to pair this with a moisturizer. For the money, Hydrating Complex should contain some notable antioxidants and at least one cell-communicating ingredient, but this is still a worthwhile serum to try if the price doesn't give you pause.

☺ GOOD **$$$ TNS Ceramide Treatment Cream** *($64 for 2 fl. oz.)* is a very good moisturizer for normal to very dry skin, save for the concerns about daily application of a product that contains multiple growth factors (that's what SkinMedica's human fibroblast conditioned media is, though there isn't much of it used here). This moisturizer's blend of peptides, non-volatile plant oils, and antioxidants is, along with the omission of fragrance, praiseworthy, but the growth factor issues keep this from earning a Best Product rating.

☺ GOOD $$$ **Uplifting Eye Serum** *($55 for 0.5 fl. oz.)* cannot diminish puffy eyes or dark circles any better than any other serum because antioxidants and plant extracts cannot address these eye-weary woes effectively. Some of the plant extracts in this water-based serum have an anti-inflammatory action, and that can help alleviate some puffiness caused by irritation (such as from smoke or allergies). However, that's not the type of under-eye puffiness related to aging, which is what most readers who write to us about this condition are dealing with. Age-related puffiness under the eyes has to do with skin slackening and the fat pads beneath it loosening, causing a droopy, pouched look. This type of puffiness cannot be addressed by skin-care products; the only remedy is cosmetic surgery, where the results are often remarkable. This Eye Serum still has merit for use on slightly dry skin anywhere on the face. Despite this product offering little hope for those struggling with age-related puffiness, it's an overall impressive, fragrance-free formula that can make skin feel smoother and (temporarily) tighter due to the amount of film-forming agent it contains. But even so, you don't need to use a special eye-area serum to gain those benefits—a facial serum with these types of ingredients would work just as well.

☺ GOOD $$$ **Vitamin C + E Complex Age Defense** *($95 for 1 fl. oz.)* consists of silicones blended with two types of stabilized vitamin C and lesser amounts of vitamin E. Although this silky, fragrance-free serum is a good way to see how your skin will respond to an efficacious amount of vitamin C, the formula isn't as impressive as that of the Hydra-Pure Vitamin C Serum from Dr. Dennis Gross Skincare. His version costs a few dollars more for the same amount of product, but it also contains a better array of antioxidants and adds cell-communicating ingredients to the mix. For even less money but an equally superior formula, consider Paula's Choice RESIST Super Antioxidant Concentrate Serum.

☹ AVERAGE $$$ **15% AHA/BHA Face Cream** *($40 for 2 fl. oz.)* contains a blend of fruit and sugar extracts, which the company uses to ramp up its claim about the AHA content in an effort to make consumers think they're getting a potent exfoliant. The bad news is that bilberry, sugarcane, and citrus extracts don't function in the same manner as tried-and-true AHAs such as glycolic or lactic acids. This Face Cream does contain salicylic acid as well, but not in an amount that would prove efficacious, despite the fact that the pH of this product would allow exfoliation to occur. At best, this is worthwhile as a lightweight moisturizer with antioxidants, and is best for normal to dry skin.

☹ AVERAGE $$$ **Dermal Repair Cream** *($120 for 1.7 fl. oz.)* has a major weakness (well beyond its high price): jar packaging. With antioxidants so central in this formula, jar packaging is absolutely not what you want to see (refer to the Appendix to find out more).

☹ AVERAGE $$$ **Redness Relief CalmPlex** *($80 for 1.6 fl. oz.)* is a surprisingly basic, overpriced moisturizer that is all but void of state-of-the-art ingredients proven to reduce redness. Where are the anti-irritants and skin-repairing ingredients? Glycerin is present (and it's a great repairing ingredient), but hundreds of moisturizers use glycerin. SkinMedica uses an ingredient known as 4-ethoxybenzaldehyde to reduce facial redness, yet research on this compound is limited, to say the least. The single study attesting to the redness-reducing effects of 4-ethoxybenzaldehyde examined daily use of a product with 1% of this ingredient (likely the amount SkinMedica uses) over a 4-week period. The study was done double-blind (always good, because neither the participants nor the evaluators know who got which product), but the improvements weren't all that spectacular. Of particular curiosity is that all the subjects had rosacea that was classified as "stable," which likely means they were using other products to control their symptoms. In the end, we cannot say for certain if the study's results were from the combination of 4-ethoxybenazaldehyde with a prescription topical treatment or if the ingredient itself really helped (Source: *Dermatologic Surgery*, July 2005, pages 881–885). At best, this is an OK option for those with slightly dry skin. The fact that it's fragrance-free makes it good for sensitive skin, too, but really, sensitive skin needs more than what this can provide.

☺ AVERAGE **$$$ TNS Ultimate Daily Moisturizer + SPF 20** *($85 for 2 fl. oz.)*. This in-part zinc oxide sunscreen for normal to dry skin contains an interesting blend of ingredients. Included are novel water-binding agents, antioxidants, and skin-identical ceramides. The amount of SkinMedica's questionable human fibroblast conditioned media is potentially cause for concern because we simply don't know (nor does SkinMedica, at least not with a strong degree of certainty) how safe growth factors are when used as part of a daily anti-aging skin-care routine on healthy, intact skin. For now, all that can be reasonably concluded is that there are too many unknowns about topical use of growth factors to deem it advisable to seek this group of ingredients when shopping for anti-aging products.

☹ POOR **TNS Essential Serum** *($260 for 1 fl. oz.)*. SkinMedica sells many serums, but because TNS Essential is their most expensive serum, they wanted to let you know it is "unparalleled" for anti-aging, which of course begs the question as to why do they keep selling their other products? Shouldn't this be the only one you need? This product is neither unparalleled nor the serum to beat, but we must say that it contains some outstanding ingredients and is beautifully packaged. It is brimming with antioxidants and includes a potentially effective amount of the skin-lightening agent alpha-arbutin. All of that is good news, but it doesn't justify the price. For this amount of money, you may as well have your skin discolorations treated with any of the light-emitting devices that have proven successful, from Intense Pulsed Light to Fraxel, assuming you're a good candidate for these procedures. Despite the beneficial ingredients in this product there is a major caveat. It is, in fact, what SkinMedica is known for: "human fibroblast conditioned media." The human fibroblast conditioned media/TNS complex present in many of SkinMedica anti-aging products is a cocktail of growth factors, none of which have a history of safety when used as part of a daily anti-aging skin-care routine on healthy, intact skin. A detailed report on human fibroblast conditioned media is presented in the introductory summary for SkinMedica, which is available for free on CosmeticsCop.com. For now, all that can be reasonably concluded is that there are too many unknowns about topical use of growth factors to deem it advisable to seek products with this group of ingredients when shopping for anti-aging products. Conceivably, it's a promising field, but your skin doesn't need to be the guinea pig for what may prove to be problematic with ongoing use. The large amount of human fibroblast conditioned media in this serum (it is the first ingredient) is why, despite several positives, it is not rated favorably. Of lesser concern but still worthy of mention is that the formula contains several fragrance ingredients that pose a risk of irritation (and that's not what you want your anti-aging products to do).

☹ POOR **TNS Eye Repair** *($95 for 0.5 fl. oz.)*. It is a shame that jar packaging was chosen because this fragrance-free eye cream is brimming with potent antioxidants (all of which will break down and become ineffective with repeated exposure to light and air). Impressive ingredients abound, while emollients provide smoothing relief for normal or slightly dry skin. Aside from the disappointing packaging, you also have to consider SkinMedica's unique ingredient, human fibroblast conditioned media. Considering the unknowns surrounding topical use of this growth factor blend and the amount present, this eye cream is not recommended. For more information on this topic, please refer to the summary of the SkinMedica brand on CosmeticsCop.com. The same comments and concerns apply to SkinMedica's **TNS Illuminating Eye Cream** ($85 for 0.5 fl. oz.).

☹ POOR **TNS Recovery Complex** *($165 for 0.63 fl. oz.)* is among the most heavily hyped product in the SkinMedica line but as it turns out, there's not much to this fuchsia-tinted, water-based serum except for the TNS complex of growth factors (human fibroblast conditioned media). This complex is the first ingredient, but before you get excited that your aging concerns are over, please refer to the summary for SkinMedica at CosmeticsCop.com. There you will find information on what's behind this ingredient complex as well as a discussion of the potential risks associated with using a cocktail of growth factors daily on healthy skin. These risks are compounded when you're using multiple products with growth factors, and especially one such as this, where the growth factors are the predominant ingredient. This product also contains several fragrance ingredients that put your skin at risk for irritation. The bottom line: There is no reason to consider this serum over many others, whose formulas treat skin to a blend of proven ingredients that can improve its appearance, which includes making wrinkles less apparent and improving discolorations. You'll find such serums in the Best Products chapter at the end of this book.

SKINMEDICA SUN CARE

☺ GOOD $$$ **Daily Physical Defense SPF 30+** *($45 for 3 fl. oz.)* is a good, though somewhat pricey, sunscreen for normal to oily or sensitive skin. Broad-spectrum sun protection is provided from gentle mineral actives titanium dioxide and zinc oxide, and the formula is fragrance-free. It has a light, silky texture that, true to claim, wears well under makeup. It's also great for use around the eyes because the mineral actives are unlikely to cause irritation or stinging. The inactive ingredients are listed in alphabetical rather than descending order, which is permitted by the FDA because sunscreens are regulated as over-the-counter drugs. This sunscreen would be rated higher if it contained a greater range of antioxidants and repairing ingredients. The caffeine and green tea will be helpful, but for the money more antioxidants would propel this to a Best rating.

☺ GOOD $$$ **Environmental Defense Sunscreen SPF 50+** *($45 for 3 fl. oz.)*. This fragrance-free, water-resistant sunscreen provides critical UVA (think anti-aging) protection with its in-part zinc oxide sunscreen. The base formula has a silky lotion texture that's best for normal to oily skin. It's not a slam-dunk for breakout-prone skin, but as is the case with most sunscreens, you need to experiment to see how this texture feels to you. The amount of zinc oxide is unlikely to cause or worsen breakouts. SkinMedica included some notable antioxidants, which is always a plus for any SPF-rated product. All in all, though pricey, this is a very good sunscreen to consider.

SKINMEDICA LIP CARE

☹ POOR **TNS LipPlump System** *($55)* makes claims that it will restore lip volume and fullness in minutes, seemingly replacing what aging takes away and, of course, allowing you to avoid lip injections; however, lip injections really do make a difference (tsk, tsk… and to think a dermatologist is behind this silliness). Step 1 involves applying **Lip Renewal**, which is a standard lip balm in most respects, except for the TNS complex of growth factors (listed as human fibroblast conditioned media). The collagen and elastin in this product cannot plump lips from the outside in, but they're effective water-binding agents. There is no research anywhere demonstrating that any growth factor, lab-engineered or not, can restore fullness to lips that have thinned over the years; so this is just a good lip balm with a potentially questionable ingredient (i.e., TNS complex). Step 2 is the **Lip Plumper**, a lip gloss-type product that causes a feeling of warmth and increased circulation to lips because it contains benzyl nicotinate. This B-vitamin derivative isn't as irritating as the potent menthol and pepper combinations often seen in lip plumpers, and it works to an extent—just don't expect the full, pouty lips you've dreamed of. Although the Lip Plumper is fairly innocuous, the unknowns about frequent use of growth hormones on lips is frightening, especially if you consider that you're going to be ingesting at least a small amount of these hormones.

SKINMEDICA SPECIALTY SKIN-CARE PRODUCTS

☺ GOOD $$$ **Acne Treatment Lotion** *($52 for 2 fl. oz.)* is a very expensive, but effective, topical disinfectant for acne-prone skin. It contains 2.5% benzoyl peroxide as the active ingredient, and is in a lightweight base suitable for all skin types. The only cause for concern is the witch hazel and sage extract, though we suspect these ingredients don't comprise much of the total formula. This will help with acne, but given the range of less expensive benzoyl peroxide products, it's a tough sell.

☹ POOR **TNS Line Refine** *($75 for 0.12 fl. oz.)* is sold as a product that can rapidly fill in and smooth wrinkles around the mouth and eye, two spots where most women absolutely don't want to see signs of aging. Of course, you won't actually see your wrinkles reduced, at least not to the extent you may be hoping. The texture of this product means it has a mild, spackle-like effect on skin. It contains a lot of film-forming agent that works to temporarily fill superficial (not etched) wrinkles, though how long the visual trickery lasts depends on how expressive you are. As for long-term benefits, although this product contains some intriguing ingredients, none are capable of making skin look progressively younger. Like most of the leave-on products from SkinMedica, this contains their TNS complex, built around their human fibroblast conditioned media ingredient. TNS is a blend of human growth factors that present unknown risks to skin, and are a big reason why this product isn't recommended. (For more information about TNS complex, please refer to the brand summary for SkinMedica at CosmeticsCop.com). The other reason TNS Line Refine isn't recommended is because it contains the irritating menthol derivative menthyl lactate. Clearly, SkinMedica doesn't really believe this works or why else would they need to include an ingredient that gives consumers the impression the product is doing something? Unfortunately, routine irritation from this menthol derivative won't help skin of any age improve (see the Appendix to learn how irritation hurts your skin).

SMASHBOX (MAKEUP ONLY)

Strengths: A unique Anti-Shine product for very oily skin; mostly good foundations with a neutral range of shades; the powder eyeshadows; Photo Finish Lipstick; a lash primer that really makes a difference; well-constructed makeup brushes that cost less than the department store competition.

Weaknesses: Many products are priced higher than they should be; a couple of products contain irritants that have no benefit for skin; several lackluster makeup categories, including concealer, blush, eye pencils, and brow shapers; the Cream Eyeliner is a mistake if you expect any amount of longevity; several specialty products that should offer more for the money.

For more information and the latest Smashbox reviews, visit CosmeticsCop.com.

SMASHBOX FOUNDATIONS & PRIMERS

☺ GOOD $$$ **Camera Ready Full Coverage Foundation SPF 15** *($38)* is a cream-to-powder foundation that provides almost opaque coverage. It applies creamy but sets to a satin finish that can feel slightly moist. The titanium dioxide sunscreen provides excellent UVA/UVB protection without making skin look chalky. Those with normal to dry skin will find this an excellent option; the formula is too creamy for anyone with combination or oily skin and the waxes are not for anyone with acne-prone skin. Ignore the included too-rough-to-use brush, it's useless. The shade range is limited to options for those with fair to medium skin tones. Watch out for Medium M3 and M4 and for Dark D1, which are too yellow and orange for most to use convincingly. If not for the cumbersome, difficult-to-open compact, this would have rated a Best Product.

☺ GOOD $$$ **Camera Ready BB Cream SPF 35** *($39)*. Smashbox is on the BB cream bandwagon, and although their contribution is a good one, it bears repeating that BB creams are not miraculous or must-have products. Essentially, they're just tinted moisturizers (most include sunscreen) that usually contain a few extra ingredients that may or may not benefit your skin. This provides decent broad-spectrum sun protection that includes titanium dioxide for sufficient UVA protection, though the amount is on the low side for optimum protection, which makes this a bit less desirable from a sun protection standpoint. This fragrance-free formula has a slightly thick yet creamy-soft texture that blends easily and meshes well with skin. It provides sheer to light coverage and a natural-looking matte finish that helps keep excess shine in check, at least for a few hours (this won't replace a mattifier or other oil-absorbing product you may be using). The five shades offer a greater range than most BB creams (two shades are what's typically offered) and all of them are workable. Note that the Medium shade is darker than what usually passes for "medium" and the Dark shade is slightly copper but still worth checking out. In terms of the claims, this doesn't provide an "ethereal effect," nor is it hydrating enough to please those with dry skin. It is best for normal to combination or oily skin. As for enhancing makeup wear, this works—but no better than a lightweight serum or moisturizer that's compatible with your skin type.

☺ GOOD $$$ **High Definition Healthy F/X Foundation SPF 15** *($38)* is said to be packed with anti-aging and firming ingredients that revitalize skin. The in-part titanium dioxide sunscreen deserves most of the credit for anti-aging (assuming you apply this daily and liberally), but nothing in this product will revitalize or firm skin. The silky, fluid texture is built around no fewer than six forms of silicone, and they ensure a smooth, even application that meshes well with skin, which is this foundation's strongest point. Blending takes longer than usual but is OK, and this sets to a soft satin finish appropriate for normal to slightly dry skin (even if it's prone to blemishes). You'll get medium coverage that looks surprisingly skin-like, and this wears quite well. Among the mostly neutral shades, the only ones to consider carefully are Light L3 and Medium M3. There are no shades for fair skin tones, but everyone in between (including darker skin tones) should find a good match.

☺ GOOD $$$ **Photo Finish Foundation Primer Light** *($36 for 1 fl. oz.)* contains nothing to combat blemishes and has minimal ability to (temporarily) fill in large pores, but it doesn't contain ingredients that aggravate or encourage blemishes, which is a plus. The water-based serum is fragrance-free and contains a tiny amount of vitamin C. It works well under foundation, but

---

♠ Irritating ingredients are a problem for all skin types. Find out why in the Appendix.

if your skin is oily and you're using a matte-finish foundation, this won't provide a significant boost in terms of wear-time. It makes application smoother, but that's a tactile sensation rather than a legitimate need (your foundation should go on smoothly if you're using a good one and taking care of your skin). Still, primers have their proponents, and this is one more to consider.

☺ GOOD $$$ **Photo Finish Luminizing Foundation Primer** *($38)*. This bronze-tinted primer looks dark in the bottle, but on application it sheers out to leave your skin with a soft, peachy tan sheen laced with a golden copper shimmer. The silky, weightless texture feels great and it has a dry matte (in feel) finish suitable for normal to oily skin, assuming those with oily skin don't mind adding more shine. As claimed, this primer contains some notable antioxidants; however, the clear pump bottle packaging demands careful storage away from light to preserve their efficacy. This primer isn't a superior replacement for a matte-finish serum loaded with beneficial ingredients, but just like such a serum, it facilitates makeup application and has a minor, temporary filling effect on large pores and superficial lines.

☺ GOOD $$$ **Photo Finish Targeted Pore & Line Primer** *($32)*. This silicone-based primer is sold as being able to reduce wrinkles while filling in pores. To some extent, it does this because of its spackle-like texture. It dispenses as a thick, translucent paste that you pat into and over lines and large pores. Once set, you'll notice a slight filling effect, just like you'll get from many other primers with this texture. As for the anti-aging peptides, they're barely present, and there's no substantiated research proving they're an ace solution for wrinkles. Whether used under or over makeup, this primer and its powdery matte finish help fill in superficial wrinkles and pores, at least for a few hours.

☺ GOOD $$$ **Sheer Focus Tinted Moisturizer SPF 15** *($30)* is so sheer that any coverage you get will be accidental! That makes choosing from among the four shades (plus a shimmer shade labeled "Luminous") as easy as figuring out which one comes closest to the depth of your skin tone. The sunscreen includes zinc oxide for sufficient UVA protection, and the fluid, moist texture has good slip so blending is easy. Sheer Focus sets to a satin-matte finish. The vitamins and anti-aging peptides Smashbox refers to are barely present—all of them are listed after the preservative—so they don't even come close to qualifying as "packed." Still, this is a good, very sheer tinted moisturizer for normal to dry skin.

☹ AVERAGE $$$ **Photo Finish Foundation Primer** *($36 for 1 fl. oz.)* is a colorless, silicone-based serum that has little going for it other than being a fairly standard silicone-enriched primer that makes your skin feel smooth. Applying this can help ensure a semi-matte finish when paired with a matte-finish liquid or powder foundation. That's good for normal to oily or combination skin, but the formula isn't as elegant as several serums that function like primers but provide skin with a wide complement of beneficial ingredients. This contains some great antioxidants, but the clear bottle packaging means this must be stored away from light to ensure the potency of these beneficial ingredients.

☹ AVERAGE $$$ **Photo Finish Foundation Primer SPF 15 & Dermaxyl** *($42 for 1 fl. oz.)* does not provide sufficient UVA protection, so the sun protection claims cannot be relied on, and that's never a good sign for an anti-aging product (see the Appendix to learn which UVA-protecting ingredients to look for). This silicone-based primer does contain several antioxidants, but the translucent glass packaging won't help keep them stable, so that's a loss as well. The Dermaxyl complex is a trademark of ingredient manufacturer Sederma. The key ingredient is palmitoyl oligopeptide and although this has potentially intriguing benefits for skin, the amount Smashbox includes doesn't measure up to the quantity Sederma recommends for efficacy. That means, at best, that the peptide functions as a water-binding agent, making this Smashbox primer slightly more hydrating than the other Smashbox primers—but the price is unwarranted.

☺ AVERAGE $$$ **Photo Finish Color Correcting Foundation Primer** *($38)* is a pure silicone-based primer that, like others, can make skin feel very silky and appear matte. Such an even canvas can facilitate makeup application, but this Smashbox product offers a few strangely tinted shades meant to correct uneven skin tones (such as redness, sallowness, and so on). Thankfully, the peach and lavender shades are so sheer the color change is minimal, meaning that your foundation won't look strange when used with them. However, the green shade has too much color and gives skin an odd, alien hue that substitutes one problem for another. These are not preferred to Smashbox's other Photo Finish primers.

☺ AVERAGE $$$ **Studio Skin 15 Hour Wear Foundation SPF 10** *($42)*. This fragrance-free liquid foundation blends on well and sets to a matte finish that stays put throughout the day, but the 15-hour claim is really pushing it; after 15 hours, there isn't going to be much foundation left. With over 10 shades, ranging from fair to deep, you're likely to find a color that suits your skin tone. Coverage is in the medium range, which makes it ideal for minor skin tone issues or small imperfections. Although this provides broad-spectrum sun protection, the low SPF rating is disappointing, and demands that you pair this foundation with a product rated SPF 15 or greater underneath.

SMASHBOX CONCEALERS

☺ AVERAGE $$$ **Camera Ready Full Coverage Concealer** *($20)* is a creamy, twist-up stick concealer that applies smoothly and blends well, though it remains moist and quickly settles into lines around the eye. Despite the name, this provides full coverage only if you pile it on—and that causes it to crease even more. This is still worth considering if you want a cream concealer and the eight shades are nearly impeccable (shade 1 is too white for just about anyone), but it must be set with powder to minimize the creasing.

☺ AVERAGE $$$ **Eye Beam Double-Ended Brightener** *($22)*. This dual-sided pencil offers two flesh-toned shades, each needing routine sharpening to maintain a fine point. The texture of both is smooth and they glide over skin, being initially creamy but setting to a dry finish that stays put better than expected (thanks to talc, which is the third ingredient). This pencil brightens the eye area with each shade's soft, pearlescent finish. When applied sparingly and softly blended with a brush, the effect can be flattering. This is worth a look if you don't mind pencils that require regular sharpening.

☺ AVERAGE $$$ **High Definition Concealer** *($20)* is a water- and silicone-based concealer that has a slightly creamy texture and decent slip for controlled blending. It provides nearly full coverage, but its smooth matte finish has a tendency to look chalky. Another issue is that although it's a squeeze tube, the opening readily dispenses too much product, and putting it back in is a messy endeavor. One more comment: Other than the fact that all the shades except Medium/Dark are good, this concealer contains angelica root extract, which can cause contact dermatitis (Source: naturaldatabase.com).

☺ AVERAGE $$$ **Photo Op Under Eye Brightener** *($19)* is a concealer/highlighter combination product applied with a brush. It imparts sheer to light coverage for minor flaws and leaves obvious sparkles on skin (that's the "brightening" part). Smashbox recommends using this with a concealer, which is a good idea if you need more than meager coverage. In photographs, the amount of shine this leaves behind may prove to be too much, and it's definitely overkill for daytime makeup.

SMASHBOX POWDERS

✓☺ BEST **$$$ Photo Set Finishing Powder SPF 15** *($28)* is a lightweight, fragrance-free loose-powder that feels luxuriously smooth and sheers out onto skin for a nearly imperceptible finish, although those with dark skin tones may notice a slight whitish tint. Best of all, it sets makeup, absorbs oil, and protects skin with reliable broad-spectrum sun protection from the sun's harmful rays. Although this provides reliable broad-spectrum sun protection, it is not wise to rely on any powder as your sole source of sunscreen. That's because you need to apply sunscreen liberally to obtain the SPF rating on the label of a product, and most people are unlikely to apply a powder liberally enough, especially one at this price, to get the needed level of protection. For best results, use powders with sunscreen as an add-on to your moisturizer or foundation with sunscreen.

✓☺ BEST **$$$ Photo Set Pressed Powder** *($29)* has a lightweight texture that goes on satin smooth to even out your skin tone. Four neutral shades (ranging from fair to dark) are offered, each of which initially goes on sheer, but layers well for medium coverage without looking powdery and cakey.

SMASHBOX BLUSHES & BRONZERS

✓☺ BEST **$$$ Bronze Lights** *($29)* is one of the best talc-based pressed bronzing powders around. It has a wonderfully smooth texture that makes application nearly foolproof, plus it looks incredibly natural on skin. Even better, both shades (Suntan Matte is preferred, Sunkissed Matte is more peachy than bronze) offer a matte finish! It's definitely a consideration if you love bronzing powder but are tired of those with sparkles.

☺ GOOD **$$$ Blush Rush** *($24)* is a sheer powder blush whose suede-smooth texture applies beautifully. Each shade is infused with some shimmer, but the product application is so sheer that it doesn't pose a problem for daytime wear. Ignore the long-wearing claims because this will wear just as well, but not better than, any other similarly formulated powder blush. The Flush shade is a beautiful pale pink that also works great as a highlighter.

☺ GOOD **$$$ Halo Hydrating Perfecting Bronzer** *($39)* is a powder bronzer that comes in semi-solid form, but the method of application turns it into a loose powder. The component includes a metal sifter mechanism that shaves off powder from the disc below, pushing it up and out so it's ready for application. This isn't a packaging or formulary necessity, but it's a clever, relatively clean way to use loose powder. As for the powder, it has a soft, silky texture and imparts low-glow radiance to skin. The color is a beautiful golden bronze that looks great on all but very dark skin tones. Smashbox mentions that this loose bronzing powder reduces signs of aging, but the formula's trace amounts of beneficial extras cannot do that, not to mention that the finish isn't much for taking the focus away from wrinkles. The 48 minerals allegedly in this powder are nowhere to be found on the ingredient list, so consider that and the anti-aging claims to be bogus. Still, this is a very good, loose bronzing powder if the cost doesn't give you pause.

☺ AVERAGE **$$$ O-Glow** *($26)* Remember mood rings? The jewelry that changed color after being in contact with your skin? Smashbox tries to recapture that idea with a silicone-based clear blush they refer to as "intuitive" because "this clear gel reacts with your personal skin chemistry to turn cheeks the exact color you blush, naturally in just seconds!" Sounds like the perfect "natural blush," but the claim is bogus. Yes, this goes on clear and changes color as it blends—but it turns into the same translucent fuchsia hue on everyone. The Paula's Choice staff represents skin tones from fair to dark. We asked several staffers to sample this blush and let us know what color it turned on their skin, and did they think it matches how they blush naturally. All of them had the same color response (fuchsia) and none of them claimed to blush this shade (no one does). We admit, it's cool to watch a clear gel turn into a vibrant pink shade as you blend, and this has a smooth powder finish that lasts, but the color itself isn't personalized and the strong color isn't going to work for everyone.

SMASHBOX EYESHADOWS & EYE PRIMER

✓☺ BEST $$$ **Photo Op Eye Shadow Trio** *($28)* is a pressed-powder eyeshadow that comes in a flip-cap compact with three shades separated by plastic dividers (a nice touch). The texture is inordinately smooth and the color payoff (how much color you get with a single swipe of the brush) is great. Blending is almost effortless, too, and the colors tend to go on true. The drawback, at least if you want a matte finish, is that every trio is shiny. Depending on the set the shine can range from soft to obvious sparkles but at least it doesn't flake all over. The best trios for workable shine and a good combination of colors include Shutterspeed, Multi-Flash, Filter (this one is almost matte), Cover Shot, and Auto Expose.

☺ GOOD $$$ **Photo Finish Lid Primer** *($20)*. Sold as "an ultra-luxurious lid primer" (we guess when you're offering a superfluous makeup item you need a good adjective to make it sound important), this is merely a peach-tinged liquid concealer that offers slight camouflage and sets quickly to a dry matte finish. The finish has a subtle tackiness to it that doesn't make eyeshadow application easier, but it's not a deal-breaker. The best reason to consider this is if you have oily eyelids and you're not satisfied with the results you get using a regular concealer with a strong matte finish. If that's not your dilemma, this is easy to pass up.

☺ GOOD $$$ **Single Eye Shadow** *($16)* has an impressively smooth texture that applies evenly, and only the shiniest shades are mildly prone to flaking (every color has some amount of shine). The only drawback (and for some this may be a plus) is that even the darkest shades tend to go on sheer, so building intensity takes some effort.

SMASHBOX EYE & BROW LINERS

☺ GOOD $$$ **Limitless Eye Liner** *($19)*. If you don't mind spending more than you need to for a basic eyeliner, this automatic, retractable pencil with a built-in sharpener (should you decide you need it) is very good. The silicone- and wax-based formula goes on smoothly and a bit creamy, but sets to a budge-proof finish. Once set, the liner remains tacky to the touch, but that isn't an issue that you'll notice unless you routinely rub your eyes, which is a great way to ruin your nicely applied eye makeup—so don't do that! Other than the metallic blue Peacock shade, the colors are rich and ideal for dramatic eye lining.

☺ GOOD $$$ **Jet Set Waterproof Eye Liner** *($22)* is waterproof, comes in a range of classic and trendy colors (of which Teal is not recommended), and wears beautifully. We couldn't fault anyone for using this eyeliner, but we'd be sure to tell them they spent too much money! Note: Like most long-wearing gel liners, this one has a tendency to dry out unless you replace the cap tightly after each and every use. Forgetting to do this even once can make this eyeliner unusable.

☺ AVERAGE $$$ **Brow Tech** *($24)* is described by Smashbox as "the answer to everyone's prayers," but before you reconsider your pleas for world peace or that new car you've always wanted, consider that this is merely a split-pan compact with a shine-infused brow powder that you mix with the other half, which is a clear, thick wax. But no one needs shiny eyebrows, and the wax can look heavy and thick, not a look everyone will appreciate.

☺ AVERAGE **$$$ Brow Tech Trio** *($24)* comes with two pressed-powder brow colors and a wax to set them in place. In each set, the lighter shade is meant to fill brows and the darker shade is supposed to be used to define them, or you can mix them together to customize your ideal shade. There are good options for blonde, brunette, or auburn-colored brows. The wax helps hold brow shape without leaving hairs stiff, but we wish they included a brush or comb to apply it (especially at this price). As is, you're left with using your fingertips, which doesn't offer the most precision or control. All in all, this is a decent product, but at this price we expected more.

☺ AVERAGE **$$$ Brow Tech To Go** *($26)* comes with a creamy, waxy brow pencil on one end and a brush-on clear brow gel on the other. The brush is useful for sweeping hairs into place, and the gel helps them stay put with a soft, flexible hold. The automatic pencil's tip is wider than some may prefer, which makes it difficult to draw thin strokes to fill in between brow hairs. We also noticed that it was prone to crumbling, so application can get a bit messy and waste product. Color-wise, the two shades (Taupe and Brunette) are natural-looking and last all day, but all things considered, this brow enhancer has too many flaws to be worth your time and money.

☺ AVERAGE **$$$ Limitless Waterproof Liquid Liner Pen** *($22)*. Perhaps it's because alcohol is the fourth ingredient, but this felt-tip pen–style liquid eyeliner is prone to fading with little provocation. On application, the color is intense and spreads in a controlled, fluid fashion along the upper lash line. Dry time is, not surprisingly, quite fast, but it's disappointing that the intensity doesn't last long, although at least it isn't prone to flaking. A better choice for strong color and stay-put results is M.A.C.'s Fluidline.

☹ POOR **Cream Eye Liner** *($22)* is an interesting notion that sounds better than it ends up being. In the pro column, these do go on very smoothly and intensely. The cons include their tendency to fade, smear, and run with the slightest blink or smile, which makes them not worth the effort, especially at this price. For a superior version of this product, consider the silicone-enhanced gel eyeliners available from Bobbi Brown, Stila, M.A.C., or L'Oreal.

SMASHBOX LIP COLOR & LIPLINER

✓☺ BEST **$$$ Limitless Long Wear Lip Gloss SPF 15** *($22)* is an excellent lip gloss that includes an in-part avobenzone sunscreen. The shade range is pleasing and each shade goes on sheer, leaving a high-gloss finish that feels sticky. The stickiness is a trade-off for the tenacious wear you get from this gloss. It also has minimal slickness so it's a good choice for those who find that gloss barely stays on their lips before they're out the door.

✓☺ BEST **$$$ Lip Enhancing Gloss** *($18)*. Although you don't need to spend this much to get a great lip gloss, this is an excellent option that also happens to be fragrance-free. It has an unusually moist but sheer texture that hydrates lips while providing a non-sticky, beautifully glossy finish. The sponge-tip applicator is simple to use and the shade range offers an enticing mix of soft and dramatic colors. The selection is plentiful without being overwhelming—not a bad shade in the bunch!

✓☺ BEST **$$$ Reflection High Shine Lip Gloss** *($19)* is an excellent emollient lip gloss. It has a smooth application and highly reflective, dimensional finish that works alone or applied over any shade of lipstick, and it's only minimally sticky.

☺ GOOD **$$$ Be Legendary Lipstick** *($19)*. This creamy lipstick goes on slightly thick and melts into lips for a moisturizing, smooth feel. The shade range is extensive and includes attractive options for most skin tones. Colors go on opaque with a creamy, ever-so-slightly shiny finish. Beware of the texture of this lipstick. It lends itself to bleeding into fines lines around the mouth, but if that's not an issue, this is a nice lipstick option.

☺ GOOD $$$ **Limitless Lip Stain & Color Seal Balm** *($23)*. This version of what looks like a magic marker–style lip stain comes dual-ended. In addition to the lip stain on one end, you get a lip balm in the same shade as the stain on the other end. This might seem like a good way to combat the inherent dryness of a lip stain, but, unfortunately, using the balm over the stain breaks down the color faster, affecting its longevity, and there goes the benefit of using a lip stain. We got about three hours of wear (nowhere near the eight hours Smashbox claims) before it started to show significant signs of wear. If you're willing to compromise on long wear, you'll find this a very good lip stain that doesn't grab on dry spots or bleed into lines around the mouth. The shades are all bright or bold (Sangria is a juicy red) and opaque, so your lips really make a statement!

☹ AVERAGE $$$ **The Nude Lip Liner** *($16)*. This standard, needs-sharpening pencil has a silicone base that helps create a soft, creamy texture that glides on and sets to a slightly tacky, but budge-proof finish. As the name states, the small group of colors are nude/lip-toned shades, each with a brown undertone many will find versatile. The shades correspond with different skin tones from fair to dark, and it's a good way to determine which shade will work best for you. For example, the Dark shade is close to a chocolate brown, and looks much better against a darker skin tone than it does on someone with fair skin. This would earn a higher rating if not for the need to routinely sharpen.

☹ POOR **O-Gloss** *($22)*. The original pink O-Gloss Intuitive Lip Gloss has now expanded to include a Noir version and a Gold version, each claiming to transform to your lip's own perfect shade. Hardly an "intuitive" gloss, each version turns nearly the same shade on everyone, with slight differences depending on the natural color of your lips. The original O-Gloss dispenses clear and turns a sheer shade of pink when applied to your lips. The Noir version dispenses as a dark blackberry color and turns to a sheer berry shade. The Gold version dispenses as a shimmering gold color and turns shimmering peach as you apply. Each gloss has a smooth but somewhat sticky texture with a high-shine finish. Despite the novelty, there are several ingredients in this gloss that cause irritation (peppermint oil among them), and as such it is not recommended.

SMASHBOX MASCARAS

✓☺ BEST $$$ **Bionic Mascara** *($19)* has a silly name and makes even sillier claims (ions do not make eyelashes stronger or longer), but wow: does this mascara deliver dramatic results! With just a few strokes, lashes are thickened, incredibly long, and beautifully defined. The formula is water-resistant (it'll withstand slight tearing or a light mist of rain), but not waterproof. It removes with a water-soluble cleanser and wears all day without flaking or smearing, which is just more to love about Smashbox's best mascara.

✓☺ BEST $$$ **Layer Lash Primer** *($17)* is one of a handful of lash primers that actually do make a difference, even when used with an already-outstanding mascara. The effect (especially with the best mascaras) isn't night-and-day, but if you're looking to eke a bit more out of your usual mascara, this product is a decent add-on—and that's a refreshing change of pace! One of the reasons it works where others fail is that its conditioning formula keeps lashes soft and flexible, while at the same time allowing a regular mascara to adhere evenly to already-pumped-up lashes.

☹ POOR **Full Exposure Mascara** *($19)* allows you to create thick, long lashes with just a couple of strokes, but this impressive feat comes with significant drawbacks: The brush is oversized and difficult to maneuver around the eyes without getting mascara on the eyelid and under-brow area (even if you're being exceptionally careful); the formula tends to smear quickly and takes longer than usual to set; and some flaking occurs during wear, leading to red, irritated eyes. In the end, if the concept of a big brush for big results appeals to you, consider any of the Diorshow mascaras from Dior.

☹ POOR **Hyperlash Mascara** *($21)*. This mascara's selling point is that the applicator features standard rubber bristles on one side and comb-like vertical bristles on the other. The brush side is said to build and thicken while the comb side defines and lengthens. Unfortunately, neither side results in beautiful lashes. Whether you use one side followed by the other or pay no attention to which side you're using, you'll get an uneven, slightly too wet application that takes considerable effort to make lashes look separated and dramatic. Once set, lashes tend to stick together and look slightly bent, requiring repair work. You'll also be dealing with smearing and flaking before you can say "Well, that was a waste of money!" Don't bother.

SMASHBOX FACE & BODY ILLUMINATORS

☺ GOOD **$$$ Fusion Soft Lights** *($30)* are nearly identical to the regular Soft Lights reviewed below, but feature individual strips of color in one unit that can be applied separately or swirled together for a high-shine effect that appears almost glossy (but feels powder dry).

☺ GOOD **$$$ Soft Lights** *($29)* is a smooth-textured pressed shimmer powder that blends beautifully and clings better than expected. The shine ranges from subtle (Glow and Hue) to Las Vegas–caliber glitz.

☺ AVERAGE **$$$ Artificial Light Luminizing Lotion** *($26)* has a very silky, fluid feel and produces a shimmer that's softly metallic. It's an OK option for shine, but because this stays moist it is prone to rubbing off and fading. For this amount of money, there should be no drawbacks, and overall this isn't worth considering over better, longer-lasting options from Lorac or Make Up For Ever.

☺ AVERAGE **$$$ Artificial Light Luminizing Powder** *($20)* comes in an inconveniently small tube into which you must dip the sponge-like tip applicator in order to pick up the color so you can apply the loose powder. The applicator makes it difficult to use, especially on larger areas. On the plus side, the shimmering, creamy gold color imparts a beautiful glow, ideal for highlighting areas such as the brow bone or cheekbone. However, you only get 0.035 ounces, so you're really overpaying for such a small amount of product, especially given that the applicator doesn't help and, in fact, makes it harder to use.

SMASHBOX BRUSHES

✓☺ BEST **$$$ #13 Foundation Brush** *($29)*. For those so inclined, Smashbox's synthetic-hair #13 Foundation Brush is one of the better brushes of its type available and the price is comparable to those of most other lines. Other ☺ GOOD **$$$ Smashbox Brushes** ($18–$52) are more realistically priced than those of other artistry-based lines, and there are some expert options to consider, all with snazzy red lacquered handles that visually set them apart from the standard black of other lines. The ones to consider are **#12 Angle Brow** ($20), **#15 Definer Brush** ($24), **#10 Crease Brush** ($24), **#19 Face & Body Brush** ($52), and **#9 Cream Eye Liner Brush** ($20), the last being one of the better types of this brush around because it's thin enough to use for both upper and lower lashlines and you can make the line as thin or thick as you like using almost any eyeshadow.

SMASHBOX SPECIALTY MAKEUP PRODUCTS

✓☺ BEST **$$$ Anti-Shine** *($27 for 1 fl. oz.)* remains an intriguing product for anyone with very oily skin. Its colorless formula contains mostly water and absorbent magnesium. Magnesium (as in Phillips' Milk of Magnesia) absorbs oil very well and does not feel as heavy on the skin as clays do. This formula goes on extremely matte and dry and has great staying power; it is definitely worth trying if you have oily to very oily skin, and it works well with a matte-finish foundation. Anti-Shine may be applied under or over foundation to keep oiliness in check. Another option with a more elegant texture is Paula's Choice Shine Stopper Instant Matte Finish.

SONIA KASHUK (MAKEUP ONLY)

Strengths: Affordable and widely available (though exclusive to Target stores); good makeup remover; the makeup is the star attraction, with impressive options for foundation, powder, blush, lip color, eyeliner, and especially makeup brushes.

Weaknesses: The concealers, eye pencil, and brow shapers are a letdown; the makeup palettes may seem convenient, but several of the included products perform poorly.

For more information and reviews of the latest Sonia Kashuk products, visit CosmeticsCop.com.

SONIA KASHUK EYE-MAKEUP REMOVER

✓☺ BEST **Remove Eye Makeup Remover** *($10.19 for 4 fl. oz.)* is a simple, water- and silicone-based makeup remover, but it works beautifully to remove all types of long-wearing makeup and wins extra points for being fragrance-free and including no extraneous ingredients except a tiny amount of coloring agent. The small amount of benzoyl alcohol is part of the preservative system and should not pose a risk of irritation. However, like all preservatives, this may cause minor stinging if you get the product in the eye itself.

SONIA KASHUK FOUNDATIONS & PRIMER

☺ GOOD **Perfecting Luminous Foundation** *($9.99)* has very sheer to light coverage with a dewy finish. This liquid foundation for someone with normal to dry skin has a great soft texture thanks to the significant amounts of silicone and mineral oil. Most of the shades are nicely neutral and worth considering by light to medium skin tones. Camel is an OK option that may be too orange for some medium skin tones. Note: The color visible through the bottle does not resemble the product after it has dried on skin, which makes choosing the best shade a bit tricky.

☺ GOOD **Radiant Tinted Moisturizer SPF 15** *($13.69)* is a lightweight tinted moisturizer with an in-part avobenzone sunscreen. It has a cushiony, moist texture on application, but sets to a soft matte finish with the tiniest hint of shine. You'll achieve soft color and very sheer coverage from each of the shades, all of them outstanding. This formula is best for normal to dry skin. Those with oily or blemish-prone skin will not appreciate the short-lived matte finish, and the thickeners and waxes aren't the best over breakout-prone areas.

☺ AVERAGE **$$$ Primer Vitamin Serum** *($18.99 for 0.5 fl. oz.)* is a fragrance-free foundation primer that has a serum-like texture, but so do most primers that don't mention "serum" in the name. And, for the most part, using a well-formulated serum rather than a primer is better for your skin because you're getting the beneficial ingredients a serum contains along with the smoothing effect primers provide. This isn't recommended over others because it contains a potentially irritating amount of witch hazel distillate. As the most concentrated form of this plant, its alcohol content puts skin at risk for irritation—and if you have oily skin (and the texture of this product makes it best for that skin type), the witch hazel's irritation can stimulate more oil production at the base of the pores. Although this primer contains some beneficial ingredients, it isn't worth considering over other options, whether labeled "primer" or "serum"—you don't need both. This contains salicylic acid, but the product's pH is not within range for this ingredient to function as an exfoliant.

SONIA KASHUK CONCEALERS

☺ AVERAGE **Confidential Concealer with Brightening Pencil** *($6.99)* is a liquid concealer that's so sheer it barely makes a difference if covering dark circles is your goal. It blends well but leaves a shiny finish and is only appropriate for highlighting. The opposite end of this brush-applied concealer is a creamy, retractable pencil that's flesh-toned and loaded with shine. It doesn't so much brighten skin as add sparkles, although they do tend to stay in place.

☺ AVERAGE **Hidden Agenda Concealer Palette** *($10.99)* provides three shades of creamy concealer and one shade of pressed powder in a single compact. The concealer is slightly thick but applies smoothly and covers well. It would be better if it didn't look so heavy with the supplied powder applied over it; a sheerer powder would have worked much better (and the concealer needs to be set with powder to minimize creasing and fading). You'll find only one of the concealer shades are needed, but the range of shades is workable for fair to light/ medium skin tones.

☹ POOR **Take Cover Concealing Stick** *($7.99)* is a lipstick-style concealer that offers four shades, but you cannot see the color without breaking the product open, and the shade swatches at the Kashuk display aren't that accurate. Not only does this have an unpleasantly thick texture, it also finishes slightly sticky and creases almost instantly. Getting back to the shades, the only acceptable color is Dusk; the others are too pink, peach, or olive to consider.

SONIA KASHUK POWDERS

✓☺ BEST **Bare Minimum Pressed Powder** *($9.39)* comes in three soft, neutral colors best for fair to light skin tones, and it has a sublimely silky texture and seamless application. This is one of those rare talc-based powders that look very natural and enhances the complexion rather than dulling it or making skin look too matte and powdery.

☺ GOOD **Barely There Loose Powder** *($8.99)* remains one of the most elegant and gossamer loose powders you'll find in this price range. Its finely milled, silky texture blends beautifully on skin and it comes in three very good colors, best for fair to light skin tones. One small caveat: This features a slightly shiny finish, which isn't ideal if you're using powder to temper shine. This powder is best for normal to dry skin.

☺ GOOD **Brightening Powder** *($10.39)* is a weightless, talc-based loose powder that adds a soft finish to makeup while imparting subtle shine. It's finely milled, which means it picks up easily with a brush and adheres well to skin. In the package the powder appears to be stark white, but it dissipates over skin, creating a softening effect that imparts faint shimmer and luminosity. The well-designed compact twists the sifter closed to keep powder from spilling out.

☺ AVERAGE **Sheer Magic Mineral Face Powder** *($14.79)* offers a **Mineral Concealer**, **Sheer Mineral Powder Foundation**, and **Sheer Mineral Blush** in one cleverly stacked component. The creamy concealer's main ingredient is titanium dioxide, so it goes on opaque and drags a bit during blending. It can easily look too heavy and has a tendency to crease into lines around the eyes and to magnify large pores. The Sheer Mineral Powder Foundation contains only mica and zinc oxide. The mica provides a silky texture and soft glow finish while the zinc oxide provides opacity, giving this loose-powder foundation medium coverage. With the exception of the peachy Honey, all the shades are soft and neutral and include options for fair skin tones. The Sheer Mineral Blush is almost identical to the Sheer Mineral Powder Foundation, but includes a token amount of gemstones that have no effect on skin. For a loose-powder blush, the pigmentation is stronger than expected, so this is best brushed on lightly. Overall, this earns an average rating due to the concealer's drawbacks and the inherent mess that comes with applying foundation and blush in loose-powder form. The packaging lacks conveniences to minimize the mess, while the openings are too small for many full-size brushes. The "mineral" in the names is mere hype, just like it is for the rest of the industry.

SONIA KASHUK BLUSHES & BRONZERS

✓☺ BEST **Beautifying Blush** *($8.99)* is a pressed-powder blush with a super-smooth, non-powdery application and a collection of mostly sheer colors. Building intensity with this blush requires effort, but it's a good option for a hint of color. The matte shades include Flamingo and Pink.

✓☺ BEST **Creme Blush** *($9.89)* is housed in a slim compact and best described as cream-to-powder rather than cream. It's initially creamy, but sets to a soft powder finish that adds an enlivening, non-shimmering glow to cheeks. This is fantastically easy to blend and it lasts longer than a true cream blush. Every shade is beautiful, too!

✓☺ BEST **Super Sheer Liquid Tint** *($9.99)* is a liquid blush that is aptly named! The silky formula imparts super sheer color that gives cheeks a healthy transparent flush. This has a slightly tacky finish, but is much easier to blend than most gel blushes; you get more playtime with Kashuk's tint, whereas a traditional gel blush sets almost immediately. The shade range is small but impressive, and none go on as dark as the packaging may imply. Fans of gel blush, take note!

☺ GOOD **Shimmering Loose Mineral Blush** *($8.79)* is a very sheer, feather-light loose-powder blush that leaves a sparkling finish on skin. Definitely more for adding shine than color to cheeks, it is best dusted on to highlight skin for evening makeup. The sparkles are a bit much for casual or professional daytime makeup, though they cling to skin reasonably well.

☺ AVERAGE **Bare Minimum Pressed Bronzer** *($9.99)* has a big golden yellow "S" in the middle of it; the "S" is for "Sonia." When combined with the darker bronzing powder that surrounds it, however, the result on skin is more golden peach with shimmer than anything resembling a tan. This is an OK option if you want a warm-toned blush, but that's about it.

☺ AVERAGE **Shimmering Loose Mineral Bronzer** *($8.69)* has a subtle shimmering effect to give skin a healthy glow. The color is a natural-looking, medium bronze shade that will show up well on light to medium skin tones. The downside is that the lightweight, fluffy texture of the powder has a tendency to cling more prominently to normal areas of skin (not too oily or too dry), which can lead to uneven results.

SONIA KASHUK EYESHADOWS

☺ GOOD **Eye Shadow Duo** *($6.99)* has a slightly creamy texture and applies smoothly and softly. One shade in each duo is shiny (many duos feature two shiny shades), but it's subtle (more subtle than it appears in the compact) and doesn't flake.

☺ GOOD **Eyeshadow Palette** *($14.29)* provides six shades of Kashuk's powder eyeshadow along with a sheer cream concealer and a dual-sided sponge-tip applicator, which you should toss out (Kashuk's eyeshadow brushes are preferred). Each powder shadow applies smoothly

The Reviews S

but quite sheer. They layer well, so you can achieve more dramatic shaping and shading, and the shades offer both matte and shimmer finishes. The concealer is described as an eyeshadow base, and it has a soft powder finish that works well to enhance application while evening out minor discolorations on the eyelids.

☺ GOOD **Eye Shadow Quad** *($13.69)* offers four coordinated eyeshadows in one compact, and has a slightly creamy texture that applies smoothly and softly. The colors include options for highlighting, contouring, and eyelining, making these practical kits. Most of the sets have at least one shiny shade, but it's low-key and suitable for daytime makeup.

SONIA KASHUK EYE & BROW LINERS

✓☺ BEST **Eyeliner Palette** *($13.29)* contains five shades of ultra-pigmented powder eyeshadow meant to be used as eyeliner. Applying this smooth-textured powder dry imparts a soft smokey effect (though still very pigmented); using it wet with a thin eyeliner brush creates more intense drama that doesn't flake away. The shades—black, brown, olive, plum, and navy—are rich, vibrant, and leave a soft matte finish. The attractive white compact includes a small, well-made lining brush that could work on the go, but you'll need a full-size brush to get the most out of this palette.

☺ AVERAGE **Brow Definer** *($5.99)* is a very standard, but good, brow pencil available in two shades suitable for dark blonde to medium brown brows. Why Kashuk didn't offer more shades is a mystery, but what's here is workable and it has a soft powder finish. This would receive a higher rating if it didn't require routine sharpening.

☺ AVERAGE **Brow Kit Arch Alert Palette** *($9.99)* includes four shades of creamy, sheer brow wax (for blondes, redheads, and brunettes) and two unbelievably small applicators: a wedge brow brush to apply the wax and a mascara-type wand to groom brows. The wax doesn't do much to enhance brows and the colors are too soft for any real definition, while the tools are difficult to work with when compared to full-size brushes. If you try this you'll most likely only need one shade; why these weren't offered as stand-alone colors (without the nearly useless applicators) is a mystery.

☺ AVERAGE **Jet Set Liquid Liner** *($5.99)* takes an inordinately long amount of time to dry! This is a problem for any liquid liner because if you open your eyes too soon—Bam!—you've got eyeliner on your upper eyelid, and you're starting all over with your eye makeup design. Beyond that issue, this also dries to a glossy finish, which can accentuate eyelid wrinkles. The color stays rich and true, unless you encounter even a bit of moisture, then it's prone to smearing.

☹ POOR **Eye Definer** *($5.99)* is a substandard pencil that needs routine sharpening, and the oil–based formula tends to fade and smudge without much provocation.

SONIA KASHUK LIP COLOR & LIPLINERS

✓☺ BEST **Ultra Shine Sheer Lip Gloss** *($8.99)* is a commendable lip gloss with an elegant brush applicator that doesn't splay. It feels emollient without being too slick or greasy, and has a soft gloss finish that's barely sticky. The shade range presents sheer and juicy hues, and all of them are recommended.

✓☺ BEST **Velvety Matte Lip Crayon** *($7.59)* is a thick pencil for lip color and if you want an opaque matte finish that feels virtually weightless, this is outstanding. The palette of shades is soft and wearable—we can't imagine most women balking at any of the colors—and all apply with enviable smoothness. For a lipstick in pencil form, the tip stays impressively pointed and isn't prone to becoming smushed down unless you apply with a lot of pressure.

The finish is truly matte, and can begin to feel dry, but if you're OK with that then you'll likely love this product. We normally downgrade any lip pencil that needs routine sharpening, as Velvety Matte Lip Crayon does. However, we made an exception because this lip color's attributes are otherwise excellent.

☺ GOOD **Satin Luxe Lip Color SPF 16 Sunscreen** *($9.99)* is aptly named for its luxuriously smooth texture and satin finish. The creamy formula glides on and imparts a hint of shine in an array of richly-pigmented, attractive shades. Added bonus: It contains broad-spectrum sun protection that includes avobenzone for reliable UVA screening! This lipstick can bleed into the lines around your mouth (if you have them), but that's typical of creamy lipsticks. Our only (minor) complaint is that the formula includes potentially irritating flavoring ingredients. The flavoring is subtle so there isn't huge cause for concern, but this lipstick would have been better off without it.

☺ AVERAGE **Lip Definer** *($5.99)* has a creamy, oil–based formula, but the creaminess is not a problem unless you have an issue with lipstick feathering into lines around the mouth. There aren't many colors available, but they cover the basics and are versatile.

SONIA KASHUK MASCARA

☺ GOOD **Lashify Mascara** *($6.99)* is worth considering if you need a mascara that's better at lengthening than thickening and that wears well without a flake or smear. The packaging now includes a built-in metal lash comb that, while not our personal favorite (plastic combs are safer), works well to add separation to lashes.

SONIA KASHUK BRUSHES

✓☺ BEST **Sonia Kashuk Brushes** *($1.99-$20.99)* offer several professional makeup brush options. Some have an ergonomically designed handle and a polished, futuristic look that's eye-catching (with a slightly higher price point), and the more basic options have a slim white handle (and lower price tags). There are plenty of natural and synthetic hair options (each are clearly marked), but almost all of them are recommended and a bona fide beauty bargain. With so many options and at these prices you can experiment with specialty brushes to see what works for you.

☺ GOOD **Synthetic Flat Top Multipurpose Brush** *($15.79)* doesn't have the shape or profile of a traditional brush (synthetic or natural hair), but it's an interesting departure that produces similar results, as long as you use the flat side of the brush rather than "dotting" with the cut-straight-across brush head. For a synthetic hair brush, this feels remarkably soft and has superior density, which is ideal for holding and applying powder of all kinds.

SONIA KASHUK SPECIALTY PRODUCT

✓☺ BEST **Matte, Oil Blotting Papers** *($6.69 for 100 sheets)* work quite well and are sized larger than most, which means they aren't the most discrete option to tuck into an evening bag. However, you can mop up more shine with a single sheet, so that may make these more appealing—and the price is right!

☺ AVERAGE **Perfecting Transparent Mattifier** *($14.99)* is touted as being able to combat shine throughout the day, but it didn't meet our expectations (we did a split face test to be sure). While this colorless primer temporarily smoothes over pores, the mattifying effect quickly dissipates and your skin is left looking just as oily as if you hadn't used it. On the plus side, the velvety thick texture blends out to a silky-dry finish suitable for those with oily skin. It wears well under makeup and is fragrance-free. All in all, this could be used as a basic primer but there's nothing special about it.

ST. IVES (SKIN CARE ONLY)

Strengths: A couple of water-soluble cleansers, a gentle microdermabrasion alternative.

Weaknesses: Overly abrasive scrubs; ineffective anti-acne products; dated moisturizers; overall, the facial-care products are substandard, even if they are inexpensive.

For more information and reviews of the latest St. Ives products, visit CosmeticsCop.com.

ST. IVES CLEANSERS

☺ GOOD **Moisturizing Olive Cleanser** *($7.99 for 5 fl. oz.)* is a basic water-soluble cleanser for normal to slightly dry or slightly oily skin. An olive oil–derived ingredient is part of the formula, but any potential benefit from the antioxidants in olives is rinsed down the drain. Still, the oil portion will help dissolve makeup while keeping skin smooth and soft during cleansing.

☹ AVERAGE **Apricot Cleanser Blemish-Fighting** *($5.49 for 6.5 fl. oz.)* contains salicylic acid, tea tree extract, and cornmeal to make it a cleanser/scrub. The salicylic acid won't do a thing to fight blemishes because it is rinsed from the skin too soon and the amount included is too small. However, if used gently, this has merit as a cleansing scrub for those with normal to dry skin. Note that using a topical scrub over acne lesions is not a good idea. Acne cannot be scrubbed away, and scrub-like ingredients can irritate already inflamed lesions, prolonging their stay when the objective is to heal them.

☹ AVERAGE **Makeup Remover & Facial Cleanser** *($5.49 for 6 fl. oz.)* is a somewhat greasy cleansing lotion that certainly removes makeup, but the residue it leaves behind doesn't make this preferred to a water-soluble cleanser unless you have very dry skin.

☹ POOR **Apricot Face Wash, Blemish & Blackhead Control** *($5.49 for 6.5 fl. oz.)* would have been a good option for normal to oily skin had it not been for the inclusion of menthyl lactate, which is an irritant that has no benefit for skin. See the Appendix to learn how irritants like this hurt skin.

☹ POOR **Naturally Clear Green Tea Cleanser** *($6.59 for 6.75 fl. oz.)* differs little from lots of others anti-acne cleansers: It contains 2% salicylic acid as the active ingredient and a menthol derivative to make skin tingle as it's cleansed. The tingling isn't helpful—it's the type of irritation that can trigger oil production at the base of your pores—and the salicylic acid's brief contact with skin means your acne isn't likely to improve. There are other problematic ingredients in this cleanser, too, making it one to leave at the drugstore.

ST. IVES SCRUBS

☺ GOOD **Moisturizing Olive Scrub** *($7.99 for 5 fl. oz.)* is a very good cleansing scrub for normal to very dry skin. The abrasive agent is jojoba beads, and they are cushioned by fatty acids, oil, and paraffin (wax). The cleansing agent helps this rinse better than it would without them, but this is not a product for those who are looking for a scrub that doesn't leave a hint of residue. The antioxidants in this scrub look good on the label, but they're rinsed from skin before they have a chance to work.

☺ GOOD **Naturally Clear Green Tea Scrub** *($6.50 for 4.5 fl. oz.)* is medicated with 1% salicylic acid, but it will have no effect on your acne because the product's pH is too high. Even if the pH were within an efficacious range, salicylic acid is mostly wasted in rinse-off products. Silica beads serve as the scrub agent, and they're supported by detergent cleansing

---

🌷 Highly fragranced products smell good, but won't help your skin! See the Appendix for details.

agents. As long as you don't expect this scrub to clear your skin, it is a good option for normal to oily skin—just be sure to not use it over acne lesions, because acne cannot be scrubbed away.

☺ AVERAGE **Apricot Scrub Gentle, for Sensitive Skin** *($4.29 for 6 fl. oz.)* is abrasive enough to not be preferred over gentler facial scrubs or a washcloth with a gentle, water-soluble cleanser. Although they're natural, walnut shells can scratch and tear at skin

☺ AVERAGE **Apricot Scrub Renew & Firm** *($4.29 for 6 fl. oz.)* is a fairly gentle scrub primarily because it contains just a tiny amount of abrasive walnut shell powder and because what's listed before it on the ingredient list provides a buffering effect. This can be an OK scrub for normal to dry skin. Note that the tiny amount of AHA glycolic acid has no impact on the exfoliating properties of this scrub.

☹ POOR **Apricot Scrub Blemish & Blackhead Control** *($4.29 for 6 fl. oz.)* has too many negatives to make it a worthy contender in the facial scrub category. Walnut shells and cornmeal can be too abrasive and tear skin, not to mention rupture acne lesions and prolong healing time, increasing the chances you'll end up with red marks once the blemish heals. This scrub also contains the fragrance ingredient limonene, which can cause irritation that makes oily skin worse. Please keep in mind that blackheads cannot be scrubbed away. Because a blackhead begins deep in the pore lining, you need an exfoliant that penetrates the buildup to dissolve the clog that leads to a blackhead. That's not possible from any scrub; you need to use a well-formulated BHA exfoliant medicated with salicylic acid (you'll find recommended options in our Best Products chapter).

☹ POOR **Apricot Scrub Invigorating, for All Skin Types** *($4.29 for 6 fl. oz.)* has too many negatives to make it a worthy contender in the facial scrub category. Walnut shells and cornmeal can be too abrasive and tear skin, and the amount of sodium lauryl sulfate can cause dryness and a tight feeling after you rinse. A scrub should not make your skin dry and irritated; instead, it should gently reveal the glowing skin beneath old, dull skin. Research shows the gentlest (and most state-of-the-art) way to exfoliate is with a well-formulated AHA or BHA product, not scrubs.

ST. IVES MOISTURIZERS

☺ AVERAGE **Collagen Elastin Facial Moisturizer** *($5.99 for 10 fl. oz.)* is about as basic a facial moisturizer for normal to dry skin as you're likely to find at the drugstore. Most cosmetics companies have long since given up claiming that collagen and elastin can reduce wrinkles when applied topically. Why hasn't St. Ives? Besides, even if these two ingredients could fuse with the collagen and elastin in skin, St. Ives uses only a fractional amount of each. This moisturizer also contains small amounts of fragrance ingredients known to irritate skin.

☺ AVERAGE **Timeless Skin Collagen Elastin Facial Moisturizer** *($5.99 for 10 fl. oz.)* Although this facial moisturizer has a great price and unusually generous size, its formula is a big step backward. In many ways, moisturizers don't get more dated than this. Instead of a sophisticated mix of repairing ingredients and antioxidants, you're left with mostly water, mineral oil, and slip agents. That's OK, but not great and your skin deserves great! The tiny amounts of collagen and elastin in this moisturizer won't provide timeless results. Neither ingredient can fuse with or shore up these supportive substances in skin, even when they're used in greater amounts. Normally we'd comment on the jar packaging being a problem for the light- and air-sensitive ingredients, but in this case the formula is so bare bones, the packaging is mostly a hygiene issue. This moisturizer does contain a small amount of fragrance ingredients known to cause irritation.

STILA (MAKEUP ONLY)

Strengths: Inexpensive for a department-store/boutique line; the foundations are remarkable in most respects, especially shade selection and texture; bronzing powder with sunscreen; very good options for blush and eyeshadow; the Brow Polish and Lip Shine are standouts; several attractive, versatile shimmer products; great makeup brushes.

Weaknesses: Convertible Eye Color and Kajal Eye Liner have too many weaknesses; some problematic lip glosses; the lip pencils are average at best.

For more information and the latest Stila reviews, visit CosmeticsCop.com.

STILA FOUNDATIONS & PRIMERS

✓☺ BEST **$$$ Illuminating Liquid Foundation** *($38)* is a creamy, mineral oil–based makeup that's very good for dry skin seeking light to medium coverage with a satin-smooth, shimmer finish. The shine is noticeable, and with a sheer powder dusted over it this can lend a radiant glow to the skin. All the shades are soft and neutral whether skin is fair or dark (but not very dark).

✓☺ BEST **$$$ Natural Finish Oil-Free Makeup** *($38)* is an outstanding liquid foundation with an exceedingly silky application that blends beautifully and provides light to medium coverage with a satin-matte finish. The formula is oil-free and an excellent choice for normal to oily skin prone to blemishes. The shades available include options for fair to dark skin tones.

✓☺ BEST **$$$ Sheer Color Tinted Moisturizer Oil-Free SPF 20** *($34 for 1.7 fl. oz.)* is a great fragrance-free tinted moisturizer for all skin types but particularly for sensitive skin. The active ingredients are gentle minerals titanium dioxide and zinc oxide, so this is unlikely to cause stinging or be a problem for use around the eyes. The soft, lightweight cream texture glides over skin, providing sheer to light coverage and a soft, satin-matte finish that looks natural. Even better are Stila's mostly neutral shades, with good options for fair to medium skin tones. The darker shades are trickier, but Deep and especially Bronze are worth an audition by those with dark skin; neither shade looks too copper or ashen. As much as we applaud this tinted moisturizer with sunscreen, it must be said that the product is extremely similar to Paula's Choice Barely There Sheer Matte Tint SPF 20. The Paula's Choice option doesn't have the extensive shade range Stila does, but it also costs significantly less money per ounce. With Stila's version you get 1.7 ounces; Paula's Choice Barely There Sheer Matte Tint is offered in a 1-ounce size.

☺ GOOD **$$$ Illuminating Powder Foundation SPF 12** *($28)* deserves its rating even though its titanium dioxide–based sunscreen is below the minimum SPF 15. This is recommended with the caveat that it be used over a regular sunscreen or foundation with sunscreen rated SPF 15 or higher. This talc-based powder foundation is extraordinarily silky and applies seamlessly, offering light, non-powdery coverage and a barely there, slightly shiny finish. The shades are terrific and not to be missed if you prefer this type of foundation and don't mind the initially high price.

☺ AVERAGE **$$$ Illuminating Tinted Moisturizer Oil-Free SPF 20** *($32)* contains the pure mineral sunscreens titanium dioxide and zinc oxide and has a lightweight, fragrance-free lotion consistency that glides over skin for easy application. Once blended, the result is a sheer, luminescent finish. Unfortunately, there are only two shades and both have a slightly peach undertone, which is unflattering if used all over the face. It's also important to keep in mind that any sunscreen must be applied liberally to get the stated protection, and in this case that would leave you with a peachy glow that won't look like real skin.

☺ AVERAGE **$$$ One Step Correct** *($36)*. Stila claims that One Step Correct "instantly makes Imperfections disappear" and "reduces fine lines, wrinkles, pores and pigmentation." In reality, the formula is far too sheer to provide color correction or to camouflage even minor imperfections. All you have to do is test this at the store and you'll see exactly what we mean. Once it sets, skin has a slight sheen (and, thankfully, no odd overtones of purple, peach, or mint green), but that's it. What you're hoping to hide is still glaringly obvious. This product also is advertised as an anti-aging primer trademarked with Stila's "Youth Revival Bio-Available Mineral Complex," but a look at the ingredient list reveals that it is about as state-of-the-art as a typewriter. In terms of anti-aging, this contains some standard vitamins, but nothing that's present in an appreciable amount—and the minerals are scant, not to mention that minerals have no special benefit for your skin. You're left with a tacky, gel-like serum with little benefit beyond looking cool in the bottle. Why bother?

☺ AVERAGE **$$$ Perfect & Correct Foundation** *($44)* is an unusual mix of ingredients whose moist and dry finishes are seemingly at war with each other. The result is a sheer- to light-coverage foundation that makes skin feel tacky, even after it has been removed. The slightly creamy, soft texture feels more like moisturizer than makeup and it leaves a dewy finish that is best for normal to dry skin. As usual with Stila, the shades are mostly exemplary neutrals, with options for fair to dark (but not very dark) skin tones. Only Warm should be considered carefully due to its orange-ish tint. This pump-dispensed liquid foundation has its strong points, but you definitely want to experiment with it before making a purchase—many will find the tacky finish isn't pleasant to live with.

☺ AVERAGE **$$$ Stay All Day 10-in-1 HD Beauty Balm** *($38)*. We're surprised that a BB cream claiming to be "10-in-1" doesn't even contain sunscreen as part of its benefit. Most BB creams offer this critical anti-aging benefit, but not this one. So what does it do? Let's go over the nine (yes nine, not ten) claims Stila lists on their site:

"*Luxurious beauty balm glides onto skin and leaves a silky, powdery finish.*" This is true!

"*High-definition formula helps reduce pore size and provides oil and blemish control.*" It doesn't reduce pore size or blemishes, but the matte finish helps minimize oily shine.

"*Contains innovative micro spheres, which have been shown to hide skin imperfections and reduce wrinkle depth by up to 84%.*" This is marketing mumbo jumbo, and the finish is too sheer to hide anything more than minor imperfections.

"*Features an exclusive complex, which helps reduce redness and skin irritation.*" Unfortunately this actually contains irritants such as linalool and fragrance!

"*Enriched with Tripeptide-37, bamboo and pea extracts, which help diminish the appearance of fine lines and wrinkles.*" The concentrations of these ingredients are too low to have any benefit.

"*Infused with natural, skin-protecting emollients which have been shown to increase anti oxidant activity by up to 89.7%.*" Ignore this unsubstantiated claim.

"*Uses the smallest particle size of coated pigments for seamless, smooth coverage.*" The coverage is indeed seamless and smooth.

"*Ideal for all skin types and skin tones.*" Not true. This is best for normal to oily skin, and the sole peachy-cream shade would only work for medium-light skin tones.

"*Oil-free, paraben-free and dermatologist tested.*" Those are meaningless terms. Oil and parabens aren't anything to be afraid of, and "dermatologist tested" doesn't have any bearing on how well this product performs or its safety.

In the end, this is an over-hyped BB cream that turns out to be mediocre. The fact that it also contains small amounts of fragrance and other irritating ingredients cancels out any other beneficial ingredients.

STILA CONCEALERS

☺ AVERAGE **$$$ Brighten & Correct Concealer** *($28)* has a slightly creamy liquid texture and is supposed to camouflage and brighten while correcting dark circles and wrinkles around the eyes. It contains no ingredients proven to help improve dark circles, though the coverage and finish this has will significantly reduce their appearance, just as any good concealer will do. As for wrinkles, the formula contains tiny amounts of a few peptides, but whether used in low or high amounts it takes more than peptides to improve wrinkles. Best considered for its concealing benefits, the product is packaged in a click pen–style component that feeds concealer onto a synthetic brush for easy application. The texture is slightly thick but quite silky, and it blends readily. It sets to a soft matte finish and provides moderate to full coverage. Each shade offers some degree of brightening and this is accomplished without adding sparkles to the under-eye area. If only the shades were better! Among the options, only Fair is worth serious consideration. Medium, Tan, and Deep all suffer from noticeable peach to orange tones. To some extent the peachiness can counteract bluish or purple dark circles, but your blending must be precise and you run the risk of replacing one color problem with another. This is best applied in sheer layers; overdoing this causes the concealer to look obvious and accentuate lines around the eyes.

☺ AVERAGE **$$$ Perfecting Concealer** *($23)* has a slightly thick, greasy formula that's a step backward when compared to many other modern concealers. You'll get full coverage with an opacity that camouflages redness and dark circles, but it's tricky to blend and is so emollient it will crease into lines no matter how much powder you use for setting. If you decide to try this, avoid shades H and K, which are too ash and copper for dark skin. The other shades are predominantly neutral and there are some good options for fair skin.

STILA POWDERS

☺ GOOD **$$$ Hydrating Finishing Powder** *($32)* is a powder with water that goes on slightly damp and then dries. This has more movement then traditional powders, and can adhere to skin slightly better. We disagree that the water adds hydration though, because water in and of itself isn't going to add or hold moisture to skin (if it did, taking a bath should be all skin needs to be free from dryness and that is absolutely not the case). The main ingredient in here is the very absorbent mineral silica. The texture is nearly weightless and silky, yet, as expected, the silica lends a dry finish. Therefore, this powder and its sole translucent shade (suitable for light to medium skin tones) is best for normal to oily skin.

☺ GOOD **Sheer Pressed Powder** *($28)* does indeed go on quite sheer. This talc-based powder doesn't feel the least bit heavy, nor is it too dry or powdery. It goes on lightly and has a silky matte finish, yet manages to keep excess oil in check without making skin look flat and dull. The palette of shades is a bit odd: Light and Medium are suitable for fair skin tones only, while Dark is best for light to medium skin tones. Finding your best match isn't as easy as it should be, but this pressed powder is still recommended for all skin types.

STILA BLUSHES & BRONZERS

☺ GOOD **$$$ Convertible Color** *($25)* is a find for dry skin. This is basically a sheer, emollient blush that feels more like a lipstick in compact form. This is intended for use on lips and cheeks for a simple, easy, "finger-painted" look. The texture is creamy bordering on greasy (akin to traditional lipstick), and the large color range is exceptional, with a few eye-catching sheer, but bright, hues. The color of each compact is a very good representation of how the shade appears on skin, though of course the product itself is more translucent.

☺ GOOD **$$$ One Step Bronze** *($36)* is merely a good lotion-like bronzer for normal to dry skin, even though it's billed as a bronzing serum and packaged to showcase it's "triple helix" swirl fill. The fragrance-free formula has a cream-gel texture that slips easily over skin, so blending isn't an issue. This sets to a sheer, slightly moist finish that leaves a soft wash of peachy-tan color infused with gold sparkles. A real tan doesn't shine, but with this product you're stuck with obvious sparkles that can look distracting when worn during daylight hours. This works best to add a golden gleam to skin at night. Contrary to claim, the sparkling finish doesn't reduce the appearance of wrinkles. In truth, shine magnifies wrinkles so products like this are best used over smooth, unlined areas. Good news: the sparkling finish doesn't flake.

☺ GOOD **$$$ Stila Sun Bronzer** *($28)* is a fragrance-free pressed bronzing powder with a silky, almost creamy texture that applies soft and even. It's best to begin with a sheer application and build intensity from there, and this builds beautifully when richer color is desired. The finish is soft satin with a hint of shimmer from each of the two shades. Shade 02 is preferred because it's a soft tan color that's great for fair to light skin tones. Shade 01 is too peachy to pass as bronzer, and doesn't look all that great as a blush, either. This bronzing powder isn't dark enough for women of color.

☹ AVERAGE **One Step Bronze Skin Tone Illuminating Bronzing Serum** *($36)*. Stila claims this product can "improve skin tone, even out the complexion, and smooth the appearance of fine lines and wrinkles." While it does have some interesting ingredients for skin, the benefits don't outweigh the negatives. In the long run, this is merely a gel-cream bronzer with a high amount of shimmer that's shiny enough to accentuate fine lines and wrinkles. Plus, the single bronze shade has undertones of copper and orange, making this an extremely limited color choice for a natural tan look on light and most medium skin tones. The gel-creamy texture blends on smoothly and dries to a lightweight finish, but that isn't reason enough to buy this otherwise disappointing bronzing serum.

☹ POOR **Custom Color Blush** *($20)* has to be one of the silliest marketing contrivances for a makeup product we've seen in a while! Stila claims this powder blush "reacts with your skin's pH to create a one-of-a-kind, customized shade," but that simply isn't true, at least not any more than it is for any other product you buy that interacts with your skin. Even if it were true and the color really did alter based on the pH of your skin, that could make it turn into a color you hate. Don't worry, that's not the case here—you just might hate the color, but that is only because the shade selection is limited and it won't work for everyone. This has a velvety powder texture with a soft matte finish that blends smoothly, yet it's expensive given the number of excellent blushes at the drugstore that out-perform it.

☹ POOR **Bronzing Tinted Moisturizer SPF 20** *($32)* doesn't provide sufficient UVA sun protection so it's a poor choice in that regard (see the Appendix for details). In addition, it requires quite a bit of blending to ensure even application and it contains a potentially drying amount of salt (sodium chloride). This tinted moisturizer imparts a flattering sheer bronze color, geared for light to medium skin tones.

STILA EYESHADOWS & PRIMERS

✓☺ GOOD **$$$ Eye Shadow Pan** *($18)* has a gorgeous, smooth, suitably dry texture that blends well. Shine rules the roost here, but at least these apply easily, cling well, and aren't garish. These single eyeshadows are now sold in refillable, biodegradable magnetic compacts rather than in a pan alone. The shade selection is nearly as large as your imagination, with plenty of shades to love and even a few to avoid.

☺ GOOD $$$ **Baked Eye Shadow Trio** *($28)*. If you can get past the domed shape (which makes the lack of dividers between the three colors more apparent and a bit awkward to use) and you want more shiny eyeshadows, then this is an outstanding, beautifully silky trio to consider. The powder-based formula glides over lids and practically blends itself, and its strong shimmer finish doesn't flake. In short, it's an ideal find for those with unwrinkled, smooth eyes looking to really make them sparkle. All the sets are predominantly warm-toned and are highly recommended—just be sure to use shadow brushes that fit within the borders of each color to avoid turning each trio into a smudgy mess in the container.

☺ GOOD $$$ **Eye Shadow Trio** *($20)* presents its colors in one compact without dividers, which can make using just one shade tricky (unless your shadow brushes aren't too wide). The texture is smooth and application fairly even with a strong color deposit. Almost as strong as the color is the shine, which is present in each color in every trio. "Subtle" isn't on this eyeshadow's list of attributes. Still, those looking for shine will find it clings well and can make for a dramatic departure from sheer, demure daytime shades. Bella, Venus, and Rocker are the most workable trios. The rest have at least one shade that either isn't flattering or is just plain difficult to blend with the others.

☹ AVERAGE $$$ **Prime Pot Waterproof Eye Shadow Primer** *($20)* has a smooth, creamy consistency that blends evenly without excessive slip. Although the finish definitely helps keep eyeshadows in place, it also remains tacky. Surprisingly, the tacky finish doesn't hinder eyeshadow application; however, this primer's strong colors (Taffy is pink-peach and Caramel is strongly peach) affect how the eyeshadows "read" on your skin. For better results, and without the need to add an extra product to your makeup bag, use a liquid or cream concealer as your eyeshadow base. If needed, set it with a dusting of powder before applying shadows and you should be all set!

☹ POOR **Convertible Eye Color** *($22)* is a dual-ended product that gives you an automatic, retractable eye pencil along with an iridescent powder eyeshadow dispensed from a sponge tip. The pencil is a breeze to work with, but the powder eyeshadow tends to apply unevenly and flakes no matter how careful you are. For that reason alone, this product isn't recommended.

STILA EYE & BROW LINERS

✓☺ BEST $$$ **Stay All Day Waterproof Brow Color** *($22)* is an excellent liquid brow color whose formula is housed in a pen-like component outfitted with a built-in fine-tipped brush. The brush makes it easy to apply soft color between brow hairs for fuller, more defined brows. The water-based formula sets quickly and once it does, it's there to stay. It holds up through sweat and exposure to water, yet removes easily with a regular cleanser. Two brunette shades are available, making this best for those with light to medium or medium-dark brown brows. For a less expensive but equally good alternative to this product, consider Paula's Choice Browlistic Long-Wearing Precision Brow Color.

☺ GOOD $$$ **Smudge Pots** *($20)* is able to stand up to oily eyelids without fading, smearing, or running. This is a slightly moist gel-cream eyeliner that sets to a long-wearing matte finish. The color intensity does not build as quickly as other well-formulated gel eyeliners, going on more sheer and requiring you to layer if you want a solid, more dramatic line, but it's still worth a look. How thin or thick a line you create depends entirely on the type of brush you use; a pointed eyeliner brush produces a thin line, while a wedge brush can easily create a thicker line. The only reason to choose Stila's version over similar products is if you're looking for a sheer application rather than for a dramatic one. The shade selection consists of basic shades of black, brown, and gray as well as some wilder hues.

☺ GOOD $$$ **Smudge Stick Waterproof Eye Liner** *($20)*. If an automatic, nonretractable eye pencil that offers rich colors with a metallic, glitter-infused sheen is what you're after, then this waterproof liner is worth considering. The texture is creamy and application is smooth, and it sets quickly to a long-wearing finish, so smudge fast If you're going for a smokey look. Although the glitter isn't the best look for wrinkled eyes, it doesn't flake.

☹ AVERAGE $$$ **Sparkle Waterproof Liquid Eye Liner** *($22)*. If you have the need for a glitter-infused liquid eyeliner that's waterproof, this is an option to check out, though it's not without some drawbacks. Chief among them is the unharmonious marriage of brush and liquid liner formula. We're not sure if it's the formula or the brush, but it's impossible to get a single clean line with this product. You're forced to layer or you end up with a line that looks streaky and uneven. Along with a trickier application, the formula takes its time to set—more time than it should, which increases the risk of smearing as you wait for this to dry. Once set, it's quite tenacious and, true to product name, waterproof. Note that the formula is also prone to flaking before it dries, especially if you blink a lot before it sets. As for the finish, the color (when successive layers are applied) is rich and has a glittery, metallic sheen. The shades combine classics like black and brown with brighter, shock-value hues so which one you choose depends on the look you're after. On balance, this liquid eyeliner has more cons than pros, and for the money should be much better than it is.

☹ AVERAGE $$$ **Stay All Day Waterproof Liquid Eye Liner** *($20)*. Although this liquid eyeliner isn't waterproof (even a slight mist of water will cause it to break down and run), the felt-tip brush applicator and even-flow liquid formula make this a cinch to apply evenly. The brush tip doesn't allow for a thin line, but if you want a moderate to thick line with minimal effort, this works great, it sets quickly, and it doesn't smudge, unless your eye area gets wet. We were torn on how to rate this product because there is much to like about it. Ultimately, because of the name and the fact that it isn't waterproof, we determined an Average rating was most appropriate.

☹ POOR **Kajal Eye Liner** *($18)* is a rare misstep from Stila, because this is one disappointing, needs-sharpening pencil. It does have a super-soft texture that makes it easy to apply, but it's so creamy (and stays that way) that smearing and fading are inevitable. Yes, you can enhance this pencil's longevity by setting it with a powder eyeshadow, but why not use a pencil (or powder eyeshadow) that lasts well to begin with?

STILA LIP COLOR & LIPLINERS

☺ GOOD $$$ **Lip Enamel Luxe Gloss** *($22)* is a richly pigmented lip gloss that imparts a remarkable amount of color with a shiny, high-gloss finish. The creamy gloss texture creates a velvety smooth layer that leaves lips feeling moisturized but not sticky. The attractive shade range offers a variety of richly pigmented colors, from plum to pink to red.

☺ GOOD $$$ **Lip & Cheek Stain** *($24)* is much easier to apply to lips than cheeks, but because the formula is a cross between a gel and a cream blush you don't get a very moist finish, so you might end up reaching for lip gloss anyway. Applied to cheeks, this produces a nice flush and it blends well, though the smaller brush-on applicator is best for lips.

☺ GOOD $$$ **Lip Glaze** *($22)* is a moderately thick, smooth lip gloss with a minimally sticky finish and a glaze-like shine. It's packaged in a click-pen component with a built-in brush applicator and the brush itself is nicely cut to fit the contours of the mouth. Numerous shades are available, ranging from translucent with shimmer to glossy reds and berry tones.

☺ GOOD **$$$ Long Wear Lip Color** *($20)*. This slim, twist-up lipstick with a rounded tip (rather than angled) goes on slick and stays that way. It feels very light and its staying power comes from the stain effect it has on lips. It's an intriguing way to get lip color that lasts longer than traditional lipstick, but it doesn't take as long as the two-step lip paint/top coat products. This is worth a try if you don't like the lip paint/top coat options, and Stila offers some enticing shades.

☺ GOOD **$$$ Long Wear Liquid Lip Color** *($22)* is deeply pigmented and has the look and texture of an opaque stain, but it has enough slip to make application easier than your typical long-wearing lip product. Packaged in a sturdy tube with a wand applicator, some shades contain shimmer (and there are some bright hues), but the finish is matte—really matte. In addition, there is no question that this formula is drying, so exfoliating and moisturizing your lips beforehand helps keep things comfortable. Although this lip color doesn't budge or transfer, after a couple of hours, it does make any lines on your lips more noticeable. Applying balm or gloss over it will cause the color to deteriorate somewhat (as will exposure to greasy foods), but otherwise this holds up for several hours before you need a touch-up.

☺ AVERAGE **$$$ Long Wear Lip Liner** *($18)* stays put, blends on easily, and has rich pigmentation. It's a decent option for those who need a lipliner that lasts past their morning coffee, though it does require sharpening and the selection of shades is limited.

STILA MASCARAS

☺ GOOD **$$$ MAJOR Major Lash Mascara** *($22)* is meant to build on the success and stellar results from Stila's original (discontinued) Major Lash Mascara, which sold for one-third the cost of this. Performance-wise, both "Majors" are nearly equal in that they build thick, long lashes without clumps. However, the brush on MAJOR Major Lash Mascara is enormous and difficult to maneuver into the inner corner of the eye. No matter how we applied this, we got dots of mascara near our tear ducts and also on our eyelids above the outer corner. This was not an issue with the regular Major Lash Mascara, and given that one's convenience and lower price, it's a shame Stila let it go.

☺ AVERAGE **$$$ Glamoureyes Mascara** *($22)* adds volume, but it fails to define lashes and tends to flake as the day wears on. Why bother with this, given there are far superior mascaras from brands like L'Oreal or Maybelline at the drugstore?

STILA FACE AND BODY ILLUMINATORS

✓☺ BEST **$$$ All Over Shimmer Liquid Luminizer** *($20)* is packaged in a glass bottle and includes a brush applicator. It is more fluid, less slick, and less powdery at dry-down than its predecessor (All Over Shimmer), and is overall a significant improvement. This stays in place, dries quickly after blending, and looks natural. Its shimmer is more glow-y than shiny and the shade selection best suits fair to medium skin tones. A little goes a long way, so the price is somewhat justified, not to mention that this product is versatile. This is Stila's best shine-enhancing option.

☺ AVERAGE **$$$ All Over Shimmer Duo** *($22)* is a single product with one light pink shade and one golden beige shade, both of which work well to highlight features by adding a touch of glowing luminosity to your skin. It's easy to apply and goes on soft and smooth, setting to a silky-dry texture that adheres well. The two shades are flattering for fair to medium skin tones, and this highlights areas without looking overly shiny or glaring.

STILA BRUSHES

✓☺ BEST **Stila Brushes** *($20–$50)*. Stila provides several great brushes, most with a soft but firm feel and excellent shapes. There are even a few unique dual-sided and retractable options, and almost every brush is available in long- or short-handled versions. Stop by and check these out if you are shopping for brushes, especially the following: **#9 All Over Blend Brush** ($24), **#15 Double Sided Brush** ($32), **#17 Retractable Bronzing Brush** ($26), and **#20 Eye Enhancer Brush** ($32).

STRIVECTIN (SKIN CARE ONLY)

Strengths: A good cleanser and a couple of moisturizers are worth a look.

Weaknesses: Expensive; the original (and now the "improved" StriVectin-SD product (and every other product sold under this brand name) is absolutely not better than Botox or other cosmetic corrective procedures; some of the products contain irritant peppermint oil.

For more information and reviews of the latest StriVectin products, visit CosmeticsCop.com.

STRIVECTIN CLEANSER

☺ GOOD $$$ **StriVectin-SH Replenishing Cleanser** *($29 for 4 fl. oz.)* is an expensive cleanser that has some great qualities that make it an option for dry to very dry skin. One of its weaknesses (other than the sticker shock—no question that there are less expensive cleansers available that work better than this one) is that some of the oils and emollients it contains don't rinse well, so expect to use a washcloth to avoid leaving an oily residue on your skin. The residue issue isn't a big problem and, in fact, can be helpful for extra dry skin, but it's something we want to make you aware of because not everyone with dry skin will like how this makes your skin feel after it's rinsed. The NIA-114 ingredient mentioned in the claims is myristyl nicotinate. This ingredient is similar to niacinamide, the B vitamin that helps improve the skin's barrier function among several other benefits. There isn't much NIA-114 in this cleanser, however, and it's rinsed down the drain before it can have much benefit, but more important, the emollient ingredients play a much greater part in helping to preserve the skin's protective barrier during cleansing. This cleanser is provisionally recommended assuming you don't mind its high price. Also, despite not listing "fragrance," this contains two ingredients (methyldihydrojasmonate and hexamethylindanopyran) whose sole function is fragrance. Their inclusion makes this cleanser a poor choice for extra-sensitive skin. For other skin types, it's okay because the amount of these ingredients is low and it's a rinse-off product.

STRIVECTIN SCRUB

☹ POOR **StriVectin SD Instant Retexturizing Scrub** *($45 for 5 fl. oz.)* polishes skin with polyethylene (plastic) beads and jojoba beads. It has a smooth, cushiony texture that rinses well, so at least StriVectin got the aesthetics right. Where they went wrong was adding peppermint and citrus oils, both of which are highly irritating for your skin (see the Appendix to find out how irritation damages skin). Had this been better formulated, outside of the outrageous price, it would've been an excellent scrub.

STRIVECTIN MOISTURIZERS (DAYTIME & NIGHTTIME), EYE CREAMS, & SERUMS

☺ GOOD $$$ **Instant Moisture Repair** *($59 for 2 fl. oz.)* is not a traditional moisturizer, according to the claims for this product, but the description from there states what any well-formulated moisturizer does: "Works on the surface of skin and in the underlying uppermost layers to add and help keep moisture in skin, thus reversing the look and feel of dryness." And that is exactly what you get, an impressive moisturizer for normal to dry skin. It contains a broad complement of ingredients skin needs to repair its barrier, resist moisture loss, and be able to function in a more normal, healthy manner. This would earn our top rating if the formula did not contain fragrance ingredients known to cause irritation. Their presence is minor compared with the wealth of helpful ingredients in this moisturizer, but without question the formula would be better off without them.

☺ GOOD $$$ **StriVectin-SH Age Protect SPF 30** *($49 for 2 fl. oz.)* is a very good daytime moisturizer with sunscreen for normal to oily skin. It provides broad-spectrum sun protection and includes stabilized avobenzone for critical UVA (think anti-aging) protection. Other beneficial ingredients in this silky moisturizer with sunscreen include myristyl nicotinate (a derivative of niacinamide), several antioxidants, and skin-repairing ingredients such as ceramides and glycerin. These are the types of ingredients all skin types need to look and act younger, and the antioxidants help boost the skin's environmental defenses. This would be rated higher if it did not contain several fragrance ingredients that pose a slight risk of irritation. On balance, though, it's a well-formulated product that cannot truly reverse aging, but will protect your skin from sun damage and help repair some signs of aging.

☹ AVERAGE **StriVectin-TL Tightening Neck Cream** *($89 for 1.7 fl. oz.)* is part of StriVectin's marketing ploy making a big deal out of their NIA-114 ingredient, which is patented and included in this and a few of their other products. First, in terms of patented ingredients, a patent has nothing to do with efficacy. A patent is obtained without any proof that what you're patenting actually works. The "patented" claim always sounds impressive to unsuspecting consumers, which is why lots of companies use that claim, but it isn't proof of anything; it merely means that you have laid claim to the use of an ingredient for a specific purpose. Back to the NIA-114: It's the exact same ingredient (listed as myristyl nicotinate) included in the Nia24 brand of products reviewed elsewhere on CosmeticsCop.com. StriVectin claims they're the only company that uses this ingredient, but clearly that's not true. Here are the key details: Myristyl nicotinate is a derivative of nicotinic acid, a component of vitamin B3 (niacin). It isn't the same ingredient as niacinamide, but it functions in nearly the same manner (Source: naturaldatabase.com). Just like niacinamide, there is research on myristyl nicotinate's ability to improve the skin's barrier function, mitigate signs of sun damage, and reduce the incidence of atopic dermatitis, commonly known as dry skin. Niacinamide and myristyl nicotinate are both compatible with several prescription drugs used to treat various skin conditions and are believed to enhance their efficacy and/or minimize the negative side effects. Myristyl nicotinate is stabilized to prevent the release of, or quick conversion to, nicotinic acid, which can cause facial flushing, particularly in those dealing with rosacea (Sources: *Journal of Pharmaceutical and Biomedical Analysis*, February 2007, pages 893–899; *Drug Development and Industrial Pharmacy*, November 2007, pages 1176–1182; and *Experimental Dermatology*, November 2007, pages 927–935, and June 2007, pages 490–499). Is there any research proving NIA-114 can tighten or lift skin on the neck to reduce signs of sagging? No, none. It's a very good ingredient for all skin types, but it isn't the solution for a thinning, lax neck or sagging jawline. And, given that this ingredient functions identically to niacinamide, which is included in other products from Estee Lauder, Olay, and Paula's Choice, you don't need to spend this kind of money to get the benefit from this ingredient. Without the claims coming true to the extent you may be hoping, is there reason to consider this moisturizer? Other than the fact that you don't need a neck cream, you should apply a well-formulated facial moisturizer and/or serum to your neck, too, as there isn't a shred of research showing that skin on the neck or chest needs anything different from the skin our your face. Although this contains a range of intriguing antioxidants, plant extracts, and smoothing ingredients, most of them will not remain stable and effective because this moisturizer is packaged in a jar See the Appendix for details on the problems jar packaging presents.

☹ AVERAGE **StriVectin-TL Tightening Face Serum** *($89 for 1.7 fl. oz.)* is part of StriVectin's marketing campaign that makes a big deal out of their NIA-114 ingredient, discussed above in the review for StriVectin-TL Tightening Neck Cream. Although the lifting claims won't come true to the extent you may be hoping, there are reasons to consider this serum, although they're not quite compelling enough to go ahead with a purchase. Beyond the NIA-114 ingredient, most of the other anti-aging ingredients are present in tiny amounts. Meanwhile, this contains lots of film-forming agents to make skin feel tighter (but keep in mind that skin feeling tighter is not the same as loose skin actually becoming tighter). It has a lightweight texture and silky finish, but it also contains hidden sources of fragrance (such as methyldihydrojasmonate) as well as fragrant orange oil, which poses a risk of irritation (see the Appendix for details).

☹ AVERAGE $$$ **StriVectin Overnight Facial Resurfacing Serum** *($59 for 0.9 fl. oz.)* is sold as a liquid exfoliant that differs from harsh scrubs because it gently dissolves dead skin cells while you sleep. But none of the ingredients in this water-based fluid are capable of exfoliating skin! The formula contains some good anti-irritants and antioxidants, but some are of the fragrant variety so they aren't as stellar as many others. (Fragrance isn't a skin-care benefit, but it can be a skin-care detriment because fragrance can cause irritation, which has a negative effect on collagen and hurts skin's ability to heal.) The only ingredient that comes close to functioning as an exfoliant is willow bark extract, and here's why: Willow bark contains salicin, a substance that when taken orally is converted by the digestive process to salicylic acid (BHA). The process of converting the salicin in willow bark to salicylic acid requires the presence of enzymes, and is a complex digestive process; because skin doesn't have a digestive system, it is unlikely that salicin applied to the skin will be converted to salicylic acid. Further, salicin, much like salicylic acid, is stable only under acidic conditions. The likelihood that this product can mimic the effectiveness of salicylic acid is at best questionable, and in all likelihood impossible—and the pH of this serum wouldn't keep the willow bark in the acidic environment it needs to work.

☹ AVERAGE $$$ **StriVectin-SD Eye Concentrate for Wrinkles** *($59 for 1 fl. oz.)* asks you to pin your antiwrinkle hopes on a derivative of the cell-communicating ingredient niacinamide. This derivative is myristyl nicotinate, a derivative of nicotinic acid, which is a component of vitamin B3 (niacin). Technically, it isn't the same as niacinamide, but it functions in nearly the same manner (Source: naturaldatabase.com). There isn't any research indicating myristyl nicotinate Is a critical ingredient for the eye area, nor is it a boon for those struggling with dark circles or puffy eyes. Also, there are lots of products containing niacinamide that don't cost as much as this one. There are several other beneficial ingredients present, but none in a significant amount that would justify the claims on the label. At best, this is an OK, but overpriced, option for normal to dry skin. It contains fragrant plants and fragrance ingredients that make it ill advised for use close to the eyes. Last, don't forget that you don't need an eye cream (we explain why that's true in the Appendix).

🖋 Exposing oily skin to irritating ingredients makes it worse! See the Appendix to learn more.

☺ AVERAGE $$$ **StriVectin-SD Intensive Concentrate for Stretch Marks and Wrinkles, for Sensitive Skin** *($79 for 2 fl. oz.)* has half of its most beneficial ingredients listed after the preservative, so they don't count for much as far as "anti-aging power" goes. When it comes to sensitive skin, generally speaking, fewer ingredients per product are better, but this product has an unusually long ingredient list, which makes it riskier for someone with truly sensitive skin. StriVectin mentions that this contains "none of the oils or fragrances that can cause irritation," yet this absolutely contains fragrant components known to cause irritation. For example, methyldihydrojasmonate is a form of fragrance, as is the ingredient hexamethylindanopyran. These tongue-twisters aren't commonly known sources of fragrance, but that is precisely how they function in cosmetics. This also contains fragrant rose extract, so clearly, the claim is misleadjust like the original StriVectin formula, the sensitive-skin version isn't capable of improving these marks to a significant degree. Stretch marks occur when skin is abnormally stretched and expanded for a period of time. Typically, this occurs during pregnancy, weight gain, and weight loss. The abnormal stretching causes the skin's support structure of collagen and elastin to break down or rupture. In fact, the visible curled ends of stretch marks beneath the skin are actually bands of broken elastin. (Think of elastin as rubber bands beneath the skin that give it spring and the ability to snap back into place.) Essentially, stretch marks are scars that have formed from the inside out, rather than scarring that occurs when skin is externally wounded. Regrettably, stretch marks are among the toughest skin-care concerns to treat because there are no cosmetic ingredients or products that can make much of a difference in their appearance. It is impossible for any cosmetic to raise the indentations back to where the skin level used to be or to repair snapped elastin fibers. You can choose to believe the ads if you like, but it will simply be money thrown down the drain. All this leaves you with a moisturizer that's marketed as being great for sensitive skin and stretch marks, but that won't help either concern. Although this contains several beneficial ingredients (including myristyl nicotinate, an ingredient that works like niacinamide) as well as some good emollients for dry skin, there are plenty of other moisturizers that cost less and whose claims won't leave you disappointed.

☹ POOR **StriVectin Instant Facial Sculpting Cream** *($79 for 1.7 fl. oz.)* claims you won't be disappointed if your goal is to lift facial contours, but don't count on that benefit. Looking past the fact that StriVectin's parent company has launched numerous products that make outlandish, impossible claims (remember the "Works Like Botox?" ads, which no product can do and that was challenged by the FDA with warning letters?), this moisturizer can't help but be disappointing. Nothing in the formula is capable of lifting skin, improving a sagging jawline, or even ameliorating those bothersome "ear wrinkles" the company refers to in the claims. This moisturizer contains some helpful ingredients (though nowhere near the amount your skin deserves), but the few antioxidants won't remain potent for long due to the jar packaging. Just in case you have dry skin and are still considering this, please know that it contains an oriental plant extract (*Anemarrhenae asphodeloides*) that has proven to be phototoxic (Source: *Journal of Ethnopharmacology*, January 2010, pages 11–18) and offers no benefit to skin. This also contains a form of resorcinol that increases the irritant potential. In short, there's no compelling reason to consider this moisturizer over several others with far more beneficial ingredients that are proven to make a difference in aging skin, although not sagging, which can't be changed with any skin-care product. If sagging or lost facial contours are your chief concern, those can be successfully remedied only with cosmetic surgery or cosmetic corrective procedures, but do check out the Appendix to see to what extent good skin care can help (not solve) this issue.

☹ POOR **StriVectin-HS Hydro-Thermal Deep Wrinkle Serum** *($153 for 0.9 fl. oz.)* is a cosmetics rip-off that is a must to avoid. That's not only because it doesn't work as claimed, but because it includes an inaccurate ingredient statement (there's no such ingredient as "Tripeptide"; it should be followed by a number). For over $150, you're getting a water-based serum that temporarily tightens skin because of the amount of sodium polystyrene sulfonate (a film-former) and egg white (albumen) it contains. It cannot penetrate to the dermal/epidermal junction and plump deep wrinkles from the bottom up. Wasting money on a few bottles of this would only match the cost for a series of facial peels or Intense Pulsed Light (IPL) treatments, options proven to make a positive difference in skin. (Though even so, neither of these treatments will significantly improve the appearance of deep wrinkles—for that, more invasive procedures are needed, not to mention a daily commitment to protecting skin from sun damage).

STRIVECTIN SPECIALTY SKIN-CARE PRODUCTS

☹ POOR **StriVectin-EV Get Even Brightening Serum** *($89 for 1.7 fl. oz.)* is a water-based serum containing a range of ingredients that can improve brown spots and an uneven skin tone. Chief among them is a form of niacinamide (myristyl nicotinate, what StriVectin refers to as "NIA-114") and ascorbyl glucoside, a form of vitamin C that shows up in numerous other skin-lightening and brightening products. Both of these ingredients have some solid research proving their worth for discolorations—and this formula appears to contain an efficacious amount of them, too. We like that StriVectin included some skin-repairing and soothing ingredients, yet wish they hadn't thrown fragrant oils and fragrance ingredients into the mix. It is particularly ironic that one of the fragrance ingredients (limonene) is known to cause skin discolorations when skin is exposed to sunlight (Source: naturaldatabase.com). Between the limonene and citrus oils plus other fragrance ingredients, this serum becomes difficult to recommend. All these ingredients can cause irritation that hurts skin's healing and ability to repair damage. Given the number of skin-lightening products that omit these problematic ingredients (and cost less), there's not much reason to go with StriVectin's contribution to the fray.

☹ POOR **StriVectin-EV Get Even Spot Repair** *($49 for 0.14 fl. oz.)* is essentially a smaller, portable version of StriVectin-EV Get Even Brightening Serum above. It is packaged in a pen-style component with a built-in targeted applicator so you can hone in on dark spots. Otherwise, the formula has the same pluses and minuses as its "big sister."

☹ POOR **StriVectin-SD Intensive Concentrate for Stretch Marks and Wrinkles** *($135 for 5 fl. oz.)* has irritants such as peppermint oil as its major weakness. You will feel the tingling sensation as soon as you apply this emollient, slightly greasy cream, and it doesn't dissipate. That's not good news because it means your skin is telling you loud and clear that it is being damaged. This type of irritation causes collagen breakdown and hurts the skin's ability to repair itself. On the other hand, this formula does contain several beneficial ingredients that would help stimulate healthy collagen production. Another issue is that in addition to the problematic peppermint oil, this also contains clary and bergamot oils. The latter is capable of causing a phototoxic reaction when skin is exposed to sunlight. All the anti-aging ingredients, proven or not, mean little if to get them on your skin you're exposing it to irritants that hurt its ability to look and act younger. The bottom line is that despite adding some intriguing extras that the original StriVectin-SD lacked (meaning it wasn't as special as originally touted), the replacement isn't going to net the improvements you're trying to achieve.

TARTE COSMETICS

Strengths: Excellent foundation; great cheek stain and powder blush; superior pressed powder and eyelining pencils; unique, innovative, beautiful packaging; complete ingredient lists on the company's website; great mascaras.

Weaknesses: Expensive; some gimmicky products and claims (such as those for Amazonian clay); lacks matte eyeshadow options.

For more information and the latest reviews of Tarte Cosmetics, visit CosmeticsCop.com

TARTE COSMETICS SERUM

☺ AVERAGE **$$$ Smooth Operator Amazonian Clay Illuminating Serum** *($32 for 1.7 fl. oz.)*. We must state up front that the claims made for the clay in this serum are without scientific support. Whether sourced from the banks of the Amazon or the shores of the Mississippi River or your backyard, clay cannot "neutralize any negative skin condition." Actually, that's an incredibly broad statement that's open to interpretation: What does it mean to "neutralize" a skin condition anyway? Stop it from getting worse? Make it go away? Either way, clay is not the answer to a broad range of skin concerns. Even if clay were a powerhouse ingredient for skin (it isn't; at best, clay is a good absorbent ingredient for oily skin), the amount of it in this serum is so small your skin isn't likely to notice. Instead, you're getting a lot of standard (and synthetic) ingredients, which is all well and good, but it's not able to give you the dream complexion this serum promises. This product is closer to a foundation primer than a serum; it has a sheer tint and a silky lotion texture that leaves skin feeling moist and with a subtle glow. The formula contains two sunscreen ingredients (ethylhexyl methoxycinnamate and benzophenone-3), but does not list an SPF rating, so you cannot rely on it for sun protection. A mix of antioxidants is present, but for the most part the amounts aren't all that impressive. Note that the sunscreen ingredients in this product can make it a problem for use around the eyes; some people may experience a stinging or burning sensation, which is true for many synthetic sunscreen actives. We mention this here because this product is more like makeup and, therefore, likely to be applied close to the eyes.

TARTE COSMETICS LIP CARE

☺ GOOD **FRxtion Sugar Lip Exfoliator & Soothing Balm** *($15)*. This two-sided lipstick-shaped product provides a lip exfoliator on one side and lip balm on the other. The sugar exfoliator works well, gently removing dry skin from the lips, and the balm is moisturizing. The two-sided design of this product makes it convenient to use, but you must be prepared to use each side equally or the dual benefit becomes a moot point. The lipstick case in which FRxtion is packaged features a convenient pop-up mirror that appears when you pull off the top.

TARTE COSMETICS FOUNDATIONS & PRIMERS

☺ GOOD **$$$ Amazonian Clay 12-Hour Full Coverage Foundation SPF 15** *($38)* is a fragrance-free foundation that promises full coverage, sun protection, and a weightless texture—and it essentially delivers on all three. Dispensed from its squeeze tube, this has an initially thick, almost toothpaste-like texture that belies how silky and light it feels as it's blended. It melds convincingly with skin, providing medium to full coverage and a soft-focus, powdery finish best for normal to oily skin. This foundation's finish is the kind that will magnify the slightest hint of dry skin, so be sure skin is sufficiently prepped before applying. Also, take care to apply this lightly around the eyes if you have wrinkles, because this foundation, like many others, will magnify these signs of aging. Sun protection is provided by gentle mineral actives titanium dioxide and zinc oxide, making this a good choice for sensitive skin, too. As for the cons, this has a tendency to ball up slightly as you blend. It's not a deal-breaker because this effect goes away with further blending—but consider whether you want to take as much time to blend as this foundation demands. Also consider whether you really need this much coverage. Flaws are hidden but no question this looks like makeup, not natural skin. In terms of longevity, this goes the distance—maybe not for 12 hours as claimed, but most with oily skin will find this delivers several hours of wear without breaking up, fading, or looking spotty. The shades present some beautiful, soft colors for fair to medium skin tones. The best among them are Fair, Ivory (both excellent for very light skin tones), Light, Tan, and Tan Deep. Light Medium is slightly peach while Medium has a yellow tinge that requires careful inspection in daylight to ensure it matches well. The darkest shade (Deep) is slightly orange but workable.

☺ GOOD $$$ **Amazonian Clay Pressed Mineral Powder with SPF 8** *($30)* works well when applied after foundation or on its own worn as a mineral foundation. It works better dry than wet; dry application provides sheer coverage and a natural matte finish that is excellent at controlling shine for hours without turning cakey. This applies equally well with a powder brush or the included latex sponge, depending on how much coverage you desire. The SPF 8 provides broad-spectrum protection but the low rating is a letdown. It means that you must combine this with a SPF 15 or higher sunscreen, but that doesn't keep this from being an impressive, though pricey, powder worth considering. Almost all the shades are good and geared toward those with light to tan skin tones. Consider Honey 12 carefully, as it can turn slightly peach.

☺ GOOD $$$ **Smooth Operator Amazonian Clay Tinted Moisturizer with SPF 20** *($36)* is lightweight and blends easily, providing sheer coverage without feeling oily or appearing obvious on the skin. The moisturizing formula leaves a satin finish that wears well for hours. Adding to this, Smooth Operator includes a mineral-based broad-spectrum sunscreen. This is highly recommended for those with normal to slightly dry or slightly oily skin. The shade range favors fair to medium skin tones; there are only a couple of options for darker skin tones. One caution: The citrus extracts have a small potential to be irritating, but this effect should be offset by the soothing agents that are also in this antioxidant-rich foundation. Tarte changed the packaging on this product from opaque tube to a clear tube, thus allowing light to degrade the antioxidants in this product. As such, it is no longer a Best product.

☹ AVERAGE $$$ **Clean Slate 360 Poreless 12-hr Perfecting Primer** *($30)* is a standard clear silicone gel with some plant oil—it won't "perfect" any large, problematic pores, but its smoothing effect on skin texture and its silky finish will give your foundation more staying power. The smoothing effect of this product will also help reduce the appearance of minor dryness or flaky skin. This primer offers a good blend of antioxidants, but contains some fragrant plant oils that are potentially risky for all skin types, especially if you have sensitive skin. The inclusion of fragrant plants keeps this otherwise well-formulated primer from earning a higher rating. In terms of reducing pore size, try using a BHA exfoliant instead, such as those from the Paula's Choice line.

☹ POOR **Clean Slate Flawless 12-hr Brightening Primer** *($30)* isn't the brightest or most exciting formula in its class, but it has a creamy texture that will make skin feel softer upon application and the formula contains antioxidants for added benefit. The sheer, enlivening pink shimmer plus the creamy feel of this primer makes it a good option for those with dry skin; no question it makes a dull complexion appear more radiant. Those with oily skin should definitely leave this product on the shelf—it will make you look and feel greasy, especially when used under makeup. Although there's much to like about this primer, it's all for naught because it contains skin-irritant grapefruit oil. The citrus scent may seem uplifting, but fragrance isn't skin care (see the Appendix for details). What a shame!

☹ POOR **ReCreate Anti-Aging Foundation with Wrinkle Rewind Technology SPF 15** *($37)* used to get our highest rating, but its reformulation went downhill. First of all, the anti-aging claims Tarte makes about ReCreate's Wrinkle Rewind Technology are far-fetched; this foundation won't increase skin elasticity, firmness, or resiliency. The amount of peptide is practically nonexistent, and no peptide is the sole solution for the multiple signs of aging skin. In fact, because ReCreate no longer provides broad-spectrum protection, you're leaving your skin vulnerable to the sun's most damaging, aging rays. In terms of performance, ReCreate provides medium coverage but not all the colors are workable; some are a bit on the orangey side. The finish errs a bit on the chalky side, too. All in all, this foundation went from a stud to a dud.

TARTE COSMETICS CONCEALERS

✓☺ BEST $$$ **Maracuja Creaseless Waterproof Concealer** *($24)* is a quadruple-threat winner if you're waging war against dry skin around the eyes plus dark circles; it's moisturizing, provides full coverage, is fragrance-free and also waterproof! The smooth texture allows for easy blending and—despite the great coverage—this has a natural-looking finish (when properly blended). We suggest setting this concealer with a powder to help keep it creaseless. As for the colors, the fair shade is too pink—however, the other four shades are very natural and provide workable options for light to dark (but not very dark) skin. This type of concealer is too emollient to apply over breakouts, at least if you want to discourage them from getting worse. It's best applied around the eyes.

☺ AVERAGE $$$ **Dark Circle Defense Natural Under Eye Corrector and Brush** *($32)* is a creamy, borderline greasy, and very thick concealer in a compact that's sold with a full-size, synthetic-bristled brush. The brush is great and works well to apply this type of product. The problem is the concealer, which provides outstanding coverage for the darkest of dark circles, but it remains creamy and creases easily. The opacity of this product coupled with its texture adds up to obvious camouflage, but again—Wow!—does this ever cover dark circles! Also worth mentioning is that both shades have a peachy pink cast that doesn't help this look any better once blended. What about the claim that this reduced puffy eyes by 56% in four weeks? There isn't any ingredient in here that can solve that problem, whether over a year or in less than a month.

☺ AVERAGE $$$ **Smooth Operator Amazonian Clay Waterproof Concealer** *($22)* definitely has a smooth application but it's likely to leave you bumpy and broken out if you prone to blemishes. This cream-to-powder concealer is best suited for those with normal to dry skin—who have very little to conceal. Although the product feels thick, the coverage is medium at best, and tends to cake when layered for more coverage. The emollient nature of this concealer causes it to settle into lines around the eyes—unless you take care to blend well, and then set with powder. Four shades are available, all of which are neutral and suitable for light to tan skin tones. To avoid streaky or cakey application, resist applying this product directly from the twist-up container. Instead, use your fingertip to tap and blend the concealer over the area you wish to cover, or use a concealer brush. This stuff sets very quickly, so you'll want to make sure to get the placement right on the first try.

TARTE COSMETICS POWDER

☺ GOOD **$$$ Smooth Operator Amazonian Clay Finishing Powder** *($28)* has an incredibly soft and smooth texture. The lightweight, fragrance-free loose-powder formula sheers out onto skin for a nearly imperceptible finish, although those with dark skin tones may notice a slight whitish tint. This can be used to set makeup and refine your complexion. Although this temporarily absorbs oil, don't count on it to stay matte for long. By the way, you can ignore the claims Tarte makes about Amazonian clay. That's just marketing mumbo jumbo.

TARTE COSMETICS BLUSHES & BRONZERS

✓☺ BEST **$$$ Amazonian Clay 12-Hour Blush** *($25)*. The hook with this pressed-powder blush is that it's made with clay from the banks of the Amazon River. Supposedly, this clay is nutrient rich and the nutrients are said to help your skin, but they don't. Not only is clay devoid of the kind of ingredients skin needs to look its best, but also the amount of it in this blush is minuscule at best. Where this excels is with its beautifully silky, talc-based texture that meshes well with skin. The colors look bold and bright in their compacts, but go on easily, leaving a translucent, blushing-from-within look that's very impressive. Although pricey, you get lasting color (although 12 hours is stretching it; those with oily skin will find this doesn't last quite that long) that enlivens cheeks, and—surprise—almost all the shades have a matte finish! Blushing Bride has obvious shine, but that's it. Dollface is great for fair skin, Exposed would work on light to tan skin tones, and Flush is a beautiful deep plum for women of color. If you're up for a blush color that's not the typical pink or rose, consider the coral-hued Tipsy for a change of pace.

✓☺ BEST **$$$ Cheek Stain** *($30)* is outstanding! The creamy formulation in stick form gives you more blending time than standard gel or liquid stains, making application easier. The colors, which appear darker than they apply, blend down to sheer, natural-looking flush that wears well for hours. All this, and the shade range is beautiful. This type of blush is best for normal to dry skin not prone to blemishes.

☺ GOOD **$$$ Smooth Operator Amazonian Clay Finishing Powder in Bronze** *($28)* has an incredibly soft and smooth texture. The lightweight, fragrance-free loose-powder formula imparts a sparkling sheer bronze color. Sparkles don't exactly equal a natural tan look, but if you want your bronzer to glow, this will do the trick. By the way, you can ignore the claims Tarte makes about Amazonian clay. That's just marketing mumbo jumbo and perhaps Tarte's way of justifying the hefty price tag.

☺ GOOD **$$$ Amazonian Clay Bronzer** *($29)*. This talc-free pressed bronzing powder has a dry but smooth texture and soft color payoff of sheer golden tan. The gold, faux leather compact is attractive, but it's what's inside that counts, and users will be rewarded with an even application and an almost-matte finish—there's just a hint of shine, and it's suitable for daytime wear. As for the mineral claim, the minerals used in this bronzing powder are no different from those that show up in numerous other powders.

☹ POOR **Amazonian Clay 12-Hour Shimmering Blush** *($25)* is flooded with sparkles that don't cling very well to skin. Instead of adding a subtle luminosity, they look overdone and distracting. The shades themselves are richly pigmented and come in some attractive colors, but that can't make up for this pressed-powder blush's other shortcomings.

TARTE COSMETICS EYESHADOWS & EYE PRIMER

✓☺ BEST **$$$ Amazonian Clay Waterproof Cream Eyeshadow** *($19)* is a simple and stylish solution if you're looking for a smudge-proof, long-wearing eyeshadow that can take the heat (and the water). Finding such a great shade selection in a one-and-done eyeshadow—that actually has staying power—is rare, yet this comes through: This wears for hours without creasing or budging! It goes on nearly opaque and packs a pleasing pop of high shimmer in each shade. It's smooth enough to apply with your finger, but we suggest using a small, flat, eyeshadow brush (for hygiene!) and more control over placement. You'll want to get the application right, because even though this cream shadow goes on easily, it dries to a silky finish quickly, making any post-application adjustments difficult. This cream eyeshadow is fragrance-free.

☺ AVERAGE $$$ Eye Couture Day-to-Night Eyeshadow Palette ($44). These shimmery shadows (there are no matte options) apply and blend well, but that's where the good news ends. The double-ended eyeshadow brush isn't properly shaped to allow for precise application of the color. Part of the palette includes an eyelining pencil, but it is too creamy, prone to smearing, and needs sharpening. For this price, you're better off buying separate eyeshadows, eyeliner, and brushes to get what you really need to go from day-to-night looking beautiful; after all, that is the goal, right?

☹ POOR Clean Slate 360 Creaseless 12-hour Smoothing Eye Primer ($19) means well but causes more problems than it solves. The biggest negative is that it sets to an ashy white cast that will leave your eyelids looking more like a dirty chalkboard than a clean slate. As for the 12 hour creaseless wear claim, expect closer to four or five hours of worry-free wear—if worn with a powder eyeshadow (a cream eyeshadow causes this primer to crease and smudge). The amount of film-forming agent and dry-finish ingredients can also feel uncomfortable around the eyes. There are definitely less drying and more effective eye primers available for a lower price, or you can eliminate the need for this type of product by prepping your eyelid area with a liquid concealer that has a matte finish.

TARTE COSMETICS EYE & BROW LINERS

✓☺ BEST $$$ emphasEYES Amazonian Clay Waterproof Liner ($22). This long-wearing gel eyeliner is sold with a full-size, dual-sided eyeliner brush. The brush works great and gives you the option of easily drawing a thick or thin line. The eyeliner has a smooth, creamy texture that slides on easily and quickly sets to a slightly tacky finish. The tackiness doesn't get in the way of this product's ability to wear without smearing or fading, although the "micronized clay" from the Amazon River is mainly hype. Clay won't have an effect on how well eyeliner lasts, although it can help absorb excess oil. Among the shades, stick with Black, Brown, and Bronze for classic eye designs. The blue and green shades are more trend-driven and do little to shape or shade the eye, but depending on the look you're after (and your profession), you may find them appealing.

✓☺ BEST $$$ emphasEYES Aqua-Gel Eyeliner ($18). This automatic, retractable eye pencil does in fact have a water-based formula (most pencils are silicone-, oil-, or wax-based). Luckily, the water is joined by a slip agent, which helps this pencil apply smoothly, while the water itself creates a slight cooling sensation. The formula doesn't contain irritants such as peppermint, so no worries there. Although the texture is slick, it doesn't feel greasy. It needs a minute or so to set but once it does, you're rewarded with a budge-proof finish that really lasts. We're partial to classic shades like Black, Brown, Charcoal, and for a fun evening look, the sexy sheen that Bronze adds. But if you want brighter, trendy colors, they're here, too.

✓☺ BEST $$$ emphasEYES Eyeliner High Definition Inner Rim Eyeliner Pencil ($18). These ultrafine-tipped pencils are great for getting liner close to and in between the lash line and lashes. The creamy formula makes it easy to precisely line the eye or smudge the color for a smokier look. Despite the creaminess that enhances application, the color wears well for hours, with minimal fading. These pencils are only made more attractive by the fact that they never need sharpening. Tarte recommends using this for lining the inner rim of the eyes, but just for the health of your eye, that's not a good idea on a daily basis

☺ GOOD $$$ **EmphasEYES Amazonian Clay Waterproof Brow Pencil** *($19.50)* is a good, very slim, automatic, nonretractable brow pencil. It has a smooth, dry texture and a soft application that layers well for added depth. Its powder-like finish stays put and is waterproof, but will smear if you rub your brows while they're damp, so be careful. The two shades are best for dark blonde to medium brown brows.

TARTE COSMETICS LIP COLOR & LIPLINERS

☹ POOR **LipSurgence Natural Lip Luster Lip Tint** *($24)*. This chunky, twist-up lip pencil contains peppermint oil. The irritation this oil causes can lead to chapped lips and other problems. Given the number of sheer, glossy lip tints that omit irritants, there's no reason to settle for one that presents this risk (and costs a lot, too, plus you have to sharpen it, which is a pain).

☹ POOR **LipSurgence Natural Matte Lip Tint** *($24)* is the matte version of the Lip-Surgence products above, and also contains the problematic ingredient peppermint oil, which encourages dryness and irritation. What a pity considering this would have been a fabulous option otherwise!

TARTE COSMETICS MASCARA

✓☺ BEST $$$ **Lights, Camera, Lashes! 4-in-1 Natural Mascara** *($19)*. Tarte claims this mascara lengthens, curls, volumizes, and conditions, and for the most part, they're right. The conditioning claim is negligible (no mascara functions in this manner), but this gives lashes lots of length, volume, and curl, with minimal clumping and no flaking or smearing. You can apply just one coat for a natural look or layer it for more dramatic lashes. This is a great mascara, and unquestionably the best one Tarte Cosmetics offers.

☺ GOOD $$$ **Gifted Amazonian Clay Smart Mascara** *($19)* has a slightly wet application that can lead to smearing during application, so take it slow. The well-designed brush allows for good length and lets you build a decent amount of thickness, too. The best part of the brush is how easily it separates lashes for a clean, fringed look. Each lash is defined without clumps and once set, this has minimal tendency to flake. This requires a silicone- or oil–based makeup remover; it doesn't come off easily with a water-soluble cleanser alone. Note that the claims that this mascara strengthens and repairs lashes are not supported by its formula. This contains the same basic ingredients seen in most mascaras, though it does leave lashes feeling soft. Tarte Cosmetics claims that the Amazonian clay hydrates lashes, but that's a complete falsehood! Regardless of where it is sourced, clay *absorbs* oil and moisture—it doesn't provide hydration and it cannot "nourish" lashes any more than rubbing milk over your arm will supply calcium to your bones!

☺ GOOD $$$ **Lights, Camera, Splashes! 4-in-1 Waterproof Mascara** *($19)* doesn't have the same dramatic impact as its non-waterproof counterpart above, but it's good nonetheless. You won't get much volume from this (which is typical of most waterproof mascaras), but it does separate, curl, and lengthen nicely with minimal clumping and no smearing or flaking. It wears well and you definitely need an eye-makeup remover to get it off, another indicator of this mascara's tenacity.

☺ GOOD $$$ **MultiplEYE Clinically-Proven Natural Lash Enhancing Mascara** *($24)*. As you can tell by the name of this mascara, like dozens of others being launched of late, Tarte wants you to believe it can grow lashes just like Lattise, the prescription-only eyelash–growing medication being advertised on television and in fashion magazine ads. This product can't do anything more than work like a mascara. Taking this on its own merits as a mascara is another story: It is excellent, providing dramatically enhanced lashes. This sweeps on with ease, doesn't clump, and quickly builds long, thick lashes that get more voluminous with each stroke. All this, plus the formula doesn't flake, but is easy to remove with a water-soluble cleanser! The only letdown is the price because, quite simply, you can find equally outstanding mascaras at the drugstore for less money. Formula-wise, this differs little from most mascaras. Tarte included some intriguing water-binding agents and a peptide, but there is no evidence these ingredients stimulate the growth of longer, thicker lashes. As for the clinical proof, Tarte doesn't make this information available. Even if they did, it isn't difficult to prove that a good mascara (which this definitely is) increases the appearance of lash length and thickness—that's why we wear mascara!

TARTE COSMETICS FACE & BODY ILLUMINATOR

☺ GOOD $$$ **Provocateur Amazonian Clay Shimmering Powder** *($30)* is an intriguing option because it gives the optical illusion of dewy, radiant skin when in reality this powder has a drier matte texture. It's an appealing combination of effects that adds an attractive glow to skin and can be applied all over or used as a highlighter. Although its drier texture and matte feel may appeal to those with oily skin, the radiant shine will make oily areas look shinier. Therefore, unless you don't mind adding shine to your oily skin, this powder is best for normal to dry skin or you can dust it over areas that aren't oil-prone. It has a soft, lightweight texture that sets just as well over a bare face as it does over foundation. The generous pan size is also a plus; you're getting more product to play with, and enough room for a big fluffy brush—which is the tool we suggest for achieving an even distribution of soft color and shine. For lighter skin, the Rose shade may be too deep to use for an all-over color, but is still fabulous to dust on as a bronzer/highlighter with an angled brush. The Amazonian clay is merely kaolin, a standard absorbent clay that shows up in lots of products. Sourcing this from the Amazon doesn't make it special for skin—it's just a good marketing story.

☺ AVERAGE $$$ **Maracuja Blush & Glow Brightening Luminizer and Cheek Tint** *($32)*. The idea of a 2-in-1 blush/illuminator is intriguing, but what was meant to be convenient is ultimately disappointing. The Maracuja Blush that this product is named for is confined to the thimble-sized cap area and comes across as an afterthought. The awkward size difference between this cream blush and the illuminator in the tube beneath it makes these two look more like an odd couple than a good pair. There's only a measly .06 fl. oz. of blush compared to 1.7 fl. oz. of illuminator (which is only supposed to be used "a few drops" at a time). We struggled on how to rate this product because although the illuminator is very good and holds its own against other similar products—you're paying for two products, yet you're really only getting one plus a smidgen of another. If you decide to try this and want to get the blush to last longer, consider using the illuminator first and then blending the blush on top of it—this method of application provides a soft pop of color on top of an attractive glow, and helps the blush portion blend better over the cheeks.

TARTE COSMETICS BRUSHES

☺ GOOD **$$$ Glam on the Go Kabuki Brush** *($29).* Tarte doesn't skimp on packaging and Glam on the Go Kabuki Brush is no exception. The quilted purple case that holds this goat-hair brush is beautiful, and the short-handled kabuki brush inside isn't bad either. The soft goat-hair brush is slightly domed and works well to apply loose powder, pressed powder, blush, and bronzer. The handle may to be too stubby for some, but if you're not concerned about that, give it an audition!

☹ POOR **Brush with Greatness Double-Ended Eyeshadow Brush** *($24)* is soft enough to be usable for blending, but the surprising shapelessness of both ends doesn't make it a great option for precise and even eyeshadow application.

TARTE COSMETICS SPECIALTY MAKEUP PRODUCTS

☺ AVERAGE **$$$ MultiplEYE Lash Enhancer** *($65)* is essentially being sold as a non-prescription alternative to Latisse, the prescription-only product from Allergan that contains an active ingredient that really does make lashes longer, thicker, and darker. MultiplEYE Lash Enhancer from Tarte, on the other hand, doesn't contain anything that can help grow lashes—it's really that simple—which makes this product not worth your money or time. The company claims they're including a proprietary plant peptide to make lashes 152% longer (which would result in preposterously long lashes if it were true), but they're actually including one of the same peptides (myristoyl pentpeptide-17) that Jan Marini includes in her expensive Marini Lash product (reviewed on CosmeticsCop.com), which also doesn't work. The other ingredients in Tarte's product, such as soy protein and vitamin C, don't stand a chance of growing lashes either. There's no research proving any ingredient in this product works to grow lashes, so unless the company is using a drug ingredient and not identifying it, this isn't a product you can rely on for the kind of results that Latisse provides.

THE BODY SHOP

Strengths: Lists complete product ingredients on its website; affordable; the Aloe products for Sensitive Skin are appropriate for that skin type; good selection of eye-makeup removers; one of the best pressed-powder foundations around; great pressed powder; liquid eyeliner; lip gloss; nice selection of affordable makeup brushes and specialty products.

Weaknesses: The Tea Tree Oil collection; subcategories that focus on one beneficial ingredient (vitamin E, vitamin C, etc.) to the exclusion of others, making for several collections of one-note products; no effective routine to address blemishes; poor skin-lightening products; some lackluster to poor liquid foundations and concealers.

For more information and reviews of the latest The Body Shop products, visit CosmeticsCop.com.

THE BODY SHOP CLEANSERS

✓☺ BEST **Aloe Calming Facial Cleanser, for Sensitive Skin** *($14 for 6.75 fl. oz.)* is a good, gentle cleansing lotion for normal to dry or sensitive skin. It is fragrance-free and does not contain detergent cleansing agents. The oil content may require the use of a washcloth for complete removal.

✓☺ BEST **Aloe Gentle Facial Wash, for Sensitive Skin** *($16 for 4.2 fl. oz.)* is a very good, fragrance-free, gentle water-soluble cleanser for its intended skin type. In fact, this is great for all but very oily skin and rinses cleanly while removing makeup easily.

☺ GOOD **Seaweed Purifying Facial Cleanser, for Combination/Oily Skin** *($14 for 6.76 fl. oz.)* is a good cleansing lotion that omits detergent cleansing agents in favor of silicone and emollients. It is best for normal to slightly dry skin and rinses surprisingly well without the aid of a washcloth. This cleanser isn't more purifying than any other, so ignore that claim.

☺ GOOD **Vitamin E Cream Cleanser** *($14 for 6.7 fl. oz.)* is a very standard, cold cream–style cleanser for normal to dry skin. It does contain fragrance and fragrance ingredients that are potentially irritating, though less so in a rinse-off product like this. The amount of vitamin E is insignificant.

☺ GOOD $$$ **Natrulift Softening Cream Cleanser** *($14.50 for 6.76 fl. oz.)* is a silky, slightly greasy cleansing lotion that's best for normal to dry skin not prone to breakouts. It contains a paltry amount of anti-aging ingredients such as antioxidants, but they're wasted in a cleanser because they are rinsed down the drain. This does a thorough job of removing makeup, but you may find you need to use a washcloth with this for complete removal.

☺ GOOD $$$ **Natrulift Softening Facial Wash** *($14.50 for 3.38 fl. oz.)* is a water-soluble cleanser for normal to oily skin that won't minimize signs of aging (and, of course, it won't lift your skin). Its refreshing, clean-rinsing formula removes makeup and the tiny amount of plant oils shouldn't pose problems for those with blemish-prone skin. The small amount of antioxidants isn't going to exert an anti-aging effect, especially not in a cleanser that is rinsed off the skin. Note that this ends up being very expensive for the tiny amount of product, especially for what amounts to a very basic cleanser.

☺ AVERAGE **Nutriganics Foaming Facial Wash** *($14 for 5 fl. oz.)* has a Nutriganics name that implies nutrition and organic, two buzzwords that likely will attract lots of attention. As it turns out, there isn't anything about this cleanser that's particularly organic, natural, or nutritious. It's a liquid-to-foam water-soluble cleanser that contains gentle detergent cleansing agents and more fragrance than beneficial plant oils and extracts. A high amount of fragrance in a cleanser isn't good news for your skin; however, because a cleanser is rinsed quickly, it's less an issue than it would be for a leave-on product. This is an OK option for normal to dry skin.

☹ POOR **Nutriganics Softening Cleansing Gel** *($14.50 for 3.3 fl. oz.)* is an emollient cleanser that looks like a gel, but feels quite creamy, almost greasy, making it preferred for dry skin. Although the formula contains some beneficial ingredients to protect dry skin as you cleanse, it ends up being a problem for all skin types due to the numerous fragrant oils. All these fragrant oils are potent irritants, and not good to use around the eyes. Given the irritants, it really doesn't matter that the formula contains Community Fair Trade ingredients. Helping communities farm and profit from sustainable ingredients is great, but the ingredients don't have to be those that cause irritation. See the Appendix to learn how fragrant irritants hurt skin.

☹ POOR **Seaweed Deep Cleansing Facial Wash, for Combination/Oily Skin** *($13 for 3.3 fl. oz.)* has merit as a water-soluble cleanser for its intended skin type, but doesn't make it across the finish line because it contains irritating menthol. See the Appendix to learn how irritants like menthol make oily skin worse.

☹ POOR **Tea Tree Cleansing Wipes** *($12 for 25 wipes)* are below-standard wipes that have minimal cleansing ability and don't remove excess oil and makeup as well as most water-soluble cleansers. They're pricey for what you get too: These work out to be $0.48 per wipe and you'll be replacing them in less than a month! The amount of tea tree oil is too low to function as a disinfectant, while this contains fragrant oils and fragrance ingredients that cause irritation and are definitely not for use around the eyes.

The Reviews T

☹ POOR **Tea Tree Skin Clearing Facial Wash** *($11 for 8.4 fl. oz.)* has the makings of a very good water-soluble cleansing option for normal to oily skin, but things get problematic due to the inclusion of menthol and *Calophyllum inophyllum* seed oil, which is derived from a species of evergreen tree. Research has shown this ingredient is cytotoxic (kills cells) and although it may have antibacterial properties for acne, there are better ingredients to use for this purpose (Sources: *Journal of Photochemistry and Photobiology*, September 2009, pages 216–222; and *Phytochemistry*, October 2004, pages 2789–2795). The tea tree oil adds a medicinal scent, but the amount in this cleanser isn't great enough to combat acne-causing bacteria, not to mention it's rinsed from skin before it can be of much benefit.

☹ POOR **Tea Tree Skin Clearing Foaming Cleanser** *($13 for 5 fl. oz.)* is a liquid-to-foam cleanser that contains a hefty amount of tea tree oil, but also includes menthol, making it too irritating for any skin type. The seed oil from the *Calophyllum inophyllum* plant is also a problem for skin due to its irritating chemical constituents. See the Appendix to learn how irritating ingredients make oily, acne-prone skin worse, not better.

☹ POOR **Vitamin E Gentle Cleansing Wipes** *($14 for 25 wipes)* are water- and castor oil–based cleansing wipes that, while effective for removing makeup, contain the fragrant irritants of linalool, eugenol, and limonene, among others. With the abundance of cleansing wipes available, most for less money, there is no reason to use these and subject skin to irritation.

THE BODY SHOP EYE-MAKEUP REMOVERS

✓☺ BEST **Camomile Waterproof Eye Make-Up Remover** *($14.50 for 3.3 fl. oz.)* doesn't contain much chamomile, but is in fact an excellent lotion-type eye-makeup remover for all skin types. It works swiftly to remove even stubborn waterproof mascara, and is fragrance-free. This is best applied before washing with a water-soluble cleanser.

☺ GOOD **Camomile Gentle Eye Make-Up Remover** *($15 for 8.4 fl. oz.)* is a basic, fragrance-free makeup remover that contains silicone and a small amount of detergent cleansing agents to help dissolve eye makeup and other long-wearing makeup. The amount of chamomile is likely too small to have a soothing effect. The size is larger than most makeup removers, which makes the price easier to accept. Still, despite being a good formula, this isn't as effective as makeup removers from Almay, Neutrogena, or Paula's Choice.

THE BODY SHOP TONERS

☹ AVERAGE **Aloe Calming Toner, for Sensitive Skin** *($12 for 6.75 fl. oz.)* is a really boring concoction of just water, aloe, slip agents, and glycerin. It doesn't provide much benefit to skin other than slight moisture and helping to remove last traces of makeup. Sensitive skin needs more than what this provides.

☹ AVERAGE **Vitamin E Face Mist** *($16 for 3.2 fl. oz.)* is a very basic toner with a minor amount of vitamin E, almost to the point of making the name embarrassing. It's an OK option for normal to dry skin, and contains fragrance in the form of rose water.

☹ AVERAGE **$$$ Vitamin C Energizing Face Spritz** *($18 for 3.3 fl. oz.)* is a very basic, spray-on toner whose vitamin C content (it's listed as magnesium ascorbyl phosphate) is minimal given the product's name. It's an OK option for normal to slightly dry skin, but it's disappointing that a small amount of fragrance ingredients was included. Fragrance isn't skin care and the fragrance ingredients in this toner put your skin at risk of irritation (see the Appendix for details). This toner is not "ideal" for setting makeup as claimed. The main ingredients will end up causing makeup meltdown (or streaking), not prolonging its wear.

☹ POOR **Seaweed Clarifying Toner, for Combination/Oily Skin** *($12.50 for 6.76 fl. oz.)* contains menthol and that additive is made more irritating by the presence of fragrance ingredients such as linalool and citronellol. See the Appendix to learn how irritating ingredients make oily skin worse.

☹ POOR **Natrulift Softening Toner** *($14.50 for 6.76 fl. oz.)* lists alcohol as its second ingredient so it is not going to help skin of any age. Alcohol causes dryness, irritation, and free-radical damage, which leads to collagen breakdown. The result is skin that looks older than it is and is less able to maintain itself in a healthy manner. Almost equally stinging is that this toner contains more fragrance than state-of-the-art anti-aging ingredients.

☹ POOR **Nutriganics Refreshing Toner** *($14.50 for 6.75 fl. oz.)*. There isn't anything about this toner that's particularly organic, natural, or nutritious. The second ingredient is witch hazel water, which can be irritating; after that it's mostly glycerin, a thickener, and preservative. This toner won't do much for skin beyond causing a lot of irritation. The witch hazel water is bad enough, but The Body Shop added several fragrant plant oils and extracts that will sabotage rather than enhance healthy skin. See the Appendix to learn how daily use of fragrant products damages skin.

☹ POOR **Tea Tree Skin Clearing Toner** *($11 for 8.4 fl. oz.)* lists alcohol as the second ingredient and also contains a host of other problematic ingredients that won't improve matters for blemish-prone skin. Alcohol in this amount causes dryness, free-radical damage, and irritation that can stimulate more oil production at the base of your pores. The anti-irritants this contains won't be of much help due to the irritating ingredients that dull their impact.

☹ POOR **Vitamin E Hydrating Toner** *($12.50 for 7 fl. oz.)* is an exceptionally basic toner that is an average formula for normal to dry skin. The amount of vitamin E is OK, but what earns this product its low rating is the inclusion of numerous fragrance ingredients capable of causing irritation. With so little positives (it contains more preservative than beneficial ingredients), there is no reason to consider this. Plus, the irritation this toner causes hurts your skin's healing process and impairs healthy collagen production.

THE BODY SHOP EXFOLIANTS & SCRUBS

☺ GOOD **Aloe Gentle Exfoliator, for Sensitive Skin** *($15 for 2.5 fl. oz.)* exfoliates skin with a small amount of mildly abrasive diatomaceous earth derived from tiny sea creatures. This ingredient is cushioned in a slightly creamy base of water, aloe, slip agents, and thickeners. It is a workable option for dry skin and is fragrance-free.

☺ GOOD **Honey & Oat 3-In-1 Scrub Mask** *($17 for 3.6 fl. oz.)* has natural ingredients such as oat bran for its scrub action, kaolin (clay) for its absorbency when used as a mask, and honey for its moisture-binding ability (though this will be minimal due to the inclusion of clay). It's a novel option for those with normal to dry skin looking for a close-to-natural scrub. Used as a mask, it may end up confusing skin because it is overall too emollient for oily skin and too absorbent for dry skin. It's not a "triple action" time-saving product, but when used gently is a serviceable scrub.

☺ GOOD **Seaweed Pore-Cleansing Facial Exfoliator, for Combination/Oily Skin** *($15 for 2.5 fl. oz.)* is a cleanser and topical scrub in one that uses olive seed powder as the abrasive agent. The jojoba oil is inappropriate for oily areas, but this is an acceptable scrub for normal to slightly dry skin.

☀ Sunscreens must provide reliable UVA (anti-aging) protection. See the Appendix for details.

☺ AVERAGE **Vitamin E Cream Exfoliator** *($15 for 2.5 fl. oz.)* contains some problematic fragrance ingredients (eugenol among them) that downgrade an otherwise excellent topical scrub for dry to very dry skin. This is still worth considering since it is rinsed from skin so quickly.

☺ GOOD $$$ **Vitamin C Facial Cleansing Polish** *($16 for 3.3 fl. oz.)* contains vitamin C as touted in the product name, but its presence in this standard scrub is little more than window dressing. Besides, what little vitamin C this contains is rinsed from your skin anyway. This is worth considering if you have normal to oily skin and prefer scrubs that also function as cleansers. If you're not a fan of scrubs, no worries: A well-formulated AHA or BHA exfoliant is a better way to go!

☺ AVERAGE $$$ **Tea Tree Skin Clearing Exfoliating Pads** *($15 for 40 pads)* are water-steeped pads that also contain salicylic acid, but the amount is too low and the pH is way outside the narrow range this exfoliating ingredient needs for efficacy. The other plant oils in these pads do not have reliable research proving their worth for skin, whether breakouts are the issue or not. In short, these pads do little more than add an extra cleansing step and leave skin scented with medicinal tea tree oil. Despite the economic stewardship that comes from sourcing tea tree oil from a community in Kenya, the fact remains that these anti-acne pads cannot exfoliate skin and the amount of tea tree oil isn't enough to function as a topical disinfectant capable of killing acne-causing bacteria.

☺ AVERAGE $$$ **Vitamin C Microdermabrasion** *($20 for 2.5 fl. oz.)* contains diatomaceous earth (listed as solum diatomae) as the main abrasive agent. This is not the ingredient you get from professional microdermabrasion treatments, which typically use aluminum or magnesium oxide crystals. The problem with diatomaceous earth (a fancy way to describe the fossilized remains of algae and shells) is that the individual particles are rough and have a tendency to scratch and tear at your skin. In contrast, polyethylene or jojoba beads are spherical and a much gentler way to polish your skin. Regardless of the abrasive agent, scrubs aren't preferred to well-formulated AHA or BHA exfoliants, especially if signs of aging or acne are your concern. As for the vitamin C, its presence in this scrub is so minor that it's seemingly an afterthought, not to mention that its benefit is rinsed down the drain.

☹ POOR **Tea Tree Blackhead Exfoliating Wash** *($13 for 3.3 fl. oz.)* is a slightly creamy scrub that essentially claims you can scrub blackheads away, which absolutely isn't true. A facial scrub can help remove the top portion of the blackhead, but since you're not doing anything about the underlying cause, the blackhead is back before you know it. Moreover, because this uses apricot seed powder as one of the abrasive agents, it can be rougher on skin than a well-formulated scrub should be. The amount of tea tree oil is too low to have an antibacterial effect against acne, and blackheads have nothing to do with bacteria. This contains the seed oil from the *Calophyllum inophyllum* plant which is also a problem for skin due to its irritating chemical constituents.

THE BODY SHOP MOISTURIZERS (DAYTIME & NIGHTTIME), EYE CREAMS, & SERUMS

☺ GOOD **Aloe Protective Serum, for Sensitive Skin** *($21 for 1 fl. oz.)* is an aloe-based serum that has some intriguing ingredients for slightly dry sensitive skin, though many of them are present in amounts too small for skin to notice. Still, this gel-like serum is fragrance-free and provides antioxidant benefit via its soybean oil content. Although not a true state-of-the-art serum, it is a worthy choice for those with sensitive skin.

☺ GOOD **Aloe Soothing Moisture Lotion SPF 15, for Sensitive Skin** *($18 for 1.7 fl. oz.)* is worth considering as a fragrance-free daytime moisturizer for normal to slightly dry skin.

It includes an in-part avobenzone sunscreen and lightweight moisturizing ingredients plus a tiny amount of anti-irritants.

☺ AVERAGE **Aloe Eye Defense** *($18 for 0.5 fl. oz.)* is a good, though relatively unexciting, lightweight moisturizer for slightly dry skin anywhere on the face. Aloe has anti-inflammatory properties, but a product intended to soothe signs of sensitivity should contain more than just aloe as its anti-irritant backbone. This contains a tiny amount of soothing allantoin and some respectable water-binding agents, so it's certainly not a waste-of-time product, but the truth is you don't need to bother with eye cream (see the Appendix to find out why).

☺ AVERAGE **Aloe Soothing Day Cream, for Sensitive Skin** *($16.50 for 1.7 fl. oz.)* isn't the most soothing moisturizer around, and the tiny amount of oat flour in this fragrance-free moisturizer will barely register on skin. It's just a basic moisturizer for normal to slightly dry skin. Sensitive skin needs more than what this provides!

☺ AVERAGE **Aloe Soothing Night Cream, for Sensitive Skin** *($20 for 1.7 fl. oz.)* is a more emollient version of the Aloe Soothing Day Cream, for Sensitive Skin above. It contains an additional soothing agent, though not in an amount great enough for irritated skin to notice.

☺ AVERAGE **Natrulift Firming Day Lotion SPF 15** *($20 for 1.69 fl. oz.)* is a daytime moisturizer with an in-part avobenzone sunscreen that provides reliable broad-spectrum protection, which is always a primary way to achieve anti-aging benefits. The lightweight, silky texture is surprisingly moisturizing, making this best for normal to dry rather than combination or oily skin. This contains two forms of the antioxidant pomegranate. Despite pomegranate's benefits for skin, it isn't the only anti-aging ingredient to look for. Unfortunately, the lack of other beneficial ingredients (besides the sunscreens) in this moisturizer makes it a one-note product. Skin of any age does best when treated to a range of beneficial substances, and you're simply not getting enough of them here. As for firming, keeping your skin protected from further sun damage (which this does) helps prevent further loss of firmness. While pomegranate is one of many ingredients that can stimulate collagen production and repair, there are other daytime moisturizers that supply a far more impressive range of antioxidants in combination with other essential ingredients.

☺ AVERAGE **Natrulift Firming Day Cream** *($30 for 1.7 fl. oz.)* is an emollient moisturizer that is ill suited for daytime use because it lacks sunscreen. Without it, there's no sense in referring to it as a day cream. After all, skin cannot tell time, so the only difference between a day cream and a night cream should be that your day cream (or lotion) contains sunscreen, period. Although this moisturizer contains some helpful, if basic, ingredients for dry skin, the fact that it's packaged in a jar is a deal-breaker. See the Appendix to learn why jar packaging is a problem.

☺ AVERAGE **Natrulift Refreshing Eye Roll-on Eye Gel** *($10 for 0.5 fl. oz.)* is housed inside a pen-like component outfitted with a rollerball applicator. Inside is a lightweight gel-like fluid that doesn't contain anything particularly impressive for skin, whether around the eyes or elsewhere. This feels cooling and refreshing, but that's about it. The gel dispensed via the rollerball applicator won't lift skin one bit, though the massaging action can help reduce puffiness (the kind from allergies or general swelling, not age-related puffiness due to fat pads beneath the skin shifting out of place). This contains a tiny amount of antioxidants and the cell-communicating ingredient adenosine, but nothing to get excited about. Clinique All About Eyes Serum is a better version of this product in the same type of packaging. Yes, Clinique's costs more but in this case you're getting a better formula, too. Ultimately, you don't need a special serum for the eye area (see the Appendix for details), but products like this can help reduce some types of puffiness (but again, not the kind that results from aging—that requires surgery).

☺ AVERAGE **Nutriganics Smoothing Day Cream** (*$22 for 1.69 fl. oz.*) isn't suitable for daytime use because it lacks sun protection. We could concede to this being a good nighttime moisturizer for dry skin, but it isn't ideal due to the numerous fragrant plant extracts and fragrance ingredients it contains. You'd be better off mixing pure shea butter with olive or jojoba oil and applying that blend to dry skin. Both of those are far more natural than this product.

☹ AVERAGE **Nutriganics Smoothing Night Cream** (*$24 for 1.69 fl. oz.*) contains some helpful natural ingredients that are great for dry skin, but the amount of fragrance ingredients and fragrant plant extracts is cause for concern. The salicylic acid doesn't function as an exfoliant because there is only a small amount and the pH of this moisturizer is too high, although to give them credit, The Body Shop isn't making exfoliation claims. This is a tough sell because it's truly a mixed bag for dry skin.

☹ AVERAGE **Nutriganics Smoothing Eye Cream** (*$20 for 0.5 fl. oz.*). There isn't anything about this eye cream that's particularly organic or nutritious. It's a rather basic formula that comes in a soothing cornflower water base and includes thickeners, plant oil, and wax. There's also a good deal of mica for shine, but shine isn't skin care. This eye cream is tough to recommend, not only because it has a mundane formula, but also because it contains several fragrance ingredients known to irritate skin, which can be even more of a problem if used near the eyes. See the Appendix to find out why, in truth, you don't need an eye cream.

☺ AVERAGE **Seaweed Mattifying Day Cream, for Combination/Oily Skin** (*$16.50 for 1.7 fl. oz.*) offers skin slightly more than the Seaweed Clarifying Night Treatment reviewed below, but that's not saying much. This is an average water- and silicone-based moisturizer for its intended skin type. Its finish is minimally matte.

☺ AVERAGE **Seaweed Mattifying Moisture Lotion SPF 15, for Combination/Oily Skin** (*$18 for 1.69 fl. oz.*) provides an in-part avobenzone sunscreen in a lightweight lotion base suitable for its intended skin type. What's missing are several essential elements necessary to create a great moisturizer, making this an effective, though average, option.

☺ AVERAGE **Vitamin C Daily Moisturizer SPF 30, Dull Skin** (*$20 for 1.69 fl. oz.*) is a daytime moisturizer with an in-part avobenzone sunscreen. The lightweight, silky texture is deceptively moisturizing, making this best for normal to dry rather than combination or oily skin. As for the vitamin C, it's present as tetrahexyldecyl ascorbate, but not in an amount that's going to cause dull skin to do an about-face or look more even-toned. Despite vitamin C's benefits for skin, it isn't the only anti-aging ingredient to look for, and more to the point, it takes more than any one ingredient can provide to improve the skin's appearance. This moisturizer is a one-note product with sunscreen, but skin of any age does best when treated to a range of beneficial substances, and that's simply not what you're getting here.

☺ AVERAGE **Vitamin E Illuminating Moisture Cream** (*$18.50 for 1.7 fl. oz.*) is an average moisturizer for normal to dry skin. Its jar packaging won't help keep the meager amount of vitamin E stable once you've opened it (see the Appendix for details).

☺ AVERAGE **Vitamin E Moisture Cream** (*$16.50 for 1.7 fl. oz.*) is nearly identical to the Vitamin E Illuminating Moisture Cream above, and the same review applies.

☺ AVERAGE **Vitamin E Moisture Serum** (*$21 for 1 fl. oz.*) shortchanges skin on vitamin E and other antioxidants, and ends up being a basic, lightweight, water- and silicone-based serum that's an acceptable, though hardly exciting, option for normal to dry skin. There is nothing about this serum that is not easily replaced by myriad alternatives.

☺ AVERAGE **Vitamin E Nourishing Night Cream** (*$20 for 1.7 fl. oz.*) covers some of the basics in terms of what makes a great moisturizer, but some isn't enough, and the jar packaging won't keep the tiny amount of vitamin E in here stable once the product is opened. See the Appendix to find out why jar packaging is a problem.

☺ AVERAGE **$$$ Natrulift Firming Serum** *($36 for 1 fl. oz.)* is a serum that claims to help your skin look and act younger; however, the formula is mostly disappointing. It is lightly hydrating and OK for normal to slightly dry skin, but most of the intriguing ingredients are listed after the preservative, which means you're not getting much to help your skin look younger, and your skin deserves those ingredients in abundance! This cannot lift your skin in the least, and it's disappointing that it also contains several fragrance ingredients known to cause irritation.

☺ AVERAGE **$$$ Vitamin C Facial Radiance Powder** *($28 for 0.61 fl. oz.)* consists of a vitamin C powder (containing 5% ascorbic acid, the chemical name for vitamin C) packaged with a water-based serum. You're supposed to mix a small amount of the powder with the serum before applying it to your face—a step that's more gimmicky than necessary, although the packaging definitely has a medicinal look. Vitamin C doesn't need to be in powder form to be efficacious, nor does it need to be packaged separately from other ingredients. For the most part, this is a one-note product. Vitamin C has multiple benefits for your skin, but your skin deserves more than one great ingredient. Just like a healthy diet features a variety of nutritious foods, a healthy skin-care routine should encompass a variety of beneficial ingredients. What keeps this from earning a better rating is the inclusion of fragrance ingredients known to be irritating. Products such as Paula's Choice RESIST Super Antioxidant Concentrate Serum supply your skin with a range of beneficial ingredients (including vitamin C) in a silky, fragrance-free formula.

☺ AVERAGE **$$$ Wise Woman Eye Cream** *($24 for 0.5 fl. oz.)* is an aloe-based moisturizer that contains more witch hazel than beneficial ingredients, though not enough to be irritating. This is an OK, slightly emollient formula whose most intriguing ingredients are listed after the preservative, so they don't count for much. See the Appendix to learn why, in truth, you don't need an eye cream.

☺ AVERAGE **$$$ Wise Woman Regenerating Day Cream** *($32 for 1.7 fl. oz.)* isn't suitable for daytime because it does not carry an SPF rating (though sunscreen agents are the second- and fifth-listed ingredients). Why The Body Shop included broad-spectrum protection without going through the testing necessary to establish an SPF rating is a mystery, and leaves this as an unwise choice for any woman. Moisturizer-wise, it doesn't break any new ground and is best suited for normal to dry skin. The antioxidants are sullied by jar packaging (see the Appendix for details).

☺ AVERAGE **$$$ Wise Woman Vitality Serum** *($36 for 1 fl. oz.)* is built around the ingredient lactobacillus clover flower extract. Lactobacillus is a type of aerobic bacteria that produces large amounts of lactic acid as it ferments with carbohydrate sources. There is some research indicating that taking supplements of lactobacillus (it is also considered a probiotic) may help reduce skin allergies and forms of dermatitis. However, substantiated research on topical application of lactobacillus is nonexistent, though it likely functions as a water-binding agent. Clover flower has no research proving its mettle for aging skin, and it may be sensitizing. There is little reason to consider this serum compared to superior options from Olay, Clinique, and Paula's Choice.

☻ POOR **Nutriganics Smoothing Serum** *($24 for 1 fl. oz.)* contains many of the same ingredients seen in The Body Shop's Nutriganics moisturizers. You'd think the serum would take a different approach, using complementary ingredients, but instead it's more of the same, and that's a mixed bag of good and problematic ingredients. This serum contains as many helpful ingredients as potentially irritating ingredients, including numerous fragrance ingredients that no one's skin needs. Ultimately, it's the fragrant, irritating plant oils and other forms of fragrance that keep this serum from being worth serious consideration. See the Appendix to find out how daily use of highly fragrant products hurts your skin.

☹ POOR **Seaweed Clarifying Night Treatment, for Combination/Oily Skin** *($20 for 1 fl. oz.)* is a boring moisturizer. Despite enticing claims, this product is primarily water, thickener, and preservative. Lots of ingredients follow these basics, but none of them are intriguing for skin and leave it shortchanged yet highly fragranced.

☹ POOR **Tea Tree Skin Clearing Lotion** *($13 for 1.69 fl. oz.)* is a lightweight moisturizer that has a silicone-enriched, silky texture, but the amount of tea tree oil is too low to function as a topical disinfectant for acne. Moreover, this contains some problematic fragrance ingredients and fragrant oils, all of which can make oily, acne-prone skin worse (see the Appendix for details).

☹ POOR **Wise Woman Regenerating Night Cream** *($36 for 1.7 fl. oz.)* would have been a slam-dunk for dry to very dry skin were it not for jar packaging that hinders the effectiveness of the antioxidant-rich plant oils and the inclusion of irritating lavender oil. See the Appendix to learn why jar packaging and lavender oil are bad news for your skin.

☹ POOR **Vitamin C Eye Reviver Duo** *($22 for 0.5 fl. oz.)* is a dual-sided product housed as an eye cream on one end and an eye gel on the other. Claims of reviving the delicate skin around the eyes and relieving dark circles are standard for this kind of product, but neither formula contains anything capable of doing that. The two formulas are utterly basic and unimpressive. The **Eye Cream** is lightly hydrating, but lacks a significant amount of state-of-the-art ingredients; in fact, there is more preservative in this product than beneficial ingredients. It includes two sunscreen ingredients (ethylhexyl methoxycinnamate and avobenzone, listed by its chemical name butyl methoxydibenzoylmethane), but because neither is listed as an active ingredient you cannot rely on this for sun protection. The Eye Cream also contains mica for shine, but shine isn't skin care. Turning to the **Eye Gel**, you're getting little more than water and the irritant witch hazel distillate. A small amount of alcohol is also present. The irritation from the Eye Gel can impair skin's healing process and hinder healthy collagen production—both of which can make dark circles look worse. Save your money and take superior care of your eye area by using your face product, if it is well formulated and appropriate for the skin type around your eyes!

☹ POOR **Vitamin C Facial Radiance Capsules** *($28 for 28 capsules)* is a serum that features individual capsules containing a mix of silicones with vitamin C (ascorbic acid) and plant oils, some of which are fragrant and capable of causing irritation. This is also true of the fragrance ingredients this contains. A well-formulated vitamin C serum need not smell like an orange grove to be effective. In fact, the fragrant citrus oil can cause irritation that hurts your skin's healing process and impairs healthy collagen production—so much for radiant, younger-looking skin!

☹ POOR **Vitamin C Skin Boost** *($26 for 1 fl. oz.)* is a silicone-based serum that contains more fragrance than vitamin C (listed as ascorbic acid). In addition to the fragrance, this also contains several fragrance ingredients that only add to the irritation the fragrance presents. Fragrance isn't skin care and there are plenty of serums with vitamin C that either omit fragrance entirely or contain a much lower amount. This isn't the serum to choose if you're keen on vitamin C, especially because there are precious few other beneficial ingredients to be found here. For the money, if you're concerned about signs of aging and want a serum with vitamin C and lots of other youth-enhancing ingredients, look no further than Paula's Choice RESIST Super Antioxidant Concentrate Serum.

THE BODY SHOP LIP CARE

✓☺ BEST **Cocoa Butter Lip Care Stick** *($8 for 0.15 fl. oz.)* is an excellent lip balm that contains a thoughtful blend of nut oils, wax, olive oil, and, as the name states, cocoa butter. An added bonus is several anti-irritants, which makes this lip balm a step above most others.

☺ GOOD **Aloe Lip Treatment** *($9.50 for 0.5 fl. oz.)* is a good lip balm packaged in a tube for convenient, take-along use. The simple blend of castor oil and coconut oil does a great job of preventing chapped lips, and The Body Shop was wise to not include any extraneous irritants like mint or menthol as so many other companies do. As for the aloe, its presence is so meager your lips won't notice—but that's OK, because everything that precedes it on the list is helpful.

☺ GOOD **Born Lippy Balms** *($6 for 0.3 fl. oz.)* are standard castor oil– and lanolin-based lip balms that are available in a variety of fruit flavors. Never mind the fact that fruit-flavored balms encourage lip-licking and create the need to reapply the product frequently. More important is that not all the flavors are recommended. The one to avoid due to irritating fragrant components is **Strawberry**. The **Raspberry** and **Watermelon** balms do not contain these problematic ingredients and are recommended.

☺ GOOD **Delipscious Tinted Lip Conditioner** *($10)* is a highly fragranced tinted lip balm that definitely delivers plenty of moisturizing ingredients and a subtle wash of color to lips. All shades have a fruity scent and lightly sweet flavor, which makes it tempting to lick this balm off your lips, although doing so is not recommended because it will promote chapping (this is a tinted lip balm, not dessert).

☹ AVERAGE **Hemp Lip Protector** *($8 for 0.15 fl. oz.)* contains some fragrance ingredients (linalool, limonene, and geraniol) that pose a risk of irritation with each use. This is disappointing because dry, chapped lips are less likely to improve with so much fragrance. It still contains some very good plant-based emollients that protect lips from moisture loss, but it's just not a sure bet.

☹ POOR **Lip Butter** *($6 for 0.3 fl. oz.)* has a buttery-smooth texture and can ably take care of dry, chapped lips. However, it is available in several flavors and all but one of them contains irritating fragrant components. The flavor to consider is **Coconut**; none of the others is recommended.

☹ POOR **Vitamin E Lip Care Stick SPF 15** *($8 for 0.15 fl. oz.)* does not contain the UVA-protecting ingredients of titanium dioxide, zinc oxide, avobenzone, Tinosorb, or Mexoryl SX, and is not recommended.

☹ POOR **Lip Scuff** *($12 for 0.14 fl. oz.)* is an oil–based, lipstick-style exfoliant that contains spearmint and peppermint oils along with the irritating menthol derivative menthyl lactate. As is, chapping will be diminished due to the scrub particles but lips will be irritated, which, surprise, leads to more chapping.

THE BODY SHOP SPECIALTY SKIN-CARE PRODUCTS

☹ AVERAGE **Aloe Protective Restoring Mask, for Sensitive Skin** *($22 for 3.3 fl. oz.)* contains one substantial emollient and a small amount of nonfragrant plant oil; however, this is a boring mask for those with normal to dry or sensitive skin. Aloe isn't a protective ingredient, at least not when it comes to shielding skin from further irritation or helping to improve its barrier function (though that's not to say it doesn't have benefit for skin). A greater concentration of soothing agents and non-jar packaging would have made this mask a much better product.

☹ AVERAGE **Seaweed Pore Perfector, for Combination/Oily Skin** *($21 for 0.5 fl. oz.)* contains mostly water, silicone, and alcohol. It's doubtful the alcohol will have a detrimental effect on skin given that the amount is likely less than 5%, but its prominence is definitely a red flag. Plus, this contains lots of fragrance ingredients that have no positive effect on blemishes, and that may cause irritation. See the Appendix to find out how irritating ingredients make oily skin worse.

☺ AVERAGE **Tea Tree Blemish Gel** *($9 for 0.08 fl. oz.)* lists alcohol as the second ingredient and also contains a host of other problematic ingredients that won't improve matters for blemish-prone skin. See the Appendix to learn why alcohol is a big problem, especially for oily, acne-prone skin.

☺ AVERAGE **Vitamin E Sink-In Moisture Mask** *($22 for 3.38 fl. oz.)* is worth considering by those with dry to very dry skin due to its effective blend of glycerin, silicone, plant oils, and skin-identical ingredients. It's a shame the jar packaging doesn't help keep the vitamin E stable, but without question this will make dry skin look and feel better, and it does not need to be rinsed from skin.

☺ AVERAGE $$$ **Seaweed Ionic Clay Mask** *($22 for 4.2 fl. oz.)* contains several types of seaweed, but seaweed cannot detoxify skin. The ionic properties attributed to the clay content are bizarre because clay is merely an absorbent, whether ions are involved or not. This mask is an OK yet needlessly pricey option to use on oily skin or oily areas. The amount of alcohol (it's the fifth ingredient) is not likely to be problematic.

☹ POOR **Nutriganics Smoothing Mask** *($22 for 3.98 fl. oz.)* is a below-standard clay-based mask whose appeal to those with oily, blemished skin is marred by the inclusion of numerous fragrance ingredients and fragrant oils. The combined irritation these cause will lead to increased oil production at the base of your pores. Also worth noting is that this mask's blend of clay and nonfragrant plant oils is bound to be confusing for those with oily skin, yet too drying for those with dry skin.

☹ POOR **Tea Tree Blemish Fade Night Lotion** *($18 for 1 fl. oz.)* is a lightweight moisturizer that contains barely any tea tree oil, instead relying on laurelwood oil (listed as *Calophyllum inophyllum* and also known as tamanu oil) for its alleged anti-blemish properties. We wrote "alleged" because there is insufficient evidence available to gauge the effectiveness of this oil for blemishes and it is an irritant (it kills skin cells) (Source: naturaldatabase.com). It might work to some extent against blemishes due to its potential antibacterial action and fatty acid composition, but wouldn't you rather spend your money experimenting with proven anti-acne ingredients?

☹ POOR **Tea Tree Face Mask** *($15 for 3.85 fl. oz.)* is a clay mask that isn't recommended because it contains *Calophyllum inophyllum* seed oil, which is derived from a species of evergreen tree. Research has shown this ingredient is cytotoxic (kills cells) and although it may have antibacterial properties for acne, there are better ingredients to use for this purpose (Sources: *Journal of Photochemistry and Photobiology*, September 2009, pages 216–222; and *Phytochemistry*, October 2004, pages 2789–2795).

THE BODY SHOP FOUNDATIONS & PRIMERS

✓☺ BEST **All in One Face Base** *($22)*. This talc-based, pressed-powder foundation has an amazingly silky application that provides a natural matte finish and light coverage. Few powders look this natural on skin, and it does a great job of minimizing pores and controlling excess oil. The six shades are best for fair to medium skin tones and all of them are soft and neutral. All in One Face Base is best for normal to slightly dry or slightly oily skin.

☺ GOOD **Extra Virgin Minerals Liquid Foundation** *($25)* is a lightweight, fragrance-free liquid foundation that provides normal to dry skin with light to medium coverage. It also blends far better than The Body Shop's cream compact version of this foundation. Although the texture is silky-soft, allowing for easy application with your fingertips, a brush, or a sponge, the finish is definitely dewy, so you'll want to experiment to see if it will work well for your skin type. If wrinkles are an issue, be advised that this did settle slightly into lines around the eyes. Among the many shades there are options for fair to dark skin tones, though you'd do best to avoid Rose Beige and Golden Vanilla because, despite their names, they have ashy undertones that can make the complexion look grayish. As for the mineral makeup angle, it's more marketing buzz than a beauty breakthrough.

☺ GOOD **Extra Virgin Minerals Powder Foundation** *($25)* is a wonderful soft, finely milled loose-powder foundation that feels nearly weightless on skin, and it is indeed a mineral-based powder (like countless others). Housed in a screw-top jar with a sifter, application requires the standard "mineral makeup method" of shaking out some powder into the lid, swirling the brush in the contents, then applying to your face. That technique works well enough (though it's messy), but unlike many loose mineral foundations, this one cannot provide full coverage without looking cakey. If you prefer sheer to light coverage and have normal to oily or combination skin, you're in luck, but that assumes you don't mind a soft shimmer finish. Of all the Extra Virgin foundations, this one has the most neutral shades that will suit the widest range of fair to tan skin tones. As for the mineral makeup angle, it's more marketing buzz than a beauty breakthrough.

☺ GOOD **Skin Primer Matte It** *($14)* is a fragrance-free, silicone-based primer that has a slightly viscous texture that melts into skin, leaving a silky, imperceptible soft matte finish. It is an option for normal to oily skin and aids with foundation application. Despite our enthusiasm, there are other lightweight moisturizers and serums whose ingredient rosters best this one and that supply skin with a wide range of ingredients that it needs to look its best. Those with sensitive, oily skin may want to check this out, though.

☹ AVERAGE **Extra Virgin Minerals Compact Foundation** *($25)* is a very good cream-to-powder foundation for dry skin. The butter-smooth texture glides on—although blending takes some effort because this has a tendency to streak and splotch. You'll immediately see medium coverage that you can easily build to full without looking cakey. The Body Shop claims this is a matte finish, yet it feels and looks significantly dewy, which makes sense given the emollient formula. Once it sets, the shininess of the finish dissipates to a satin matte look, but we noticed that it tended to pool slightly, accentuating pores. The half moon-shaped synthetic brush included in the compact worked surprisingly well, but you'll need a small sponge to blend or get into smaller parts of the face, like under the eye or around the nose. Among the many shades, there are options for fair to dark skin tones, but in a foundation with this much pigment there's very little room for a shade to be "off," so experiment in the store and check the results on your skin in daylight before you buy. As for the mineral makeup angle, it's more marketing buzz than a beauty breakthrough.

☹ AVERAGE **Oil-Free Foundation SPF 15** *($23)* gets its sunscreen partly from titanium dioxide. Although that's great news for this matte finish foundation, the high amount (and likely the grade) of titanium dioxide used lends a slightly chalky finish that is difficult to soften. If you want an oil-free, medium to full coverage foundation and are amenable to this one's finish (the chalkiness is coupled with a soft shimmer), it may be worth a look. The predominantly yellow-based shades are good and include options for fair to dark skin tones.

☹ AVERAGE **Skin Primer Moisturize It** *($14)* is not the least bit moisturizing, although it does leave a very smooth finish. This has a very thin texture that's easy to apply, and it sets quickly to a subtle glow finish. Given the lack of intriguing ingredients in the formula, this isn't worth strong consideration over several other primers or, better yet, a serum loaded with beneficial ingredients.

☺ AVERAGE **$$$ Moisture Foundation SPF 15** *($23)* certainly delivers on its promise of moisture and, therefore, is definitely too emollient for skin that's even slightly oily. The silky consistency is that of any good rich moisturizer and it won't run or dribble out of its airtight pump. Once applied, you'll see a dewy finish, but then, unfortunately, it turns greasy and settles into lines within minutes. As if that weren't issue enough, the limited shade range provides suitable options only for lighter skin tones, because Shade 6 wears too orange (incidentally, the darker Shades 7 and 8 aren't even available in most stores, but can be found online). There's no question that this foundation will deliver moisture and UVA protection in the form of zinc oxide, but with such light coverage and that unpleasantly greasy finish, it's doubtful this will do more to flatter and even your complexion.

THE BODY SHOP CONCEALER

☹ POOR **Concealer Pencil** *($11 for 0.13 fl. oz.)* is a thick, creamy concealer packaged as a chunky pencil that needs regular sharpening. This covers well and blends better than expected, but the greasepaint-like texture creases easily and the shades aren't anything to get excited about. Considering the number of amazing concealers available in all price ranges, this isn't worth an audition.

THE BODY SHOP POWDERS

✓☺ BEST **Pressed Face Powder** *($18.50)* has an admirably silky, talc-based texture that is minimally dry. In fact, the oils in this pressed powder and the smooth, non-powdery finish it provides make it a good choice for those with normal to dry skin. The shades are remarkably neutral and meant for light to medium skin tones only.

☺ GOOD **Loose Face Powder** *($16 for 0.49 fl. oz.)* has a silky, airy, talc-based texture and a drier-than-usual finish that is ideal for normal to very oily skin. Shades 01, 02, and 03 are neutral flesh tones perfect for fair to medium skin, while shade 05 is a sheer bronze color with gold shimmer, which tends to flake.

THE BODY SHOP BLUSHES & BRONZERS

☺ GOOD **Baked-To-Last Bronzer** *($22)* is a pressed bronzing powder that comes in two flattering shades that blend evenly on skin for a believable medium or dark tan effect. Each shade imparts a shiny finish that is luminescent rather than overly shiny, so your skin is left with a radiant glow. This is a good option for anyone looking for a sun-kissed appearance with a hint of shimmer.

☺ GOOD **Pearly Lip & Cheek Stain** *($14)* is a dual-purpose product that produces a soft, natural color beneath a slightly moist, pearly finish that can be applied to either lips or cheeks. It's available in only one shade: a gold-flecked pink. As a lip color, it's nothing extraordinary, but it's workable as a cheek stain. Surprisingly, the sole color option proves flattering on most skin tones and sets nicely without any greasiness beyond its intended luminescence. The product has a thicker, more manageable consistency than water-based cheek stains, but the sponge-tip wand applicator makes it tricky to use for application on the face; however, it's a huge improvement over fast-drying stains with brush-tip applicators that are very difficult to work with. With some practice, this is a unique option for anyone who finds liquid cheek stains too bright or too unruly.

☺ GOOD **$$$ Baked-To-Last Blush** *($18)* is a dual-sided, pressed-powder blush that goes on smooth. One part of the container is a blush shade and the other half is a shiny peachy shade. They can be applied together or separately. The color goes on sheer and imparts a slight shimmering effect that is luminescent, leaving your skin with a healthy, flushed glow.

☺ AVERAGE **Cheek Color** *($16)* is a large-size traditional powder blush, reminiscent of the size and packaging of M.A.C.'s powder blushes. This has a soft texture and a dry but smooth application that imparts very sheer, see-through color. All the shades shine, but Golden Pink is ultra-shiny and is not recommended for daytime. The shine among the remaining understated shades is, well, understated!

☹ POOR **Honey Bronze Brilliance Powder** *($22)* is an illuminating bronzer housed in a tube that's outfitted with a built-in brush. The packaging makes this difficult to dispense through the attached brush which, in turn, makes it tricky to control the amount of loose powder that comes out. The shades go on sheer yet uneven and are laced with so much glitter that you can hardly see any color through the sparkling flecks. Worse yet, the Copper shade has a strong burgundy undertone, making it an unflattering choice for almost any skin color. This isn't such a brilliant option after all!

☹ POOR **Honey Bronze Bronzing Gel** *($14)* has a lightweight, liquid-gel texture that must be blended well for even results. The major issue is that the sole shade is an unnatural tan color: orange-y bronze with reddish undertones. Fortunately, it goes on sheer so you aren't overwhelmed with color, but it's still unflattering.

THE BODY SHOP EYESHADOWS

☺ AVERAGE **Baked Eye Color** *($12.50)* is a shimmery pressed-powder eyeshadow that offers two marbleized shades in one compact, without a divider. The eight shades available consist of jewel and earth tones. The texture is soft, making it easy to apply and blend, but depending on the depth of color you're going for, you may be disappointed with how sheer this shadow is. In short, you'll see more shimmer than color, but the shimmer stays put with minimal flaking. The powder is soft pressed in its compact, watch out for crumbling if this jostles around in your makeup bag.

☺ AVERAGE **Eye Colors** *($9 for 0.06 fl. oz.)* feel silky and blend beautifully, but here's the frustration: All the shades, even the dark ones, go on extremely sheer. Talk about subtle color! And these do not build that well, so you're pretty much stuck with no intensity and a light wash of color that stands a good chance of fading even before you leave your house. If you're looking for very soft color, these are worth a peek, but watch out for the glittery shades because they do not apply as smoothly and the glitter tends to flake. The non-glittery but still shiny shades don't have this trait. If you're shopping for matte options, you'll need to look elsewhere.

☺ AVERAGE **Eye Shimmer** *($9 for 0.05 fl. oz.)* doesn't apply as smoothly as the Eye Colors above, but it's not worth downgrading to a Poor rating. The small selection of shades is all about shine, and they serve their purpose with minimal flaking despite slightly uneven application.

THE BODY SHOP EYE & BROW LINERS

✓☺ BEST **Liquid Eyeliner** *($13.50)* has an excellent soft, but firm, brush that is adept at drawing a thin, continuous line and has a fast-drying formula that minimizes the risk of smearing, plus it wears beautifully.

☺ GOOD **$$$ Brow & Liner Kit** *($18)* combines a brow powder and powder eyeshadow to use as liner in one petite compact. The circular component houses a cleverly designed dual-sided brush, but regrettably the brow brush is too stiff (and deposits too much product if your brows are thin) and the eyeliner brush is too floppy for precise control. Still, both powders go on smoothly and are pigment-rich. Each also has a touch of shine, but it's barely noticeable on skin. The three duos include options for all brow colors except shades of red or auburn.

☺ AVERAGE **Brow & Lash Gel** *($15 for 0.33 fl. oz.)* is a standard clear gel that works to groom brows and barely enhance lashes. It will feel sticky unless applied lightly, but it doesn't take much to achieve a groomed look.

☺ AVERAGE **Eye Definer** *($11 for 0.04 fl. oz.)* is a routine pencil in terms of the inevitable sharpening, but it does glide on and is minimally creamy, which means there's a low risk of smudging or fading.

☹ POOR **Brow Definer** *($10)* has a smooth, not-too-stiff texture but applies unevenly, first depositing even color followed by dots and specks of color, plus the tip breaks off quickly. Under the assumption that we were experimenting with old testers, we tried this pencil at other Body Shop stores, all with the same result. That's reason enough to avoid it.

THE BODY SHOP LIP COLOR & LIPLINERS

✓☺ BEST **Lip Liner Fixer** *($11)* remains a very good automatic, retractable lip pencil whose colorless formula puts an invisible border around the mouth that stops lipstick from feathering into lines. Keep in mind that as effective as this pencil is, it won't completely stop greasy, overly slick lipsticks or lip glosses from traveling into lines around the mouth.

☺ GOOD **Colourglide Lip Color** *($12.50)* is an emollient, creamy lipstick whose colors have a good stain, but you really need to layer them to get much impact. They're best for someone who wants light to moderate coverage and a slightly glossy finish. The oil–based formula will quickly move into lines around the mouth so if that describes your predicament, move on to other lipsticks. Otherwise, the shade range is extensive, with a pleasing array of cream and shimmer finishes.

☺ GOOD **Hi-Shine Lip Treatment** *($10 for 0.4 fl. oz.)* is billed as a treatment because it contains marula oil, but this plant oil isn't a special or essential ingredient for lip care, it's just another emollient plant oil. This is otherwise a standard viscous gloss that offers a wet-looking, high-shine finish with a slightly sticky feel. All the colors are very sheer.

☺ GOOD **Love Gloss** *($10)* is a very good, affordable lip gloss! It applies easily thanks to a hollow, petal-shaped sponge-tip applicator that helps disperse the gloss evenly onto lips, and the high-shine finish is minimally sticky. The shimmer shades impart sheer color with flecks of shine; the cream shades leave a more vibrant wash of color.

☺ AVERAGE **Lip Care** *($14)* is a very ordinary, but nevertheless emollient, lipstick-type lip balm that has a particularly glossy finish. It will soothe dry lips quite nicely.

☺ AVERAGE **Lip Liner** *($10)* is a standard, but quite workable, lip pencil that features some versatile colors. If this did not need to be sharpened it would earn a Best rating for its texture and application. If you don't mind sharpening, consider this a top pick.

☹ POOR **Lip & Cheek Stain** *($14 for 0.2 fl. oz.)* is an exceptionally sheer, gel-based stain whose single shade stays sticky on the skin, so this isn't preferred to superior versions from Origins or BeneFit.

⊘ Think "hypoallergenic" means safe for sensitive skin? See the Appendix to find out the truth.

THE BODY SHOP MASCARAS

☺ GOOD **Super Volume Mascara** *($15)* doesn't fall into the "super" category. It builds average length and thickness in equal measures, and has a slightly uneven application that requires a bit more patience—but the results may be worth it if you want a reliable mascara that doesn't take lashes too far.

☹ AVERAGE $$$ **Big & Curvy Mascara** *($18)* is disappointing for a mascara that claims to be all about thickening lashes. The thin brush with short bristles leads to clumping, and it requires multiple coats to build volume. On the plus side, it does hold curl, lengthens lashes, and offers a flake-free finish, but the wet-formula application can be messy, and it doesn't compare well to others on our list of Best Mascaras at the end of this book.

☹ AVERAGE $$$ **Big & Curvy Waterproof Mascara** *($18)* is a cleverly named waterproof mascara that holds up extremely well, whether you're swimming in the ocean or having a good cry. In fact, it stays on almost too well, requiring an extra application of makeup remover to get it off. It's such a shame this tenacious mascara has a thin brush with short bristles that causes clumping, even though the formula delivers length and holds curl well. Your lashes will feel stiff and there will be some flaking, but you can count on a waterproof, smudge-free finish. Ultimately, this mascara's faults and price don't make it a worthy consideration.

☹ AVERAGE $$$ **Divide & Multiply Mascara** *($18)* has a sleek, conical brush with rubber bristles. It goes on slightly wet but without a hint of smearing or clumping. With several strokes (and some patience) you can build beautifully defined, slightly thickened lashes with a soft, fringed finish with near-perfect lash separation. With all that praise, why the average rating? In a word, wearability. We regret to report that this mascara doesn't go the distance for worry-free wear. Throughout the day we found signs of flaking and more than once our tear duct area had what can only be described as "globs of black goo" from this mascara breaking down. For what this costs, you should expect better wear.

THE BODY SHOP FACE & BODY ILLUMINATORS

☺ GOOD **Shimmer Waves** *($22)* presents "waves" of shiny pressed-powder colors in one compact. Although the powder has a dry, grainy feel, it goes on smoothly and clings better than expected. The finish is best described as moderate shimmer, and is an option for evening glamour.

☹ AVERAGE $$$ **Brush-On Beads** *($21)* has been part of The Body Shop makeup line for years, but we don't understand why these shiny bronzing powder beads have maintained such an indispensable status in this line. In any event, this is still the same as it ever was, and it works well for a sparkling peachy brown effect. The beads allow for very sheer color application, but if they break you're left with an uneven application with chunks of powder.

☹ AVERAGE $$$ **Brush on Radiance** *($21)* consists of small, loose beads of powder, each in varying pearlescent shades of shimmery peach, pink, and golden beige, which combine on your powder brush to create a warm, flattering glow. Unfortunately, this shimmer powder flakes easily and doesn't adhere to the brush or skin very well, making application and wearability below any acceptable standard.

☹ AVERAGE **Lightening Touch** *($14)* has been around for years and is available in three sheer shades. It's an OK highlighting option with a soft shimmer finish, but doesn't illuminate the skin in the same beguiling way as superior options from Giorgio Armani and Lorac (the latter brand is reviewed on CosmeticsCop.com).

☹ AVERAGE **Radiant Highlighter** *($14)* has a glimmering finish that's not subtle and not a great way to softly highlight skin. If you're looking to add an ethereal, whitish sparkling shine to skin, this is a product to consider; however, it doesn't make wrinkles less apparent as claimed. The formula is fragrance-free.

THE BODY SHOP BRUSHES

✓☺ BEST **Extra Virgin Minerals Foundation Brush** *($25)* is a fantastic kabuki-style brush! The ultra-dense, super-soft synthetic hair picks up powder easily and feels extremely luxurious on skin. The rounded shape makes it versatile enough to blend the edges of foundation along the jaw line and to maneuver in hard-to-reach places, like the side of the nose. What makes this brush best for foundation application is that its synthetic bristles won't absorb the moisture in liquid foundation the way that natural hair can, so you get a more even application and your brush retains its shape.

☺ GOOD **The Body Shop Brushes** *($10.50–$26)* are each composed of synthetic hair and most of them are supremely soft and beautifully shaped. The best of the bunch (notable for their ability to hold and accurately deposit color) include **Face & Body Brush** ($26), **Foundation Brush** ($23), **Kabuki Bronzing Brush** ($23), **Slanted Brush** ($18), **Retractable Blusher Brush** ($22), and **Blusher Brush** ($24). The less appealing or unnecessary brushes include the rubber-tipped **Line Softener** ($10.50), **Brow & Lash Comb** ($10.50), **Lipstick/Concealer Brush** ($14.50), and **Eyeshadow Blender Brush** ($18), which is nicely shaped but doesn't have enough give to apply color evenly. The **Mini Brush Kit** ($18.50) is a small, portable brush set that includes a built-in mirror and a brush to apply powder, blush, eyeshadow, and lipstick. It's not the best to tote for applying a full makeup, but is ideal to keep in your purse or office for quick touch-ups.

TOO FACED

Strengths: website has complete ingredient lists; nice range of bronzing powders and a self-tanner; Full Bloom Lip & Cheek Creme Color is exceptional; good powder eyeshadows if you want shine; great BB cream (which is really just a tinted moisturizer with sunscreen).

Weaknesses: An irritating concealer; lacks matte eyeshadow options; terrible mascaras; dismal selection of eyeliners; Lip Injection lip plumpers contain irritating ingredients.

For more information and reviews of the latest Too Faced products, visit CosmeticsCop.com.

TOO FACED EYE-MAKEUP REMOVER

☺ AVERAGE $$$ **Lash Injection Antidote** *($21.15 for 3 fl. oz.)* is a water-based eye-makeup remover that contains a silicone and wax blend to effectively dissolve any type of eye makeup, including waterproof mascara. The amount of alcohol makes it questionable and potentially irritating; however, as a solvent, it can play a role in makeup removal. It's just that there's no need to risk it causing problems, not when there are plenty of better silicone-enhanced makeup removers available for half the price.

TOO FACED SUN CARE

✓☺ BEST $$$ **Tanning Bed In A Tube** *($28 for 6 fl. oz.)* is an excellent self-tanning lotion for normal to dry skin! The emollient formula is easy to smooth on, and the formula contains more than a dusting of antioxidants, which is more than most self-tanners can claim! This is tinted so you can see where it has been placed (and get some instant color gratification), plus it contains mineral pigments for a soft shine.

TOO FACED LIP CARE

☹ POOR **Love Lisa Luxury Lip Balm SPF 15** *($16)* fails miserably for two reasons: It's loaded with irritating ingredients that are a problem for lips and it does not supply sufficient broad-spectrum sun protection. See the Appendix to find out why any sunscreen product should provide reliable protection from the sun's aging UVA rays and why irritation is so bad for your lips.

☹ POOR **Lip Injection** *($19)* is in no way a cosmetic lip treatment as Too Faced claims. It contains the irritating ingredients benzyl nicotinate and *Capsicum frutescens* (pepper extract), which make your lips swell. This will temporarily plump your lips but it also leaves them stinging and irritated. This is one injection you'll definitely feel and it won't make things better afterward.

☹ POOR **Lip Injection Extreme** *($28)* is very similar to but even more irritating than Too Faced's Lip Injection reviewed above, and is not recommended.

TOO FACED FOUNDATIONS & PRIMERS

✓☺ BEST $$$ **Amazing Face Oil Free Close-Up Coverage Foundation** *($36)* is a liquid foundation that earns the "amazing" part of its name! It has a dewy finish without looking or feeling greasy, plus the lightweight texture blends on smoothly and offers medium coverage in flattering, neutral shades, ranging from fair to deep. This is a great option for anyone who doesn't need full coverage and wants a natural look complete with a more even skin tone.

✓☺ BEST $$$ **Tinted Beauty Balm SPF 20** *($32)* is an excellent option if you're curious to find out what all the fuss over BB creams is about. But before you get too caught up in the hype, know that for the most part, BB creams are little more than tinted moisturizers, often with sunscreen. Most include some beneficial ingredients that may or may not be present in tinted moisturizers, but that's where the excitement stops. BB creams hold no advantage in terms of multi-tasking beyond what the best tinted moisturizers with sunscreen provide. And despite their names, they're not particularly beneficial for blemishes (think acne, red marks, white bumps, etc.). This earns its rating due to its gentle mineral sunscreens that provide broad-spectrum protection and because its formula, packaged in an opaque tube, is chock-full of plant and vitamin-based antioxidants. Also worth noting is the 1.5-ounce size, which is larger than the normal 1-ounce fill. This has a lightweight, slightly moisturizing texture that slips smoothly over skin, making even application easy. It provides sheer coverage and sets to a satin finish that leaves a healthy, enlivened glow. The fragrance-free formula is best for normal to dry skin and is also suitable for sensitive or rosacea-affected skin (though if you have pronounced redness, this won't provide satisfactory coverage). Those looking for a less expensive, lighter-weight version of this product may want to consider Paula's Choice Barely There Sheer Matte Tint SPF 20. Three of the four shades are great: Be careful with Beach Glow, which is on the peachy side. Also, the lightest shade (Vanilla Glow) is a bit too yellow for fair skin but still deserving of an audition in the store.

☺ GOOD $$$ **Primed & Poreless Skin Smoothing Face Primer** *($30)* does an impressive job of temporarily smoothing superficial wrinkles and filling in pores thanks to its silicone-rich formula. The texture is thick and the finish dry, making it ideal for those with oily skin. This primer could conceivably be worn alone because it comes in only one shade, Light Beige, which virtually disappears on all but the deepest skin tones, where it can look ashen. This product isn't a slam-dunk, however, because it contains ivy extract, which can be irritating to sensitive skin. The amount of ivy is likely too small to be concerned about, but it's a plant extract skin is better off without. One more note: Take care not to overdo application, because applying anything more than a thin layer causes this to ball up when you apply other products over it.

☺ GOOD $$$ **Primed & Poreless Pure Skin Smoothing Face Primer for Sensitive Skin** *($30)*. This colorless primer temporarily smoothes over pores and superficial wrinkles thanks to the silicone-rich formula. The velvety texture is thick but blends out to a silky-dry finish suitable for those with oily skin (just don't expect the mattifying effect to last very long). Too Faced included some skin beneficial ingredients, but the amount of retinol is next to nothing. Still, the formula is irritant- and fragrance-free, making it an ideal primer for sensitive skin as claimed. One more note: Take care not to overdo application, because applying anything more than a thin layer causes this to ball up when you apply other products over it.

☺ GOOD $$$ **Wrinkle Injection Primer** *($28)* is a waterless primer with a few token antioxidants thrown in for bragging rights. Like most primers, it makes skin feel silky and the silicones help temporarily fill in and reduce the appearance of superficial lines. That's helpful under makeup, but don't be misled by the name. This is a very good foundation primer, but in no way does it mimic the results obtained from Botox or filler injections, and it will not change one wrinkle on your face.

☺ AVERAGE $$$ **Amazing Face SPF 15 Foundation Powder** *($32)* doesn't provide sufficient UVA protection (see the Appendix for details). That's a shame because this has a supremely smooth texture that blends readily, and sets to a gorgeous skin-like, fresh matte finish that's ideal for normal to oily skin. This talc-based powder foundation doesn't look the least bit dry or chalky, either. All five shades are great, although Warm Honey will appear slightly peach for some medium skin tones; there are no shades for fair or dark skin. If this provided reliable UVA protection, it would be truly amazing and easily earn our highest rating. As is, because the sunscreen is lacking, an Average rating is what it deserves.

☺ AVERAGE $$$ **Magic Wand Illuminating Foundation** *($29.25)* comes with horrible packaging. The push-button bottom dispenses too much product and the brush-tipped applicator is useless for blending. If you're able to overlook the Magic Wand problems, this liquid foundation has some good features: Its creamy texture closely resembles that of a tinted moisturizer and blends easily into the skin, providing sheer coverage and a satin finish. The shade range is very small and favors light-to-medium skin tones with normal to dry skin; someone with oily skin will not be happy with this formula. Caribbean Cocoa should be avoided altogether because it is too orange.

☺ AVERAGE $$$ **Primed & Poreless SPF 20 Bronze Tint** *($30)* has a thick but pleasant texture that blends on velvety smooth and sets to a soft, dry finish. The sheer bronze tint is a natural tan color and wears well under makeup or can be worn alone. The problems? The sole bronze shade isn't going to work for all skin tones (it's too dark for fair skin) plus this loses points because it contains ivy extract, a known skin irritant. The concentration of ivy extract is likely low enough that you don't need to be too concerned about it, but regardless, it's a plant extract your skin is better off without. Last, the sunscreen portion lacks the ingredients needed to shield your skin from the sun's entire range of damaging UVA rays, which is essential for anti-aging benefits (see the Appendix for details).

TOO FACED CONCEALERS

☺ AVERAGE $$$ **Absolutely Flawless Concealer** *($20)* is a very concentrated, full-coverage concealer that comes in a squeeze tube and has some problems that most won't be able to overlook. Yes, you get instant opaque coverage for even the darkest of dark circles or brown spots, but the emollient, thick texture stays creamy. That means you'll be dealing with fading, smearing, and creasing into lines around the eye, even if you set this with powder, which won't be all that flattering when applied over this concealer. The colors go from neutral to slightly peach, but, really, if you need this much coverage, check out the superior options from Make Up For Ever and Laura Mercier before purchasing this.

☹ POOR **Herbal Eye Concealer** *($19.50)* would have been rated better without the herbal ingredients. The inclusion of potentially irritating ingredients like lavender and bitter orange flower extracts means that you shouldn't use this cream concealer around the eyes, or anywhere on the face for that matter. Ironically, in terms of colors, the shade called Hollywood Medium is too orange for any skin type.

TOO FACED POWDERS

☺ GOOD **$$$ Absolutely Invisible Candlelight Softly Illuminating Translucent Powder** *($27)* has a lightweight, nearly imperceptible finish, except for one thing: It is littered with fine specks of glitter, which is anything but invisible. Although we don't recommend this much glitter all over your face, you can use this powder to add a glittering golden color to highlight specific features, like the cheekbone or collarbone, and the glitter clings surprisingly well.

☺ GOOD **$$$ Primed and Poreless Powder** *($28)* won't make your pores disappear, but its sole translucent shade makes skin look invisibly polished and smooth. By "invisible," we mean that once applied, you can't see this powder on your skin, but you'll see what it does, which is make your skin look polished and matte. It is best for normal to oily skin.

☺ AVERAGE **$$$ Absolutely Invisible** *($27)* is a talc- and mica-based pressed powder. Too Faced claims this powder is translucent, but it definitely has a whitish cast to it that's visible on skin. Absolutely Invisible is sheer, but even so the chalky texture and whitish finish tend to wash out the complexion.

TOO FACED BLUSHES & BRONZERS

✓☺ BEST **$$$ Chocolate Soleil Matte Bronzing Powder** *($29)* is a truly matte, and beautiful, bronzer. Who would have guessed that Too Faced, a shimmer-rific line if ever there was one, would create such a product! A light dusting of this smooth and strongly pigmented brown powder is all you need to give yourself a healthy glow. The color is not orange-y in the least, but be sure to apply sparingly, as a little goes a long way. The inclusion of cocoa powder gives this bronzer a rich chocolaty scent that may not please your nose, so be sure to get a whiff before you purchase.

✓☺ BEST **$$$ Full Bloom Lip & Cheek Creme Color** *($21)* is a creamy cheek blush that applies evenly and lasts throughout the day. The creamy texture requires a good amount of blending, but it doesn't look greasy or settle unevenly into pores. The formula sets to a finish that looks matte but feels creamy, and it stays put. When used as a lip color, the same review applies; however, it tends to rub off more easily, sort of like a semi-matte lipstick doesn't stick around all day or hold up to eating and drinking.

☺ GOOD **$$$ Peach Leopard Brightening & Perfecting Bronzer** *($29)* imparts a rich tan hue on application, and blends on smoothly without looking cakey or overdone. The leopard part of the name comes from the spotted pattern of brown and peach colors meant to be brushed on together to add a slight peach undertone to the bronzing effect. The powder's finish is primarily matte, but it contains small portions of shimmer that add a subtle glow.

☺ AVERAGE **$$$ Full Bloom Ultra Flush Blush** *($19)* is a standard pressed-powder blush that isn't worth its price, especially given that you get an unusually small amount of product. Of the shades offered, Sweet Pink and Who's Your Poppy have a glittery finish, and

Cocoa Rose is matte. The texture adheres nicely to your skin and imparts an adequate amount of color, but there are less expensive options available at the drugstore that out-perform this.

☺ AVERAGE $$$ **Pink Leopard Bronzing Powder** *($29)* certainly has an eye-catching pattern. This type of multicolored product isn't as easy to use as separately colored powders that are side-by-side. Still, this bronzer/highlighter hybrid has its positive aspects, though limited. It has a smooth texture and strong color deposit, but the pink undertones aren't flattering on everyone, so test this before buying. The shimmer factor is also very high, making this bronzer best for use as a highlighting powder rather than as an all-over bronzer.

☹ POOR **Aqua Bunny Cream to Powder Splash Proof Bronzer** *($29)* has a pleasantly smooth and lightweight texture that sets to a dry finish with subtle shine. Unfortunately, this praise doesn't extend to the color, which is an unflattering shade of orange rather than tan or bronze. It's also a bit difficult to blend without disturbing your foundation, and it contains fragrance ingredients known to cause irritation.

TOO FACED EYESHADOWS & EYE PRIMER

☺ GOOD $$$ **Duo Shadow** *($17)* has no matte options; some have strong shimmer some have subtle shimmer, and some have flecks of glitter. If you're in the market for shimmer, these powder shadows have excellent pigmentation. They apply and blend easily and wear well throughout the day. Unfortunately, the shimmer factor keeps them from being a good option for anyone who has lines around their eyes or who prefers a matte finish. Also, be careful with the glittery duos because the glitter tends to flake.

☺ GOOD $$$ **Exotic Color Intense Eye Shadow Singles** *($18)* deliver deeply pigmented color in an array of bold, trendy, and classic colors. Each has a hint of iridescence and finely milled glitter particles for added glamour, assuming you want glittery eye makeup. The velvety smooth pressed-powder texture blends on beautifully without flaking. Although not for everyone, this is a great option if you are looking to experiment with unique, fun colors.

☺ GOOD $$$ **Shadow Insurance Anti-Crease Eye Shadow Primer** *($18)* stems from the success of the original beige-colored Shadow Insurance Anti-Crease Eye Shadow Primer. Too Faced created three more versions including **Candlelight** (sparkly, shimmery cream color), **Lemon Drop** (imparts a creamy yellow hue that is intended to neutralize redness but is too sheer to do so), and **Glitter Glue** (translucent cream formula that holds loose glitter and powders in place). These eyeshadow primers work well to prevent fading and creasing. The smooth, dry finish is excellent for applying and blending shadow and permits shadows to wear beautifully for hours, except in the case of the Glitter Glue version. Glitter Glue has a tacky finish that does an excellent job of making loose powder eyeshadow or glitter adhere, but it can also result in a slightly uneven application that isn't as easy to blend. Plus, the tacky finish doesn't feel great on your eyelids and who wants to worry about that when they're out and about?

TOO FACED EYE & BROW LINERS

☺ AVERAGE $$$ **Brow Envy Brow Shaping & Defining Kit** *($35)* is a mixed bag of average and good products. The case itself is well organized, although it's too large to fit conveniently in most on-the-go cosmetic bags. The sheer brow powders are matte and work to fill in the brow and create a natural look, but the included brow brush is a bit too soft, making it more difficult than it should be to apply the powders. The wax portion works well to set the brows, but isn't as convenient as a brow gel, especially when traveling. The brow pencil is creamy and works okay, but needs sharpening. The small tweezers are decent, but the stencils are likely too thin for most people's preferences. So, for the cost, you're better off buying the brow products you need separately and leaving the rest behind.

☺ AVERAGE **$$$ Brow-nie Eye Brow Pencil** *($20)* is a standard, needs-sharpening brow pencil. It works to fill in and color the brows, but the texture is harder than most and it can be trickier to apply. For the money there are less expensive brow pencils at the drugstore that out-perform it.

☺ AVERAGE **$$$ Foiled Liners** *($16.50)* are standard, creamy, need-sharpening pencils whose characteristics can be duplicated by products from lines at the drugstore for less money. Too Faced claims that these liners are waterproof, but that's just not so. The creaminess of these pencils means that they apply easily with no tugging or pulling, and while the wear-time is decent, the color begins to fade after a few hours, and it definitely smudges and comes off in the water.

☺ AVERAGE **$$$ Liquif-Eye** *($18)* is touted as a "state of the art beauty breakthrough product that allows you to instantly transform your favorite eyeshadow into a water resistant, smudge-proof liquid liner." (A chemist told Paula about this type of product several years ago and she responded that, "Water does the same thing." He said he knew that, but that someone would probably buy this product from him— he was right.) So, although Liquif-Eye does turn powder shadows into liquid liner, so does water. The fine brush makes liner application easy, but the way the eyeshadow goes on is all about the color itself; neither water nor this Liquif-Eye change the tone. There are other drawbacks as well: Liquif-Eye applies wet, takes longer than it should to dry, and doesn't layer well (plain water actually works far better).

☺ AVERAGE **$$$ Long Stemmed Lashes Lash Enhancing Serum & Eyeliner Duo** *($38)* contains eyeliner on one end and a "lash enhancing" serum on the other. The eyeliner performs like any other standard, black, liquid liner and comes with a thin brush for precise application. It's good, but you can find better, less expensive liquid liners in drugstore lines. The lash-enhancing serum is the big disappointment. Not a single ingredient in this product has a shred of published research showing it can grow longer, thicker lashes as claimed. The rating for this product pertains to its lack of impressive results, especially given the high price when the only reliable portion is what amounts to a basic liquid eyeliner.

☺ AVERAGE **$$$ Perfect Eyes Waterproof Liner** *($18)* is a needs-sharpening eye pencil (hence the rating) whose creamy texture glides effortlessly around the eyes. Considering the initially creamy texture, this sets to a surprisingly smudge-proof finish and it wears well. On the flipside, the waterproof claim doesn't hold up, but for normal wear it gets the job done. The shades go on with bold intensity and come in a range of classic and trendy bold, yet deep, colors.

☹ POOR **Lava Gloss Eyeliner** *($16.50)* is a standard, creamy, need-sharpening eyeliner pencil. This pencil's creamy texture means it applies easily, but it also smudges easily and wears away quickly.

☹ POOR **Lava Matte Eyeliner** *($16.50)* is a fat eyeliner pencil that needs routine sharpening. Its creamy texture means that it smudges and wears away easily.

☹ POOR **Starry-Eyed Liquid Eyeliner** *($17.50)* is more scary-eyed than starry-eyed. It is nothing more than standard liquid eyeliner, and each color is packed with different shades of sparkle that resemble a runny version of glitter glue. The liner applies in sloppy globs of glitter that easily pool and clump, and so they have to be pushed around and smoothed out to create anything resembling an even line. Once the product finally dries, the result is definitely sparkly, but it's also incredibly messy—good luck not getting glitter in your eyes.

TOO FACED LIP COLOR & LIPLINERS

☺ GOOD $$$ **Glamour Gloss** *($19)* is a creamy lipstick/gloss hybrid with a sheer, shiny finish that's beautiful on lips. The wear time of Glamour Gloss is the same as for most glosses: It won't last as long as a lipstick, and it needs to be reapplied often. The color range tends toward more natural-looking pinks and brown tones, making this a great option for daytime wear.

☺ GOOD $$$ **Lip of Luxury** *($20)* is an ordinary moisturizing cream lipstick that comes in a small but attractive array of shades. There are both shimmer and matte finishes available. If color feathering into lines around the mouth is an issue for you, we highly recommend you use a lipliner.

☺ GOOD $$$ **Lip Primer Lip Insurance** *($19 for 0.15 fl. oz.)* is designed to fill in crevices on the lips and ensure long wear for lipstick, and this lightweight, silky lip primer is something you might want to consider. The slightly creamy texture glides on and quickly morphs to a smooth, semi-matte finish. To some extent, this serves as a mild soft spackle for lines on and around the mouth. The powdery finish helps keep lipstick in place, but isn't enough of a barrier to keep gloss from traveling into lines. The most compelling reason to consider this is for its slight filling effect. No, it doesn't make lips look bigger, but it does improve lipstick application and appearance without being greasy or slick. If lipstick bleeding into lines around the mouth is a constant struggle, this primer will help, but not as much as the Long-Lasting Anti-Feather Lipliner from Paula's Choice.

☹ AVERAGE $$$ **Borderline Lip Pencil** *($18.50)* is a Vaseline- and wax-based pencil. Nothing about the chubby pencil makes it special or more effective at keeping lip gloss and lipstick from creeping into lip lines; if anything, the formula could make matters worse. If you're looking for a clear lipliner to keep lipstick from traveling into lines around the mouth, Long-Lasting Anti-Feather Lipliner from Paula's Choice works beautifully, too.

☹ AVERAGE $$$ **Mood Swing Emotionally Activated Lip Gloss** *($18.50)* is a shiny, sticky gloss that dispenses clear and turns a sheer, hot pink shade when applied to the lips. Hardly an "emotionally activated" gloss, it turns nearly the same shade on everyone, and only those who favor hot pink lip gloss will find the shade flattering. The slight difference in how the shade appears on the lips has to do with the natural color of your lips, not with your mood. Despite the novelty, there is nothing in this gimmicky gloss to justify its price.

☹ AVERAGE $$$ **Perfect Lips Universal Liner** *($18.50)* glides on for smooth, even application, and the "universal" shade Perfect Nude is a pretty, rosy-nude hue, although it's not universal by any means. All in all, you're paying more than you need to for a basic lipliner that comes in only one shade, with the added inconvenience of routine sharpening.

TOO FACED MASCARAS

☺ GOOD $$$ **Lashlight a Mascara That Lights Up Your Lashes** *($25)* comes in a chunky square component that features a push button on the cap. When you're ready to apply, you click the button and the underside of the cap (where the mascara wand is attached) lights up. The effect is like holding a tiny LED-based flashlight next to your lashes. The illumination can make it easier to see every lash, but it's bright enough to distort your vision so that application isn't as seamless as it would be with good overhead or side lighting from standard bulbs. We preferred using this with the built-in lights turned off. Whichever method you go for, this mascara builds length and thickness equally and without clumping. The results aren't very dramatic, but they're still impressive. The formula is imbued with crystalline sparkling particles. They're supposed to make eyes look brighter, but the effect is really subtle.

☺ AVERAGE **$$$ Lashgasm Voluptuous Fluffing Mascara** *($21)* is taking a cue from NARS's popular Orgasm powder blush. Too Faced must be hoping you'll be just as elated after using this mascara, but don't light up a cigarette just yet. Forgive the analogy, but considering the name and the claims, this is a mascara that isn't nearly stimulating enough to stir such excitement. If anything, it goes on far too wet and uneven to produce shout-worthy results. You'll encounter some clumping and minor flaking before it sets, and you will absolutely need a lash comb or brush handy to create appealing results. Considering the cost, this isn't worth strong consideration over countless other mascaras that work better with much less effort.

☺ AVERAGE **$$$ Size Queen Mascara** *($21)*. This mascara's wand is so large and wide that it is nearly impossible to apply without getting it on the surrounding skin, which is a hassle you don't need to tolerate. Another disappointment is that the bristles are widely spaced, making it difficult to achieve defined lashes. While the formula itself does a good job of lengthening and thickening lashes, the applicator has too many downfalls to make it worthy of recommendation.

☹ POOR **Lash Injection** *($21)*. Not only does this mascara fail to plump lashes as promised, but also the merely average amount of length you get is accompanied by clumping and flaking. This mascara flakes horribly around the eyes!

☹ POOR **Lash Injection Pinpoint Mascara** *($21)* suffers from the same problems as the original large-brushed Lash Injection mascara above. Although the smaller brush Lash Injection Pinpoint has makes it easier to apply, the mascara formulation itself is dismal. Instead of defining and lengthening lashes as promised, it clumps and flakes easily, while giving lashes only a minimal amount of length.

TOO FACED BRUSHES

☺ GOOD **$$$ Retractable Kabuki Brush** *($32)* is a soft-bristled brush that is a great option for applying powder, blush, and bronzer. The large shape makes it best suited for covering larger areas of the face, and the fact that it's retractable makes it a great option for travel. Another bonus, the soft bristles are synthetic, so animal lovers will not have to miss out on giving this a try. The price is high but this is a top-quality brush, so the investment is a sound one, although there are less expensive versions that work just as well.

☺ AVERAGE **$$$ Teddy Bear Hairs** *($65)* is a five-piece brush set that is a good option for those who prefer softer cosmetic brushes. The softness of these brushes isn't an issue when using the powder/blush brush, which works great. But the softness of the eyeshadow, brow, and liner brushes means they don't pick up as much product as a stiffer-bristled brush does. If that's not an issue for you, and you prefer to use synthetic-hair cosmetic brushes, the Teddy Bear Hairs collection is worth a look. The same softness comments apply to Too Faced's **Shadow Brushes Essential 3-Piece Set** ($39).

URBAN DECAY

Strengths: Workable options in almost every category; excellent cheek tint; bonanza for anyone who wants lots of shiny eyeshadows; bronzing powder; good mattifier; brow products; makeup brushes.

Weaknesses: Mostly average to poor mascaras; limited foundation shades and some disappointing lip glosses; the products designed to help makeup last longer don't help.

For more information and reviews of the latest Urban Decay products, visit CosmeticsCop.com.

URBAN DECAY EYE-MAKEUP REMOVER

☺ AVERAGE **Meltdown Makeup Remover** *($24 for 2.5 fl. oz.)* is an expensive, though exceptionally ordinary, makeup remover that works quickly to break down all types of makeup (including waterproof formulas), but it contains enough oils to leave a slightly greasy residue. Best used prior to cleansing, this is an OK option for removing long-wearing foundation, blush, and lip color. It isn't ideal for use around the eyes because it contains fragrant plant extracts. The amount of fragrant plants isn't large, but if there's one area where you should be using fragrance-free products, it's around the eyes. (For the record, skin anywhere on the body does better when fragrance-free products are used.)

URBAN DECAY SPECIALTY SKIN-CARE PRODUCTS

☺ GOOD **$$$ De-Slick in a Tube Mattifying Gel** *($28)* is a very good way to help control and minimize the appearance of excess shine when skin is oily. This weightless gel contains absorbent magnesium aluminum silicate along with a slip agent, anti-irritant, preservatives, and fragrance (the fragrance is subtle). This helps stop shine whether applied under or over makeup, should you wish to absorb shine before touching up your powder.

☹ POOR **Guardian Angel Spray Moisturizer SPF 8** *($26 for 4 fl. oz.)* lacks the UVA-protecting ingredients of titanium dioxide, zinc oxide, avobenzone (also known as butyl methoxydibenzoylmethane), ecamsule, or Tinosorb and is not recommended. Moreover, given the standard of SPF 15 established by medical boards around the world, SPF 8 is a pathetic rating for anyone concerned with protecting their skin from sun damage, including wrinkles.

URBAN DECAY FOUNDATIONS & PRIMERS

✓☺ BEST **$$$ Complexion Primer Potion-Brightening** *($31)* is a good primer that's essentially a lightweight gel-textured fluid that has some beneficial ingredients. It smoothes on easily and makes skin feel silky, while leaving a slightly tacky finish that dissipates once makeup is applied. The formula goes above and beyond that of most primers by offering skin a plentiful range of antioxidants, water-binding agents, and cell-communicating ingredients, and it's also fragrance-free. This product is suitable for all skin types, but best for oily skin.

☺ GOOD **$$$ Complexion Primer Potion-Pore Perfecting** *($31 for 1 fl. oz.)* is a slightly thick, silicone-based primer that goes on slightly white and leaves a faint white cast. We suppose you could consider that a brightening effect, but it's basically canceled once you apply foundation over it. This primer's silky texture can slightly fill in large pores, but not to the extent that you'll look air-brushed to poreless perfection. It feels light and is compatible with oily skin.

☺ GOOD **$$$ Surreal Skin Cream to Powder Foundation** *($35)* is described as an ultra-lightweight formula, and it is. The texture is practically weightless and very silky and application is easy. As you blend, this quickly goes from a creamy glide to a soft powder finish that leaves a bit of a sheen. The drawback is that unless you blend it impeccably and touch it up during the day, it settles into lines and large pores, but that goes for many cream-to-powder foundations, so Urban Decay is hardly alone. The nonaqueous formula comes in neutral shades, with options for light to tan skin tones. If you decide to try this, toss the mini foundation brush that's included because using it produces a streaky, striped result. You can blend it away, but results are faster and more natural-looking using a sponge.

☺ AVERAGE **$$$ Surreal Skin Mineral Makeup** *($31)* is a loose-powder foundation packaged in a jar with a sponge affixed to the cap. Once opened, the powder is shaken onto the sponge, where it poofs out, allowing you to blend it over your skin. The formula is based on mica and bismuth oxychloride (the same as most mineral foundations and powders), and this product shares the same traits typical for this category of makeup, meaning it offers shine, reliable coverage, and a dry finish that can become uncomfortably dry during the day depending on your skin type. This has a decidedly light texture, and most of the shades are attractive, but you have to accept a slight sparkling effect and the drawbacks of mineral makeup to really enjoy this product. Mineral makeup is not a good choice if you have any degree of dry skin because the ingredients absorb oil (and your moisturizer), making dry skin drier. For someone with very oily skin the makeup typically separates on your skin and pools into pores, which is as unbecoming as it sounds. Getting back to the colors, there are some enticing options for dark (but not very dark) skin tones, but consider Fortune carefully due to its slight orange cast. Fantasy is too copper for most dark skin tones.

☺ AVERAGE $$$ **Urban Defense Tinted Moisturizer SPF 20** *($30)* is a letdown because the sunscreen portion of this tinted moisturizer fails to provide sufficient UVA protection (see the Appendix for details). The packaging is cute and the pump applicator is fairly easy to control, but what's inside isn't up to par with today's best tinted moisturizers. The texture leans to the greasy side of creamy and it sets to a sheer but moist finish that's only for normal to dry skin. Some good antioxidants and anti-irritants are included, and the packaging will help keep them stable, but that still doesn't change the fact that this isn't nearly as modern as it could be. As for the shades—they're good and include options for light to tan skin.

URBAN DECAY CONCEALERS

☺ GOOD $$$ **Surreal Skin Creamy Concealer** *($16)* is a liquid concealer with a slightly runny consistency that makes blending tricky and provides coverage that is more sheer than what most who use concealer want. Still, the two shades (reserved for those with fair to light skin) are good, and this is an OK option if you want sheer coverage and a satin-matte finish. The formula is appropriate for use over blemishes, but don't expect much in the way of camouflage.

☺ AVERAGE $$$ **24/7 Concealer** *($18)* is a needs-sharpening pencil, so if you don't mind routine sharpening, this creamy pencil concealer has a blendable, slightly silky texture that provides substantial coverage without looking too thick or feeling greasy. It is slightly prone to creasing into lines around the eye, but tends to stay put once it's set, so fading isn't an issue. The thickeners and wax-like ingredients in this concealer make it not well suited for use on acne.

☺ AVERAGE $$$ **Urbanglow Cream Highlight** *($24)* is a fragrance-free cream highlighter that comes in a small compact. Its initially slick texture blends over skin smoothly without being excessively slippery. Each of the shades set to a powder-like finish laced with obvious sparkles and a touch of low-glow shimmer. Although it serves its purpose as a highlighter, the formula tends to settle into lines and large pores, magnifying each.

URBAN DECAY POWDERS

✓☺ BEST $$$ **Razor Sharp Ultra Definition Finishing Powder** *($31)* is supposed to provide a stunning, soft-focus effect, even under bright and unforgiving light. It does that and more thanks to its super-fine texture and translucent color. This powder has an unusually slippery texture, but it adheres well to skin and leaves a soft, non-powdery matte finish that feels weightless yet makes skin look smooth and polished. We tested this under the bright lights at Sephora and in natural daylight (on a sunny day) and the result was impressive. This works beautifully over foundation, although the single shade won't work for everyone; it's best for fair to medium skin tones. Whether you apply this with a powder brush (sheer results) or buff it on with the built-in sponge applicator (which provides greater coverage without looking cakey), this powder exemplifies the concept of high-definition makeup.

☺ AVERAGE $$$ **De-Slick Mattifying Powder** *($32)*. One-shade-fits-all powders rarely work for everyone, and that's the case with this pale option. The talc-based formula contains a high amount of absorbent calcium carbonate, so it does a good job of absorbing excess oil to keep skin matte. The texture is smooth yet dry, plus it is difficult to pick up enough powder on your brush to sufficiently temper shine. All told, there are far better, less expensive pressed powders for oily skin.

URBAN DECAY BLUSH & BRONZER

✓☺ BEST $$$ **Afterglow Glide-On Cheek Tint** *($24)* is amazing; it goes on soft and sheer and does a great job of duplicating a lit-from-within glow. You'll look fresh-faced and radiant, at least once you get the hang of applying this product. It blends easily and leaves a subtle sparkle that's suitable for daytime wear. Even better, the texture and finish aren't too slick or the least bit greasy. The shade range offers an attractive mix of pink, rose, tan, and plum tones that work for fair to medium skin tones.

☺ GOOD $$$ **Baked Bronzing Powder** *($26)* is a talc-based pressed bronzing powder that goes on smoothly and has a sheer, dry finish. The shades would be more convincing without shine, but if a shiny tan effect is what you want, it clings well.

URBAN DECAY EYESHADOWS & EYE PRIMERS

☺ GOOD $$$ **Deluxe Eyeshadow** *($18)* has different packaging but formula-wise is quite similar to Urban Decay's regular Eyeshadows, save for an application that's a touch smoother due to the silicone content. The small selection of shades favors strong metallic colors, few of which make for an effective eye design unless you're doing eye makeup for shock value. Still, these apply and blend well and the shine stays put, so they're a consideration.

☺ GOOD $$$ **Eyeshadow Primer Potion** *($20)* promises to make eyeshadows last longer while keeping them from creasing, and it works. In addition, it facilitates a smoother application and makes blending even easier. The problem is you can get the same results from a good matte-finish concealer that's silicone-based like this one. Because most of today's best concealers follow this format, a product like this, though it works, seems superfluous (unless you don't use a silicone-based type of concealer).

☺ GOOD $$$ **Eyeshadow Primer Potion, Eden** *($20)* is similar to the Eyeshadow Primer Potion above, except this has more movement and takes longer to set.

☺ GOOD $$$ **Eyeshadow Primer Potion, Greed** *($20)* leaves a gleaming, pale gold shimmer that definitely magnifies wrinkles, but otherwise this fragrance-free primer is similar to the others from Urban Decay.

☺ GOOD $$$ **Eyeshadow Primer Potion, Sin** *($20)* is a sparkling champagne-colored version of Urban Decay's original Eyeshadow Primer Potion. It's a welcome addition for anyone who wants shimmer and doesn't already use a silicone-based foundation or concealer, which would work similarly to this primer, producing the same shadow-enhancing effect, only with shine added to the application.

☺ GOOD $$$ **Eyeshadows** *($17)* were reformulated in spring 2012, but still feature a rainbow of unusual, sometimes shocking colors sold as singles. Most of them have a superior smooth texture that applies and blends wonderfully. Every shade has some degree of shine, but the good news is that except for the colors with glitter (easily identified), the shine clings well.

☺ AVERAGE **24/7 Glide-On Shadow Pencil** *($20)* does not glide on as claimed and needs routine sharpening. We encountered a good amount of tugging and resistance to application and blending, and for those with larger lids or those looking for a dramatic eye design, it can mean a lot of wear and tear on your lids. However, some shades seem to apply more smoothly than others: Rehab, Lit, and Wasteland had the smoothest textures, while Delinquent and Barracuda were troublesome. If you're somehow able to apply and blend this product easily, you will find that it doesn't crease and stays put until you decide to take it off.

☹ POOR **Cream Eyeshadow** *($17)* boasts gel-based silicone technology, which sets to a vibrant, film-like waterproof finish. What a shame that it's a complete mess to apply using the wand applicator. If that weren't drawback enough, the product also thickens up in the tube so easily we can't see how anyone could use it for more than several applications before having to throw it away. Even with a sponge or brush, the product's consistency is goopy, making it a difficult product to blend evenly; and the pigmentation is so deep, there's little room for error.

☹ POOR **Stardust Eyeshadow** *($20)* is Urban Decay's attempt to create an ultra-glittery powder eyeshadow, and they've failed miserably! The texture is sandpaper-dry, and, not surprisingly, application is uneven and the glitter flakes all over your face. The smaller shine particles have decent cling, but the glitter is a mess and the varying shades are, for lack of a better word, ugly.

URBAN EYE & BROW LINERS

✓☺ BEST **$$$ Brow Box** *($29)* contains everything you need to get your brows in tip-top shape. There are two sets of brow powder offered: Honey Pot (blonde) and Brown Sugar (dark brown). Each kit comes with a dark and light shade so you can vary the intensity and blend the complementary colors to exactly match your brows. The kit also contains a small pot of wax to set your brows, tame stray hairs, and give them extra definition. Brow Box comes complete with a pair of tiny tweezers and a mini brush to apply the brow powder. The small size of the tweezers and brush make them difficult to use, so you'd be better off using your own tools, although they'll do the trick if you're in a pinch. On balance, there's more to like than dislike about Brow Box: The price is fair for the amount you get and the product performs!

✓☺ BEST **$$$ Urbanbrow Precision-Tip Brow Tint** *($20)* is a liquid brow tint housed in an ingenious pen-style applicator outfitted with a flexible brush tip. The brow tint is dispensed via the brush tip, which allows you to make soft, hair-like strokes between your natural brow hairs. The result is greater brow definition without the heavy look brow pencils often provide. Because this sets to a sheer, non-sticky matte finish, the results last, even through perspiration or other sources of moisture. It's a great way to softly accent your brows. Urban Decay offers two shades, which are best for dark blonde to medium brown brows. There are no shades for light blonde or red brows. Note: As much as we liked this product, we should mention that Paula's Choice Browlistic Long-Wearing Precision Brow Color is nearly identical, but costs less.

☺ GOOD **$$$ 24/7 Waterproof Liquid Eyeliner** *($19)* is waterproof, but the truth is most are, and without question the gel eyeliners (typically sold in tiny jars) are waterproof, too. Whether you want to keep your eyeliner on for 24 hours is up to you, but this option lasts all day once it sets. The fluid texture is slightly runny, so application tends to be uneven (the thin, long brush doesn't help this go on any easier, either). Still, with practice, you can build a thin or thick line that, once set, won't budge. As is typical of Urban Decay, they offer some unconventional colors. Black and brown are represented, but there also are bolder hues, so select depending on your personal preference and the look you're going for.

☺ GOOD $$$ **Urbanbrow Styling Brush and Setting Gel** *($20)* is a basic clear brow gel whose only point of distinction from less expensive brow gels is its unique brush. Rather than being a softer, "spoolie"-type brush like those often used for mascara, this brush looks more like a tiny toothbrush with firm, dense bristles that work well to groom stray or stubborn brow hairs. Whether you prefer this type of brush or the traditional style comes down to experimentation, but Urbanbrow's brush is worth considering by those who find standard brow gel brushes too wimpy. The brow gel formula holds well without feeling sticky or gummy, and provides a soft gloss to brows without making them look matted or greasy. The formula doesn't flake during wear, either.

☹ POOR **24/7 Glide-On Eye Pencil** *($19)* glides on, but this needs-sharpening pencil has a soft tip that's prone to breaking off and a finish that is creamy enough to smudge. It doesn't last all night and isn't the best fit for anyone's "on-the-go" lifestyle, and the colors are mostly clownish.

URBAN DECAY LIP COLOR & LIPLINER

☺ GOOD $$$ **Lip Envy** *($17)* is a water-based stain. The angled applicator makes it easy to be accurate, which is critical with a product like this because mistakes aren't easily wiped away. The two sheer shades (each looks quite dark before applying) are attractive.

☺ GOOD $$$ **Lip Primer Potion SPF 15** *($20)* is a colorless lipstick meant to "lay a silky foundation for your favorite lipstick or gloss." It has a silky, thick texture that feels waxy, but it's these wax ingredients that help fill lip lines for a smoother appearance. It leaves a moist yet non-glossy finish that's compatible with most standard lipsticks and glosses. The main letdown is that the sunscreen does not provide sufficient UVA protection. Well, that and the fact that using this to stop lipstick from bleeding into lines around the mouth doesn't work that well.

☺ GOOD $$$ **Lipstick** *($22)* is a very good cream lipstick whose best qualities are undermined by the fact that almost all the shades are infused with glitter. What a way to make an elegant lipstick look silly rather than beautiful. Glittery lipsticks can be fun on occasion, but you can find such options at the drugstore for a lot less money. By the way, Gash, one of the few non-glittery shades, remains a riveting red that's sure to attract attention.

☺ AVERAGE $$$ **24/7 Glide-On Lip Pencil** *($19)* is a lip pencil with a silicone-based formula. The result is an application that glides over lips without being too slick and a long-wearing finish that feels slightly tacky, although the tackiness is barely noticeable when paired with lipstick. This requires routine sharpening, hence, it doesn't have a higher rating.

☺ AVERAGE $$$ **Pocket Rocket Lip Gloss** *($19)* is a silly, gimmicky product. This packaging has images of good-looking men you can "strip" by tilting the container from side to side. The provocative package is also supposed to come laced with man-attracting pheromones, which you can (according to the company) emit simply by rubbing the flattened tube; that's really gimmicky, but if you're a teen or twenty-something it would be hard to not giggle the entire time you were testing it at the counter, and probably buying it as well. It's that kind of silly product. As for the product itself, it's pretty standard lip gloss fare: slightly sticky with a tendency to bleed, and a wand brush applicator that easily splays. The iridescent colors are chock-full of sparkle, but the creams and sheers go on quite nicely. Also worth noting is the unpleasantly strong dessert-like fragrance, which lingers far longer than the gloss does.

☺ AVERAGE **$$$ Super Saturated High Gloss Lip Color** *($19)* is a chunky, needs-sharpening lipstick that's really greasy. This goes on unusually thick and imparts rich, riveting color, and the finish is wet-look glossy, but the greasy feel is not good. The best way to use this product, if you're still inclined, is as a lip stain. Apply, then blot, and you'll be left with a strong tint without the excess greasy feel. The shade range is small and favors bold, bright colors, some of which are infused with glitter that doesn't feel grainy.

☹ POOR **Lip Junkie Lip Gloss** *($19)* is a high-shine gloss whose tingle you'll feel when you first apply. The tingle comes from peppermint oil, which is indeed an irritant, and frequent use can lead to dry, chapped lips. In the long run, this will leave your lips in worse shape than they were when you started, not to mention you likely won't see a significant plumping effect.

URBAN DECAY MASCARAS

☺ GOOD **$$$ Lush Lash Mascara Growth Serum-Infused Conditioning Mascara** *($20)* has a slightly hourglass-shaped, rubber-bristled brush that works like miniature teeth, "grabbing" each lash to elongate it. The brush also allows you to deposit extra mascara at the base of the lashes for more dramatic, eyeliner-like impact. Definitely best for length rather than thickness, you can achieve surprisingly long lashes with only minor clumping along the way. You may notice some minor smearing until this sets, but it's easily cleaned with a dry cotton swab. On balance, this is a good mascara, but it's worth mentioning that there are equally good options at the drugstore. Note: The "growth serum" this mascara contains is little more than conditioning agents and a peptide, and there is not a shred of published research proving it makes lashes grow longer, stronger, or darker. You can safely ignore this claim; this product is not mascara with the power to grow your lashes.

☺ GOOD **$$$ Skyscraper Multi-Benefit Mascara** *($20)* is positioned as an improved version of Urban Decay's original Skyscraper Mascara. We praised the original formula for its lengthening prowess and its ability to keep lashes soft and attractively fringed. This update performs almost identically, except you get a bit of thickness. Clumping is completely absent, and this separates lashes easily. The shape of the rubber-bristled brush makes it easy to reach every lash, though those with small eyes may find it a bit cumbersome.

☺ AVERAGE **$$$ Big Fatty Mascara** *($20)* purports to thicken and lengthen lashes, and its gigantic brush achieves that, though not to the same impressive extent as mascaras with smaller brushes and more variegated bristles. You may think that a big brush equals big results, but that's not the case here, nor has it been with any other enlarged mascara brush we've ever tried, with one exception: Dior's Mascara Diorshow. If you're curious to see how a large mascara brush will work for you, try Dior's version instead.

☺ AVERAGE **$$$ Cannonball Ultra Waterproof Mascara** *($20)* doesn't do a lot to justify its price. Yes, it is waterproof but so are lots of other mascaras that cost less and offer stronger performance. The formula tends to go on a bit wet, but does add instant impact and leaves lashes reasonably long with just a few short strokes from the tiny but well-designed brush. Thickness isn't much, but that's true for most waterproof mascaras because the ingredients that make the formula waterproof tend to result in a thinner texture, thus a thinner application. On the plus side, this leaves lashes soft rather than brittle, and it doesn't flake. Despite that bit of good news, if you're not extra-careful during application this will smear (a lot) before it sets.

☺ AVERAGE **$$$ Supercurl Curling Mascara** *($20)* has a curved brush that some may find helps application because, if your eyes are larger, it makes it a bit easier to reach the base of lashes without contorting your hand as you sweep the brush through lashes. Although some may find the shape of the brush an advantage, the mascara itself disappoints. It goes on inky-black but also unevenly, requiring you to comb through lashes with a separate brush for smooth results. This builds modest length and a hint of thickness but absolutely does not curl lashes. The curling benefit is the main selling point of this mascara, so the fact that lashes won't look the least bit curled or softly fringed is a letdown.

URBAN DECAY FACE & BODY ILLUMINATORS

☺ AVERAGE $$$ **Sparkling Lickable Body Powder** *($20 for 0.53 fl. oz.)* should be sold at other retail establishments, but there it was, sitting in Sephora, waiting to be dusted on someone's skin and then be kissed, or licked, off—they're flavored and scented to smell like food. The loose powder provides a strong shimmer finish, but wearing it becomes increasingly bothersome because it makes skin feel sticky, especially if you apply it near areas where you perspire.

☹ POOR **Midnight Cowboy Shimmer Body Lotion** *($28)* is a very standard body lotion imbued with a metallic shimmer. Although the shiny finish clings well, application can be tricky; it's way too easy to go from subtle glow to blinding shimmer in a flash. There's also the fact that this product contains the preservative methylisothiazolinone, which is not recommended for use in leave-on products due to its high risk of causing a sensitized reaction (Sources: *Contact Dermatitis*, November 2001, pages 257–264; and *European Journal of Dermatology*, March 1999, pages 144–160). Overall, this falls short as a shine product and is only a little better than boring as a body moisturizer.

URBAN DECAY BRUSHES

☺ GOOD $$$ **Good Karma Brushes** *($20–$39)* are worth an audition! These synthetic-hair, expertly crafted brushes are a distinct highlight and value of this line. Each one has merit depending on your needs and preferences, but generally speaking the standouts are the **Powder Brush** ($36), **Shadow Brush** ($26), and **Blending Brush** ($26).

URBAN DECAY SPECIALTY MAKEUP PRODUCTS

☺ GOOD $$$ **Eyeshadow Transforming Potion** *($18)* is said to transform eyeshadow into a liquid eye color. This water-based solution is housed in a dual-sided component that provides a synthetic brush meant for drawing wide lines and another for drawing thin, precise lines. Both work well and deepen powder eyeshadow colors, though this requires successive layers because initially the solution causes the color to go on sheer. Once set it wears reasonably well, but it's neither budge-proof nor completely waterproof. The thicker brush tends to dispense too much liquid, so be sure to remove some of it before using with a powder eyeshadow.

☺ AVERAGE $$$ **All Nighter Long Lasting Makeup Setting Spray** *($29 for 4 fl. oz.)* is sold as a makeup-setting spray for long (really long) nights out on the town. You're supposed to mist this post-makeup and enjoy worry-free wear for an impressive 16 hours. What this ends up being is hairspray for the face. The amount of alcohol means it dries quickly, allowing the film-forming agent to form a seal on skin that helps prevent makeup from fading or smearing, but that also can have a tacky feel on skin. The claim that this has temperature-control technology is silly because it doesn't do anything that plain water or alcohol wouldn't—talk about overwrought claims! This product contains completely ordinary ingredients that are incapable of protecting your makeup from body temperature changes. Overall, given the cost and formulation issues, this is not great for your skin or your makeup.

☺ AVERAGE **$$$ De-Slick Oil Control Makeup Setting Spray** *($29 for 4 fl. oz.)* is similar to the All Nighter Long Lasting Makeup Setting Spray above, and the same review applies. Overall, this is not worth the cost or effort, but you can always give it a test run next time you pass an Urban Decay counter.

☺ AVERAGE **$$$ Dew Me Moisturizing Makeup Setting Spray** *($29 for 4 fl. oz.)* is nearly identical to Urban Decay's other makeup setting sprays and is not moisturizing. As such, the same review applies.

VICHY (SKIN CARE ONLY)

Strengths: Some fragrance-free products; all the sunscreens but one contain either avobenzone or titanium dioxide for sufficient UVA protection; some good moisturizers with sunscreen; some good, inexpensive cleansers, and scrubs for dry skin.

Weaknesses: Repetitive moisturizer formulas that rarely rise above the median for excellence; jar packaging is pervasive; the at-home peel/scrub kit is mostly disappointing; a couple of irritating moisturizers; no effective products for those with skin discolorations; limited options for oily skin.

For more information and reviews of the latest Vichy products, visit CosmeticsCop.com.

VICHY CLEANSERS

☺ GOOD **Purete Thermale 3-in-1 One-Step Cleanser** *($18 for 6.7 fl. oz.)* is a standard, detergent-free cleansing lotion for normal to dry skin. It will require more than one step because this doesn't rinse well without the aid of a washcloth.

☺ GOOD **Normaderm Daily Exfoliating Cleansing Gel** *($18 for 4.2 fl. oz.)* is similar to the Normaderm Deep Cleansing Gel below, except without the witch hazel and with the inclusion of polyethylene beads, which makes this a good cleansing scrub for normal to oily skin.

☺ GOOD **Normaderm Deep Cleansing Gel, for Clear Skin** *($17 for 6.7 fl. oz.)* is medicated with a small amount of salicylic acid. Unfortunately, this tried-and-true anti-acne ingredient needs to be left on skin in order to have the most benefit—yet that's not how cleansers are designed to be used. This is still a good cleanser for normal to oily skin, and it's fine for acne-prone skin, too (as long as you understand it's going to take more than this cleanser to achieve clear skin).

☺ GOOD **Purete Thermale Purifying Foam Cream Cleanser** *($18 for 4.2 fl. oz.)* is a good, water-soluble foaming cleanser for normal to oily skin. It does a great job of removing makeup and rinses well despite a cushiony, almost creamy, texture. There is slight cause for concern that some of the potassium-based cleansing agents may be drying, which is why this cleanser is best for oilier skin rather than, say, combination skin with dry patches.

☺ GOOD **$$$ Purete Thermale Purifying Foaming Water** *($19.50 for 5.1 fl. oz.)* is a good liquid-to-foam water-soluble cleanser that's best for all skin types except sensitive (due to the fragrance it contains). It works well to remove most types of makeup and rinses cleanly. Those with oily skin may prefer a more thorough cleanser, but some of that depends on personal preference.

☺ AVERAGE **$$$ Purete Thermale Calming Cleansing Solution, for Sensitive Face and Eyes** *($16.50 for 6.76 fl. oz.)* would be much better for sensitive skin if it did not contain fragrance and rose flower extract (which just adds more fragrance). This is otherwise an exceptionally standard liquid cleanser that should not be described as "ultra-safe" or "ultra-soothing" as the company claims.

VICHY EYE-MAKEUP REMOVER

☺ GOOD **Purete Thermale Eye Make-Up Remover, for Sensitive Eyes** *($16.50 for 5.1 fl. oz.)* is a good eye-makeup remover for all skin types, though the fragrance isn't the best for sensitive skin. Still, this works well, the cleansing agents are gentle, and the amount of allantoin is soothing.

VICHY TONERS

☺ AVERAGE **Purete Thermale Hydra-Perfecting Toner for Normal and Combination Skin** *($18 for 6.76 fl. oz.)* is a good, basic, moisturizing toner that's preferred for normal to dry skin. There is no convincing research that any ingredient in this toner works like a magnet to "capture impurities." Most impurities (think dirt, dead skin cells, and traces of makeup) are removed by the sheer physical act of cleansing and/or swabbing a cotton pad over areas your cleanser may have missed, such as around the hairline. This toner also cannot detoxify your skin—no one at Vichy can explain what toxins are lurking in your skin that this toner can somehow magically remove.

☺ AVERAGE **Purete Thermale Hydra-Soothing Toner, for Dry and Sensitive Skin** *($18 for 6.7 fl. oz.)* is similar to Vichy's Purete Thermale Hydra-Perfecting Toner above, except this version is marketed to those with dry, sensitive skin. This isn't worth the expense because there are better toners that cost less and provide your skin with a broader range of beneficial ingredients.

☺ AVERAGE **Thermal Spa Water** *($13 for 5.07 fl. oz.)* is just water with nitrogen and carbon dioxide. Whether that has benefit for skin is anyone's guess because there is no research showing that to be the case. This Spa Water is nearly identical to La Roche-Posay's Thermal Spring Water; both companies are owned by L'Oreal.

☹ POOR **Normaderm 3-in-1 Unclogging Purifying Toner** *($18 for 6.7 fl. oz.)* lists alcohol as the second ingredient, which makes this too drying and irritating for all skin types. See the Appendix to learn why alcohol is a problem for all skin types.

VICHY SCRUB

☺ GOOD **Purete Thermale Purifying Exfoliating Cream** *($18 for 2.5 fl. oz.)* is an exceptionally emollient scrub that is recommended only for dry to very dry skin. The amount of shea butter, paraffin, and mineral oil makes it difficult to rinse, but it's almost impossible to use this too aggressively, which is a good thing.

VICHY MOISTURIZERS (DAYTIME & NIGHTTIME), EYE CREAMS, & SERUMS

☺ GOOD $$$ **Liftactiv CxP SPF 20 Biolifting Daily Care Anti-Wrinkle and Firming** *($46 for 1.7 fl. oz.)* includes stabilized avobenzone for reliable UVA protection. The base formula is a blend of ingredients you'll find in most moisturizers from L'Oreal-owned companies, of which Vichy is one. This has an OK formula for normal to dry skin, but not a single ingredient is capable of lifting skin or improving prominent (meaning deeply etched) wrinkles. Vichy attributes its claim to vitamin C and peptides, but the amount of vitamin C is minuscule. Even in large amounts, topical vitamin C cannot lift skin, although it can stimulate healthy collagen production and help repair sun-damaged skin for increased firmness, but lifting skin is a completely different physiological problem. This provides great sun protection and hydration, but it's overpriced considering the wealth of superior daytime moisturizers you'll find in our Best Products chapter.

☺ GOOD **Nutrilogie 1 Intensive Nourishing Moisturizer Lotion SPF 15** *($25 for 1.7 fl. oz.)* is a good daytime moisturizer with an in-part titanium dioxide sunscreen for normal to dry skin. It contains a good amount of water-binding agents and a couple of antioxidants.

☺ GOOD **$$$ Reti-C Eyes Intensive Corrective Care** *($38.50 for 0.5 fl. oz.)* is an emollient moisturizer for dry skin anywhere on the face. It contains a tiny amount of vitamin C (as ascorbic acid) and an even smaller amount of retinol, though at least the packaging will help keep these ingredients stable during use. This product is fragrance-free; see the Appendix to find out why, in truth, you don't need an eye cream.

☺ AVERAGE **Aqualia Thermal Cream Fortifying & Soothing 24Hr Hydrating Care** *($29.95 for 1.69 fl. oz.)* is an extremely ordinary moisturizer that contains mostly standard ingredients to "fortify and soothe" dry skin. The formula is typical of the moisturizers that most L'Oreal-owned lines (of which Vichy is one) launch, and that's bad news for anyone who wants brilliantly formulated anti-aging products. The "ceramide-like" polymer referred to in the claims sounds intriguing, but Vichy would've been wiser to include real ceramides because these are substances your skin can recognize and put to good use.

☺ AVERAGE **Aqualia Thermal Mineral Balm Rehydrating and Repairing Care** *($35 for 1.7 fl. oz.)*. This thick, emollient moisturizer is said to have a "bandage" effect on your skin. To some extent it does, but the ingredients Vichy chose aren't the best for repairing skin's barrier function so that it can become less dry. What's truly disappointing is the lack of state-of-the-art ingredients and the inclusion of potentially problematic alcohol. The amount of alcohol is likely too low to be cause for concern, but a moisturizer for dry, damaged skin is always better off without any of this drying and irritating ingredient. This is merely a thick-textured moisturizer that lacks truly exciting, innovative ingredients to help your dry skin look and feel its healthy best. By the way, the minerals (which appear in many Vichy products) do not have any special benefit for skin.

☺ AVERAGE **Aqualia Thermal Roll-On Eye Fortifying Hydrogel** *($28.50 for 0.5 fl. oz.)*. Here's another "eye roller"–type product that includes a lightweight moisturizer packaged in a container that dispenses its contents via a smooth metal roller-ball applicator. The massaging action of the roller ball is said to reduce puffiness. To some extent, it can do that, but no more so than massaging your eye area with your fingers. As for the formula, it's ordinary. It was actually a bit shocking to look at the ingredient list and see that it was almost entirely water, propylene glycol, and preservative. The handful of other ingredients in here is nice, but they are present in such trivial amounts they can't really help your skin.

☺ AVERAGE **Aqualia Thermal Serum Fortifying & Soothing 24Hr Hydrating Concentrate** *($35.50 for 1.01 fl. oz.)*. This water-based serum isn't concentrated with anything capable of keeping your skin hydrated for 24 hours. Alcohol, which is about as dehydrating as it gets, is high enough on the ingredient list to be a potential source of problems, including irritation, and, you guessed it, more dryness and free-radical damage (see the Appendix for more details). This serum is mostly a bust and the lack of the state-of-the-art ingredients all skin types need makes the price embarrassing.

☺ AVERAGE **Normaderm Night Daily Corrective Care for Oily Skin** *($24.50 for 1.69 fl. oz.)* is sold as a corrective option for large pores, but it's really just a lightweight moisturizer for normal to oily skin that contains one intriguing ingredient, discussed below. The silky texture has a soft matte finish and contains an OK mix of water-binding agents (including the AHA glycolic acid, though in this amount it cannot function as an exfoliant. The same is true for the form of salicylic acid this moisturizer contains). The sole intriguing ingredient is zinc PCA, which is a salt form of zinc. Although there is some research linking zinc with improving acne and reducing inflammation, no viable studies exist to support the topical use of zinc PCA for these issues or for reducing enlarged pores (Sources: *The Journal of Clinical and Aesthetic Dermatology*, September 2010, pages 20–29; and *Der Hautarzt*, January 2009, pages 42–47). This is an OK lightweight moisturizer to consider, but it's the soft matte finish that helps minimize the appearance of pores, not some special ingredient.

☹ AVERAGE **Nutrilogie 2 Intensive Nourishing Moisturizer Cream** *($32.50 for 1.69 fl. oz.)* is a basic but dry skin-soothing moisturizing cream. The amount of coriander oil is potentially irritating and the antioxidant abilities of the plant oils will be compromised due to jar packaging (see the Appendix for details).

☹ AVERAGE $$$ **Aqualia Antiox Anti-Fatigue Ice-Effect Eye Stick** *($29.50 for 0.13 fl. oz.)*. This gel-like stick moisturizer for the eye area makes the classic claims of reducing puffiness and fading dark circles. It cannot do that. If anything, this formula is a big yawn. The gel texture may feel cooling, and cold can reduce swelling if your eyes are puffy due to allergens or fluid retention, but you can get that benefit by applying a cloth-wrapped ice pack or cold eye mask. If your puffiness or under-eye bags are due to aging, this product won't help in the least; cosmetic corrective procedures and/or surgery are the only solutions for sagging skin. By the way, this contains more blue coloring agents than intriguing ingredients for your skin!

☹ AVERAGE $$$ **Aqualia Antiox "New Skin" Antioxidant Fresh Serum** *($46.50 for 0.54 fl. oz.)*. Other than making all skin types feel silky, this overpriced serum doesn't have much to offer. It contains more alcohol than antioxidants; in fact, the only antioxidant of note present is vitamin E (tocopherol), and there's only a tiny amount in this serum. The alcohol, while not present in a terribly high amount, may still cause dryness, free-radical damage, and irritation that leads to collagen breakdown. In any skin-care product, you never want to see alcohol listed before the state-of-the-art, anti-aging ingredients that all skin types need.

☹ AVERAGE **Aqualia Antiox Pro-Youth 24H Hydrating Fluid SPF 12** *($29.95 for 1.4 fl. oz.)*. Although the SPF rating on this daytime moisturizer for normal to slightly oily skin misses the benchmark of SPF 15, it does provide avobenzone for sufficient UVA protection. As for the claim that this product protects your stem cells, it doesn't contain anything special for that purpose. You could argue that simply protecting skin from sun damage will also protect stem cells in skin, so in that sense Vichy's claim is hardly unique. It's also important to point out that the base formula contains enough alcohol to potentially cause free-radical damage, which leads to collagen breakdown—so much for preserving cells of any kind in your skin! This product is also said to contain "microspheres" that burst and give skin an immediate healthy glow. Whether the microspheres are present or not, what you need to know is that this product contains coloring agents and cosmetic pigments, including those that leave skin shiny, to produce the glow. It can be attractive, but it isn't special or unique to this product; plus, shine and coloring agents are not skin care.

☹ AVERAGE **Aqualia Thermal 24Hr Hydrating Fortifying Lotion SPF 30** *($29.95 for 1.7 fl. oz.)* is short on anti-aging ingredients (beyond the sunscreen, of course), yet has a silky, lightweight texture suitable for normal to oily skin. Critical UVA protection is provided by avobenzone, which is stabilized by the sunscreen active octocrylene, and the finish of this moisturizer means it works great under makeup. If only Vichy had also included a mix of antioxidants, skin-repairing ingredients, and cell-communicating ingredients! As is, despite its great aesthetics and sun protection, the formula doesn't deserve better than an average rating.

☺ AVERAGE **$$$ Liftactiv CxP Eyes Anti-Wrinkle Eyelid Lifting Care** *($40 for 0.5 fl. oz.)* has a silky texture and will definitely moisturize dry skin, but it won't lift sagging around the eyes or anywhere else on the face. Eye-area sagging cannot be addressed by skin-care products, no matter how well formulated they are (we wish they could; see the Appendix for more info). For the money, you're not getting a state-of-the-art product. The tiny amounts of vitamin C cannot tighten or lift skin; even in large amounts, topical vitamin C cannot lift skin, although it can stimulate healthy collagen production and help repair sun-damaged skin for increased firmness. As for the caffeine, it may help in a small way to reduce morning puffiness, but it won't affect the puffiness that results from aging and sagging, which is likely what you're concerned about if you're reading this review. As for this product treating dark circles, don't count on even slight results because there isn't an ingredient in here that can have that kind of impact. Check out the Appendix to find out why, in truth, you don't need an eye cream.

☺ AVERAGE **$$$ LiftActiv CxP Total Serum** *($46 for 1 fl. oz.).* This citrus-scented, water-based serum is made to seem more medicinal than it is. The claim of it being able to stimulate fibroblasts (cells that generate collagen in your skin) is dubious because the amount of ingredients that impact this (such as vitamin C) is negligible. In fact, there's more yellow coloring agent in here than state-of-the-art ingredients! Although the formula is suitable for normal to slightly oily skin, this isn't an anti-aging serum to bank on.

☺ AVERAGE **$$$ LiftActiv Retinol HA Eyes Total Anti-Wrinkle Renovating Care** *($42 for 0.5 fl. oz.).* You may be tempted to try this eye cream based on the claims that it can "fight permanent, reversible, and programmed wrinkles," but that just isn't possible, so put your wallet away. Vichy's overblown claim is insulting and completely false; it's merely an attempt to classify different types of wrinkles (at least that's what we think they are trying to do). According to Vichy "Permanent" wrinkles are the deep, etched lines that won't go away no matter what you put on your face; "Reversible" wrinkles are fine lines caused by dryness, irritation, or thickened skin due to sun damage; "Programmed" lines, well, we're not sure what Vichy means by this. Our best guess is that these are the wrinkles you don't see now, but because of cumulative sun damage or just growing older, they're "programmed" to appear in the future (think of the sun damage you got in your 20s not showing up as wrinkles until you hit your 40s). Of course, Vichy wants you to think this is the antiwrinkle product that can take care of all these types of wrinkles, but it just isn't possible, so be prepared to be disappointed if you buy this. As it turns out, this is just a good emollient moisturizer for dry skin anywhere on the face. It contains a teeny-tiny amount of anti-aging ingredients, but does not contain retinol as claimed. Rather it contains retinyl palmitate, which is not the same as pure retinol. Retinyl palmitate requires an extra conversion step by enzymes in your skin for it to become effective and have a benefit for skin. Last, you don't need an eye cream, and we explain why in the Appendix.

☺ AVERAGE **$$$ Liftactiv Retinol HA Night** *($42 for 1 fl. oz.)* makes the same wrinkle-related claims as the LiftActiv Retinol HA Eyes Total Anti-Wrinkle Renovating Care above, and is equally disappointing. This is just a good but basic emollient moisturizer for dry skin. It doesn't contain much more than thickeners and emollient plant oils yet for what this costs, it should be loaded with antioxidants, skin-repairing ingredients, and cell-communicating ingredients that can help your skin look and act younger. Some of those ingredients (for example, retinol) are present, but in very small amounts the company certainly shouldn't be boasting about.

☺ AVERAGE **$$$ Liftactiv Retinol HA SPF 18 Total Anti-Wrinkle Intervention** *($47 for 1.35 fl. oz.)* has two things going for it, assuming the price doesn't give you pause (and it is overpriced for what you get): (1) The sunscreen actives include avobenzone for reliable UVA protection and (2) the base formula contains retinol to improve wrinkles and other signs of aging. The amount of retinol and the skin-repairing ingredient sodium hyaluronate (the salt form of hyaluronic acid; that's the "HA" in the product name) isn't too impressive, but this has a lightweight, smoothing texture for those with normal to slightly dry skin. Before considering this, take a look at the sunscreens with retinol from RoC; they cost less and include more retinol, which means it's more likely to benefit your skin.

☺ AVERAGE $$$ **Liftactiv Serum 10** (*$52 for 1 fl. oz.*). Without question this serum's claims stretch the bounds of what's possible from a skin-care product to the breaking point. This so-called "powerful" anti-aging treatment is said to lift skin as it improves wrinkles and pores, and essentially transform your skin. Unfortunately, its formula cannot support most of those claims (especially the lifting claim; sagging skin cannot be addressed by a product like this; see the Appendix to find out why). This serum is said to contain 10% rhamnose, a plant sugar. Vichy maintains they have research (in vitro, meaning it wasn't done to an actual person's skin but in a petri dish) proving that this plant sugar does all sorts of marvelous anti-aging things. Although they wouldn't share their research details with us, it turns out there is some compelling published research on how rhamnose may help skin do what it should be doing before it was damaged. It's important to point out rhamnose is not the only ingredient in town for anti-aging (clearly Vichy doesn't think so either or they wouldn't be selling so many other anti-aging products with similar claims). It's intriguing to note that although the carbohydrate (sugar) portion of rhamnose seems helpful for skin, the lipid portion (known as rhamnolipids) is toxic to skin cells. It seems rhamnose sugars (technically known as polysaccharides) function as cell-communicating ingredients. They have an affinity for cells that produce fibroblasts. Since fibroblasts are cells that create collagen, this is good news for wrinkles, because, at least in theory and in controlled lab settings, rhamnose can "tell" misbehaving fibroblast cells to begin producing normal, healthier cells (Sources: *Clinics in Plastic Surgery*, January 2012, pages 1–8; *Amino Acids*, May 2011, Epbulication; *Biochimica et Biophysica Acta*, December 2008, pages 1388–1394; and *Pathologie-Biologie*, September 2006, pages 420–425). It seems there's reason to be excited about rhamnose, but not more so than lots of other ingredients, including vitamin C, retinol, and niacinamide. Rhamnose is but one more option, not a complete solution for aging skin. Besides, given this serum's alcohol content, your skin is likely getting a dose of irritation and free-radical damage the good ingredients must fight before they can help your skin. It contains a small amount of other repairing and cell-communicating ingredients, but the majority of them are listed after the alcohol, which is disappointing. In short, this serum isn't the be-all, end-all and its alcohol content makes it less desirable than many other serums that omit this problematic ingredient.

☺ AVERAGE $$$ **LiftActiv with Rhamnose 5% Day for Normal Combination Skin** (*$49 for 1.7 fl. oz.*). This moisturizer is merely a lighter version of Vichy's LiftActiv with Rhamnose 5% Night, reviewed below. It's a bit too slick for the oily areas of combination skin, but otherwise the same comments apply. As for the rhamnose, it's discussed in the review above for LiftActiv Serum 10.

☺ AVERAGE $$$ **LiftActiv with Rhamnose 5% Dry** (*$49 for 1.7 fl. oz.*). This moisturizer for dry skin contains 5% rhamnose, a plant sugar. Vichy maintains they have research (in vitro, meaning it wasn't done to an actual person's skin but in a petri dish) proving that this plant sugar does all sorts of marvelous anti-aging things, all discussed in the review for LiftActiv Serum 10 above. Because this moisturizer is packaged in a jar, which hinders the effectiveness of all plant-based ingredients, not to mention the hygiene issue it presents when you stick your finger into the jar every day, the rhamnose likely won't remain stable. At best, this moisturizer will make dry skin look and feel better, just like lots of other emollient moisturizers. It cannot lift skin, though the mineral pigments mica and titanium dioxide will leave a radiant finish.

☺ AVERAGE **$$$ LiftActiv with Rhamnose 5% Night** *($49 for 1.7 fl. oz.)* will make dry skin look and feel better, just like lots of other emollient moisturizers. It cannot lift skin, not even a little bit, but in better packaging you may have seen a subtle difference in skin's firmness.

☺ AVERAGE **$$$ Neovadiol GF Day Densifying Re-Sculpting Care Normal/Combination** *($51 for 1.7 fl. oz.)*. There is nothing, and we mean nothing, in this very standard moisturizer that can lift sagging skin on the neck or along the jaw line. We wish this wasn't the case, but no skin-care products can address the multiple factors that cause skin to sag and lose its youthful contours (see the Appendix for more info). About all this jar-packaged moisturizer for normal to dry skin can do is make your skin feel smoother and softer, just like thousands of other moisturizers. And the jar packaging is actually a problem, which we discuss in the Appendix.

☺ AVERAGE **$$$ Neovadiol GF Day Densifying Re-Sculpting Care Dry Skin** *($51 for 1.7 fl. oz.)* is ill suited for use during daylight hours because it doesn't contain sunscreen. The claim of it being able to redefine your jaw line (presumably because sagging is evident) is completely without merit and in fact impossible from a skin-care product. We wish that wasn't the case but there are no skin-care products that can address the multiple causes of sagging. Knowing this won't work to lift anything, you're left with a standard emollient moisturizer whose few intriguing ingredients will degrade due to jar packaging (see the Appendix for details).

☺ AVERAGE **$$$ Neovadiol GF Night Densifying Re-Sculpting Care** *($54.50 for 1.7 fl. oz.)*. All you're getting with this night cream is a boring formula that's marginally acceptable for slightly dry skin. The fact that it's packaged in a jar means the beneficial ingredients won't remain stable once it is opened. See the Appendix for details and to find out why products like this offer no hope for sagging skin.

☹ POOR **Normaderm Pro Mat Ultra-Mattifying Oil-Free Lotion SPF 15** *($22 for 1.1 fl. oz.)*. "Terrible" is the best word to describe this daytime moisturizer with sunscreen! The active ingredients fail to supply sufficient UVA protection, leaving your skin vulnerable to signs of aging. Almost as bad is that the amount of alcohol is high enough to cause serious irritation. Irritation anywhere on the face causes dryness, collagen breakdown, and impairs healing. Although it's true that alcohol can de-grease oily skin, the irritation it causes stimulates more oil production at the base of the pore, leaving your skin worse than before you began using this product.

☹ POOR **Reti-C Intensive Corrective Care SPF 15** *($42.50 for 1.01 fl. oz.)* lacks the UVA-protecting ingredients of titanium dioxide, zinc oxide, avobenzone, Mexoryl SX, or Tinosorb, and is not recommended.

VICHY SUN CARE

☺ AVERAGE **$$$ UV Activ Daily Moisturizer Cream with Sunscreen SPF 15** *($32 for 3.4 fl. oz.)*. This sunscreen contains the L'Oreal-patented UVA-protecting ingredient Mexoryl SX, listed by its chemical name of ecamsule. Along with the other sunscreen actives, it provides reliable broad-spectrum sun protection. That's the good news. The not-so-good news is that this sunscreen is overpriced for what you're not getting, namely, antioxidants and skin-repairing ingredients. The base formula is stunningly ordinary and devoid of any state-of-the-art ingredients. Although ecamsule is a great UVA filter, there are others (such as avobenzone, titanium dioxide, and zinc oxide) formulated in sunscreens designed to take even better care of your skin. If you decide to try this, it is best for normal to oily skin.

The Reviews V

VICHY SPECIALTY SKIN-CARE PRODUCTS

☺ AVERAGE **Normaderm Anti-Blemish Intensive Treatment Cream** (*$18 for 1.01 fl. oz.*) is a water-based lotion with absorbent ingredients and 2% salicylic acid. The pH of this lotion is too high for the salicylic acid to effectively exfoliate, while the oil and thickeners this contains may make blemished skin worse. All told, this product is more confusing than helpful to skin.

☺ AVERAGE $$$ **ProEVEN Total Dark Spot Corrector** (*$43.50 for 1 fl. oz.*). Despite claims that promise the end of dark spots whether they're from sun damage or acne marks, ProEVEN Total Dark Spot Corrector isn't the total solution. First, an essential element of any discoloration-fighting routine is sunscreen, which this product lacks. We're not saying a skin-lightening product must contain sunscreen; rather, we're taking issue with the "total" portion of the name because it implies this is all you need to fight dark spots, when that's not the case. Daily sunscreen application is critical to helping dark spots fade, and of course for preventing new ones related to cumulative sun damage. This lightly fragranced, lotion-like spot corrector's main ingredient of interest is a form of vitamin C known as ascorbyl glucoside. The amount this contains is on par with what published research has shown is effective for inhibiting excess melanin (skin pigment) production. That's great, yet this product contains little else of interest for those fighting dark spots. It contains enough of the mineral pigment titanium dioxide for a subtle brightening effect, but that's cosmetic, not a treatment per se. Although this contains salicylic acid, the amount is too low and this product's pH is well above the ideal range for efficacy. That's a shame, because the exfoliation salicylic (or glycolic) acid provides definitely helps reduce the appearance of dark spots and red marks from acne. In the end, this is an OK option for normal to dry skin, but there are better skin-lightening products that cost less and contain a range of intriguing ingredients to help improve discolorations. You'll find those in our Best Products chapter at the end of this book.

☹ POOR **Normaderm Triple Action Anti-Acne Hydrating Lotion** (*$23.99 for 1.7 fl. oz.*) is an overly fragranced BHA exfoliant with salicylic acid as its active ingredient. Although the amount of salicylic acid is great, the pH is over 6, meaning this is incapable of exfoliating skin or helping to improve blackheads or other types of breakouts. The matte finish this leaves is partly due to the amount of skin-damaging alcohol this contains followed by the aluminum starch. This is absolutely not greasy but the fragrance is nearly overpowering and the alcohol is definitely concerning (see the Appendix to learn why). This cannot hydrate for 24 hours; in fact, it's minimally moisturizing at best and won't do a thing to make dry, flaky skin look or feel better.

WET 'N WILD (MAKEUP ONLY)

Strengths: Inexpensive (with some truly great beauty bargains), good tinted moisturizer with sunscreen; attractive powder bronzers; mostly good eyeshadow and lipstick options.

Weaknesses: Unimpressive concealers; large assortment of average to poor eyelining products; the mascaras do little to impress; some lip products suffer from the inclusion of irritants; the makeup brushes.

For more information and the latest reviews of Wet 'n Wild, visit CosmeticsCop.com

WET 'N WILD FOUNDATIONS

☺ GOOD Ultimate Sheer Tinted Moisturizer SPF 15 ($3.99) wins instant points for listing titanium dioxide plus avobenzone among its active ingredients, so sufficient UVA protection is assured. It has a slightly fluid, thin texture that blends decently and sets to a nearly matte finish suitable for normal to slightly oily skin. True to its name, coverage is sheer and definitely more akin to a tint than a true foundation. All four colors are excellent and there are options for light to tan skin. The formula is fragrance-free.

☺ AVERAGE **Ultimate Match SPF 15 Foundation** *($4.99)* is a sheer liquid foundation containing an in-part avobenzone sunscreen, although we're surprised the low amount of active ingredients achieved an SPF 15 rating. We're not disputing the rating, but if you're using this foundation as your sole source of sunscreen you may want to reconsider, just to be on the safe side. Although the price is attractive, this foundation has an antiquated feel and doesn't provide meaningful coverage. Oddly, the shades look much more neutral in the bottle than they appear on skin; most take on a slight peach cast that's difficult to soften, and the formula makes lines and pores more apparent.

☹ POOR **Intuitive Blend Shade Adjusting Foundation + Primer** *($5.99)* is little more than clever marketing because it adds up to a poor foundation and an even poorer primer. When you dispense some of this liquid foundation from the squeeze tube packaging, what you get is a runny, white liquid with small balls of powdered pigment that burst into color when they're blended. So, make no mistake, it's not intuition at work here; the color's transformation is simply a result of that powdered pigment being released into the liquid as you blend. The problem is that these pigment spheres don't break down easily, and because coverage is sheer, the graininess and streaking left behind is noticeable. Even worse, the dry finish has a film that's uncomfortable, unflattering, and quite sticky to the touch. This product also contains several irritating fragrance ingredients, as if it needed more problems!

☹ POOR **Natural Blend Mineral Foundation** *($4.99)*. From the packaging to the application, this attempt at a "natural" mineral powder foundation is a complete mess. The coverage is so sheer and application is so difficult to control that this isn't a mineral makeup worth getting to know.

WET 'N WILD CONCEALERS

☺ AVERAGE **Cover All Liquid Concealer Wand** *($2.99)* has a creamy-smooth texture, but although it provides good coverage it's not a "cover all" solution. This is too emollient for use over blemishes, but is an OK option for under-eye use or concealing minor redness. Among the four shades, Medium, Light, and Beige are strongly pink and should be avoided. Fair is recommended for that respective skin tone.

☹ POOR **Cover All Cover Stick** *($1.99)* is a lipstick-style cream concealer that's very greasy, easily creases under the eye, and offers shades that look nothing like real skin.

WET 'N WILD POWDER

☹ POOR **Natural Blend Pressed Powder** *($4.99)* is a dry pressed powder that looks anything but natural on skin, as the shades are all way too peach or orange. It tends to streak and will certainly exaggerate any dry areas. This is a drugstore pressed powder to avoid.

WET 'N WILD POWDER BLUSH & BRONZERS

☺ GOOD **Color Icon Bronzer SPF 15** *($3.93)* might be worth checking out. Wet 'n Wild has reformulated this bronzer to include SPF 15, but you can't rely on this product for adequate sun protection. Sunscreen needs to be applied liberally, all over the face (and body!), and bronzer should be dusted on over smaller areas of the face. Otherwise, the talc-based formula has the same smooth texture as other Color Icon products, and it applies easily with a powder brush.

☺ GOOD **Ultimate Minerals Bronzer** *($3.99)* is a loose-powder bronzer containing the same mineral pigments that show up in thousands of makeup products, so it's not the "ultimate" for fans of mineral makeup. The packaging is smart because the container includes a special closure for the sifter, which minimizes mess, and the smaller holes in the sifter make controlled dispensing easier. Application with a brush is smooth, sheer, and even. The bronze effect is best described as a peachy tan color with moderate shimmer that flatters light to medium skin tones.

☹ AVERAGE **Color Icon Blusher** *($2.97)* is a pressed-powder blush that has a surprisingly smooth texture. The sparkle-free shades (Mellow Wine and Heather Silk) have an ever-so-slight satin finish that looks very natural. The tricky part with this talc-based blush is the inconsistent color payoff: It goes from super sheer to scary bright very fast, which means that you'll definitely need to employ a proper blush brush (the one included is as cheap as the flip-top packaging). This blush also tends to grab skin unevenly, especially on top of foundation, so careful blending is a must.

WET 'N WILD EYESHADOWS

✓☺ BEST **Color Icon Eyeshadow Singles** *($1.99)* are definitely worthy of attention! The texture is impressively smooth, and the pigmentation is some of the best you'll find at the drugstore—let alone for less than $2! The trade-off for this bargain price is that the packaging is cheap and somewhat temperamental, but the product inside is nonetheless outstanding. Though these do blend and wear well, they will need some touching up if you plan on wearing them from day to night. Of the shades available, there are some sophisticated options in matte, satin, and soft shimmer finishes, but take care to avoid Envy, Lagoon and gold-flecked Kitten, whose sparkles flake easily.

☺ GOOD **Color Icon Eyeshadow Collection** *($4.99)*. These pressed-powder eyeshadow sets offer eight shades with varying levels of shimmer and pigmentation. Not all the colors complement each other, but there are some attractive choices to consider, and at least Wet 'n Wild provides some guidelines on the back of the package as to how to use them together. We noticed these powders had a tendency to drip onto skin below the eyes during application, so it's wise to give your brush (use a regular eyeshadow brush, not the included applicators) a tap to dust off the excess powder. Otherwise, the silky-dry texture blends on smoothly. Our only complaint is the absence of matte shades. As is, we don't recommend these sets for anyone with wrinkly lids because their shimmery, iridescent finish will magnify them even more. If that's not an issue for you, then this is a beauty bargain!

☺ GOOD **Color Icon Eyeshadow Trio** *($2.99)* are assembled as how-to kits for a foolproof contoured eye design, and they mostly succeed. Like other Color Icon shadows, the texture is smooth and the application is easy if you use a professional brush (the included applicators are a waste of time). The pigmentation across the shades in each palette is inconsistent, so these require some experimenting to determine which of the shades go on heavier than the others. With each pressed powder eyeshadow embossed with "Eyelid," "Crease," or "Browbone," these give novice makeup-wearers some idea of where to start, though the shades are versatile enough to work outside of these placements.

☹ POOR **Idol Eyes Cream Eyeshadow** *($1.99)* is a stout, emollient pencil that needs regular sharpening. It has a very smooth, creamy texture that glides on, but because the creaminess remains, fading and smudging occur shortly after application. Each shade is infused with glitter that tends to separate from the color as the liner breaks down during wear.

WET 'N WILD EYE & BROW LINERS

☺ GOOD **H2O Proof Liquid Eyeliner** *($3.99)* has a good, firm brush that lays down a continuous line of color from a formula that not only dries quickly, but also is tenaciously waterproof. A minor issue is that the color saturation isn't as intense as it could be. This requires layering if you want more definition (and for most of the colors, you will). That's not a deal-breaker, but it's enough to keep this liquid eyeliner from earning a higher rating.

☺ GOOD **Perfect Pair Eye Wand** *($3.99)* combines a retractable, shiny eye pencil and creamy eyeshadow in one dual-sided pen component. Both ends work well, with the pencil being preferred for its powder finish. The eyeshadow is very shiny and tends to crease slightly, but this won't be a problem if you use it only to highlight the brow bone.

☺ GOOD **MegaEyes Defining Marker** *($3.99)* is a very good liquid eyeliner with a great price! It is dispensed from a felt-tip applicator that's firm yet flexible, so application can be precise. The formula flows evenly and sets quickly, minimizing the risk of smearing. Once set, this wears well, though not quite as long as gel eyeliners; some fading is apparent, but not enough to necessitate a touch-up. This is available in one shade: Blackest Black.

☻ AVERAGE **MegaLiner Liquid Eyeliner** *($2.99)* dries quickly and doesn't flake, chip, or smear once it has set, but this loses points because its long, thin, somewhat flimsy brush makes drawing an even line unusually tricky. If you're adept at handling this type of brush you may want to consider this—but avoid the green, blue, and purple shades unless it's Halloween.

☻ AVERAGE **Mega Eyes Creme Eyeliner** *($3.99)* is actually gel eyeliner and it comes packaged in a screw-top glass jar along with a small, useless brush that you're better off tossing out. Assuming you already have a proper eyeliner brush, you can count on smooth and precise (albeit wet) application that sets to a satin finish. Although this product claims to be waterproof, and it initially performed well, after a few hours out on the town, it began showing signs of wear by cracking and flaking. At the end of the night, what was left of it came off easily with eye-makeup remover.

☻ AVERAGE **Ultimate Brow Kit** *($3.99)* provides two shades of talc-based brow powder along with a colorless brow wax and very small tools. You get an angled brow brush and tweezers, neither of which is preferred to full-size versions. The brow powder is workable, with good pigmentation and an even application if applied sheer. You have to be mindful of how much powder you pick up with your brush to avoid flaking and a messy application. The brow powders are matte and present options for brunettes only.

☹ POOR **Color Icon Brow & Eye Liner** *($1)*. This needs-sharpening pencil is supposed to be a two-for-one product for brow filling and eye lining, but it isn't all that impressive for either purpose. As a brow pencil, the waxy-cream texture goes on a bit heavy and can easily look overdone. It helps set brow hairs in place as you fill them in, but it can also make them look matted down if you're overzealous during application. As eyeliner, it takes a good amount of pressure to apply smoothly. It should also be noted that, in most cases, the color that matches your eyebrows isn't going to be your top choice for eyeliner and vice versa, so the dual purpose benefit is lost.

☹ POOR **MegaLast Retractable Eyeliner** *($1.99)* has a somewhat hard texture, so it doesn't glide across the lid as smoothly as it should. It also requires a good amount of pressure in order to achieve rich, even color. The price is tempting, but with performance like this, you're not really getting a beauty bargain after all.

WET 'N WILD LIP COLOR & LIPLINERS

✓☺ BEST **Wild Shine Lip Lacquer** *($2.99)*. Naming this a lip lacquer is inaccurate because it is really a lightweight cream lipstick—albeit a smooth-textured one that gives some department store cream lipsticks a run for their money. Application is smooth, coverage and color intensity moderate, and this sets to a soft cream finish that doesn't readily move into lines around the mouth or require frequent touch-ups. The soft shimmer shades are most attractive, and for the price, you may want to try a few! One more plus: This lipstick is fragrance-free!

☺ GOOD **Diamond Brilliance Moisturizing Lip Sheen** *($2.99)* is for anyone who likes a fairly tenacious lip gloss that imparts sheer color and a blatantly glossy finish. This wand-applicator gloss competes favorably with much more expensive options, and doesn't suffer from a cloying fragrance or artificial fruit- or dessert-like flavors. The majority of colors pair well with any lipstick shade, too, though you must be able to tolerate a slightly sticky finish.

☺ GOOD **Glassy Gloss Lip Gel** *($2.99)* is a very good, fragrance-free sheer lip gloss packaged in a tube. This has a slightly runny texture so careful dispensing is needed (especially if the gloss has been kept in a warm environment), but it feels lush and smooth, and is not sticky or overly slick. The shades are sheer enough to work with a wide range of lipstick colors.

☺ GOOD **Mega Last Lip Color** *($1.97)* is a pigment-rich lipstick with an impressively durable semi-matte finish and very little slip. The shade range, while extensive, lacks sophistication, but if you can find yourself a shade that works for you (and at this price you can afford to experiment), this is definitely worth a try.

☺ GOOD **MegaSlicks Lip Color Pencil** *($2.99)* looks deceiving because you'd swear it was a pencil that needed to be sharpened. Look closer and it's a cleverly designed automatic pencil whose tip can be wound up or down. This thick pencil has a slightly dry application and semi-matte finish with nearly opaque colors. It wears longer than traditional lipsticks, but you may need to add some gloss for comfort.

☺ GOOD **MegaSlicks Lip Gloss** *($1.99)* is a good basic lip gloss that feels slightly thick, isn't too slick, and is slightly sticky. All the sheer shades have soft to moderate shimmer and are applied with a sponge-tip wand. This lip gloss has a strong fragrance.

☺ GOOD **Perfect Pair Lip Wand** *($3.99)* combines a retractable, shimmer finish lip pencil with a slim, sheer lipstick in one dual-sided unit. The pencil is standard fare in terms of application and wear (it's too creamy to last the day) and the lipstick feels light, provides moderate coverage, and imparts a frosted shimmer. This will appeal to teens more than adults, but for those who use lipliner and lipstick and like strong shimmer, it is convenient.

☺ GOOD **Silk Finish Lipstick** *($1.29)* is Wet n' Wild's most opaque lipstick, but also its greasiest. The wide shade selection has a nice stain, helping to keep the color around longer, but this is also greasy enough to immediately bleed into any lines around the mouth. If that's not an issue for you and you want full-coverage color, the price is tough to beat!

☹ AVERAGE **Color Icon Lip Liner** *($0.93)* is a standard, needs-sharpening pencil that's neither too creamy nor too dry, although the finish is slightly tacky. A few of the colors are excellent versatile shades that you really should check out if you don't mind routine sharpening. At less than a dollar, it's an indisputable value, though sharpening is always a hassle! This pencil would've earned a Good rating if it didn't require sharpening.

☹ POOR **Natural Blend Lip Shimmer** *($1.99)* is a veritable knock-off of Burt's Bees' popular Lip Shimmers (even some of the shade names are identical), and even though it's a fraction of the cost, this twist-up lip product has all the problems of the Burt's Bees version—irritating plant oils that can cause irritation and chapped lips—and is best avoided.

☹ POOR **MegaBrilliance Lip Gloss** *($1.99)* is a lightweight, minimally sticky lip gloss loaded with large flecks of glitter. As you might guess, the glitter feels grainy (almost scratchy) shortly after application, and the effect is far from sophisticated or glamorous.

WET 'N WILD MASCARA

☺ GOOD **MegaLength Mascara** *($2.99)* lives up to its name! The thin, rubber-bristled brush allows you to coat even the most hard-to-reach lashes and provides prodigious length. The only downside is that you do get some minor clumping but nothing that can't be smoothed out with a mascara comb. It also doesn't add much volume, but from the name that's no surprise. If you're looking for a flake-free, smudge-proof lengthening mascara, give this beauty bargain a try.

☺ AVERAGE **MegaLash Clinical Mascara** *($4.99)* does an adequate job of creating separation and length with a slight curl, but there's not a lot of volume or drama to this mascara, which makes it an OK choice for understated, daytime wear. The brush is nothing special, and the formula is on the dry side, although it does keep your lashes soft all day.

☺ AVERAGE **MegaPlump Mascara** *($3.99)* has a name that makes you think of thick lashes, perhaps? Well, that's what we were hoping would happen with this, but not even successive coats provided any lengthening or thickening. The only thing plump about it is the tube. It wears well, removes easily, and is an OK option if you want minimally enhanced lashes.

☺ AVERAGE **MegaProtein Mascara** *($1.99)* contains a tiny, not "mega," amount of soy protein, and protein in and of itself isn't the fast track to gorgeous lashes. This mascara, like most of those from Wet n' Wild, does little to impress. Its main accomplishment is average length; you cannot build bigger, longer lashes with this no matter how long you try.

☺ AVERAGE **MegaWink Mascara** *($2.99)* is an OK mascara for a really natural look without a hint of thickness. You'll get soft, separated lashes without clumps and a minimal curled effect.

☹ POOR **MegaVolume Mascara** *($2.99)* is a nearly do-nothing mascara that is 100% misnamed.

WET 'N WILD FACE & BODY ILLUMINATORS

☹ POOR **MegaShimmer Shimmer Dust** *($2.99)* is a loose shimmer powder that has an unappealingly dry, slightly grainy texture. It imparts subtle to glittery shine depending on the shade, but none of them cling well and they feel terrible on skin when used over large areas.

☹ POOR **MegaSparkle Confetti** *($2.99)* is loose glitter that has a dimensional, multicolored effect that can be striking in most lighting. The low rating is because this product has absolutely no ability to cling to skin, meaning the effect is short-lived and glitter gets all over the place.

WET 'N WILD BRUSHES

☺ AVERAGE **Kabuki Powder Brush** *($3.99)*. This full-size synthetic kabuki brush has adequate density for picking up powder, but the bristles are far too stiff to make applying it enjoyable. The stiff bristles are packed so tightly, they don't spread out evenly and instead gather from one side to the other. It's possible that this brush will open up over time, though synthetic bristles don't unfold or wear in the way natural hair bristles do—but for the price, it's not much of a gamble.

☹ POOR **Makeup Artistry Tool Kit** *($1.99)*. The too-tiny kit gives new meaning to the phrase "Why bother?" and the brushes are all the throwaway variety.

WET 'N WILD SPECIALTY MAKEUP PRODUCTS

☺ AVERAGE **Megalash Clinical Serum** *($6.99)*. It seems that almost every cosmetics company wants you to believe that they have a product that can help you grow longer lashes, including this one from Wet n' Wild. This lash serum doesn't contain any ingredients proven capable of growing lashes one iota. It's worth mentioning that the star ingredient in Megalash Clinical Serum (myristoyl pentapeptide-17) is one of the same star ingredients in Jan Marini's $160 lash growth serum, Marini Lash (reviewed on CosmeticsCop.com). If you want to give this product a try to see if it works for you, despite the fact that this peptide has no ability to grow lashes, skip Marini's version and give this one a spin for a fraction of the price.

YES TO (SKIN CARE ONLY)

Strengths: Inexpensive; complete ingredient lists are provided on company website; some good cleansers; an impressive selection of reasonably well-formulated moisturizers, both with and without sunscreen.

Weaknesses: No products to successfully address the needs of those with acne or skin discolorations; several products contain irritating fragrant oils; jar packaging; potentially weak preservative system compared with those of many other brands.

For more information and reviews of the latest Yes To products, visit CosmeticsCop.com.

YES TO CLEANSERS

✔☺ BEST **Yes to Cucumbers Gentle Milk Cleanser** *($8.99 for 6 fl. oz.)* is a minimally fragranced cleansing milk that is an outstanding option for normal to dry skin. Its gentle formula soothes and helps remove makeup while rinsing cleanly. The addition of cucumber doesn't count for much because this plant's benefit is mostly rinsed down the drain, but it's great Yes To didn't include fragrant plants known to cause irritation. Note that because this contains fragrance (albeit a very low amount), it isn't a top choice for those with sensitive or rosacea-affected skin. Otherwise, it comes highly recommended—and the price is great, too!

☺ GOOD **Yes to Blueberries Brightening Facial Towelettes** *($7.99 for 30 towelettes)* are fragranced cleansing cloths that are a fairly gentle way to cleanse your skin and remove makeup at home or on the go. Best for normal to dry skin, the antioxidant-rich formula replaces typical cleansing agents with emollient ingredients and plant oil. These do remove makeup, but can leave a bit of a residue you may want to rinse off with water, which defeats the purpose of using cleansing cloths; if you're going to rinse anyway, you may as well use a regular cleanser. These cloths are not recommended for sensitive skin because they contain fragrance and fragrant plant extracts.

☺ GOOD **Yes to Carrots Daily Cream Facial Cleanser** *($7.99 for 6 fl. oz.)* is a fragranced, creamy cleanser that is a good option for normal to dry skin. It feels soothing and does a good job removing most types of makeup (you'll need a makeup remover to take off waterproof mascara or long-wearing lip stains). Yes to Carrots claims this is 96% natural, and this looks to be the case, although some of the "chemical-sounding" ingredients aren't natural per se but are naturally derived. Still, fans of natural products may want to give this cleanser a go.

☺ AVERAGE **Yes To Blueberries Age Refresh Smoothing Daily Cleanser** *($9.99 for 4.5 fl. oz.)* is a good, creamy cleanser that is best for dry to very dry skin. Its rich, buttery texture helps remove makeup, but because it doesn't rinse easily, you'll want to use a washcloth with it. The lemon and apple extracts are present in teeny amounts and contrary to claim don't have benefit for skin. Lemon peel isn't the least bit cleansing and neither lemon nor apple extract are natural sources of AHA as claimed. Although lemon and apple do contain citric acid and malic acid, respectively, these do not function the same way as AHAs, even if the citric acid or malic acid is present in appropriate amounts in a product with an appropriate pH level. Even so, in a cleanser, these ingredients are rinsed down the drain, so it's all nonsense anyway.

☺ AVERAGE **Yes to Carrots Exfoliating Cleanser** *($9.99 for 3.38 fl. oz.)* contains natural scrub particles from carrot root and bamboo. That sounds appealing, but the problem with these ingredients is that they tend to have rough, uneven edges that can scratch and cause microscopic tears in skin, especially if you overdo the scrubbing. Ironically, synthetic polyethylene beads are a better choice for a scrub because they are smooth, rounded, and polish skin with minimal risk of irritation. As a cleanser, this is best for normal to dry skin. It doesn't contain detergent cleansing agents but instead relies on emollients to remove makeup and debris, along with the scrub particles.

☺ AVERAGE **Yes to Carrots Makeup Removing Cleanser** *($9.99 for 8.45 fl. oz.)* contains ingredients that swiftly remove makeup, though you may find using this with a washcloth is necessary to avoid a skin-dulling residue. Best for normal to dry skin not prone to breakouts, the only significant drawback is the amount of fragrance this contains. Fragrance isn't skin care, and since this cleanser doesn't rinse easily on its own, you're leaving traces of fragrance on skin, which can lead to irritation. Fragrance is also a problem to use around the eyes, which you're likely to do with this product, assuming you wish to remove eye makeup. For a superior cleanser that removes makeup and omits fragrance, consider Paula's Choice Skin Recovery Softening Cream Cleanser instead.

☺ AVERAGE **Yes to Cucumbers Soothing Daily Gentle Cleanser** *($9.99 for 3.38 fl. oz.)* is a fairly gentle cleanser that is overpriced due to the tiny amount of product provided. Yes To sells other cleansers that have better formulas and, ounce for ounce, cost less, too. A potential concern with this formula is the amount of salt (sodium chloride) it contains. Salt shows up in most water-soluble facial cleansers (and in shampoos) because it helps thicken and stabilize these products. Typically only a low amount is needed, which negates the concern of dryness that can occur when the salt is present in higher amounts. Although this doesn't get an enthusiastic recommendation, if you're curious it's best for normal to oily skin.

☺ AVERAGE **Yes to Cucumbers Soothing Facial Towelettes** *($5.99 for 30 towelettes)* are an OK but not-too-thorough way to cleanse skin. It's worth noting the fragrance doesn't come from cucumber extract but rather the fragrance added. The formula isn't great at removing makeup and will leave those with oily skin feeling their face isn't clean enough. These cleansing cloths are best for those with normal to dry skin who wear minimal makeup. The fragrance isn't the best to leave on skin so for best results, rinse with water after cleansing.

☺ AVERAGE **Yes to Tomatoes Daily Clarifying Cleanser** *($9.99 for 3.38 fl. oz.)* is a fairly gentle cleanser that is overpriced due to the tiny amount of product provided. Yes To sells other cleansers that have better formulas and, ounce for ounce, cost less, too. Although this cleanser doesn't get an enthusiastic recommendation, if you're curious it's suitable for normal to oily skin. As for the tomatoes and other food extracts in this cleanser, they look good on the label but their benefits are mostly rinsed down the drain.

YES TO EXFOLIANTS & SCRUBS

☺ AVERAGE **Yes to Tomatoes Acne Daily Pore Scrub** *($9.99 for 4 fl. oz.)* is not a good idea, primarily because acne cannot be scrubbed away and using abrasive products over blemishes can cause irritation that prolongs healing and increases the risk of red marks once the blemish is gone. Although this scrub is medicated with anti-acne ingredient salicylic acid, the pH of this scrub won't allow it to function as an exfoliant. Ideally, salicylic acid is best in leave-on rather than rinse-off products. In rinse-off products like this, its contact with skin is too brief for it to be of much help. This is an OK scrub to use if you have normal to dry skin and are not dealing with breakouts, but all skin types will find a well-formulated AHA or BHA exfoliant provides results that no scrub can match.

☺ AVERAGE **Yes to Tomatoes Repairing Acne Lotion** *($14.99 for 1.7 fl. oz.)* is an effective BHA exfoliant that contains 1% salicylic acid as its active ingredient. The fluid gel (it's not a lotion) is quite fragrant, that's but one of its problems. The pH of 2.9 is within range for the salicylic acid to function as an exfoliant, but it's also low enough to cause undue irritation (there's a big difference between pH 2.9 and, say 3.2, in much the same way there's a difference between a magnitude 2.9 and 3.2 earthquake). This will exfoliate and help improve acne-prone skin, but it also contains a couple of irritating ingredients that won't help anyone's skin. What a shame, as the price is attractive and this does contain some effective natural ingredients.

YES TO MOISTURIZERS (DAYTIME & NIGHTTIME), EYE CREAMS, & SERUMS

✓☺ BEST **Yes To Carrots Daily Facial Moisturizer with SPF 15** *($14.99 for 1.7 fl. oz.)* is a very good daytime moisturizer with sunscreen for normal to dry skin not prone to blemishes. The sole active ingredient is zinc oxide, and it's in an emollient formula that is cosmetically elegant and treats skin to a good mix of antioxidants. Ignore the claim that this detoxifies your skin—it doesn't—and no one at the Yes To brand could specify which toxins this product is supposed to eliminate. Hokey claim aside, this is highly recommended and, for the most part, is about as natural as you can get when it comes to moisturizers with sunscreen.

☺ GOOD **Yes to Blueberries Age Refresh Daily Facial Moisturizer SPF 30** *($19.99 for 1.4 fl. oz.)* is a very good daytime moisturizer with sunscreen for normal to dry skin that's not prone to breakouts. Because this contains fragrance, it is not recommended for sensitive skin; however, the fragrance isn't as intense as the similar product, Yes to Cucumbers Daily Calming Moisturizer SPF 30 (reviewed below). The mineral actives are the gentlest sun protection ingredients around, so this would be a boon for sensitive skin if not for the fragrance. Getting back to the mineral actives of titanium dioxide and zinc oxide, the combined amounts are what makes this product a tricky one for breakout-prone skin, because both of these ingredients have the potential to clog pores. The amount of mineral actives in this moisturizer also leaves a slight white cast, but it's not a deal-breaker, especially if you plan to follow with makeup. What's certain is that those with oily or combination skin won't like this product's heavier, moist finish. True to its name, this contains blueberry, and this antioxidant is joined by several others to help skin better defend itself against environmental causes of aging. This would earn our top rating if it contained some cell-communicating ingredients and a more sophisticated mix of repairing ingredients (both essential for skin that looks and acts younger), but it's still worth considering. Note: The tiny amount of alcohol is not cause for concern. When alcohol appears at the end of an ingredient list, it isn't present in a great enough concentration to cause irritation.

☺ GOOD **Yes To Blueberries Age Refresh Eye Firming Treatment** *($19.99 for 0.5 fl. oz.)* contains lots of natural ingredients, most of which provide antioxidant benefit without adding fragrance, which is always to your skin's benefit. The formula is best for dry skin and can leave a slightly greasy finish, so it's not the best to apply under makeup. (The finish can cause concealer to crease and eyeliner to smear.) Before you get too excited, please know that you don't need an eye cream (see the Appendix for details). This product proves it because the ingredients it contains are the same ingredients that appear in numerous facial moisturizers—it doesn't contain anything special for the eye area. This product is said to contain a floral ingredient known as paracress that supposedly can firm skin and reduce wrinkles in less than a month. There is no research supporting this claim; in fact, the only research pertaining to topical application of this plant extract on skin has shown that it penetrates skin when mixed with an alcohol or glycol ingredient, but that's it (Source: *Journal of Ethnopharmacology*, January 2010, pages 77–84). Just because it penetrates skin doesn't mean it can stimulate collagen production or has any special benefit for skin around the eyes, especially not when mixed with alcohol, which causes collagen breakdown and free-radical damage.

☺ GOOD **Yes to Cucumbers Calming Night Cream** *($14.99 for 1.7 fl. oz.)* is a good moisturizer for normal to very dry skin. It is packaged to ensure that the plant- and vitamin-based antioxidants remain stable during use, which is great! Although this is an antioxidant-rich formula, skin also needs a good range of repairing and cell-communicating ingredients to look and feel its young, healthy best. Sadly, those types of ingredients are missing and that's what keeps this moisturizer from earning our top rating.

☺ GOOD **Yes to Cucumbers Daily Calming Moisturizer SPF 30** *($14.99 for 1.4 fl. oz.)* is very similar to Yes To Blueberries Daily Repairing Moisturizer SPF 30 above, though for some reason the Yes to Cucumbers version costs less for the same amount of product. The most discernible difference is the Yes to Blueberries option contains blueberry while the Yes to Cucumbers version contains, you guessed it, cucumber. Otherwise, the same review applies.

☺ GOOD **Yes to Cucumbers Soothing Daily Calming Moisturizer** *($14.99)* is a wonderfully emollient, well-formulated facial moisturizer for dry to very dry skin. It is not recommended for dry skin that's prone to breakouts, but if that's not a concern for you, this is worth considering. The formula contains a blend of common and novel antioxidants, but all of them will benefit skin because this moisturizer is packaged to keep these sensitive ingredients stable during use. In terms of soothing skin, we wish this contained some proven anti-irritants, but without question the emollient plants and oils will help make dry skin look and feel better. This would earn our top rating if it contained a greater range of repairing ingredients and perhaps a cell-communicating ingredient or two. These types of ingredients are essential if your goal is skin that look and acts younger. This is not recommended for sensitive skin because it contains fragrance and fragrant rosemary extract.

☺ GOOD **$$$ Yes to Blueberries Brightening Eye Roller** *($19.99 for 0.5 fl. oz.)* consists of a lightweight, somewhat tacky gel housed in a small cylindrical container outfitted with a roller-ball applicator. The idea is to massage the product around tired, puffy eyes to "brighten" and "refresh." The formula is mostly water and blueberry juice with gum-based thickeners, so it has a lightweight texture—and of course the blueberries provide an antioxidant boost. The roller-ball application feels nice, and manual massage from this type of applicator can help reduce puffiness due to fluid retention or allergies, but not age-related puffiness (as in sagging or under-eye bags that you have no matter the season or your health concerns). This product does not contain anything proven to lighten dark circles, though if your eye area skin is dry, hydrating with a product such as this automatically makes dark circles look better (dryness magnifies the darkness). That benefit is hardly unique to this product; if anything, this won't be moisturizing enough if dryness around the eyes is your concern. All told, this gel-based eye-area moisturizer is a good option that treats skin anywhere on the face to some helpful ingredients.

☺ AVERAGE **Yes To Blueberries Age Refresh Daily Repairing Moisturizer** *($19.99 for 1.7 fl. oz.)* is not recommended for use during the day because it doesn't contain sunscreen. Unless you're willing to pair it with a foundation with sunscreen rated SPF 15 or greater (and apply it liberally and evenly), reserve use of this moisturizer for nighttime. That said, it's a simple, close-to-all-natural formula that is OK for normal to dry skin. However, it is neither powerful nor a special formula for skin. What is impressive is that for a mostly natural moisturizer, it doesn't contain needless irritants, such as essential oils, citrus, or other plant extracts, that can hurt skin, as so many other natural products do.

☺ AVERAGE **Yes To Blueberries Age Refresh Intensive Skin Repair Serum** *($19.99 for 1 fl. oz.)* contains 100% natural ingredients, but not all of them are beneficial for your skin. Antioxidants are present, including the blueberry juice that serves as the main ingredient, but the formula also contains alcohol—the kind that causes dryness, free-radical damage, and collagen breakdown. Because of the mix of alcohol and fragrance in this serum, the risk of irritation really makes it a no go, which makes it a less enticing option than others on our Best Serums list at the end of this book.

☺ AVERAGE **Yes To Blueberries Age Refresh Overnight Hydrating Cream** *($19.99 for 1.7 fl. oz.)* is nearly identical to the Yes to Blueberries Age Refresh Daily Repairing Moisturizer above. This nighttime version has a slightly creamier texture and a couple of novel ingredients, but that's about it. Either of these moisturizers is suitable for use at night if you have normal to dry skin, but neither is a particularly exciting option.

☺ AVERAGE **Yes to Carrots Moisturizing Eye Cream** *($14.99 for 1.7 fl. oz.)* is an emollient eye cream that contains some great ingredients for dry skin anywhere on the face, but guess what? Its fragranced formula differs in no meaningful way from Yes to Carrot's facial moisturizer for dry skin. It is further proof that you don't need an eye cream. Because this is packaged in a jar, the plant-based antioxidant ingredients will break down as soon as you open this. Those beneficial ingredients are great to see in skin-care products, but they're sensitive to light and air, not to mention the hygiene issues jar packaging presents. Ultimately, this eye cream is not only superfluous, it's also a bad investment because the most important ingredients won't remain stable, which means your skin won't see much benefit from them.

☺ AVERAGE **Yes to Carrots Repairing Night Cream** *($14.99 for 1.7 fl. oz.)* is an oil-rich moisturizer for dry to very dry skin that contains some brilliant ingredients which will ease dryness while offering antioxidant benefits. Unfortunately, because this night cream is packaged in a jar, the plant- and vitamin-based antioxidants won't remain stable during use (see the Appendix for details). The packaging is really a shame because there's a lot to like about this formula. We wish the antioxidants were present in greater amounts and the orange oil can be a source of irritation, but this, too, will lose potency once you open the product.

☺ AVERAGE **Yes to Carrots Rich Moisture Day Cream** *($14.99 for 1.7 fl. oz.)* is nearly identical to others from Yes to Carrots, including those designated as night creams. Actually, this is ill-advised for daytime use because it does not offer sun protection. Yes, you can pair this with another moisturizer or foundation that's rated SPF 15 or greater but why apply two moisturizers when only one is needed (and for daytime it should ideally contain sunscreen)? Besides, because this moisturizer is packaged in a jar, all the beneficial plant- and vitamin-based antioxidants won't remain stable (see the Appendix for details). If you still wish to consider this, the formula is best for dry to very dry skin. The amount of fragrant orange oil this contains poses a slight risk of irritation, while the amount of salicylic acid (also known as BHA) is too low to function as an exfoliant.

☺ AVERAGE **Yes to Cucumbers Soothing Eye Gel** *($14.99 for 1.01 fl. oz.)* plays to the old beauty trick of placing fresh cucumber slices over the eye to help reduce puffiness. That does work to some extent, but that's not because it's cucumber—it's because the cucumber is cold when you take it out of the refrigerator. It's the coolness of the vegetable that reduces puffiness and constricts the skin; cucumber slices just happen to fit the contours of the eye area. Although this water-based gel has potential as a lightweight moisturizer for slightly dry skin anywhere on the face, it isn't recommended for the eye area. Why? It contains some plant extracts that can be sensitizing, and that potential is even stronger when you place it near the eyes. Truly state-of-the-art skin care should never involve placing irritating ingredients anywhere on your face or body, especially when they serve no purpose other than to aggravate skin. You're better off treating occasional puffy eyes with real cucumber slices and/or cooled chamomile tea bags.

☹ POOR **Yes to Tomatoes Clear Skin Daily Balancing Moisturizer** *($14.99 for 1.7 fl. oz.)* is supposed to contain powerful ingredients to absorb oil (and it's marketed to those with breakout-prone skin) yet it contains a triglyceride (a component of skins' oil) as well as nonfragrant plant oils! What was Yes To thinking? Did anyone check the claims against the ingredient list? Apparently not because this moisturizer is way too emollient for anyone struggling with breakouts, not to mention it has zero ability to absorb excess oil! Ordinarily we'd shift gears and recommend this for normal to dry skin that's not prone to breakouts, but because the formula contains potent irritant red pepper extract, it isn't advised for anyone's skin. Red pepper causes irritation that can stimulate more oil production in the pore lining, making oily skin worse, and its irritancy is bad news for any skin type.

YES TO SUN CARE

✓☺ BEST **Yes To Carrots Hydrating Body Lotion with SPF 30** *($14.99 for 4.2 fl. oz.)* provides its broad-spectrum protection with a high amount of zinc oxide. It can feel a bit thick on skin and needs to be massaged in thoroughly to avoid a whitish cast, but this is otherwise a great way to protect your skin in the sun. The base formula is best for dry skin not prone to breakouts, and Yes To included some notable antioxidants for additional environmental protection. Because this contains fragrance, it is a tricky sunscreen to recommend for those with sensitive skin.

YES TO LIP & SMILE CARE

☹ POOR **Yes To Carrots Pomegranate Lip Butter with SPF 15** *($8.99 for 3 tubes)* offers broad-spectrum sun protection from zinc oxide but it contains several fragrance ingredients known to be irritating to skin (lips, too). One of the fragrance ingredients is eugenol, which is especially irritating because it kills skin cells and damages healthy collagen production (Source: *Toxicologic Pathology*, August 2007, pages 693–701). Note: This is also known as Conditioning Lip Butter with SPF 15.

YES TO SPECIALITY SKIN-CARE PRODUCTS

☹ POOR **Yes to Carrots Softening Facial Mask** *($14.99 for 1.7 fl. oz.)* is all but guaranteed to leave your skin confused. It contains a mix of clay (kaolin) followed by almond oil and a series of thickening agents that are too heavy for oily or combination skin. You might think this mask is a good choice for dry skin but with clay as the second ingredient, most with dry skin will find this mask too absorbent. See what we mean by leaving your skin confused?

☹ POOR **Yes to Cucumbers Calming Facial Mask** *($14.99 for 1.7 fl. oz.)* is nearly identical to the Yes to Carrots Softening Facial Mask above, except the carrot is replaced by cucumber. Otherwise, the same comments apply.

☹ POOR **Yes to Tomatoes Acne Roller Ball Spot Stick** *($9.99 for 0.5 fl. oz.)* seems to be a convenient way to spot treat the occasional breakout with a roll-on applicator. If only what was dispensed from the cute roller ball were helpful! The formula is medicated with anti-acne salicylic acid, but the pH of this blemish treatment is too high for it to function as an exfoliant, which means you won't get that significant anti-acne benefit. Most upsetting and detrimental to your skin is the inclusion of several irritants, including alcohol, witch hazel, lavender oil, and grapefruit juice. See the Appendix to find out how these irritants make oily, acne-prone skin worse.

☹ POOR **Yes To Tomatoes Clear Skin Acne Blemish Clearing Facial Towelettes** *($7.99 for 25 sheets)* are medicated with anti-acne salicylic acid and the pH of the formula is within range for it to function as an exfoliant; however, this isn't the way to go to experience the benefits salicylic acid offers. The formula contains irritants including witch hazel, red pepper, and alcohol, all of which can make inflamed, reddened, acne-prone skin worse (see the Appendix for details). These aren't the type of ingredients to leave on your face, but the fact that the cleansing solution really should be rinsed defeats the convenience of using cleaning cloths.

☹ POOR **Yes to Tomatoes Clear Skin Skin Clearing Facial Mask** *($14.99 for 1.7 fl. oz.)* is another clay-based mask for oily skin that is bound to leave its intended skin type confused. The reason is because the formula also contains a high amount of oil. The oil will keep the clay from working as well as it otherwise would, and it also makes this mask difficult to rinse. Titanium dioxide and a thickening agent only complicate the problems the high amount of oil causes—and none of this is skin-clearing. As for the tomatoes, an extract is included. That's nice and it does have antioxidant properties, but it and the other plant extracts won't remain stable because this mask is packaged in a jar. If the clay and oil issue weren't bad enough, the company also added a pepper extract that can incite redness and cause irritation. In short, this mask is minimally helpful for oily, breakout-prone skin and may just make matters worse.

☹ POOR **Yes to Tomatoes Deep Cleansing Facial Pads** *($7.99 for 50 pads)* stands a good chance of making matters worse. That's because it contains an irritating amount of alcohol along with witch hazel water and, further down the ingredient list, red pepper extract. Combined, these promote serious irritation that hurts skin's healing process and can actually stimulate more oil production at the base of the pores. The result? More breakouts due to excess oil and prolonged healing time for red marks blemishes leave behind. This contains anti-acne superstar salicylic acid, but the amount is too low to provide much benefit, not to mention the pH of these pads won't allow the salicylic acid to function as an exfoliant (which is the goal).

YVES SAINT LAURENT

Strengths: Every sunscreen includes avobenzone for sufficient UVA protection; some moisturizers with elegant textures; good makeup removers and toners; Radiant Touch is a favorite for good reason; intriguing blushes; some fantastic mascaras; very good liquid highlighter; innovative gloss/stain lip products.

Weaknesses: Expensive; no AHA or BHA products; no products to effectively manage acne or combat skin discolorations; mostly mundane moisturizers and serums; pervasive use of jar packaging; antiwrinkle claims that epitomize ridiculous, yet cost hundreds of dollars; mostly average foundations, eyeshadow quads; mostly average lipstick and gloss options.

For more information and reviews of the latest Yves Saint Laurent products, visit Cosmetics-Cop.com.

YVES SAINT LAURENT EYE-MAKEUP REMOVER

☺ GOOD $$$ **Instant Eye Make-Up Remover** *($30 for 3.3 fl. oz.)* is a standard, dual-phase eye-makeup remover that works very well to remove all types of makeup. It is fragrance-free and suitable for all skin types, and contains soothing plant extracts. The tiny amount of panthenol this contains will not help make eyelashes stronger.

YVES SAINT LAURENT TONER

☹ POOR **Top Secrets Pore Refiner Skincare Brush** *($55 for 1.3 fl. oz.)* is nothing more than an alcohol-laden toner packaged so you can dispense it via a built-in synthetic brush. The smooth-bristled brush is said to refine your pores and make your skin tone more even. It's a gimmick that will only waste your time and money. The amount of alcohol is a problem (see the Appendix for details) and the formula also contains several fragrance ingredients known to cause irritation. Salicylic acid is a very helpful ingredient for improving how the pore functions, but the pH of this product prevents it from working in this manner.

YVES SAINT LAURENT EXFOLIANT

☺ GOOD $$$ **Top Secrets Natural Action Exfoliator Granule Free** *($44 for 2.5 fl. oz.)* is a very expensive, but good, scrub for normal to dry skin. You don't need to spend anywhere near this much for a scrub, and in fact a wet washcloth used with your facial cleanser would work just as well. But if you're inclined to indulge, this is a gentle option whose granules are from sugar, not polyethylene or shells. This scrub can be tricky to rinse, and in terms of the vitamins mentioned in the claims, they're barely present in the formula (not to mention their benefit would be rinsed down the drain).

YVES SAINT LAURENT MOISTURIZERS, EYE CREAMS, & SERUMS

☺ AVERAGE $$$ **Forever Youth Liberator Eye Cream** *($95 for 0.5 fl. oz.)* has a light, silky texture that helps make wrinkles appear smoother. The thing is, lots of facial serums and moisturizers offer this too, proving once again why eye creams are unnecessary (your facial moisturizer or serum can and should be applied around the eyes, too). What's disappointing about this eye cream is the lack of state-of-the-art, anti-aging ingredients. Only a tiny amount is present and what's here won't remain stable due to jar packaging, which exposes these delicate ingredients to light and air (see the Appendix for details). Also a letdown is that there's more shine (from mica, a mineral pigment) than antioxidants—and this eye cream contains fragrance (so much for the argument that the eye area needs fragrance-free formulas). In the end, this cannot "visibly re-contour the eye" as claimed and ends up being an expense you don't need to add to your skin-care budget.

☺ AVERAGE $$$ **Temps Majeur Creme** *($345 for 1.6 fl. oz.)* has an elegantly silky texture and contains ingredients that help normal to slightly dry or slightly oily skin feel and look better, but the antioxidant activity of the mushroom extract will be lost once this ultra-pricey jar-packaged product is opened. This is prestigious in name only; for the money, it should be loaded with a range of state-of-the-art ingredients.

☺ AVERAGE $$$ **Temps Majeur Intensive Skin Supplement for the Eyes** *($135 for 0.5 fl. oz.)* is a fragrance-free, emollient eye cream that's useful for dry skin anywhere on the face. Like all eye creams, it doesn't contain anything proven to be unique or special for the eye area (see the Appendix to learn why you don't need an eye cream). Although sold as a "complete" anti-aging eye product, this is incomplete because it doesn't provide sun protection—by far priority number one when signs of aging are your concern. The company makes the usual claims of this eye cream being able to combat puffiness and dark circles, but it cannot make good on those promises. The titanium dioxide and mica provide a brightening effect with a shiny finish, but those are makeup tricks, not skin care. Although the formula contains some excellent antioxidants and plant extracts, they will not remain stable once this jar-packaged eye cream is opened.

☺ AVERAGE $$$ **Temps Majeur Serum** *($225 for 1 fl. oz.)* is only worth the price if you believe mushroom stem extract is the fountain of youth. Most species of mushroom have antioxidant capability and other various attributes that can be helpful for skin. But none of these benefits is in line with what YSL claims this serum can do, and the few other potentially intriguing ingredients are barely present. By the way, the gum base of this serum can lend a slightly sticky finish. All told, we wouldn't choose this over serums from Olay, Neutrogena, Clinique, Estee Lauder, or Paula's Choice.

☺ AVERAGE $$$ **Temps Majeur Ultra Riche Creme** *($345 for 1.6 fl. oz.)* is a suitable moisturizer for dry to very dry skin, but the workhorse ingredients in this product are found in hundreds of other moisturizers with much more realistic prices. You're not getting anything substantial for your substantial investment; if anything, it's quite a letdown to know that the jar packaging won't keep the efficacious antioxidants in this product stable during use (see the Appendix to find out why jar packaging is a no-no).

☹ POOR **Hydra Feel Fresh Hydrating Water Gel** *($62 for 1.6 fl. oz.)* lists alcohol as the second ingredient, and as such is too drying and irritating for all skin types. The amount of alcohol will also make the acrylate-based film-forming agent (think hairspray-type ingredients) that follows it irritating. What a mess for those with oily skin!

☹ POOR **Top Secrets Flash Radiance Skincare Brush** *($55 for 1.3 fl. oz.)* has absolutely nothing that will make "fatigued" skin look less tired. What you're getting is mostly packaging novelty and misleading claims. This silicone-based serum has a spackle-like texture that you brush on skin. The component comes equipped with a synthetic brush that dispenses the product onto itself. What's inside is ordinary when compared with today's genuinely state-of-the-art serums, and that includes the ones with mild wrinkle-filling effects on skin such as Estee Lauder's Perfectionist [CP +R] or Paula's Choice Antioxidant Concentrates. Perhaps most disappointing is the inclusion of menthol-derived irritants, whose tingling action is meant to convince you that this product is doing something to refresh or energize tired skin, when all it's really doing is irritating your skin, which leads to further stress, thus making your skin worse than it was before using this product.

☹ POOR **Top Secrets Flash Touch Wake-Up Eye Care** *($44 for 0.1 fl. oz.)* is YSL's offering of an eye-area product packaged with a vibrating metal roller-ball applicator. This roll-on device is somehow supposed to help the formula reduce signs of fatigue, along with puffy eyes and dark circles. Let's be clear: The ONLY type of puffiness this roller-ball applicator may be able to reduce via massage is puffiness that occurs due to fluid retention. Neither the device nor the product housed inside can do a thing for age-related puffy eyes (also known as sagging or under-eye bags) or for dark circles. This particular version's formula and needlessly high price are why it's not recommended. The amount of alcohol is cause for concern (see the Appendix for details) and the lack of state-of-the-art ingredients is disappointing, as are the irritants arnica and Italian cypress. Really, the only top secret is how YSL convinces women to spend exorbitant amounts of money on their average to poor skin-care products.

☹ POOR **Top Secrets Wake-Up Eye Care Flash Touch** *($44 for 1 tube)* is housed in a slim tube outfitted with a metal roller-ball applicator. Regrettably, this thin-textured gel/serum for the eye area doesn't contain anything unique for skin around the eyes, and is completely ineffective for reducing puffiness or dark circles. The amount of alcohol (it's the third ingredient) is cause for concern because alcohol is irritating and pro-aging. This also contains enough film-forming agent (think hairspray) to leave skin feeling a bit tacky. But by far the biggest concern and reason for this product's poor rating is the inclusion of fragrant plant extracts known to cause irritation (Source: naturaldatabase.com). Mica is present for shine and titanium dioxide helps brighten the eye area, but you can get these benefits from numerous other products that don't come with this one's high price tag and problematic formula.

YVES SAINT LAURENT FOUNDATIONS & PRIMERS

☺ GOOD **$$$ Matt Touch** *($42)* has a luxuriously silky, weightless texture that works to slightly fill in pores and make skin feel supremely smooth. Of course, this also facilitates foundation application, just as most serums and moisturizers with this kind of texture do. Its oil-control abilities aren't as good as those of similar options from Paula's Choice and Smashbox, but if you happen to come across it and want to try a sample under your makeup, go for it.

☺ GOOD **$$$ Perfect Touch Radiant Brush Foundation** *($55)* comes in a unique component that features a built-in synthetic foundation brush. Carefully squeezing the tube pushes a silky liquid foundation onto the brush, allowing you to paint it on. The foundation begins slightly thick but blends very well, providing sheer to light coverage and a luminous finish suitable for normal to dry skin. YSL offers 15 shades, and just over half are remarkably neutral. The following shades are too peach, orange, or copper for most skin tones: #6, #8, #10, #12, #13, and #14. The brush applicator is workable if you prefer this method of applying foundation, though it blends just as well using your fingertips or a makeup sponge.

☺ AVERAGE **$$$ Matt Touch Foundation SPF 10** *($52)* had great potential to be an outstanding oil-absorbing foundation with a long-lasting matte finish for very oily skin. The main problem is the lack of sufficient UVA protection and an SPF rating too low for adequate daytime protection (at least if you're concerned with following sunscreen guidelines from almost every major dermatologic association). The silicone-based texture dispenses from its tube nearly as thick as toothpaste; however, the texture quickly softens as it warms on your skin, and leaves it feeling incredibly silky with a powdery finish. It feels nearly weightless, but the finish will grossly exaggerate even a slight hint of dry skin or flaking. There are 12 shades, which is more than most of YSL's other foundations offer. All blend out softer and more neutral than they first appear, but there are definitely some colors to avoid, including #3, #10, and #11. Shade #6 is slightly peach, but may work for some medium skin tones. We wish all the elements were in place to make this a slam-dunk recommendation for very oily, acne-prone skin. As is, this unique foundation has enough drawbacks for it to not deserve better than its neutral rating.

☺ AVERAGE **$$$ Teint Majeur Luxurious Foundation SPF 18** *($99)* has an enviable, beautifully silky texture and a gorgeous skin-like finish while providing medium coverage. What a shame that the price is so out of line and that the sunscreen lacks the UVA-protecting ingredients of avobenzone, titanium dioxide, zinc oxide, Mexoryl SX, or Tinosorb. Without this key element, there is no way this otherwise terrific foundation (even the shade range is impressively neutral) can work "anti-aging miracles" for anyone's skin. See the Appendix to learn which UVA-protecting ingredients to look for in any SPF-rated product.

The Reviews Y

☺ AVERAGE $$$ **Teint Radiance Radiance-Enhancing Flawless Foundation SPF 20** *($48)* promises flawless radiance, and in most respects it delivers, albeit with some caveats. The SPF 20 is impressive and it includes titanium dioxide for reliable UVA protection. Unfortunately, the amount of titanium dioxide is less than what we'd like to see and likely low enough that you'll want to pair this foundation with an SPF-rated moisturizer that provides better UVA protection. Texture-wise, this is fluid and silky, but it takes its time to set to a soft, glow-y finish as you blend. Although the finish enlivens your skin, this foundation tends to slip into lines and magnify every pore and crease on your skin. You absolutely must use this with a serum or, yes, even a foundation primer, to look your best. There are eight shades, most of which are best for light to medium skin tones. The only one to avoid is the very rosy Amber. The unfairly named Peach is just slightly indicative of that color and, given its name, Pink Beige is surprisingly neutral.

☺ AVERAGE $$$ **Teint Resist Long Wear Endless Comfort Transfer Resistant Foundation SPF 10** *($55)* is a liquid foundation with sunscreen that does indeed live up to its long-wear name. The silky texture sets to a matte finish and offers full coverage without being too thick. This product blends smoothly and evenly, and really stays put once it dries. Though this foundation has some great elements, there are a few downfalls: Insufficient sun protection is the big one, with an SPF 10 that is too low to provide daytime protection, although you could pair this with a pressed powder with SPF 15 or greater or a moisturizer underneath; but, for the money, it should at least meet the SPF 15 or greater standard set by medical boards all over the world. Another problem is the pump applicator that's hard to control—there's no easy way to get just a little to come out and you don't want to waste a drop at $55 an ounce. Plus, many of the shades have a peachy to orange undertone, which is not the best for almost any skin tone (avoid Peach, Gold Beige, Pink Beige, Amber, and Honey).

☹ POOR **Matt Touch Compact Long Lasting Matt Finish Foundation SPF 20** *($57)* is a powder foundation that is buttery soft to the touch (thanks to the talc), but is one of the least-flattering powder foundations we've encountered, especially at this price! Forget about applying this foundation wet because it doesn't transfer to skin at all from a moist sponge. Even the YSL salesperson could not get this to adhere to her skin when wet, after she specifically recommended doing so for more coverage. Standard dry application results in sheer coverage that feels great going on, but leaves skin with a dry, oddly felt-like finish that looks unnatural and unflattering. Building to achieve medium coverage just amplifies the furry, felt effect. Factor in the lack of broad-spectrum sunscreen protection, and this product is not recommended

YVES SAINT LAURENT CONCEALERS

☺ GOOD $$$ **Touche Éclat Radiant Touch** *($40)* is the original brush-on highlighter, cleverly packaged in a pen-style component with a built-in synthetic brush. Although not much for concealing (the coverage isn't too substantial), it functions well as a highlighter or to add a subtle radiance to shadowy areas, particularly under the eyes. It is light enough to layer over a regular concealer (which you'll need if dark circles are apparent), and the best of the six shades are #1 and #2. Shade #3 is slightly peach but likely too sheer to matter, while #4 has an orange cast that limits its appeal. Shades #5 and #6 are OK options for tan skin tones, but definitely test these at the YSL counter before buying.

☹ POOR **Anti-Cernes Multi-Action Concealer** *($35)* is an expensive greasy, heavy-looking concealer that creases in no time. If for some reason you prefer this type of product, there are significantly less expensive versions available at the drugstore.

YVES SAINT LAURENT POWDER

☺ AVERAGE **$$$ Poudre Sur Mesure Semi-Loose Powder** *($60)* comes in a cake form, but the container shaves off the top layer when you twist it, creating a loose powder. It's less messy than conventional loose powder, but this clever convenience doesn't come cheap. The talc- and aluminum starch-based formula goes on sheer and has a dry finish suitable for normal to very oily skin. Each of the five colors has a bit of shine, so this is not for those who want to use powder to keep shine at bay.

YVES SAINT LAURENT BLUSHES & BRONZER

☺ GOOD **$$$ Blush Radiance** *($45)* is a powder blush that comes with a matte and shimmer shade that you blend together to create soft glow. Most of the shades go on sheer, though some have a bit more intensity. The silky texture blends on smoothly and though the shade selection is small, there are some attractive options to consider. Is it worth the hefty price tag? We'll let you decide, but here's a hint: You can find luminous blushes from the drugstore that are just as good or better but for far less money!

☺ GOOD **$$$ Blush Variation** *($45)* contains four tone-on-tone shades. Because they don't have dividers between them, it's best to simply swirl your blush brush over the entire tablet, like you would for a single shade of powder blush. The tone-on-tone effect simply ends up as one uniform shade on your cheeks anyway! This has a smooth, powdered sugar-fine texture that applies softly and leaves cheeks looking fresh and healthy. Because the formula contains emollient ingredients (including lanolin oil), it is best for normal to dry skin not prone to breakouts.

☺ GOOD **$$$ Creme de Blush Soft Blush** *($38)* is an overpriced, fragranced blush that has a sponge-like, cream-to-powder texture that must be blended quickly for best results. Inefficient blending can lead to a blotchy look, but with a deft hand, this provides a soft, flushed effect with a lasting, non-sparkling finish. The colors are on the vivid side, but they blend on much softer than they look in the package. Although this blush has its strong points, you can find similar, but much less expensive, options from Maybelline and Revlon. Cream-to-powder blush is best for normal to slightly oily skin.

☺ AVERAGE **$$$ Terre Saharienne Bronzing Powder SPF 12** *($50)* blends smoothly and imparts a subtle shimmer finish with slight hints of sparkle. Watch out for the Copper Sand shade, which has strong reddish orange undertones, but otherwise you can expect a beautiful, bronze glow. This bronzer is streak-free and has the potential to last throughout the day. YSL had good intentions by including SPF 12, but SPF 15 would have been far better. However, because it lacks the UVA-protecting ingredients of titanium dioxide, zinc oxide, avobenzone, ecamsule, or Tinosorb, this bronzer is not recommended for sun protection. The SPF rating and lack of reliable UVA protection is what ultimately earned this bronzer its rating.

YVES SAINT LAURENT EYESHADOWS

☺ GOOD **$$$ Fard Lumiere Aquaresistant Water Resistant Cream Eyeshadow** *($30)*. This cream-to-powder eyeshadow lives up to its promise of water resistance (only the Pink Sands shade broke ever-so-slightly when wet). The shades are all luminous with varying degrees of sparkles, but will set surprisingly crease-free if you allow ample drying time. The intensity of the pigment is both a blessing and a curse because the product sets so quickly, you need to work fast to apply it evenly. A little goes a long way, so rather than using your fingers, apply it with a synthetic brush, which will afford better control (and better hygiene around the eyes).

☺ GOOD **$$$ Ombres Duolumieres Eye Shadow Duo** *($41)* is worth considering (price notwithstanding) if you want lots of shine and strong colors. The pairings are much more workable than they used to be, with predominantly brown and gray tones ideal for shadowing and shaping. Avoid duos 13 and 29, whose color combinations are more for shock than allure.

☹ AVERAGE **$$$ Ombres 5 Lumieres 5 Colour Harmony for Eyes** *($58)*. Although YSL offers some truly workable color combinations, the texture of these powder eyeshadows is drier than many others, which makes them trickier to work with. As it happens, these apply and build intensity well enough, but, for the money, this isn't the eyeshadow collection to splurge on. If you simply must have YSL shadows or you happen to prefer a drier texture that isn't as smooth as many others, the best sets are Sahara, Tawny, and Bronze Gold.

☹ AVERAGE **$$$ Ombre Solo Mono Eyeshadow** *($30)* is a pressed-powder eyeshadow with a silky but dry texture that hinders application a bit and leads to some flaking. The shade selection favors strong shine, with #6 being the only matte option. If the flaking weren't an issue the shine would be tolerable, but at this price an eyeshadow should be nearly perfect in every way.

☺ AVERAGE **$$$ Pure Chromatics Wet and Dry Eye Shadow** *($48)* is a very shiny eyeshadow quad that "pushes the limits of color" with a new generation of pigments that allow for two distinctive effects: Dry application leaves a sheer satin finish and wet application leaves a bold metallic finish. Although the effect is noticeable, it's not unique—you can use most powder eyeshadows wet or dry—and the way the color looks depends on which method you choose. In the end, it's not such a big deal. Aside from the marketing claims, these powder shadows end up being more trouble than they're worth. Applied dry, they're almost too sheer and can look uneven. Wet application is better, at least if you want a strong metallic finish, but some flaking is inevitable. The quads are a mishmash of colors with little rhyme or reason to them, so they are hard to coordinate. Surveying the options, you may feel as we did: Two shades from one set would work better with two shades from another set—and at this price every shade should be one you'll use as part of your eyeshadow design.

☹ POOR **Ombres Quadralumieres Eye Shadow Quartet** *($54)* is no match for the powder eyeshadows from haute couture fashion competitor Dior, and the prices of the two lines are nearly identical. These YSL quads suffer from a dry texture that makes blending difficult (though they do have some smoothness) and especially from terribly contrasting colors that are for fantasy or high fashion, not real-world, makeup.

YVES SAINT LAURENT EYE & BROW LINERS

✓☺ BEST **$$$ Easy Liner for Eyes Automatic Eyeliner** *($32)* can proudly keep up with the best of them. The calligraphy-style brush makes application a breeze and allows for precision and detail whether you prefer a classic thin line or want to build up to a more dramatic look. The liquid texture dries in seconds and is transfer-resistant while the matte finish offers a decent amount of color, although you may need to apply a couple of layers to achieve an intense color.

✓☺ BEST **$$$ Eyeliner Effet Faux Cils Long-Wear Cream Eyeliner** *($25)* goes on super-smooth and delivers bold color along the lash line. The texture allows ample time to blend (which is great for a smoky look) before setting to a smudge-proof, water-resistant finish. It stays put so well that you'll need a good makeup remover—cleanser alone won't get all of it off. Our only (minor) complaint is that YSL didn't create more matte options; All but one shade has a metallic finish which can be overpowering and accentuate wrinkly skin. If that doesn't concern you, this is an excellent, long-wearing cream eyeliner!

☺ GOOD **$$$ Eyeliner Moire Liquid Eyeliner** *($34)* is a liquid liner with a thin, tapered brush that applies evenly, allowing you to lay down a solid line with one swift stroke. All the colors (except black) are metallic and the formula takes longer than it should to dry, but if you can endure that, it stays on marvelously well.

☻ AVERAGE **$$$ Eyebrow Pencil** *($28)* costs a mint and needs routine sharpening, but it's a good, non-greasy eyebrow pencil that won't smudge. It finishes and remains slightly tacky, but that's less of an issue if you apply this softly. Among the standard shades, #4 is puzzlingly shiny.

☺ AVERAGE **$$$ Eyeliner Effet Faux Cils Bold Felt-Tip Eyeliner Pen** *($32)* glides on smoothly to deliver bold, black color. The felt-tip pen is flexible so you can closely follow to the lash line, and it allows you to easily control whether you want a thick or thin line. The sole disappointment (beyond the too-high price) is that some of the eyeliner tends to wear off by day's end leaving an uneven finish, which is even more noticeable if you are sporting a dramatic cat-eye look.

☹ POOR **Waterproof Eye Pencil** *($28)* is only slightly waterproof, and that's just one of several problems. The tip is so soft it breaks easily during application; the width of the pencil tip allows only for a thick line, which reduces this pencil's versatility; and it's so creamy it smears readily before it sets. Two words: Don't bother.

YVES SAINT LAURENT LIP COLOR & LIPLINERS

✓☺ BEST **$$$ Gloss Pur Pure Lip Gloss** *($30)* has a decadent, slightly syrupy texture that glides over lips and provides a luscious glossy finish. The colors look quite dark and imposing in the container, but each goes on sheer and may work alone or over lipstick. The ingredient statement lists butyl methoxydibenzoylmethane (aka avobenzone), but it's not listed as active and so you cannot rely on it for UVA protection. Although pricey, this is an undeniably enticing lip gloss with a smooth, non-sticky finish.

✓☺ BEST **$$$ Rouge Pur Couture Glossy Stain** *($32)* is definitely a product that lipstick aficionados should check out! The first ingredient in this enhanced lipstain is octyldodecanol—which creates the emollient texture. It's a unique ingredient to see front and center in a lip stain, though it's not a must-have or amazing ingredient, just an emollient texture enhancer. We'll admit we were skeptical at first, but YSL got everything right! With one easy swipe-and-go application you're getting the intense color effect of using a lipliner, a lipstick, and a gloss—in a fraction of the time. If you've had trouble "coloring inside the lines" with other products, or if you're wary of lip color that tends to bleed, there is nothing to worry about with this one. The slanted applicator tip is just the right size to allow for precise, even distribution. Best of all, the shades are wonderful. Each of them will stay colorful and glossy (though, increasingly less so) for the claimed five-hour wear time!

✓☺ BEST **$$$ Touche Brilliance Sparkling Touch for Lips** *($30)* is a fantastic lip gloss that is packaged just like YSL's Touche Eclat Radiant Touch highlighter, meaning the gloss is dispensed onto a synthetic brush applicator. The texture is superb and the finish is a gleaming shine that's not the least bit sticky. As for the colors, they're an enticing mix of sheer, bright, and bold metallic.

☺ GOOD **$$$ Rouge Volupte Perle Silky Sensual Radiant Lipstick SPF 15** *($34)* is pricey, but this sheer, lightweight yet emollient lipstick provides soft color and sun protection. UVA protection is provided by avobenzone, and the shade range, although small, has a fun mix of nude and bright hues. What keeps this lipstick with sunscreen from earning our top rating is its slick texture and somewhat greasy finish. Longevity isn't this lipstick's strength, and it absolutely isn't for anyone with lines around the mouth. Otherwise, if the price and need to reapply often don't bother you, this is worth a peek.

☺ AVERAGE $$$ **Dessin des Levres Lip Liner** *($28)* is a very good standard pencil that feels slightly creamy going on, but ends up having a drier than usual finish, which helps keep it in place. The color range has been toned down and now favors browns, mauves, and reds—so there are clearly some missing links between this and Saint Laurent's lipstick palette.

☺ AVERAGE $$$ **Fard a Levres Rouge Pur Pure Lipstick** *($32)* is a very ordinary, yet extraordinarily overpriced lipstick that comes in a range of shades and finishes, all of which have an unpleasant greasiness. The packaging is gorgeous, but that doesn't make up for the lackluster product inside. The promising semi-matte Satin shades have deep, gorgeous color, but they drag across the lips, deposit color unevenly, and are far too drying. Conversely, the Cream shades are a slippery mess to apply and will smear before you can say, "Lipstick teeth." Only the Metallic shades seem to stay put, but they are all packed with highly-reflective glitter that won't flatter lips that have any degree of visible lines.

☺ AVERAGE $$$ **Gloss Volupte Sheer Sensual Gloss Stick SPF 9** *($30)* is an intriguing lip gloss/sheer lipstick hybrid. The twist-up applicator affords smooth application, yet it has the texture and moisture of a lip gloss. The finish leaves more of a balm-like sheen than true glossiness (there's no stickiness or high-mirror shine), and even though the four fruit-inspired shades may seem bright, the colors go on sheer. Unfortunately, the sunscreen protection is solely from octinoxate, which means you're not getting sufficient UVA protection (see the Appendix for details). That fact, coupled with the addition of strong fragrance, prevents this product from receiving a higher rating.

☺ AVERAGE $$$ **Rouge Pur Couture Pure Color Lipstick SPF 15** *($30)* is behind the times, mostly due to its creamy-bordering-on-greasy texture. The sunscreen does not include the ingredients needed to shield your lips from the sun's entire range of damaging UVA rays, which is essential for anti-aging benefits (see the Appendix for details). The shades are beautiful, flatter a wide range of skin tones, and go on semi-opaque. The slick finish means you'll be reapplying often and probably noticing that this creeps into any lines around your mouth. This lipstick also contains a lingering fragrance.

☺ AVERAGE $$$ **Rouge Pur Shine Sheer Lipstick SPF 15** *($32)* does not contain the UVA-protecting ingredients of titanium dioxide, zinc oxide, avobenzone, Mexoryl SX, or Tinosorb, so it is not recommended as a reliable lipstick with sunscreen. It is otherwise a slick, shimmer-infused lipstick that feels very light and features some gorgeous soft colors. Its Average rating is for not providing sufficient UVA protection.

☺ AVERAGE $$$ **Rouge Volupte Lipstick** *($34)* is a very expensive lipstick that has beautiful packaging and some rich colors that leave a lasting stain on lips. Unfortunately, it is one of the greasiest lipsticks around. This will travel into lines around the mouth before you can say "I like this color!" and it has a slick, glossy finish that's more prone to movement than any lipstick we've seen in recent memory.

YVES SAINT LAURENT MASCARAS

✓☺ BEST $$$ **Volume Effet Faux Cils Luxurious Mascara for a False Lash Effect** *($30)* doesn't quite measure up to the effect obtainable from false eyelashes, but it ranks as YSL's best mascara. That's because it builds beautifully and thickens well without clumps. The result is lashes that are dramatic without being over-the-top, and all with a soft, fringed curl. This mascara also comes off completely with a water-soluble cleanser. Note: YSL also sells a Noir

Radical shade of this mascara that they list separately on their website. All the comments above apply, except the Noir Radical shade is a rich, inky black for added drama.

☺ GOOD $$$ **Mascara Volume Effet Faux Cils Luxurious Mascara Waterproof for a False Lash Effect** *($30)* is not akin to using false eyelashes! It's just a very good, truly waterproof mascara. Its primary strength beyond holding its own when lashes get wet is how beautifully it lengthens. Thickness is slight, so this is really for creating long, separated, flutter-worthy lashes. The brush eliminates clumps and delivers a very smooth, clean application, which is great. The only drawback is the price; without question you do not need to spend anywhere near this much for a great waterproof mascara.

☺ AVERAGE $$$ **Mascara Aquaresistant Mascara Waterproof** *($30)* is expertly waterproof, even if lashes get completely soaked. Yet that's about the only exciting aspect of this otherwise ordinary mascara. Lashes get somewhat longer and there are no clumps, but for the money there are much more impressive waterproof mascaras at the drugstore.

☹ POOR **Mascara Singulier Nuit Blanche Waterproof Multi-Intensities Exaggerated Lashes** *($30)* has a long, meandering, and exaggerated name that was perhaps meant to distract you from the fact that its performance is disappointing. Not only is this only slightly waterproof (a fine mist is OK but a splash of water causes this to break down and run), but at best (and after much effort) you only get meager length, no thickness, and lashes that look minimally enhanced. You'll be left wondering why you bothered, and your lash line may be smarting due to this mascara's unusually scratchy brush (it's truly painful).

☹ POOR **Mascara Volume Effet Faux Cils Shocking** *($30)*. The only thing shocking about this mascara is the clumpy, spider-like lashes it produces. True to claim, lashes will look thicker but other mascaras can do that without the stuck-together mess. On the plus side, the formula doesn't flake or smudge, but that's not enough to earn our recommendation.

YVES SAINT LAURENT FACE & BODY ILLUMINATORS

✓☺ BEST $$$ **Teint Parfait Complexion Enhancer** *($42)* is sold as a sheer highlighter for all-over use on the face, and is ideal for this purpose. The easy-to-blend lotion texture imparts a sheer, slight shimmer finish that works under or over foundation. It sets to a matte (in feel) finish and is suitable for all skin types, particularly those with dull complexions. Shade #1 is a pale lilac that may be OK for very fair skin, but test it first; shade #6 has a peachy cast that should also be considered carefully. The five remaining shades are attractive and versatile, and the shimmer stays put.

YVES SAINT LAURENT BRUSHES

☺ GOOD $$$ **Yves Saint Laurent Brushes** *($30–$56)* consist of a small, workable collection, though in terms of overall quality and performance they lag behind most other lines (many that charge less for similar brushes), including M.A.C., Stila, and Laura Mercier.

☺ AVERAGE $$$ **Powder Brush** *($56)* is the weakest option because it's not dense enough to apply more than a sheer dusting of powder. The other brushes are all worth considering and are readily available for testing at the counter.

The Best Products

THE BIG FINALE!

All the products included on the lists that follow either met or exceeded the criteria established for their respective categories. As such, all these products deserve strong consideration, based on your skin type, concerns, personal preferences, and budget. (Speaking of budget, price was not a factor in determining whether a product was included in the lists below or not. How much to spend on any given product is up to you.)

If you turned directly to this chapter, figuring you'd just cut to the chase and make your shopping list, let us forewarn you that this approach can backfire. Although the streamlined lists below are indeed helpful, you should also read the full review of any product you're considering. In addition, there may be other options rated as GOOD that will work perfectly well for you, although they don't appear on the lists below. In response to frequent requests from our readers and from the media, we opted for shorter lists of only the products rated BEST. Neither group likes too many choices, which we understand completely. To make these shorter lists even easier to navigate, you'll find that the majority of categories are divided according to skin type, concerns, and, in the case of makeup, also according to texture.

Although this book is comprehensive, as it goes to press there are new products being created and launched, plus ongoing publication of new research unveiling the promise of ingredients that may have increased benefits or risks for skin. To keep you up to date on the latest products and corresponding ingredient research and to make it easy for you to find the best skin care and makeup products available, we urge you to visit CosmeticsCop.com. This site includes all the reviews in this book (plus thousands more), and is updated regularly with new reviews, revisions to existing reviews (e.g., when a product is discontinued), and hundreds of complete line reviews that, for reasons of space and timing, are not included in this book. In addition to CosmeticsCop.com, we offer our free Beauty Exclusives emails (sign up at CosmeticsCop.com) to keep you in the know. These two resources provide more extensive in-depth explanations and clarifications about specific topics than we could possibly provide in this book.

BEST CLEANSERS (INCLUDING CLEANSING CLOTHS)

Why do I need this product, and what results can I expect?

A gentle, water-soluble cleanser removes dirt, excess oil, and makeup. Your skin will look and act healthier, feel smoother, and be ready to receive maximum benefit from your other products.

In order to make the Best Products list, a facial cleanser must:

- Be gentle and water soluble (this is critical)
- Not contain needless irritants or drying cleansing agents
- Remove excess oil and makeup without stripping skin

- Rinse without leaving a noticeable residue
- Be fragrance-free or contain minimal fragrance

All the cleansers listed below were chosen for their exceptional formulation that's gentle yet effective for removing surface dirt, oil, perspiration, and makeup without making skin feel dry or tight. Those with normal to slightly dry, combination, or very oily skin should use a water-soluble gel or foaming cleanser; those with normal to very dry skin can use those, too, or if preferred, a cleansing lotion.

We never recommend bar soap because the ingredients that keep bar soap in its bar form can clog pores, and the cleansing agents they contain are almost always drying.

Emollient wipe-off cleansers may be the only types of cleansers that don't cause dry, sensitive skin to become drier, so we recommend them for that skin type, although in most cases such products were not rated BEST because they are inherently difficult to rinse (and you should never remove a cleanser with tissues—talk about outdated!).

We don't recommend most cleansers for blemish-prone skin because they often contain topical disinfectants such as benzoyl peroxide or the exfoliant (and mild antibacterial agent) salicylic acid. Although those are great anti-acne ingredients, in a cleanser, they're rinsed down the drain before they have a chance to affect your blemished skin for the better. Visit Cosmetics-Cop.com for our latest reviews and top picks of cleansers.

BEST CLEANSERS FOR *ALL SKIN TYPES EXCEPT VERY DRY:

Alpha Hydrox Foaming Face Wash ($7.49 for 6 fl. oz.)

Boots Expert Anti-Blemish Cleansing Foam ($5.29 for 5 fl. oz.)

Clean & Clear Foaming Facial Cleanser, Sensitive Skin ($5.29 for 8 fl. oz.)

DHC Make Off Sheet ($8 for 50 sheets)

Eucerin Redness Relief Soothing Cleanser ($8.79 for 6.8 fl. oz.)

Kiehl's Ultra Facial Cleanser, For All Skin Types ($18 for 5 fl. oz.)

M.A.C. Wipes ($15 for 30 sheets)

Merle Norman Delicate Balance Calming Cleanser ($19 for 4 fl. oz.)

Neutrogena One Step Gentle Cleanser ($6.49 for 5.2 fl. oz.)

Olay Foaming Face Wash, for Sensitive Skin ($7.99 for 7 fl. oz.) and Pro-X Restorative Cream Cleanser ($19.99 for 5 fl. oz.)

Paula's Choice CLEAR Pore Normalizing Cleanser ($10.95 for 6 fl. oz.), Earth Sourced Perfectly Natural Cleansing Gel ($16.95 for 6.7 fl. oz.), and RESIST Optimal Results Hydrating Cleanser ($16.95 for 6.4 fl. oz.)

Physicians Formula Gentle Cleansing Lotion, for Normal to Dry Skin ($7.25 for 8 fl. oz.) and Hydrating & Balancing Cleanser ($11.95 for 5 fl. oz.)

SkinCeuticals Purifying Cleanser ($32 for 8 fl. oz.)

Yes To Yes to Cucumbers Gentle Milk Cleanser ($8.99 for 6 fl. oz.)

*All the cleansers on the list above were either recommended for all skin types or are equally suited for normal to oily or normal to dry skin.

BEST CLEANSERS FOR NORMAL TO OILY/COMBINATION OR BLEMISH-PRONE SKIN:

Boots Beautifully Balanced Purifying Cleanser, for Oily/Combination Skin ($7.99 for 6.6 fl. oz.), Expert Anti-Blemish Cleansing Foam ($5.29 for 5 fl. oz.), and Expert Sensitive Gentle Cleansing Wash ($4.49 for 5 fl. oz.)

CeraVe Foaming Facial Cleanser ($11.99 for 12 fl. oz.)

Clean & Clear Daily Pore Cleanser, Oil-Free ($5.49 for 5.5 fl. oz.)

Laura Mercier Flawless Skin One-Step Cleanser ($35 for 6.8 fl. oz.)

Neutrogena Fresh Foaming Cleanser ($6.49 for 6.7 fl. oz.), Naturals Fresh Cleansing + Makeup Remover ($7.49 for 6 fl. oz.), Oil-Free Makeup Removing Cleanser for Acne Prone Skin ($5.99 for 5.2 fl. oz.), and One Step Gentle Cleanser ($6.49 for 5.2 fl. oz.)

Paula's Choice CLEAR Pore Normalizing Cleanser ($10.95 for 6 fl. oz.), Earth Sourced Perfectly Natural Cleansing Gel ($16.95 for 6.7 fl. oz.), Hydralight One Step Face Cleanser ($15.95 for 8 fl. oz.), and Skin Balancing Oil-Reducing Cleanser ($15.95 for 8 fl. oz.)

Peter Thomas Roth Gentle Foaming Cleanser ($32 for 6.7 fl. oz.)

SkinCeuticals Purifying Cleanser ($32 for 8 fl. oz.)

BEST CLEANSERS FOR NORMAL TO DRY OR VERY DRY SKIN:

Alpha Hydrox Foaming Face Wash ($7.49 for 6 fl. oz.)

CeraVe Hydrating Cleanser ($11.40 for 12 fl. oz.)

Clinique Comforting Cream Cleanser ($19.50 for 5 fl. oz.), Liquid Facial Soap Extra Mild ($16 for 6.7 fl. oz.), Redness Solutions Soothing Cleanser ($21.50 for 5 fl. oz.), Take The Day Off Cleansing Balm ($27.50 for 3.8 fl. oz.), and Take The Day Off Cleansing Milk ($26 for 6.7 fl. oz.)

DHC Cleansing Milk ($24 for 6.7 fl. oz.)

Estee Lauder Verite LightLotion Cleanser ($23.50 for 6.7 fl. oz.)

Jason Natural Red Elements Hydrating Lotion Cleanser, for Normal to Dry Skin ($12.49 for 7.25 fl. oz.)

L'Occitane Ultra Comforting Cleansing Milk ($22 for 6.7 fl. oz.)

La Roche-Posay Toleriane Dermo-Cleanser ($22.95 for 6.76 fl. oz.) and Toleriane Purifying Foaming Cream ($23.95 for 4.22 fl. oz.)

Laura Mercier Flawless Skin Oil-Free Foaming One-Step Cleaner ($35 for 6.8 fl. oz.)

Neutrogena Extra Gentle Cleanser ($6.49 for 6.7 fl. oz.) and Naturals Fresh Cleansing + Makeup Remover ($7.49 for 6 fl. oz.)

Nu Skin Creamy Cleansing Lotion, for Normal to Dry Skin ($16.60 for 5 fl. oz.)

Olay 2-in-1 Daily Facial Cloths, Sensitive ($5.99 for 33 cloths)

Paula's Choice Earth Sourced Perfectly Natural Cleansing Gel ($16.95 for 6.7 fl. oz.), Moisture Boost One Step Face Cleanser ($15.95 for 8 fl. oz.), RESIST Optimal Results Hydrating Cleanser ($16.95 for 6.4 fl. oz.), and Skin Recovery Softening Cream Cleanser ($15.95 for 8 fl. oz.)

SkinCeuticals Purifying Cleanser ($32 for 8 fl. oz.)

SkinMedica Sensitive Skin Cleanser ($34 for 6 fl. oz.)

The Body Shop Aloe Calming Facial Cleanser, for Sensitive Skin ($14 for 6.75 fl. oz.) and Aloe Gentle Facial Wash, for Sensitive Skin ($16 for 4.2 fl. oz.)

BEST TONERS

Why do I need this product, and what results can I expect?

A well-formulated toner will smooth, soften, and calm skin while removing the last traces of makeup. They also add vital skin-repairing ingredients after cleansing. Your skin will feel softer, look smoother, and redness will be reduced. Those with oily skin will see smaller pores.

A toner is only essential if it is beautifully formulated to improve your skin. All the toners on this list meet or exceed this expectation. A well-formulated toner is only added to the Best Products list if it:

- Does not contain needless irritants such as alcohol, witch hazel, peppermint, menthol, citrus, and fragrant plant extracts
- Fortifies your skin with proven antioxidants
- Drenches your skin with critical repairing ingredients
- Contains soothing anti-irritants
- Is fragrance-free

Almost without exception, the majority of toners are either boring concoctions of water and glycerin or contain irritating ingredients such as alcohol, witch hazel, and menthol. Those types of toners (they may also be labeled "fresheners," "tonics," "softening lotions," or "astringents") are NOT recommended.

Recognizing that a well-formulated toner can be an integral part of one's skin-care routine, the toners on this list supply skin with antioxidants, innovative water-binding and skin-repairing agents, and/or cell-communicating ingredients—all essential elements for creating and maintaining healthy, radiant skin and/or improving how skin looks and feels. If you've stayed away from toners due to thinking they were unnecessary, you'll be surprised at how much a well-formulated toner can improve skin concerns such as redness, flaking, and enlarged pores. Visit CosmeticsCop.com for the latest info on our top picks for toners.

Note: Some toners appear on both lists below. In those cases, the toner in question is suitable for all skin types.

BEST TONERS FOR NORMAL TO OILY/COMBINATION SKIN:

M.A.C. Lightful Softening Lotion ($30 for 6 fl. oz.)

MD Formulations Moisture Defense Antioxidant Spray ($28 for 8.3 fl. oz.)

Paula's Choice Earth Sourced Purely Natural Refreshing Toner ($16.95 for 5 fl. oz.), Hydralight Healthy Skin Refreshing Toner ($15.95 for 6.4 fl. oz.), RESIST Advanced Replenishing Toner ($18.95 for 4 fl. oz.), and Skin Balancing Pore-Reducing Toner ($15.95 for 6.4 fl. oz.)

BEST TONERS FOR NORMAL TO VERY DRY SKIN:

BeautiControl Skinlogics Platinum Plus Relaxing Tonic ($23 for 6.7 fl. oz.)

DHC CoQ10 Lotion ($35 for 5.4 fl. oz.)

M.A.C. Lightful Softening Lotion ($30 for 6 fl. oz.)

MD Formulations Moisture Defense Antioxidant Spray ($28 for 8.3 fl. oz.)

Merle Norman Daily Moisture Toner ($18 for 6 fl. oz.)

Paula's Choice Earth Sourced Purely Natural Refreshing Toner ($16.95 for 5 fl. oz.), Moisture Boost Essential Hydrating Toner ($15.95 for 6.4 fl. oz.), RESIST Advanced Replenishing Toner ($18.95 for 4 fl. oz.), and Skin Recovery Enriched Calming Toner ($15.95 for 6.4 fl. oz.)

BEST SCRUBS

Why do I need this product, and what results can I expect?

Scrubs aren't essential, but some people enjoy using them. With a well-formulated scrub, you can expect to see smoother, softer skin free from dry, flaky patches. But these same benefits plus many more can be obtained from an AHA or BHA exfoliant, which negates the need for a scrub.

As stated above, scrubs are not essential and definitely not preferred to exfoliating with a washcloth or a well-formulated alpha hydroxy acid (AHA) or beta hydroxy acid (BHA) exfoliant. For those who prefer scrubs, we offer the list below. In order to make the list, a scrub must:

- Contain a gentle yet effective scrub ingredient (typically rounded polyethylene beads)
- Rinse easily
- Be formulated without irritants such as mint, citrus, excess fragrance, or menthol
- Make skin feel smooth and look refined

Scrubs reviewed as best for normal to oily skin are typically gel-based and rinse completely, those reviewed as best for normal to dry skin provide an exfoliating benefit while also cushioning skin with emollients or other moisturizing ingredients. In addition, most of the scrubs below are either fragrance-free or contain minimal fragrance. Visit CosmeticsCop.com for the latest info on the best scrubs.

BEST SCRUBS FOR NORMAL TO OILY/COMBINATION SKIN:

Boots Expert Sensitive Gentle Smoothing Scrub ($5.49 for 3.3 fl. oz.)

Nivea Skin Refining Scrub, Normal to Combination Skin ($5.99 for 2.5 fl. oz.)

BEST SCRUBS FOR NORMAL TO DRY SKIN:

Boots Expert Sensitive Gentle Smoothing Scrub ($5.49 for 3.3 fl. oz.)

SkinMedica Skin Polisher ($40 for 2 fl. oz.)

BEST MAKEUP REMOVERS (EYES & FACE)

Why do I need this product, and what results can I expect?

You need a makeup remover to ensure every last trace of your makeup (particularly your eye makeup) is removed each night. Missing tiny bits of makeup can lead to a buildup that causes or worsens puffy, red, or irritated eyes. Regular use of a makeup remover prevents this and may even reduce puffy eyes brought on by traces of makeup.

Makeup removers can be very helpful (and sometimes absolutely necessary) for removing long-wearing or waterproof formulas. All the makeup removers on the list below:

- Are gentle and fragrance-free
- Do not contain irritating ingredients
- Work quickly and efficiently with minimal effort
- May be used before or after cleansing

If you routinely wear eye makeup, consider using a makeup remover around your eye area at least once weekly. Doing so can go a long way toward preventing eye irritation (including puffiness) from leaving tiny bits of makeup residue around your eyes each night (we're talking about the makeup you may have missed using your face cleanser). Over time, this buildup can become encrusted along the upper and lower lash line, leading to problems you may not think to blame on your eye makeup.

Keep in mind that a cotton swab soaked in makeup remover works great for taking off stubborn eyeliner or waterproof mascara at lash roots, and is easier to control than a cotton pad. Visit CosmeticsCop.com for our latest reviews and top picks of makeup removers.

BEST MAKEUP REMOVERS FOR ALL SKIN TYPES:

Bobbi Brown Instant Long-Wear Makeup Remover ($24 for 3.4 fl. oz.)

Boots Organic Face Nourishing Eye Makeup Remover ($6.99 for 2.5 fl. oz.)

Clinique Take The Day Off Makeup Remover for Lids, Lashes & Lips ($18 for 4.2 fl. oz.)

DHC Eye & Lip Makeup Remover ($12.50 for 4 fl. oz.)

L'Oreal Paris Clean Artiste Waterproof & Long Wearing Eye Makeup Remover ($6.99 for 4 fl. oz.)

Laura Mercier Flawless Skin Dual Action Eye Makeup Remover Oil-Free ($22 for 3.4 fl. oz.)

Mary Kay Oil-Free Eye Makeup Remover ($15 for 3.75 fl. oz.)

Neutrogena Eye Make-Up Remover, All Skin Types ($7.99 for 4 fl. oz.), Eye Makeup Remover Lotion-Hydrating ($6.99 for 3 fl. oz.), and Oil-Free Eye Makeup Remover ($6.99 for 5.5 fl. oz.)

Paula's Choice Gentle Touch Makeup Remover ($12.95 for 4.3 fl. oz.)

philosophy just release me dual-phase, extremely gentle, oil-free eye makeup remover ($18 for 6 fl. oz.)

Physicians Formula Eye Makeup Remover Lotion, for Normal to Dry Skin ($4.75 for 2 fl. oz.)

Sonia Kashuk Remove Eye Makeup Remover ($10.19 for 4 fl. oz.)

The Body Shop Camomile Waterproof Eye Make-Up Remover ($14.50 for 3.3 fl. oz.)

BEST ANTI-ACNE PRODUCTS WITH BENZOYL PEROXIDE

Why do I need this product, and what results can I expect?

An acne treatment with benzoyl peroxide kills acne-causing bacteria and helps reduce redness. With regular use, you'll see fewer breakouts and a reduction in large, red, swollen blemishes. Your acne may even be eliminated completely!

For someone who struggles with blemishes, a topical disinfectant medicated with benzoyl peroxide is a fundamental way to effectively treat this condition. One of the primary causes of blemishes is the presence of a bacterium, and killing this bacterium can be of great help to many of those suffering with varying degrees of acne. Benzoyl peroxide is considered the most effective topical disinfectant for the treatment of blemishes. Generally, benzoyl peroxide products come in concentrations of 2.5%, 5%, and 10%. As a general rule, it's best to start with a lower concentration to see if that works for you. If not, you can then try the next higher concentration. If you find that the higher concentrations don't work, then it may be time for you to consult a dermatologist or health care provider for a prescription topical disinfectant and/or for other topical acne treatments (e.g., Retin-A, Avita, Tazorac, or generic versions of these [active ingredient tretinoin, and, in the case of Tazorac, tazarotene]). You can read more about these options in the Expert Advice section of CosmeticsCop.com. Also see CosmeticsCop.com for the latest reviews of top-rated products with benzoyl peroxide.

BEST ANTI-ACNE PRODUCTS WITH BENZOYL PEROXIDE:

Clean & Clear Persa-Gel 10, Maximum Strength ($5.99 for 1 fl. oz.)

Clinique Acne Solutions Emergency Gel Lotion ($15 for 0.5 fl. oz.)

La Roche-Posay Effaclar Duo Dual Action Acne Treatment ($36.95 for 1.35 fl. oz.)

Kate Somerville Anti Bac Clearing Lotion ($39 for 1.7 fl. oz.)

Mary Kay Acne Treatment Gel ($7 for 1 fl. oz.)

Paula's Choice CLEAR Daily Skin Clearing Treatment, Regular Strength ($16.95 for 2.25 fl. oz.) and CLEAR Daily Skin Clearing Treatment, Extra Strength ($17.95 for 2.25 fl. oz.)

ProActiv Solution Advanced Blemish Treatment ($18 for 0.33 fl. oz.) and Repairing Treatment ($29 for 2 fl. oz.)

Serious Skin Care Clearz-It Acne Medication ($17.50 for 2 fl. oz.) and Clearz-It Nano Hydra+ On-the-Spot Treatment Acne Medication ($18.50 for 2 fl. oz.)

BEST AHA EXFOLIANTS

Why do I need this product, and what results can I expect?

AHA exfoliants gently remove built-up layers of dry, dead, sun-damaged skin to reveal fresher, brighter, more even, and smoother skin. You'll see a reduction in wrinkles, roughness, and uneven skin tone plus renewed radiance and firmer skin.

AHAs (alpha hydroxy acids) are brilliant ingredients for exfoliating normal to dry, sun-damaged skin. To earn a spot on the Best Products list, an AHA exfoliant must:

- Have the right pH range essential for efficacy
- Contain an amount of AHA(s) research has shown to be effective
- Be formulated without needless irritants such as alcohol or menthol
- Include antioxidants and other beneficial ingredients
- Not be packaged in a jar (see the Appendix for details)

An effective AHA product needs to have between 5% and 10% concentration of one or more of these ingredients: glycolic acid, lactic acid, malic acid, mandelic acid, or tartaric acid. Among those, glycolic acid is by far the most common.

A few brands sell exfoliants that use polyhydroxy acids (PHAs) such as lactobionic acid. Despite claims of superiority to AHAs, PHAs work in a similar manner and net the same results as AHAs. They're an option, but not inherently better than AHAs (or BHA/salicylic acid).

You may use an AHA product every day. Some may find that twice a day is best, while others once every other day, depending on your skin type and its response. You will find AHA products reviewed throughout this book with a happy face/GOOD rating, and these are options if your singular goal is exfoliation. However, the choices on the list below are preferred because they offer a range of beneficial ingredients such as antioxidants and repairing agents.

AHAs are not as effective for acne- or blackhead-prone skin. This is because AHAs cannot penetrate oil and, therefore, cannot get into the pore lining where clogs begin. Salicylic acid (BHA) should be considered if acne, oily skin, blackheads, or white bumps are your concern. It can penetrate oil and, therefore, can get into the pore where it can improve and repair pore function while dissolving blockages of dead skin cells and oil that contribute to blackheads and acne. Whichever exfoliant you choose, always monitor your skin's response, and remember: Irritation is never the goal. Visit CosmeticsCop.com for our latest reviews and top picks of AHA exfoliants.

BEST AHA EXFOLIANTS FOR NORMAL TO OILY/COMBINATION SKIN:

Clinique Turnaround Concentrate Radiance Renewer, All Skin Types ($42.50 for 1 fl. oz.)

MD Formulations Vit-A-Plus Night Recovery ($50 for 1 fl. oz.)

Olay Regenerist Night Resurfacing Elixir ($31.99 for 1.7 fl. oz.)

Paula's Choice RESIST Daily Smoothing Treatment 5% AHA ($25.95 for 1.7 fl. oz.), RESIST Weekly Resurfacing Treatment 10% AHA ($28.95 for 2 fl. oz.), and Skin Perfecting 8% AHA Gel ($19.95 for 3.3 fl. oz.)

BEST AHA EXFOLIANTS FOR NORMAL TO DRY SKIN:

Clinique Turnaround Concentrate Radiance Renewer, All Skin Types ($42.50 for 1 fl. oz.)

Derma E Evenly Radiant Overnight Peel ($16.95 for 2 fl. oz.)

DHC Renewing AHA Cream ($39 for 1.5 fl. oz.)

MD Formulations Moisture Defense Antioxidant Lotion ($50 for 1 fl. oz.) and Vit-A-Plus Illuminating Serum ($65 for 1 fl. oz.)

Olay Regenerist Night Resurfacing Elixir ($31.99 for 1.7 fl. oz.)

Paula's Choice RESIST Daily Smoothing Treatment 5% AHA ($25.95 for 1.7 fl. oz.), RESIST Weekly Resurfacing Treatment 10% AHA ($28.95 for 2 fl. oz.), Skin Perfecting 8% AHA Gel ($19.95 for 3.3 fl. oz.); and RESIST Remarkable Skin Lightening Lotion, 7% AHA ($18.95 for 2 fl. oz.)

Peter Thomas Roth Glycolic Acid 10% Moisturizer ($45 for 2.2 fl. oz.)

BEST BHA EXFOLIANTS (INCLUDING FOR ACNE)

Why do I need this product, and what results can I expect?

BHA exfoliants reduce redness, smooth skin's surface, and exfoliate inside the pore lining where clogs that lead to pimples, blackheads, and white bumps occur. With ongoing use, you'll see smoother, younger-looking skin free from clogged pores, enlarged pores, bumps, and breakouts. BHA also stimulates collagen production for smoother, younger-looking skin.

BHA (salicylic acid) is a superstar ingredient for exfoliating normal to oily, combination, and blemish-prone skin. In order to make the Best Products list, a BHA exfoliant must:

- Have the right pH range essential for efficacy
- Contain an amount of BHA research has shown to be effective
- Be formulated without irritants (such as sd alcohol, witch hazel, or menthol)
- Contain antioxidants and other beneficial ingredients
- Not be packaged in a jar (see the Appendix for details)

As a general rule for all forms of breakouts (including blackheads and white bumps), BHA is preferred over AHA because BHA is better at cutting through the oil inside the pore. Penetrating the pore is necessary to exfoliate the pore lining. However, some people (including those allergic to aspirin) can't use BHA, so an AHA exfoliant is the next option to consider. If that describes you, please refer to the list of Best AHA Exfoliants above.

An added benefit of salicylic acid for those struggling with acne is that it is naturally anti-inflammatory and also has a mild antibacterial action. Its anti-inflammatory action can be helpful for those struggling with the skin disorder rosacea. BHA is also best for those struggling with white bumps on the skin.

Like AHAs, BHA has anti-aging benefits. Ongoing use of a well-formulated BHA exfoliant helps smooth skin texture, improves uneven skin tone, and stimulates collagen production for firmer skin. Visit CosmeticsCop.com for our latest reviews and top picks of BHA exfoliants.

BEST BHA EXFOLIANTS FOR NORMAL TO OILY/COMBINATION SKIN:

Neutrogena Oil-Free Acne Stress Control 3-In-1 Hydrating Acne Treatment ($6.99 for 2 fl. oz.)

Paula's Choice CLEAR Anti-Redness Exfoliating Solution, Extra Strength ($19.95 for 4 fl. oz.); CLEAR Anti-Redness Exfoliating Solution, Regular Strength ($19.95 for 4 fl. oz.); RESIST Remarkable Skin Lightening Gel 2% BHA ($18.95 for 2 fl. oz.); Skin Perfecting 1% BHA Gel ($19.95 for 3.3 fl. oz.); Skin Perfecting 2% BHA Gel ($19.95 for 3.3 fl. oz.); and Skin Perfecting 2% BHA Liquid ($19.95 for 4 fl. oz.)

philosophy clear days ahead oil-free salicylic acid acne treatment & moisturizer ($39 for 2 fl. oz.)

BEST BHA EXFOLIANTS FOR NORMAL TO DRY SKIN:

Paula's Choice CLEAR Anti-Redness Exfoliating Solution, Extra Strength ($19.95 for 4 fl. oz.); CLEAR Anti-Redness Exfoliating Solution, Regular Strength ($19.95 for 4 fl. oz.); Skin Perfecting 1% BHA Lotion ($19.95 for 3.3 fl. oz.); and Skin Perfecting 2% BHA Lotion ($19.95 for 3.3 fl. oz.)

ProActiv Solution Clarifying Night Cream ($27 for 1 fl. oz.)

BEST MOISTURIZERS WITHOUT SUNSCREEN

Why do I need this product, and what results can I expect?

All skin types will benefit from a moisturizer that contains the types of ingredients research has shown help your skin look healthier and younger. When you use the right moisturizer for your skin type, you will see smoother, radiant skin that's hydrated. Dry, dull, flaky skin will be replaced by skin that looks and acts younger.

A moisturizer without sunscreen must be a state-of-the-art formula that meets the following criteria to earn a place on the Best Products list:

- Helps skin fight environmental damage
- Increases healthy collagen production
- Contains a mix of antioxidants, skin-repairing, and cell-communicating ingredients (which benefit all skin types)
- Helps skin produce younger, healthier cells

- Improves skin texture and hydration
- Contains the appropriate ingredients for your skin type
- Not be packaged in a jar (see the Appendix for details)

Moisturizers without sunscreen should only be applied at night unless your foundation contains sunscreen and is rated SPF 15 or higher (and you must apply it liberally and evenly over your entire face).

Generally, we recommend using moisturizers without sunscreen as part of your evening skin-care routine. All the moisturizers on this list include the state-of-the-art ingredients published research has proven are essential for creating and maintaining healthier, smoother, younger-looking skin.

Those with normal to dry skin should choose a moisturizer with a lotion or lightweight cream texture. If you have dry skin, look for moisturizers with a thicker, creamier texture. Those with oily skin should only use moisturizers in gel or toner (liquid) form. If your skin is prone to breakouts, including blackheads, it is best to use the moisturizer on dry areas only, and opt for the thinnest texture you can get away with. The goal is to make skin smoother and hydrate without clogging pores or creating a greasy finish. At night, moisturizer should be the last skin-care product you apply. Any of the moisturizers on the lists below may be applied around the eyes and on your neck, too. Visit CosmeticsCop.com for our latest reviews and top picks of moisturizers.

BEST LIGHTWEIGHT MOISTURIZERS FOR NORMAL TO SLIGHTLY DRY, OILY, OR COMBINATION SKIN:

Clinique Super Rescue Antioxidant Night Moisturizer, for Combination Oily to Oily Skin ($44.50 for 1.7 fl. oz.) and Super Rescue Antioxidant Night Moisturizer, for Dry Combination Skin ($44.50 for 1.7 fl. oz.)

Dermalogica Map-15 Regenerator ($85 for 0.3 fl. oz.)

Mary Kay TimeWise Night Restore & Recover Complex-Combination/Oily ($40 for 1.7 fl. oz.)

MD Formulations Moisture Defense Antioxidant Hydrating Gel ($45 for 1 fl. oz.)

Murad Time Release Retinol Concentrate for Deep Wrinkles ($65 for 0.5 fl. oz.)

Olay Pro-X Deep Wrinkle Treatment ($47 for 1 fl. oz.) and Regenerist Wrinkle Revolution Complex ($31.99 for 1.7 fl. oz.)

Paula's Choice Earth Sourced Antioxidant-Enriched Natural Moisturizer ($20.95 for 2 fl. oz.), Hydralight Moisture-Infusing Lotion ($19.95 for 2 fl. oz.), RESIST Anti-Aging Clear Skin Hydrator ($22.95 for 1.7 fl. oz.), RESIST Barrier Repair Moisturizer with Retinol ($22.95 for 1.7 fl. oz.), and Skin Balancing Invisible Finish Moisture Gel ($19.95 for 2 fl. oz.)

BEST MOISTURIZERS FOR NORMAL TO DRY SKIN:

CeraVe Facial Moisturizing Lotion PM ($13.99 for 3 fl. oz.)

Clinique Super Rescue Antioxidant Night Moisturizer, for Very Dry to Dry Skin ($44.50 for 1.7 fl. oz.)

BeautiControl Cell Block-C P.M. Cell Protection ($40 for 1 fl. oz.), Cell Block-C Intensive Brightening Elixir ($30 for 1 fl. oz.), and Skinlogics Platinum Plus Brightening Day Creme ($26 for 3.5 fl. oz.)

DDF-Doctor's Dermatologic Formula Pro-Retinol Energizing Moisturizer ($88 for 1.7 fl. oz.)

Dr. Denese New York HydroShield Ultra Moisturizing Face Serum ($65 for 1 fl. oz.)

Elizabeth Arden Ceramide Gold Ultra Restorative Capsules ($68 for 0.95 fl. oz.)

Estee Lauder Nutritious Vita-Mineral Moisture Lotion ($38 for 1.7 fl. oz.)

M.A.C. Strobe Cream ($15 for 1 fl. oz.)

Mary Kay TimeWise Night Restore & Recover Complex-Normal/Dry ($40 for 1.7 fl. oz.) and TimeWise Targeted-Action Line Reducer ($40 for 0.13 fl. oz.)

MD Formulations Moisture Defense Antioxidant Hydrating Gel ($45 for 1 fl. oz.)

Neutrogena Healthy Skin Anti-Wrinkle Cream, Night ($12.99 for 1.4 fl. oz.)

Olay Pro-X Deep Wrinkle Treatment ($47 for 1 fl. oz.) and Total Effects 7-in-1 Anti-Aging Moisturizer, Mature Skin Therapy ($22.99 for 1.7 fl. oz.)

Paula's Choice Earth Sourced Antioxidant-Enriched Natural Moisturizer ($20.95 for 2 fl. oz.), Moisture Boost Hydrating Treatment Cream ($19.95 for 2 fl. oz.), RESIST Barrier Repair Moisturizer with Retinol ($22.95 for 1.7 fl. oz.), and Skin Recovery Replenishing Moisturizer ($19.95 for 2 fl. oz.)

RoC Multi-Correxion Night Treatment ($27.99 for 1 fl. oz.)

SkinMedica Rejuvenative Moisturizer ($54 for 2 fl. oz.) and Age Defense Tri-Retinol Complex ES ($75 for 1 fl. oz.)

BEST MOISTURIZERS FOR DRY TO VERY DRY SKIN:

Boscia Restorative Night Moisture Cream ($48 for 1 fl. oz.)

Clinique Super Rescue Antioxidant Night Moisturizer for Very Dry to Dry Skin ($44.50 for 1.7 fl. oz.)

Elizabeth Arden Ceramide Gold Ultra Restorative Capsules ($68 for 0.95 fl. oz.)

Paula's Choice Earth Sourced Antioxidant-Enriched Natural Moisturizer ($20.95 for 2 fl. oz.), Moisture Boost Hydrating Treatment Cream ($19.95 for 2 fl. oz.), and Skin Recovery Replenishing Moisturizer ($19.95 for 2 fl. oz.)

philosophy miracle worker miraculous anti-aging neck cream ($45 for 2 fl. oz.)

BEST DAYTIME MOISTURIZERS WITH SUNSCREEN (SPF 15 OR GREATER)

Why do I need this product, and what results can I expect?

This essential morning step keeps your skin shielded from sun damage—the leading cause of wrinkles, rough texture, and dark spots. Protecting your skin from further sun damage allows it to generate younger, healthier skin cells. This is the critical step to having radiant skin with fewer wrinkles. You will see fewer signs of aging!

Sunscreens are essential for skin care day in and day out, 365 days a year, no matter where you live. If applied correctly (meaning liberally and reapplied as often as needed), **they are the best anti-wrinkle product you can use.** In order to make the Best Products list, a moisturizer with sunscreen must:

- Provide broad-spectrum sun protection and be rated SPF 15 or greater
- Help skin fight sun damage

- Increase healthy collagen production
- Contain a mix of antioxidants, skin-repairing ingredients, and cell-communicating ingredients (which all skin types need)
- Improve skin texture
- Contain the appropriate ingredients for your skin type
- Not be packaged in a jar (see the Appendix for details)

Most of the changes that take place on our skin over the years, such as wrinkles, brown spots, broken capillaries, loss of elasticity, texture problems, enlarged pores, and dryness, are the result of sun damage from exposure to the sun without appropriate or adequate sun protection. Sunscreens can help prevent much of this plus potentially help prevent some forms of skin cancer (and are an absolute must if you have already been treated for any type of skin cancer or have a family history of it).

If you are not using a sunscreen of some kind (lotion, cream, gel, serum, or foundation with sunscreen) with SPF 15 or greater and that contains one or more of the UVA-protecting ingredients avobenzone, zinc oxide, titanium dioxide, Mexoryl SX, or, outside the United States, Tinosorb, then you are doing nothing of lasting value for the long-term health of your skin. Really!

All the antiwrinkle, firming, anti-aging, skin tone– or dark spot–correcting or rejuvenating products in the world are completely and totally useless if you are not protecting your skin from the sun every day. It is of vital importance to the health of your skin to include a well-formulated sunscreen in your daily skin-care routine. Arguably, the most unethical thing the cosmetics industry does is sell women a plethora of anti-wrinkle products that more often than not do not include reliable sun protection.

If you have oily, blemish-prone, or sensitive skin, finding the ideal daytime moisturizer with sunscreen can be a challenge. In the last few years many cosmetics chemists have created lightweight and gentle sunscreens whose texture and typically smooth matte finish are just what someone struggling with oily skin, oily areas, or breakouts needs. Still, for the face, someone with oily skin may prefer to use a foundation with sunscreen rated SPF 15 or greater, and apply a well-formulated sunscreen from the neck down. Although it's more difficult for someone with oily skin, it still takes experimentation to figure out what product with sunscreen works best for you. Keep in mind that despite noncomedogenic or non-acnegenic claims made on labels, no sunscreen is guaranteed to be problem-free for someone struggling with acne.

All the moisturizers with sunscreen on this list are rated SPF 15 or greater and include avobenzone, zinc oxide, titanium dioxide, Mexoryl SX, or Tinosorb (the latter approved for use outside the United States) as one or more of the active ingredients (if these are listed someplace else on the ingredient list, it does not count toward reliable sun protection). Avobenzone may be listed on an ingredient label by its chemical name, butyl methoxydibenzoylmethane, and Mexoryl SX may be listed as ecamsule.

Every moisturizer with sunscreen on this list contains a range of antioxidants and also includes other skin-beneficial ingredients such as those that mimic healthy skin's structural components. These ingredients work to help skin look and act younger! Antioxidants, in particular, are proving to be an incredibly helpful addition to sunscreens because they not only boost the efficacy of the active ingredients, but also help offset free-radical damage from sun exposure.

Selecting an SPF-rated daytime moisturizer without antioxidants isn't giving your skin as much of a fighting chance against the cascade of damage that sun exposure can cause (and that can be dramatically minimized with diligent, liberal application and, when needed, reapplication of a sunscreen rated SPF 15 or greater). Visit CosmeticsCop.com for our latest reviews and top picks of daytime moisturizers with sunscreen.

Note: Daytime moisturizers with sunscreen that contain the mineral actives titanium dioxide and/or zinc oxide may leave a discernible white cast on skin. This is something to be aware of when testing or deciding to buy these products.

BEST DAYTIME MOISTURIZERS WITH SUNSCREEN FOR NORMAL TO SLIGHTLY DRY OR OILY/COMBINATION SKIN:

Avon Mark For Goodness Face Antioxidant Skin Moisturizing Lotion SPF 30 ($18 for 1.7 fl. oz.)

Dr. Denese New York SPF 30 Defense Day Cream ($49 for 2 fl. oz.)

Kate Somerville SPF 55 Serum Sunscreen ($45 for 2 fl. oz.)

M.A.C. Studio Moisture Fix SPF 15 ($30 for 1.7 fl. oz.)

Neutrogena Ageless Intensives Tone Correcting Moisture SPF 30 ($18.99 for 1 fl. oz.)

Olay Complete Ageless Skin Renewing UV Lotion SPF 20 ($22.99 for 2.5 fl. oz.), Regenerist DNA Superstructure UV Cream SPF 30 ($31.99 for 1.7 fl. oz.), and Regenerist UV Defense Regenerating Lotion SPF 50 ($31 for 1.7 fl. oz.)

Paula's Choice Moisture Boost Daily Restoring Complex, SPF 30 with Antioxidants ($20.95 for 2 fl. oz.) and Skin Balancing Daily Mattifying Lotion, SPF 15 with Antioxidants ($20.95 for 2 fl. oz.)

Peter Thomas Roth Clini-Matte All Day Oil-Control SPF 20 ($48 for 1.7 fl. oz.) and Sheer Liquid SPF 50 Anti-Aging Sunscreen ($52 for 1.7 fl. oz.)

philosophy miracle worker spf55 miraculous anti-aging fluid ($57 for 1.7 fl. oz.)

RoC Multi Correxion 4-Zone Daily Moisturizer SPF 30 ($27.99 for 1.7 fl. oz.)

BEST DAYTIME MOISTURIZERS WITH SUNSCREEN FOR NORMAL TO DRY OR VERY DRY SKIN:

BeautiControl BC Spa Facial Defend & Restore Moisture Creme SPF 20 ($32 for 2.6 fl. oz.), BC Spa Facial Defend & Restore Moisture Lotion SPF 20 ($32 for 2.6 fl. oz.), and Cell Block-C New Cell Protection SPF 20 ($30 for 1 fl. oz.)

Boscia Restorative Day Moisture Cream SPF 15 ($48 for 1 fl. oz.)

Clinique City Block Sheer Oil-Free Daily Face Protector SPF 25 ($19 for 1.4 fl. oz.), Sun SPF 30 Face Cream ($19 for 1.7 fl. oz.), and Sun SPF 50 Face Cream ($19 for 1.7 fl. oz.)

DDF-Doctor's Dermatologic Formula Protect and Correct UV Moisturizer SPF 15 ($64 for 1.7 fl. oz.)

Elizabeth Arden Extreme Conditioning Cream SPF 15 ($38.50 for 1.7 fl. oz.)

Estee Lauder Time Zone Line & Wrinkle Reducing Lotion SPF 15 ($58 for 1.7 fl. oz.)

Kiss My Face Face Factor Face + Neck SPF 30 ($12.95 for 2 fl. oz.)

MD Formulations Moisture Defense Antioxidant Moisturizer SPF 20 ($36 for 1.7 fl. oz.)

Olay Regenerist DNA Superstructure UV Cream SPF 30 ($31.99 for 1.7 fl. oz.)

Paula's Choice Moisture Boost Daily Restoring Complex, SPF 30 with Antioxidants ($20.95 for 2 fl. oz.); RESIST Cellular Defense Daily Moisturizer, SPF 25 with Antioxidants ($24.95 for 2 fl. oz.); and Skin Recovery Daily Moisturizing Lotion SPF 15 & Antioxidants ($20.95 for 2 fl. oz.)

Yes To Yes To Carrots Daily Facial Moisturizer with SPF 15 ($14.99 for 1.7 fl. oz.)

BEST "MINERAL" DAYTIME MOISTURIZERS WITH SUNSCREEN WHOSE ONLY ACTIVES ARE TITANIUM DIOXIDE AND/OR ZINC OXIDE, (BEST FOR NORMAL TO DRY OR SENSITIVE SKIN):

BeautiControl BC Spa Facial Defend & Restore Moisture Creme SPF 20 ($32 for 2.6 fl. oz.), BC Spa Facial Defend & Restore Moisture Lotion SPF 20 ($32 for 2.6 fl. oz.) and Cell Block-C New Cell Protection SPF 20 ($30 for 1 fl. oz.)

Clinique City Block Sheer Oil-Free Daily Face Protector SPF 25 ($19 for 1.4 fl. oz.) and Redness Solutions Daily Protective Base SPF 15 ($18.50 for 1.35 fl. oz.)

Obagi Nu-Derm Physical UV Block SPF 32 ($39.31 for 2 fl. oz.)

Paula's Choice RESIST Cellular Defense Daily Moisturizer, SPF 25 with Antioxidants ($24.95 for 2 fl. oz.) and Skin Recovery Daily Moisturizing Lotion SPF 15 & Antioxidants ($20.95 for 2 fl. oz.)

BEST EYE-AREA MOISTURIZERS

Why do I need this product, and what results can I expect?

You don't need an eye cream—really! See the Appendix to find out why. If you choose to use one anyway, results will be similar to what facial moisturizers provide.

Eye creams/eye-area moisturizers (including eye gels and serums) are products you can skip, but if you're intent on using one, make sure it:

- Contains an impressive mix of beneficial ingredients
- Includes antioxidants, skin-repairing ingredients, and cell-communicating ingredients
- Is able to help skin anywhere on the face look and act younger
- Is not packaged in a jar (see the Appendix for details)

The eye creams and other eye-area products below are recommended not because they're ideal for the eye area or work to reduce dark circles and puffiness. Rather, they made the list because each contains an outstanding assortment of beneficial ingredients for skin anywhere on the face. Essentially, these are moisturizer formulas designated as eye-area products, though **they contain nothing that is specific or better for skin around the eyes compared to the best facial moisturizers available.** You're definitely not getting as much for your money with these products versus moisturizers, but there's no denying that many consumers are convinced they need a separate product to treat skin around the eyes (check out the Appendix to learn why you don't need an eye cream). For those so inclined, the eye creams below are brilliant options. Please refer to each product's individual review for an assessment of claims and information on formulary specifics, such as whether or not it is fragrance-free (many on the lists below are) and, in some cases, comparisons with less expensive options. Visit CosmeticsCop.com for our latest reviews and top picks of eye creams and eye-area products.

BEST EYE-AREA MOISTURIZERS FOR NORMAL TO OILY/COMBINATION SKIN:

BeautiControl Regeneration Tight, Firm & Fill Eye Firming Serum ($44 for 0.46 fl. oz.) and Regeneration Overnight Retinol Recovery Eye Capsules ($38 for 30 capsules)

Dr. Denese New York FirmaTone Rx Eye Puff and Circle Minimizer ($36 for 0.2 fl. oz.)

Estee Lauder Verite Special EyeCare ($45 for 0.5 fl. oz.)

M.A.C. Prep + Prime Vibrancy Eye Primer ($30 for 0.5 fl. oz.)

Olay Pro-X Eye Restoration Complex ($47 for 0.5 fl. oz.), Regenerist Eye Lifting Serum ($24.99 for 0.5 fl. oz.), and Regenerist Touch of Concealer Eye Regenerating Cream ($24.99 for 0.5 fl. oz.)

BEST EYE-AREA MOISTURIZERS FOR NORMAL TO DRY SKIN:

BeautiControl Regeneration Tight, Firm & Fill Eye Firming Serum ($44 for 0.46 fl. oz.) and Regeneration Overnight Retinol Recovery Eye Capsules ($38 for 30 capsules)

DDF-Doctor's Dermatologic Formula Bio-Moisture Eye Serum ($88 for 0.5 fl. oz.)

Dr. Denese New York FirmaTone Rx Eye Puff and Circle Minimizer ($36 for 0.2 fl. oz.)

Estee Lauder Verite Special EyeCare ($45 for 0.5 fl. oz.)

Kate Somerville Line Release Under Eye Repair ($125 for 0.5 fl. oz.)

Olay Pro-X Eye Restoration Complex ($47 for 0.5 fl. oz.), Regenerist Eye Lifting Serum ($24.99 for 0.5 fl. oz.), and Regenerist Touch of Concealer Eye Regenerating Cream ($24.99 for 0.5 fl. oz.)

Nu Skin Tru Face IdealEyes Eye Refining Cream ($43.70 for 0.5 fl. oz.)

Perricone MD Cosmeceuticals Advanced Eye Area Therapy ($98 for 0.5 fl. oz.)

Shiseido Bio-Performance Super Eye Contour Cream ($55 for 0.53 fl. oz.)

BEST RETINOL PRODUCTS

Why do I need this product, and what results can I expect?

A well-formulated product with retinol treats skin to this proven anti-aging superstar as well as other critical ingredients skin needs to look and act younger. With ongoing use of a retinol product, you will see smoother, firmer, more even skin with smaller pores and reduced wrinkles.

Retinol is among the anti-aging superstar ingredients you should be looking for when shopping for skin care to help you look younger (though it is not the only anti-aging ingredient to consider). In order to make the Best Products list, a product with retinol must:

- Contain an efficacious amount of retinol
- Be packaged to ensure the retinol will remain potent and stable during use (clear or jar packaging is out; see the Appendix for details)
- Contain other anti-aging ingredients such as proven antioxidants and skin-repairing ingredients
- Contain minimal to no fragrance and no irritating ingredients

All the retinol products on this list are packaged to ensure that the retinol remains stable during use, which is absolutely essential for this light- and air-sensitive ingredient. Each also contains an amount of retinol that is within the range of what research has shown to be effective.

Whether you choose a moisturizer or serum with retinol comes down to preference and skin type. Generally, someone with dry skin is likely to prefer a moisturizer with retinol while someone with oily skin will prefer a serum with retinol, but experiment to see which texture works best with the other products in your skin-care routine. It is also fine to use a moisturizer and serum with retinol.

You can apply a retinol product once or twice daily (first-time users should apply once every other day, preferably in the evening). Generally, it is best to apply a retinol product at night. If you opt to use one during daylight hours, you must protect your skin with a well-formulated sunscreen rated SPF 15 or greater. **Skipping this step will negate any anti-aging benefits the retinol would otherwise provide.**

It is fine to combine any retinol product with an AHA or BHA product. However, because retinol can cause mild flaking and sensitivity for some people, pay attention to how your skin responds. If you notice undesirable side effects, decrease frequency of use or separate the application so you use the retinol product in the evening and the exfoliant as part of your daytime routine.

It is also OK to combine a retinol product with a prescription retinoid such as Renova, other forms of tretinoin, or other retinoids such as Differin (adapalene) or Tazorac (tazarotene). Keep in mind that doubling up may increase your risk of side effects such as redness, sensitivity, and flaking. Should this occur, stop using the over-the-counter retinol product and see how your skin responds just to the prescription retinoid.

Lastly, keep in mind that with retinol, more is not better. It doesn't take much retinol to prompt positive changes in your skin, but higher amounts (generally approaching 1% or greater) can tip the scales in favor of irritation, which is never the goal. Remember: More retinol is not better and may make matters worse! Visit CosmeticsCop.com for our latest reviews and top picks of products with retinol.

BEST MOISTURIZERS WITH RETINOL:

DDF-Doctor's Dermatologic Formula Pro-Retinol Energizing Moisturizer ($88 for 1.7 fl. oz.)

Murad Time Release Retinol Concentrate for Deep Wrinkles ($65 for 0.5 fl. oz.)

Neutrogena Healthy Skin Anti-Wrinkle Cream, Night ($12.99 for 1.4 fl. oz.)

Olay Pro-X Deep Wrinkle Treatment ($47 for 1 fl. oz.)

Paula's Choice RESIST Barrier Repair Moisturizer with Retinol ($22.95 for 1.7 fl. oz.)

RoC Multi-Correxion Night Treatment ($27.99 for 1 fl. oz.)

SkinMedica Age Defense Tri-Retinol Complex ES ($75 for 1 fl. oz.)

BEST SERUMS WITH RETINOL:

BeautiControl Regeneration Overnight Retinol Recovery Eye Capsules ($38 for 30 capsules) and Regeneration Overnight Retinol Recovery Serum ($46 for 1 fl. oz.)

Dr. Denese New York FirmaTone Rx RetinolMax Chin and Neck Firming Serum ($48.50 for 1 fl. oz.), FirmaTone Rx RetinolMax Firming Serum ($79.92 for 1 fl. oz.), HydroShield Eye Serum ($58.50 for 1 fl. oz.), and HydroShield Ultra Moisturizing Face Serum ($65 for 1 fl. oz.)

Kate Somerville Quench Hydrating Face Serum ($65 for 1 fl. oz.)

Nu Skin Clear Action Acne Medication Night Treatment ($35.50 for 1 fl. oz.)

Paula's Choice RESIST Intensive Wrinkle-Repair Retinol Serum ($29.95 for 1 fl. oz.), Skin Balancing Super Antioxidant Concentrate Serum with Retinol ($25.95 for 1 fl. oz.), and Skin Recovery Super Antioxidant Concentrate Serum with Retinol ($25.95 for 1 fl. oz.)

Peter Thomas Roth Retinol Fusion PM ($65 for 1 fl. oz.)

Serious Skin Care A-Force XR, Retinol Serum ($37.50 for 1 fl. oz.)

SkinCeuticals Retinol 0.5 Refining Night Cream with 0.5% Pure Retinol ($54 for 1 fl. oz.) and Retinol 1.0 Maximum Strength Refining Night Cream with 1.0% Pure Retinol ($59 for 1 fl. oz.)

BEST SERUMS

Why do I need this product, and what results can I expect?

Serums filled with antioxidants and other anti-aging ingredients protect your skin from environmental damage, collagen breakdown, and pollution. Immediately, your skin will feel smoother and look radiant. With twice-daily use, signs of damage will fade and your skin will look and behave healthier and younger.

Serums are an incredibly popular skin-care category and for good reason: A brilliantly formulated one can provide truly remarkable anti-aging results! In order to make the Best Products list, a serum must:

- Contain ingredients that fight environmental damage
- Be loaded with antioxidants proven to help skin become healthier
- Contain ingredients that stimulate healthy collagen production
- Treat skin to essential repairing and cell-communicating ingredients so it can look and act younger
- Contain minimal to no fragrance
- Not contain irritants such as fragrant oils or mint
- Be packaged to ensure the efficacy and stability of the ingredients

Formula-wise, the best serums not only make skin feel silky, but also contain a blend of sophisticated ingredients with substantiated research proving their benefit for skin of all ages. Such ingredients include those mentioned above, along with anti-irritants to soothe and calm skin.

Because many serums have a texture that is suitable for oily or breakout-prone skin, they can be a brilliant way for those with this skin type or concern to obtain the benefits of antioxidants and cell-communicating ingredients, including retinol (serums containing an impressive amount of retinol in stable packaging are listed above).

You will notice that the serums on this list are on the expensive side. We wish this weren't the case, but it is. There are two reasons for this: Most cosmetics companies position serums as specialty or targeted products, almost always with an anti-aging angle. Therefore, as the perceived (or the claimed) benefits increase, so does the price. The more real-world reason for the high prices is that it's expensive to create serums (most are nonaqueous, and water is the least expensive yet most pervasive skin-care ingredient around) that contain the level and range of state-of-the-art ingredients needed to improve skin.

The cost of several of the ingredients in these serums is, on a pound-for pound basis, staggering when compared to the cost of ubiquitous ingredients such as triglycerides, glycerin, or mineral oil. Although most of the best serums are costly, at least you know you're getting an intelligently formulated product whose ingredients have a proven track record of improving skin's health and appearance.

Whether you apply any serum before or after your moisturizer is a matter of personal preference. Generally, the serum can be applied before moisturizer, but experiment with order of application to see which works best for you. Those with oily or combination skin may find a serum is the only "moisturizer" they need. Also, most serums can and should be applied around the eyes, too—no need to purchase a separate serum for the eye area. Visit CosmeticsCop.com for our latest reviews and top picks of serums.

BEST SERUMS FOR ALL SKIN TYPES EXCEPT VERY OILY SKIN:

BeautiControl Regeneration Overnight Retinol Recovery Eye Capsules ($38 for 30 capsules); Regeneration Overnight Retinol Recovery Serum ($46 for 1 fl. oz.); Regeneration Platinum Plus Face Serum ($65 for 1 fl. oz.); and Regeneration Tight, Firm & Fill Eye Firming Serum ($44 for 0.46 fl. oz.)

Bobbi Brown Intensive Skin Supplement ($67 for 1 fl. oz.)

DDF-Doctor's Dermatologic Formula Mesojection Antioxidant Moisturizing Serum ($88 for 0.9 fl. oz.) and Wrinkle Resist Plus Pore Minimizer Moisturizing Serum ($85 for 1.7 fl. oz.)

Dr. Denese New York FirmaTone Rx RetinolMax Chin and Neck Firming Serum ($48.50 for 1 fl. oz.), FirmaTone Rx Eye Puff and Circle Minimizer ($36 for 0.2 fl. oz.), FirmaTone Rx RetinolMax Firming Serum ($79.92 for 1 fl. oz.), HydroShield Eye Serum ($58.50 for 1 fl. oz.), and HydroShield Ultra Moisturizing Face Serum ($65 for 1 fl. oz.)

Elizabeth Arden Ceramide Gold Ultra Restorative Capsules ($68 for 0.95 fl. oz.)

Estee Lauder Advanced Night Repair Concentrate Recovery Boosting Treatment ($85 for 1 fl. oz.), Nutritious Vita-Mineral Radiance Serum ($40 for 1 fl. oz.), Perfectionist [CP+R] Wrinkle Lifting/Firming Serum ($65 for 1 fl. oz.), and Re-Nutriv Intensive Lifting Serum ($185 for 1 fl. oz.)

Kate Somerville Quench Hydrating Face Serum ($65 for 1 fl. oz.)

Mary Kay TimeWise Even Complexion Essence ($35 for 1 fl. oz.)

Nu Skin 180º Night Complex ($62.50 for 1 fl. oz.) and Celltrex CoQ10 Complete ($45.90 for 0.5 fl. oz.)

Olay Regenerist Eye Lifting Serum ($24.99 for 0.5 fl. oz.), Regenerist Micro Sculpting Serum ($26.99 for 1.7 fl. oz.), Regenerist Regenerating Serum ($24.99 for 1.7 fl. oz.), and Regenerist Regenerating Serum Fragrance-Free ($24.99 for 1.7 fl. oz.)

Paula's Choice RESIST Super Antioxidant Concentrate Serum ($25.95 for 1 fl. oz.), RESIST Intensive Wrinkle-Repair Retinol Serum ($29.95 for 1 fl. oz.), and Skin Recovery Super Antioxidant Concentrate Serum with Retinol ($25.95 for 1 fl. oz.)

Peter Thomas Roth Retinol Fusion PM ($65 for 1 fl. oz.)

Serious Skin Care A-Force XR, Retinol Serum ($37.50 for 1 fl. oz.)

SK-II Cellumination Essence Hydrating Serum ($220 for 1 fl. oz.) and Signs Wrinkle Serum ($175 for 1 fl. oz.)

SkinCeuticals Retinol 0.5 Refining Night Cream with 0.5% Pure Retinol ($54 for 1 fl. oz.) and Retinol 1.0 Maximum Strength Refining Night Cream with 1.0% Pure Retinol ($59 for 1 fl. oz.)

BEST ULTRA-LIGHT OR MATTIFYING SERUMS FOR VERY OILY SKIN:

BeautiControl Regeneration Overnight Retinol Recovery Serum ($46 for 1 fl. oz.)

Bobbi Brown Intensive Skin Supplement ($67 for 1 fl. oz.)

Dr. Denese New York HydroShield Eye Serum ($58.50 for 1 fl. oz.)

M.A.C. Prep + Prime Skin Brightening Serum ($40 for 1 fl. oz.)

Nu Skin Celltrex CoQ10 Complete ($45.90 for 0.5 fl. oz.) and Clear Action Acne Medication Night Treatment ($35.50 for 1 fl. oz.)

Paula's Choice Skin Balancing Super Antioxidant Concentrate Serum with Retinol ($25.95 for 1 fl. oz.)

SkinCeuticals Retinol 0.5 Refining Night Cream with 0.5% Pure Retinol ($54 for 1 fl. oz.) and Retinol 1.0 Maximum Strength Refining Night Cream with 1.0% Pure Retinol ($59 for 1 fl. oz.)

BEST ALL-PURPOSE SUNSCREENS
(INCLUDING WATER-RESISTANT AND CHILDREN/BABY FORMULAS)

Why do I need this product, and what results can I expect?

Sunscreens rated SPF 15 or higher are fundamental for skin's health and appearance. Regardless of your age or where you live, daily use of a well-formulated sunscreen is a critical element of keeping your skin smooth, even, firm, and healthy. Of course, routine use of sunscreen along with sun-smart behavior will significantly reduce your risk of skin cancer and multiple signs of aging.

Sunscreens are essential for skin care day in and day out, 365 days a year. If applied correctly (meaning liberally and reapplied as often as needed), they are the best anti-wrinkle product you can use—and the best way to keep your skin acting normally and functioning in a healthy manner. In order to earn a spot on the Best Products list, a sunscreen, whether the label claims it's for adults or kids, must:

- Provide broad-spectrum sun protection and be rated SPF 15 or greater
- Protect skin from UVA damage with one or more of the right active ingredients
- Help fight sun damage while strengthening skin with antioxidants and repairing ingredients
- If labeled as such, contain ingredients that make it water-resistant
- Contain minimal to no fragrance

Note: Sunscreens marked with an asterisk (*) are water-resistant. Visit CosmeticsCop.com for our latest reviews and top picks of sunscreens.

Second note: Sunscreens that contain the mineral actives titanium dioxide and/or zinc oxide may leave a discernible white cast on skin. This is something to be aware of when testing or deciding to buy these products.

BEST SUNSCREENS FOR NORMAL TO SLIGHTLY DRY OR OILY/COMBINATION SKIN:

Clinique Sun SPF 15 Face/Body Cream ($21 for 5 fl. oz.)

Mary Kay SPF 30 Sunscreen* ($14 for 4 fl. oz.)

Neutrogena Ultra Sheer Dry-Touch Sunblock SPF 30 ($9.49 for 3 fl. oz.) and Ultra Sheer Dry-Touch Sunblock SPF 45 ($9.49 for 3 fl. oz.)

Paula's Choice Extra Care Non-Greasy Sunscreen SPF 45* ($14.95 for 5 fl. oz.) and Weightless Finish Sunscreen Spray SPF 30, Face & Body ($15.95 for 4 fl. oz.)

Peter Thomas Roth Uber-Dry Sunscreen SPF 30 ($26 for 4.2 fl. oz.) and Ultra-Lite Oil-Free Sunblock SPF 30 ($26 for 4.2 fl. oz.)

philosophy here comes the sun age-defense water-resistant SPF 30 UVA/UVB broad-spectrum sunscreen* ($26 for 4 fl. oz.) and here comes the sun age-defense water-resistant SPF 40 UVA/UVB broad-spectrum sunscreen for face* ($30 for 2 fl. oz.)

Physicians Formula Sun Shield For Faces Extra Sensitive Skin SPF 25 ($8.95 for 4 fl. oz.)

BEST SUNSCREENS FOR NORMAL TO DRY OR VERY DRY SKIN:

Alba Botanica Very Emollient Sunblock Mineral Protection, Fragrance Free SPF 30 ($10.99 for 4 fl. oz.) and Very Emollient Sunblock Mineral Protection, Kids SPF 30 ($10.99 for 4 fl. oz.)

Clinique Sun SPF 30 Body Cream ($21 for 5 fl. oz.)

Jason Natural Sunblock Mineral SPF 30 ($14.95 for 4 fl. oz.)

Kiss My Face Kids Natural Mineral Sunblock Lotion SPF 30 ($14.99 for 4 fl. oz.), Oat Protein Complex Sun Screen SPF 18 ($11.95 for 4 fl. oz.), and Sun Spray Lotion SPF 30 ($15.95 for 8 fl. oz.)

Neutrogena Sensitive Skin Sunblock SPF 30 ($8.99 for 4 fl. oz.)

Nu Skin Sunright Body Block SPF 15 ($16 for 3.4 fl. oz.) and Sunright Body Block SPF 30* ($14.40 for 3.4 fl. oz.)

Obagi Nu-Derm Physical UV Block SPF 32 ($39.31 for 2 fl. oz.)

SkinCeuticals Physical UV Defense SPF 30 ($38 for 3 fl. oz.), Sport UV Defense SPF 45* ($37 for 3 fl. oz.)

Yes To Yes To Carrots Hydrating Body Lotion with SPF 30 ($14.99 for 4.2 fl. oz.)

BEST MINERAL SUNSCREENS WHOSE ONLY ACTIVES ARE TITANIUM DIOXIDE AND/OR ZINC OXIDE, (BEST FOR NORMAL TO DRY OR SENSITIVE SKIN):

Alba Botanica Very Emollient Sunblock Mineral Protection, Fragrance Free SPF 30 ($10.99 for 4 fl. oz.)

Jason Natural Sunblock Mineral SPF 30 ($14.95 for 4 fl. oz.)

Neutrogena Sensitive Skin Sunblock SPF 30 ($8.99 for 4 fl. oz.)

SkinCeuticals Physical UV Defense SPF 30 ($38 for 3 fl. oz.)

BEST SELF-TANNERS

Why do I need this product, and what results can I expect?

Self-tanners aren't a necessary part of your skin-care routine, but they are the ONLY way to get a "tan" without damaging your skin or increasing signs of aging. A well-formulated self-tanner will leave you with a soft, natural-looking tan that fades gradually, just like a real (yet skin-damaging) tan would.

A self-tanner is the only way to get a tan without damaging your skin. There's truly no such thing as a safe tan from the sun. It's like thinking there's a safe cigarette when research has made it clear any amount of smoking damages the body. Although the majority of self-tanners have more similarities than differences, those that made the Best Products list stood out because:

- They contain a range of beneficial extras (such as antioxidants) for all skin types
- They contain minimal to no fragrance
- They omit skin irritants such as alcohol and fragrant plants
- They're easy to apply and produce a natural tan color

By and large, almost all self-tanners will work as indicated, because 99% of them contain the same "active" ingredient, dihydroxyacetone (DHA). DHA reacts with amino acids found in the top layers of skin to create a shade of brown; the effect takes place within two to six hours, and color depth can be built by reapplying. DHA has a long history of safe use, but It Is critical to keep in mind that the "tan" you get from DHA **does not provide any sun protection.** If you decide to use a self-tanner, be sure you continue to protect exposed skin every day with a well-formulated sunscreen rated SPF 15 or greater and that contains the UVA-protecting ingredients of avobenzone, zinc oxide, titanium dioxide, Mexoryl SX (ecamsule), or Tinosorb.

Although we have no doubt you will have success with any self-tanner rated with a happy face (for best results, be sure to follow the application instructions exactly), the handful of options below are the self-tanners that, for the most part, are also state-of-the-art moisturizers or gels that just happen to turn skin a beautiful shade of tan. Other brands with self-tanners worth considering include those rated with a happy face from Alba Botanica, Banana Boat, Coppertone, L'Oreal, Olay, and Neutrogena. Visit CosmeticsCop.com for our latest reviews and top picks of self-tanners.

BEST SELF-TANNERS FOR ALL SKIN TYPES:

Dr. Denese New York Glow Younger Clear Self-Tanner for Face and Body ($21 for 6 fl. oz.)

Paula's Choice Almost the Real Thing Self-Tanning Gel, Face & Body ($12.95 for 5 fl. oz.)

Too Faced Tanning Bed In A Tube ($28 for 6 fl. oz.)

BEST FACIAL MASKS

Why do I need this product, and what results can I expect?

Depending on your concerns and skin type, masks can be a helpful extra to add to your skin-care routine. They're not required for beautiful skin, but many enjoy using them and the process can be a relaxing respite from a hectic life. With an absorbent mask, you can expect to see less oil and smaller pores; with a moisturizing mask you can expect to see smooth, dewy-looking skin free from signs of dryness.

Facial masks aren't essential but they can be a pampering, relaxing interval for women. However, for good skin care, what you do daily is vastly more important than what you do once a week or once a month. For those who enjoy using facial masks, the ones that made the Best Products list contain:

- Ingredients that absorb excess oil without overdrying (for oily skin)
- Ingredients that provide hydration, suppleness, and repair (for dry skin)
- Ingredients that supply multiple benefits to make the investment (of your money and time) worth it

Many facial masks for normal to oily skin contain clay as their main ingredient, along with some thickening agents. Although that can be a benefit because it absorbs oil, the improvement is short-lived, not long term. Other masks contain clay as well, but also include water-binding agents and plant oils, and that can make them better for normal to combination or slightly dry skin.

Masks for normal to dry skin are often just moisturizers and nothing more, and don't necessarily warrant the extra time it takes to apply them. They aren't bad for skin; they just aren't a necessary step. If you opt to use such masks, try leaving them on overnight for maximum results.

There are also masks that contain a plasticizing agent that you subsequently pull or peel off your skin. These do impart a temporary soft feeling to the skin because what you're doing is pulling off a layer of skin, but that is hardly beneficial or lasting (and we do not rate this type of mask favorably because the peel-off ingredients are irritating). Visit CosmeticsCop.com for our latest reviews and top picks of facial masks.

BEST MASKS FOR NORMAL TO OILY/COMBINATION AND/OR BLEMISH-PRONE SKIN:

Clinique Acne Solutions Oil-Control Cleansing Mask ($20 for 3.4 fl. oz.)

Paula's Choice Skin Balancing Oil-Absorbing Mask ($15.95 for 4 fl. oz.)

BEST MASKS FOR NORMAL TO DRY OR VERY DRY SKIN:

Aveda Tourmaline Charged Radiance Masque ($31 for 4.2 fl. oz.)

BeautiControl Regeneration Tight, Firm & Fill Dermal Filling Moisture Masque ($40 for 5 fl. oz.)

Derma E Hyaluronic Hydrating Mask ($29.50 for 4 fl. oz.)

Estee Lauder Resilience Lift Extreme Ultra Firming Mask ($40 for 2.5 fl. oz.)

Paula's Choice Skin Recovery Hydrating Treatment Mask ($15.95 for 4 fl. oz.)

BEST SKIN-LIGHTENING PRODUCTS

Why do I need this product, and what results can I expect?

Used at least once daily and coupled with daily use of a sunscreen rated SPF 15 or greater, skin lighteners fade brown spots and discolorations. After 8–12 weeks of daily use, you will see discolorations fade or even disappear completely. Your skin tone will be more even and radiant. Ongoing use is needed to maintain results.

When sun- or hormone-induced brown skin discolorations appear, your best treatment option is a well-formulated skin-lightening product (along with diligent use of a sunscreen rated

SPF 15 or greater, and greater is better when discolorations are present). In order to make the Best Products list, a skin-lightening product must:

- Contain the active ingredient hydroquinone or other skin-lightening ingredients with research supporting their efficacy on discolorations
- Be packaged to protect the active Ingredients from light and air exposure, which cause them to break down and become ineffective
- Contain antioxidants, smoothing, and soothing ingredients to enhance skin health
- Contain minimal to no fragrance
- Not contain irritating ingredients such as alcohol

The skin-lightening products on this list either contain the time-proven, safe skin-lightening agent hydroquinone or they contain ingredients related to it, such as arbutin or other agents that research (however limited) has shown hold some promise for lightening sun- or hormone-induced brown spots. In some instances, skin lightening products with stabilized vitamin C are also worth considering.

Some of these skin-lightening products also contain an AHA or BHA at the correct pH for exfoliation to occur. The synergistic combination of hydroquinone and an AHA or BHA exfoliant not only allows the hydroquinone to work better, but also helps remove layers of uneven, sun-damaged skin (and those with BHA can help keep breakouts and blackheads at bay, so it's a double bonus).

Hydroquinone has become a controversial ingredient, despite considerable research demonstrating its safety when properly formulated (meaning following over-the-counter guidelines rather than adulterating products with compounds that can cause skin problems). For detailed information about this gold standard skin-lightening agent, please refer to our Cosmetic Ingredient Dictionary at CosmeticsCop.com.

Over-the-counter hydroquinone products are available in strengths of 1% to 2%; higher concentrations are available from dermatologists and cosmetic surgeons. There are few agreed-upon formulary standards for other skin-lightening agents such as various forms of vitamin C or niacinamide. Generally, you want to see these types of ingredients toward the beginning of a lightening product's ingredient list so they stand a good chance of working.

Keep in mind that **no skin-lightening product will work if you don't use an effective sunscreen daily.** Also, if you're using any over-the-counter product with hydroquinone and you haven't noticed any skin-lightening results after three months of daily use (plus daily use of a well-formulated sunscreen rated SPF 15 or greater), you should discontinue applying it. If this occurs, it is very likely that, for whatever reason, over-the-counter strengths of hydroquinone are not effective for you. You can try prescription-strength hydroquinone or consider various laser or light-emitting treatments from a dermatologist. In many instances, fighting brown spots requires a multi-step approach that often involves dermatologist-administered treatments for maximum results.

For best results, apply your skin-lightening product to affected areas twice daily, after cleansing and before applying moisturizer and/or serum and sunscreen (which should always go on last as part of your morning routine). Visit CosmeticsCop.com for our latest reviews and top picks of skin-lightening products.

BEST SKIN-LIGHTENING PRODUCTS THAT CONTAIN HYDROQUINONE:

Alpha Hydrox Spot Light Skin Lightener Fade Cream ($9.99 for 0.85 fl. oz.)

Kate Somerville Complexion Correction Spot Reducing Concentrate ($48 for 0.5 fl. oz.)

Paula's Choice RESIST Clearly Remarkable Skin Lightening Gel with 2% BHA ($19.95 for 2 fl. oz.) and RESIST Remarkable Skin Lightening Lotion with 7% AHA ($19.95 for 2 fl. oz.)

ProActiv Solution Dark Spot Corrector ($22 for 1 fl. oz.)

BEST SKIN-LIGHTENING PRODUCTS THAT *DON'T* CONTAIN HYDROQUI-NONE:

BeautiControl Cell Block-C Intensive Brightening Elixir ($30 for 1 fl. oz.)

Dermalogica Extreme C ($85 for 0.3 fl. oz.)

Mary Kay TimeWise Even Complexion Essence ($35 for 1 fl. oz.)

Olay Pro-X Discoloration Fighting Concentrate ($47 for 0.4 fl. oz.)

Paula's Choice RESIST Pure Radiance Skin Brightening Treatment ($26.95 for 1 fl. oz.)

philosophy miracle worker dark spot corrector ($62 for 1 fl. oz.)

BEST OIL-ABSORBING PRODUCTS (INCLUDING BLOTTING PAPERS)

Why do I need this product, and what results can I expect?

You only need this type of product if excess shine or very oily areas (such as your forehead, nose, and chin) are among your skin concerns. With an oil-absorbing product, expect to see a refined, matte complexion that isn't a constant source of frustration.

Oil-absorbing products aren't the most exciting category, but they can be an extremely helpful way to keep excess shine in check. Those that earned a spot on the Best Products list featured:

- Either an innovative absorbent ingredient or formula proven to mattify skin
- The ability to blot excess shine without removing a lot of makeup
- Non-powdery formulas (these tend to make skin look uneven)
- Minimal to no fragrance

In terms of oil-blotting papers, this category was a difficult one to pick the top options due to the basic and similar nature of these products. The ones that made the cut did so because they had a nifty convenience feature, were noticeably more absorbent than the competition, or proved to be a very cost-effective option. Keep in mind that the many oil-absorbing papers reviewed in this book are options as well, though those with added oil, powders, or clays tend to be more troublesome than oil-absorbing papers without these ingredients (they often leave an unattractive coating on skin).

Beyond oil-blotting papers, you'll find some innovative leave-on products that work to keep excess shine in check for hours. These may be used under or over makeup.

For best results, always touch up with a pressed powder after blotting. This provides a unified matte finish and makes skin look smooth and refined. Apply the powder with a brush (not a puff or sponge) to avoid a thick, cakey look. Several makeup brands sell retractable powder brushes that work great for touch-ups on the go. Visit CosmeticsCop.com for our latest reviews and top picks of oil-absorbing products.

BEST OIL-ABSORBING PAPERS:

Boscia Fresh Blotting Linens ($10 for 100 sheets)

e.l.f Shine Eraser ($1 for 50 sheets)

Paula's Choice Oil Blotting Papers ($6.95 for 100 sheets)

Sonia Kashuk Matte, Oil Blotting Papers ($6.69 for 100 sheets)

BEST OIL-ABSORBING/MATTIFYING PRODUCTS (THAT MAY BE APPLIED OVER OR UNDER MAKEUP TO CONTROL SHINE):

Laura Mercier Secret Finish Mattifying ($27 for 1 fl. oz.)

Paula's Choice Shine Stopper Instant Matte Finish with Microsponge Technology ($21.95 for 1 fl. oz.)

Smashbox Anti-Shine ($27 for 1 fl. oz.)

BEST LIP-CARE PRODUCTS (INCLUDING LIP SCRUBS)

Why do I need this product, and what results can I expect?

Lips need special care to keep them smooth, soft, and flake-free. You can eliminate dry, chapped lips with the right mix of lip scrub and lip balm (for daytime use it is advised that any lip balm you use contain sunscreen and be rated SPF 15 or greater).

Whether it's a lip balm, a lip sunscreen, or a lip scrub to remove dry, flaky skin, a lip product must meet these criteria to make the Best Products list:

- The formula must be gentle and fragrance-free
- It must be effective for its intended purpose
- It must not contain irritants such as camphor, menthol, or fragrant oils that damage lips (which reinforces chapping via irritation)
- If sunscreen is present, it must provide broad-spectrum protection and be rated SPF 15 or greater

Lips are certainly a focal point of the face, and an area that should not be ignored when it comes to sun protection and moisturizing. As it turns out, there are several outstanding products to help you take excellent care of your lips and make uncomfortable chapping a distant memory!

The lip products on this list include options to remove dry, flaky skin from chapped lips, protect lips from daily sun exposure, or prevent lips from becoming dry and chapped. And all of them are fragrance-free, because fragrance, whether natural or synthetic, is a big source of lip irritation.

Unless you apply an opaque lipstick every day, it is important to use a lip balm or lipstick with sunscreen rated SPF 15 or greater (recommended lipsticks with sunscreen appear later in this chapter). Taking the time to protect your skin from sun exposure should always include your delicate, sun-vulnerable lips, too. Visit CosmeticsCop.com for our latest reviews and top picks of lip-care products.

BEST LIP BALMS WITH SUNSCREEN (SPF 15 OR GREATER):

Alba Botanica Very Emollient Sunblock Lip Care SPF 25 ($2.50 for 0.15 fl. oz.)

BeautiControl Skinlogics Lip Balm SPF 20 ($12 for 0.06 fl. oz.)

Jane Iredale Lip Drink SPF 15 (reviewed on CosmeticsCop.com; $12 for 0.18 fl. oz.)

Mary Kay Lip Protector Sunscreen SPF 15 ($7.50 for 0.16 fl. oz.)

NARS Pure Sheer SPF 15 Lip Treatment (reviewed on CosmeticsCop.com; $25 for 0.06 fl. oz.)

Shiseido Sun Protection Lip Treatment SPF 36 PA++ ($20 for 0.14 fl. oz.)

BEST LIP BALMS WITHOUT SUNSCREEN:

BeautiControl Platinum Regeneration Age Defying Lip Treatment ($23.50 for 0.09 fl. oz.)

Boots Botanics Organic Lip Balm ($6.99 for 0.33 fl. oz.)

Eucerin Aquaphor Lip Repair ($4.29 for 0.35 fl. oz.)

L'Oreal HiP Studio Secrets Professional Jelly Balm ($9 for 0.15 fl. oz.)

La Roche-Posay Ceralip Lip Repair Cream ($17.95 for 0.51 fl. oz.)

M.A.C. Lip Conditioner ($15 for 0.5 fl. oz.)

Merle Norman Lip Revive ($20 for 0.5 fl. oz.)

Neutrogena Naturals Lip Balm ($2.99 for 0.15 fl. oz.)

Paula's Choice Lip & Body Treatment Balm ($10.95 for 0.5 fl. oz.)

SkinCeuticals Antioxidant Lip Repair Restorative Treatment, for Damaged or Aging Lips ($38 for 0.3 fl. oz.)

The Body Shop Cocoa Butter Lip Care Stick ($8 for 0.15 fl. oz.)

BEST LIP SCRUBS:

BeautiControl Lip Apeel ($22 for 1.25 fl. oz.)

Paula's Choice Lip Perfecting Gentle Scrub with Micro-Beads ($7.95 for 0.5 fl. oz.)

BEST SKIN-CARE PRODUCTS FOR SENSITIVE SKIN

The following lists of products are recommended for those with truly sensitive or rosacea-affected skin based on one primary criterion: they do not contain ingredients known to be irritating or especially problematic for sensitive skin or rosacea. That means none of these products contain fragrance of any kind (including essential oils) and none of them feature inordinately long ingredient lists (which increases the odds that your skin will suffer a negative reaction). Please be aware that even with careful consideration and adherence to usage guidelines we cannot guarantee these products will not cause problems for your sensitive or rosacea-prone skin. No product or product line can make this guarantee (at least not honestly) because of the many variables that can conspire to cause your skin to have a sensitized reaction. Rosacea, in particular, is a disorder that may cause a person's skin to flare with minimal provocation, or from even the most benign cosmetic ingredients, climate changes, hormonal fluctuation, and stress.

The goal of this list is to make it easier for persons with sensitive or rosacea-prone skin to find products that may work for them without making matters worse. Please know that managing rosacea requires the care and supervision of a physician along with careful use of skin-care products and avoidance of external triggers that worsen this condition. If you experience a lingering reaction to any skin-care product, including those from the list below, discontinue use and consult your physician for advice.

Note: Although all the products below received a BEST rating, there are other products in this book that received a lesser rating but are still suitable for sensitive skin. This was typically due to packaging concerns, but that doesn't change the fact that the formula itself is suitable for sensitive or rosacea-prone skin. Visit CosmeticsCop.com for our latest reviews and top product picks for those with sensitive skin.

CLEANSERS:

Boots Expert Sensitive Cleansing & Toning Wipes ($4.49 for 30 wipes), Expert Sensitive Gentle Cleansing Lotion ($4.49 for 6.7 fl. oz.), Expert Sensitive Gentle Cleansing Wash ($4.49 for 5 fl. oz.) and Hydrating Cleanser ($11.40 for 12 fl. oz.)

CeraVe Hydrating Cleanser ($11.40 for 12 fl. oz.) and Foaming Facial Cleanser ($11.99 for 12 fl. oz.)

Clean & Clear Foaming Facial Cleanser, Sensitive Skin ($5.29 for 8 fl. oz.)

Clinique Liquid Facial Soap Extra Mild ($16 for 6.7 fl. oz.), Redness Solutions Soothing Cleanser ($21.50 for 5 fl. oz.), Take The Day Off Cleansing Balm ($27.50 for 3.8 fl. oz.) and Take The Day Off Cleansing Milk ($26 for 6.7 fl. oz.)

DHC Cleansing Milk ($24 for 6.7 fl. oz.)

Estee Lauder Verite LightLotion Cleanser ($23.50 for 6.7 fl. oz.)

Eucerin Redness Relief Soothing Cleanser ($8.79 for 6.8 fl. oz.)

L'Occitane Ultra Comforting Cleansing Milk ($22 for 6.7 fl. oz.)

La Roche-Posay Toleriane Dermo-Cleanser ($22.95 for 6.76 fl. oz.)

Merle Norman Delicate Balance Calming Cleanser ($19 for 4 fl. oz.)

Neutrogena Extra Gentle Cleanser ($6.49 for 6.7 fl. oz.)

Olay 2-in-1 Daily Facial Cloths, Sensitive ($5.99 for 33 cloths); Foaming Face Wash, for Sensitive Skin ($7.99 for 7 fl. oz.); and Pro-X Restorative Cream Cleanser ($19.99 for 5 fl. oz.)

Paula's Choice cleansers (all types; see PaulasChoice.com for details)

SkinCeuticals Purifying Cleanser ($32 for 8 fl. oz.)

SkinMedica Sensitive Skin Cleanser ($34 for 6 fl. oz.)

The Body Shop Aloe Calming Facial Cleanser, for Sensitive Skin ($14 for 6.75 fl. oz.) and Aloe Gentle Facial Wash, for Sensitive Skin ($16 for 4.2 fl. oz.)

EYE-MAKEUP REMOVERS:

Bobbi Brown Instant Long Wear Makeup Remover ($24 for 3.4 fl. oz.)

Boots Organic Face Nourishing Eye Makeup Remover ($6.99 for 2.5 fl. oz.)

Clinique Take the Day Off Makeup Remover for Lids, Lashes, & Lips ($18 for 4.2 fl. oz.)

Neutrogena Oil-Free Eye Makeup Remover ($6.99 for 5.5 fl. oz.) and Eye Makeup Remover Lotion–Hydrating ($6.99 for 3 fl. oz.)

Nivea Eye Makeup Remover, All Skin Types ($7.99 for 4 fl. oz.)

Paula's Choice Gentle Touch Makeup Remover ($12.95 for 4.3 fl. oz.)

TONERS:

Paula's Choice toners (all types, particularly RESIST Advanced Replenishing Toner ($18.95 for 4 fl. oz.) and Skin Recovery Enriched Calming Toner ($15.95 for 6.4 fl. oz.); see PaulasChoice.com for details).

SCRUBS:

Boots Expert Sensitive Gentle Smoothing Scrub ($5.49 for 3.3 fl. oz.)

AHA EXFOLIANTS:

Olay Regenerist Night Resurfacing Elixir ($31.99 for 1.7 fl. oz.)

Paula's Choice RESIST Daily Smoothing Treatment ($25.95 for 1.7 fl. oz.)

BHA EXFOLIANTS:

Paula's Choice CLEAR and Skin Perfecting BHA exfoliants (various formulas, prices, and sizes; see PaulasChoice.com for details).

MOISTURIZERS WITHOUT SUNSCREEN:

Boscia Restorative Night Moisture Cream ($48 for 1 fl. oz.)

CeraVe Facial Moisturizing Lotion PM ($13.99 for 3 fl. oz.)

MD Formulations Moisture Defense Antioxidant Hydrating Gel ($45 for 1 fl. oz.)

Olay Pro-X Deep Wrinkle Treatment ($47 for 1 fl. oz.)

Paula's Choice Hydralight Moisture-Infusing Lotion ($19.95 for 2 fl. oz.), Moisture Boost Hydrating Treatment Cream ($19.95 for 2 fl. oz.), RESIST Anti-Aging Clear Skin Hydrator ($22.95 for 1.7 fl. oz.), Skin Balancing Invisible Finish Moisture Gel ($19.95 for 2 fl. oz.), and Skin Recovery Replenishing Moisturizer ($19.95 for 2 fl. oz.)

MOISTURIZERS WITH SUNSCREEN:

BeautiControl Cell Block-C New Cell Protection SPF 20 ($30 for 1 fl. oz.), BC Spa Facial Defend & Restore Moisture Creme SPF 20 ($32 for 2.6 fl. oz.), and BC Spa Facial Defend & Restore Moisture Lotion SPF 20 ($32 for 2.6 fl. oz.)

Clinique City Block Sheer Oil-Free Daily Face Protector SPF 25 ($19 for 1.4 fl. oz.) and Redness Solutions Daily Protective Base SPF 15 ($18.50 for 1.35 fl. oz.)

Obagi Nu-Derm Physical UV Block SPF 32 ($39.31 for 2 fl. oz.)

Paula's Choice RESIST Cellular Defense Daily Moisturizer SPF 25 ($24.95 for 2 fl. oz.) and Skin Recovery Daily Moisturizing Lotion SPF 15 & Antioxidants ($20.95 for 2 fl. oz.)

EYE-AREA MOISTURIZERS:

Estee Lauder Verite Special EyeCare ($45 for 0.5 fl. oz.)

SERUMS:

Elizabeth Arden Ceramide Gold Ultra Restorative Capsules ($68 for 0.95 fl. oz.)

Olay Regenerist Regenerating Serum Fragrance-Free ($24.99 for 1.7 fl. oz.)

Paula's Choice RESIST Super Antioxidant Concentrate Serum ($25.95 for 1 fl. oz.)

SK-II Signs Wrinkle Serum ($175 for 1 fl. oz.)

FACIAL MASKS:

Paula's Choice Skin Recovery Hydrating Treatment Mask ($15.95 for 4 fl. oz.)

ALL-PURPOSE SUNSCREENS:

Alba Botanica Very Emollient Sunblock Mineral Protection, Fragrance Free SPF 30 ($10.99 for 4 fl. oz.)

Jason Natural Sunblock Mineral SPF 30 ($14.95 for 4 fl. oz.)

Kiss My Face Oat Protein Complex Sun Screen SPF 18 ($11.95 for 4 fl. oz.)

Neutrogena Sensitive Skin Sunblock SPF 30 ($8.99 for 4 fl. oz.)

Obagi Nu-Derm Physical UV Block SPF 32 ($39.31 for 2 fl. oz.)

Physician's Formula Sun Shield for Faces Extra Sensitive Skin SPF 25 ($8.95 for 4 fl. oz.)

SkinCeuticals Physical UV Defense SPF 30 ($38 for 3 fl. oz.)

SPECIALTY PRODUCTS:

Paula's Choice Redness Relief Treatment, for All Skin Types ($15.95 for 4 fl. oz.) and RESIST Pure Radiance Skin Brightening Treatment ($26.95 for 1 fl. oz.)

BEST FOUNDATIONS WITH SUNSCREEN

If you have stayed away from foundation because of a previous negative experience, there has never been a safer time to try it again; the right one can make a huge difference in the appearance of your skin. And if you have oily to very oily skin, choosing a foundation with sunscreen is a great idea because it will help keep excess shine in check while eliminating the need for you to apply two products (when it comes to very oily skin, fewer products is better). In order for a foundation with sunscreen to make the Best Products list, it must:

- Be rated SPF 15 or greater and provide sufficient UVA protection
- Have an exemplary texture that blends beautifully
- Come in a range of neutral colors that look like real skin
- Wear with minimal to no signs of problems

The foundations on this list, whether cream, liquid, cream-to-powder, or powder all have exemplary, class-leading textures, beautiful finishes, reliable coverage, and a selection of neutral shades that match real skin tones (rather than masking skin with an odd shade of pink, rose, or peach). All of them also provide reliable sun protection that includes one or more of these critical UVA sunscreens: titanium dioxide, zinc oxide, or avobenzone (we have yet to see a foundation with sunscreen that contains ecamsule, otherwise known as Mexoryl SX, or outside the U.S., Tinosorb).

Choosing the right foundation color is not only time-consuming, but also exceedingly frustrating. The only way to discover your ideal match is to apply the foundation on your facial skin, perhaps two different colors on either side of your face, and then check it in daylight. If the color isn't an exact match, you have to go back in and try again.

Another hurdle is to find a foundation with a pleasing texture, one that feels soft and silky, but doesn't streak, cake, or look thick, and that takes experimentation, too.

Determining how much coverage you want is another factor, and then there's what type of foundation (liquid, powder, cream, or stick formulas). Now tell us that isn't a challenge!

Financially, if you can splurge on only one cosmetic product, foundation is it. This is the one category where spending a little bit more is the best option, not because expensive means better, but because it's just way too risky to buy a foundation you can't try on first, either with a tester at the cosmetics counter or with samples you can take home or, in some cases, order online.

Still, many mass-market outlets and drugstores have very good hassle-free return policies for used makeup, and it's wise to inquire about that before purchasing makeup in these environments (Note: all of them require you to keep your receipt as proof of purchase). Do not keep a foundation that ends up being the wrong color—return it and keep trying until you get it right.

Note: Several foundations with sunscreen reviewed in this book would have earned a Paula's Pick rating had their SPF value been higher. Because it is widely accepted that SPF 15 is the minimum amount of daytime protection needed, we made the decision (with occasional exceptions) to not give foundations with sunscreen below SPF 15 a rating above average. However, if you are willing to pair such a foundation with another product rated SPF 15 or greater, then you may in fact want to consider those foundations as well. This is one more reason why, depending on your needs and preferences, shopping from the Best Products list alone may not be the perfect approach. Visit CosmeticsCop.com for our latest reviews and top picks of foundations with sunscreen.

BEST FOUNDATIONS WITH SUNSCREEN (SPF 15 OR GREATER) FOR VERY OILY SKIN:

LIQUID:

Boots Stay Perfect Foundation SPF 15 ($13.99)

L'Oreal Paris True Match Super-Blendable Makeup SPF 17 Sunscreen ($10.95)

Paula's Choice Best Face Forward Foundation SPF 15 ($14.95)

Shiseido Sun Protection Liquid Foundation SPF 42 PA+++ ($35)

BEST FOUNDATIONS WITH SUNSCREEN (SPF 15 OR GREATER) FOR NORMAL TO OILY/COMBINATION SKIN:

LIQUID:

Almay Nearly Naked Liquid Makeup SPF 15 ($10.99), TLC Truly Lasting Color 16 Hour Makeup SPF 15 ($12.49), and Smart Shade Smart Balance Skin Balancing Makeup SPF 15 ($13.99)

Benefit "Hello Flawless" Oxygen Wow Liquid Foundation SPF 25 ($34)

Boots Stay Perfect Foundation SPF 15 ($13.99)

Chanel Mat Lumiere Long Lasting Luminous Matte Fluid Makeup SPF 15 ($54)

Clinique Even Better Makeup SPF 15 ($26)

L'Oreal Paris Visible Lift Serum Absolute Advanced Age-Reversing Makeup SPF 17 ($12.48)

M.A.C. Matchmaster SPF 15 Foundation ($33) and Studio Sculpt SPF 15 Foundation ($30)

Paula's Choice Best Face Forward Foundation SPF 15 ($14.95)

Shiseido Dual Balancing Foundation SPF 17 ($38.50), Perfect Smoothing Compact Foundation SPF 15 ($31), and Sun Protection Liquid Foundation SPF 42 PA+++ ($35)

PRESSED POWDER:

Bobbi Brown Skin Foundation Mineral Makeup SPF 15 ($38)

Clinique Almost Powder Makeup SPF 15 ($24)

Shiseido Sheer Mattifying Compact SPF 22 ($30) and Sun Protection Compact Foundation SPF 34 PA+++ ($27)

LOOSE POWDER:

Jane Iredale Amazing Base Loose Minerals SPF 20 ($42)

CREAM-TO-POWDER:
Cover Girl CG Smoothers AquaSmooth Compact Makeup SPF 15 ($9.99)
Revlon PhotoReady Compact Makeup SPF 20 ($13.99)
Shiseido Stick Foundation SPF 15-18 ($38.50)

BEST FOUNDATIONS WITH SUNSCREEN (SPF 15 OR GREATER) FOR NORMAL TO DRY SKIN:

LIQUID:
Almay Line Smoothing Makeup SPF 15 ($13.99)
Chanel Mat Lumiere Long Lasting Luminous Matte Fluid Makeup SPF 15 ($54)
Estee Lauder Resilience Lift Extreme Radiant Lifting Makeup SPF 15 ($37.50)
M.A.C. Studio Sculpt SPF 15 Foundation ($30)
Paula's Choice All Bases Covered Foundation SPF 15 ($14.95)
Revlon ColorStay Makeup with Softflex for Normal to Dry Skin SPF 15 ($12.99)

PRESSED POWDER:
Bobbi Brown Skin Foundation Mineral Makeup SPF 15 ($38)
Giorgio Armani Lasting Silk UV Compact SPF 34 ($59)
Jane Iredale PurePressed Base Mineral Foundation SPF 20 ($40–$52)
Physicians Formula Healthy Wear SPF 50 Powder Foundation ($14.95)
Shiseido Perfect Smoothing Compact Foundation SPF 15 ($31)

LOOSE POWDER:
Jane Iredale Amazing Base Loose Minerals SPF 20 ($42)
Korres Natural Wild Rose Mineral Foundation SPF 30 ($28)
Laura Mercier Mineral Powder SPF 15 ($35 for 0.34 fl. oz.)

CREAM-TO-POWDER AND/OR STICK:
Estee Lauder Resilience Lift Extreme Ultra Firming Creme Compact Makeup SPF 15 ($37.50)
Giorgio Armani Designer Shaping Cream Foundation SPF 20 ($65)
Revlon New Complexion One Step Compact Makeup SPF 15 ($12.99)
Shiseido Stick Foundation SPF 15-18 ($38.50)

BEST FOUNDATIONS WITH SUNSCREEN (SPF 15 OR GREATER) FOR DRY TO VERY DRY SKIN:

LIQUID:
Revlon Age Defying Makeup with Botafirm SPF 15 Dry Skin ($11.99) and Age Defying Makeup with Botafirm SPF 20 ($13.99)

BEST SHEER FOUNDATIONS/TINTED MOISTURIZERS WITH SUNSCREEN (SPF 15 OR GREATER) FOR ALL SKIN TYPES EXCEPT VERY OILY:

Aveda Inner Light Mineral Tinted Moisture SPF 15 ($28)
BeautiControl BC Color Tinted Moisturizer SPF 15 ($22)

Bobbi Brown SPF 15 Tinted Moisturizer ($40)

Boots Soft & Sheer Tinted Moisturiser SPF 15 ($11.99)

Dr. Denese New York SPF 30 Defense Day Cream ($49 for 2 fl. oz.)

Elizabeth Arden Pure Finish Mineral Tinted Moisturizer SPF 15 ($30)

Laura Mercier Illuminating Tinted Moisturizer SPF 20 ($42)

Laura Geller Barely There Tinted Moisturizer SPF 20 ($30)

Neutrogena Healthy Skin Enhancer SPF 20 ($10.49), Healthy Skin Glow Sheers SPF 30 ($10.99) and Mineral Sheers Powder Foundation SPF 20 ($11.99)

Paula's Choice Barely There Sheer Matte Tint SPF 20 ($14.95)

Stila Sheer Color Tinted Moisturizer Oil-Free SPF 20 ($34 for 1.7 fl. oz.)

BEST BB CREAMS:

Note: Please visit CosmeticsCop.com for other highly-rated BB creams from brands not included in this book.

Too Faced Tinted Beauty Balm SPF 20 ($32)

BEST FOUNDATIONS WITHOUT SUNSCREEN

The same standards mentioned for foundations with sunscreen above apply to this category, too, minus the sunscreen comments. If you opt to use a foundation without sunscreen during the day, it is critical for the health of your skin that you apply a moisturizer rated SPF 15 or greater prior to applying your foundation. Neglecting sun protection, even when it's cloudy and even when your time outdoors may be limited to walking to get the mail, sun protection is skin care priority number one—especially if your goal is younger-looking skin free from wrinkles, sagging, and brown spots. Visit CosmeticsCop.com for our latest reviews and top picks of foundations without sunscreen.

BEST FOUNDATIONS WITHOUT SUNSCREEN FOR VERY OILY SKIN:

LIQUID:

Almay Clear Complexion Makeup ($13.99)

Clinique Stay-Matte Oil-Free Makeup ($23)

Make Up For Ever HD Invisible Cover Foundation ($40)

Maybelline Superstay Makeup 24HR ($10.99)

NARS Sheer Matte Foundation ($42)

PRESSED POWDER:

Avon Smooth Minerals Pressed Foundation ($11)

Make Up For Ever Duo Mat Powder Foundation ($32)

CREAM-TO-POWDER:

Boots Intelligent Balance Mousse Foundation ($13.99)

Maybelline Dream Matte Mousse Foundation ($9.79)

BEST FOUNDATIONS WITHOUT SUNSCREEN FOR NORMAL TO OILY/COM-BINATION SKIN:

LIQUID:

Almay Clear Complexion Makeup ($13.99)

Clinique Perfectly Real Makeup ($24)

Estee Lauder Invisible Fluid Makeup ($35)

Make Up For Ever HD Invisible Cover Foundation ($40)

Maybelline Dream Liquid Mousse Airbrush Finish ($9.79)

NARS Sheer Glow Foundation ($42) and Sheer Matte Foundation ($42)

Stila Natural Finish Oil-Free Makeup ($38)

Too Faced Amazing Face Oil Free Close-Up Coverage Foundation ($36)

PRESSED POWDER:

Avon Smooth Minerals Pressed Foundation ($11)

Clinique Perfectly Real Compact Makeup ($24)

Laura Mercier Powder Foundation ($40)

M.A.C. Studio Fix Powder Plus Foundation ($27)

Make Up For Ever Duo Mat Powder Foundation ($32)

Sephora Matifying Compact Foundation ($20)

The Body Shop All in One Face Base ($22)

CREAM-TO-POWDER:

Boots Intelligent Balance Mousse Foundation ($13.99)

Maybelline Dream Smooth Mousse Foundation ($9.79)

BEST FOUNDATIONS WITHOUT SUNSCREEN FOR NORMAL TO DRY SKIN:

LIQUID:

Estee Lauder Invisible Fluid Makeup ($35)

Maybelline Dream Liquid Mousse Airbrush Finish ($9.79)

Stila Illuminating Liquid Foundation ($38)

Too Faced Amazing Face Oil Free Close-Up Coverage Foundation ($36)

PRESSED POWDER:

Avon Smooth Minerals Pressed Foundation ($11)

Lancome Dual Finish Versatile Powder Makeup ($36.50)

M.A.C. Studio Fix Powder Plus Foundation ($27)

The Body Shop All in One Face Base ($22)

LOOSE POWDER:

Mary Kay Mineral Powder Foundation ($18)

CREAM-TO-POWDER:

Bobbi Brown Oil-Free Even Finish Compact Foundation ($42)

BEST LIQUID FOUNDATIONS WITHOUT SUNSCREEN FOR DRY TO VERY DRY SKIN:

LIQUID:

Stila Illuminating Liquid Foundation ($38)

CREAM-TO-POWDER:

Bobbi Brown Oil-Free Even Finish Compact Foundation ($42)

BEST FOUNDATIONS WITH MAXIMUM COVERAGE, REGARDLESS OF SKIN TYPE, WITH AND WITHOUT SUNSCREEN:

BeautiControl Secret AGEnt Undercover Makeup ($18)

Laura Mercier Silk Creme Foundation ($42)

BEST FOUNDATION PRIMERS

Foundation primers are not essential to beautiful makeup application, but we've chosen some favorites for those curious about this superfluous category. A foundation primer should:

- Be lightweight and apply smoothly
- Enhance makeup application
- For oily skin, help keep excess shine in check
- Not change the color of your skin

If you're among those who believe foundation primers are a must, the truth is most of us are already priming our skin for makeup by virtue of following a good skin-care routine beforehand. You don't need a special product labeled "primer" before applying foundation, and there is nothing in foundation that skin needs to be protected from, so let's put that myth to rest!

The primers on this list are included not only because their formulas surpass standard primers but also because our readers continue to ask us for our favorites in this group.

Although all the recommendations below are great, you can achieve similar results by applying a state-of-the-art serum or lightweight moisturizer instead. You definitely don't need a well-formulated moisturizer, serum, and a primer. That's going overboard and can cause your makeup to not last as long—just the opposite of what primers are said to do. Visit Cosmetics-Cop.com for our latest reviews and top picks for foundation primers.

Note: If you decide to use a primer, it should be applied after your regular skin-care routine but before your daytime moisturizer with sunscreen.

BEST FOUNDATION PRIMERS:

Estee Lauder Matte Perfecting Primer ($32 for 1 fl. oz.)

Giorgio Armani Light Master Primer ($57 for 1 fl. oz.)

M.A.C. Prep + Prime Line Filler ($20 for 0.5 fl. oz.)

Tarte Cosmetics Smooth Operator Amazonian Clay Illuminating Serum ($32 for 1.7 fl. oz.)

Urban Decay Complexion Primer Potion-Brightening ($31 for 1 fl. oz.)

BEST CONCEALERS

Most makeup artists will tell you that a great concealer is essential, and they're right! Concealers are a makeup staple and in order to make the Best Products list they must:

- Have a smooth texture that's easy to blend
- Set to a long-wearing finish
- Not (or minimally) crease into lines around the eyes
- Come in a range of neutral colors for a range of skin tones
- Provide good coverage that doesn't fade after several hours

Although there are lots of good concealers available in all price ranges, the options on this list represent the elite, whether you prefer a liquid formula (generally best for normal to oily skin or for use on blemishes) or cream formula (generally best for normal to dry skin not prone to blemishes or for under-eye use).

Each concealer on this list has a beautiful texture, provides moderate to significant coverage without looking thick or cakey, and has an impressive wear-time with minimal to no risk of creasing into lines around the eye. Concealers with sunscreen on this list include UVA-protecting ingredients and are an excellent way to apply extra sun protection around your eyes.

We have no doubt you will be pleased with almost any concealer on this list, but please refer to each individual review for details before making your final decision.

The highlighters listed below are best used, not surprisingly, to highlight key features or brighten shadowed areas. Generally, these do not provide much, if any, coverage and are best applied over a liquid or cream concealer. Visit CosmeticsCop.com for our latest reviews and top picks of concealers.

Note: We do not recommend color-correcting concealers because they rarely (if ever) look convincing in natural light, and they often substitute one visible discoloration for another.

BEST LIQUID CONCEALERS:

Chanel Correcteur Perfection Long Lasting Concealer ($40)

Dior DiorSkin Sculpt Lifting Smoothing Concealer ($35)

L'Oreal Paris True Match Concealer ($8.95) and Visible Lift Serum Age-Reversing Concealer SPF 20 ($12.95)

Lancome Maquicomplet Complete Coverage Concealer ($29.50)

M.A.C. Select Cover-Up ($17)

Make Up For Ever Full Cover Concealer ($30)

Mary Kay Concealer ($10)

Origins Quick, Hide! Long-wearing Concealer ($15)

BEST CREAM, CREAM-TO-POWDER, AND STICK CONCEALERS:

Clinique All About Eyes Concealer ($16)

Elizabeth Arden Ceramide Ultra Lift and Firm Concealer ($19.50)

Paula's Choice Soft Cream Concealer ($9.95)

Shiseido Natural Finish Cream Concealer ($25)

Tarte Cosmetics Maracuja Creaseless Waterproof Concealer ($24)

BEST HIGHLIGTERS:

Avon Mark GetBright Hook Up Highlighter ($6.50)

Chanel Eclat Lumiere Highlighter Face Pen ($40)

Maybelline Dream Lumi Touch Highlighting Concealer ($7.99)

BEST POWDERS

Whether you prefer loose or pressed powder or a powder with sunscreen, in order to make the Best Products list, a face powder must:

- Have a beautifully silky texture that surpasses the norm
- Provide a smooth, polished finish that accentuates skin
- Not look or feel heavy, cakey, or dull
- Contain minimal to no fragrance
- For powders with sunscreen, be rated SPF 15 or greater and provide broad-spectrum sun protection

It is truly difficult to find a bad loose or pressed powder. For the most part, all of them have an appreciable degree of silkiness and do their jobs of setting makeup, absorbing excess oil, and helping skin look finished. Because of this, we were extra picky about which powders made the cut for inclusion on the Best Products list.

Those who find the list below too limiting should know that any powder rated "GOOD" is also worth considering (but, for various reasons, isn't in the same league as the powders on this list). Depending on your preferences and expectations, the powder field is mostly wide open and includes options from the palest porcelain to the deepest ebony skin.

Expense does not distinguish powders; there are equally beautiful options at the drugstore as there are at the department store. For example, L'Oreal and Lancome (owned by L'Oreal) have equally impressive powders for normal to dry skin. Lancome's has more elegant packaging, but that doesn't affect how it applies or looks on your face.

A separate category of pressed powders are those that contain sunscreen with an SPF 15 and the mineral-based UVA-protecting ingredients of titanium dioxide or zinc oxide. These are excellent options to touch up makeup and add sun protection over your foundation to be sure you have lasting coverage. Because of their thicker texture, these can also double as powder foundation, though they are best used over a regular sunscreen or over a foundation with sunscreen to boost sun protection. Visit CosmeticsCop.com for our latest reviews and top picks of all types of powder.

BEST LOOSE POWDERS FOR NORMAL TO OILY/COMBINATION OR VERY OILY SKIN:

Almay Nearly Naked Loose Powder ($11.99)

Bobbi Brown Sheer Finish Loose Powder ($35)

Boots Perfect Light Loose Powder ($11.99) and Perfect Light Portable Loose Powder ($12.99)

Chanel Poudre Universelle Libre Natural Finish Loose Powder ($52)

Make Up For Ever Super Matte Loose Powder ($24) and Multi Loose Powder ($34)

Smashbox Photo Set Finishing Powder SPF 15 ($28)

Sonia Kashuk Bare Minimum Pressed Powder ($9.39)

Urban Decay Razor Sharp Ultra Definition Finishing Powder ($31)

BEST LOOSE POWDERS FOR NORMAL TO DRY SKIN:

Almay Nearly Naked Loose Powder ($11.99)

Avon Ideal Shade Loose Powder ($9)

Bobbi Brown Sheer Finish Loose Powder ($35)

Chanel Poudre Universelle Libre Natural Finish Loose Powder ($52)

Clarins Loose Powder ($35)

Clinique Blended Face Powder & Brush ($21)

DHC Q10 Face Powder ($17)

Giorgio Armani Micro-fil Loose Powder ($49)

L'Oreal Paris Translucide Naturally Luminous Powder ($11.79) and True Match Naturale Soft-Focus Mineral Finish ($15.25)

La Mer The Powder ($65)

Lancome Absolue Powder Radiant Smoothing Powder ($56) and Ageless Minerale Perfecting and Setting Mineral Powder with White Sapphire Complex ($36)

Laura Mercier Loose Setting Powder ($34)

M.A.C. Select Sheer Loose Powder ($23)

Paula's Choice Healthy Finish Pressed Powder SPF 15 ($14.95)

Smashbox Photo Set Finishing Powder SPF 15 ($28)

Urban Decay Razor Sharp Ultra Definition Finishing Powder ($31)

BEST PRESSED POWDERS FOR NORMAL TO OILY/COMBINATION OR VERY OILY SKIN:

Avon ExtraLasting Pressed Powder SPF 15 ($11) and Ideal Shade Pressed Powder ($9)

Bobbi Brown Sheer Finish Pressed Powder ($34)

Cover Girl TruBlend Pressed Powder ($7.79) and Advanced Radiance Age-Defying Pressed Powder ($7.79)

Giorgio Armani Luminous Silk Powder ($47)

L'Oreal Paris True Match Super-Blendable Powder ($10.95)

M.A.C. Mineralize Skinfinish ($29) and Select Sheer Pressed Powder ($23)

Maybelline Dream Matte Face Powder ($8.23), Fit Me! Pressed Powder ($7.99), and Instant Age Rewind Protector Finishing Powder SPF 25 ($9.25)

Physicians Formula Mineral Wear Talc-Free Mineral Face Powder SPF 16 ($13.95)

Revlon Age Defying with DNA Advantage Powder ($13.99)

Shiseido Pureness Matifying Compact Oil-Free SPF 16 ($20.50)

Smashbox Photo Set Pressed Powder ($29)

Sonia Kashuk Bare Minimum Pressed Powder ($9.39)

Urban Decay Razor Sharp Ultra Definition Finishing Powder ($31)

BEST PRESSED POWDERS FOR NORMAL TO DRY SKIN:

Almay Line Smoothing Pressed Powder ($13.49)

Avon ExtraLasting Pressed Powder SPF 15 ($11)

Bobbi Brown Sheer Finish Pressed Powder ($34)

Cover Girl TruBlend Pressed Powder ($7.79) and Advanced Radiance Age-Defying Pressed Powder ($7.79)

Giorgio Armani Luminous Silk Powder ($47)

L'Oreal Paris True Match Super-Blendable Powder ($10.95)

Lancome Translucence Mattifying Silky Matte Powder ($29)

Laura Mercier Pressed Setting Powder ($30)

M.A.C. Mineralize Skinfinish ($29), Select Sheer Pressed Powder ($23), and Studio Careblend Pressed Powder ($23)

Mary Kay Sheer Mineral Pressed Powder ($16)

Maybelline Fit Me! Pressed Powder ($7.99)

N.Y.C. (New York Color) Smooth Skin Pressed Face Powder ($2.99)

Neutrogena Healthy Skin Pressed Powder SPF 20 ($11.99)

Physicians Formula Mineral Wear Talc-Free Mineral Face Powder SPF 16 ($13.95) and Youthful Wear Cosmeceutical Youth-Boosting Illuminating Face Powder ($13.95)

Sonia Kashuk Bare Minimum Pressed Powder ($9.39)

The Body Shop Pressed Face Powder ($18.50)

Urban Decay Razor Sharp Ultra Definition Finishing Powder ($31)

BEST PRESSED POWDERS WITH SUNSCREEN FOR ALL SKIN TYPES:

Avon ExtraLasting Pressed Powder SPF 15 ($11)

Maybelline Instant Age Rewind Protector Finishing Powder SPF 25 ($9.25)

Neutrogena Healthy Skin Pressed Powder SPF 20 ($11.99)

Paula's Choice Healthy Finish Pressed Powder SPF 15 ($14.95)

Physicians Formula Mineral Wear Talc-Free Mineral Face Powder SPF 16 ($13.95)

Shiseido Pureness Matifying Compact Oil-Free SPF 16 ($20.50)

BEST BRONZING POWDERS, GELS, AND LIQUIDS

In order for a bronzing product to make the Best Products list, it must (regardless of the type):

- Have a superior texture that ensures even application
- Not streak or look blotchy
- Offer at least one convincing tan color
- Have minimal to no shine (a real tan isn't shiny)
- Look natural and be compatible with blush for a dimensional look

The bronzers on this list are those we found to be the top-performing options, whether you prefer powder (the predominant form), liquid, cream-to-powder, or a bronzing gel, the latter of which is ideal for oily, breakout-prone skin.

Those looking for a bronzing powder or liquid with noticeable shine should refer to the list of Best Face & Body Illuminating/Shimmer Products. The bronzing powders on this list have a matte or semi-matte finish, which is far more natural (at least for daytime) than trying to create a fake tan that glistens. A small amount of sheen is fine, but it should produce a soft glow, not obvious sparkles. Visit CosmeticsCop.com for our latest reviews and top picks of bronzing products.

BEST PRESSED BRONZING POWDERS:

Avon Mark Bronze Pro Bronzing Powder ($10)

Dior Bronze Harmonie de Blush ($44) and Dior Bronze Matte Sunshine SPF 20 ($46)

M.A.C. Bronzing Powder ($23)

Neutrogena Healthy Skin Custom Glow Blush & Bronzer ($11.49)

Rimmel Natural Bronzer ($5.79)

Smashbox Bronze Lights ($29)

Too Faced Chocolate Soleil Matte Bronzing Powder ($29)

BEST BRONZING CREAM:

NARS Multiple Bronzer ($38)

BEST BLUSHES

In order to make the Best Product list, a blush must:

- Have a smooth texture and even application
- Be easy to blend
- Enliven cheeks with soft to moderate color
- Have a matte to minimally shiny finish
- Come in an array of workable colors for multiple skin tones

For the most part, blush is probably one of the easiest cosmetics to get right because it is nearly impossible to buy a bad blush. Not that there aren't some real losers out there, but there are far more winners. The problem with blush is usually in application, and that is where good brushes come into play.

Using the proper brush is essential for getting blush to go on correctly. With very few exceptions, you should just discard the mini-brushes that come packaged with a powder blush in favor of an elegant, professional-size blush brush.

Powder blush is by far the most popular form of this makeup staple, but for variety's sake many lines offer cream, cream-to-powder, and liquid or gel blushes. Those that proved particularly impressive (or easier than usual to work with) earned our top rating.

Because most blushes in all forms have some degree of shine (clearly, many women must want shiny cheeks), we did not take a true matte finish into strong consideration. There are some terrific matte blushes available, but, for the most part, what passes for matte today still has a hint of shine. Please refer to each blush's individual review for comments on its finish (matte, almost matte, or level of shine). Visit CosmeticsCop.com for our latest reviews and top picks of all types of blush.

Note: The cream blushes on the lists below are recommended only for dry to very dry skin that is not prone to blemishes. Cream-to-powder blushes, whether in stick or compact form, are best for normal to slightly dry or slightly oily skin not prone to breakouts. Those prone to breakouts, even if dry skin is also an issue, should stick with powder, liquid, or gel blushes.

BEST POWDER BLUSHES:

Avon Mark Good Glowing Mosaic Blush ($8)

BeautiControl BC Color Mineral Blush ($16)

Dior Bronze Harmonie de Blush ($44) and DiorBlush ($42)

e.l.f. Studio Blush ($3)

Estee Lauder Pure Color Blush ($28)

Jane Iredale PurePressed Blush ($27)

Korres Natural Zea Mays Blush ($24)

L'Oreal Paris True Match Super-Blendable Blush ($10.95)

Laura Mercier Second Skin Cheek Colour ($24)

NARS Blush ($27)

NYX Cosmetics Blush ($6)

Sonia Kashuk Beautifying Blush ($8.99)

Tarte Cosmetics Amazonian Clay 12-Hour Blush ($25)

BEST CREAM, CREAM-TO-POWDER, OR STICK BLUSHES:

Avon Mark Just Pinched Instant Blush Tint ($8)

Boots Cheek Tint ($9.99)

Clarins Multi-Blush ($28.50)

Clinique Blushwear Cream Stick ($21)

e.l.f. Studio Cream Blush ($6)

Elizabeth Arden Ceramide Cream Blush ($24)

Estee Lauder Signature Satin Creme Blush ($26)

Laura Mercier Creme Cheek Colour ($22)

L'Oreal Paris Magic Smooth Soufflé Blush ($12.95)

Laura Geller Air Whipped Blush ($26)

Mary Kay Cream Blush ($13)

NYX Cosmetics Stick Blush ($6)

Revlon Cream Blush ($9.79)

Sonia Kashuk Creme Blush ($9.89)

Tarte Cosmetics Cheek Stain ($30)

Too Faced Full Bloom Lip & Cheek Creme Color ($21)

Urban Decay Afterglow Glide-On Cheek Tint ($24)

BEST LIQUID OR GEL BLUSHES:

Benefit Benetint ($29) and Cha Cha Tint ($29)

Make Up For Ever HD Microfinish Blush ($25)

Sonia Kashuk Super Sheer Liquid Tint ($9.99)

BEST EYESHADOWS & EYESHADOW PRIMERS

Eyeshadows are essential to a full makeup application. Most women state that their eyes are their best feature, so naturally playing up your best feature makes sense! In order to earn a spot on the Best Products list, an eyeshadow must:

- Have a smooth texture that applies easily
- Blend well and offer a good color payoff
- Not flake, easily smudge, or quickly fade
- Come in a range of classic and neutral shades
- Not contain shine particles that look distracting or flake into the eye

The eyeshadows we rate as the best have enviable silky textures, apply seamlessly, blend and build well, and have staying power.

You can shop in both the drugstores and the department stores and find wonderful textures and colors, although when it comes to variety of matte shades, the scales remain tipped in favor of the department stores (primarily in the makeup artist–driven lines such as M.A.C., Laura Mercier, and Bobbi Brown).

Those of you who love eyeshadow with some shine will find the options almost limitless, regardless of where you shop. The good news is that today's best shiny eyeshadows add more glow than glitter to your eyes, and the shine clings much better than in the past (though there are still plenty of shiny eyeshadows that flake, none of which are on this list).

Eyeshadows on this list include singles, duos, trios, and quads. Please keep in mind that purchasing multiple eyeshadows as part of a set only makes sense if you'll really use the color combinations provided (and in many cases, you won't want to, at least not if you want to create a classic, understated eye design). Visit CosmeticsCop.com for our latest reviews and top picks of all types of eyeshadow.

Note: Without question, brushes are a must for smooth, flawless application of eyeshadows. Do NOT use the tiny, sponge-tip applicators included with many shadows. They tend to make the results choppy and are not adept at blending multiple shades for a subtle gradation of color. Your shadows will apply and blend so much better with brushes!

In terms of eyeshadow primers, although many women enjoy using them, they're not an essential step to flawless eye makeup. They can help enhance shadow application and wear, but really are no better than prepping the eyelid and under-brow area with a good matte finish concealer and light dusting of powder. Still, for those intent on using a product labeled "eyeshadow primer," we've included our favorites in this group.

BEST POWDER EYESHADOWS (INCLUDING SINGLES, DUOS, TRIOS AND QUADS):

Clinique Colour Surge Eye Shadow Duo ($18), Colour Surge Eye Shadow Quad ($25.50), Colour Surge Eye Shadow Soft Shimmer ($15), and Colour Surge Eye Shadow Stay Matte ($15)

DHC Eye Shadow Moon ($6)

Dior 1-Couleur Eyeshadow ($29) and 5-Couleur Eyeshadow Palette ($59)

Elizabeth Arden Color Intrigue Eyeshadow ($15) and Color Intrigue Eyeshadow Duo ($24.50)

Estee Lauder Pure Color EyeShadow ($20) and Pure Color EyeShadow Duo ($30)

Giorgio Armani Maestro Eye Shadow Quads ($59)

Jane Iredale PurePressed Eye Shadows ($19)

L'Oreal Paris HiP Studio Secrets Professional Concentrated Shadow Duo ($7.99), HiP Studio Secrets Professional Matte Shadow Duo ($9.99), Studio Secrets Professional Color Smokes Eye Shadow ($5.99), and Studio Secrets Professional Eye Shadow Singles ($4.48)

Laura Mercier Luster Eye Colour ($22) and Matte Eye Colour ($22)

M.A.C. Eye Shadow Veluxe ($15), Matte2 Eye Shadow ($15), and Paint Pot ($17.50)

Mary Kay Mineral Eye Color ($6.50) and Mineral Eye Color Bundle ($19.50)

NARS Eyeshadow ($24)

NYX Cosmetics Eyeshadow ($5)

Physicians Formula Bright Collection Shimmery Quads Eye Shadow ($6.75), Matte Collection Quad Eye Shadow ($6.75), and Shimmer Strips Custom Eye Enhancing Shadow & Liner ($10.95)

Revlon CustomEyes Shadow & Liner ($8.99)

Sephora Colorful Mono Eyeshadow ($12)

Smashbox Photo Op Eye Shadow Trio ($28)

Stila Eye Shadow Pan ($18)

Wet 'n Wild Color Icon Eyeshadow Singles ($1.99)

BEST CREAM-TO-POWDER, STICK, GEL, AND CREAM EYESHADOWS:

Bobbi Brown Long-Wear Cream Shadow ($24) and Metallic Long-Wear Cream Shadow ($24)

L'Oreal Paris Infallible 24 HR Eye Shadow ($7.95)

Revlon Illuminance Creme Eyeshadow ($6.50)

Shiseido Shimmering Cream Eye Color ($25)

Tarte Cosmetics Amazonian Clay Waterproof Cream Eyeshadow ($19)

BEST EYESHADOW PRIMERS:

Estee Lauder Double Wear Stay in Place Eyeshadow Base ($16)

M.A.C. Prep + Prime Eye ($17)

NARS Smudge Proof Eyeshadow Base ($24)

BEST EYE AND BROW LINERS (INCLUDING BROW TINTS/GELS)

There are numerous options to line eyes and define the brows, depending on your mood, makeup style, and the amount of time you have to apply such products.

We remain fond of lining eyes with a matte-powder eyeshadow, used wet or dry (with wet application producing a more intense effect). However, the various gel-type eyeliners are also a great way to go, especially for those with oily eyelids. There also are some incredible liquid eyeliners to consider.

When it comes to eye and brow pencils, those rated as standard tend to have more similarities than differences. We did not rate any pencil that needed routine sharpening a BEST because there are enough excellent automatic (no sharpening required) pencils available; we just can't understand why anyone would bother with the other kind, though this is still the dominant version both at drugstores and department stores. The eye and brow pencils on the lists below have quick, smooth applications and a long-wearing finish. The eye pencils tend to be creamier but don't smear, while the brow pencils have a drier texture and powder-like finish.

Several companies sell tinted eyebrow gels as a way to fill, groom, and define the brow. There are also a few companies that make a clear brow gel that isn't much different from using hairspray on a toothbrush and brushing it through the brow. For the most part, the natural-colored brow gels are great, and we strongly recommend them as another way to make eyebrows look fuller but not artificial. The brow gels listed below are those that keep brows groomed while not feeling sticky or making brow hairs feel stiff or look obviously coated. Visit CosmeticsCop.com for our latest reviews and top picks of eyeliners and brow products.

BEST LIQUID, CAKE, OR GEL EYELINERS:

Almay Liquid Eyeliner ($7.29)

Avon Mark Keep It Going Longwear Eyeliner & Shadow ($11)

BeautiControl Liquid Eye Liner ($12)

Bobbi Brown Long-Wear Gel Eyeliner ($22)

Clinique Brush-On Cream Liner ($15)

Dior Liquid Eyeliner ($34)

e.l.f Essential Waterproof Eyeliner Pen ($1) and Studio Cream Eyeliner ($3)

Estee Lauder Double Wear Stay-in-Place Gel Eyeliner ($21.50) and Double Wear Zero-Smudge Liquid Eyeliner ($21.50)

L'Oreal Paris HiP Studio Secrets Professional Color Truth Cream Eyeliner ($10.19), Lineur Intense Felt Tip Liquid Eyeliner ($6.50), and Voluminous Mistake-Proof Marker Eyeliner ($7.29)

Lancome Artliner Precision Point EyeLiner ($29.50)

M.A.C. Fluidline ($15) and Penultimate Eyeliner ($18.50)

Maybelline Line Stiletto Ultimate Precision Liquid Eyeliner ($7.25)

Physicians Formula Eye Booster 2-in-1 Lash Boosting Eyeliner + Serum ($10.95) and Eye Definer Felt-Tip Eye Marker ($6.95)

Revlon ColorStay Liquid Eye Pen ($8.99) and ColorStay Liquid Liner ($7.29)

Sephora Doe Eyed Felt Eyeliner ($12)

Sonia Kashuk Dramatically Defining Long Wearing Gel Liner ($8.99) and Eyeliner Palette ($13.29)

Tarte Cosmetics emphasEYES Amazonian Clay Waterproof Liner ($22)

The Body Shop Liquid Eyeliner ($13.50)

Yves Saint Laurent Eyeliner Effet Faux Cils Long-Wear Cream Eyeliner($25)

BEST AUTOMATIC EYE PENCILS:

DHC Eyeliner Perfect Pro Pencil ($7)

M.A.C. Technakohl Liner ($15)

Maybelline Line Stylist Eyeliner ($7.25) and Unstoppable Smudge-Proof Waterproof Eyeliner ($7.23)

NARS Larger Than Life Long-Wear Eyeliner ($23)

Rimmel Exaggerate Waterproof Eye Definer ($5.67)

Tarte Cosmetics emphasEYES Aqua-Gel Eyeliner ($18) and emphasEYES Eyeliner High Definition Inner Rim Eyeliner Pencil ($18)

Yves Saint Laurent Easy Liner for Eyes Automatic Eyeliner ($32)

BEST AUTOMATIC EYEBROW PENCILS:

Clinique Instant Lift for Brows ($15)

M.A.C. Eye Brow Pencils ($15)

Origins Fill in the Blanks Eyebrow Enhancer ($15)

Physicians Formula Brow Definer Automatic Brow Pencil ($5.95)

Sephora Retractable Brow Pencil Waterproof ($12)

BEST EYEBROW GELS, WAXES, AND BROW TINTS:

Laura Geller Eyebrow Tint & Tamer ($21.50)

Paula's Choice Brow/Hair Tint ($9.95) and Browlistic Long-Wearing Precision Brow Color ($9.95)

Sephora Arch It Brow Kit ($35)

Stila Stay All Day Waterproof Brow Color ($22)

Urban Decay Brow Box ($29) and Urbanbrow Precision-Tip Brow Tint ($20)

BEST LIPSTICKS (INCLUDING LIPSTICKS WITH SUNSCREEN, LIP STAINS, AND LONG-WEARING LIPCOLOR)

Lipstick is essential to a complete makeup application, and is one cosmetic few women are ever without! In order to make the Best Products list, a lipstick, regardless of texture (cream, matte, sheer, and so on) had to:

- Apply smoothly and evenly
- Feel comfortable and have an attractive finish
- Come in a range of basic and dramatic colors
- Offer reasonable to excellent staying power
- If it contained sunscreen, it must be rated SPF 15 or greater and contain UVA-protecting ingredients
- Not contain irritants or excessive fragrance

Given the number of lipsticks available and women's wide range of preferences for this essential cosmetic (some like sheer with a glossy finish, others want moderate coverage with a satin finish, or semi-matte textures with shimmer, and on and on and on...), it was a struggle to determine the best. The top picks listed below include all those traits and more, with the widest range of choice being the cream lipsticks. Cream lipsticks are middle-of-the-road options that balance what most women want from a lipstick (comfort, moisture, and color that lasts at least a couple of hours) with what they don't like but are willing to tolerate (slippery feel, routine touch-ups, and lipstick coming off on coffee cups and significant others).

The color range for each was taken into consideration as well, keeping in mind a balance of classic, bold, and trendy shades. That being said, it must be noted that the numerous lipsticks rated "GOOD" with a happy face are also worth considering. It all depends on your preferences; that's why it was so difficult to narrow down the list of the best options in this category. Despite the struggle, we feel confident that after all the lipsticks we tested, those listed below are exemplary in their category and worthy of must-try status. Visit CosmeticsCop.com for our latest reviews and top picks of all types of lipstick.

BEST MATTE OR SEMI-MATTE LIPSTICKS:

Cover Girl Lip Perfection Lipstick ($6.99)

Elizabeth Arden Color Intrigue Effects Lipstick ($19.50)

Estee Lauder Double Wear Stay-in-Place Lipstick ($25)

Laura Mercier Satin Lip Colour ($32)

M.A.C. Matte Lipstick ($14.50)

NARS Pure Matte Lipstick ($25) and Semi Matte Lipstick ($24)

NYX Cosmetics Matte Lipstick ($6) and Soft Matte Lip Cream ($6)

Revlon Super Lustrous Matte Lipstick ($7.99)

Sephora Rouge Cream Lipstick ($12)

Sonia Kashuk Velvety Matte Lip Crayon ($7.59)

Too Faced Full Bloom Lip & Cheek Creme Color ($21)

BEST CREAM LIPSTICKS:

Chanel Rouge Coco Hydrating Creme Lip Colour ($32.50)

Clarins Joli Rouge ($24.50) and Rouge Prodige True Colour & Shine Lipstick ($24.50)

Clinique Long Last Soft Shine Lipstick ($15) and Vitamin C Smoothie Antioxidant Lip Colour ($17.50)

Cover Girl Blast Flipstick Blendable Lip Duo ($7.99) and Lip Perfection Lipstick ($6.99)

DHC Lip Color Perfect Pro Creme ($11) and Moisture Care Lipstick ($14.50)

e.l.f. Mineral Lipstick ($5)

Elizabeth Arden Color Intrigue Effects Lipstick ($19.50)

Estee Lauder Signature Hydra Lustre Lipstick ($22.50)

Giorgio Armani Rouge D'Armani Lipstick ($30)

L'Oreal Paris Intensely Moisturizing Lipcolor ($10)

Lancome Color Design Sensational Effects Lipcolor ($22)

Laura Geller Creme Couture Soft Touch Matte Lipstick ($18)

M.A.C. Lipsticks (Amplified Cremes, Mattes, and Satins $14.50)

Make Up For Ever Rouge Artist Intense ($19)

Mary Kay Creme Lipstick ($13)

Maybelline Color Sensational Lipcolor ($7.49)

N.Y.C. (New York Color) Ultra Moist Lip Wear ($0.99)

Revlon Super Lustrous Lipstick ($7.99)

Rimmel Lasting Finish Lipstick ($4.92)

Sephora Rouge Cream Lipstick ($12)

Shiseido Perfect Rouge Lipstick ($25)

Wet 'n Wild Wild Shine Lip Lacquer ($2.99)

BEST SHEER LIPSTICKS:

Boots Sheer Temptation Lipstick ($9.99)

Revlon Colorburst Lip Butters ($5.99)

Shiseido Perfect Rouge Lipstick ($25)

BEST LIPSTICK WITH SUNSCREEN RATED SPF 15 OR GREATER:

Clinique High Impact Lipstick SPF 15 ($15)

Paula's Choice Sheer Cream Lipstick SPF 15 ($10.95)

BEST LIP PAINTS/STAINS LONG-WEARING LIPCOLOR:

e.l.f. Studio Lip Stain ($3)

Estee Lauder Double Wear Stay-in-Place Lip Duo ($25)

L'Oreal Paris HiP Studio Secrets Professional Shine Struck Liquid Lipcolor ($12)

M.A.C. Pro Longwear Lipcolour ($22) and Pro Longwear Lustre Lipcolour ($22)

Make Up For Ever Liquid Lip Color ($20)

Maybelline SuperStay 24 Color ($9.99)

N.Y.C. (New York Color) Smooch Proof LIPStain 16H ($4.99)

Yves Saint Laurent Rouge Pur Couture Glossy Stain ($32)

BEST LIP GLOSSES

Next to mascara, lip gloss is quite possibly the most beloved makeup product among women. We understand why, and in order for a lip gloss to make the Best Product list, it had to:

- Offer a smooth, even application
- Have a comfortable texture and non-sticky finish
- Not slip right off lips or fade within minutes
- Not contain needless irritants such as menthol or mint
- Come in a range of enticing colors

Lip gloss is an incredibly popular item for women of all ages. Regardless of where we went or what line we were checking out, if there was one makeup item that made women gleeful, it was lip gloss. We don't know whether it's the low-commitment sheer colors or the glossy finish reminiscent of youth and sex appeal, but lip gloss is a big deal!

The lip glosses on this list feature sheer and opaque options. Sheer lip glosses may be worn alone or over a lipstick; opaque or nearly opaque lip glosses (also known as liquid lipsticks) may be worn alone or over a bold lipstick for added depth and color impact.

Spending a lot on lip gloss isn't the best idea because it's fleeting, but for those so inclined, there are some great expensive options, too. Where applicable, we have noted which lip glosses offer varying finishes, such as shimmer, metallic, or sparkling. Visit CosmeticsCop.com for our latest reviews and top picks of lip glosses.

Note: Lip glosses that are on the sheer and pigmented/opaque lists include a mix of soft/ sheer, and bold/opaque colors. Choose based on the look you're after.

BEST SHEER (COLOR) LIP GLOSSES:

BeautiControl Lip Gloss ($16)

Boots Botanics Lip Gloss ($7.99)

Clinique Superbalm Moisturizing Gloss ($15)

Cover Girl Queen Collection Lip Gloss ($5.49)

e.l.f. Mineral Lip Gloss ($3)

Giorgio Armani Lip Shimmer ($27)

Korres Natural Lip Butter Glaze ($14)

L'Oreal Paris Colour Riche Lip Gloss ($8.95)

Make Up For Ever Super Lip Gloss ($16)

Neutrogena MoistureShine Gloss ($7.99)

NYX Cosmetics Mega Shine Lip Gloss ($5.50)

Smashbox Lip Enhancing Gloss ($18)

Sonia Kashuk Ultra Shine Sheer Lip Gloss ($8.99)

BEST PIGMENTED/OPAQUE LIP GLOSSES:

Chanel Rouge Allure Laque Luminous Satin Lip Colour ($32.50)

Korres Natural Cherry Full Color Gloss ($17)

L'Oreal Paris Colour Riche Le Gloss ($7.95) and HiP Studio Secrets Professional Shine Struck Liquid Lipcolor ($12)

M.A.C. Cremesheen Glass ($19.50)

Make Up For Ever Liquid Lip Color ($20)

Mary Kay Nourishine Plus Lip Gloss ($14)

Maybelline Color Sensational Lip Gloss ($6.49)

NARS Larger Than Life Lip Gloss ($26)

NYX Cosmetics Mega Shine Lip Gloss ($5.50)

Rimmel Stay Glossy Long-Lasting Lipgloss ($4.99)

Smashbox Limitless Long Wear Lip Gloss SPF 15 ($22), Lip Enhancing Gloss ($18), and Reflection High Shine Lip Gloss ($19)

Yves Saint Laurent Gloss Pur Pure Lip Gloss ($30) and Touche Brilliance Sparkling Touch for Lips ($30)

BEST LIP GLOSSES WITH SUNSCREEN RATED SPF 15 OR GREATER:

Laura Geller Shine & Shield SPF 15 Lip Gloss ($18)

Smashbox Limitless Long Wear Lip Gloss SPF 15 ($22)

BEST LIP PENCILS (INCLUDING ANTI-FEATHER OPTIONS)

Using a lip pencil is a matter of personal preference. It can help shape and shade the mouth for stronger emphasis, particularly with bold colors, and can also serve as a base for lip gloss (so you still have some color after the gloss wears off). In order to make the Best Products list, a lip pencil must:

- Not require routine sharpening
- Have a firm yet smooth texture
- Apply easily and set to a long-wearing finish
- Not fade quickly or bleed into lines around the mouth

Automatic lip pencils (those that do not need sharpening) are the only ones that earned a BEST rating. If you don't mind routinely sharpening pencils, there are some good ones to consider outside of the short list presented here.

For best results, apply lip pencil prior to your lipstick, following the natural outline of your mouth. Once lipstick is applied, you can use the pencil to further define the lip line, particularly the "cupid's bow" at the center of your upper lip.

Avoid trying to enlarge your mouth with lip pencil. Up close and in person, this rarely looks convincing … it just looks like you missed your mouth! Also avoid using a lip liner that is markedly darker than your lipstick or gloss. This never looked good when it was popular (and who knows why it was ever in fashion) and merely makes the mouth look odd. Visit CosmeticsCop.com for our latest reviews and top picks of lip pencils.

BEST AUTOMATIC LIP PENCILS:

BeautiControl BC Color Lip Perfecting Pencil ($12)

Clinique Quickliner for Lips ($15)

Dior RougeLiner Automatic Lip Liner ($29)

e.l.f. Studio Lip Lock Pencil ($3)

Lancome Le Crayon Lip Contour ($23.50)

Mary Kay Lip Liner ($12)

Origins Automagically Lip Lining Pencil ($15)

Paula's Choice Long-Lasting Anti-Feather Lipliner ($7.95)

L'Oreal Paris Infallible Never Fail Lipliner ($8.99)

Revlon ColorStay Lipliner ($7.99)

Sephora Retractable Waterproof Lip Liner ($12)

BEST MASCARAS (INCLUDING LASH PRIMERS)

Mascara is a makeup staple, and we've found the best ones out there so you can make the most of your lashes. In order to make the Best Products list, a mascara must:

- Have a wow-factor feature that provides superior results
- Quickly enhance lashes, whether from lengthening, thickening, separating, or any combination of these and other features
- Not smudge, smear, flake, or contain eye irritants (such as strong fragrance)
- If waterproof, the formula must hold up when lashes get wet

The sheer number of mascaras available is nothing short of astounding! We should also mention the wide variety of mascara brushes that are available, from a thin comb with serrated edges to a tightly packed full row of nylon or rubber bristles, each providing different effects and each deserving of experimentation to see if you prefer the results from one type of brush over another.

Performance of any mascara comes down to the perfect marriage of brush and formula, with packaging components (such as the wiper that "cleans" the brush as you remove it from the tube) coming in a close second. The rest is preference-related depending on the lash look you want.

There are excellent mascaras in all price ranges, so it's not logical to buy the most expensive mascara when reasonably priced ones are equally good. Given that this is one product you can't readily test at the counters, purchase a few of the inexpensive ones first and see what you think!

Because the mascaras on this list are only those rated BEST, you'll find that each has its own wow factor; that is, they offer impressive results quickly and go the distance when it comes to superior application and wear. Although there are plenty of formidable options here, you should also know that the mascaras rated with a happy face in this book are worth considering, too, depending on your preferences. Visit CosmeticsCop.com for our latest reviews and top picks of regular and waterproof mascaras plus lash primers.

BEST REGULAR MASCARAS:

Almay One Coat Lengthening Mascara ($5.99) and One Coat Nourishing Mascara Triple Effect ($7.99)

Bare Escentuals bareMinerals Flawless Definition Curl & Lengthen Mascara ($18) and bareMinerals Flawless Definition Volumizing Mascara ($18)

BeautiControl SpectacuLash Mascara ($10)

Boots Exceptional Definition Nutrient Enriched Mascara ($7.99)

Clarins Wonder Perfect Mascara ($24)

Clinique High Impact Mascara ($15) and Lash Doubling Mascara ($15)

Cover Girl Lash Blast Length ($7.79) and Lash Blast Volume ($7.79)

DHC Mascara Perfect Pro Double Protection ($17.50)

Dior DiorShow Iconic Mascara ($28.50)

e.l.f. Studio Lash Extending Mascara ($3) and Wet Gloss Lash & Brow Clear Mascara ($1)

Elizabeth Arden Ceramide Lash Extending Treatment Mascara ($20)

Estee Lauder Double Wear Zero-Smudge Lengthening Mascara ($21) and Sumptuous Bold Volume Lifting Mascara ($21)

Giorgio Armani Eyes to Kill Exceptional Volume Mascara ($30) and Eyes to Kill Lash Stretching Mascara ($30)

Guerlain Le2 de Guerlain Two Brush Mascara ($36)

L'Oreal Paris Double Extend with Lash Boosting Serum Mascara ($12.99), Double Extend Lash Fortifier & Extender Mascara ($10.99), Telescopic Explosion Mascara ($9.49), Voluminous Full Definition Volume Building Mascara ($7.29), and Voluminous Naturale Natural-Looking Volume & Definition Mascara ($7.29)

Lancome L'Extreme Instant Extensions Lengthening Mascara ($26) and Definicils High Definition Mascara ($26)

Laura Mercier Long Lash Mascara ($24) and Thickening and Building Mascara ($20)

M.A.C. Haute & Naughty Lash ($19), Studio Fix Lash ($15), and Zoom Lash Mascara ($15)

Mary Kay Lash Love Mascara ($15)

Maybelline Full 'n Soft Mascara ($7.77), Lash Discovery Mini Brush Mascara ($6.99), The Colossal Volum' Express Mascara ($7.77), Volum' Express Mascara 3X, Curved Brush ($7.77), Volum' Express The Falsies Mascara Black Drama ($7.39), and Volum' Express Turbo Boost Mascara 7X ($7.77)

N.Y.C. (New York Color) Big Bold Ultra Volumizing Mascara ($2.99), City Curls Curling Mascara ($2.99), High Definition Separating Mascara ($4.99), and Sky Rise Lengthening Mascara ($1.99)

NYX Cosmetics Doll Eye Mascara Longlash ($9); Doll Eye Mascara Volume ($9); and Provocateur 1 Brush, 2 Styles ($6)

Paula's Choice Great Big Lashes Mascara ($9.95) and Illicit Lash Maximum Impact Mascara ($10.95)

Peter Thomas Roth Lashes to Die For The Mascara ($22)

Revlon Fabulash Mascara ($6.79)

Rimmel The Max Volume Flash Mascara ($6.83)

Sephora Atomic Volume Mascara ($15) and Lash Plumper ($12)

Smashbox Bionic Mascara ($19)

Tarte Cosmetics Lights, Camera, Lashes! 4-in-1 Natural Mascara ($19)

Yves Saint Laurent Volume Effet Faux Cils Luxurious Mascara for a False Lash Effect ($30)

BEST WATERPROOF MASCARAS:

Bobbi Brown No Smudge Mascara ($24)

Chanel Inimitable Waterproof Mascara ($30)

Dior DiorShow Waterproof Mascara ($25)

Estee Lauder Sumptuous Waterproof Bold Volume Lifting Mascara ($21)

Lancome Definicils Waterproof High Definition Mascara ($26)

M.A.C. Zoom Waterfast Lash ($15)

Make Up For Ever Lengthening Waterproof Mascara ($23)

Maybelline Define-A-Lash Volume Waterproof Mascara ($7.49), Lash Discovery Waterproof Mascara ($7.77), Lash Stiletto Voluptuous Mascara Waterproof ($8.95), One by One Volum' Express Waterproof Mascara ($8.15), The Colossal Volum' Express Waterproof Mascara ($7.77), and Volum' Express The Falsies Mascara Waterproof ($7.39)

BEST MASCARA PRIMERS:

BeautiControl SpectacuLash Thickening Primer and Maximum Length Mascara ($20; *this is a dual-sided product with primer on one end and mascara on the other*)

Smashbox Layer Lash Primer ($17)

BEST FACE AND BODY ILLUMINATING/SHIMMER PRODUCTS

Shine is a makeup trend that's here to stay. There are many ways to add shine to your makeup routine, and those that take a subtle approach tend to be the most flattering. In order to make the Best Products list, face and body illuminating/shimmer products must:

- Be easy to apply and mesh well with skin
- Give skin a fresh, radiant finish rather than glaring sparkles
- Offer workable, non-clownish colors for various skin tones
- Mix well with and blend over other makeup products

The options on this list favor liquid shimmer products because they not only tend to be the most versatile, but also tend to have the most flattering finishes and shine that cling well to skin.

These products are recommended for evening or special-occasion makeup (except weddings if you're the bride; shimmer and shine tend to register as greasy, glossy skin in photographs). For best results, use sparingly (remember, you can always add more if the level of shine isn't to your liking). These products, especially the liquids, may be applied over or under your foundation or tinted moisturizer. Visit CosmeticsCop.com for our latest reviews and top picks of face and body illuminating/shimmer products.

BEST LIQUID, CREAM, CREAM-TO-POWDER, OR GEL SHIMMER PRODUCTS:

Avon Mark Get Bright Hook Up Highlighter ($6.50)

Chanel Eclat Lumiere Highlighter Face Pen ($40)

Giorgio Armani Fluid Sheer ($59)

Maybelline Dream Lumi Touch Highlighting Concealer ($7.99)

Stila All Over Shimmer Liquid Luminizer ($20)

Yves Saint Laurent Teint Parfait Complexion Enhancer ($42)

BEST PRESSED POWDERS WITH SHIMMER:

Benefit 10 ($28)

Dior DiorSkin Ultra Shimmering All Over Face Powder ($44)

e.l.f. Mineral Glow ($8)

Estee Lauder Signature 5-Tone Shimmer Powder for Eyes, Cheeks, Face ($38)

Laura Mercier Shimmer Bloc ($38)

BEST MINERAL MAKEUP

Mineral makeup is seemingly here to stay. Clearly, many women enjoy this type of makeup, though it definitely has its limitations and isn't nearly as awe-inspiring as companies selling it want you to believe. In order for a mineral makeup product to make the Best Products list, it must:

- Feature a smooth, lightweight texture
- Blend easily without streaking or caking
- Not make skin look unnaturally dry, flat, or powdered
- Contain minimal to no fragrance
- For loose powders, be packaged to minimize mess

Note: All the SPF-rated mineral makeup products below provide sufficient UVA protection. The powders can be an excellent adjunct to your daytime moisturizer or liquid foundation with sunscreen, and this is how we advise using them in terms of sun protection. It is highly unlikely you'll apply any loose or pressed mineral powder liberally enough by itself to get the amount of sun protection stated on the label. Visit CosmeticsCop.com for our latest reviews and top picks of mineral makeup.

BEST MINERAL FOUNDATIONS:

Avon Smooth Minerals Pressed Foundation ($11)

Bobbi Brown Skin Foundation Mineral Makeup SPF 15 ($38)

Elizabeth Arden Pure Finish Mineral Tinted Moisturizer SPF 15 ($30)

Jane Iredale Amazing Base Loose Minerals SPF 20 ($42) and PurePressed Base Mineral Foundation SPF 20 ($40-$52)

Korres Natural Wild Rose Mineral Foundation SPF 30 ($28)

Mary Kay Mineral Powder Foundation ($18)

Neutrogena Mineral Sheers Powder Foundation SPF 20 ($11.99)

BEST MINERAL POWDERS:

e.l.f. Mineral Glow ($8)

L'Oreal Paris True Match Naturale Soft-Focus Mineral Finish ($15.25)

Lancome Ageless Minerale Perfecting and Setting Mineral Powder with White Sapphire Complex ($36)

Laura Mercier Mineral Powder SPF 15 ($35 for 0.34 fl. oz.)

M.A.C. Mineralize Skinfinish ($29)

Physician's Formula Mineral Wear Talc-Free Mineral Face Powder SPF 16 ($13.95)

BEST MINERAL BLUSHES, EYESHADOWS, AND LIP COLORS:

BeautiControl BC Color Mineral Blush ($16)

e.l.f. Mineral Lipstick ($5) and Mineral Lip Gloss ($3)

Jane Iredale PurePressed Eye Shadows ($19)

Mary Kay Mineral Eye Color ($6.50) and Mineral Eye Color Bundle ($19.50)

BEST MAKEUP BRUSHES

Brushes are essential to beautiful makeup application. In order to make the Best Products list, brushes, whether sold singly or in sets, must:

- Be well designed for their intended purpose
- Be soft and well shaped, not floppy, for expert control
- Feel exquisite and be easy to use
- Be built to last through years of daily use

Professional-size brushes are available in all price ranges. Keep in mind that the density, shape, and cut of the brush is more important than the source of the bristles.

Although many cosmetics companies love to brag about the type and grade of animal hair used for their brushes, remember, you are not buying a mink coat. Hair softness, brush shape, and firmness (which affect application) are what matters the most, no matter the source.

Many cosmetics lines are offering synthetic brushes that are often exquisite replications of natural-hair brushes and must be felt to be believed. These synthetic brushes are excellent, and an easy solution for anyone conflicted about using animal-hair brushes for applying makeup.

Please note that not every single brush from the brands on the list was rated BEST. For comments on individual brushes, please refer to the respective brand's review in Chapter 14. A brush collection that rates BEST represents a superior combination of performance, craftsmanship, and value. Visit CosmeticsCop.com for our latest reviews and top picks of brushes, both individual and brush sets.

BEST MAKEUP BRUSHES (INCLUDING INDIVIDUALS AND BRUSH SETS):

Aveda Flax Sticks ($55–$65) and Inner Light Foundation Brush ($40)

Avon Mark All Over Eye Shadow Brush ($8) and Concealer Brush ($7)

Benefit Foundation Brush ($24)

Chanel The Eyeshadow Brushes ($28–$38) and Face/Cheek Brushes ($32–$65)

e.l.f. 11-Piece Studio Brush Collection ($30)

Elizabeth Arden Face Powder Brush ($28)

Estee Lauder Brushes ($20–$42)

Jane Iredale Deluxe Eye Shader ($24)

Lancome Mineral Powder Foundation Brush ($37.50)

M.A.C. Brushes ($11–$71)

Make Up For Ever Make Up For Ever Brushes ($13–$54)

NARS Brushes ($26–$75)

Origins Brushes ($16.50–$35)

Paula's Choice Makeup Application Sponges ($5.95 for 10 sponges) and Mini Brush Set ($38.95)

Sephora Brushes ($10–$41)

Smashbox #13 Foundation Brush ($29)

Stila Brushes ($20–$50)

Sonia Kashuk Brushes ($1.99–$20.99)

The Body Shop Extra Virgin Minerals Foundation Brush ($25)

BEST SPECIALTY PRODUCTS (INCLUDING WRINKLE FILLERS)

Following is a list of miscellaneous products that have interesting effects or have an intriguing premise that just doesn't fit squarely into the above categories. For details about these products, please refer to the individual reviews in this book.

Note that we also include wrinkle fillers on this list because a few of those products are impressive to the extent that cosmetic ingredients allow. None of the wrinkle fillers recommended last all day or are going to make a women in her 50s look like she's in her 20s, but they can help and the best ones treat skin to a range of beneficial ingredients.

BEST SPECIALTY PRODUCTS, ALL TYPES:

BeautiControl Regeneration Tight, Firm & Fill Extreme Wrinkle Concentrate ($40 for 0.04 fl. oz.)

Eucerin Aquaphor Healing Ointment ($5.99 for 1.75 fl. oz.) and Aquaphor Baby Healing Ointment ($8.28 for 3 fl. oz.)

La Prairie Cellular Lip Line Plumper ($130 for 0.08 fl. oz.)

Laura Mercier Secret Finish Mattifying ($27 for 1 fl. oz.)

M.A.C. Prep + Prime Lip ($15)

Mary Kay TimeWise Age-Fighting Lip Primer ($22.50 for 0.5 oz.)

NYX Cosmetics Pore Filler ($13)

Paula's Choice Brighten Up 2-Minute Teeth Whitener ($14.95 for 2.5 grams)

Paula's Choice Cuticle & Nail Treatment ($10.95 for 0.06 fl. oz.)

Paula's Choice First Class Refillable Travel Kit ($12.95)

Paula's Choice Redness Relief Treatment ($15.95 for 4 fl. oz.)

Peter Thomas Roth Lashes to Die For Platinum ($125 for 0.16 fl. oz.)

The Body Shop Lip Line Fixer ($11)

CHAPTER SIXTEEN

Cosmetic Ingredient Dictionary Online

You can access our comprehensive Cosmetic Ingredient Dictionary online in the Expert Advice section at CosmeticsCop.com. This unique, online resource is a great way to find reliable information and succinct ratings for over 1,600 common cosmetic ingredients ranging from antioxidants and antiwrinkle ingredients to anti-acne ingredients, hundreds of plant extracts, vitamins, minerals, cleansing agents, preservatives, and on and on.

The conclusions reached for all the skin-care product reviews in this book are based around the product's formulation and what the published scientific research and literature shows to be true about those ingredients. All the details for almost every ingredient can be found in our online Cosmetic Ingredient Dictionary. Use this dictionary to gain an understanding of the significance of an ingredient in terms of its claims and its potential (if any) for irritation. You can then use this information to make comparisons among products before you make a purchase.

My team routinely updates this dictionary with new terms and changes to existing terms as new research is published. We hope it helps you demystify the exaggerated and over-hyped claims you've been bombarded with by the cosmetics industry.

CHAPTER SEVENTEEN

Appendix

This section, which is referred to in product reviews throughout this book, is where you will find essential information that we opted to put in one place rather than repeating it endlessly throughout the reviews. Let this appendix serve as a handy reference and reminder of the issues associated with numerous skin-care and makeup products. Keeping these issues in mind will allow you to shop smarter and more easily find the best products for your skin type and concerns.

WHY JAR PACKAGING IS A PROBLEM

Jar packaging is a problem for any state-of-the-art cosmetic formula. All plant extracts, vitamins, antioxidants, and other state-of-the-art ingredients break down in the presence of air, so once a jar is opened and air enters, these important ingredients begin to deteriorate.

Jars also are unsanitary because you're dipping your fingers into them with each use, adding bacteria that further deteriorate the beneficial ingredients.

Sources: *Free Radical Biology and Medicine*, September 2007, pages 818–829; *Ageing Research Reviews*, December 2007, pages 271–288; *Dermatologic Therapy*, September-October 2007, pages 314–321; *International Journal of Pharmaceutics*, June 12, 2005, pages 197–203; *Pharmaceutical Development and Technology*, January 2002, pages 1–32; *International Society for Horticultural Science*, actahort.org/members/showpdf?booknrarnr=778_5; Beautypackaging.com, and beautypackaging.com/articles/2007/03/airless-packaging.php.

WHY YOU DON'T NEED AN EYE CREAM

We know it's hard to believe, but the truth is you don't need a special product for the eye area, whether labeled eye cream or something else. Although there is much you can do to improve the skin around your eyes, the ingredients capable of doing that don't need to come from, and often aren't even included in, an eye cream. For example, most eye creams don't contain sunscreen, and that is a serious problem because it leaves the skin around your eyes vulnerable to sun damage, which will make dark circles and wrinkling worse!

You can save money and take superior care of your eye area by using your face product, if it is well formulated and appropriate for the skin type around your eyes!

WHY IRRITATION IS BAD FOR EVERYONE'S SKIN

Irritation, whether you see it on the surface of your skin or not, causes inflammation and as a result impairs healing, damages collagen, and depletes the vital substances your skin needs to stay young. For this reason, it is best to eliminate, or minimize as much as possible, your exposure to known skin irritants, especially when there are brilliant formulas available that do not include these types of problematic ingredients.

Sources: *Inflammation Research*, December 2008, pages 558–563; *Skin Pharmacology and Physiology*, June 2008, pages 124–135 and November-December 2000, pages 358–371; *Journal of Investigative Dermatology*, April 2008, pages 15–19; *Journal of Cosmetic Dermatology*, March 2008, pages 78–82; *Mechanisms of Ageing and Development*, January 2007, pages 92–105; and *British Journal of Dermatology*, December 2005, pages S13–S22.

❧ WHY HIGHLY FRAGRANCED PRODUCTS ARE A PROBLEM

Daily use of products that contain a high amount of fragrance, whether the fragrance in-gredients are synthetic or natural, causes chronic irritation that can damage healthy collagen production, lead to or worsen dryness, and impair your skin's ability to heal. Fragrance-free is the best way to go for all skin types.

If fragrance in your skin-care products is important to you, it should be a very low amount to minimize the risk to your skin. Minimizing skin's exposure to fragrance is one of the best things to do to keep skin young, smooth, and healthy.

Sources: *Inflammation Research*, December 2008, pages 558–563; *Skin Pharmacology and Physiology*, June 2008, pages 124–135 and November-December 2000, pages 358–371; *Journal of Investigative Dermatology*, April 2008, pages 15–19; *Journal of Cosmetic Dermatology*, March 2008, pages 78–82; *Mechanisms of Ageing and Development*, January 2007, pages 92–105; and *British Journal of Dermatology*, December 2005, pages S13–S22.)

⚸ WHY IRRITATION MAKES OILY, BREAKOUT-PRONE SKIN WORSE

Applying irritating ingredients to oily skin is a surefire way to make matters worse, not bet-ter. The irritating ingredients, be they alcohol, menthol, citrus, or numerous others, stimulate excess oil production at the base of the pores, so skin ends up being oilier and pores become (or stay) enlarged.

Treating oily skin gently with effective products designed to absorb excess oil, exfoliate inside the pore, and help normalize pore function is the best approach to see improvements.

Sources: *Clinical Dermatology*, September-October 2004, pages 360–366; and *Dermatol-ogy*, January 2003, pages 17–23.

☀ WHY THE RIGHT UVA-PROTECTING INGREDIENTS MATTER

SPF-rated products must include active ingredients capable of protecting your skin not only from the sun's UVB rays (which cause sunburn), but also UVA rays. The sun's UVA rays put skin at increased risk for wrinkles, brown spots, sagging, and a host of other problems, including skin cancer. Sufficient UVA and UVB protection is needed every day of your life, rain or shine, and even indoors (the bad rays of the sun come through windows). You may be shocked to learn that sun damage begins the first minute unprotected skin sees daylight (not just sunshine, but daylight itself, even on cloudy days)! The SPF rating on a product's label reflects the protection it provides from sunburn caused by the sun's UVB rays, but there is no agreed-upon rating for the sun's silent though more penetrating (and in many ways more damaging) UVA rays. Because of this, you need to be sure any sunscreen you're considering contains one or more of these UVA-protecting ingredients listed as one of the "actives" to assure you are getting sufficient UVA protection: **avobenzone**, **titanium dioxide**, **zinc oxide**, **Mexoryl SX (ecamsule)**, or **Tinosorb**.

Sources: *Photochemical and Photobiological Sciences*, December 2011, pages 81–90; *Cosmetic Dermatology*, Second Edition, Baumann, Leslie MD, McGraw Hill, 2009, pages 246–252; *American Journal of Clinical Dermatology*, Supplement, 2009, pages 19–24; *The Encyclopedia of Ultraviolet Filters*, Shaath, Nadim A., Allured Publishing, 2007; and *Photodermatology, Photoimmunology, and Photomedicine*, October 2003, pages 242–253.

⊘ WHY THE "HYPOALLERGENIC" CLAIM IS MEANINGLESS

"Hypoallergenic" is little more than a nonsense word meant to make products seem safer or somehow better for sensitive skin. Don't believe it, because shopping for products with this claim is not a guarantee of a gentle or safer formula.

There are no accepted testing methods, ingredient restrictions, regulations, guidelines, rules, or procedures of any kind, anywhere in the world, for determining whether or not a product qualifies as being hypoallergenic. A company can label their product "hypoallergenic" because there is no regulation that says they can't, no matter what proof they may point to—and what proof can they provide given there is no standard to measure against?

Because there are no regulations governing this supposed category that was made up by the cosmetics industry, there are plenty of products labeled "hypoallergenic" that contain problematic ingredients and that could indeed trigger allergic reactions, even for those with no previous history of skin sensitivity. The word "hypoallergenic" gives you no reliable understanding of what you are or aren't putting on your skin.

Sources: fda.gov; *Clinical and Experimental Dermatology*, May 2004, pages 325–327; and *Ostomy and Wound Management*, March 2003, pages 20–21.

⍦ WHY ALCOHOL IN COSMETIC PRODUCTS IS A PROBLEM

The types of alcohol to watch out for in cosmetic products include those listed as "sd alcohol" followed by a number (such as SD Alcohol 40), "Alcohol Denatured" (may be abbreviated as "Denat"), "Isopropyl Alcohol," and plain "Alcohol." These types of alcohol cause dryness and free-radical damage, and impair skin's ability to heal.

The irritation it causes damages healthy collagen production and can stimulate oil production at the base of the pore, making oily skin worse.

Ingredients such as cetyl alcohol or stearyl alcohol are not irritating. These and similar ingredients are known as fatty alcohols, and they are benign ingredients for skin, not to mention beneficial for dry skin.

Sources: "Skin Care—From the Inside Out and Outside In," *Tufts Daily*, April 1, 2002; eMedicine Journal, May 8, 2002, volume 3, number 5, emedicine.com; *Cutis*, February 2001, pages 25–27; *Contact Dermatitis*, January 1996, pages 12–16; and http://pubs.niaaa.nih.gov/publications/arh27-4/277-284.htm.

♥ WHY PRODUCTS CLAIMING TO LIFT SAGGING SKIN DON'T WORK

Many skin-care products claim they can firm and lift skin, but none of them work, at least not to the extent claimed. A face-lift-in-a-bottle isn't possible, but with the right mix of products, you will see firmer skin that has a more lifted appearance—and that's exciting!

In order to gain these youthful benefits, you must protect skin from any and all sun damage every day, use an AHA (glycolic acid or lactic acid) or BHA (salicylic acid) exfoliant, and use products that have a wide range of antioxidants and skin-repairing ingredients. This combination of products (remember, one product doesn't do it all) has extensive research showing how they can significantly improve many of the signs of aging such as firming skin, reducing wrinkles and brown spots, and eliminating dullness. You'll find them on our list of Best Anti-Aging/Antiwrinkle Products on CosmeticsCop.com and listed in Chapter 15, *The Best Products*, under Best Toners, Best AHA Exfoliants, Best BHA Exfoliants, Best Moisturizers Without Sunscreen, Best Daytime Moisturizers With Sunscreen, Best Retinol Products, and Best Serums.

WHY LAVENDER OIL IS A PROBLEM FOR EVERYONE'S SKIN

Research indicates that components of lavender, specifically linalool, can be cytotoxic, which means that topical application causes skin-cell death. Lavender leaves contain camphor, which is a known skin irritant.

Because the fragrance constituents in lavender oil oxidize when exposed to air, lavender oil is a pro-oxidant, and this enhanced oxidation increases its irritancy on skin. Lavender oil is the most potent form, and even small amounts of it (0.25% or less) are problematic. It is a must to avoid in skin-care products, but is fine as an aromatherapy agent for inhalation or relaxation.

Sources: *Contact Dermatitis*, September 2008, pages 143–150; *Psychiatry Research*, February 2007, pages 89–96; *Cell Proliferation*, June 2004, pages 221–229; and naturaldatabase.com.

FEB 2013